OBESITY

Epidemiology, Pathophysiology, and Prevention

Second Edition

Edited by

Debasis Bagchi and Harry G. Preuss

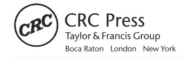

CRC Press
Taylor & Francis Group
Boca Raton   London   New York

CRC Press is an imprint of the
Taylor & Francis Group, an **informa** business

CRC Press
Taylor & Francis Group
6000 Broken Sound Parkway NW, Suite 300
Boca Raton, FL 33487-2742

© 2013 by Taylor & Francis Group, LLC
CRC Press is an imprint of Taylor & Francis Group, an Informa business

No claim to original U.S. Government works

Printed in the United States of America on acid-free paper
Version Date: 20120328

International Standard Book Number: 978-1-4398-5425-9 (Hardback)

Library of Congress Cataloging-in-Publication Data

Obesity : epidemiology, pathophysiology, and prevention / edited by Debasis Bagchi, Harry G. Preuss. -- 2nd ed.
     p. cm.
     Summary: "The spread of obesity has been declared a worldwide epidemic by the World Health Organization (WHO). In fact, a new term, globesity, has been coined to describe the recent upsurge of overweight and obesity throughout the world's population. How severe is the problem? According to WHO, worldwide obesity has more than double since 1980. In 2008, 1.5 billion adults, 20 and older, were overweight [1]. Of these over 200 million men and 300 million women were obese. 65% of the world's population live in countries where overweight and obesity kills more people than underweight [1]. Furthermore, nearly 43 million children under the age of five were underweight in 2010 [1]"-- Provided by publisher.
     Includes bibliographical references and index.
     ISBN 978-1-4398-5425-9 (hardback)
     1. Obesity--Epidemiology. 2. Obesity--Pathophysiology. I. Bagchi, Debasis, 1954- II. Preuss, Harry G.

RC645.O23O2465 2011
616.3'98--dc23   2012000311

Visit the Taylor & Francis Web site at
http://www.taylorandfrancis.com

and the CRC Press Web site at
http://www.crcpress.com

*Dedicated to my beloved father, the late Tarak Chandra Bagchi, MSc, AIC,
and my beloved father-in-law, the late Nakuleshwar Bardhan, BA.*

Debasis Bagchi

*Dedicated to my teachers, especially the late Rachel B. Lott (third grade),
the late MSG Thomas Hannon (CCD), and the late Dr. Robert F. Pitts
(postdoctoral training). They along with many others prepared me for my career.*

Harry G. Preuss

Contents

PART I Introduction

PART II Pathophysiology of Obesity

PART III   Obesity and Degenerative Diseases

PART IV Novel Concept in Obesity Drug Development

PART V Safety of Obesity Drugs

PART VI Natural, Nutritional, and Physical Approaches of Weight Management

Contents

PART VII Child Obesity and Prevention

PART VIII   Bariatric Surgery in Weight Management

Preface

The spread of obesity has been declared a worldwide epidemic by the World Health Organization (WHO). In fact, a new term, globesity, has been coined to describe the recent upsurge of overweight and obesity throughout the world's population. How severe is the problem? According to WHO, worldwide obesity has more than doubled since 1980. In 2008, 1.5 billion adults, 20 years and older, were overweight [1]. Of these, more than 200 million men and 300 million women were obese. Sixty-five percent of the world's population live in countries where overweight and obesity kills more people than underweight [1]. Furthermore, nearly 43 million children under the age of five were overweight in 2010 [1].

To make matters worse, overweight and obesity in children are significant public health problems in the United States. It has been estimated that between 16% and 33% of children and adolescents are obese [2]. The number of adolescents who are overweight has tripled since 1980, and the prevalence of obesity among younger children has more than doubled [2]. According to the 1999–2002 National Health and Nutrition Examination Survey (NHANES), 16% of children aged between 6 and 19 years are overweight. Not only have the rates of overweight in children increased, but also the heaviest children in a recent NHANES were markedly heavier than those in previous surveys [2]. In addition to type 2 diabetes, obesity has also been linked to other broad-spectrum, degenerative diseases, including other metabolic disorders and certain forms of cancer. It has been reported that 80% of type 2 diabetes, 70% of cardiovascular diseases, and 42% of breast and colon cancers are related to obesity [3]. Obesity is the major factor behind 30% of gallbladder perturbations, leading to surgery, and 26% of incidences of high blood pressure.

This unfortunate outcome has generated an unlimited array of weight loss strategies. Products and programs that induce rapid weight loss and disturb metabolic homeostasis dominate the focus of marketers and consumers alike; however, rapid weight loss is potentially unhealthy and frequently induces undesirable rebound weight gain consequences. In addition, many antiobesity pharmaceuticals are accompanied by adverse reactions, making the cure worse than the disorder itself; thus, it is very important to develop a strategic therapeutic intervention using safe, novel, and natural supplements supported by credible research. This book, intended for practicing medical professionals, clinical nutritionists, dieticians, and researchers, addresses many issues relevant to obesity: the molecular mechanism and pathophysiology leading to obesity and metabolic disorders, the safety of obesity drugs, drug development strategies, the influences of physical activity and nutrition, and the benefits of research-supported nutraceutical supplements.

The 63 chapters in this book have been written by experts in their respective fields and have been divided into 8 parts. Part I provides a general introduction. Chapter 1, written by a world-renowned nutritionist and a health professional, provides an overview on the epidemiology of obesity. Chapter 2 explains the relationship between obesity and type 2 diabetes. Part II deals with the pathophysiology of obesity. Chapter 3 by Professor Karl-Heinz Wagner and Helmut Brath demonstrates the global view on noncommunicable diseases and where we all are going. This part demonstrates the evidence for refined food addiction; correlates obesity with environmental estrogens and endocrine disruption, cigarette smoking, and inflammatory responses; and elaborates the roles of neurotransmitters, neurobiology, leptin, ghrelin (the hunger hormone), DNA methylation, and sleep. Part III correlates obesity with diverse degenerative diseases, including metabolic syndrome, type 2 diabetes, and diverse inflammatory responses such as wound healing and angiogenesis. Professor George Corcoran, immediate past president of the Society of Toxicology, discusses the role of drug and chemical toxicities in overweight and obesity in Chapter 18. Finally, Professor Merlin Butler emphasizes the genomic imprinting disorders in obesity in Chapter 19.

Part IV starts with Dr. Olivier Boss et al.'s chapter covering new concepts in obesity drug development. This is followed by Dr. Susan Schwartz and Dr. David Savastano's chapter on the history and regulation of prescription and over-the-counter weight loss drugs. The world-renowned Pennington Biomedical Research Center scientists Dr. Alok Gupta and Dr. Frank Greenway discuss the safety of obesity drugs in Part V. This part is further expanded to discuss the historical perspective of obesity drugs, efficacy of current obesity drugs, and future directions. Part VI consists of 33 chapters on natural, nutritional, and physical approaches of weight management. The roles of exercise and physical activity in weight management and weight loss, the usefulness of pedometers, the nutritional and dietary approaches for weight control, gender effects of adiposity, and antiaging effects of caloric restrictions are thoroughly demonstrated by experts in the field. This part also covers carbohydrate blocks; vegetarian, plant-based, and Atkins diets; the concept of the glycemic index; as well as the roles of chromium (III), (–)-hydroxycitric acid, bitter orange (*Citrus aurantium* and *p*-synephrine), conjugated linoleic acid, curcumin, tea, chitosan, *Caralluma fimbriata*, glucomannan, medium chain triglycerides, marine lipids, calcium and dairy products, the banned weight loss ingredient ephedra, *Coleus forskohlii* extract, and *Lagerstroemia speciosa* (coroslic acid) in weight management. There are also two interesting chapters, including a review on weight loss and a chapter providing the reflections of a practicing dietician regarding weight loss supplements. Part VII deals with child obesity—a most challenging issue in the new millennium. Five chapters highlight the intricate aspects of this problem and possible strategies for prevention. Part VIII discusses bariatric surgery and how this may help in weight management and in reversing metabolic disorders.

Finally, we extend our special thanks and gratitude to all the authors for their invaluable contributions and to Randy Brehm and Jill Jurgensen for their continued support.

REFERENCES

1. Obesity and overweight, Fact Sheet No 311, Updated March 2011, http://www.who.int/mediacentre/factsheets/fs311/en/ (dated October 12, 2011).
2. Childhood obesity statistics and trends, http://www.stop-childhood-obesity.com/childhood-obesity-statistics.html (dated October 12, 2011).
3. Obesity statistics: Weight statistics—Adults, children, obesity-related diseases, 2006, http://www.annecollins.com/obesity/statistics-obesity.htm (dated October 12, 2011).

Debasis Bagchi, PhD, MACN, CNS, MAIChE
College of Pharmacy, University of Houston
Houston, Texas

Harry G. Preuss, MD, MACN, CNS
Georgetown University Medical Center
Washington, District of Columbia

Editors

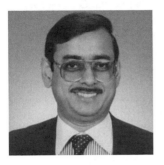

Debasis Bagchi, PhD, MACN, CNS, MAIChE, received his PhD in medicinal chemistry in 1982. He is a professor in the Department of Pharmacological and Pharmaceutical Sciences at the University of Houston, Houston, Texas. Dr. Bagchi is also the director of Innovation & Clinical Affairs at Iovate Health Research Sciences Inc., Oakville, Ontario, Canada. He is the immediate past president of the American College of Nutrition (ACN), Clearwater, Florida, and immediate past chairman of the Nutraceuticals and Functional Foods Division at the Institute of Food Technologists, Chicago, Illinois. Dr. Bagchi is the vice-chair of the International Society of Nutraceuticals and Functional Foods (ISNFF). He also serves as a distinguished advisor at the Japanese Institute for Health Food Standards, Tokyo, Japan. Dr. Bagchi received the Master of American College of Nutrition Award in October 2010. His research interests include free radicals, human diseases, carcinogenesis, pathophysiology, mechanistic aspects of cytoprotection by antioxidants, and regulatory pathways in obesity, diabetes, and gene expression.

Dr. Bagchi has authored 12 books and 278 papers in peer-reviewed journals and has 15 patents to his credit. He has delivered invited lectures at various national and international scientific conferences and has organized workshops and group discussion sessions. He is a fellow of the ACN and the Nutrition Research Academy and a member of the Society of Toxicology, the New York Academy of Sciences, and the TCE Stakeholder Committee of the Wright Patterson Air Force Base, Ohio. Dr. Bagchi is a member of the Study Section and Peer Review Committee of the National Institutes of Health, Bethesda, Maryland, the associate editor of the *Journal of Functional Foods* and the *Journal of the American College of Nutrition*, and also serves as an editorial board member of numerous peer-reviewed journals, including *Antioxidants and Redox Signaling*, *Cancer Letters*, *Toxicology Mechanisms and Methods*, and other scientific and medical journals. He is also a consulting editor of CRC Press/Taylor & Francis.

Dr. Bagchi received funding from various institutions and agencies, including the U.S. Air Force Office of Scientific Research, Nebraska State Department of Health, Biomedical Research Support Grant from the National Institutes of Health (NIH), National Cancer Institute (NCI), Health Future Foundation, the Procter & Gamble Company, and Abbott Laboratories.

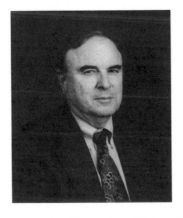

Harry G. Preuss, MD, MACN, CNS, received his BA and MD from Cornell University, Ithaca, New York, and Cornell University Medical Center, New York City, New York, respectively; trained for three years in internal medicine at Vanderbilt University Medical Center Nashville, Tennessee, under Dr. David E. Rogers; studied for two years as a fellow in renal physiology at Cornell University Medical Center under Dr. Robert F. Pitts; and spent two years in clinical and research training in nephrology at Georgetown University Medical Center Washington, DC, under Dr. George E. Schreiner. During his training years, he was a special research fellow of the NIH. After working for five years as an assistant and associate (tenured) professor of medicine at the University of Pittsburgh Medical Center, where he became an established investigator of the American Heart Association, Dr. Preuss returned to Georgetown University Medical Center and is now a tenured professor in four departments—biochemistry, physiology, medicine, and pathology. He subsequently performed a six-month sabbatical in molecular biology at the NIH in the laboratories of Dr. Maurice Burg.

Dr. Preuss' bibliography includes more than 220 peer-reviewed medical research papers, 190 general medical contributions (chapters, reviews, etc.), 7 patents, and more than 250 abstracts. He has written, edited, or coedited nine books and three symposia published in well-established journals. He has recently published two books: one coauthored for the lay public entitled *The Natural Fat Loss Pharmacy* (Broadway Books/Rodale Press), which has sold over 120,000 copies, and a second coedited for the academic community entitled *Obesity: Epidemiology, Pathophysiology, and Prevention* (CRC Press), which received outstanding reviews from the *New England Journal of Medicine* and the *Journal of American Medical Association*. In 1976, Dr. Preuss was elected as a member to the American Society for Clinical Investigations, a prestigious research group. He is currently an advisory editor for six journals. His previous government appointments included four years on the advisory council for the National Institute on Aging, two years on the advisory council of the director of the NIH (NIA representative), and two years on the advisory council for the Office of Alternative Medicine of the NIH. He has been a member of many other peer research review committees for the NIH and American Heart Association and was a member of the National Cholesterol Education Program of the NHLBI (NIH).

Dr. Preuss was elected the ninth Master of the ACN. He is a former chairman of two ACN councils—the Cardiovascular and Aging Council and the Council on Dietary Supplements, Nutraceuticals, and Functional Foods. After a brief stint on the board of directors of the ACN, Dr. Preuss spent three years as secretary–treasurer and three consecutive years as vice president, president-elect, and, finally, as president in 1998. In 2008 and 2011, he was reelected president of the ACN—the only person to hold this office more than once. Dr. Preuss is a member of the board of directors for the Alliance for Natural Health (ANH-USA) and has also served as their treasurer. He wrote the nutrition section for the *Encyclopedia Americana* and is the past president of the Certification Board for Nutrition Specialists (CBNS) that gives the CNS certification. He was chairman of the Institutional Review Board (IRB) at Georgetown University, which reviews all clinical protocols at Georgetown University Medical Center, for over 20 years. He is the recipient of the William B. Peck, James Lind, and Bieber Awards for his research and activities in the medical and nutrition field. His current research, both laboratory and clinical, centers on the use of dietary supplements and nutraceuticals to favorably influence or even prevent a variety of medical perturbations, especially those related to obesity, insulin resistance, and cardiovascular disorders. Lately, he has also researched the ability of many essential oils and fats to overcome various infections, including those resistant to antibiotics. He recently won, through a vote of his peers, the coveted Charles E. Ragus Award of the ACN for publishing the best research paper in their journal for the year 2006 and the ACN Award for 2010 given to an outstanding senior investigator in nutrition.

Contributors

Sanjiv Agarwal, PhD, FACN
Campbell Soup Company
Camden, New Jersey

Bharat B. Aggarwal, PhD
Department of Experimental Therapeutics
MD Anderson Cancer Center
The University of Texas
Houston, Texas

Akhtar Afshan Ali, PhD
Division of Systems Biology
Center of Excellence for Hepatotoxicity
National Center for Toxicological Research
U.S. Food and Drug Administration
Jefferson, Arkansas

Rakesh Amin, JD, LLM
AminTalati, LLC
Chicago, Illinois

Brittany M. Angle, BS
Division of Biological Sciences
University of Missouri-Columbia
Columbia, Missouri

Livia S.A. Augustin, PhD
Clinical Nutrition and Risk Factor
   Modification Center
St. Michael's Hospital
and
Faculty of Medicine
Department of Nutritional Sciences
University of Toronto
Toronto, Ontario, Canada

David J. Baer, MS, PhD
Diet and Human Performance Laboratory
Beltsville Human Nutrition Research Center
and
Food Components and Health Laboratory
United States Department of Agriculture
Beltsville, Maryland

Debasis Bagchi, PhD, MACN, CNS, MAIChE
Department of Pharmacological
   and Pharmaceutical Sciences
College of Pharmacy
University of Houston
Houston, Texas

and

Iovate Health Sciences International, Inc.
Oakville, Ontario, Canada

Manashi Bagchi, PhD
Nutri Today LLC
Boston, Massachusetts

Marilyn L. Barrett, PhD
Pharmacognosy Consulting Services
Mill Valley, California

Stacey J. Bell, DSc, RD
Consultant
Boston, Massachusetts

Saibal K. Biswas, PhD
Department of Biochemistry
Dr. Ambedkar College
Nagpur, India

Dawn Blatt, PT, DPT, MS
Division of Rehabilitation Sciences
School of Health Technology and Management
Stony Brook University
Stony Brook, New York

**Jeffrey B. Blumberg, PhD, FASN,
   FACN, CNS**
Antioxidants Research Laboratory
Jean Mayer USDA Human Nutrition Research
   Center on Aging
Tufts University
Boston, Massachusetts

Olivier Boss, PhD
Energesis Pharmaceuticals, Inc.
Cambridge, Massachusetts

Anne Bouloumié, PhD
Institut National de la Santé et de la Recherche
    Médicale
Toulouse, France

Helmut Brath, MD
Diabetes Outpatient Clinic
Vienna, Austria

Antje Bruckbauer, MD, PhD
NuMeta Sciences, Inc.
Knoxville, Tennessee

Hien T. Bui, PharmD
Department of Pharmaceutical Sciences
School of Pharmacy
Loma Linda University
Loma Linda, California

Corinne Bush, MS, CNS
Far Hills Wellness Center
Bedminster, New Jersey

Merlin G. Butler, MD, PhD, FFACMG
Department of Psychiatry and Behavioral
    Sciences and Pediatrics
Kansas University Medical Center
Kansas City, Kansas

Monina S. Cabrera, MD
Children's Hospital and Medical Center
University of Nebraska Medical Center
Omaha, Nebraska

Hayden T. Cale, BS
Department of Chemistry and Biochemistry
La Sierra University
Riverside, California

**Francesco P. Cappuccio, FRCP, FFPH,
    FAHA**
Division of Metabolic and Vascular Health
Warwick Medical School
University of Warwick
Coventry, United Kingdom

Hellas Cena, MD
Department of Public Health,
    Neuroscience, Experimental and
    Forensic Medicine
Section of Human Nutrition
School of Medicine
University of Pavia
Pavia, Italy

Archana Chatterjee, MD, PhD
Division of Pediatric Infectious Diseases
School of Medicine
Creighton University
Omaha, Nebraska

Shampa Chatterjee, PhD
Institute for Environmental Medicine
University of Pennsylvania Medical Center
Philadelphia, Pennsylvania

C.-Y. Oliver Chen, PhD
Antioxidants Research Laboratory
Jean Mayer USDA Human Nutrition
    Research Center on Aging
Tufts University
Boston, Massachusetts

Laura Chiavaroli, MSc
Risk Factor Modification Center
and
Li Ka Shing Institute
St. Michael's Hospital
and
Faculty of Medicine
Department of Nutritional Sciences
University of Toronto
Toronto, Ontario, Canada

Benjamin L. Coe, MS
Division of Biological Sciences
University of Missouri-Columbia
Columbia, Missouri

George B. Corcoran, PhD, ATS
Department of Pharmaceutical Sciences
Eugene Applebaum College of Pharmacy
    and Health Sciences
Wayne State University
Detroit, Michigan

Kevin Corley, MD
Children's Hospital and Medical Center
University of Nebraska Medical Center
Omaha, Nebraska

Cyrile Anne Curat, PhD
Institut National de la Santé et de la Recherche
    Médicale
Toulouse, France

Sanja Cvitkusic, BS
Department of Food, Bioprocessing
    and Nutrition Science
North Carolina State University
Raleigh, North Carolina

Jean Claude Desmangles, MD, FAAP
Children's Hospital and Medical Center
University of Nebraska Mcdical Center
Omaha, Nebraska

Bernard W. Downs, BSc
LifeGen Research
Lederach, Pennsylvania

Courtenay Dunn-Lewis, MA
Human Performance Laboratory
Department of Kinesiology
University of Connecticut
Storrs, Connecticut

Anand Dusad, MD
College of Pharmacy
University of Nebraska Medical Center
and
Veterans Affairs Medical Center
Omaha, Nebraska

Rama S. Dwivedi, PhD
Division of Cardiovascular and Renal
    Products
U.S. Food and Drug Administration
Silver Spring, Maryland

Nina Eikelis, PhD
Human Neurotransmitters Laboratory
Baker IDI Heart and Diabetes Institute
Melbourne, Victoria, Australia

Mary G. Enig, PhD, FACN, MACN, CNS
Enig Associates, Inc
Silver Spring, Maryland

Lisa M. Esposito, MS, RD, CSSD, LN
Sanford University of South Dakota
    Medical Center
Sioux Falls, South Dakota

Paul W. Esposito, MD
University of Nebraska Medical Center
Omaha, Nebraska

Cristina Fernandez, MD
Department of Pediatrics
Creighton University
and
Children's Hospital and Medical Center
University of Nebraska Medical Center
Omaha, Nebraska

Rafael Fernández-Fernández, PhD
Department of Cell Biology, Physiology
    and Immunology
University of Córdoba
Córdoba, Spain

Dilip Ghosh, PhD, FACN
Nutriconnect
Sydney, New South Wales, Australia

Jean-Paul Giacobino, PhD
University of Geneva Medical Center
Geneva, Switzerland

Shirley Gonzalez, MD, FAAP
Division of General Pediatrics
St. Elizabeth's Medical Center
Brighton, Massachusetts

and

Tufts University School of Medicine
Boston, Massachusetts

Cheri L. Gostic, PT, DPT, MS
Division of Rehabilitation Sciences
School of Health Technology and Management
Stony Brook University
Stony Brook, New York

Frank L. Greenway, MD
Department of Clinical Trials
Pennington Biomedical Research Center
Louisiana State University System
Baton Rouge, Louisiana

Alok K. Gupta, MD, FAAFP, FASH
Pennington Biomedical Research Center
Louisiana State University System
Baton Rouge, Louisiana

Gabriel Keith Harris, MS, PhD
Department of Food, Bioprocessing
    and Nutrition Science
North Carolina State University
Raleigh, North Carolina

Sandra G. Hassink, MD
Thomas Jefferson University
Philadelphia, Pennsylvania

and

Department of Pediatrics
Alfred I. DuPont Hospital for Children
Wilmington, Delaware

Robert P. Heaney, MD
Creighton University
Omaha, Nebraska

Masashi Hosokawa, PhD
Hokkaido University
Hokkaido, Japan

J.R. Ifland, PhD
Refined Food Addiction Research
    Foundation
Houston, Texas

Sushil K. Jain, PhD
Department of Pediatrics
Health Sciences Center
Louisiana State University
Shreveport, Louisiana

Sarah S. Jaser, PhD
School of Nursing
Yale University
New Haven, Connecticut

David J.A. Jenkins, MD, PhD, DSc
Risk Factor Modification Center
and
Li Ka Shing Institute
St. Michael's Hospital
and
Faculty of Medicine
Department of Nutritional Sciences
University of Toronto
Toronto, Ontario, Canada

Gilbert R. Kaats, PhD, FACN
Integrative Health Technologies, Inc.
Health and Research Center
San Antonio, Texas

Chithan Kandaswami, PhD, FACN, CNS
Castle Hills Health
Saskatoon, Saskatchewan, Canada

Joyce K. Keithley, DNSc, RN, FAAN
College of Nursing
Rush University
Chicago, Illinois

Cyril W.C. Kendall, PhD
Clinical Nutrition and Risk Factor
    Modification Center
St. Michael's Hospital
and
Faculty of Medicine
Department of Nutritional Sciences
University of Toronto
Toronto, Ontario, Canada

and

College of Pharmacy and Nutrition
University of Saskatchewan
Saskatoon, Saskatchewan, Canada

Birgit Khandalavala, MD
Department of Family Medicine
School of Medicine
Creighton University
Omaha, Nebraska

Yu-Sik Kim, MS
Department of Medical Science
College of Medicine
Yonsei University
Seoul, Korea

Kathryn T. Knecht, PhD
Department of Pharmaceutical Sciences
School of Pharmacy
Loma Linda University
Loma Linda, California

Richard Zwe-Ling Kong, PhD
Department of Food Science
National Taiwan Ocean University
Keelung, Taiwan

William J. Kraemer, PhD, FACSM, FNSCA, FISSN, FACN
Human Performance Laboratory
Department of Kinesiology
University of Connecticut
Storrs, Connecticut

Madhura Kulkarni, MPharm
Department of Pharmaceutical Sciences
College of Pharmacy and Health Sciences
Texas Southern University
Houston, Texas

Julian E. Leakey, PhD, DABT
Office of Scientific Coordination
National Center for Toxicological Research
Jefferson, Arkansas

Young Sup Lee, PhD
School of life Sciences
College of Natural Sciences
Kyungpook National University
Daegu, Korea

Lorenz Lehr, PhD
Department of Cell Physiology and Metabolism
University of Geneva Medical School
Geneva, Switzerland

Marty Lerner, PhD
Milestone Treatment Center
Dallas, Texas

Karla Lester, MD
Community Pediatrician
Lincoln, Nebraska

Sherry M. Lewis, PhD
Office of Scientific Coordination
National Center for Toxicological Research
Jefferson, Arkansas

Karine Lolmède, PhD
Institut National de la Santé et de la Recherche Médicale
Toulouse, France

Hui-Ying Luk, MS
Human Performance Laboratory
Department of Kinesiology
University of Connecticut
Storrs, Connecticut

Muhammed Majeed, PhD
Sabinsa Corporation
East Windsor, New Jersey

Melania Manco, MD, PhD, FACN
Liver Unit
Bambino Gesù Pediatric Hospital and Research Institute
Rome, Italy

Marianne T. Marcus, EdD, RN, FAAN
Department of Nursing Systems
School of Nursing
University of Texas Health Science Center
Houston, Texas

Ian L. Megson, PhD
Department of Diabetes and Cardiovascular Science
Centre for Health Science
University of the Highlands and Islands
Inverness, United Kingdom

Howard Miller, MS
Nutratech Inc.
West Caldwell, New Jersey

Michelle A. Miller, PhD, MAcadMEd, FFPH
Division of Metabolic and Vascular Health
Warwick Medical School
University of Warwick
Coventry, United Kingdom

Alexandra Miranville, PhD
Institut National de la Santé et de la Recherche Médicale
Toulouse, France

Arash Mirrahimi, MSc
Risk Factor Modification Center
and
Li Ka Shing Institute
St. Michael's Hospital
and
Faculty of Medicine
Department of Nutritional Sciences
University of Toronto
Toronto, Ontario, Canada

Sumeet K. Mittal, MD
School of Medicine
Creighton University
Omaha, Nebraska

Kazuo Miyashita, PhD
Hokkaido University
Hokkaido, Japan

Jacob D. Mulligan, PhD
Department of Medicine
The University of Wisconsin-Madison
Madison, Wisconsin

Ya Fatou Njie-Mbye, PhD
Department of Pharmaceutical Sciences
College of Pharmacy and Health Sciences
Texas Southern University
Houston, Texas

Sunny E. Ohia, PhD
Department of Pharmaceutical Sciences
College of Pharmacy and Health Sciences
Texas Southern University
Houston, Texas

Catherine A. Opere, PhD
Department of Pharmacy Sciences
School of Pharmacy and Health Professions
Creighton University
Omaha, Nebraska

Sridevi Patchva, PhD
Department of Experimental Therapeutics
MD Anderson Cancer Center
The University of Texas
Houston, Texas

Sahdeo Prasad, PhD
Department of Experimental Therapeutics
MD Anderson Cancer Center
The University of Texas
Houston, Texas

Harry G. Preuss, MD, MACN, CNS
Georgetown University Medical Center
Washington, District of Columbia

Ruben E. Quiros-Tejeira, MD
Pediatric Gastroenterology, Hepatology
    & Nutrition Clinic
and
Pediatric Liver and Intestinal Transplantation
    Center
and
Division of Pediatrics and Surgery
University of Nebraska Medical Center
Omaha, Nebraska

Irfan Rahman, PhD
Department of Environmental Medicine
University of Rochester Medical Center
Rochester, New York

Dominic S. Raj, MD
Division of Renal Diseases and
    Hypertension
Department of Medicine
The George Washington University
Washington, District of Columbia

Ramaswamy Rajendran, MSc
Green Chem Herbal Extracts & Formulations
Bangalore, India

Betsy Ramsey, MS, RD, CDE, LDN
George L. Tully III, MD Diabetes Care Center
St. Elizabeth's Medical Center
Brighton, Massachusetts

Geetanjali Rathore, MD
Department of Pediatrics
and
Children's Hospital and Medical Center
University of Nebraska Medical Center
Omaha, Nebraska

Dana Reed, MS, CNS, CDN
Reed Nutrition
New York, New York

Ariel Robarge, RD
Department of Nutrition
Nutritious Lifestyles, Inc.
Orlando, Florida

K.M. Rourke, PhD
Refined Food Addiction Research
    Foundation
Houston, Texas

Sashwati Roy, PhD
Department of Surgery
Comprehensive Wound Center
Davis Heart and Lung Research Institute
Wexner Medical Center at the Ohio State
    University
Columbus, Ohio

Joan Sabate, MD, PhD
Department of Nutrition
and
Department of Epidemiology
School of Public Health
Loma Linda University
Loma Linda, California

William Frederick Salminen, PhD, DABT
Division of Systems Biology
Food and Drug Administration
Center of Excellence for Hepatotoxicity
National Center for Toxicological Research
Jefferson, Arkansas

Kurt W. Saupe, PhD
Department of Medicine
The University of Wisconsin-Madison
Madison, Wisconsin

David M. Savastano, PhD
GlaxoSmithKline Consumer Healthcare
Parsippany, New Jersey

Susan M. Schwartz, PhD
GlaxoSmithKline Consumer Healthcare
Parsippany, New Jersey

Chandan K. Sen, PhD
Department of Surgery
Davis Heart and Lung Research Institute
Wexner Medical Center at The Ohio State
    University
Columbus, Ohio

Coralie Sengenès, PhD
Institut National de la Santé et de la Recherche
    Médicale
Toulouse, France

Mohd Shara, PhD, PharmD, FACN
Faculty of Pharmacy
Jordan University of Science and
    Technology
Irbid, Jordan

Catherine A. Shaw, PhD
Centre for Cardiovascular Science
Queen's Medical Research Institute
University of Edinburgh
Edinburgh, United Kingdom

Adeeb Shehzad, PhD
Laboratory of Cellular Biochemistry
School of Life Sciences
College of Natural Sciences
Kyungpook National University
Daegu, South Korea

Kantha Shelke, PhD
Corvus Blue LLC
Chicago, Illinois

John L. Sievenpiper, MD, PhD
Department of Pathology and Molecular
    Medicine
McMaster University
Hamilton, Ontario, Canada

Na-Young Song, PhD
Tumor Microenvironment Global Core
    Research Center
College of Pharmacy
Seoul National University
Seoul, South Korea

Madhusudan G. Soni, PhD, FACN, FATS
Soni & Associates Inc.
Vero Beach, Florida

Krobua Srichaikul, MSc
Risk Factor Modification Center
and
Li Ka Shing Institute
St. Michael's Hospital
and
Department of Nutritional Sciences
Comprehensive Wound Center
University of Toronto
Toronto, Ontario, Canada

and

Medical School
University of Ottawa
Ottawa, Ontario, Canada

**Sidney J. Stohs, PhD, FACN, CNS, ATS,
   FASAHP**
Creighton University Medical Center
Omaha, Nebraska

Sang-Hoon Suh, PhD
Department of Physical Education
Yonsei University
and
Korea Institute of Sport Science
Seoul, Korea

Young-Joon Surh, PhD
Tumor Microenvironment Global Core
   Research Center
College of Pharmacy
Seoul National University
Seoul, Korea

Barbara Swanson, PhD, RN, ACRN
College of Nursing
Rush University
Chicago, Illinois

Ashish Talati, JD, MS
AminTalati, LLC
Chicago, Illinois

Julia A. Taylor, PhD
Division of Biological Sciences
University of Missouri-Columbia
Columbia, Missouri

W.C. Taylor, PhD
School of Public Health
The University of Texas
Houston, Texas

Manuel Tena-Sempere, MD, PhD
Department of Cell Biology, Physiology
   and Immunology
University of Córdoba
and
Centro de Investigación Biomédica en Red de
   Fisiopatologia de la Obesidad y Nutrición
Instituto de Salud Carlos III
Córdoba, Spain

Beverly B. Teter, MACN, CNS
Department of Animal and Avian Sciences
University of Maryland
College Park, Maryland

Don K. Tran, PharmD
Department of Pharmaceutical Sciences
School of Pharmacy
Loma Linda University
Loma Linda, California

Giovanna Turconi, PhD
Department of Public Health, Neuroscience,
   Experimental and Forensic Medicine
Section of Human Nutrition
School of Medicine
University of Pavia
Pavia, Italy

Jay K. Udani, MD
Medicus Research LLC
Northridge, California

and

Northridge Hospital Integrative Medicine
   Program
Los Angeles, California

Ramasamy V. Venkatesh, BSc, PGDIT
Gencor Pacific Limited
Discovery Bay, Hong Kong

Frederick S. vom Saal, PhD
Division of Biological Sciences
University of Missouri-Columbia
Columbia, Missouri

Karl-Heinz Wagner, PhD
Department of Nutritional Sciences
University of Vienna
Vienna, Austria

Betty Wedman-St. Louis, PhD, RD, LD
Private Practice
Disc & Spine Center
Pinellas Park, Florida

and

Department of Health Sciences
South University
Tampa, Florida

Maria R. Wing, PhD
Division of Renal Diseases and
   Hypertension
Department of Medicine
School of Medicine and Health Sciences
The George Washington University
Washington, District of Columbia

Xi Yang, PhD
Division of Systems Biology
Food and Drug Administration
Center of Excellence for Hepatotoxicity
National Center for Toxicological Research
Jefferson, Arkansas

Subhashini Yaturu, MD, FACE
Endocrinology Section
Stratton VA Medical Center
and
Department of Medicine
Albany Medical College
Albany, New York

Shirley Zafra-Stone, BS
Products Solution Research Inc.
Davis, California

Fernando Zapata, MD
Division of Pediatric Gastroenterology
and
Children's Hospital and Medical Center
University of Nebraska Medical Center
Omaha, Nebraska

Michael B. Zemel, PhD
Department of Nutrition
The University of Tennessee, Knoxville
and
NuMeta Sciences, Inc.
Knoxville, Tennessee

Part I

Introduction

1 Epidemiology of Obesity
Current Status

Giovanna Turconi, PhD and Hellas Cena, MD

CONTENTS

INTRODUCTION

Obesity is a complex, multifactorial chronic disease involving environmental (social and cultural), genetic, physiologic, metabolic, behavioral, and psychological components.

It has been increasing at an alarming rate throughout the world over the past two decades to the extent that it is now a pandemic, affecting millions of people globally, and it is the second leading cause of preventable death in the United States [1].

The 2010 International Obesity Task Force (IOTF) analysis [2] estimates that approximately 1.0 billion adults are currently overweight (body mass index [BMI] 25–29.9 kg/m²) and a further 475 million are obese. When Asian-specific cutoff points for the definition of obesity (BMI > 28 kg/m²) are taken into account, the number of adults considered obese globally is over 600 million. The IOTF estimates that up to 200 million school-age children are either overweight or obese, 40–50 million of which are classified as obese. In the European Union—27 member states—approximately 60% of adults and over 20% of school-age children are overweight or obese. This equates to around 260 million adults and over 12 million children being either overweight or obese.

Obesity is defined as a condition of excess body fat, and it is associated with a large number of debilitating and life-threatening disorders, such as a major increase in associated cardiovascular, metabolic, and other noncommunicable diseases [3]. It also contributes to increased mortality rates from all causes, including cardiovascular diseases (CVD) and cancer.

The obesity prevalence rate increase is evident in Westernized countries, where obesity has been present for decades, but today, it is also particularly noticeable in less developed countries that previously have not experienced problems with overweight and obesity. For example, the prevalence of obesity has increased by about 10%–40% in the majority of European countries in the last decade, and it currently affects nearly one-third of the adult American population, as well as more than half of the adult population living in urban areas of Western Samoa in the Pacific [4].

Between 1980 and 2004, the prevalence of obesity in the United States increased from 15% to 33% among adults and the prevalence of overweight in children increased from more than 6% to 19% [5]. Obesity is a complex condition, and prevention and treatment are difficult.

Obesity in the developing world reflects the profound changes in society over the past 20–30 years that have created an environment that promotes a sedentary lifestyle and the consumption of a high-fat, energy-dense diet, collectively known as the "nutrition transition." As poor countries become more prosperous, they acquire some of the benefits along with some of the problems of industrialized nations, including obesity (Figure 1.1) [6].

Because the direct measurement of body fat is difficult, the BMI, a simple weight-to-height ratio (kg/m^2), is typically used to classify overweight and obese adults. Consistent with this, the WHO has published international standards for classifying overweight and obesity in adults (Table 1.1). Obesity is defined as a BMI $\geq$ 30 kg/m^2 but can be further subdivided on the basis of the severity of the obesity [1].

The interpretation of BMI in terms of body fatness and in comparison with weight standards (or definitions of obesity) varies by sex, age, and other factors [7]. Only if the same body weight standards are considered to be appropriate for both men and women does a given value of BMI have the same meaning in terms of relative weight. A given value of BMI may be numerically the same for men and women and for people of different ages, but may not represent the same percentage of body fat, the same degree of risk or, even necessarily, the same degree of overweight relative to a weight standard [5].

Although the BMI provides a simple, convenient measurement of obesity, a more important aspect of obesity is the regional distribution of excess body fat. Visceral or intra-abdominal obesity, in contrast to subcutaneous or lower body obesity, carries the greatest risk of a number of chronic-degenerative diseases, including CVD and noninsulin-dependent diabetes mellitus (NIDDM). The importance of central obesity is clear in populations (e.g., Asian) who tend to have relatively low BMI values but high

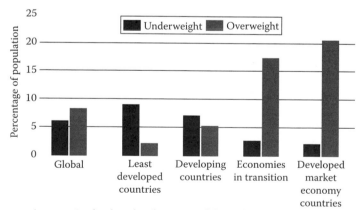

As countries develop, they face many of the problems common in industrialized nations. Obesity is one of the most worrisome.
Source: WHO, 2000.

FIGURE 1.1 From least to most developed countries: overweight is on the rise. (From FAO, The developing world's new burden: Obesity, food and agricultural organization, United Nations, Geneva, Switzerland, 2002, http://www.fao.org/FOCUS/E/obesity/obes2.htm, accessed on October 12, 2011.)

TABLE 1.1

WHO Standard Classification of Obesity

	BMI (kg/m²)	Risk of Comorbidities
Normal range	18.5–24.9	Average
Overweight	25.0–29.9	Mildly increased
Obesity class I	30.0–34.9	Moderate
Obesity class II	35.0–39.9	Severe
Obesity class III	≥40	Very severe

Source: WHO, Obesity: Preventing and managing the global epidemic, Report of a WHO consultation on obesity, Technical Report Series, No. 894, World Health Organization, Geneva, Switzerland, 2000, p. 256.

levels of abdominal fat and are particularly prone to NIDDM, hypertension, and CVD. Methods for evaluating abdominal fat include measuring waist circumference. Changes in waist circumference reflect changes in risk for CVD and other chronic diseases. As with the BMI, cutoff values have been set to identify increased risk, but for waist circumference, these must be sex and population specific (Table 1.2) [1].

In children, "overweight, obesity, and at risk for overweight" are the terminologies for different levels of weight or BMI [8]. For adults, the currently used definitions of overweight and obesity are related to functional outcomes of mortality and morbidity and are based on fixed values of BMI, not varying by age or sex; in children, there are no risk-based fixed values of BMI used to determine overweight because it is unclear what risk-related criteria should be used.

A variety of reference data sets for BMI in childhood exist. One reference set of BMI values that has been widely used consists of sex-specific smoothed 85th and 95th percentiles for single year of age from 6 to 19 years based on data from the first NHANES I, 1971–1974, in the United States [9]. In 1995, a WHO Expert Committee recommended the use of these reference values [10].

TABLE 1.2

Sex-Specific Waist Circumferences for "Increased Risk" and "Substantially Increased Risk" of Metabolic Complications Associated with Obesity in Caucasians

	Risk of Obesity-Associated Metabolic Complications	
	Increased	Substantially Increased
Men	≥94 cm	≥102 cm
Women	≥80 cm	≥88 cm

Source: WHO, Obesity: Preventing and managing the global epidemic, Report of a WHO consultation on obesity, Technical Report Series, No. 894, World Health Organization, Geneva, Switzerland, 2000, p. 256.

Note: The figures are population specific, and the relative risk also depends on the levels of obesity (BMI) and other risk factors for CVD and NIDDM.

In 2000, Cole et al. [11] published a set of smoothed sex-specific BMI cutoff values based on six nationally representative data sets from Brazil, Great Britain, Hong Kong, the Netherlands, Singapore, and the United States. These values, often referred to as the IOTF cutoff values, represent cutoff points chosen as the percentiles that matched the adult cutoffs of BMI 25 and 30 at age 18 years. The IOTF cutoffs were not intended as clinical definitions and were not aimed at replacing the national reference data, but rather to provide a common set of definitions that researchers and policy makers in different countries could use for descriptive and comparative purposes internationally. The IOTF's

TABLE 1.3
All-Cause and Disease-Specific Cause of Death from Several Epidemiological Studies in Relation to BMI

Study and BMI Criteria (kg/m²)	All-Cause Mortality[a]	
	Male	Female
Nurses Health Study (age 30–55 years, with 16 years' follow-up)		
19.0–21.9	—	2.46
22.0–24.9	—	2.46
25.0–26.9	—	2.61
27–28.9	—	3.35
29–31.9	—	3.90
>32	—	4.64
British Regional Heart Study[8] (age 40–59 years, with 13.8 years' follow-up)		
20–21.9	12.6	—
22–23.9	11.5	—
24–25.9	11.8	—
26–27.9	11.8	—
28–29.9	13.3	—
>30	16.8	—
Gothenburg Birth Cohort[9] (age 47–55 years, with 19.7 years' follow-up)		
20.0–22.5	15.5	—
22.5–25.0	13.9	—
25.0–27.5	14.3	—
27.5–30	16.6	—
>30	21.1	—
Cancer Prevention Study II (age 65–74 years)[10]		
22.0–23.4	8.54	4.98
23.5–24.9	8.98	5.95
25.0–26.4	9.41	5.98
26.5–27.9	10.38	6.36
28.0–29.9	12.70	7.96
30.0–31.9	13.70	8.36
32.0–34.9	17.98	11.11
>35.0	27.67	12.99

Source: Caterson, I.D. et al., *Circulation*, 110, e476, 2004.
[a] Deaths/thousand patient-years.

international standard for analyzing childhood overweight and obesity data has been widely adopted, and it enables more realistic comparisons to be made between data from different countries.

However, we must still recognize that overweight and obesity are part of a continuum and that health risks increase with increasing weight in the individual.

It has been estimated that the costs of obesity account for up to 8% of the total health-care costs in Western countries, and they represent an enormous burden with regard to individual illness, disability, and early mortality as well as in terms of the costs to employers, tax payers, and society.

The mortality associated with excess weight increases as the degree of obesity and overweight increases. One study estimated that between 280,000 and 325,000 deaths annually in the United States could be attributed to overweight and obesity [12]. More than 80% of these deaths occur among people with a BMI > 30 kg/m². The increase in deaths due to obesity has been documented in a number of studies from around the world (Table 1.3) [13–17].

PREVALENCE OF OBESITY IN THE ADULT POPULATION

It should be noted that it is often difficult to make a direct comparison of the prevalence of obesity between countries due to the inconsistent classifications used for obesity. This problem may be overcome with the adoption in future surveys of the WHO standardized classification for obesity.

From available data, the worldwide prevalence of obesity has been found to range from less than 5% in rural China, Japan, and some African countries to levels as high as 55% of the adult population in urban Samoa. Table 1.4 shows the prevalence estimates of overweight and obesity within the world in 2002 and projections for 2005 and 2010, by sex, in the adults aged 15 and over provided by the WHO in 2005 [18].

Obesity levels also vary depending on ethnic origin. In the United States, particularly among women, large differences exist in the prevalence of obesity among populations of different ethnic origins within the same country.

EUROPE

Obesity is relatively common in Europe, especially among women and in Southern and Eastern European countries. A marked trend toward increasing levels of adult overweight and obesity can be found throughout Europe, although prevalence rates differ. Data from WHO (2005) [18] suggest that the range of obesity prevalence in European countries in 2002 is 2.5% 26.2% for men and up to 33% for women. When judged on obesity alone, at least 21 European countries have female obesity rates above 20%, including Malta and Turkey (>30%).

The prevalence of obesity has increased by about 10%–40% in most of the European countries in the last decade. In France, obesity rose from 8.0% to 11.3% and from 8.4% to 11.4% in women and men, respectively, in self-reported survey conducted between 1997 and 2003. In the Netherlands, obesity rose gradually from 6.2% to 9.3% and from 4.9% to 8.5% in women and men, respectively, from the late 1970s to the mid-1990s. The most dramatic increase was recorded in the United Kingdom, where the obesity rate rose from 13.2% to 22.2% in men and from 16.4% to 23.0% in women respectively in just 10 years, up to 2003, this compared with an obesity rate of 6%–7% in 1980 [19].

Figure 1.2 shows the prevalence of adult obesity in Europe provided by the IOTF 2003 [20].

UNITED STATES

National survey data from the United States show that the prevalence of overweight and obesity among adults remained relatively constant over the 20 year period from 1960 to 1980. It began to increase around the mid-1980s, and the past 25 years have witnessed a dramatic increase. In 1985, only a few states participated in and provided obesity data to the Behavioral Risk Factor Surveillance System (BRFSS) of the Centers for Disease Control and Prevention (CDC). In 1991, four states reported obesity prevalence rates of 15%–19%, and no states had rates at or above 20%. In 2004, 7 states had

TABLE 1.4
Prevalence Estimates of Overweight and Obesity for 2002, and Projections for 2005 and 2010, by Sex, Adults Aged 15 and over, around the World

	Prevalence of Overweight Male			Prevalence of Overweight Female			Prevalence of Obesity Male %			Prevalence of Obesity Female %		
	2002	2005	2010	2002	2005	2010	2002	2005	2010	2002	2005	2010
WHO African region												
Angola	19.9	21.3	23.8	31.4	33.6	37.2	1.6	1.9	2.4	5.9	6.9	8.7
Benin	15.8	17.9	21.9	32.8	39.1	43.8	0.7	1.0	1.5	6.2	9.3	12.1
Botswana	35.5	37.8	41.6	46.9	49.4	53.5	4.6	5.4	6.9	12.9	14.6	17.7
Burkina Faso	10.6	12.1	15.1	15.8	16.0	19.4	0.3	0.4	0.6	1.1	1.1	1.7
Burundi	7.0	7.8	9.1	16.3	18.1	21.1	0.1	0.1	0.2	1.2	1.5	2.2
Cameroon	35.7	38.7	43.9	38.3	41.1	45.8	6.3	7.5	10.1	9.2	10.8	13.8
Cape Verde	30.5	32.4	35.6	41.8	44.1	48.0	4.0	4.6	5.8	11.0	12.5	15.1
Central African Republic	6.7	7.2	8.0	17.7	18.5	20.0	0.1	0.1	0.1	1.1	1.3	1.5
Chad	10.4	12.0	15.0	17.1	19.2	22.9	0.3	0.4	0.6	1.3	1.7	2.6
Comoros	17.7	20.0	24.3	33.1	35.9	40.7	0.9	1.2	1.9	5.8	7.1	9.6
Congo, Democratic Republic of	4.3	4.8	5.7	11.9	13.3	15.8	0.0	0.0	0.1	0.6	0.8	1.1
Congo, Republic of	12.0	12.7	13.8	24.2	25.2	26.8	0.4	0.4	0.5	2.7	3.0	3.5
Côte d'Ivoire	10.9	11.6	12.7	32.5	34.2	36.0	0.2	0.2	0.3	4.8	5.4	6.2
Djibouti	17.6	18.9	21.2	28.8	31.0	34.5	1.2	1.4	1.8	5.0	5.8	7.4
Equatorial Guinea	35.4	37.5	41.0	46.1	48.5	52.3	5.6	6.4	7.9	13.8	15.4	18.4
Eritrea	2.9	3.1	3.5	5.9	5.7	6.3	0.0	0.0	0.0	0.1	0.1	0.1
Ethiopia	7.4	7.8	8.6	3.1	3.3	3.7	0.1	0.2	0.2	0.0	0.0	0.0
Gabon	22.7	25.4	30.2	45.0	47.7	52.2	1.8	2.3	3.4	13.5	15.5	19.2
Gambia	9.0	10.3	12.8	20.5	22.8	27.0	0.2	0.3	0.5	1.9	2.5	3.6
Ghana	27.3	30.3	35.6	26.2	28.1	32.5	2.6	3.3	4.8	3.5	4.2	5.9
Guinea	14.5	16.5	20.3	27.8	30.4	34.9	0.6	0.8	1.3	4.2	5.2	7.1
Guinea-Bissau	10.5	11.4	12.9	20.3	22.1	25.1	0.4	0.5	0.6	2.4	2.8	3.7
Kenya	6.5	6.9	7.7	21.3	21.7	23.3	0.1	0.1	0.1	1.8	1.9	2.2
Lesotho	26.3	27.5	29.5	68.7	69.5	70.8	1.7	1.9	2.3	33.2	34.3	36.1
Liberia	27.8	29.6	32.7	39.2	41.6	45.4	3.3	3.8	4.8	9.6	11.0	13.4

Madagascar	12.9	4.5	17.5	18.1	20.2	24.1	0.7	1.0	1.5	1.5	1.9	2.9
Malawi	14.3	5.1	16.4	21.6	23.5	25.2	0.6	0.7	0.8	1.6	2.0	2.4
Mali	12.8	14.6	13.1	26.1	33.6	38.4	0.4	0.6	1.0	3.4	6.2	8.4
Mauritania	27.5	30.4	35.4	52.2	54.6	58.6	2.9	3.7	5.3	20.6	22.9	26.9
Mozambique	8.7	9.3	12.3	24.3	25.3	26.9	0.1	0.2	0.2	2.7	3.0	3.4
Namibia	11.6	12.3	13.5	31.5	32.6	34.4	0.2	0.3	0.4	4.9	5.3	6.1
Niger	12.1	13.9	17.2	19.6	21.3	25.1	0.4	0.6	0.9	1.9	2.3	3.4
Nigeria	19.6	21.9	26.0	29.6	32.2	36.8	1.6	2.0	3.0	4.9	6.0	8.1
Rwanda	6.8	7.3	8.1	19.2	20.1	21.7	0.1	0.1	0.1	1.2	1.3	1.6
Sao Tome and Principe	14.4	15.5	17.5	25.2	27.2	30.5	0.8	0.9	1.2	3.7	4.4	5.7
Senegal	14.4	16.1	19.2	34.1	36.7	41.0	1.0	1.3	2.0	7.8	9.2	11.8
Seychelles	55.1	58.5	65.8	68.6	70.7	73.8	14.2	16.7	21.3	35.8	38.6	43.2
Sierra Leone	20.2	22.4	26.3	41.6	44.5	49.1	1.9	2.4	3.5	10.9	12.7	16.0
Somalia	9.8	10.6	12.1	19.3	21.1	24.0	0.3	0.4	0.6	2.1	2.6	3.4
South Africa	38.2	39.3	41.3	66.4	67.2	68.5	6.2	6.7	7.6	34.3	35.2	36.8
Sudan	16.0	17.2	19.3	27.0	29.1	32.5	1.0	1.2	1.5	4.3	5.1	6.5
Swaziland	33.6	35.8	39.5	45.2	47.8	51.9	4.0	4.7	6.1	11.8	13.5	16.5
Tanzania, United Republic of	14.7	15.4	16.8	26.0	27.0	28.7	0.6	0.7	0.8	2.8	3.1	3.6
Togo	15.0	17.1	20.9	28.3	30.9	35.5	0.6	0.9	1.4	4.3	5.3	7.3
Uganda	6.9	7.4	3.2	20.1	22.2	23.9	0.1	0.1	0.1	1.3	1.6	1.9
Zambia	7.0	7.5	3.3	20.2	18.6	20.0	0.1	0.1	0.1	1.6	1.3	1.5
Zimbabwe	14.5	15.3	13.7	47.2	48.9	50.6	0.5	0.6	0.8	14.1	15.3	16.7
WHO Eastern Mediterranean and Middle East region												
Afghanistan	11.2	12.7	15.6	15.6	17.4	20.8	0.3	0.5	0.7	1.1	1.4	2.1
Algeria	32.1	34.1	37.4	43.2	45.6	49.4	4.5	5.2	6.4	11.9	13.4	16.2
Armenia	53.9	53.9	53.9	52.8	52.8	52.8	12.1	12.1	12.1	19.8	19.8	19.8
Bahrain	60.9	60.9	60.9	66.0	67.3	69.5	21.2	21.2	21.2	33.5	35.2	37.9
Brunei Darussalam	55.3	56.4	58.1	61.9	63.2	65.2	14.4	15.2	16.6	25.9	27.4	29.7
Egypt	64.5	64.5	69.7	69.7	74.2	76.0	22.0	22.0	22.0	39.3	45.5	48.0
Iran, Islamic Republic of	47.3	48.5	48.5	55.7	57.8	60.2	9.4	10.0	10.0	25.0	27.0	29.5
Iraq	38.7	40.1	42.4	49.0	50.8	53.6	6.6	7.2	8.3	15.5	16.8	19.1
Jordan	57.5	57.5	57.5	63.4	63.4	65.4	19.6	19.6	19.6	40.2	35.6	37.9
Kuwait	69.5	69.5	69.5	76.6	79.0	80.4	29.6	29.6	29.6	49.2	52.9	55.2
Lebanon	51.7	51.7	51.7	52.9	54.3	56.7	14.9	14.9	14.9	23.9	25.2	27.4

(continued)

TABLE 1.4 (continued)

Prevalence Estimates of Overweight and Obesity for 2002, and Projections for 2005 and 2010, by Sex, Adults Aged 15 and over, around the World

	Prevalence of Overweight Male			Prevalence of Overweight Female			Prevalence of Obesity Male %			Prevalence of Obesity Female %		
	2002	2005	2010	2002	2005	2010	2002	2005	2010	2002	2005	2010
Libyan Arab Jamahiriya	47.6	48.8	50.8	56.0	57.5	59.8	10.7	11.4	12.7	21.1	22.5	24.9
Morocco	31.1	31.1	31.1	53.0	54.7	57.5	3.7	3.7	3.7	19.0	20.5	23.1
Oman	43.4	43.4	43.4	46.0	47.8	50.8	7.7	7.7	7.7	13.5	14.8	17.0
Pakistan	16.7	18.8	22.8	23.2	25.5	29.5	0.8	1.0	1.6	2.9	3.6	5.0
Qatar	56.9	57.9	59.5	62.9	64.1	65.9	16.6	17.4	18.7	27.9	29.3	31.6
Saudi Arabia	62.4	63.1	63.1	63.0	63.8	65.9	22.3	23.0	23.0	32.8	33.8	36.4
Syrian Arab Republic	47.2	48.4	50.4	55.7	57.2	59.6	10.5	11.2	12.4	20.8	22.2	24.6
Tunisia	42.8	42.8	42.8	57.9	59.2	61.4	7.7	7.7	7.7	28.8	30.2	32.6
United Arab Emirates	66.9	66.9	66.9	68.4	69.6	71.6	24.5	24.5	24.5	37.9	39.4	42.0
Yemen	24.6	24.6	24.6	27.8	29.4	32.2	2.0	2.0	2.0	4.4	5.1	6.2
WHO European region												
Albania	57.2	57.2	57.2	52.5	52.5	52.5	18.6	18.6	18.6	23.8	23.8	23.8
Andorra	59.8	60.9	62.5	65.5	66.8	68.7	14.9	15.8	17.1	27.3	28.8	31.2
Austria	59.0	61.0	62.9	53.4	53.2	55.2	19.5	21.3	23.1	20.4	20.3	21.8
Azerbaijan	57.4	57.4	57.4	56.8	56.8	56.8	15.4	15.4	15.4	24.9	24.9	24.9
Belarus	63.7	63.7	63.7	69.9	69.9	69.9	16.2	16.2	16.2	32.2	32.2	32.2
Belgium	49.0	51.9	54.1	40.7	40.7	42.9	11.4	13.3	14.8	9.5	9.5	10.7
Bosnia and Herzegovina	56.6	56.6	56.6	51.0	51.0	51.0	13.8	13.8	13.8	21.5	21.5	21.5
Bulgaria	62.8	62.8	62.8	45.5	45.5	45.5	17.0	17.0	17.0	19.0	19.0	19.0
Croatia	60.0	61.3	63.5	45.3	46.4	48.3	17.1	18.2	20.1	15.4	16.2	17.6
Cyprus	50.4	51.7	53.9	59.0	60.6	63.0	9.4	10.1	11.4	20.7	22.2	24.7
Czech Republic	56.7	58.1	60.1	47.0	47.8	49.3	17.4	18.5	20.2	20.0	20.7	22.1
Denmark	50.7	52.5	55.0	37.5	39.1	41.4	9.6	10.6	12.0	6.4	7.1	8.3
Estonia	50.7	50.7	50.7	33.8	33.8	33.8	8.6	8.6	8.6	8.4	8.4	8.4
Finland	63.8	64.9	67.1	52.0	52.4	54.5	18.0	18.9	20.9	17.5	17.8	19.4

Country												
France	44.1	45.5	48.0	33.4	34.7	36.9	7.2	7.8	9.0	6.1	6.6	7.6
Georgia	37.4	38.9	41.5	48.9	50.8	53.8	4.7	5.2	6.1	13.4	14.7	17.1
Germany	63.7	65.1	67.2	53.6	55.1	57.1	19.7	20.9	22.9	19.2	20.4	22.1
Greece	74.6	75.7	77.5	60.1	61.3	63.2	26.2	27.7	30.3	23.4	24.5	26.4
Hungary	55.9	55.9	55.9	47.4	47.4	47.4	15.8	15.8	15.8	16.1	16.1	16.1
Iceland	57.7	59.0	61.2	50.5	61.7	63.7	15.7	16.7	18.5	22.0	23.2	25.3
Ireland	50.0	51.5	53.9	40.3	41.7	43.9	9.5	10.3	11.7	8.4	9.1	10.4
Israel	55.9	57.2	59.4	56.3	57.5	59.3	15.2	16.2	17.9	23.3	24.3	25.9
Italy	51.9	52.7	55.0	37.8	38.3	40.0	12.2	12.9	14.4	12.2	12.6	13.7
Kazakhstan	43.9	43.9	43.9	41.9	38.9	38.9	7.9	7.9	7.9	13.1	11.0	11.0
Kyrgyzstan	34.5	34.5	34.5	43.9	43.9	43.9	5.0	5.0	5.0	14.2	14.2	14.2
Latvia	49.9	49.9	49.9	44.7	44.7	44.7	9.7	9.7	9.7	15.0	15.0	15.0
Lithuania	62.3	62.3	62.3	43.9	43.9	43.9	16.8	16.8	16.8	13.9	13.9	13.9
Luxembourg	53.0	54.4	56.9	52.6	54.0	56.2	11.2	12.1	13.6	15.0	16.0	17.8
Macedonia, FYR	37.1	37.1	37.1	57.4	57.4	57.4	5.9	5.9	5.9	24.3	24.3	24.3
Malta	70.2	71.4	73.3	65.1	66.1	67.6	24.6	25.9	28.1	33.8	34.8	36.5
Moldova, Republic of	33.3	34.8	37.5	45.4	47.4	50.7	3.5	4.0	4.8	11.2	12.5	14.8
Monaco	58.0	59.1	50.9	64.3	65.6	67.6	13.7	14.5	15.9	26.0	27.5	29.9
Netherlands	46.7	48.0	50.2	42.6	44.0	46.1	9.6	10.4	11.7	10.7	11.5	12.9
Norway	53.3	54.8	57.2	42.0	43.4	45.8	10.4	11.3	12.8	8.6	9.3	10.7
Poland	50.7	50.7	50.7	44.3	44.3	44.3	12.9	12.9	12.9	18.0	18.0	18.0
Portugal	55.5	58.5	60.9	27.6	49.2	51.2	13.1	13.7	15.5	14.6	16.1	17.7
Romania	37.7	37.7	37.7	40.6	40.6	40.6	5.5	5.5	5.5	12.0	12.0	12.0
Russian Federation	46.5	46.5	46.5	51.7	51.7	51.7	9.6	9.6	9.6	23.6	23.6	23.6
San Marino	57.6	58.8	60.5	64.1	65.4	67.4	13.5	14.3	15.7	25.7	27.2	29.7
Serbia and Montenegro	61.2	61.2	61.2	48.5	48.5	48.5	17.7	17.7	17.7	20.6	20.6	20.6
Slovakia	50.7	52.0	54.0	59.1	60.6	62.9	10.1	10.8	12.0	21.3	22.8	25.3
Slovenia	54.8	56.0	57.9	62.1	63.5	65.7	11.8	12.5	13.9	23.7	25.2	27.6
Spain	55.7	55.8	57.9	45.7	47.7	49.8	15.6	15.6	17.3	14.5	15.8	17.3
Sweden	51.7	54.5	57.0	43.3	44.9	47.2	10.1	11.8	13.3	10.0	10.9	12.4
Switzerland	52.4	54.1	56.5	53.8	56.7	58.9	11.4	12.4	13.9	16.4	18.7	20.6
Tajikistan	29.2	30.8	33.5	41.8	43.9	47.4	2.5	2.9	3.6	9.2	10.4	12.6
Turkey	47.9	47.9	47.9	65.4	65.7	55.7	10.8	10.8	10.8	32.1	32.5	32.5

(continued)

TABLE 1.4 (continued)

Prevalence Estimates of Overweight and Obesity for 2002, and Projections for 2005 and 2010, by Sex, Adults Aged 15 and over, around the World

	Prevalence of Overweight Male			Prevalence of Overweight Female			Prevalence of Obesity Male %			Prevalence of Obesity Female %		
	2002	2005	2010	2002	2005	2010	2002	2005	2010	2002	2005	2010
Turkmenistan	48.1	48.1	48.1	45.5	45.5	45.5	9.3	9.3	9.3	15.0	15.0	15.0
Ukraine	41.2	41.2	41.2	48.5	48.5	48.5	7.4	7.4	7.4	19.4	19.4	19.4
United Kingdom	62.5	65.7	67.8	58.8	61.9	63.8	18.7	21.6	23.7	21.3	24.2	26.3
Uzbekistan	42.0	42.0	42.0	44.3	49.9	49.9	7.1	7.1	7.1	13.5	17.6	17.6
WHO North American region												
Antigua and Barbuda	50.0	51.2	53.2	58.3	59.8	62.1	10.4	11.2	12.4	21.5	22.9	25.3
Bahamas	55.9	57.0	58.7	62.5	63.8	65.9	13.9	14.7	16.0	25.6	27.1	29.5
Barbados	55.5	59.2	65.1	77.8	80.1	83.3	14.1	16.8	22.0	46.7	50.8	57.2
Belize	43.3	44.7	47.0	53.3	54.9	57.6	7.3	7.9	9.0	17.2	18.6	21.0
Canada	64.5	65.1	66.9	55.9	57.1	59.5	23.1	23.7	25.5	22.2	23.2	25.7
Dominica	61.5	65.1	70.8	74.4	77.1	80.8	16.9	20.0	25.8	41.8	46.0	52.6
Grenada	47.4	48.7	50.8	56.4	58.0	60.4	9.1	9.8	11.0	19.8	21.2	23.6
Guyana	40.6	42.1	44.4	51.2	52.9	55.8	6.3	6.8	7.9	15.6	17.0	19.4
Haiti	13.0	15.1	19.0	39.8	50.6	57.7	0.5	0.7	1.3	8.2	15.0	21.1
Jamaica	36.0	40.0	46.8	71.8	74.7	79.0	3.8	5.1	7.7	36.4	41.0	48.3
Mexico	64.6	68.4	73.6	65.6	67.9	73.0	20.3	24.0	30.1	31.6	34.3	41.0
Saint Kitts and Nevis	50.7	52.0	53.9	58.9	60.3	62.6	10.8	11.6	12.8	22.0	23.4	25.8
Saint Lucia	41.3	45.5	52.5	65.7	69.1	74.1	5.0	6.6	9.8	30.5	34.7	41.7
Saint Vincent and the Grenadines	44.3	45.6	47.9	54.0	55.7	58.3	7.7	8.4	9.5	17.8	19.2	21.6
Trinidad and Tobago	54.8	58.9	65.2	74.4	77.0	80.8	11.3	14.0	19.1	41.9	46.1	52.7
United States of America	72.2	75.6	80.5	69.8	72.6	76.7	32.0	36.5	44.2	37.8	41.8	48.3
WHO South and Central American region												
Argentina	70.1	73.1	77.7	62.1	65.7	71.2	28.0	31.4	37.4	27.1	31.0	37.8
Bolivia	52.5	56.3	62.4	64.4	68.0	73.2	12.2	14.7	19.4	28.8	33.1	40.2
Brazil	43.4	47.4	54.0	49.2	53.5	60.3	6.9	8.7	12.4	15.0	18.3	24.5
Chile	58.9	62.6	68.4	64.4	68.0	73.3	16.1	19.0	24.3	27.2	31.6	39.1

Colombia	52.7	56.5	62.6	55.1	54.6	61.1	12.4	14.9	19.6	20.3	19.9	26.1
Costa Rica	49.8	53.9	60.1	56.2	57.8	63.8	10.6	13.0	17.5	22.7	24.2	30.5
Cuba	55.2	59.2	65.4	57.0	61.1	67.2	12.3	14.9	20.1	20.7	24.6	31.5
Dominican Republic	42.5	46.6	53.4	62.8	66.4	71.7	6.0	7.7	11.2	27.8	31.8	38.7
Ecuador	40.2	41.7	44.0	50.9	52.6	55.5	6.1	6.7	7.7	15.4	16.7	19.1
El Salvador	42.1	43.5	45.8	52.3	54.0	56.8	6.8	7.4	8.5	16.5	17.8	20.2
Guatemala	53.2	56.9	62.9	61.1	65.4	70.9	13.1	15.7	20.5	25.0	29.7	36.8
Honduras	36.2	37.6	40.1	47.5	49.4	52.5	4.7	5.2	6.2	13.1	14.4	16.7
Nicaragua	48.9	52.9	59.4	62.9	68.1	73.1	9.3	11.5	15.9	28.3	34.3	41.1
Panama	45.2	46.5	48.7	54.7	56.3	58.9	8.1	8.8	9.9	18.3	19.8	22.2
Paraguay	40.9	42.3	44.7	51.4	53.2	56.0	6.4	7.0	8.0	15.8	17.2	19.6
Peru	50.8	54.6	60.9	62.7	64.7	70.1	10.8	13.2	17.7	28.9	31.1	37.7
Suriname	41.0	42.4	44.8	51.5	53.2	56.1	6.4	7.0	8.1	15.8	17.2	19.6
Uruguay	60.0	63.6	69.3	54.1	58.1	64.4	17.1	20.1	25.7	19.6	23.3	29.8
Venezuela	65.6	69.1	74.4	57.5	61.4	67.3	19.7	23.2	29.5	22.4	26.2	33.0
WHO Southeast Asian region												
Bangladesh	5.9	6.7	8.4	4.3	5.4	6.7	0.1	0.1	0.2	0.1	0.2	0.2
Bhutan	34.0	35.3	37.7	44.7	46.5	49.6	5.3	5.8	6.7	13.1	14.3	16.5
India	15.0	16.8	20.1	13.7	15.2	18.1	0.9	1.1	1.7	1.1	1.4	2.0
Maldives	29.7	32.3	36.6	45.7	47.6	50.8	4.7	5.7	7.7	20.2	22.0	25.0
Mauritius	35.6	39.0	44.8	49.5	52.3	56.8	4.5	5.6	8.0	16.1	18.3	22.3
Nepal	7.7	8.8	11.0	8.0	8.0	9.9	0.1	0.2	0.3	0.2	0.2	0.3
Sri Lanka	8.8	8.9	9.1	5.0	5.9	7.9	0.2	0.2	0.2	0.1	0.1	0.2
WHO Western Pacific region												
Australia	69.7	72.1	75.7	60.2	62.7	66.5	21.2	23.8	28.4	22.5	24.9	29.1
Cambodia	9.6	13.3	21.4	7.1	9.3	13.8	0.1	0.2	0.5	0.1	0.1	0.4
China	27.5	33.1	45.0	22.7	24.7	32.0	1.0	1.6	4.1	1.5	1.9	3.6
Cook Islands	92.0	92.6	93.4	88.5	89.2	90.3	67.9	69.5	72.1	69.0	70.8	73.4
Fiji	42.7	43.9	47.5	63.4	65.6	69.5	7.8	8.7	10.7	29.8	32.5	37.1
Indonesia	9.6	9.7	9.9	20.3	22.7	27.1	0.2	0.2	0.2	2.0	2.6	3.9
Japan	25.3	27.0	29.8	18.6	18.1	16.2	1.5	1.8	2.3	1.5	1.5	1.1
Kiribati	71.4	73.2	76.1	71.9	73.9	77.1	27.6	29.8	33.6	37.9	41.0	46.1
Korea, Democratic People's Republic of	31.0	32.7	35.5	44.0	46.2	49.7	2.4	2.7	3.4	9.5	10.7	12.9
Korea, Republic of	32.8	40.2	55.5	38.2	43.8	51.0	2.3	4.1	8.3	7.2	10.1	14.6

(continued)

TABLE 1.4 (continued)
Prevalence Estimates of Overweight and Obesity for 2002, and Projections for 2005 and 2010, by Sex, Adults Aged 15 and over, around the World

	Prevalence of Overweight Male			Prevalence of Overweight Female			Prevalence of Obesity Male %			Prevalence of Obesity Female %		
	2002	2005	2010	2002	2005	2010	2002	2005	2010	2002	2005	2010
Lao People's Democratic Republic	30.4	32.1	34.9	43.5	45.6	49.2	2.3	2.6	3.3	9.2	10.4	12.6
Malaysia	22.5	22.7	23.0	34.2	37.2	42.2	1.6	1.6	1.7	6.8	8.2	11.0
Marshall Islands	39.1	40.6	43.0	50.0	51.8	54.7	5.7	6.3	7.3	14.8	16.1	18.5
Micronesia, Federated States of	91.5	92.1	93.1	89.5	90.1	91.1	64.3	66.2	69.1	71.3	72.9	75.3
Mongolia	46.0	53.0	64.1	65.8	69.3	74.4	5.2	7.9	14.5	24.6	29.0	36.6
Myanmar	27.8	29.4	32.3	41.1	43.3	47.0	1.8	2.1	2.7	8.0	9.1	11.3
Nauru	96.3	96.5	96.9	92.0	92.4	93.0	82.3	83.2	84.6	77.7	78.8	80.5
New Zealand	65.2	68.7	73.9	64.0	68.2	74.2	19.7	23.0	28.9	26.7	31.5	39.9
Niue	76.9	78.5	80.9	83.8	85.0	86.7	34.4	36.8	40.7	58.6	61.0	64.7
Palau	72.7	74.5	77.2	81.0	82.4	84.5	29.0	31.2	35.0	52.2	55.0	59.4
Papua New Guinea	29.2	31.5	35.3	26.1	29.0	34.0	2.0	2.5	3.4	3.2	4.2	6.1
Philippines	21.7	21.9	22.2	25.4	28.5	33.6	1.1	1.1	1.1	2.8	3.7	5.5
Samoa	77.2	78.7	81.1	80.7	82.1	84.1	36.2	38.4	42.2	55.0	57.3	60.9
Singapore	23.6	23.8	24.1	20.7	22.0	26.7	1.3	1.3	1.4	1.6	1.8	2.9
Solomon Islands	36.8	38.2	40.7	48.0	49.9	52.9	4.9	5.4	6.4	13.4	14.7	17.1
Thailand	27.7	27.9	28.3	32.5	35.2	39.9	2.5	2.5	2.6	7.0	8.4	11.1
Timor-Leste, Democratic Republic of	35.9	37.2	39.5	46.4	48.2	51.1	6.0	6.5	7.5	14.2	15.4	17.7
Tonga	89.5	90.3	91.4	90.9	91.4	92.1	58.7	60.7	64.0	74.8	76.1	78.1
Tuvalu	51.2	52.5	54.4	59.2	60.7	62.9	11.1	11.9	13.1	22.3	23.8	26.2
Vanuatu	54.0	56.3	60.2	60.1	62.9	67.2	11.9	13.4	16.2	23.4	26.3	31.4
Vietnam	2.7	4.1	7.5	7.0	8.7	12.2	0.0	0.0	0.0	0.2	0.3	0.7

Source: British Hearth Foundation Statistics website, Prevalence estimates of overweight and obesity for 2002, and projections for 2005 and 2010, by sex, adults aged 15 and over, the world. From The SuRF Report 2, Surveillance of chronic risk factors: Country-level data and comparable estimates, pp. 66–72, 73–79, 2005 WHO, Geneva, Switzerland, January 29, 2009, http://www.heartstats.org and https://apps.who.int/infobase/publicfiles/SuRF2.pdf

Notes: Values are age standardized to the WHO Standard Population. Overweight is defined as BMI ≥ 25 kg/m². Obese is defined as BMI ≥ 30 kg/m². Estimates for 2005 and 2010 are projections only.

Males

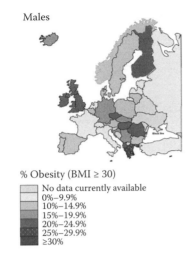

Females

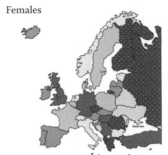

% Obesity (BMI ≥ 30)

- No data currently available
- 0%–9.9%
- 10%–14.9%
- 15%–19.9%
- 20%–24.9%
- 25%–29.9%
- ≥30%

Maps are not presented to scale
This International Obesity Task Force assessment of
obesity prevalence is based on published surveys or
unpublished data provided to the IOTF for its WHO global
burden of disease research. If you would like to discuss
or offer additional data, please email rleach@iotf.org.

© Prepared by Rachel Jackson Leach and Neville Rigby,
International Obesity Task Force, 231 North Gower Street,
London NW1 2NS email: obesity@iotf.org
www.iotf.org the IOTF is a part of the International
Association for the Study of Obesity.

FIGURE 1.2 Prevalence of adult obesity in Europe (BMI ≥ 30 kg/m²). (From Rigby, N. and James, P., Waiting for a green light for health? Europe at the crossroads for diet and disease, IOTF Position Paper, International Obesity Task Force, London, U.K., 2003, http://www.iotf.org/media/euobesity2.pdf, accessed on November 24, 2011.)

obesity prevalence rates of 15%–19%, 33 states had rates of 20%–24%, and 9 states had rates higher than 25% (no data for one state). A IOTF report [19] shows that obesity stands at 28% in men and 34% in women, although this rate rises to as high as 50% among black women and includes a very significant component of morbid obesity. The data shown in Figure 1.3 [21] were collected through the CDC's BRFSS. Each year, state health departments use standard procedures to collect data through a series of monthly telephone interviews with U.S. adults.

Obesity trends* among U.S. adults
BRFSS, 1991, 1996, 2004
(*BMI ≥ 30, or about 30 lb overweight for 5′4″ person.)

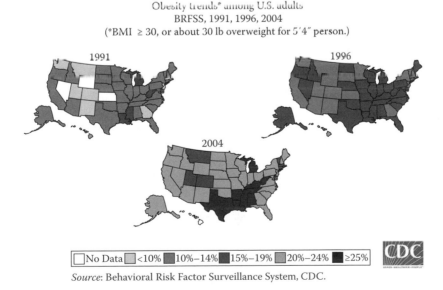

No Data | <10% | 10%–14% | 15%–19% | 20%–24% | ≥25%

Source: Behavioral Risk Factor Surveillance System, CDC.

FIGURE 1.3 Trends in U.S. adults obesity from 1991 to 2004. (From CDC, Overweight and Obesity: Obesity Trends: U.S. Obesity trends 1985–2004, Centers for Disease Control and Prevention, Washington, DC, 2005, http://www.cdc.gov/nccdphp/dnpa/obesity/trend/maps/index.htm).

TABLE 1.5

Age-Adjusted Prevalence of Overweight, Obesity, and Extreme Obesity among U.S. Adults Aged 20–74

Sample Size and Weight Status	NHANES I 1960–1962	NHANES I 1971–1974	NHANES II 1976–1980	NHANES III 1988–1994	NHANES 1999–2000	NHANES 2001–2002	NHANES 2003–2004	NHANES 2005–2006	NHANES 2007–2008
Sample (n)	6,126	12,911	11,765	14,468	3,603	3,916	3,756	3,835	4,881
Overweight (25 ≤ BMI < 30)	31.5	32.3	32.1	32.7	33.6	34.4	33.4	32.2	33.6
Obese (BMI ≥ 30)	13.4	14.5	15.0	23.2	30.9	31.3	32.9	35.1	34.3
Extremely obese (BMI ≥ 40)	0.9	1.3	1.4	3.0	5.0	5.4	5.1	6.2	6.0

Source: Ogden, C.L. and Carroll, M.D., Prevalence of overweight, obesity, and extreme obesity among adults: United States, trends 1976–1980 through 2007–2008, http://www.cdc.gov/nchs/data/hestat/obesity_adult_07_08/obesity_adult_07_08.hm. (accessed on November 24, 2011).

Notes: NHES is National Health Examination Survey. NHANES is National Health and Nutrition Examination Survey, and BMI is body mass index. Age adjusted by the direct method to the year 2000 U.S. Census Bureau estimates using the age groups 20–39, 40–59, and 60–74 years. NHES included adults aged 18–79, and NHANES I and II did not include individuals over age 74, so trend estimates are based on ages 20–74. Pregnant females were excluded from the analysis.

Prevalence estimates generated for the maps may vary slightly from those generated for the states by the BRFSS, as slightly different analytic methods are used.

Results from the 2007–2008 National Health and Nutrition Examination Survey (NHANES), using measured heights and weights, indicate that an estimated 34.2% of U.S. adults aged 20 years and over are overweight, 33.8% are obese, and 5.7% are extremely obese [22].

The NHANES 2007–2008 data for adults aged 20 years and over suggest an increase in obesity between the late 1980s and today in the United States, with the estimated age-adjusted prevalence moving upward from a previous level of 23% in NHANES III (1988–1994) to approximately 34% in 2007–2008 [22]. Among women, however, there was no significant change between 1999–2000 and 2007–2008. Among men, there was a significant linear increase between 1999–2000 and 2007–2008, but no change between 2003–2004 and 2007–2008. It is possible to examine trends since 1960 among adults aged 20–74. These estimates are shown in Table 1.5 and Figure 1.4 [22]. Although the prevalence of obesity more than doubled between 1976–1980 and 2007–2008, the prevalence of overweight remained stable during the same period.

A recent study [23] that analyzes BMI values among U.S. adults in 1999–2000 and 2007–2008 shows that, for both men and women, the estimated median BMI (50th percentile) tended to be slightly higher in 2007–2008 than in 1999–2000 within all age groups; however, some of the differences were extremely small. In 1999–2000, the median BMI for men aged 20–39 years was 26.0 vs. 26.6 in 2007–2008 and for women 25.6 vs. 26.5; for men aged 40–59 years, 27.4 vs. 28.3 and for women 27.6 vs. 27.7; and finally for men aged 60 years or older, 27.5 vs. 28.3 and for women 27.4 vs. 27.6.

It must be noted that overweight and obesity in the United States occur at higher rates among racial or ethnic minority populations such as African Americans and Hispanic Americans, compared with Caucasian Americans. Asian Americans have a relatively low prevalence for obesity. Women and persons of low socioeconomic status within minority populations appear to be particularly affected by overweight and obesity. Cultural factors that influence dietary and exercise behaviors are reported to play a major role in the development of excess weight in minority groups [24].

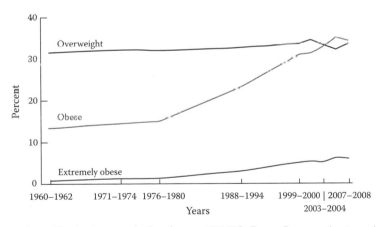

Note: Age-adjusted by the direct method to the year 2000 U.S. Census Bureau estimates, using the age groups 20–39, 40–59, and 60–74 years. Pregnant females were excluded. Overweight is defined as a body mass index (BMI) of 25 or greater but less than 30; obesity is a BMI greater than or equal to 30; extreme obesity is a BMI greater than or equal to 40.

Source: CDC/NCHS, National Health Examination Survey cycle I (1960–1962); National Health and Nutrition Examination Survey I (1971–1974), II (1976–1980), and III (1988–1994), 1999–2000, 2001–2002, 2003–2004, 2005–2006, and 2007–2008.

FIGURE 1.4 Trends in overweight, obesity, and extreme obesity among adults aged 20–74 years: the United States 1960–2008. (From Ogden, C.L. and Carroll, M.D., Prevalence of overweight, obesity, and extreme obesity among adults: United States, trends 1976–1980 through 2007–2008, http://www.cdc.gov/nchs/data/hestat/obesity_adult_07_08/obesity_adult_07_08.hm, accessed on November 24, 2011.)

TABLE 1.6

Prevalence of Obesity among U.S. Adults Aged 20 and over, by Sex and Race/Ethnicity, for Selected Years 1988–1994 through 2007–2008

Characteristic	NHANES 1988–1994	NHANES 1999–2000	NHANES 2001–2002	NHANES 2003–2004	NHANES 2005–2006	NHANES 2007–2008
Men, all	20.2	27.5	27.8	31.1	33.3	32.2
Men, non-Hispanic white	20.3	27.3	29.1	31.1	33.1	31.9
Men, non-Hispanic black	21.1	28.1	27.9	34.0	37.2	37.3
Men, Mexican American	23.9	28.9	25.9	31.6	27.0	35.9
Women[a], all	25.4	33.4	33.3	33.2	35.3	35.5
Women[a], non-Hispanic white	22.9	30.1	31.3	30.2	32.9	33.0
Women[a], non-Hispanic black	38.2	49.7	48.3	53.9	52.9	49.6
Women[a], Mexican American	35.3	39.7	37.0	42.3	42.1	45.1

Source: Ogden, C.L. and Carroll, M.D., Prevalence of overweight, obesity, and extreme obesity among adults: United States, trends 1976–1980 through 2007–2008, http://www.cdc.gov/nchs/data/hestat/obesity_adult_07_08/obesity_adult_07_08.hm, (accessed on November 24, 2011).

Notes: NHANES is National Health and Nutrition Examination Survey. Age adjusted by the direct method to the year 2000 U.S. Census Bureau estimates using the age groups 20–39, 40–59, and 60 years and over. Obesity is defined as having a BMI greater than or equal to 30.

[a] Excludes pregnant females.

The prevalence of overweight and obesity increased over the last years among the various racial and ethnic groups. Table 1.6 [22] shows the estimates in obesity prevalence by race or ethnicity for men and women since NHANES III (1988–1994).

Between 1988–1994 and 2007–2008, the prevalence of obesity among men increased from 20.3% to 31.9% among non-Hispanic white men, from 21.1% to 37.3% among non-Hispanic black men, and from 23.9% to 35.9% among Mexican American men.

Among women in 2007–2008, non-Hispanic black women were significantly more likely to be obese (49.6%) than non-Hispanic white women (33.0%). Similarly, Mexican American women were more likely to be obese (45.1%) than non-Hispanic white women (33.0%). Similar disparities existed in 1988–1994 (22.9% of non-Hispanic white women, 38.3% of non-Hispanic black women, and 35.3% of Mexican American women were obese).

The American Indian population also has high prevalence rates of overweight (where overweight is defined as a BMI of ≥27.8 for men and ≥27.3 for women). The highest rates for American Indians are 80% for women and 67% for men in Arizona, according to researchers of the 1995 Strong Heart Study.

The prevalence of overweight, obesity, and severe obesity (BMI of 40 or more) has increased for both men and women in the various racial and ethnic groups in the United States over the last decade [24].

LATIN AMERICA AND CARIBBEAN

Evidence of the impact of the nutrition transition is clear in the growing levels of obesity throughout this region. Obesity rates are reported to vary for men from about 7% in El Salvador and Brazil to 28% in Argentina, but among women, rates rise as high as 29% in Bolivia and Perù (Table 1.4).

Obesity is a significant problem in the Caribbean and affects women more than men. Abdominal obesity, using WHO waist circumference limits, ranged from 3% of men in St. Lucia to 8% in Barbados, but among women was found to be as high as 34% in Jamaica, 41% in St. Lucia, and 45% in Barbados [25].

In Brazil, the problem of dietary deficit appears to be rapidly shifting to one of dietary excess [4]. Obesity is rising, especially among lower-income groups.

Africa

In contrast to most Western countries, the emphasis in Africa has been on undernutrition and food security rather than overweight and obesity. Regional studies, however, do indicate a growing prevalence of overweight and obesity in certain socioeconomic groups.

Women show prevalence rates of obesity higher than men. In 2002, prevalence value of 33.2% was observed in Lesotho, 35.8% in Seychelles, and 34.3% in South Africa (Table 1.4).

Wide disparities in levels of obesity can be found. In South Africa, where mean BMI values for men and women are 22.9 and 27.1 kg/m^2, respectively, overweight rate in women is 66.4% and levels of central obesity have been assessed at 42% [26]. The South African Health Review 2000 indicated obesity rates from 8% among black men to 20% among Caucasian men, but among women, the rates ranged from 20% for Indian/Asians women to 30.5% for black women.

From the 1960s until the 1980s, the notion of "healthy" or "benign" obesity was propagated in South Africa. Not surprisingly, this led to ignorance around the problem of obesity, and the treatment of some of the comorbid diseases was neglected. Fortunately, as an increasing number of seminal studies draw us closer to reality, the misperception of benign obesity is being corrected [27].

In North Africa the prevalence of overweight among women is high (Table 1.4). Half of all women are overweight (BMI > 25), with rates of 57.9% in Tunisia and 53.0% in Morocco, and obesity rates (BMI > 30) of 28.8% in Tunisia and 19.0% in Morocco are found, a threefold increase over 20 years [28]. High rates of overweight among women were also observed in Botswana (46.9%), Equatorial Guinea (46.1%), Gabon (45.0%), Lesotho (68.7%), Mauritania (52.2%), and Seychelles (68.6%). In parts of sub-Saharan Africa, obesity often exists alongside undernutrition [29].

Japan, China, and Western Pacific Countries

In Japan, obesity in men has doubled since 1982, whereas its rise in women has been restricted to the younger age group (20–29 years) for which it has increased 1.8 times since 1976 [4]. Using the obesity cutoff at BMI > 25 as standard, adult obesity in Japan would average 25%, rising to 30% in men over 30 years old, and in women over 40 years old, thus representing a three- to fourfold increase over the last 40 years [30].

In the Chinese population [31], it has long been suggested that the BMI-based definition for obesity should be lower than that for European or North American populations [32], where obesity is defined as a BMI of 30 kg/m^2 or greater. The reason for this [33] is because obesity-associated metabolic complications occur at lower BMIs in Chinese people compared to Europeans/North Americans. Overall, the consensus is that BMI cutoffs for obesity should be lower in China whereby overweight was defined as BMI of 24–27.9 kg/m^2 and obesity was defined as BMI > 28 kg/m^2 [34,35].

Obesity is increasing in China and is more common in urban areas and among women. One out of five persons with obesity in the world is Chinese [36].

Between 1992 and 2002, the prevalence of overweight and obesity increased in all genders and age groups and in all geographic areas. The Chinese obesity standard shows an increase from 20.0% to 29.9%. The annual increase rate was highest in men aged 18–44 years and women aged 45–59 years (approximately 1.6% and 1.0% points, respectively). In general, male subjects, urban residents, and high-income groups had a greater increase [37].

Today there are more than 200 million people in China who are overweight or obese. By 2020, it is predicted that there will be more obese population in China than in the United States [38].

Obesity is not new to the Pacific and has long been regarded by Polynesian and Micronesian societies of this region as a symbol of high social status and prosperity. The prevalence has risen dramatically, however, in the last 20 years. The link between obesity and type 2 diabetes is most manifest in this region which has some of the highest levels of adult obesity. Obesity prevalence rates (Table 1.4) of between 55% and 80% can be observed among men and women in some islands including Samoa and Nauru. In Tonga, a high percentage of the adults (59% of men and 75% of women) are obese, and recently, 12% of men and nearly 18% of women were identified with type 2 diabetes, a doubling of the rate over 25 years. A further 20% were found to be at risk due to elevated blood sugar levels [39].

PREVALENCE OF OBESITY IN CHILDREN AND ADOLESCENTS

The prevalence of childhood overweight has increased in almost all countries for which data are available. Exceptions are also found among infant preschool children in some lower-income countries. Obesity and overweight have increased more dramatically in economically developed countries and in urbanized populations [40].

As shown in a review [40], secular trends for school-age children show that prevalence of overweight and obesity is increasing in all countries. The exceptions are Russia and to a lesser extent Poland, where the prevalence of overweight showed a decline across the period indicated. For some countries, such as the former East Germany, New Zealand, the Netherlands, and Canada, the prevalence of overweight has been rising by more than 1% each year.

IOTF has published estimates of the prevalence of overweight and obesity among children on a global and regional basis. Table 1.7 [41] shows the prevalence data, by sex and different ranges of years, in the latest available years, of overweight and obese children within the world by WHO regions and countries [41].

EUROPE

Recent concern has focused on children and adolescent obesity, which is a rapidly growing problem in many countries. The concern is not only that young people, who are already overweight and obese, are destined to remain so throughout their adult lives with heightened risks to health, but also that youngsters are already developing diseases of old age, such as type 2 diabetes.

Surveys show overweight and obesity levels among children in Southern Europe to be higher than their Northern European counterparts as the traditional Mediterranean diet gives way to more processed foods rich in fat, sugar, and salt.

The 2005 IOTF European Union platform briefing paper [19] shows that the Mediterranean islands of Malta, Sicily, Gibraltar, and Crete as well as the countries of Spain, Portugal, and Italy report overweight and obesity levels exceeding 30% among children aged 7–11 as illustrated in Figure 1.5 [19].

In addition, England, Ireland, Cyprus, and Greece report levels above 20%, while France, Switzerland, Poland, the Czech Republic, Hungary, Germany, Denmark, the Netherlands, and even Bulgaria report overweight and obesity levels of 10%–20% among this same age group [19].

For teenagers (aged 13–17), seven countries indicate overweight and obesity levels above 20% with Crete peaking at 35% as shown in Figure 1.6 [19]. The data in both Figures 1.5 and 1.6 are from available surveys, so comparisons require caution as the survey years may differ.

Childhood overweight and obesity are accelerating rapidly in some countries. The rise has been particularly marked in the recent years. IOTF estimates [19] prepared for WHO show that one out of five children in Europe is overweight. An additional 400,000 children each year are becoming overweight, and at least 3 million are obese. Annual increases in prevalence of around 0.2% during the 1970s rose to 0.6% during the 1980s, and up to 0.8% in the early 1990s, reaching as high as 2.0% in some cases by the 2000s.

UNITED STATES

Overweight and obesity for children and adolescents are defined respectively as being at or above the 85th and 95th percentile of the gender-specific BMI for age growth charts [9].

TABLE 1.7
Prevalence of Overweight and Obese Children by WHO Region and Country, by Sex, Latest Available Year, around the World

	Year of Survey	Age Range Years (Inclusive)	Overweight (Including Obesity)		
			Boys	Girls	Cutoff
WHO African region					
Algeria	2003	7–17	6.0	5.6	IOTF
Ethiopia	1987–1995	5–17	0.1	0.4	IOTF
Mali	1993	5–17	0.2	0.5	IOTF
Senegal	1992	5–17	0.1	0.5	IOTF
Seychelles	1999	5,9,12, and 16	9.2	15.8	IOTF
Zimbabwe	1990–1994	5–17	1.7	2.4	IOTF
WHO American region					
Bolivia (urban)	2003	14–17	15.6	27.5	IOTF
Brazil	2002	7–10	23.0	21.1	IOTF
Canada	1996	7–13	33.0	27.0	IOTF
Chile	2000	6	26.0	27.1	IOTF
Mexico	1995	5–17	32.3	31.1	IOTF
Trinidad and Tobago	1999	5,6,9, and 10	8.1	8.8	IOTF
United States	1988–1994	5–17	26.8	28.1	IOTF
Venezuela	1976–1982	10 and 15	21.1	17.2	IOTF
WHO Eastern Mediterranean region					
Bahrain	2000	12–17	29.9	38.5	IOTF
Iran	1995	6	24.7	26.8	IOTF
Kuwait	1999–2000	10–14	30.0	31.8	85/95th percentile
Lebanon	1996	5–17	23.4	19.7	IOTF
Saudi Arabia	2002	5–17	16.7	19.4	IOTF
WHO European region					
Austria	2003	8–12	22.5	16.7	90/97th percentile
Belgium	1998–1999	5–15	27.7	26.8	85/95th percentile
Bulgaria	1998	7–17	18.9	16.1	IOTF
Cyprus	1999–2000	6–17	25.4	22.6	IOTF
Czech Republic	2001	5–17	14.7	13.4	IOTF
Denmark	1996/1997	6–16	14.1	15.3	IOTF
Finland (self-report)	1999	12–17	19.4	11.2	IOTF
France	2000 (12 years 2001)	7,8,9, and 12	19.1	19.3	IOTF
Germany	1995	5–17	14.1	14.0	IOTF
Greece	2003	13–17	29.6	16.1	IOTF
Hungary	1993–1994	10 and 15	17.8	15.9	IOTF
Iceland	1998	9	22.0	25.5	IOTF
Italy	1993–2001	5–17	26.6	24.8	IOTF
Macedonia, FYR	1995–2002	6–17	18.6	16.7	85/95th percentile
Malta	1992	10	32.7	38.5	IOTF
Netherlands	1997	5–17	8.8	11.8	IOTF
Poland	1996	5–17	16.7	13.6	IOTF
Portugal	2002/2003	7–9	29.5	34.3	IOTF
Russian Federation	1992	5–17	24.2	19.7	IOTF

(*continued*)

TABLE 1.7 (continued)

Prevalence of Overweight and Obese Children by WHO Region and Country, by Sex, Latest Available Year, around the World

	Year of Survey	Age Range Years (Inclusive)	Overweight (Including Obesity)		
			Boys	Girls	Cutoff
Slovakia	1995–1999	11–17	9.8	8.2	IOTF
Spain	1998–2000	5–16	31.0	19.5	IOTF
Sweden	2001	6–11	17.6	27.4	IOTF
Switzerland	2002	6–12	21.0	23.2	IOTF
Turkey	2001	12–17	11.4	10.3	IOTF
United Kingdom (England)	2001	5–17	21.8	27.1	IOTF
WHO Southeast Asia region					
India	2002 approximately	5–17 boys, 5–15 girls	12.9	8.2	IOTF
Nepal	1997	5–17	0.0	0.0	IOTF
Thailand	1997	5–15	21.1	12.6	IOTF
WHO Western Pacific region					
Australia	1995	7–17	21.1	21.3	IOTF
Japan	1996–2000	6–14	16.2	14.3	IOTF
Singapore	1993	10 and 15	20.4	14.6	IOTF
China	1999–2000	11 and 15	14.9	8.0	IOTF
New Zealand	2000	11 and 12	30.0	30.0	IOTF

Source: British Hearth Foundation Statistics website, Prevalence of overweight and obese children by WHO region and country, by sex, latest available years, the world. From The International Obesity Task Force, (2006), IOTF, August 5, 2008, http://www.heartstats.org, http://www.iotf.org/database/ChildhoodTablebyRegionFeb06.htm

Results from the 2007–2008 NHANES [42], using measured heights and weights, indicate that an estimated 16.9% of children and adolescents aged 2–19 years are obese. Between 1976–1980 and 1999–2000, the prevalence of obesity increased. Between 1999–2000 and 2007–2008, there was a discontinuous trend in obesity prevalence for any age group, except for adolescents aged 12–19 years for whom a slight increasing trend was observed.

There was an increase between NAHNES II and NAHNES III and a further increase between NHANES III and NANHES 2003–2004. By 2003–2004, more than 17% of teenagers (12–19 years old) were overweight. The prevalence of overweight among boys and girls increased significantly during the 6 year time period from 1999 to 2004 [5].

In 2007–2008 [43], 9.5% of infants and toddlers were at above the 95th percentile. Among children and adolescents aged 2–19 years, 11.9% were at or above the 97th percentile, 16.9% were at or above the 95th percentile, and 31.7% were at or above the 85th percentile.

Table 1.8 [42] shows the increase in obesity that has occurred since 1971–1974. Among preschool children aged 2–5, obesity increased from 5.0% to 10.4% between 1976–1980 and 2007–2008 and from 6.5% to 19.6% among those aged 6–11. Among adolescents aged 12–19, obesity increased from 5.0% to 18.1% during the same period.

Figure 1.7 [42] shows the trends since the 1960s by age group.

There are significant racial and ethnic disparities in obesity prevalence among U.S. children and adolescents. Table 1.9 [42] shows the estimates in obesity prevalence by race/ethnicity for boys and girls since NHANES III (1988–1994).

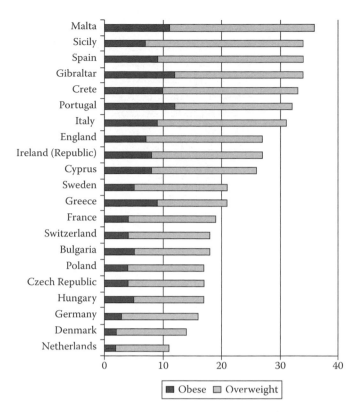

FIGURE 1.5 Percentage of schoolchildren aged 7–11 obese or overweight. (From Lobstein, T., Rigby, N., and Leach, R., EU platform on diet, physical activity and health, IOTF EU Platform Briefing Paper, in collaboration with the European Association for the Study of Obesity, International Obesity Task Force, London, U.K., 2005, http://ec.europa.eu/comm/health/ph_determinants/life_style/nutrition/documents/iotf_en.pdf)

In 2007–2008, the prevalence of obesity was significantly higher among Mexican American adolescent boys (26.8%) than among non-Hispanic white adolescent boys (16.7%). In NHANES III (1988–1994), there was no significant difference in prevalence between Mexican American and non-Hispanic white adolescent boys.

Between 1988–1994 and 2007–2008, the prevalence of obesity increased from 11.6% to 16.7% among non-Hispanic white boys, from 10.7% to 19.8% among non-Hispanic black boys, and from 14.1% to 26.8% among Mexican American boys.

Among girls in the period 2007–2008, non-Hispanic black adolescents (29.2%) were significantly more likely to be obese compared with non-Hispanic white adolescents (14.5%). Similarly, non-Hispanic black adolescent girls (16.3%) were more likely to be obese compared with non-Hispanic white adolescent girls (8.9%) in the period 1988–1994.

Between 1988–1994 and 2007–2008, the prevalence of obesity increased from 8.9% to 14.5% among non-Hispanic white girls, from 16.3% to 29.2% among non-Hispanic black girls, and from 13.4% to 17.4% among Mexican American girls.

Prevalence estimates differed by age and by race/ethnic group [43]. Trend analyses indicate no significant trend between 1999–2000 and 2007–2008 except at the highest BMI cutoff point (BMI $\geq$97th percentile) among all 6–19 year old boys and among non-Hispanic white boys of the same age.

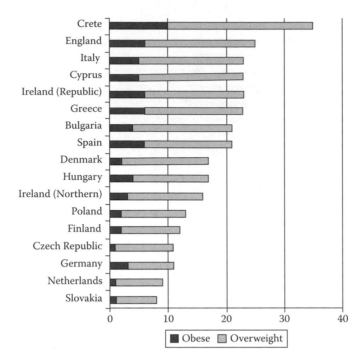

FIGURE 1.6 Percentage of schoolchildren aged 13–17 obese or overweight. (From Lobstein, T., Rigby, N., and Leach, R., EU platform on diet, physical activity and health, IOTF EU Platform Briefing Paper, in collaboration with the European Association for the Study of Obesity, International Obesity Task Force, London, U.K., 2005, http://ec.europa.eu/comm/health/ph_determinants/life_style/nutrition/documents/iotf_en.pdf)

TABLE 1.8

Prevalence of Obesity among U.S. Children and Adolescents Aged 2–19, for Selected Years 1963–1965 through 2007–2008

Age (in Years)[a]	NHANES 1963–1965 1966–1970[b]	NHANES 1971–1974	NHANES 1976–1980	NHANES 1988–1994	NHANES 1999–2000	NHANES 2001–2002	NHANES 2003–2004	NHANES 2005–2006	NHANES 2007–2008
Total	c	5.0	5.5	10.0	13.9	15.4	17.1	15.5	16.9
2–5	c	5.0	5.0	7.2	10.3	10.6	13.9	11.0	10.4
6–11	4.2	4.0	6.5	11.3	15.1	16.3	18.8	15.1	19.6
12–19	4.6	6.1	5.0	10.5	14.8	16.7	17.4	17.8	18.1

Source: Ogden, C.L. and Carroll, M.D., Prevalence of obesity among children and adolescents: United States, trends 1963–1965 through 2007–2008, http://www.cdc.gov/nchs/data/hestat/obesity_child_07_08/obesity_child_07_08.htm, accessed on December 12, 2011.

Note: Obesity defined as BMI greater than or equal to sex- and age-specific 95th percentile from the 2000 CDC Growth Charts.

[a] Excludes pregnant women starting with 1971–1974. Pregnancy status not available for 1963–1965 and 1966–1970.

[b] Data for 1963–1965 are for children aged 6–11; data for 1966–1970 are for adolescents aged 12–17, not 12–19 years.

[c] Children aged 2–5 were not included in the surveys undertaken in the 1960s.

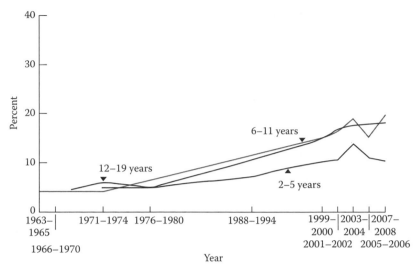

Note: Obesity is defined as body mass index (BMI) greater than or equal to sex- and age-specific 95th percentile from the 2000 CDC Growth Charts.

Sources: CDC/NCHS, National Health Examination Surveys II (ages 6–11), III (ages 12–17), and National Health and Nutrition Examination Surveys (NHANES) I–III, and NHANES 1999–2000, 2001–2002, 2003–2004, 2005–2006, and 2007–2008.

FIGURE 1.7 Trends in obesity among children and adolescents: the United States 1963–2008. (From Ogden, C.L. and Carroll, M.D., Prevalence of obesity among children and adolescents: United States, Trends 1963–1965 through 2007–2008, http://www.cdc.gov/nchs/data/hestat/obesity_child_07_08/obesity_child_07_08.htm, accessed on December 12, 2011.)

TABLE 1.9
Prevalence of Obesity among U.S. Adolescents Aged 12–19, for Selected Years 1988–1994 through 2007–2008

	NHANES 1988–1994	NHANES 1999–2000	NHANES 2001–2002	NHANES 2003–2004	NHANES 2005–2006	NHANES 2007–2008
Boys, all	11.3	14.8	17.6	18.2	18.2	19.3
Boys, non-Hispanic white	11.6	11.8	16.6	19.1	15.5	16.7
Boys, non-Hispanic black	10.7	21.1	16.7	18.4	18.4	19.8
Boys, Mexican American	14.1	27.2	21.8	18.3	25.6	26.8
Girls[a], all	9.7	14.8	15.7	16.4	17.3	16.8
Girls[a], non-Hispanic white	8.9	11.0	13.7	15.4	13.5	14.5
Girls[a], non-Hispanic black	16.3	25.2	22.0	25.4	29.8	29.2
Girls[a], Mexican American	13.4	19.3	20.3	14.1	25.4	17.4

Source: Ogden, C.L. and Carroll, M.D., Prevalence of obesity among children and adolescents: United States, Trends 1963–1965 through 2007–2008, http://www.cdc.gov/nchs/data/hestat/obesity_child_07_08/obesity_child_07_08.htm, accessed on December 12, 2011.

Note: Obesity defined as BMI greater than or equal to sex- and age-specific 95th percentile from the 2000 CDC Growth Charts.

[a] Excludes pregnant females.

AUSTRALIA, CHINA, ASIAN/PACIFIC ISLANDERS, AND NEW DELHI

In Australia, between 1985 and 1995, the prevalence of obesity among children aged 7–15 years increased 4.6-fold among girls and 3.4-fold among boys [44]. Countries undergoing rapid urbanization and economic development are experiencing double challenges: they have to fight both childhood undernutrition and a growing tide of obesity [45–47]. For example, in China, the prevalence of overweight and obesity among children aged 7–9 years increased from 1% to 2% in 1985 to 17% among girls and 25% among boys in 2000 [47]. In addition, obesity prevalence varies across socioeconomic strata. In developed countries, children of low socioeconomic status are more affected than their wealthy counterparts [48–50]. The opposite is observed in developing countries, where children in the upper socioeconomic status are more likely than poor children to be obese [51,52].

The overall prevalence of obesity among Asian/Pacific Islander adolescents [53] in 2006–2007 was 22.9% and was 19.4% for overweight. The prevalence of obesity was markedly different between Asians and Pacific Islanders (12.1% vs. 35.6%). Obesity also differed noticeably among ethnic subgroups, ranging from 8.4% to 17.5% among Asians and from 17.2% to 48.6% among Pacific Islanders. The prevalence of overweight students ranged from 12.8% to 17.3% among Asians and from 16.4% to 21.1% among Pacific Islanders.

Recent data indicate a rise in obesity both in children and in adolescents in developing countries. The overall prevalence of overweight/obesity in urban children in New Delhi has shown an increase from 16% in 2002 to about 24% in 2006–2007 [54].

HEALTH CONSEQUENCES OF OBESITY AND MORBIDITY

Obesity has a great number of negative health, social, and economic consequences, as evidenced by the higher mortality and morbidity rates among overweight and obese individuals than lean people. Obese subjects have a 50%–100% increased risk of premature death from all causes, compared to individuals with a healthy weight.

In addition, childhood obesity seems to increase the risk of subsequent morbidity, whether or not obesity persists into adulthood. Indeed, higher BMI among children is associated with higher levels of blood pressure and serum lipids [43,55], factors that in adults are associated with higher cardiovascular risk. One concern is the emerging risk of type 2 diabetes mellitus among children and adolescents [56]. Nevertheless, it should be noted that among youth this is a very low prevalence condition, occurring primarily in children with a strong family history of diabetes who are from certain ethnic groups, who are markedly obese by adult standards, or both [57–63].

The health consequences of obesity range from a number of nonfatal complaints that impact the quality of life, such as respiratory difficulties, musculoskeletal disorders like osteoarthritis, skin problems, infertility, and increased risk of high levels of disability, to complaints that lead to an increased risk of premature death including NIDDM, gallbladder disease, cardiovascular problems (hypertension, stroke, and CHD), and certain cancers (endometrial, breast, and colon). These conditions cause premature death and substantial disability. Hypertension, diabetes, and raised serum cholesterol are between two and six times more prevalent among heavier women. Severe obesity is associated with a 12-fold increase in mortality in 25–35 year olds when compared to lean individuals.

The psychological consequences of obesity can range from lowered self-esteem to clinical depression; rates of anxiety and depression are three to four times higher among obese individuals [4]. In addition to its physical consequences, obesity creates a massive social burden in that negative attitudes toward the obese can lead to discrimination in many areas of their life, including health care and employment [4].

TABLE 1.10
Benefits of Weight Loss (IOTF, WHO, 1998)

Obesity Comorbidity	Weight Loss	Benefits of Weight Loss
Mortality	10 kg	>20% reduction in total mortality
		>30% reduction in diabetes-related death
		Reduction in obesity-related cancer death
Diabetes	10 kg	50% reduction in fasting glucose
Blood pressure	10 kg	10 mmHg reduction in systolic pressure
		20 mmHg reduction in diastolic pressure
Blood lipids	10 kg	10% reduction in TOT cholesterol
		15% reduction in LDL cholesterol
		30% reduction in triglycerides
		8% increase in HDL cholesterol
Blood clotting indices		Reduced red cell aggregability
		Improved fibrinolytic capacity
Physical complication	5–10 kg	Improved back and joint pain
		Improved lung function
		Decreased breathlessness
		Reduced frequency of sleep apnea
Ovarian function	>5% weight loss	Improved ovarian function

BENEFITS OF WEIGHT LOSS

Modest weight reduction can significantly reduce the risk of these serious health conditions. Weight loss in overweight and obese individuals improves physical, metabolic, and endocrinological complications, often dramatically. Weight loss in obese persons can also improve depression, anxiety, psychosocial functioning, mood, and quality of life.

In a 12 year study in the United States, intentional weight loss of 0.5–9.0 kg in overweight women with existing obesity-related disease led to a 20% reduction in total mortality, a 40%–50% reduction in mortality from obesity-related cancers, and a 30%–40% reduction in diabetes-related deaths [4]. Table 1.10 shows the major benefits of weight loss on health status (IOTF, WHO, 1998).

ECONOMIC COSTS OF OBESITY

Often overshadowed by the health and social consequences of obesity is the economic cost to society and to the individual. The direct cost of diagnosis, treatment, and management of obesity within national health-care systems have been assessed in a few countries to date. Although the methodology varied considerably between studies, making it difficult to compare costs across countries and to extrapolate the results from one country to another, these estimates suggest that between 2% and 8% of the total health-care costs in Western countries can be attributed to obesity [4]. This represents a major fraction of national health-care budgets comparable with, for example, the total cost of cancer therapy. The potential impact on health-care resources in the less-developed health-care systems of developing countries is likely to be even more severe.

In addition to the direct costs of obesity are costs in terms of the individuals (including the intangible costs of poor health and reduced quality of life) and society (such as the indirect costs of loss of productivity due to sick leave and premature pensions). Being able to determine the indirect costs of obesity that arise from, for example, the loss of wages and productivity would raise the total cost of obesity even higher.

TABLE 1.11
Examples of Direct Costs in EU Compared with the United States

Country	Direct Costs in Euros (Millions)	% Health Expenditure
England (1995)	816 (+3.270 indirect)	1.5%
France (1992)	640–1320	1.5%
Germany (1996)	10.600	—
Portugal (1996)	230	3.5%
Netherlands (1981–1989)	454	4.0%
United States	US$92.000	7.0%

Source: IOTF/EASO, Obesity in Europe: The case for action, International Obesity Task Force and European Association for the Study of Obesity, London, U.K., 2002, http://www.iotf.org/media/euobesity.pdf, accessed on December 18, 2011, from IOTF collected data, Converted January 2002—unadjusted for inflation.

The direct medical costs of obesity in the United States have been estimated as more than $70 billion in 1995 dollars [64] and more than $92 billion in 2002 dollars [65]. The costs of treatment are also high. For example, it has been estimated that in 1989 alone, Americans spent more than $30 billion trying to lose weight [66].

The IOTF is planning to investigate further the direct and indirect costs of obesity worldwide as part of its implementation plan. Data collected by the IOTF in 2002 are summarized in Table 1.11 [67].

Prevention is clearly more cost effective than treatment, in terms of both economic and personal costs.

NEED FOR ACTION

Obesity is a serious medical condition which needs urgent attention throughout the world.

Despite its high prevalence and our improved understanding of how the disease develops, only limited effective obesity management systems are in place in national health-care services around the world. This is in contrast with other chronic diseases, such as diabetes and coronary heart disease, where integrated care is frequently provided.

It is clear therefore that the rational development of coordinated health-care services for the management of overweight and obese patients is needed in most countries.

Primary health-care services should play the dominant role, although hospital and specialist services are also required for dealing with more severe cases and the associated major life-threatening complications.

There is an urgent need for expanded training of all health-care workers to improve their levels of knowledge and skills with regard to obesity management strategies.

The IOTF was established in May 1996 to tackle the emerging global epidemic of obesity. The IOTF is a part of the International Association for the Study of Obesity (IASO), an organization that represents 43 National Obesity Associations across the globe. The IOTF is composed of world experts in the field of obesity and related diseases from around the world, including China, Japan, Chile, Australia, Brazil, the United States, Canada, and Europe. The IOTF collaborates closely with the WHO and is engaged with other international health organizations and national governments to raise awareness and help develop solutions to the global epidemic of obesity.

The IOTF aims to achieve action on the prevention and management of overweight and obesity and endeavors to create an environment that encourages and supports the development of appropriate public and health policies and programs for prevention and management of obesity.

The IOTF initiative on the prevention and management of obesity has four main goals:

1. Increase the awareness among governments, health-care professionals, and the community that obesity is a serious medical condition and a major health problem with substantial economic costs.
2. Provide evidence and guidance for the development of better prevention and management strategies.
3. Secure the commitment of policy makers to take action.
4. Foster the development of national, regional, and international structures that will enable and support the implementation of taking action on the problems of overweight and obesity.

Management strategies are shown in Figure 1.8 (IOTF, WHO, 1998).

In 1997, the WHO, together with the IOTF, held an expert consultation on obesity to review the extent of the obesity problem and examine the need to develop public health policies and programs to tackle the global problem of obesity. The consultation resulted in the publication of an interim report: "Obesity: preventing and managing the global epidemic" [4] and the subsequent WHO Technical Report Series 894.

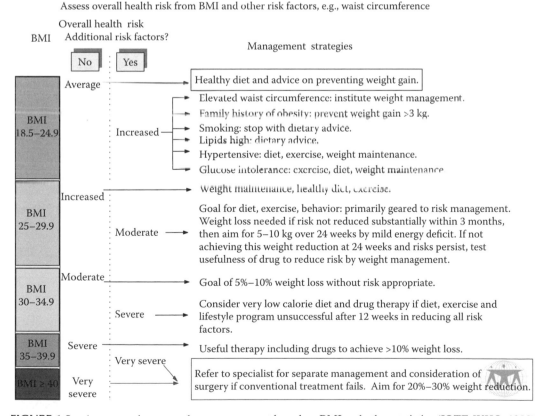

FIGURE 1.8 A systematic approach to management based on BMI and other statistics (IOTF, WHO, 1998). (From WHO, Obesity: Preventing and managing the global epidemic, Report of a WHO consultation on obesity, World Health Organization, Geneva, Switzerland, 1998.)

The IOTF has identified a number of areas where our understanding of overweight and obesity must be improved. Specific working groups have examined the following issues: childhood obesity, economic costs of obesity, management of obesity, public health approaches to the prevention of obesity, and, finally, training of health professionals.

ACKNOWLEDGMENT

The authors wish to thank Dr. Micaela Viganò for her help in updating this chapter.

REFERENCES

1. WHO, Obesity: Preventing and managing the global epidemic. Report of a WHO consultation on obesity, Technical Report Series, No. 894, World Health Organization, Geneva, Switzerland, 2000, p. 256.
2. International Obesity Task Force (IOTF), The global epidemic, 2009, http://www.iaso.org/iotf/obesity/obesitytheglobalepidemic/ (accessed on October 12, 2011).
3. Must, A., Spadano, J., Coakley, E.H. et al., The disease burden associated with overweight and obesity, *JAMA*, 282, 1523–1529, 1999.
4. WHO, Obesity: Preventing and managing the global epidemic. Report of a WHO consultation on obesity, World Health Organization, Geneva, Switzerland, 1998.
5. Ogden, C.L., Yanovski, S.Z., Carrol, M.D. et al., The epidemiology of obesity, *Gastroenterology*, 132, 2087–2102, 2007.
6. FAO, The developing world's new burden: Obesity, Food and Agricultural Organization, United Nations, Geneva, Switzerland, 2002, http://www.fao.org/FOCUS/E/obesity/obes2.htm (accessed on October 12, 2011).
7. Baumgartner, R.N., Heymsfield, S.B., and Roche, A.F., Human body composition and the epidemiology of chronic disease, *Obes. Res.*, 3, 73–95, 1995.
8. Flegal, K.M., Tabak, C.J., and Ogden, C.L., Overweight in children: Definitions and interpretation, *Health Educ. Res.*, 21, 755–760, 2006.
9. Must, A., Dallal, G.E., and Dietz, W.H., Reference data for obesity: 85th and 95th percentiles of body mass index (wt/ht^2) and triceps skinfold thickness, *Am. J. Clin. Nutr.*, 53, 839–846, 1991. [Erratum in: *Am J Clin Nutr* 1991; 54: 773].
10. World Health Organization. Physical status: The use and interpretation of anthropometry. Report of the WHO Expert Committee. WHO Technical Report Series 854. World Health Organization, Geneva, Switzerland, 1995.
11. IOTF Childhood Obesity Working Group—Cole, T.J., Bellizzi, M.C., Flegal, K.M. et al., Establishing a standard definition for child overweight and obesity worldwide: International survey, *BMJ*, 320, 1240–1243, 2000.
12. Allison, D.B., Fontaine, K.R., Manso, J.E. et al., Annual deaths attributable to obesity in the United States, *JAMA*, 282, 1530–1538, 1999.
13. Caterson, I.D., Hubbard, V., Bray, G.A. et al., AHA conference proceedings: Obesity, a worldwide epidemic related to heart disease and stroke: Group III: Worldwide Comorbidities of Obesity, *Circulation*, 110, e476–e483, 2004.
14. Manson, J.E., Willett, W.C., Stampfer, M.J. et al., Body weight and mortality among women, *N. Engl. J. Med.*, 333, 677–685, 1995.
15. Shaper, A.G., Wannamethee, S.G., and Walker, M., Body weight: Implications for the prevention of coronary heart disease, stroke, and diabetes mellitus in a cohort study of middle aged men, *BMJ*, 314, 1311–1317, 1997.
16. Rosengren, A., Wedel, J., and Wilhelmsen, L., Body weight and weight gain during adult life in men in relationship to coronary heart disease and mortality. A prospective population study, *Eur. Heart. J.*, 20, 269–277, 1999.
17. Calle, E.E., Thun, M.J., Petrelli, J.M. et al., Body-mass index and mortality in a prospective cohort of U.S. adults, *N. Engl. J. Med.*, 341, 1097–1105, 1999.
18. British Hearth Foundation Statistics website, Prevalence estimates of overweight and obesity for 2002, and projections for 2005 and 2010, by sex, adults aged 15 and over, the World. From The SuRF Report 2, Surveillance of chronic disease risk factors: Country-level data and comparable estimates, pp. 66–72, 73–79, 2005 WHO, Geneva, Switzerland, January 29, 2009, http://www.heartstats.org and https://apps.who.int/infobase/publicfiles/SuRF2.pdf

19. Lobstein, T., Rigby, N., and Leach, R., EU platform on diet, physical activity and health. IOTF EU platform briefing paper, in collaboration with the European Association for the Study of Obesity, International Obesity Task Force, London, U.K., 2005, http://ec.europa.eu/comm/health/ph_determinants/life_style/nutrition/documents/iotf_en.pdf

20. Rigby, N. and James, P., Waiting for a green light for health? Europe at the crossroads for diet and disease, IOTF position paper, International Obesity Task Force, London, U.K., 2003, http://www.iotf.org/media/euobesity2.pdf (accessed on November 24, 2011).

21. CDC, Overweight and obesity: Obesity trends: U.S. obesity trends 1985–2004, Centers for Disease Control and Prevention, Washington, DC, 2005, http://www.cdc.gov/nccdphp/dnpa/obesity/trend/maps/index.htm (accessed on November 24, 2011).

22. Ogden, C.L. and Carroll, M.D., Prevalence of overweight, obesity, and extreme obesity among adults: United States, trends 1976–1980 through 2007–2008, http://www.cdc.gov/nchs/data/hestat/obesity_adult_07_08/obesity_adult_07_08.hm (accessed on November 24, 2011).

23. Flegal, K.M., Carrol, M.D., Ogden, C.L. et al., Prevalence trends in obesity among US adults, 1999–2008, *JAMA*, 303(3), 235–241, 2010.

24. AOA, Obesity in minority populations, AOA fact sheet. American Obesity Association, Washington, DC, 2002, http://www.obesity.org/subs/fastfacts/Obesity_Minority_Pop,shtml (accessed on November 30, 2011).

25. Okosun, I.S., Forrester, T.E., Rotimi, C.N. et al., Abdominal adiposity in six populations of West African descent: Prevalence and population attributable fraction of hypertension, *Obes. Res.*, 7(5), 453–462, 1999.

26. Puoane, T., Steyn, K., Bradshaw, D. et al., Obesity in South Africa: The South African demographic and health survey, *Obes. Res.*, 10(10), 1038–1048, 2002.

27. Van der Merwe, M.T. and Pepper, M.S., Obesity in South Africa. The international Association for the Study of Obesity, *Obes. Rev.*, 7(4), 315–322, 2006.

28. Mokhtar, N., Elati, J., Chabir, R. et al., Diet culture and obesity in Northern Africa, *J. Nutr.*, 131(3), 887S–892S, 2001.

29. Maire, B., Delpeuch, F., Cornu, A. et al., Urbanization and nutritional transition in sub-Saharan Africa: Exemplified by Congo and Senegal [in French], *Rev. Epidemiol. Sante Publique*, 40(4), 252–258, 1992.

30. Kanazawa, M., Yoshiike, N., Osaka, T. et al., Criteria and classification of obesity in Japan and Asia-Oceania, *World Rev. Nutr. Diet*, 94, 1–12, 2005.

31. Shiwaku, K., Anuurad, E., Enkhmaa, B. et al., Appropriate BMI for Asian populations, *Lancet*, 363, 1077, 2004.

32. Razak, F., Anand, S.S., Shannon, H. et al., Defining obesity cut points in a multiethnic population, *Circulation*, 115, 2111–2118, 2007.

33. Zhang, X.F., Atlla, J., D'Este, K. et al., Prevalence and magnitude of classical risk factors for coronary heart disease in a cohort of 4400 Chinese steelworkers over 13.5 years follow-up, *Eur. J. Cardiovasc. Prev. Rehabil.*, 11, 113–120, 2004.

34. Zhou, B.F., Predictive values of body mass index and waist circumference for risk factors of certain related diseases in Chinese adults—Study on optimal cut-off points of body mass index and waist circumference in Chinese adults, *Biomed. Environ. Sci.*, 15, 83–96, 2002.

35. Zhou, B.F., Effect of body mass index on all-cause mortality and incidence of cardiovascular diseases—Report for meta-analysis of prospective studies open optimal cut-off points of body mass index in Chinese adults, *Biomed. Environ. Sci.*, 15, 245–252, 2002.

36. Wu, Y., Editorial: Overweight and obesity in China, *BMJ*, 333, 362–363, 2006.

37. Wang, Y., Popkin, B.M., Wang, X. et al., Is China facing an obesity epidemic and the consequences? The trends in obesity and chronic disease in China, *Int. J. Obes.*, 31, 177–188, 2006.

38. Levine., J.A., Medical progress. Obesity in China: Causes and solutions, *Chinese Med. J.*, 120(11), 1043–1050, 2007.

39. Colagiuri, S., Colagiuri, R., Na'ati, S. et al., The prevalence of diabetes in the kingdom of Tonga, *Diabetes Care*, 25(8), 1378–1383, 2002.

40. Wang, Y. and Lobstein, T., Worldwide trends in childhood overweight and obesity, *Int. J. Pediatr. Obes.*, 1, 11–25, 2006.

41. British Hearth Foundation Statistics website, Prevalence of overweight and obese children by WHO region and country, by sex, latest available years, the world. From The International Obesity task Force, (2006), IOTF, August 5, 2008, http://www.heartstats.org

42. Ogden, C.L. and Carroll, M.D., Prevalence of obesity among children and adolescents: United States, trends 1963–1965 through 2007–2008, http://www.cdc.gov/nchs/data/hestat/obesity_child_07_08/obesity_child_07_08.htm (accessed on December 12, 2011).

43. Ogden, C.L., Carrol, M.D., Curtin, L.R. et al., Prevalence of high body mass index in US children and adolescents, 2007–2008, *JAMA*, 303(3), 242–249, 2010.

44. Magarey, A.M., Daniels, L.A., and Boulton, T.J., Prevalence of overweight and obesity in Australian children and adolescents: Reassessment of 1985 and 1995 data against new standard international definitions, *Med. J. Aust.*, 174(11), 561–564, 2001.

45. de Onis, M. and Blossner, M., Prevalence and trends of overweight among preschool children in developing countries, *Am. J. Clin. Nutr.*, 72(4), 1032–1039, 2000.

46. Ebbeling, C.B., Pawlak, D.B., and Ludwig, D.S., Childhood obesity: Public-health crisis, common sense cure, *Lancet*, 360(9331), 473–482, 2002.

47. Wang, L., Kong, L., Wu, F. et al., Preventing chronic diseases in China, *Lancet*, 366, 1821–1824, 2005.

48. Stamatakis, E., Primatesta, P., Chinn, S. et al., Overweight and obesity trends from 1974 to 2003 in English children: What is the role of socioeconomic factors? *Arch. Dis. Child*, 90(10), 999–1004, 2005.

49. Strauss, R.S. and Pollack, H.A., Epidemic increase in childhood overweight, 1986–1998, *JAMA*, 286(22), 2845–2848, 2001.

50. Strauss, R.S., Childhood obesity, Pediatr, *Clin. North Am.*, 49(1), 175–201, 2002.

51. Salmon, J., Timperio, A., Cleland, V. et al., Trends in children's physical activity and weight status in high and low socio-economic status areas of Melbourne, Victoria, 1985–2001, *Aust. N.Z. J. Public Health*, 29(4), 337–342, 2005.

52. Chatwal, J., Verma, M., and Riar, S.K., Obesity among pre-adolescent and adolescents of a developing country (India), *Asia Pac. J. Clin. Nutr.*, 13(3), 231–235, 2004.

53. Shabbir, S., Kwan, D., Wang, M.C. et al., Asians and Pacific Islanders and the growing childhood obesity epidemic, *Ethn. Dis.*, 20(2), 129–135, 2010.

54. Bhardwaj, S., Misra, A., Khurana, L. et al., Childhood obesity in Asian Indians: A burgeoning cause of insulin resistance, diabetes and sub-clinical inflammation, *Asia Pac. J. Clin. Nutr.*, 17(1), 172–175, 2008.

55. Freedman, D.S., Dietz, W.H., Srinivasan, S.R. et al., The relation of overweight to cardiovascular risk factors among children and adolescents: The Bogalusa Heart Study, *Pediatrics*, 103, 1175–1182, 1999.

56. Fagot-Campagna, A., Emergence of type 2 diabetes mellitus in children: Epidemiological evidence, *J. Pediatr. Endocrinol. Metab.*, 13, 1395–1402, 2000.

57. American Diabetes Association, Type 2 diabetes in children and adolescents. Consensus statement, American Diabetes Association, *Diabetes Care*, 23, 381–389, 2000.

58. Sinha, R., Fisch, G., Teague, B. et al., Prevalence of impaired glucose tolerance among children and adolescents with marked obesity, *N. Engl. J. Med.*, 346, 802–810, 2002.

59. Fagot-Campagna, A., Saaddine, J.B., Flegal, K.M. et al., Diabetes, impaired fasting glucose, and elevated HbA1c in U.S. adolescents: The Third National Health and Nutrition Examination Survey, *Diabetes Care*, 24, 834–837, 2001.

60. Ehtisham, S., Barrett, T.G., and Shaw, N.J., Type 2 diabetes mellitus in UK children—An emerging problem, *Diabet. Med.*, 17, 867–871, 2000.

61. Drake, A.J., Smith, A., Betts, P.R. et al., Type 2 diabetes in obese white children. *Arch. Dis. Child.*, 86, 207–208, 2002.

62. Wabitsch, M., Hauner, H., Hertrampf, M. et al., Type II diabetes mellitus and impaired glucose regulation in Caucasian children and adolescents with obesity living in Germany, *Int. J. Obes. Relat. Metab. Disord.*, 28, 307–313, 2004.

63. Wiegand, S., Maikowsk, U., Blankenstein, O. et al., Type 2 diabetes and impaired glucose tolerance in European children and adolescents with obesity—A problem that is no longer restricted to minority groups, *Eur. J. Endocrinol.*, 151, 199–206, 2004.

64. Colditz, G.A., Economic costs of obesity and inactivity, *Med. Sci. Sports Exerc.*, 31, S663–S667, 1999.

65. Finkelstein, E.A., Flebelkorn, I.C., and Wang, G., National medical spending attributable to overweight and obesity: How much, and who's paying? Health Aff (Millwood), *Suppl Web Exclusives*, W3, 219–226, 2003.

66. National Task Force on the Prevention and Treatment of Obesity/National Institutes of Health, Very low-calorie diets, *JAMA*, 270, 967–974, 1993.

67. IOTF/EASO, Obesity in Europe: The case for action, International Obesity Task Force and European Association for the Study of Obesity, London, U.K., 2002, http://www.iotf.org/media/euobesity.pdf (accessed on December 18, 2011).

2 Epidemiology of Type 2 Diabetes and Obesity

Kevin Corley, MD, Monina S. Cabrera, MD,
Jean Claude Desmangles, MD, FAAP,
Cristina Fernandez, MD, and Archana Chatterjee, MD, PhD

CONTENTS

INTRODUCTION

Type 2 diabetes has been viewed as a disorder in middle-aged adults and the elderly. However, in the last few decades, type 2 diabetes has appeared in younger adults and adolescents. It is an emerging problem around the world, particularly among people of minority ethnicity. In North America, type 2 diabetes mellitus comprises 30% of all newly diagnosed diabetes in patients 10–20 years of age [1]. This epidemic is closely associated with the prevalence of obesity among youth of all backgrounds. There is a clear relationship between insulin resistance, type 2 diabetes, metabolic syndrome, increased visceral adipose tissue, and obesity [2].

PREVALENCE OF TYPE 2 DIABETES AND OBESITY

In the 1990s, type 2 diabetes started increasing, particularly in African Americans (AAs), Mexicans, and Mexican American populations. Studies from the United States estimated 70%–75% of type 2 diabetes mellitus was in AAs, and in Texas and California, one-third of the patients were Mexican

American [3]. In 1977, the first evidence of the association between diabetes and obesity was noted in Pima Indians (0.9%) along with cardiovascular complications [4]. The incidence of diabetes increased four times over the next two decades in the same population [5]. From 1994 to 1997, 682 5–19 year old children were diagnosed with diabetes; 14% of these patients had type 2 diabetes mellitus, and of those, 63% were female [6]. The risk of developing type 2 diabetes mellitus was 3 times greater for AA adolescents and 5.5 times greater for Hispanics than whites [2]. In another study of adolescents, the odds ratio for the development of type 2 diabetes in AAs compared to Caucasians was 2.8 [7].

In 1988 and 1994, the National Health and Nutrition Examination Survey (NHANES) found 20% of children 12–17 years old with a BMI above the 85th percentile, and 8%–17% of these children were obese. The frequency of childhood obesity had doubled since 1980, along with the severity of obesity and its complications [2]. The Bogalusa Heart Study showed an increase of obesity in patients 5–24 years of age living in Louisiana, over a 20 year period; overweight increased from 15% to 30% and obesity from 5% to 11% in those 5–14 years old and from 5% to 15% for those 15–17 years old [2].

The prevalence of type 2 diabetes mellitus in children and adolescents has increased over the last 20 years in many countries and several ethnic groups [8]. In the United States, it has been identified as an epidemic. While 90% of Caucasian diabetic children over 10 years old had type 1 diabetes mellitus, 21%–76% of AA, Hispanic, Asian/Pacific Islander, and Native American children in the same age group had been diagnosed with type 2 diabetes mellitus [9]. In Japan, 80% of all the new diabetes in children and adolescents in 2000 was type 2 diabetes mellitus [10]. The incidence of type 2 diabetes increased from 0.2 per 100,000 in 1976 to 2 per 100,000 in 1995. Adolescent diabetes incidence doubled for type 2 diabetes mellitus associated with high obesity rates [10]. Similar increases have been observed in Thailand, China, India, New Zealand, and Australia [2]. In Europe and South America, the prevalence of type 2 diabetes in children and adolescents is lower [11,12]. Public health experts suggest that the early appearance of type 2 diabetes will result in a major social health burden to the next generation, in large part, because of debilitating cardiovascular complications [13].

OBESITY AND OTHER RISK FACTORS FOR TYPE 2 DIABETES

Multiple factors have been identified for adult type 2 diabetes and obesity which also apply to children and adolescents. Risk factors for young people to develop type 2 diabetes include family history, race, ethnicity, obesity, and a sedentary lifestyle. The risk of developing type 2 diabetes is five times higher for individuals with first-degree relatives with type 2 diabetes as compared to controls of the same gender, age, and weight with no family history of diabetes [14]. The risk of metabolic syndrome during childhood was higher in neonates large or small for gestational age and in those who had mothers with gestational diabetes [15]. In the United States, type 2 diabetes is two to six times more prevalent among children of AA, Hispanic, Asian, and Native American descent than in non-Hispanic Caucasian children [16]. Lifestyle choices such as high-calorie diets and reduced physical activity are also correlated with type 2 diabetes [17].

FAMILY HISTORY

Forty-five to eighty percent of affected youth have at least one parent with diabetes and 74%–100% have a first- or second-degree relative with type 2 diabetes [18]. Children with diabetes are also more likely to have a family history of cardiovascular disease (CVD), with one study showing that up to 28% have a positive family history of CVD [19]. The Bogalusa Heart Study has shown that children of individuals with type 2 diabetes were more likely to be obese and have higher blood pressures, fasting insulin, glucose, and triglycerides [20]. In a study among Pima Indians, it was shown that the cumulative incidence of type 2 diabetes was highest in offspring if both parents had diabetes [2].

Genetic Considerations

Family clustering and segregation analysis indicate that siblings of affected individuals have 3.5 times the general population risk of developing type 2 diabetes mellitus [21]. Over 20 loci have been linked to type 2 diabetes mellitus in adults, the most important being non-insulin-dependent diabetes mellitus (NIDDM1), described among Mexican American siblings in Starr County Texas [21]. This county, which is 97% Mexican American, has the highest disease-specific diabetes mortality in Texas. Four hundred and twenty-four siblings were evaluated, and 16 X-linked markers were examined. Identified as linked to type 2 diabetes mellitus was the NIDDM1 site on chromosome 2, accounting for approximately 30% of the family clustering [22].

Ethnicity

Ethnicity is widely recognized as an important risk factor in the development of type 2 diabetes in adults. The data suggest that the influence of ethnicity is even stronger for youth-onset than for adult-onset type 2 diabetes. Higher prevalence has been seen in Asians, Hispanics, indigenous people (United States, Canada, Australia), and AAs, with some of the highest rates in the world being observed among Pima Indians [23]. Lipolysis is significantly less in AA children than in European American children, suggesting an energy conservation phenotype that would have survival value in times of famine, but is detrimental with excess nutrition (thrifty genotype) [23].

Diet and Activity

A close association between obesity and diabetes has been seen in the last decade. A Japanese study reflects the influence of Westernized diets consumed by Japanese Americans on the development of obesity and diabetes [24]. In the United States, the National Longitudinal Survey of Youth, a prospective cohort study conducted from 1986 to 1998, showed that over this period, the overweight prevalence increased annually by 3.2% in non-Hispanic whites (NHWs), 5.8% in AAs, and 4.3% of Hispanics, and 12.3% of NHWs were overweight [25]. Another study of nearly 5000 children in the United States has shown that during 1999–2000, 15% of 6–19 year olds were overweight, compared with 11% in 1994–1998. A two- to fourfold increase in the prevalence of obesity from 1985 to 1997 has also been reported in Australian children aged 7–15 years [23]. In India, a study found that the age-adjusted prevalence of being overweight among 13–18 year olds was around 18% [26]. Prevalence rates increased with age and decreasing physical activity and with higher socioeconomic status. Other factors, also thought to be important among Indian Asians, are low birth weight (LBW) and insulin resistance. In Canada, 48%–51% of indigenous children aged 4–19 years were found to have a weight >90th percentile [23].

Obese children have been shown to have many of the proinflammatory, proatherogenic changes associated with insulin resistance, hepatic steatosis, elevated total-low-density lipoprotein-cholesterol (LDL-C), and elevated levels of vascular adhesion molecules, tumor necrosis factor (TNF-α), C-reactive protein, interleukin-6 (IL-6), and fibrinogen, while the high-density lipoprotein-cholesterol (HDL-C) is reduced [26]. The increase in childhood obesity and type 2 diabetes precedes CVD which develops over several years. Obese children have approximately 40% lower insulin-stimulated glucose metabolism compared with nonobese children [2]. AA 5–10 year olds, especially girls, have reduced insulin sensitivity, and this correlates with increases in blood pressure, triglycerides, subcutaneous fat, percentage of total body fat, and stage of sexual maturation. Insulin-stimulated glucose metabolism decreases while fasting insulinemia increases with increasing BMI [27].

Overall in the United States, only 50% of young people aged 12–21 years are involved in physical activity, with almost 25% admitting to no physical activity at all [28]. Even in schools, there is a decline in physical education, with participation rates down from 41.6% in 1991 to 24.5% in 1995. A study of 1732 9–15 year olds showed that the risk of having an elevated metabolic score only began to fall when more than 60 min/day of moderate activity was accumulated, suggesting that the current targets of 30 min/day may be inadequate [29].

INTRAUTERINE ENVIRONMENT

The intrauterine environment has been recognized as being an important contributor to disease in adult life. Both LBW (<2500 g) and high birth weight are associated with the development of type 2 diabetes in later life [30]. Both genetic and environmental factors are likely to be involved. The fetal response to intrauterine malnutrition leads to insulin resistance and impaired beta-cell development, increasing the risk of diabetes later in life. Studies of monozygotic and dizygotic twins have shown that the lower-birth-weight twin has a greater risk of diabetes in adulthood [23]. Birth weight may also be influenced by genetic factors, with a recent study suggesting that paternal type 2 diabetes may play a role [31]. Children born to a father with type 2 diabetes weighed an average of 86 g less than children from a nondiabetic parent.

ROLE OF MATERNAL DIABETES

Exposure to maternal diabetes in utero is a significant risk factor for obesity, IGT, and type 2 diabetes in youth. Silverman et al. followed a cohort of offspring of diabetic mothers and found that although neonatal macrosomia disappears after the 1st year of life, by the age of 8, almost half of the children have obesity [32]. The exposure to maternal diabetes in utero as well as maternal obesity accounts for the development of type 2 diabetes in other populations, such as the Pima Indians and others [23]. In another study of maternal diabetes, fetal beta-cell function was assessed in 88 pregnancies with pregestational or gestational diabetes by measuring amniotic fluid insulin (AFI) concentration at 32–38 weeks of gestation and performing oral glucose tolerance tests annually in the offspring from 18 months of age. Only one of 27 adolescents with normal AFI had IGT, in contrast to one-third of those with elevated AFI [32]. These studies suggest a generation to generation accumulation of risk for type 2 diabetes mellitus.

ROLE OF BREASTFEEDING

Early childhood nutrition also plays a role in the development of insulin resistance. High-protein intake in infancy and later obesity has been suggested. Breast-feeding results in a more appropriate caloric intake at a critical stage in development than bottle feeding, which is more likely to be associated with overfeeding and obesity. Glucose tolerance testing was carried out in 720 Pima Indians aged 10–39 years, including 325 who had been exclusively bottle fed as infants, 144 who were exclusively breast fed, and the rest partially breast fed for the first 2 months of life [33]. The breast-fed children had significantly lower rates of type 2 diabetes mellitus than those exclusively bottle fed for each age decade, with an odds ratio of 0.41 [33]. Prolonged breast-feeding markedly reduced the risk of overweight in nearly 10,000 5–6 year old German children; 3.8% of those exclusively breast fed for 2 months were overweight versus 0.8% of those breast fed for longer than 12 months [2]. This finding may be due to the lower insulin responses and the lower energy and protein intake in breast-fed infants versus bottle-fed infants. The frequent overweight of the bottle-fed infant may contribute to insulin resistance and obesity in adolescence and young adulthood.

ROLE OF PUBERTY

Diagnosis of type 2 diabetes mellitus peaks at approximately 13.5 years of age, corresponding to the time of peak adolescent growth and development. Puberty is associated with relative insulin resistance [34]. Insulin-mediated glucose metabolism is approximately 30% lower in adolescents than in prepubertal children in young adults. The physiologic insulin resistance of puberty is of no consequence in the presence of adequate beta-cell function. The cause of this resistance is the transitory increased activity of the growth hormone-insulin growth factor, which coincides with insulin resistance of adolescence [2].

PATHOPHYSIOLOGY

The etiology of type 2 diabetes in children and adolescents is multifactorial, similar to adults, involving genetics and environmental factors. Type 2 diabetes results from the combination of insulin resistance and β-cell function failure. Insulin resistance is strongly associated with obesity, particularly central adiposity. This is believed to be the first abnormality in diabetes, preceding insulin secretion failure [35]. Insulin resistance in adults has been recognized for decades as a main feature in the development of type 2 diabetes and has been associated with obesity, the metabolic syndrome, hypertension, and heart disease [36]. In children, insulin resistance is also significantly related to obesity and cardiometabolic risk [37].

DEFINITION: INSULIN RESISTANCE

Insulin resistance is defined as the decreased tissue response to insulin-mediated cellular action and is the inverse of insulin sensitivity. It refers to the reduced glucose uptake in the whole body in response to physiological insulin levels and its effects on glucose and insulin metabolism. Insulin resistance is determined primarily by the response of skeletal muscle with over 75% of infused glucose taken up by muscle and only 2%–3% by adipose tissue [38].

IMPORTANCE OF INSULIN RESISTANCE

Insulin resistance is associated with obesity, although not all obese people are insulin resistant, and insulin resistance may occur in nonobese children and adults. It can occur in normal physiological conditions, such as puberty and pregnancy [39]. The adverse effects related to insulin resistance are mediated by compensatory hyperinsulinemia [40]. Standards for insulin levels in children have not been established due to the use of different techniques to measure insulin, lack of cohort studies, and long-term outcome studies. Clinical features such as acanthosis nigricans can predict but cannot define it. Fasting insulin is not an optimal tool to assess peripheral insulin sensitivity, but it provides information regarding compensatory hyperinsulinemia and liver metabolism [41]. Fasting insulin as an index of insulin resistance may be applicable in some studies that involve a large population of children. The glucose tolerance test has high correlation with insulin resistance in adult studies compared to other tests. The oral glucose tolerance test has also been studied in obese 8–18 year olds [42].

Obesity is a complex disorder that is affected by many interacting genetic and nongenetic factors. Leptin signaling is the key biological pathway controlling energy balance. Insulin and leptin are secreted in proportion to body fat and serve as an adiposity signal, acting on the same neurons of the hypothalamic arcuate nucleus to regulate energy homeostasis. Ghrelin, which is secreted by the stomach and duodenum, serves as a hunger signal at the hypothalamus and brain stem, whereas other peptides secreted by the gastrointestinal tract, including neuropeptide Y, act as satiation signals. The ligands leptin, proopiomelanocortin, cocaine-amphetamine-related transcript, and brain-derived neurotrophic factors; the receptors for leptin; and the enzyme prohormone convertase 1 have function-changing mutations that are associated with obesity in children [43].

Puberty is associated with increased fat mass in girls compared to boys. This increase in fat mass results in increased insulin resistance during puberty, as well as worsening changes in leptin in girls compared to boys [44]. Abdominal obesity promotes insulin resistance due to the increase of free fatty acids, increased gluconeogenesis, and decreased insulin clearance by the liver [45]. Insulin resistance is associated with obesity and central adiposity, as noted earlier. This is followed by failure of insulin secretion [46]. In adolescents at risk of diabetes, the transition from normal tolerance to IGT or prediabetes is associated with rapid weight gain and decrease in the insulinogenic index, reduced insulin sensitivity, and long-term, decreased insulin secretion. In one study, the decrease of β-cell function in type 2 diabetes, observed over 6 years of follow-up, was approximately 15% per year [47]. This loss of function is faster than what was observed in adults in the UKPDS study, which was 7% per year [14].

CLASSIFICATION AND DIAGNOSIS OF TYPE 2 DIABETES IN CHILDHOOD

The criteria for diagnosis of diabetes in childhood are based on glucose levels and symptoms:

- Fasting glucose ≥126 mg/dL
- Glucose test tolerance—glucose ≥200 mg/dL
- Classic symptoms of diabetes and casual glucose ≥200 mg/dL, plus polyuria, polydipsia, and unexplainable weight loss [48]

Plasma C-peptide levels over 1 ng/mL are suggestive of type 2 diabetes [49]. In patients with risk factors such as family history, ethnicity, acanthosis nigricans, hypertension, dyslipidemia, and polycystic ovarian syndrome starting at 10 years of age, it is recommended that fasting glucose be repeated every 2 years, by the American Diabetes Association [50].

CLINICAL FEATURES

Usually, children and adolescents with type 2 diabetes have similar but fewer symptoms than adults. Obesity is predominantly visceral associated with hypertension, hyperlipidemia, sleep apnea, polycystic ovary syndrome, and acanthosis nigricans. The initial presentation of type 2 diabetes in children and adolescents may be of hyperosmolar coma. This coma affects 4% of all type 2 diabetics and has mortality rates from 14% to 43% [51]. Symptoms are change in level of consciousness (average Glasgow coma score 9–15), average osmolality of 400 mOsm, and glucose level of 600 mg/dL. Only 5%–50% of type 2 diabetes mellitus presents with diabetic ketoacidosis. Typically, 85%–98% of individuals with type 1 diabetes mellitus are positive for specific auto antibodies to insulin, glutamic acid decarboxylase (GAD), or the tyrosine phosphate insulin antibodies [52]. Overweight or obesity, family history of type 2 diabetes mellitus, acanthosis nigricans, polycystic ovary syndrome, lipid disorder, and hypertension occur in children with type 2 diabetes mellitus. Most of the children with type 2 diabetes mellitus present in middle to late puberty. During puberty, there is ~25%–50% decline in insulin sensitivity with recovery when puberty is completed [39]. Fasting insulin and C-peptide are usually normal or elevated, but not as elevated as might be expected for the degree of hyperglycemia. IGT is a high predictor of type 2 diabetes mellitus and CVD [53]. Source studies have reported 25% IGT in obese children and silent diabetes in 4% of obese adolescents [54]. IGT can be reversible in both adults and adolescents [55]. Insulin sensitivity is inversely associated with BMI and percentage of body fat [56]. Nonalcoholic fatty liver is associated with hepatic and peripheral insulin resistance. Polycystic ovarian syndrome (amenorrhea, hirsutism, obesity, and diabetes) is known to be associated with IGT and insulin resistance [39].

COMPLICATIONS

Adolescents with type 2 diabetes may present with various comorbidities. Microvascular chronic complications include retinopathy, microalbuminuria, and peripheral neuropathy [57]. Macrovascular complications also occur. Arterial hypertension and dyslipidemia are more common than in type 1 diabetics that have had the disease for the same period of time. A multicenter study observed hypertension in 10%–32% of type 2 diabetic teenagers, eight times more frequent than in type 1 diabetes [58]. Lipid disorders were present in 24%–44% of the cases of type 2 diabetes mellitus, and only 1% of the children with type 1 diabetes mellitus were treated with medication for dyslipidemia [58]. Microalbuminuria is present in 14%–25% at the time of diagnosis, worsens with time, and is associated with poor glucose control and can progress to renal failure [59]. The risk of hepatic steatosis, cirrhosis, and portal hypertension are five times higher in children with metabolic syndrome secondary to type 2 diabetes mellitus [60]. Hypertension associated with obesity has underlying mechanisms associated with insulin resistance. Sodium retention occurs due to the antinatriuretic effect of insulin, increased aldosterone, and increased adrenal cortical activity. Leptin adipokines and rennin angio-tensin, impaired vascular endothelial function, and other vascular mechanisms are also associated with insulin resistance. Treatment with lifestyle changes, diet, and orlistat improves symptoms, but more studies are needed on the use of diuretics, ACE inhibitors, and possibly angiotensin II receptor inhibitors to increase insulin sensitivity and reduce diabetes risks [61]. Neuropsychiatric disease is more prevalent in teenagers with type 2 diabetes, including depression, ADHD, hyperactivity, neuro-psychomotor disorder, or bipolar disorder. Sixty-three percent of these patients have been reported to be using antipsychotic drugs, increasing the possibility of weight gain [62].

PREVENTION

- Maternal obesity, gestational diabetes, smoking in pregnancy, and maternal malnutrition should be targeted to decrease obesity and insulin resistance in children [32].
- Breast-feeding reduces obesity, but no specific data are available on its impact on insulin resistance.
- Early diagnosis of preschool children at risk for obesity is a target along with preventing excessive weight gain with combined intervention programs [63].

Early detection of insulin resistance, obesity, and type 2 diabetes is important to decrease complications for young patients. The value to the health-care system is significant as it increases the quality of life and decreases the cost of long-term complications [64].

REFERENCES

1. American Diabetes Association. Type 2 diabetes in children and adolescents. American Diabetes Association. *Diabetes Care* 2000;23:381–389.
2. Rosenbloom AL, Silverstein JH, Amemiya S, Seitler P, Klingensmith GJ. Type 2 diabetes in children and adolescents. *Pediatr Diabetes* 2009;10(Suppl 12):17–32.
3. Upchurch SL, Brosnan CA, Meininger JC et al. Characteristics of 98 children and adolescents diagnosed with type 2 diabetes by their health care provider at initial presentation. *Diabetes Care* 2003;26:2209.
4. Savage PJ, Bennett PH, Senter RG, Miller M. High prevalence of diabetes in young Pima Indians: Evidence of phenotypic variation in a genetically isolated population. *Diabetes* 1979;28:937–942.
5. Pinhas-Hamiel O, Dolan LM, Daniels SR, Standiford D, Khoury PR, Zeitler P. Increased incidence of non-insulin dependent diabetes mellitus among adolescents. *J Pediatr* 1996;128:608–615.
6. Macaluso CJ, Bauer UE, Deeb LC et al. Type 2 diabetes mellitus among Florida children and adolescents, 1994 through 1998. *Public Health Rep* 2002,117.373–379.
7. Signorello LB, Schlundt DG, Cohen SS et al. Comparing diabetes prevalence between African American and Whites of similar socioeconomic status. *Am J Public Health* 2007;97:2260–2267.
8. Libman I, Arslanian SA. Type 2 Diabetes mellitus: No longer just in adults. *Pediatr Ann* 1999;28:589–593.
9. Liase AD, D'Agostino RB, Hamman RF, Kilgo PD, Lawrence JM, Liu LL, Loots B, Linder B, Marcovina S, Rodriguez B, Standiford D, Williams DE. The burden of diabetes mellitus among US youth: Prevalence estimates from the SEARCH for diabetes in youth study. *Pediatrics* 2006;118:1510–1518.
10. Urakami T, Morimoto S, Nitadori Y, Harada K, Owada M, Kitagawa T. Urine glucose screening program at schools in Japan to detect children with diabetes and its outcome-incidence and clinical characteristics of childhood type 2 diabetes in Japan. *Pediatr Res* 2007;61(2):141–145.
11. Ortega-Rodriguez E, Levy-Marchal C, Tubiana N, Czernichow P, Polak M. Emergence of type 2 diabetes in a hospital based cohort in children with diabetes mellitus. *Diabetes Metab* 2001;27:574–578.
12. Rami B, Schober E, Nachbauer E, Waldhor T. Type 2 diabetes is rare but not absent in children under 15 years of age in Austria. *Eur J Pediatr* 2003;162:850–852.
13. Short K, Blackett P, Gardner A, Copeland K. Vascular health in children and adolescents: Effects of obesity and diabetes. *Vasc Health Risk Manag* 2009;5:973–990.
14. Mathews DR, Cull CA, Stratton IM, Holman RR, Turner RC. UKPDS 26: Sulphonylurea failure in non-insulin dependent diabetic patients over 6 years. UK Prospective Diabetes Study (UKPDS) group. *Diabet Med* 1998;15:297–303.

15. Klein BE, Klein R, Moss SE, Cruickshanks KJ. Parental history of diabetes in population-based study. *Diabetes Care* 1996;19:827–830.
16. Boney CM, Verma A, Tucker R et al. Metabolic syndrome in childhood; association with birth weight, maternal obesity and gestational diabetes mellitus. *Pediatrics* 2005;115:e290–e296.
17. Carter J, Pugh JA, Monterrosa A. Non–insulin-dependent diabetes mellitus in minorities in the United States. *Ann Intern Med* 1996;125:221–232.
18. Sinha AK, O'Rourke SO, Leonard D, Yarker S. Early onset type 2 diabetes (T2DM) in the indigenous communities of far north Queensland (FNQ). In: *Australian Diabetes Society Annual Scientific Meeting*, Cairns, Queensland, Australia, 2000, p. 90.
19. Glowinska B, Urban M, Koput A. Cardiovascular risk factors in children with obesity, hypertension and diabetes: Lipoprotein (a) levels and body mass index correlate with family history of cardiovascular disease. *Eur J Pediatr* 2002;161:511–518.
20. Nguyen QM, Srinivasan SR, Xu JH, Chen W, Berenson GS. Changes in risk variables of metabolic syndrome since childhood in pre-diabetic and type 2 diabetic subjects: The Bogalusa Heart Study. *Diabetes Care* 2008;31(10):2044–2049.
21. Hallman DM, Boerwinkle E, Gonzalez VH, Klein BE, Klein R, Hanis CL. A genome-wide linkage scan for diabetic retinopathy susceptibility genes in Mexican Americans with type 2 diabetes from Starr County, Texas. *Diabetes* 2007;56(4):1167–1173.
22. Hanis CL, Boerwinkle E, Chakraborty R et al. A genome-wide search for human non-insulin-dependent (type 2) diabetes genes reveals a major susceptibility locus on chromosome 2. *Nat Genet* 1996;13:161–166.
23. Shaw J. Epidemiology of childhood type 2 diabetes and obesity. *Pediatr Diabetes* 2007;8:7–15.
24. Hara H, Egusa G, Yamakido M. Incidence of non-insulin-dependent diabetes mellitus and its risk factors in Japanese-Americans living in Hawaii and Los Angeles. *Diabet Med* 1996;13(9 Suppl 6):S133–S142.
25. Strauss RS, Pollack HA. Epidemic increase in childhood overweight. *JAMA* 2001;286(22):2845–2848.
26. Jain S, Pant B, Chopra H, Tiwari R. Obesity among adolescents of affluent public schools in Meerut. *Indian J Public Health* 2010;54(3):158–160.
27. Caprio S, Tamborlane WV. Metabolic impact of obesity in childhood. *Endocrinol Metab Clin North Am* 1999;28:731–747.
28. Nesmith JD. Type 2 diabetes mellitus in children and adolescents. *Pediatr Rev* 2001;22:147–152.
29. Andersen LB, Harro M, Sardinha LB et al. Physical activity and clustered cardiovascular risk in children: A cross-sectional study (The European Youth Heart Study). *Lancet* 2006;368:299–304.
30. Ozanne SE, Hales CN. Early programming of glucose-insulin metabolism. *Trends Endocrinol Metab* 2002;13:368–373.
31. Koebnick C, Kelly LA, Lane CJ, Roberts CK, Shaibi GQ, Toledo-Corral CM, Davis JN, Weigensberg MJ, Goran MI. Combined association of maternal and paternal family history of diabetes with plasma leptin and adiponectin in overweight Hispanic children. *Diabet Med* 2008;25(9):1043–1048.
32. Silverman BL, Metzger BE, Cho NH, Loeb CA. Impaired glucose tolerance in adolescent offspring of diabetic mothers. Relationship to fetal hyperinsulinism. *Diabetes Care* 1995;18:611–617.
33. Pettitt DJ, Forman MR, Hanson RL, Knowler WC, Bennet PH. Breastfeeding and incidence of non-insulin-dependent diabetes mellitus in Pima Indians. *Lancet* 1997;350:166–168.
34. Rosenbloom AL, Wheeler L, Bianchi R, Chin FT, Tiwary CM, Grgic A. Age adjusted analysis of insulin responses during normal and abnormal glucose tolerance tests in children and adolescents. *Diabetes* 1975;24:820–828.
35. Gungor N, Bacha F, Saad R, Janosky J, Arslanian S. Youth type 2 diabetes: Insulin resistance, beta cell failure, or both? *Diabetes Care* 2005;28:638–644.
36. Reaven GM. Banting lecture 1988. Role of insulin resistance in human disease. *Diabetes* 1988;37:1595–1607.
37. Ten S, Maclaren N. Insulin resistance syndrome in children. *J Clin Endocrinol Metab* 2004;89:2526–2539.
38. DeFronzo RA. Pathogenesis of type 2 (non-insulin dependent) diabetes mellitus: A balanced overview. *Diabetologia* 1992;35:389–397.
39. Levy-Marchal C, Arslanian S, Cutfield W, Sinaiko A, Druet C, Marcovecchio ML, Chiarelli F, ESPE-LWPES-ISPAD-APPES-APEG-SLEP-JSPE, Insulin Resistance in Children Consensus Conference Group. Insulin resistance in children: Consensus, perspective, and future directions. *J Clin Endocrinol Metab* 2010;95(12):5189–5198.
40. Goran MI, Gower BA. Longitudinal study on pubertal insulin resistance. *Diabetes* 2001;50:2444–2450.
41. Ferrannini E, Galvan AQ, Gastaldelli A, Camastra S, Sironi AM, Toschi E, Baldi S, Fraserra S, Monzani F, Antonelli A, Nannipieri M, Mari A, Seghieri G, Natali A. Insulin: New roles for an ancient hormone. *Eur J Clin Invest* 1999;29:842–852.

42. Schwartz B, Jacobs DR Jr., Moran A, Steinberger J, Hong CP, Sinaiko AR. Measurement of insulin sensitivity in children: Comparison between the euglycemic-hyperinsulinemic clamp and surrogate measures. *Diabetes Care* 2008;31:783–788.

43. Yeckel CW, Weiss R, Dziura J, Taksali SE, Dufour S, Burgert TS, Tamborlane WV, Caprio S. Validation of insulin sensitivity indices from oral glucose tolerance test parameters in obese children and adolescents. *J Clin Endocrinol Metab* 2004;89:1096–1101.

44. Han JC, Lawlor D, Kimm SY. Childhood obesity. *Lancet* 2010;375:1737–1748.

45. Biro FM, Huang B, Morrison JA, Horn PS, Daniels SR. Body mass index and waist-to-height changes during teen years in girls are influenced by childhood body mass index. *J Adolesc Health* 2010;46:245–250.

46. Ferrannini E, Balkau B, Coppack SW et al. Insulin resistance, insulin response and obesity are indicators of metabolic risk. *J Clin Endocrinology Metab* 2007;92:2885–2892.

47. Gungor N, Arslanian S. Progressive beta cell failure in type 2 diabetes of youth. *J Pediatr* 2004;44:656–659.

48. Report of the Expert Committee on the diagnosis and classification of diabetes mellitus. *Diabetes Care* 1997;20:1183–1197.

49. Hannon TS, Rao G, Arslanian SA. Childhood obesity and type 2 diabetes mellitus. *Pediatrics* 2005;116:473–480.

50. Invitti C, Guzzaloni G, Girardini L, Morabito F, Viberti G. Prevalence and concomitants of glucose intolerance in European obese children and adolescents. *Diabetes Care* 2003;26:118–124.

51. Rosenbloom AL. Hyperglycemic crises and their complications in children. *J Pediatr Endocrinol Metab* 2007;20:5–18.

52. Reinehr T, Schober E, Wiegand S et al. Beta-cell autoantibodies in children with type 2 diabetes mellitus: Subgroup or misclassification? *Arch Dis Child* 2006;91:473–477.

53. Polonsky KS, Sturis J, Bell GI. Seminars in Medicine of the Beth Israel Hospital, Boston. Non-insulin-dependent diabetes mellitus: A genetically programmed failure of the beta cell to compensate for insulin resistance. *N Eng J Med* 1996;334:777–783.

54. Sinha R, Fisch G, Teague B et al. Prevalence of impaired glucose tolerance among children and adolescents with marked obesity. *N Engl J Med* 2002;346:802–810.

55. Knowler WC, Barrett-Connor E, Fowler SE et al. Reduction in the incidence of type 2 diabetes with lifestyle intervention or metformin. *N Eng J Med* 2002;346:393–403.

56. Perseghin G, Bonfanti R, Magni S, Lattuada G et al. Insulin resistance and whole body energy homeostasis in obese adolescents with fatty liver disease. *Am J Physiol Endocrin Metab* 2006;291:E697–E703.

57. Pinhas-Hamiel O, Zeitler P. Acute and chronic complications of type 2 diabetes mellitus in children and adolescents. *Lancet* 2007;369:1823–1831.

58. Kershnar AK, Daniels SR, Imperatore G, Palla SL, Petitti DB, Pettit DJ, Marcovina S, Dolan LM, Hamman RF, Liese AD, Pihoker C, Rodriguez BL. Lipid abnormalities are prevalent in youth with type 1 and type 2 diabetes: The SEARCH for diabetes in youth study. *J Pediatr* 2006;149:314–319.

59. Rodriguez BL, Fuijimoto WY, Mayer-Davis EJ, Imperatore G, Williams DE, Bell RA, Wadwa RP, Palla SL, Liu LL, Kershnar A, Daniels SR, Linder B. Prevalence of cardiovascular disease risk factors in U.S. children and adolescents with diabetes: The SEARCH for diabetes in youth study. *Diabetes Care* 2006;29:1891–1896.

60. McGavock J, Sellers E, Dean H. Physical activity for the prevention and management of youth-onset type 2 diabetes mellitus: Focus on cardiovascular complications. *Diab Vasc Dis Res* 2007;4:305–310.

61. Kotchen T. Obesity-related hypertension: Epidemiology, pathophysiology and clinical management. *Am J Hypertens* 2010;23:1170–1178.

62. Buchholz S, Morrow AF, Coleman PL. Atypical antipsychotic-induced diabetes mellitus: An update on epidemiology and postulated mechanisms. *Intern Med J* 2008;38:602–606.

63. Bhargava SK, Sachdev HS, Fall CH, Osmond C et al. Relation of serial changes in childhood body-mass index impaired glucose tolerance in young adulthood. *N Eng J Med* 2004;350:865–875.

64. Colagiuri S, Davies D. The value of early detection of type 2 diabetes. *Curr Opin Endocrinol Diabetes Obes* 2009;16:95–99.

Part II

Pathophysiology of Obesity

3 Global View on the Development of Noncommunicable Diseases
Where Are We Going?

Karl-Heinz Wagner, PhD and Helmut Brath, MD

CONTENTS

PRESENT GLOBAL SITUATION OF NONCOMMUNICABLE DISEASES

Of the 57 million global deaths in 2008, 63% or 36 million were due to noncommunicable diseases (NCDs) (Alwan et al., 2010), and annual NCD deaths are projected to further rise worldwide. NCDs mainly comprise cardiovascular diseases (CVDs), diabetes, cancers, and chronic respiratory diseases. Decades ago, as popular belief presumes, they were typically found in developed countries due to the predominantly sedentary lifestyle (WHO, 2010a).

However, the greatest increase is expected to be seen in highly populated low- and middle-income regions, such as China, India, Pakistan, or Indonesia. Nearly 80% of NCD deaths (over 80% of cardiovascular and diabetes deaths, almost 90% of deaths from chronic obstructive pulmonary disease [COPD] and more than two-thirds of all cancers) occur in low- and middle-income countries, and NCDs are the most frequent causes of death in most countries in the Americas, the Eastern Mediterranean, Europe, Southeast Asia, and the Western Pacific, except in Africa. Even in African nations, NCDs are rising rapidly and are projected to exceed communicable, maternal, perinatal, and nutritional diseases as the most common causes of death by 2030 (WHO, 2008, 2010a).

NCDs also lead to death at a younger age in low- and middle-income countries, where 29% of NCD deaths occur among people under the age of 60, compared to 13% in high-income countries. For cancer incidence, the estimated percentage increase by 2030, compared with 2008, will be greater in low- (82%) and lower-middle-income countries (70%) compared with the upper-middle- (58%) and high-income countries (40%). The same tendency is true for CVD and type 2 diabetes. The NCD epidemic strikes disproportionately among people of lower social levels. NCDs and poverty create a vicious cycle whereby poverty exposes people to behavioral risk factors for NCDs, and, in turn, the resulting NCDs may become an important driver to the downward spiral that leads families toward poverty. The rapidly growing burden of NCDs in low- and middle-income countries is accelerated by the negative effects of globalization, rapid unplanned urbanization, and increasingly sedentary lives (see Section 3.4) (Farmer et al., 2010; Ferlay et al., 2010; WHO, 2010a).

RISK FACTORS FOR THE NCDs

The main risk factors for NCDs for individuals have been well known for decades and are similar in almost all countries. Tobacco use; unhealthy diet with foods high in saturated and trans fats, salt, and sugar (especially in sweetened drinks); physical inactivity; and the harmful consumption of alcohol cause more than two-thirds of all new cases of NCDs and increase the risk of complications in people with NCDs. At least 80% of heart disease, stroke, and type 2 diabetes, as well as 40% of cancer, could be avoided by healthy diet, regular physical activity, and avoidance of tobacco use (World Cancer Research Fund, 1997; WHO, 2002).

Consumption of foods high in saturated and industrially produced trans fats, salt, and sugar is the cause of at least 14 million deaths or 40% of all deaths every year from NCDs (WHO, 2004). Overconsumption of salt causes up to 30% of all cases of hypertension. Physical inactivity causes about 3 million or 8% of all deaths per year from NCDs. Alcohol consumption leads to 2.3 million deaths each year, 60% of which are due to NCDs, and has adverse health, social, and economic effects, not only for the people who drink (Leon et al., 2007; Casswell et al., 2011).

Almost 6 million people die from tobacco use each year, both from direct tobacco use and from second-hand smoke. By 2020, this number will increase to 7.5 million, accounting for 10% of all deaths (WHO, 2010a). The exposure to second-hand smoke accounts for about 1.0% of the worldwide mortality (Oberg et al., 2011). These risk factors lead to metabolic conditions which are linked to NCDs such as raised blood pressure, raised cholesterol and glucose, overweight/obesity, and cancer-associated infections. Raised blood pressure is estimated to cause 7.5 million deaths, about 12.8% of all, and is a major risk factor for CVD. Raised cholesterol is estimated to cause 2.6 million deaths annually (WHO, 2010a), increasing the risks of heart disease and stroke. Raised cholesterol is highest in high-income countries. Risks of heart disease, stroke, and diabetes increase steadily with increasing body mass index (BMI). Estimated 35.8 million (2.3%) of global disability adjusted life years (DALYs) are caused by overweight or obesity (WHO, 2009). In 2008, 35% of adults aged 20 years and older were overweight (BMI > $25\,\text{kg/m}^2$) (34% men or 205 million and 35% of women or 297 million) (Table 3.1). This is presumably the first time in history of mankind that there are more overweight than underweight individuals. The worldwide prevalence of obesity has nearly doubled between 1980 and 2008 (Stuckler, 2008). The prevalence of overweight and obesity was highest in the WHO region of the Americas (62% for overweight in both sexes and 26% for obesity) and lowest in the WHO region of Southeast Asia (14% overweight in both sexes and 3% for obesity). However, the highest prevalence of overweight among infants and young children is in upper-middle-income populations, while the fastest rise in overweight is in the lower-middle-income group. At present, more than 1.3 billion people globally are overweight or obese. Urban and rural areas in all countries have more than 5%–10% of their populations overweight. This is a globe where more than 25% of Chinese adults are now overweight or obese and about two-thirds of the adult populations in countries as diverse as the low- to middle-income countries of Egypt, Mexico, and South Africa as well as higher income countries such as Australia, the United Kingdom, and the United States (Popkin, 2007).

TABLE 3.1

Comparable Estimates of Prevalence of Overweight and Obesity in Adults Aged +20 Years

Country	Overweight (≥25 kg/m²)	Obesity (≥30 kg/m²)
Australia[a]	63.7 (60.5–66.7)	26.8 (24.1–29.4)
Brazil[b]	51.7 (47.4–55.7)	18.8 (16.0–21.6)
China[b]	25.4 (21.7–29.0)	5.7 (4.4–7.0)
Egypt[c]	67.9 (63.2–72.0)	33.1 (29.8–36.4)
Germany[a]	60.5 (55.9–64.8)	25.1 (21.5–28.8)
Mexico[c]	68.3 (64.8–71.5)	32.1 (28.7–35.3)
Russia[c]	59.8 (56.5–63.0)	26.5 (23.7–29.3)
Tonga[c]	87.0 (84.1–89.6)	57.6 (52.2–62.9)
UAE[b]	71.3 (65.9–76.0)	32.7 (27.8–37.8)
UK[a]	64.2 (61.3–66.9)	26.9 (24.3–29.4)
USA[a]	70.8 (68.5–73.1)	33.0 (30.6–35.6)

Source: WHO, Global status report on non communi-cable diseases, World Health Organization, Geneva, Switzerland, 2010a.

[a] Men > women.

[b] Men almost the same BMI as women.

[c] Women > men.

GLOBAL DEVELOPMENTS OF NCDs

In 2008, the overall NCD age-standardized death rates in low- and middle-income countries were 756 per 100,000 for males and 565 per 100,000 for females—respectively, 65% and 85% higher than for men and women in high-income countries. Age-standardized NCD mortality rates for all ages were highest in the African Region for males (844 per 100,000) and for females (724 per 100,000). The leading causes of NCD deaths in 2008 were CVDs (17 million deaths, or 48% of NCD deaths), cancers (7.6 million, or 21% of NCD deaths), and respiratory diseases, including asthma and COPD (4.2 million, or 12% of NCD deaths). Over 80% of cardiovascular and diabetes deaths, almost 90% of deaths from COPD and almost two-thirds of all cancer deaths occurred in low- and middle-income countries.

This development has also a significant impact on economy. In 2005, the estimated losses in national income from heart disease, stroke, and diabetes were 18 billion dollars in China, 11 billion dollars in the Russian Federation, 9 billion dollars in India, and 3 billion dollars in Brazil. These losses accumulate over time because each year more people die (WHO, 2005).

Estimates for 2015 for the same countries are between approximately three and six times those of 2005. If nothing is done to reduce the risk of chronic diseases, an estimated US$84 billion of economic production will be lost by heart disease, stroke, and diabetes alone in those 23 countries which account for around 80% of the total chronic disease mortality burden, between 2006 and 2015 (Abegunde et al., 2007). For the latter, this would be a percentage reduction of the GDP of over 5%, for many other countries up to 1% (WHO, 2010a).

As stated before, many highly populated regions are in a period of change. In Southeast Asia, where almost 600 million people are living, NCDs are responsible for 60% of death in the region. In terms of disability, chronic NCDs were estimated to account for 61% of total DALYs in people aged 15–59 years and 84% of the burden in those aged 60 years and older in 2008. The burden is expected to rise to 74% and 89%, respectively, by the year 2030 (WHO, 2008; Dans et al., 2011).

Also in Brazil, a country in transition with almost 200 million people, NCDs have become a major health priority. In 2007, about 72% of all deaths in Brazil were attributable to NCDs, 10% to infectious or parasitic diseases, and 5% to maternal and child health disorders. The only favorable observation is a positive trend. Although the crude NCD mortality increased by 5% between 1996 and 2007, age-standardized mortality declined by 20%. This is primarily caused by declines in cardiovascular and chronic respiratory diseases, in association with the successful implementation of health policies that lead to decreases in smoking and the expansion of access to primary health care. However, overweight and obesity are still in rise with more than 60% of the population affected (Schmidt et al., 2011).

CARDIOVASCULAR DISEASES

Coronary heart disease (CHD) is the leading cause of CVD death, the single largest cause of death in developed countries, and one of the leading causes of disease burden in developing countries. High-income countries have CVD death rates of approximately 38% (Gaziano et al., 2010). While the overall rate of CVD deaths (28%) is collectively less in low- and middle-income countries, there is a great range from 58% in Eastern Europe to as low as 10% in sub-Saharan Africa. Most other developing regions appear to be following a similar pattern as the developed countries, with an initial rise in stroke and then a predominance of CHD, but the transition has occurred at a more compressed rate than in the high-income countries. Between 1990 and 2020, CHD alone is anticipated to increase by 120% for women and 137% for men in developing countries, compared with age-related increases of between 30% and 60% in developed countries (Leeder et al., 2004).

Whereas in developed countries, despite the overall increase in CHD burden, the age-adjusted death rates for CHD are declining, there is a reverse trend in developing countries, largely a result of an increase in the prevalence of the risk factors mentioned earlier, a relative lack of access to preventive interventions, and limited access to medical care.

Population growth and improved longevity are leading to increasing numbers and proportions of older people, with population aging emerging as a significant trend in many parts of the world. As populations age, annual NCD deaths are projected to rise substantially to 52 million in 2030. Annual CVD mortality is projected to increase by 6 million, and annual cancer deaths by 4 million. Detailed information of the CVD development in the different WHO regions can be found elsewhere (Gaziano et al., 2010).

CANCER

In 1970, 15% of newly reported cancers occurred in developing countries, compared with 56% in 2008. By 2030, the proportion is expected to be 70%. Almost two-thirds of the 7.6 million annual cancer deaths worldwide occur in low-income and middle-income countries, making cancer a leading cause of mortality in these settings (Boyle et al., 2008; Ferlay et al. 2010). Furthermore, increases in age-adjusted mortality rates have been recorded in certain developing regions and for specific cancers, such as breast cancer (Lozano-Ascencio et al., 2009).

Lung, breast, colorectal, stomach, and liver cancers cause the majority of cancer deaths. Within upper-middle-income and high-income countries, prostate and breast cancers are the most commonly diagnosed in males and females, respectively, with lung and colorectal cancers representing the next most common types in both sexes. These cancers also represent the most frequent types of cancer-related deaths in these countries although lung cancer is the most common cause of cancer death in both sexes, mostly attributed to tobacco smoking. In low- and middle-income countries, cancer levels vary according to the prevailing underlying risks. In sub-Saharan Africa, for example, cervical cancer is the leading cause of cancer death among women (WHO, 2010a,b).

Low survival rates in poor countries and improved survival in developed countries contribute to the disparity in the burden of cancer deaths.

Overall, case fatality from cancer (calculated as an approximation from the ratio of incidence to mortality in a specific year) is estimated to be 75% in countries of low income, 72% in countries of low-middle income, 64% in countries of high-middle income, and 46% in countries of high income (Farmer et al., 2010).

In many low- and middle-income countries, access to care, medication, oral morphine, and staff trained in palliative care is limited, so most cancer patients die without adequate pain relief. In addition to the general risk factors for NCDs mentioned earlier, infections such as hepatitis B, hepatitis C (liver cancer), human papillomavirus (HPV; cervical cancer), and *Helicobacter pylori* (stomach cancer) also cause up to 18% of cancer burden (Parkin, 2006). Furthermore, cancers are also caused by radiation and a variety of environmental and occupational exposures of varying importance, depending on the specific geographical region and cancer site.

DIABETES MELLITUS

A very recent 199 country analysis, including 2.7 million individuals, estimated that the number of adults with diabetes has doubled within the past three decades—up from 153 million in 1980 to 347 million in 2008. Although 70% of the observed increase is attributed to population growth and aging, the number also reflects the unfortunate global shift toward a Western lifestyle of unhealthy diet and physical inactivity, with obesity as the outcome (Danaei et al., 2011). Approximately 90% of those with DM have type 2 DM (WHO, 2011a). In the same time span, cardiovascular mortality of diabetes patients decreased in highly developed countries by about 50% (Carstensen et al., 2008; Gulliford and Charlton 2009; Preis et al., 2009) On the other hand, there are signs that cancer mortality has increased in diabetics.

About 80% of this population currently lives in low- and middle-income countries. Future prevalence rates will be highest in developing regions such as Asia, Latin America and Caribbean, and sub-Saharan Africa, where growth rates will exceed 104%–162%, compared with about 72% in the United States and 32% in Europe (Wild et al., 2004; Hossain et al. 2007; WHO, 2011).

Rising rates of obesity as well as aging and urbanization of the population have been linked to the DM epidemic. Nearly 90% of type 2 DM cases are estimated to be related to obesity. In reverse, DM and its related complications are the costliest consequence of obesity. Mortality from DM is also on the rise. In 2004, an estimated 3.4 million people died from consequences of high blood sugar (WHO, 2011) Diabetes is one of the leading causes of visual impairment and blindness in developed countries (Resnikoff et al., 2004). People with diabetes require at least two to three times the health-care resources compared to people without, and diabetes care may account for up to 15% of national health-care budgets (Zhang et al., 2010). Interestingly, Asian countries face a relatively larger burden of DM. Between 1970 and 2005, the prevalence of diabetes quadrupled in Indonesia, Thailand, India, and China compared with an increase of only 1.5 times in the United States (Yoon et al., 2006). India and China house the largest number of diabetics in the world with 32 million and 21 million, respectively. As well, Indonesia, Pakistan, and Bangladesh are in the top 10 in high absolute number of type 2 DM (Wild et al. 2004).

SOME REASONS FOR THIS GLOBAL DEVELOPMENT

The rapidly growing burden of NCDs in low- and middle-income countries seems to be mainly due to the negative effects of globalization, rapid urbanization, and increasingly sedentary lifestyles. These countries are in various phases of the epidemiologic transition. As countries progress from agrarian to industrial to postindustrial states, there are a series of environmental, social, and structural changes that occur, some that lead to increase longevity, others that result in exposure to risk factors for chronic diseases (Popkin 2006).

There is strong evidence on the links between poverty and lower life expectancy, and on the associations between various social determinants, especially education, and prevalent levels of NCDs, showing that people of lower social and economic positions suffer far more in countries at all levels of development. In some countries, the lowest income households have the highest levels of NCD risk factors, with negative consequences on household income (WHO, 2010a). Poverty at household level is triggered by unhealthy behavior, poor physical status, premature death, and high costs of health care.

Globalization, with its free movement of capital, technology, goods, and services, has significant effects on lifestyles. Other factors are the worldwide shifts in the trade of technology innovations that affect energy expenditures during leisure, transportation, and work; the globalization of modern food processing, marketing, and distribution techniques (most frequently linked with Westernization of the world's diet); and the vast expansion of the global mass media (Mendez and Popkin, 2005).

One global trend is the replacement of fresh markets by multinational, regional, or local large supermarkets, which are usually part of larger chains. In Latin America, the supermarkets' share of all retail food sales increased from 15% in 1990 to 60% by 2000 (Reardon et al., 2004). Supermarket use has spread across both large and small countries, from capital cities to rural villages, and from upper- and middle-class families to the working class (Hu et al. 2004). This same process is also occurring at varying rates and different stages in Asia, Eastern Europe, and Africa. Supermarkets are large providers of processed higher-fat, sugar-added, and salt-laden foods in developing countries.

Global agricultural policies have built-in a long-term focus on creating cheaper grains and animal-source foods. One good example is beef, where price is now, in the United States, around 20% of the price four decades ago (Popkin, 2006). In China, there is a shift toward great increases in the production, importation, and consumption of animal-source foods (Du et al., 2002). Nowadays, about two-thirds of the Chinese population obtain more than 15% of their energy from saturated fats, mainly from meat, dairy, and egg products. This represents a doubling over the past two decades and is expected to increase even further to about 80% of the Chinese population by 2025 (Lopez and Murray, 1998).

By 2020, lower income countries are projected to produce 63% of meat products and 50% of all cow's milk (Popkin, 2007).

Global mass media access has shifted in an equally impressive manner, but is discussed elsewhere. Further putative factors include insufficient quantity or quality of sleep, endocrine disruptors—lipophilic, environmentally stable, industrially produced substances that can affect endocrine function—reduction in variability in ambient temperature, or intrauterine and intergenerational effects (Keith et al., 2006).

CONCLUSION

NCDs represent a significant and unfortunately growing burden worldwide. During the past decades, they were mainly a topic of developed countries; nowadays, they represent the main health problem of the developing world. These trends reflect the growing societies, rapid unplanned urbanization, increasingly sedentary lives, but also a higher degree of poverty. Currently, the main focus of health care for NCDs in many low- and middle-income countries is hospital-centered acute care. To ensure early detection and timely treatment, NCDs need to be integrated into primary health care. Expanding the package of primary health-care services to include essential NCD interventions is central to any health system strengthening initiative. One global strategy to overcome this development was the launch of the WHO Action Plan for the Global Strategy for the Prevention and Control of NCDs (WHO, 2008). This offers a global vision to respond to the epidemic by integrating disease prevention and control into local policies, promote research and intervention to reduce risk factors, strengthen partnerships for prevention, and monitor NCDs and their determinants.

REFERENCES

Abegunde, D.O., Mathers, C.D., Adam, T., Ortegon, M., and Strong, K. 2007. The burden and costs of chronic diseases in low-income and middle-income countries. *Lancet* 370:1929–1938.

Alwan, A., Maclean, D.R., Riley, L.M., d'Espaignet, E.T., Mathers, C.D., Stevens, G.A., and Bettcher, D. 2010. Monitoring and surveillance of chronic noncommunicable diseases: Progress and capacity in high-burden countries. *Lancet* 376:1861–1868.

Boyle, P., Boffetta, P., and Autier, P., 2008. Diet, nutrition and cancer: Public, media and scientific confusion. *Annals of Oncology*, 19(10): 1665–1667.

Carstensen, B., Kristensen, J.K., Ottosen, P., and Borch-Johnsen, K., Steering Group of the National Diabetes Register. 2008. The Danish National Diabetes Register: Trends in incidence, prevalence and mortality. *Diabetologia* 51:2187–2196.

Casswell, S., You, R.Q., and Huckle, T. 2011. Alcohol's harm to others: Reduced wellbeing and health status for those with heavy drinkers in their lives. *Addiction* 106:1087–1094.

Danaei, G., Finucane, M.M., Lu, Y., Singh, G.M., Cowan, M.J., Paciorek, C.J., Lin, J.K., Farzadfar, F., Khang, Y.H., Stevens, G.A., Rao, M., Ali, M.K., Riley, L.M., Robinson, C.A., and Ezzati, M., Global Burden of Metabolic Risk Factors of Chronic Diseases Collaborating Group (Blood Glucose). 2011. National, regional, and global trends in fasting plasma glucose and diabetes prevalence since 1980: Systematic analysis of health examination surveys and epidemiological studies with 370 country-years and 2·7 million participants. *Lancet* 378:31–40.

Dans, A., Ng, N., Varghese, C., Tai, E.S., Firestone, R., and Bonita, R. 2011. The rise of chronic non-communicable diseases in southeast Asia: Time for action. *Lancet* 377:680–689.

Du, S., Lu, B., Zhai, F., and Popkin, B. 2002. The nutrition transition in China: A new stage of the Chinese diet. In *The Nutrition Transition: Diet and Disease in the Developing World*, eds. B. Caballero and B. Popkin, pp. 205–222. Academic Press, London, U.K.

Farmer, P., Frenk, J., Knaul, F.M., Shulman, L.N., Alleyne, G., Armstrong, L., Atun, R., Blayney, D., Chen, L., Feachem, R., Gospodarowicz, M., Gralow, J., Gupta, S., Langer, A., Lob-Levyt, J., Neal, C., Mbewu, A., Mired, D., Piot, P., Reddy, K.S., Sachs, J.D., Sarhan, M., and Seffrin, J.R. 2010. Expansion of cancer care and control in countries of low and middle income: A call to action. *Lancet* 376:1186–1193.

Ferlay, J., Shin, H.R., Bray, F., Forman, D., Mathers, C., and Parkin, D.M. 2010. GLOBOCAN 2008: Cancer incidence and mortality worldwide. Lyon, France: International Agency for Research on Cancer.

Gaziano, T.A., Bitton, A., Anand, S., Abrahams-Gessel, S., and Murphy, A. 2010. Growing epidemic of coronary heart disease in low- and middle-income countries. *Curr. Probl. Cardiol.* 35:72–115.

Gulliford, M.C. and Charlton, J. 2009. Is relative mortality of type 2 diabetes mellitus decreasing? *Am. J. Epidemiol.* 169:455–461.

Hossain, P., Kawar, B., and El Nahas, M. 2007. Obesity and diabetes in the developing world—A growing challenge. *N. Engl. J. Med.* 356:213–215.

Hu, D., Reardon, T., Rozelle, S., Timmer, P., and Wang. H. 2004. The emergence of supermarkets with Chinese characteristics: Challenges and opportunities for China's agricultural development. *Dev. Policy Rev.* 22:557–586.

Keith, S.W., Redden, D.T., Katzmarzyk, P.T., Boggiano, M.M., Hanlon, E.C., Benca, R.M., Ruden, D., Pietrobelli, A., Barger, J.L., Fontaine, K.R., Wang, C., Aronne, L.J., Wright, S.M., Baskin, M., Dhurandhar, N.V., Lijoi, M.C., Grilo, C.M., DeLuca, M., Westfall, A.O., and Allison, D.B. 2006. Putative contributors to the secular increase in obesity: Exploring the roads less travelled. *Int. J. Obes.* 30:1585–1594.

Leeder, S., Raymond, S., Greenberg, H., Liu, H., and Esson, K. 2004. *A Race Against Time: The Challenge of Cardiovascular Disease in Developing Countries*. New York: Trustees of Columbia University.

Leon, D.A., Saburova, L., Tomkins, S., Andreev, E., Kiryanov, N., McKee, M., and Shkolnikov, V.M. 2007. Hazardous alcohol drinking and premature mortality in Russia: A population based case-control study. *Lancet* 369:2001–2009.

Lopez, A.D. and Murray, C.C. 1998. The global burden of disease, 1990–2020. *Nat. Med.* 4:1241–1243.

Lozano-Ascencio, R., Gómez-Dantés, H., Lewis, S., Torres-Sánchez, L., and López-Carrillo, L. 2009. Tendencias del cáncer de mama en América Latina y El Caribe. *Salud Pública Méx* 51:S147–S156.

Mendez, M.A. and Popkin, B. 2005. Globalization, urbanization and nutritional change in the developing world. *J. Agric. Dev. Econ.* 1:220–241.

Oberg, M., Jaakkola, M.S., Woodward, A., Peruga, A., and Prüss-Ustün, A. 2011. Worldwide burden of disease from exposure to second-hand smoke: A retrospective analysis of data from 192 countries. *Lancet* 377:139–146.

Parkin, D.M. 2006. The global health burden of infection-associated cancers in the year 2002. *Int. J. Cancer* 118:3030–3044.

Popkin, B.M. 2006. Global nutrition dynamics: The world is shifting rapidly toward a diet linked with noncommunicable diseases. *Am. J. Clin. Nutr.* 84:289–298.

Popkin, B.M. 2007. Understanding global nutrition dynamics as a step towards controlling cancer incidence. *Nat. Rev. Cancer* 7:61–67.

Preis, S.R., Pencina, M.J., Hwang, S.J., D'Agostino, R.B.Sr., Savage, P.J., Levy, D., and Fox, C.S. 2009. Trends in cardiovascular disease risk factors in individuals with and without diabetes mellitus in the Framingham Heart Study. *Circulation* 21:212–220.

Reardon, T., Timmer, P., and Berdegue, J. 2004. The rapid rise of supermarkets in developing countries: Induced organizational, institutional, and technological change in agrifood systems. *J. Agric. Dev. Econ.* 1:168–183.

Resnikoff, S., Pascolini, D., Etya'ale, D., Kocur, I., Pararajasegaram, R., Pokharel, G.P., and Mariotti, S.P. 2004. Global data on visual impairment in the year 2002. *Community Eye Health J.* 17:61.

Schmidt, M.I., Duncan, B.B., Azevedo e Silva, G., Menezes, A.M., Monteiro, C.A., Barreto, S.M., Chor, D., and Menezes, P.R. 2011. Chronic non-communicable diseases in Brazil: Burden and current challenges. *Lancet* 377:1949–1961.

Stuckler, D. 2008. Population causes and consequences of leading chronic diseases: A comparative analysis of prevailing explanations. *Milbank Q.* 86:273–326.

WHO. 2002. Diet, nutrition, and the prevention of chronic diseases: WHO Technical Report Series 916. Geneva: World Health Organization.

WHO. Risk factor estimates for 2004. www.who.int/healthinfo/global_burden_disease/risk_factors/en/index. html (accessed July 22, 2011).

WHO. 2005. Preventing chronic diseases: A vital investment: WHO global report. Geneva, Switzerland: World Health Organization.

WHO. 2008. Action plan for the global strategy for the prevention and control of noncommunicable diseases. Geneva, Switzerland: World Health Organization (document A61/8).

WHO. 2009. Global health risks: Mortality and burden of disease attributable to selected major risks. Geneva, Switzerland: World Health Organization.

WHO. 2010a. Global status report on non communicable diseases. Geneva, Switzerland: World Health Organization.

WHO. 2010b. The global burden of disease: 2004 update. Geneva, Switzerland: World Health Organization.

WHO. 2011. Diabetes factsheet 2011. http://www.who.int/mediacentre/factsheets/fs312/en/ (accessed July 26, 2011).

Wild, S., Roglic, G., Green, A., Sicree, R., and King, H. 2004. Global prevalence of diabetes: Estimates for the year 2000 and projections for 2030. *Diabetes Care* 27:1047–1053.

World Cancer Research Fund and American Institute for Cancer Research. 1997. Food, nutrition, and the prevention of cancer: A global perspective, Washington, DC: American Institute for Cancer Research.

Yoon, K.H., Lee, J.H., Kim, J.W., Cho, J.H., Choi, Y.H., Ko, S.H., Zimmet, P., and Son, H.Y. 2006. Epidemic obesity and type 2 diabetes in Asia. *Lancet* 368:1681–1688.

Zhang, P., Zhang, X., Brown, J., Vistisen, D., Sicree, R., Shaw, J., and Nichols, G. 2010. Global healthcare expenditure on diabetes for 2010 and 2030. *Diabetes Res. Clin. Pract.* 87:293–301.

4 Evidence for Refined Food Addiction

J.R. Ifland, PhD, Harry G. Preuss, MD, MACN, CNS,
Marianne T. Marcus, EdD, RN, FAAN, K.M. Rourke, PhD,
W.C. Taylor, PhD, and Marty Lerner, PhD

CONTENTS

INTRODUCTION

In spite of obesity-related sequelae such as diabetes, cardiovascular disease, and hypertension, public health experts suggest that we have a worldwide obesity epidemic that seems resistant to solution. In this chapter, we examine one plausible explanation for the epidemic: that obesity is in part a symptom of the consequences of an addiction to refined foods such as sugars, artificial sweeteners, flour, salt, caffeine, processed fats, and dairy products. This hypothesis can be framed by asking several key questions: (a) How is overeating similar to other chemical dependencies, such as drug and alcohol addiction? (b) does the evidence support the concept that overeating is a kind of addiction? and (c) are today's refined foods and highly processed commercial food products addictive in nature, thereby contributing to the spread of obesity and eating disorders?

Evaluating the evidence for refined food addiction is important for a number of reasons. For individuals, adapting an addiction treatment or recovery model to overeating could open the door to employing several different, yet similar, protocols with a history of successful outcomes for sufferers of chemical dependencies. For example, a common denominator among addiction treatment programs is complete abstinence from the offending substances. This includes abstinence from alcohol for the alcoholic, abstinence from cocaine for the cocaine addict, abstinence from all forms of tobacco for the smoker, and so forth. Further, more recent research within the addiction treatment field suggests that addictions can be process-oriented, such as gambling, sex addiction, and compulsive shopping, despite the absence of an identified substance but rather an "addictive behavior," which requires refraining from any and all such behaviors as a tenet of the recovery process. Congruent with these treatment principles is limiting the addict's exposure to cues (triggers) that add to the physical and psychological craving associated with the offending substance or behavior(s). If an addictive mechanism is at work in overeating, abstinence from particular refined foods and associated cues could help reduce pathological behavior.

On the macrolevel, public education, particularly of children and adolescents, can impact vast segments of our society and encourage us to change consumption patterns as was the case with tobacco. In summary, the net effect of education could well impact the economic, social, and physical well-being of all segments of our society, obese and nonobese alike. In particular, the emphasis should be on those elements that have been successful in curbing tobacco use, such as the limitations and regulatory efforts made regarding alcohol, controlled substances, and similar prevention programs aimed at youth.

Evidence for refined food addiction is varied with findings supporting both physiological and cognitive mediators providing support for this phenomenon. Pathological overeating and resultant obesity and the more familiar forms of chemical dependencies are both physical and mental states with highly complex and extensive trait characteristics. Almost every aspect of the individual, family, and society at large is affected. As a result, the evidence for pathological overeating as mediated in large part by a physical addictive process might be best approached from different angles. Because the literature for addiction etiology and treatment as well as pathological overeating is extensive, a comprehensive approach permits in-depth comparisons across a variety of dimensions. We will therefore examine the diversity of the literature on both substance dependency (addiction) and pathological overeating with reference to individuals, including neurological functioning, behavior patterns, morbidity, genetic variations, and fetal syndromes. The influence within family systems is also explored. Last, comparisons between refined foods and tobacco are made regarding socioeconomic and political influences within the food industry, crop subsidy policies, marketing and media incentives, and demographic/epidemiological patterns.

Because the literature with respect to the topics of addiction and pathological overeating is vast, the evidence is initially presented as a list of elements in support of the foregoing hypothesis, rather than a detailed discussion of each element, as the latter is beyond the scope of this chapter. Moreover, the evidence presented is not intended to be exhaustive; rather it is representative of the kinds of research that support the hypothesis that overeating is a kind of addiction. These are limitations of this chapter which are discussed in more detail in Section 4.4.3. Discussion includes citing the evidence for refined food as an addictive substance for many individuals suffering with obesity and related eating disorders according to the very criteria published by the American Psychiatric Association (APA) in the Diagnostic and Statistical Manual (DSM) for Mental Illness [DSM IV] for substance dependency. Moreover, using the criteria for the Surgeon General's 1964 landmark decision to categorize tobacco as an harmful substance due to the strong association between tobacco and lung cancer, we evaluate an association between obesity and refined food products.

Although the evidence is presented methodically, we point out that addiction syndromes in general and especially food addiction are controversial. Because addicts can adjust their behavior when rewards are offered, even when substances of abuse are available, some observers say loss of control does not exist (Peele 1992). There is also a concept that overeating occurs because of social and culture mores, and not because of an addictive mechanism (Rogers and Smit 2000). Resolving this controversy is important because if overeating is found to be the result of addiction pathology, addiction treatment protocols and public policies could be helpful as applied to overeating.

METHODOLOGY

We searched Pubmed; a handbook of food addiction, *Food Cravings and Addiction* (Hetherington 2001); a book on the tobacco experience, *Cigarette Century* (Brandt 2007); a book on the politics of food, *Food Politics* (Nestle 1996); and the 12-step literature using search terms addiction, drug abuse, overeating, cueing, cravings, fast food, and obesity.

RESULTS

A broad review of the addiction and overeating literature reveals that researchers have made similar findings in 19 types of research. The types of research range from brain imaging research to genetic and behavioral studies. Similarities were also found in characteristics of family systems, a broad syndrome of consequences, and a fetal syndrome. Macroevidence was found in corporate business practices, a great cost to society, epidemiological patterns, and government subsidies.

1. *Neurofunctioning*: The neurological evidence for overeating as an addiction is extensive as researchers have been searching for ways to intervene in both addictions and overeating even before the advent of neuroimaging techniques at the end of the twentieth century. In addition to neuroimaging, research methods include microdialysis of rat brains and observance of behaviors, such as lever pressing in response to the introduction of known transmitter agonists. Because of the depth of the field, a handbook has been published (Hetherington 2001) as well as a number of review articles (Pelchat et al. 2004; Blumenthal and Gold 2010; Frascella et al. 2010; Liu et al. 2010; Gearhardt et al. 2011). Key findings of the research are activation of the same reward/pleasure/addiction pathways for both addiction and overeating, which include dopamine, opiate, serotonin, endorphin, and endocannabinoid pathways. Downregulation in the receptor fields for dopamine is found in both methamphetamine abusers and the obese (Wang et al. 2004). In addition, reduced cognitive functioning during cravings has been found in both addictions and overeating (Volkow et al. 2008). Impaired inhibition has been found for both alcohol in alcoholics and food in overeaters (Batterink et al. 2010; Filbey et al. 2011).

   The neurofunctioning literature is the strongest category of evidence that overeating functions as an addiction. The breadth and consistency of research support the concept.

2. *Neuroresponses to environmental cueing*: Many researchers have examined the brain's response to drug and food cues in laboratory animals as well as humans (Kelley et al. 2005; Cota et al. 2006; Cornier et al. 2007; Petrovich and Gallagher 2007; Anderson 2009; Stice et al. 2011). The evidence shows that very little exposure to either drug or refined food cues is required to stimulate a global response of neurotransmitter release in the addictive pathways. For example, mere thoughts of a food or drug can create an addictive response (Stice et al. 2008; Volkow et al. 2010). Other characteristics of cueing that appear in both drug addiction and overeating include heightened response to compounding of cues (Weiss 2005; Rolls and McCabe 2007), persistence of heightened reactivity after abstinence (Grimm et al. 2002), heightened reactivity in the early stages of abstinence (Lu et al. 2004; Grimm et al. 2005), heightened sensitivity in past abusers (Ranaldi et al. 2009), and place triggers (Schroeder et al. 2001; Hetherington 2007). Sensitivities to food cues but not drug cues are augmented by peripheral signaling in orexin, leptin, and insulin (Holland and Petrovich 2005; Blumenthal and Gold 2010). Leptin resistance is also a factor in uninhibited overeating in spite of satiety (Berthoud 2007).

   Like the neurofunctioning literature, the cueing literature is broad and consistent. It functions as collateral evidence that would support public policy measure such as reduced advertising for refined foods.

3. *Cognitive impairment*: During the use of both drugs of abuse and foods, changes in cognitive function are found (Esch and Stefano 2004; Stefano et al. 2007), and compromised thinking during cravings has also been observed (Kemps et al. 2008; Volkow et al. 2008). This body of evidence is not extensive. However, it offers insight into why people do not make good food decisions under craving conditions.

4. *Repeated exposure*: There is evidence that repeated exposure to both drug and refined food use and cues leads to the development of both addiction and overeating (McAuliffe et al. 2006; Mahar and Duizer 2007; Corwin and Grigson 2009). This is thought to occur via the

pathological mechanism of Pavlovian conditioning of reward pathways to produce excessive neurotransmitters in response to cues and use. Repeated cues and use heighten reward
sensitivity and cravings in both addiction and overeating. Although this is not an extensive
body of literature, it contributes to the hypotheses of the etiology of the obesity epidemic
as the result of increased advertising and number of outlets for obesogenic food as sources
of repeated exposure to cues.

5. *Genetics*: Researchers have found genetic anomalies in both drug addicts and overeaters at
the TaqA1 allele (Noble et al. 1994; Blum et al. 1996; Stice and Dagher 2010). The TaqA1
allele has additionally been correlated with heightened reward sensitivity (Lee et al. 2007).
This evidence is strong as the correlations are straightforward and replicated.

6. *Conformance to DSM-IV criteria for addiction*: Several research reports have found that
the diagnostic criteria for addiction (American Psychiatric Association 2000) are valid
when applied to overeating. These criteria include withdrawal, progression, unintended
use, failed attempts to cut back, time spent, reduction in social activities, and use in spite
of knowledge of consequences (Cassin and von Ranson 2007; Gearhardt and Corbin
2009; Ifland et al. 2009). Historically, these criteria have formed the basis for determining
that a substance is addictive. This category of evidence is consistent, but not extensive.
Nonetheless, it is an important body of evidence as these criteria are the "gold standard"
for diagnosing addictions.

7. *Behavioral syndromes*: Both addicts and overeaters display a syndrome of behavior,
including poor impulse control, numbing, blaming, shame, denial, minimizing, normalizing, and emotional avoidance (Barry et al. 2009). Both addictions and overeating exhibit
relapse and cravings (Mercer and Holder 1997; Kalra and Kalra 2004; Rosenberg 2009).
When taken with the neurofunction evidence, behavioral syndromes provide important
corroborating evidence.

8. *Muted sense of taste*: Both soft drink (Sartor et al. 2011) and tobacco use (Suliburska et al.
2004) result in a muted sense of taste.

9. *Interchangeability of drugs of abuse for food*: In addiction recovery centers, clinicians
have observed that when individuals withdraw from drugs of abuse and alcohol, they substitute food (Hodgkins et al. 2004; Kleiner et al. 2004; Kendzor et al. 2008; Cocores and
Gold 2009; Gearhardt and Corbin 2009). Smokers gain weight when they quit smoking
(Epstein and Leddy 2006). In an animal study, conditioned rats chose sugar over cocaine
(Lenoir et al. 2007). This evidence is fairly conclusive as it is a widely observed clinical
phenomenon.

10. *Family system patterns*: Researchers have shown that obesity and addictions both manifest in family systems. For example, children raised in alcoholic families are more likely
to become alcoholics, children raised in families that abuse both drugs and alcohol are
more likely to abuse both, and children raised by obese parents are more likely to become
obese (Ellis et al. 1997; Raimo et al. 2000; Kampov-Polevoy et al. 2003; Krahnstoever
Davison et al. 2005; Bayol et al. 2007; Seliske et al. 2009). Interestingly, women with a
family history of alcoholism crave sugar more than women without this history (Pepino
and Mennella 2007), and children of alcoholics crave sugar more than children of nonalcoholic parents (Mennella et al. 2010). Family patterns constitute a strong body of ancillary evidence, but do not necessarily demonstrate the core functioning of overeating as an
addiction.

11. *Fetal syndrome*: Offspring of laboratory rats fed obesogenic foods develop the metabolic
syndrome, including neuroimprinting (Armitage et al. 2005) and fatty livers (Bayol et al.
2010). Babies of mothers who abuse alcohol and those who overeat to the point of obesity
suffer from congenital defects (Stothard et al. 2009; Mattson et al. 2010; Riley et al. 2011)
including fatty liver. This body of evidence would be stronger with specific studies of compromised neurofunctioning in offspring of obese mothers.

12. *Epidemiological pattern*: Similar to addictions, overeating and obesity are more likely to occur in undereducated, lower income, Hispanic and African American populations. Analogous to tobacco use, obesity has reached about 2/3 of the population, but whereas 2/3 of smokers were men, 2/3 of overeaters are women (Giovino et al. 1995; Ellis et al. 1997; Caetano and Clark 1998; Ogden et al. 2007). Most importantly, fast-food outlets are more highly clustered around low-income neighborhoods (Day and Pearce 2011), and the proximity of food outlets is more of a factor in obesity in low-income schools (Mellor et al. 2010). The epidemiological evidence shows parallels between overeating and addiction but is tangential to the key issue of whether overeating is a kind of addiction.

13. *Consequences*: Both addictions and overeating are characterized by a range of dysfunctions as measured by the Addiction Severity Index (McLellan et al. 1992) including a propensity for physical illnesses, mental illness, financial difficulties, relationship problems, social problems, and employment problems (McLellan et al. 1992; Ouyang et al. 2008; Lim et al. 2010; Lustig 2010; Nseir et al. 2010; Ifland et al. 2012). This research makes a case for the broad devastation of overeating and supports the idea that overeating is a kind of addiction.

14. *Treatment approach*: In both drug addiction and overeating, the same approaches to treatment are found: Both conditions respond to abstinence from the substances or foods associated with loss of control (Ries 2009; Food Addicts Anonymous 2010). While abused substances are fairly easy to identify in drug and alcohol treatment, in refined food addiction, the situation is more complex with a number of foods recommended for abstinence by food addiction professionals and 12-step recovery groups. These include sugar and all other sweeteners, flour, excess salt, fatty foods, and caffeine. Treatment protocols for recovery from both addiction and overeating call for long-term support and avoidance of external triggers, such as people, places, and things (Ayyad and Andersen 2000; McNatt et al. 2007; Leombruni et al. 2009; McIver et al. 2009; Ries 2009; Food Addicts Anonymous 2010). Treatment of overeating through abstinence from particular refined foods has not been investigated. Evidence cited here is from self-endorsed food addiction recovery 12-step groups. This evidence needs further research.

15. *Psychoactive characteristics of refined foods*: There is general acceptance that foods high in sugar, fat, or salt are a factor in the obesity epidemic (Harper and Mooney 2010). The evidence for sugar addiction has been demonstrated in rats showing progressive use and a withdrawal syndrome (Avena et al. 2008). Sugar is also associated with opioid stimulation (Olszewski and Levine 2007) and numbs pain in children (Pepino and Mennella 2005), while fat consumption in rats is attenuated by pharmaceuticals used in drug treatment (Islam and Bodnar 1990; Rao et al. 2008). Chocolate has been demonstrated to possess psychoactive elements, including methylxanthines, biogenic amines, and cannabinoid-like fatty acids (Bruinsma and Taren 1999), as has caffeine (Hughes et al. 1992). Moreover, the psychoactive element of theobromine in combination with caffeine affects mood (Smit et al. 2004). Salt can be used addictively (Cocores and Gold 2009), and dairy products contain naturally occurring morphine (Meisel 1986) that can produce a numbing effect in rats (Blass et al. 1989). The numbing reaction in rats is similar to wheat gluten, which contains an opioid peptide (Fanciulli et al. 2005). In conclusion, food refinement processes are similar to drug and alcohol processing (Ifland et al. 2009) and include distillation, particle size reduction (powdering), extraction, concentration, and heating to high temperatures.

    The strength of the evidence in this category is uneven from substance to substance. It is perhaps strongest for sugar, dairy, processed fat, and caffeine; moderately strong for salt; and weakest for flour.

16. *Polysubstance use patterns*: In both addiction and overeating, addictions are stronger when more than one substance is concurrently abused. Thus, families that abuse both alcohol and drugs are more dysfunctional than alcoholic families (Raimo et al. 2000),

and polysubstance abusers have more substance problems than single substance abusers (Schuckit et al. 2001). Chocolate is thought to be addictive because of the presence of both sugar and fat (Bruinsma and Taren 1999) as it is known that combinations of sugar and fat activate endocannabinoid circuits (DiPatrizio and Simansky 2008) and encourage overeating in rats (Berner et al. 2008). This category of evidence lacks research into the myriad combinations of refined foods as they are offered commercially.

17. *Business practices*: Refined food and tobacco corporations use deceptive advertising to impute social values and health to promote their products with advertising especially aimed at younger audiences. Other business practices include affordable pricing and availability through vending machines and numerous retail outlets (Nestle 1996; Lewin et al. 2006; Brandt 2007; Brownell and Warner 2009). The evidence for these practices in the tobacco industry is strong due to the availability of documents discovered during tobacco litigation. By contrast, evidence of the food industry practices is observed.

18. *Cost to society*: Overeating, drug abuse, alcoholism, and tobacco create a significant cost to the societies in which these epidemics are present (Harwood et al. 1998; Wang et al. 2008). Although this concept is well documented, it is peripheral evidence for overeating as an addiction.

19. *Government subsidies*: Government subsidies were present in tobacco production and continue to be present in crop production that supports obesity, including wheat, corn, dairy products, and sugar (Tillotson 2004; Glynn et al. 2010). This evidence is straightforward and conclusive. It is somewhat central to the overeating as addiction argument because subsidies lower the price of refined foods making them easy to obtain and increasing the frequency of their use which is tied to increased reward sensitivity and the development of loss of control.

The results show consistent similarities between overeating and drug addiction in all features examined, particularly in regard to the hypothesis that "overeating is like drug and alcohol addiction." In physical manifestations, we found similar abnormalities in brain function across a range of pleasure circuits including prominently the dopamine and opiate circuits. Genetic anomalies in the TaqA1 allele are similar. Overeating also conforms to the DSM-IV criteria for drug addiction showing progressive use and a withdrawal syndrome. Similar syndromes of abnormal behavior appear, including poor impulse control and normalization.

We found the same patterns in family use—specifically the increased likelihood that children of adults with the syndrome are more likely to develop the same syndrome. The same wide-ranging consequences as measured by the Addiction Severity Index are also apparent. Both overeating and addiction demonstrate patterns of polysubstance use. Similarities in production methods for both drugs of abuse and refined foods also occur, including distillation, concentration, and powdering. Moreover, treatment approaches of abstinence and support were also similar in both conditions.

Worldwide, the same business practices for refined foods are present as for tobacco in terms of advertising, availability and affordable pricing. Epidemiological studies found the same disadvantaged populations suffering disproportionately from both overeating and addictions. We also found a great cost to society and government subsidies for both tobacco and the refined foods used in overeating.

DISCUSSION

The evidence for overeating as a kind of drug addiction is extensive and consistent across many fields.

While it can be difficult to "prove" causal relationships between consumption of a substance and subsequent addiction because so many factors are involved, it is widely accepted today that tobacco consumption is linked to addiction. However, as was shown in the history of evidence gathering regarding nicotine addiction and the harmful consequences of smoking, evidence is often in the eye of the beholder when special interests are at stake. If food industry executives follow the example of tobacco executives, they will always answer "no" to the addiction theory regardless of the evidence. On the other hand, a recovering food addict or food addiction professional will answer "yes" because of their clinical observations of refined food addiction, particularly a withdrawal syndrome and progressive use.

However, there are scientific standards for the evaluation of the evidence for refined food addiction as a factor in the obesity epidemic as discussed in the following text.

Evaluation of the Evidence for Refined Food Addiction

In the history of tobacco, a pivotal point occurred in 1964 when a group of scientists evaluated the evidence for a causal association between tobacco and lung cancer. They found enough evidence to support the Surgeon General's warning that smoking is hazardous (Brandt 2007). The five criteria used to determine that the association exists between tobacco and cancer were consistency, strength, specificity, temporal relationship, and logic. For our purposes, we use the five criteria to evaluate two associations: (a) Is addiction pathology, specifically heightened reward sensitivity and cravings, a factor in the epidemic of overeating/obesity? and (b) are refined foods the substances of abuse used in the addiction?

Consistency of the Association

"Comparable results are found utilizing a wide range of methods and data" (Brandt 2007). Section 4.3 describes a wide range of methods and data related to how overeating resembles drug addiction. There is a consistent association between aspects of drug abuse and overeating ranging from gene anomalies, to pleasure and signaling neurotransmitters, to patterns of consequence, behavior, diagnostic criteria, a fetal syndrome, and family dynamics, as well as macroelements of epidemiological patterns, business practices, a cost to society, and government subsidies. The evidence seems to show that addictive properties in overeating are present using a wide range of methods and data.

Two key elements of the neuro-pathology of addiction warrant closer attention. These are the increase in reward sensitivity and cravings leading to overeating, and reduced cognitive ability during cravings. Increased reward sensitivity in cravings and overeating has been found using seven different methods: MRI research demonstrates increased sensitivity and cravings in association with overeating (Beaver et al. 2006; Stice et al. 2011); dopamine agonists affect reward sensitivity (Blum et al. 2009); craving questionnaires associate cravings with overeating (Franken and Muris 2005; Davis et al. 2007); reward questionnaires associate reward sensitivity with overeating (Loxton and Dawe 2006); calorie intake during a taste test (monotonous vs. varied food) showed that increased reward correlates with increased overeating (Guerrieri et al. 2008); genetic anomalies associated with obesity correlate with a higher reward sensitivity in a questionnaire study (Lee et al. 2007); and cueing research shows the persistence of reward sensitivity in lever pressing by rats to sugar cues after abstinence (Panlilio et al. 1998).

Evidence for impaired cognitive ability during anticipation of food has been observed using two distinct methods. Positron emission tomography demonstrated that *during exposure to the reinforcer or to conditioned cues, the expected reward (processed by memory circuits) overactivates the reward and motivation circuits while inhibiting the cognitive control circuit, resulting in an inability to inhibit the drive to consume the drug or food despite attempts to do so* (Volkow et al. 2008). The second method demonstrating impaired cognitive control used a cognitive task: *simple reaction time (experiment 1) and an established measure of working memory capacity, the operation span task (experiment 2).* In this experiment, chocolate cravers had diminished ability to perform in the presence of chocolate without consuming it (Kemps et al. 2008).

Is there also consistency in the association between refined foods and addiction? The foods that elicit heightened reward responses in the brain are consistent across a range of research methods including animal behavior, animal neurotransmitter releases, substitution of foods for drugs, overlapping neurocircuits, similar responses to receptor agonists, human brain imaging, and human questionnaires. In this research, foods associated with addictive behavior and activation of addictive responses in the brain include chocolate, French fries, chocolate milkshakes, salt, palatable foods, hedonic foods, breakfast cereal (e.g., Froot Loops), snacks (e.g., Cheetohs), sweet baked goods, dairy products, processed fats, flour, and pizza. Bland foods and tasteless solutions do not provoke these responses, and study participants do not report cravings for or overuse of unrefined foods, such as fruits and vegetables, nor animal products, such as fish, poultry, and red meats.

Further, the foods showing the greatest increase in use in national consumption statistics are also foods that activate pathological reward responses. These include sweeteners, flour, processed fat, French fries, and high-fat dairy products (Ifland et al. 2009). The foods listed in Section 4.3 as having psychoactive properties are also the foods mentioned by overeaters as eliciting cravings. Finally, food addiction 12-step groups have observed clinically that eliminating sweeteners, flour, excessive salt, processed fats, and caffeine relieves cravings and precedes normal eating (Food Addicts Anonymous 2010).

Thus, the evidence appears to show that refined foods are associated with symptoms of addiction, including cravings and overuse across a wide range of methods and data, and thus supports the criterion of consistency.

Strength of the Association

"The cause and effect has a dose response, the greater the exposure, the more likely the effect" (Brandt 2007). This criterion can be translated into the proposition that greater exposure to food cues and refined foods results in greater neural reward sensitivity (the neurological pathology of addictions), whose consequences include greater overeating and obesity. Neurologically, studies show that exposure to food advertising, imagination, anticipation, and even just thoughts cause addiction-type reward and craving reactions. Research also indicates that there is a dose response to the amount of reactivity in the brain as measured by reward neurotransmitter release by the degree of overeating. Stated a different way, the greater the cueing, the greater the neurological response. Research also supports cause-and-effect of the greater the craving, the greater the overeating and the higher the BMI (Beaver et al. 2006; Stoeckel et al. 2008, 2009; Schienle et al. 2009; Burger and Stice 2011).

The strength of the association between refined foods, refined food cues, and greater overeating/obesity also bears examination. A study of chocolate cues and cravings noted that the greater the cravings, the greater the consumption of chocolate (Tuomisto et al. 1999). National statistics also indicate a strong association between consumption of refined foods and national weight gain (Popkin and Nielsen 2003; Bray et al. 2004; Ifland et al. 2009). Additionally, a survey of Australian households found that the greater the consumption of sweetened beverages, the greater the incidence of childhood obesity (Sanigorski et al. 2007).

Further, a number of studies suggest specific causes and effects: More visits to fast-food restaurants are associated with more overweight persons (Nelson et al. 2006); more television watching and exposure to television food advertising is associated with being overweight (Wiecha et al. 2006b); the greater the number of fast-food outlets per square mile, the greater the number of obese residents (Maddock 2004); the greater the ratio of fast food and convenience stores to grocery and specialty stores, the greater the incidence of obesity (Spence et al. 2009); the closer convenience stores are to high schools, the greater the obesity in ninth graders (Howard et al. 2011); and the closer schools are to fast food, the greater the incidence of obesity (Davis et al. 2007; Davis and Carpenter 2009).

Specificity of Association

"The effect is typically and powerfully associated with the cause. (90% of all lung cancers were found to occur among smokers.)" (Brandt 2007). The supposition that addictive mechanisms are typically and powerfully associated with overeating and obesity appears to be the case in a number of research methods. For example, the addiction gene anomaly is found in obese and not lean populations (Noble et al. 1994); research consistently finds greater reward sensitivity to food cues in higher BMI, not lower BMI populations (Burton et al. 2007); the addictive personality syndrome is found to be more prevalent in obese than lean people (Barry et al. 2009); the fetal syndrome is found in babies born of obese but not normally weighted mothers (Queisser-Luft et al. 1998); more severe food addiction behavior correlates with higher BMI (Gearhardt et al. 2011); a craving and withdrawal syndrome is found in obese but not lean rats (Pickering et al. 2009); obese 5–7 year olds but not lean children eat more in response to food commercials but not nonfood commercials (Halford et al. 2007); and even overfed, thin people respond more to photographs of hedonic than nonhedonic foods in MRI research (Cornier et al. 2007).

There is additional evidence in national consumption statistics that refined foods are typically and powerfully associated with overeating. Americans eat on average 1 lb per person per day of sweeteners, flour, processed fat, French fries, and high-fat dairy products but not fruits and vegetables (Putnam and Allshouse 1999). In addition, other studies support this type of association: Refined food overconsumption and underconsumption of fruits and vegetables correlate with obesity (Kayrooz et al. 1998; Krzyszycha and Szponar 2009); neighborhoods with greater numbers of fast-food outlets and convenience stores than sources of fresh fruits and vegetables have greater rates of obesity (Spence et al. 2009); and schools serving French fries and desserts more often have a greater percent of obese students (Fox et al. 2009). Moreover, sweetened beverages are associated with higher BMI (Hu and Malik 2010), especially those containing fructose (Stanhope et al. 2009). Last, MRI research demonstrates that chocolate cake, pizza, and chocolate milkshakes activate reward pathways in contrast to bland foods and tasteless solutions (Pelchat et al. 2004; Beaver et al. 2006; Guerrieri et al. 2008; Stice et al. 2008).

Temporal Relationship of Associated Variables

"The cause must precede the effect. For the smoking population, this meant that cancer appeared after people started to smoke" (Brandt 2007). Temporal relationships in refined food addiction range from less than seconds for brain dopamine in rats to respond to a cue for sugar (Roitman et al. 2004) to decades for the development of consequential disease states such as diabetes and heart disease. Research indicates that refined food cues precede activation of reward pathways in the brain in rats (Schroeder et al. 2001), especially after repeated overeating of palatable foods and exposure to cues (Volkow et al. 2008), and activation of these reward pathways in the brain precedes overeating (Stice et al. 2011).

Does exposure to refined food cueing and consumption of refined foods precede the development of obesity? This sequence of proposed cause and effect is apparent in the number of refined food advertisements shown to children during Saturday morning hours in which researchers counted refined food advertisements of 160 in 1987, 264 in 1992, and 564 in 1994 (Nestle 2002, p. 181). During the same period of time, childhood obesity doubled to 11% (Dehghan et al. 2005).

The availability of refined foods also seems to precede the development of obesity. Thus, one study indicated that an increase in visits to fast-food outlets coincided with increases in BMI 3 years later (Duffey et al. 2007). Bray also noted that increases in the consumption of HFCS (high-fructose corn syrup) preceded increases in obesity (Bray et al. 2004), and the density of food outlets around schools correlates with obesity at the schools (Fraser and Edwards 2010). The development of a variety of corn extracts precedes the obesity epidemic (BeMiller 2009). Other consumption trends show that significant increases in sweeteners, flour, French fries, processed fats, and caffeine are associated with the epidemic of obesity (Ifland et al. 2009).

Coherence of the Association

"There must be an overall logic to the cause-and-effect relationship. The 1964 Surgeon General's Report, for example, demonstrated that the epidemiological findings made sense in light of the animal experiments and knowledge of the pathology of cancer" (Brandt 2007).

The key for this criterion is to show that there is an overall logic to the cause-and-effect relationship between the pathology of addictive overeating and obesity and more importantly whether obesity epidemiological findings make sense in light of knowledge of heightened reward sensitivity, which causes cravings, which in turn lead to overeating. Another facet is whether it is logical that two sensitization mechanisms—exposure to increased cueing of refined foods and frequent use of refined foods—can heighten reward sensitivity and cravings as well as diminish cognitive ability to the point of being a significant factor in the obesity epidemic. The spread of fast food provides evidence for heightened reward sensitivity from these two sources.

In 1959, the total number of fast-food outlets (McDonald's) in the United States was over 100. By 1990, there were almost 21,822 hamburger/fast-food establishments (McDonald's, Burger King, and Wendy's) (http://www.globaled.org/curriculum/ffood4.html 2011). As shown in many studies, fast-food outlets are associated with obesity. Thus, it is logical that increases in fast-food advertising, availability of fast foods, and cheap prices would create more frequent anticipation, which has been shown to increase reward sensitivity (Stice et al. 2008). Repeated exposure to refined food cues, such as advertising images on television, billboards, and place-specific images (e.g., the Golden Arches and "The Colonel"), could also sensitize reward pathways and contribute to the development of refined food addiction. The introduction of value meals starting in 1988 contributed to increased energy intake (Ello-Martin et al. 2005). In 1997, McDonald's spent $66 million to promote a value meal (Mcdowell 1997) which would have increased visual cueing from advertising as well as increased availability by lowering price.

As to the role of refined foods, HFCS, caffeine, salt, flour, processed fats, and dairy products, especially high-fat dairy products, have all been shown to have addictive properties. When used together in "polysubstance" mode, addictive substances are synergistic in terms of addictive reactivity compared to the sum of single substances. For example, a hamburger/fast-food outlet might offer six addictive ingredients: sweetened (especially with HFCS), caffeinated beverages; fatty, salted potato products offered with sweetened catsup; wheat flour buns; and sweet, fatty sauces and cheese on fatty hamburgers. In a pizza outlet, all six ingredients are also present. Sweetened, caffeinated beverages are offered along with pizza, which contains wheat flour, processed fat, salt, and cheese. Similarly, doughnut and coffee outlets offer caffeinated coffee with cream and sugar along with pastries of wheat flour, sugar, salt, and processed fats. Fried chicken contains fat, salt, and flour; biscuits contain flour, salt, milk, and sugar; and the beverage contains caffeine and HFCS. Finally, popular ice cream stores often offer all six ingredients in ice cream cones and cakes. A thoughtful perusal of convenience stores reveals that almost all food products offered contain combinations of these six ingredients, as well as alcohol in some cases.

It is logical to think that compounded cueing in fast-food environments reinforces the development of heightened reward sensitivity and cravings. Choices, smells, bright colors, and distractions, such as clowns, toys, and playgrounds, are all factors in the development of heightened and persistent reward sensitivity, addiction, and overeating. Thus, it seems logical that the growth of fast-food outlets could have supported the development of heightened reward sensitivity and refined food addiction as a factor in the growth of obesity in the 1980s.

In addition to fast food, in the mid-1980s, the tobacco company, Philip Morris, bought Kraft Foods and General Foods, and RJ Reynolds bought Nabisco. The tobacco companies had researchers who were expert at enhancing the addictive properties of cigarettes by adding back nicotine, advertising heavily in general but especially to youngsters, and making cigarettes widely and cheaply available to encourage repeated use, all of which contribute to heightened cravings and the establishment of the addiction (Brandt 2007).

To increase sales, it is logical that tobacco companies would have instilled addictive practices in their acquired food companies to enhance reward sensitivity through repeated exposure to photographs of food through advertising, especially to children. Indeed, the sharp increase in Saturday morning sugary, fatty-food television commercials in the early 1990s would logically be the result of tobacco marketing practices extended to refined foods. The commercials, plus repeated exposure to the use of polysubstance formulations of sugary breakfast cereals and milk, sweetened fruit juices, and flour products, such as toaster snacks, (e.g., Pop Tarts, Waffles), syrup, donuts, and pancakes, would logically heighten reward sensitivity, cravings, and addictive overeating.

As discussed in Section 4.3, reward sensitivities are also heightened in multiple-cued environments. Grocery stores might be considered to be a multicued environment. During the years when tobacco companies owned refined food manufacturers, grocery stores increased their square footage and stayed open 24 hours per day. Bright lights and colorful packaging became prominent along with smells of baking, frying, and coffee brewing. In addition, other cues often present in grocery stores are tastes of free samples, party music, announcements of urgent specials, and lots of choices. There may also be reward sensitization in the form of anticipation from clipping coupons or reading about specials before the visit. In consequence, it is not unreasonable to suggest that the compounding of sight, smell, sound, taste, and anticipation cues increased reward sensitization and cravings, which lead to overeating.

The presence of crop subsidies for corn, wheat, and sugar also implies that the price of refined foods that are composed of these ingredients could be low enough that most people in the United States could afford to buy refined foods frequently enough to increase reward sensitivities.

In summary, these food industry business practices taken together might be effective enough through the pathological process of increasing exposure to food cues to increase sensitivity of responses and corresponding cravings, which lead to overeating and obesity.

At the same time, there is also evidence for a decreased ability to resist overuse of food: *naturally occurring leptin resistance allowed temporary neutralization of satiety mechanisms and evolved as a response to survive subsequent periods of famine. With today's continuous and abundant food availability for a segment of the population, the powerful cognitive processes to eat and the resulting overweight condition can partially escape negative feedback control* (Berthoud 2007). There is also evidence of impaired cognitive ability that might reasonably contribute to the inability of the individual to think through an overwhelming craving and decide not to use the refined food (Kemps et al. 2008; Volkow et al. 2008).

The foregoing evidence suggests that the association of an addictive mechanism with overeating has been demonstrated according to the 1964 criteria used to determine that an association exists between tobacco and cancer. Also, the association of refined foods with the addictive mechanism has been demonstrated according to these criteria.

BEYOND REASONABLE DOUBT

In 1964, the Surgeon General's study committee found that "The sum total of scientific evidence establishes beyond reasonable doubt that cigarette smoking is a causative factor in the rapidly increasing incidence of human epidermoid carcinoma of the lung" (Brandt 2007). In light of the evidence presented earlier, while we may not be at the point that we can state beyond a reasonable doubt that addictive mechanisms related to refined foods are a causative factor in the rapidly increasing incidence of human obesity, the evidence is extensive and growing. What may be plausibly stated, is that Americans, and especially American children, have been exposed to intense refined food cueing and interactions with fast-food chains and refined food manufacturers since the beginning of the 1980s and that this is associated with an epidemic of pathological reward sensitivity, cravings, and overeating.

As a corollary, the 1964 Surgeon General's committee also found that "The evidence of a cause-effect relationship is adequate for consideration of initiation of public health measures" (Brandt 2007). General acceptance of an addictive mechanism as an explanation for overeating might seem to bring a degree of relief and closure to the mystery surrounding the self-destructive behavior of overeating. However, the history of the United States' struggle to contain the tobacco industry suggests that containing refined food addiction will be difficult. Short of public policy changes, a senior official at the National Institute of Drug Addiction argues that there is enough evidence to support a diagnosis of food addiction in the DSM published by the APA (Frascella et al. 2010).

LIMITATIONS

This chapter is about the evidence for food addiction and is not a critical analysis of all of the literature. Thus, a limitation of this chapter is that it does not explore or attempt to explain the implications of the inconsistencies between drug addiction and overeating nor inconsistencies between the majority of research results and exceptions. Examples of the former include the role of peripheral signaling in response to food and food cues that does not exist in drug signaling (Blumenthal and Gold 2010) and the finding of diminishing reward sensitivity in moderate and extreme obesity (Davis and Fox 2008). The latter includes a study that did not find a correlation between proximity of fast food and obesity in a high school (Crawford et al. 2008) and a study which found that dairy contributes to weight loss (Dougkas et al. 2011). Although an examination of these anomalies could well contribute to our understanding of refined food addiction, they are beyond the scope of this chapter.

FUTURE RESEARCH

Due to the advent of neuroimaging, addiction research has undergone a transformation which impacts the degree and type of research required for an addiction diagnosis to be included in the DSM published by the American Psychiatric Association (APA 2000). As an indication of how far addiction diagnoses have advanced, in 1964, cigarettes were not thought to be addictive for the sole reason that smokers were not socially deviant (Brandt 2007). The science of diagnosing addictions is not straightforward as can been seen in the volumes published by the APA that describe the evidence considered in task force decisions made for and against including substance dependence diagnoses in the DSM (APA 1997).

Historically, evaluation of proposed addiction diagnoses was helped by findings of behaviors that conform to the seven DSM-IV addiction criteria, particularly progression and withdrawal syndromes. For example, conformance of caffeine use to DSM-IV criteria was researched by a telephone survey (Hughes et al. 1998). Establishment of a withdrawal syndrome was considered to be important to the study of opium and cannabis addiction (Wesson and Ling 2003; Budney et al. 2004).

The finding of the psychotropic element in the substance such as nicotine in cigarettes was also thought to help prove the addictive nature of smoking (Brandt 2007).

However, with the experience of over 20 years of neuroimaging research, several prominent addiction researchers have argued that the key evidence in the finding of an addiction has become activation of the addictive pathways in the brain. For example, Mark Gold, president *emeritus* of the American Society of Addiction Medicine, writes, "Work presented in this review strongly supports the notion that food addiction is a real phenomenon" (Blumenthal and Gold 2010). Joseph Frascella, Deputy Director of the National Institute of Drug Abuse, writes, "For more than half a century, since the beginning of formal diagnostics, our psychiatric nosology has compartmentalized the compulsive pursuit of substance (e.g., alcohol, cocaine, heroin, nicotine) from nonsubstance (e.g., gambling, food, sex) rewards. Emerging brain, behavioral, and genetic findings challenge this diagnostic boundary, pointing to shared vulnerabilities underlying the pathological pursuit of substance and nonsubstance rewards" (Frascella et al. 2010).

Arguments for the existence of food addiction do not depend on the neurological research alone. Rather, they are discussed in the context of corroborating evidence of the nature presented in this chapter. However, evidence from neuroimaging research may strengthen the plausibility of the existence of refined food addiction. As such, it may somewhat diminish the need for classic addiction research that has historically supported addiction diagnoses.

The availability of strong neuroimaging evidence brings into question the need for traditional complicated, time-consuming, and expensive research for the establishment of a finding of refined food addiction, especially a withdrawal syndrome. The first challenge in researching a withdrawal syndrome for refined foods would be establishing baseline conditions in "sober" study subjects. Study subjects would need to be "sober" from a broad range of refined foods including at least sugars and sweeteners, flour, salt, processed fats, dairy, and caffeine. Other suspect foods might also need to be eliminated. For example, foods often recommended for elimination by food addiction recovery groups, 12-step groups, also include dried fruit, nuts, olives, popcorn, and grits. Each of these substances would need to be reintroduced alone for a period of time and then withheld to examine withdrawal from that substance alone. The course of symptomology would then need to be recorded. The procedures would need to be conducted for a long period of time in large populations in controlled environments that would exclude exposure to confounding, destabilizing food cues such as food advertising.

In classic terms, refined food withdrawal research is further complicated by the polysubstance nature of refined food use. Refined food products are typically sold and used in combinations (coffee with cream and sugar and a doughnut; and taco with salt, cheese, corn flour and fatty tortilla, consumed with caffeinated sweetened soft drink). This suggests that each combination would need to be reintroduced to "sober" study subjects to generate practical knowledge about withdrawal from common commercial food products. Ideally, this research would take place at several sites for corroboration.

In summary, the question of needed research is in transition in the field of addictions in general. As the field progresses, it is to be hoped that the need for and nature of refined food addiction research will be clarified.

CONCLUSION

The evidence for overeating as refined food addiction is broad and consistently supportive of the concept. Similarities between overeating and drug abuse include neural disease mechanisms, behavior syndromes, conformance with addiction diagnostic criteria, the presence of psychotropic elements in refined foods, family patterns, and the presence of macroforces such as crop subsidies, epidemiological patterns, and corporate business practices in both refined foods and tobacco.

The evidence for an addictive mechanism related to refined foods as a significant factor in the obesity epidemic seems to meet the criteria used in determining a cause-and-effect relation between tobacco and smoking. The evidence is consistent across many types of research. It is specific insofar as the pathology occurs in obese but not in normal weight individuals and dose-dependent as more cueing results in more craving and overeating. It is also temporal as both cues and use precede heightened sensitivity, which precedes overeating, and as the appearance of fast-food and addiction-type business practices by refined food manufactures has preceded the obesity epidemic. It is logical that in light of reward and craving research, the presence of refined food cues and availability could result in an epidemic of overeating and obesity.

Given the severity of consequences, it would seem prudent to err on the side of relatively more aggressive approaches to protect vulnerable populations such as children, the elderly, the undereducated, the chronically obese, and the mentally ill from refined food cueing and use. For the individual, the family, and society as a whole, firm policy approaches to protect them from tobacco-style business practices related to refined food and refined food cueing would seem to be substantiated and warranted.

One episode in epidemiological history that might help inform treatment and policy decisions is the Broad Street pump decision made during the cholera epidemic in London in 1854. While the Broad Street pump produced popular water, a survey of the locations of cholera deaths found that the pump was at the epicenter of the epidemic. Based on this evidence, the local health council made the courageous but unpopular decision to take the handle off of the pump. Similarly, our public health officials and treatment professionals could make courageous decisions to protect the public from refined foods through implementation of tobacco-style public policies and abstinence treatment protocols.

Further research will provide evidence to confirm and continue the debate. In the meantime, vigorous discussion and education are needed. Popular information channels, such as Internet educational sites and social media sites, as well as messages about the dangers of refined foods and techniques for achieving abstinence delivered by 12-step groups may offer hope for educating people who suffer from overeating.

REFERENCES

American Psychiatric Association (1997). *DSM-IV Sourcebook*. Washington, DC, American Psychiatric Association.

American Psychiatric Association (2000). *Diagnostic and Statistical Manual of Mental Disorders Fourth Edition Text Revision (DSM-IV-TR)*. Washington, DC, American Psychiatric Association.

Anderson, P. (2009). Is it time to ban alcohol advertising? *Clin Med* **9**(2): 121–124.

Armitage, J. A., P. D. Taylor et al. (2005). Experimental models of developmental programming: Consequences of exposure to an energy rich diet during development. *J Physiol* **565**(Pt 1): 3–8.

Avena, N. M., P. Rada et al. (2008). Evidence for sugar addiction: Behavioral and neurochemical effects of intermittent, excessive sugar intake. *Neurosci Biobehav Rev* **32**(1): 20–39.

Ayyad, C. and T. Andersen (2000). Long-term efficacy of dietary treatment of obesity: A systematic review of studies published between 1931 and 1999. *Obes Rev* **1**(2): 113–119.

Barry, D., M. Clarke et al. (2009). Obesity and its relationship to addictions: Is overeating a form of addictive behavior? *Am J Addict* **18**(6): 439–451.

Batterink, L., S. Yokum et al. (2010). Body mass correlates inversely with inhibitory control in response to food among adolescent girls: An fMRI study. *Neuroimage* **52**(4): 1696–1703.

Bayol, S. A., S. J. Farrington et al. (2007). A maternal 'junk food' diet in pregnancy and lactation promotes an exacerbated taste for 'junk food' and a greater propensity for obesity in rat offspring. *Br J Nutr* **98**(4): 843–851.

Bayol, S. A., B. H. Simbi et al. (2010). A maternal "junk food" diet in pregnancy and lactation promotes nonalcoholic fatty liver disease in rat offspring. *Endocrinology* **151**(4): 1451–1461.

Beaver, J. D., A. D. Lawrence et al. (2006). Individual differences in reward drive predict neural responses to images of food. *J Neurosci* **26**(19): 5160–5166.

BeMiller, J. N. (2009). One hundred years of commercial food carbohydrates in the United States. *J Agric Food Chem* **57**(18): 8125–8129.

Berner, L. A., N. M. Avena et al. (2008). Bingeing, self-restriction, and increased body weight in rats with limited access to a sweet-fat diet. *Obesity (Silver Spring)* **16**(9): 1998–2002.

Berthoud, H. R. (2007). Interactions between the "cognitive" and "metabolic" brain in the control of food intake. *Physiol Behav* **91**(5): 486–498.

Blass, E. M., D. J. Shide et al. (1989). Stress-reducing effects of ingesting milk, sugars, and fats. A developmental perspective. *Ann N Y Acad Sci* **575**: 292–305; discussion 305–296.

Blum, K., E. R. Braverman et al. (1996). Increased prevalence of the Taq I A1 allele of the dopamine receptor gene (DRD2) in obesity with comorbid substance use disorder: A preliminary report. *Pharmacogenetics* **6**(4): 297–305.

Blum, K., T. J. Chen et al. (2009). Neurogenetics of dopaminergic receptor supersensitivity in activation of brain reward circuitry and relapse: Proposing "deprivation-amplification relapse therapy" (DART). *Postgrad Med* **121**(6): 176–196.

Blumenthal, D. M. and M. S. Gold (2010). Neurobiology of food addiction. *Curr Opin Clin Nutr Metab Care* **13**(4): 359–365.

Brandt, A. (2007). *The Cigarette Century: The Rise, Fall, and Deadly Persistence for the Product That Defined America*. New York, Basic Books.

Bray, G. A., S. J. Nielsen et al. (2004). Consumption of high-fructose corn syrup in beverages may play a role in the epidemic of obesity. *Am J Clin Nutr* **79**(4): 537–543.

Brownell, K. D. and K. E. Warner (2009). The perils of ignoring history: Big Tobacco played dirty and millions died. How similar is Big Food? *Milbank Q* **87**(1): 259–294.

Bruinsma, K. and D. L. Taren (1999). Chocolate: Food or drug? *J Am Diet Assoc* **99**(10): 1249–1256.

Budney, A. J., J. R. Hughes et al. (2004). Review of the validity and significance of cannabis withdrawal syndrome. *Am J Psychiatry* **161**(11): 1967–1977.

Burger, K. S. and E. Stice (2011). Relation of dietary restraint scores to activation of reward-related brain regions in response to food intake, anticipated intake, and food pictures. *Neuroimage* **55**(1): 233–239.

Burton, P., H. J. Smit et al. (2007). The influence of restrained and external eating patterns on overeating. *Appetite* **49**(1): 191–197.

Caetano, R. and C. L. Clark (1998). Trends in alcohol consumption patterns among whites, blacks and Hispanics: 1984 and 1995. *J Stud Alcohol* **59**(6): 659–668.

Cassin, S. E. and K. M. von Ranson (2007). Is binge eating experienced as an addiction? *Appetite* **49**(3): 687–690.

Cocores, J. A. and M. S. Gold (2009). The salted food addiction hypothesis may explain overeating and the obesity epidemic. *Med Hypotheses* **73**(6): 892–899.

Cornier, M. A., S. S. Von Kaenel et al. (2007). Effects of overfeeding on the neuronal response to visual food cues. *Am J Clin Nutr* **86**(4): 965–971.

Corwin, R. L. and P. S. Grigson (2009). Symposium overview—Food addiction: Fact or fiction? *J Nutr* **139**(3): 617–619.

Cota, D., M. H. Tschop et al. (2006). Cannabinoids, opioids and eating behavior: The molecular face of hedonism? *Brain Res Rev* **51**(1): 85–107.

Crawford, D. A., A. F. Timperio et al. (2008). Neighbourhood fast food outlets and obesity in children and adults: The CLAN Study. *Int J Pediatr Obes* **3**(4): 249–256.

Davis, B. and C. Carpenter (2009). Proximity of fast-food restaurants to schools and adolescent obesity. *Am J Public Health* **99**(3): 505–510.

Davis, C., C. Curtis et al. (2007). Psychological factors associated with ratings of portion size: Relevance to the risk profile for obesity. *Eat Behav* **8**(2): 170–176.

Davis, C. and J. Fox (2008). Sensitivity to reward and body mass index (BMI): Evidence for a non-linear relationship. *Appetite* **50**(1): 43–49.

Day, P. L. and J. Pearce (2011). Obesity-promoting food environments and the spatial clustering of food outlets around schools. *Am J Prev Med* **40**(2): 113–121.

Dehghan, M., N. Akhtar-Danesh et al. (2005). Childhood obesity, prevalence and prevention. *Nutr J* **4**: 24.

DiPatrizio, N. V. and K. J. Simansky (2008). Activating parabrachial cannabinoid CB1 receptors selectively stimulates feeding of palatable foods in rats. *J Neurosci* **28**(39): 9702–9709.

Dougkas, A., C. K. Reynolds et al. (2011). Associations between dairy consumption and body weight: A review of the evidence and underlying mechanisms. *Nutr Res Rev*: 1–24.

Duffey, K. J., P. Gordon-Larsen et al. (2007). Differential associations of fast food and restaurant food consumption with 3-y change in body mass index: The Coronary Artery Risk Development in Young Adults Study. *Am J Clin Nutr* **85**(1): 201–208.

Ellis, D. A., R. A. Zucker et al. (1997). The role of family influences in development and risk. *Alcohol Health Res World* **21**(3): 218–226.

Ello-Martin, J. A., J. H. Ledikwe et al. (2005). The influence of food portion size and energy density on energy intake: Implications for weight management. *Am J Clin Nutr* **82**(1 Suppl): 236S–241S.

Epstein, L. H. and J. J. Leddy (2006). Food reinforcement. *Appetite* **46**(1): 22–25.

Esch, T. and G. B. Stefano (2004). The neurobiology of pleasure, reward processes, addiction and their health implications. *Neuro Endocrinol Lett* **25**(4): 235–251.

Fanciulli, G., A. Dettori et al. (2005). Gluten exorphin B5 stimulates prolactin secretion through opioid receptors located outside the blood-brain barrier. *Life Sci* **76**(15): 1713–1719.

Filbey, F. M., E. D. Claus et al. (2011). Dopaminergic genes modulate response inhibition in alcohol abusing adults. *Addict Biol*. doi: 10.1111j. 1369–1600.

Food Addicts Anonymous (2010). Welcome newcomers to food addicts anonymous (FAA). Food Addicts Anonymous, Port St. Lucie, FL, Food Addicts Anonymous World Service Office.

Fox, M. K., A. H. Dodd et al. (2009). Association between school food environment and practices and body mass index of US public school children. *J Am Diet Assoc* **109**(2 Suppl): S108–S117.

Franken, I. H. and P. Muris (2005). Individual differences in reward sensitivity are related to food craving and relative body weight in healthy women. *Appetite* **45**(2): 198–201.

Frascella, J., M. N. Potenza et al. (2010). Shared brain vulnerabilities open the way for nonsubstance addictions: Carving addiction at a new joint? *Ann N Y Acad Sci* **1187**: 294–315.

Fraser, L. K. and K. L. Edwards (2010). The association between the geography of fast food outlets and childhood obesity rates in Leeds, UK. *Health Place* **16**(6): 1124–1128.

Gearhardt, A. N. and W. R. Corbin (2009). Body mass index and alcohol consumption: Family history of alcoholism as a moderator. *Psychol Addict Behav* **23**(2): 216–225.

Gearhardt, A. N., S. Yokum et al. (2011). Neural correlates of food addiction. *Arch Gen Psychiatry* **68**(8): 808–816.

Giovino, G. A., J. E. Henningfield et al. (1995). Epidemiology of tobacco use and dependence. *Epidemiol Rev* **17**(1): 48–65.

Glynn, T., J. R. Seffrin et al. (2010). The globalization of tobacco use: 21 challenges for the 21st century. *CA Cancer J Clin* **60**(1): 50–61.

Grimm, J. W., A. M. Fyall et al. (2005). Incubation of sucrose craving: Effects of reduced training and sucrose pre-loading. *Physiol Behav* **84**(1): 73–79.

Grimm, J. W., Y. Shaham et al. (2002). Effect of cocaine and sucrose withdrawal period on extinction behavior, cue-induced reinstatement, and protein levels of the dopamine transporter and tyrosine hydroxylase in limbic and cortical areas in rats. *Behav Pharmacol* **13**(5–6): 379–388.

Guerrieri, R., C. Nederkoorn et al. (2008). The interaction between impulsivity and a varied food environment: Its influence on food intake and overweight. *Int J Obes (Lond)* **32**(4): 708–714.

Halford, J. C., E. J. Boyland et al. (2007). Beyond-brand effect of television (TV) food advertisements/commercials on caloric intake and food choice of 5–7-year-old children. *Appetite* **49**(1): 263–267.

Harper, T. A. and G. Mooney (2010). Prevention before profits: A levy on food and alcohol advertising. *Med J Aust* **192**(7): 400–402.

Harwood, H. J., D. Fountain et al. (1998). Economic costs of alcohol abuse and alcoholism. *Recent Dev Alcohol* **14**: 307–330.

Hetherington, M., Ed. (2001). *Food Cravings and Addiction*. Leatherhead, Surrey, U.K., Leatherhead Food Research Association.

Hetherington, M. M. (2007). Cues to overeat: Psychological factors influencing overconsumption. *Proc Nutr Soc* **66**(1): 113–123.

Hodgkins, C. C., K. S. Cahill et al. (2004). Adolescent drug addiction treatment and weight gain. *J Addict Dis* **23**(3): 55–65.

Holland, P. C. and G. D. Petrovich (2005). A neural systems analysis of the potentiation of feeding by conditioned stimuli. *Physiol Behav* **86**(5): 747–761.

Howard, P. H., M. Fitzpatrick et al. (2011). Proximity of food retailers to schools and rates of overweight ninth grade students: An ecological study in California. *BMC Public Health* **11**(1): 68.

http://www.globaled.org/curriculum/ffood4.html (2011), accessed on February 16, 2012. Handout #4: Mcfast-food Conquers America, *Global Perspective on Fast-Food History*. The American Forum for Global Education.

Hu, F. B. and V. S. Malik (2010). Sugar-sweetened beverages and risk of obesity and type 2 diabetes: Epidemiologic evidence. *Physiol Behav* **100**(1): 47–54.

Hughes, J. R., A. H. Oliveto et al. (1992). Should caffeine abuse, dependence, or withdrawal be added to DSM-IV and ICD-10? *Am J Psychiatry* **149**(1): 33–40.

Hughes, J. R., A. H. Oliveto et al. (1998). Endorsement of DSM-IV dependence criteria among caffeine users. *Drug Alcohol Depend* **52**(2): 99–107.

Ifland, J. R., H. G. Preuss et al. (2009). Refined food addiction: A classic substance use disorder. *Med Hypotheses* **72**(5): 518–526.

Ifland, J., K. Sheppard et al. (2012). From the front lines: The impact of refined food addiction on the individual. *Food and Addiction*, K. Brownell and M. Gold (eds.), Oxford University Press (in press).

Islam, A. K. and R. J. Bodnar (1990). Selective opioid receptor antagonist effects upon intake of a high-fat diet in rats. *Brain Res* **508**(2): 293–296.

Kalra, S. P. and P. S. Kalra (2004). Overlapping and interactive pathways regulating appetite and craving. *J Addict Dis* **23**(3): 5–21.

Kampov-Polevoy, A. B., J. C. Garbutt et al. (2003). Family history of alcoholism and response to sweets. *Alcohol Clin Exp Res* **27**(11): 1743–1749.

Kayrooz, K., T. F. Moy et al. (1998). Dietary fat patterns in urban African American women. *J Community Health* **23**(6): 453–469.

Kelley, A. E., C. A. Schiltz et al. (2005). Neural systems recruited by drug- and food-related cues: Studies of gene activation in corticolimbic regions. *Physiol Behav* **86**(1–2): 11–14.

Kemps, E., M. Tiggemann et al. (2008). Food cravings consume limited cognitive resources. *J Exp Psychol Appl* **14**(3): 247–254.

Kendzor, D. E., L. E. Baillie et al. (2008). The effect of food deprivation on cigarette smoking in females. *Addict Behav* **33**(10): 1353–1359.

Kleiner, K. D., M. S. Gold et al. (2004). Body mass index and alcohol use. *J Addict Dis* **23**(3): 105–118.

Krahnstoever Davison, K., L. A. Francis et al. (2005). Reexamining obesigenic families: Parents' obesity-related behaviors predict girls' change in BMI. *Obes Res* **13**(11): 1980–1990.

Krzyszycha, R. and B. Szponar (2009). Body mass index (BMI) and dietary preferences of women living in rural areas. *Rocz Panstw Zakl Hig* **60**(1): 75–77.

Lee, S. H., B. J. Ham et al. (2007). Association study of dopamine receptor D2 TaqI A polymorphism and reward-related personality traits in healthy Korean young females. *Neuropsychobiology* **56**(2–3): 146–151.

Lenoir, M., F. Serre et al. (2007). Intense sweetness surpasses cocaine reward. *PLoS ONE* **2**(1): e698.

Leombruni, P., L. Lavagnino et al. (2009). Duloxetine in obese binge eater outpatients: Preliminary results from a 12-week open trial. *Hum Psychopharmacol* **24**(6): 483–488.

Lewin, A., L. Lindstrom et al. (2006). Food industry promises to address childhood obesity: Preliminary evaluation. *J Public Health Policy* **27**(4): 327–348.

Lim, J. S., M. Mietus-Snyder et al. (2010). The role of fructose in the pathogenesis of NAFLD and the metabolic syndrome. *Nat Rev Gastroenterol Hepatol* **7**(5): 251–264.

Liu, Y., K. M. von Deneen et al. (2010). Food addiction and obesity: Evidence from bench to bedside. *J Psychoactive Drugs* **42**(2): 133–145.

Loxton, N. J. and S. Dawe (2006). Reward and punishment sensitivity in dysfunctional eating and hazardous drinking women: Associations with family risk. *Appetite* **47**(3): 361–371.

Lu, L., J. W. Grimm et al. (2004). Incubation of cocaine craving after withdrawal: A review of preclinical data. *Neuropharmacology* **47**(Suppl 1): 214–226.

Lustig, R. H. (2010). Fructose: Metabolic, hedonic, and societal parallels with ethanol. *J Am Diet Assoc* **110**(9): 1307–1321.

Maddock, J. (2004). The relationship between obesity and the prevalence of fast food restaurants: State-level analysis. *Am J Health Promot* **19**(2): 137–143.

Mahar, A. and L. M. Duizer (2007). The effect of frequency of consumption of artificial sweeteners on sweetness liking by women. *J Food Sci* **72**(9): S714–S718.

Mattson, S. N., S. C. Roesch et al. (2010). Toward a neurobehavioral profile of fetal alcohol spectrum disorders. *Alcohol Clin Exp Res* **34**(9): 1640–1650.

McAuliffe, P. F., M. S. Gold et al. (2006). Second-hand exposure to aerosolized intravenous anesthetics propofol and fentanyl may cause sensitization and subsequent opiate addiction among anesthesiologists and surgeons. *Med Hypotheses* **66**(5): 874–882.

Mcdowell, B. (1997). McDonald's to feed value-price move with $66 mill in ads. In *Advertising Age*. New York, Crain Communications.

McIver, S., P. O'Halloran et al. (2009). Yoga as a treatment for binge eating disorder: A preliminary study. *Complement Ther Med* **17**(4): 196–202.

McLellan, A. T., H. Kushner et al. (1992). The fifth edition of the addiction severity index. *J Subst Abuse Treat* **9**(3): 199–213.

McNatt, S. S., J. J. Longhi et al. (2007). Surgery for obesity: A review of the current state of the art and future directions. *J Gastrointest Surg* **11**(3): 377–397.

Meisel, H. (1986). Chemical characterization and opioid activity of an exorphin isolated from in vivo digests of casein. *FEBS Lett* **196**(2): 223–227.

Mellor, J. M., C. B. Dolan et al. (2010). Child body mass index, obesity, and proximity to fast food restaurants. *Int J Pediatr Obes* **6**(1): 60–68.

Mennella, J. A., M. Y. Pepino et al. (2010). Sweet preferences and analgesia during childhood: Effects of family history of alcoholism and depression. *Addiction* **105**(4): 666–675.

Mercer, M. E. and M. D. Holder (1997). Food cravings, endogenous opioid peptides, and food intake: A review. *Appetite* **29**(3): 325–352.

Nelson, M. C., P. Gordon-Larsen et al. (2006). Body mass index gain, fast food, and physical activity: Effects of shared environments over time. *Obesity (Silver Spring)* **14**(4): 701–709.

Nestle, M. (1996). *Food Politics*. New York, Random House.

Nestle, M. (2002). *Food Politics*. Berkeley, CA, University of California Press.

Noble, E. P., R. E. Noble et al. (1994). D2 dopamine receptor gene and obesity. *Int J Eat Disord* **15**(3): 205–217.

Nseir, W., F. Nassar et al. (2010). Soft drinks consumption and nonalcoholic fatty liver disease. *World J Gastroenterol* **16**(21): 2579–2588.

Ogden, C. L., S. Z. Yanovski et al. (2007). The epidemiology of obesity. *Gastroenterology* **132**(6): 2087–2102.

Olszewski, P. K. and A. S. Levine (2007). Central opioids and consumption of sweet tastants: When reward outweighs homeostasis. *Physiol Behav* **91**(5): 506–512.

intrauterine growth followed by accelerated postnatal growth is referred to as "centile crossing" [24]. Recent evidence suggests that the age at which the rapid body weight increase occurs during postnatal life is a critical factor in the eventual health status of a person [23].

Estrogen and the Differentiation and Regulation of Adipose Tissue

Hormones are major regulators of adipose tissue and are critical for adipocyte development and function. An extensive array of hormones and growth factors modulate adipocyte development and activity, including growth hormone, thyroid hormone, catecholamines, glucagon, insulin and insulin-like growth factors, glucocorticoids, and, relevant to this discussion, estradiol and thus chemicals with estrogenic activity [18,33,34]. In humans, differentiation of preadipocytes into adipocytes begins prior to birth, but the majority of preadipocytes differentiate postnatally. Adipocyte number increases markedly between birth and 18 months of age, then continues to increase more slowly throughout early childhood [35]. The developmental sequence by which the adipocyte phenotype arises from undifferentiated connective tissue cells has been described in detail [36]. The adipocyte lineage arises from undifferentiated mesenchymal cells, which can also give rise to other connective tissue lineages. Mesenchymal cells become committed to an adipogenic lineage and give rise to preadipocytes, which can remain undifferentiated and quiescent, proliferate but remain undifferentiated, or differentiate as a postmitotic adipocyte [11].

While preadipocytes in mice do not begin to differentiate into adipocytes prior to birth [37], mouse preadipocytes develop from mesenchymal cells and proliferate during fetal life, and, as discussed further in the following section, they express estrogen receptors [15]. Mouse preadipocytes continue to proliferate rapidly at birth, but then the majority enters the differentiation pathway neonatally to give rise to postmitotic adipocytes. By approximately 3 weeks of age, the basic adult number of adipocytes has been established in most mouse strains [38]. A preadipocyte population still remains in adults and can give rise to new adipocytes at any time during life in both mice and humans [39].

The genes critical for inducing adipocyte differentiation, as well as their temporal sequence of expression during adipocyte differentiation, are being actively investigated [40]. For example, it is known that CCAAT/enhancer-binding proteins, such as C/EBPα, along with PPARγ play critical roles in adipocyte differentiation from the preadipocyte to the fully functional, postmitotic adipocyte [41] and that the transcription factor CREB plays an important role in regulating these genes [42]. In humans, C/EBPα mRNA levels in adipocyte tissue are elevated in those with an obese relative to lean phenotype [43]. PPARγ is expressed in adult adipocytes. PPARγ and C/EBPα are regulators of lipogenesis in addition to regulating adipocyte differentiation, and PPARγ activators result in increased fat deposition [41,42,44]. Although obesity typically involves adipocyte hypertrophy, adipocyte hyperplasia is also seen in certain types of human obesity, and similar results have been obtained in rodents with various types of obesity resulting from dietary modification or gene knockouts [36,38].

In abdominal fat, mitochondrial glycerol-3-phosphate acyltransferase (GPAT) catalyzes the initial step in glycerolipid synthesis [45]. Mice deficient in diglyceride acyltransferase (DGAT1) are resistant to diet-induced obesity and have increased insulin and leptin sensitivity [46]. The presence of the enzyme Cyp19 (aromatase) in adipocytes provides a source of intracellular estradiol via aromatization of testosterone, and aromatase activity in tissues is influenced by estrogen, including the estrogenic chemical bisphenol A (BPA) [47,48]. In aromatase knockout mice, an increase in adipocyte volume and number was observed [22,49]. Lipoprotein lipase (LPL) is a key enzyme in regulating lipids. Adipocytes express LPL, which attaches to the luminal surface of endothelial cells in capillaries. LPL binds lipid particles such as chylomicrons and very low-density lipoprotein (LDL) and breaks down the triglyceride core into free fatty acids. This step is rate limiting and necessary for formation of LDLs, high-density lipoproteins (HDLs), and free fatty acids from lipid particles. Free fatty acids can cross membranes into cells, while triglycerides cannot. As a result, LPL in capillaries of a tissue, including adipose tissue, is necessary for the uptake of lipid. Adipose tissue with a lower level of endothelial LPL will not uptake lipid as rapidly. LPL is subject to regulation by estrogen [49]. Estradiol was reported to markedly decrease the amounts of LPL mRNA as well as triglyceride accumulation in 3T3-L1 adipocytes [50].

A critical question to consider when postulating potential effects on adipocyte number and subsequent function generated during development is whether such effects would be permanent or transitory and reversible once the stimulus inducing the change in adipocyte is removed. In summary, the fetal period is a time in the mouse when changes in circulating estrogen (either exogenous or endogenous) could result in changes in adipose tissue function during later life, and changes in the methylation pattern of genes are one potential mechanism. This prediction is consistent with the evidence from other systems that exposure to sex hormones and estrogenic endocrine-disrupting chemicals during fetal life can have latent effects on the functioning of tissues after birth [33,51].

In recent years, the focus on obesity has involved the "big two" factors thought to be primarily responsible for the dramatic increase in obesity over the last two decades: reduced physical activity and overconsumption of "junk" food associated with food marketing practices [29]. However, it seems likely that environmental factors are also involved, and sorting out which factors are most important has not received much attention [7]. Thus, few epidemiological studies have examined the role of environmental estrogens in the human obesity epidemic [5,6], although data from studies with experimental animals as well as cell culture studies indicate that such studies are needed.

Estrogen is known to play an important role in regulating adipose deposition in males, and estrogen regulates key developmental events in adipogenesis [22]. Thus, while the factors regulating whether preadipocytes proliferate or differentiate are not well understood, estrogen appears to be one factor involved in their development. Adipose tissue expresses both ERα and ERβ. ERα is expressed in adipocytes, preadipocytes, and stromal vascular cells, indicating that almost all cells in adipose tissue are potentially estrogen responsive [52,53]. Estrogens appear to play a crucial role in establishment of adult adipocyte number, although effects of estrogens on adipose tissue are complex, and may vary with cell type. A number of papers have shown that estradiol increases proliferation in preconfluent 3T3-L1 preadipocyte cells or in human or rat preadipocytes *in vitro* [54–56]. Estradiol treatment of cultured preadipocytes induces increased release of mitogenic substances into the media [57]. Adipocyte hyperplasia is a particular problem because the increased adipocyte population appears to make it very difficult to ever overcome the obesity and maintain a normal weight. It is thus possible that during fetal life, exposure to estrogenic chemicals may facilitate a particularly intractable type of obesity, and this may occur via epigenetic "programming" of genes during "critical periods" in development, which results in permanent changes in gene activity [15].

ESTROGENIC CHEMICAL BPA AND OBESITY

BPA is one of the highest volume chemicals in worldwide production, with production capacity exceeding 6 billion pounds per year for use in manufacturing polycarbonate plastic, the resin that lines metal cans, and as an additive in many other types of plastic [58]. All human fetuses that have been examined have measurable blood levels of BPA [59–62], and mean or median levels found in humans are higher than levels in fetal and neonatal mice in response to maternal doses that increase postnatal growth [17,63,64].

Exposure during gestation and lactation to BPA has been shown to result in a wide range of effects observed during postnatal life in mice, rats, and a wide range of other vertebrates and invertebrate species [65,66]. We initially reported [17], and other studies have confirmed [67–71], that prenatal exposure to very low doses of BPA increases the rate of postnatal growth in mice and rats. In addition, neonatal exposure to a low dose (1 μg/kg/day) of the estrogenic drug diethylstilbestrol (DES) stimulated a subsequent increase in body weight and an increase in body fat in mice [72].

There are a number of genes that are likely to be involved in the effects of estrogenic chemicals such as BPA on adipocyte differentiation and function. The genes critical for inducing adipocyte differentiation, as well as their temporal sequence of expression during adipocyte differentiation, are being actively investigated [40,73]. We have preliminary evidence that expression of a number of genes is permanently altered as a result of differential fetal growth (based on comparisons of intrauterine growth restricted [IUGR] and macrosomic male mice), and some of the same genes are also permanently altered due to developmental exposure to BPA [34].

We are examining expression and the DNA methylation profile of these candidate genes, which are implicated in adipocyte differentiation, function, and obesity, such as PPARγ, C/EBPα, LPL, GLUT4, Cyp19 (aromatase), GPAT, and DGAT. In rats, developmental exposure to approximately 70 µg/kg/day BPA resulted in upregulation of a number of genes in abdominal adipocytes, including PPARγ and C/EBPα and LPL [34]. In mouse 3T3-L1 cells, BPA increased LPL activity and triacylglycerol accumulation; BPA resulted in the presence of larger lipid droplets in the differentiated cells [74]. Insulin and BPA interacted synergistically to further accelerate these processes. BPA also stimulated an increase in the glucose transporter GLUT4 and glucose uptake into 3T3-F442A adipocytes in cell culture [75]. In a separate study, upregulation of GLUT4 increased basal and insulin-induced glucose uptake into adipocytes [76]. In addition, low doses of BPA stimulated rapid secretion of insulin in mouse pancreatic β cells in primary culture through a nonclassical, nongenomic estrogen-response system, and the magnitude of the response was the same at equal doses of BPA and estradiol. In contrast, prolonged exposure to a low oral dose of BPA (10 µg/kg/day) resulted in stimulation of insulin secretion in adult mice that was mediated by the classical nuclear estrogen receptors; the prolonged hypersecretion of insulin was followed by insulin resistance [77]. In a subsequent study [8], these investigators reported that mice exposed during fetal life to a low dose (10 µg/kg/day) were heavier at birth relative to controls, and at 6 months of age, males prenatally exposed to BPA displayed glucose intolerance, insulin resistance, and altered insulin release from pancreatic β cells compared with control mice. It required exposure to a higher dose of BPA (100 µg/kg/day) to have a subsequent effect on the pregnant mice that displayed glucose intolerance and altered insulin sensitivity compared with unexposed controls. Furthermore, 4 months after delivery, the pregnant mice treated with BPA were heavier than control unexposed mice and had decreased insulin sensitivity and glucose intolerance. This finding stands in contrast to the typical assumption that exposure to chemicals such as BPA in adulthood alters metabolic systems during the time of exposure (activational effects), but that the consequences of exposure are not permanent. This observation suggests that BPA exposure during pregnancy in women may affect body weight and glucose metabolism later in life. Consistent with the prediction that fetuses are more sensitive to environmental chemicals than adults, the permanent effects of BPA on offspring metabolic systems occurred at a dose 10-fold lower than the dose required to cause effects in the adult mother [8].

ADULT PHENOTYPE DUE TO INTRAUTERINE GROWTH RESTRICTION IS SIMILAR TO DEVELOPMENTAL EXPOSURE TO BPA

There is extensive epidemiological evidence showing that babies with IUGR who then experience a rapid "catch-up" growth spurt during childhood are at high risk for adult obesity and type 2 diabetes, consistent with the "fetal basis of adult disease" hypothesis [27]. Thus, fetal growth rate interacts with childhood growth rate in terms of whether IUGR leads to adult obesity and other metabolic diseases. We have developed a novel crowded uterine horn mouse model that results in siblings that range from growth restricted to macrosomic due to differences in placental blood flow based on location in the crowded uterus (Figure 5.2). Importantly, the IUGR mice experience a rapid period of catch-up growth: IUGR mice experience about a 90% increase in body weight, while macrosomic males have about a 30% increase in body weight during the first week after weaning. Adult IUGR male mice show marked similarities to IUGR humans in terms of glucose intolerance and elevated insulin as well as an increase in total abdominal fat weight [78]. Importantly, while both IUGR and macrosomic males remained significantly heavier than male mice with a median body weight at birth, we have found significant differences in adipocyte gene

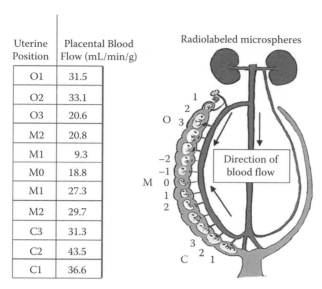

Uterine Position	Placental Blood Flow (mL/min/g)
O1	31.5
O2	33.1
O3	20.6
M2	20.8
M1	9.3
M0	18.8
M1	27.3
M2	29.7
C3	31.3
C2	43.5
C1	36.6

FIGURE 5.2 Blood flow (indicated by arrows) into the loop uterine artery is bidirectional from both the ovarian (O) and cervical (C) ends of the uterine horn, which leads to greater placental blood flow at the ends relative to the middle (M) of each uterine horn. The data shown are placental blood flow measurements taken from a hemiovariectomized pregnant female CD-1 mouse on gestation day 18; the female was injected with radiolabeled microspheres to measure blood flow [86]. Removing the left ovary prior to pregnancy results in double the number of oocytes being ovulated from the remaining right ovary and crowding in the right uterine horn, which is separate from the left uterine horn in mice and rats.

expression and number in adult male gonadal fat. There is thus a markedly different etiology of obesity in these two overweight subpopulations of mice relating to differences in both fetal and postweaning growth (B.L. Coe, unpublished observation).

As noted earlier, our initial studies show that there are some interesting parallels between the effect of perinatal exposure to BPA in a preliminary study and the consequence of a mouse pup being IUGR: in each case, there is a greater rate of weight gain during the week following weaning, and in adulthood, there are significantly fewer adipocytes, although the adipocytes are significantly larger (B.L. Coe, unpublished observation). BPA exposed developing mouse pups thus appears to have traits similar to those of IUGR pups. This is interesting in that a recent occupational study from China reported data suggesting that maternal exposure to BPA was related to IUGR [79]. In addition, there are similarities in gonadal adipocyte gene expression in comparisons of IUGR vs. macrosomic animals and the effects of BPA vs. controls, since similar to IUGR, BPA elevates PPARγ, C/EBPα, and LPL in abdominal adipocytes [34].

ENDOCRINE DISRUPTOR TRIBUTYLTIN AND OBESITY

Recent publications have implicated some other environmental chemicals with changes in adipocyte function. For example, organotin compounds were used for many years to protect the bottom of boats, and these persistent compounds remain a health problem even though their use has been restricted in recent years. In addition, organotin compounds are used as stabilizers in polyvinylchloride (PVC) plastic, which is used to manufacture the pipes that carry water into homes, and organotin compounds leach out of PVC into water [80–82].

Tributyltin (TBT) is an organotin compound and is an endocrine-disrupting chemical that results in imposex in gastropod mollusks. This is a condition in which abnormal masculinization of females occurs due to the inhibition of the estrogen-synthesizing enzyme aromatase, which results in an increase in testosterone; testosterone is the substrate that is aromatized by aromatase to form estradiol-17β [83]. TBT also inhibits aromatase activity in human granulose cells in culture [84]. TBT is a ligand for PPARγ as well as for retinoic X receptors (RXRs), which, along with estrogen receptors and PPARs, are members of the nuclear receptor superfamily. In mice, treatment of pregnant females with TBT stimulated adipocyte differentiation and increased fat mass in offspring (number and volume of adipocytes were not reported). This finding is thus consistent with other findings described earlier regarding PPARγ activation during adipogenesis and adds to other evidence that activation of RXRs are also involved [11,85].

CONCLUSIONS

At this time, there is limited human data relating obesity with environmental chemicals and specifically environmental chemicals that are estrogenic or otherwise disrupt estrogen homeostasis. However, there has been an increase in research relating environmental chemicals with obesity, insulin and glucose dysregulation, and type 2 diabetes. Findings from these studies have led to an increased awareness that energy expenditure and components of a person's diet, while important, likely do not explain the rate of increase in obesity that has been documented over the last two decades [28,29]. While the contribution of environmental chemicals to the obesity epidemic remains a largely unexamined issue, the dramatic increase in the incidence of obesity has occurred in parallel with a dramatic increase in the use of plastic. Plastic materials contain many types of endocrine-disrupting compounds in addition to BPA. The animal experiments showing a relationship between accelerated postnatal growth, altered insulin secretion, and glucose sensitivity due to developmental exposure to daily doses of BPA within the range of human exposure provide a strong argument for further research into the possibility that developmental exposure to BPA, as well as other endocrine-disrupting chemicals, is contributing to the development of obesity later in life.

ACKNOWLEDGMENT

Support during the preparation of this chapter was provided by a grant from NIEHS (ES018764) to FvS.

REFERENCES

1. Colborn T et al., Developmental effects of endocrine-disrupting chemicals in wildlife and humans. *Environ Health Perspect*, 101, 378–384, 1993.
2. Welshons WV et al., Large effects from small exposures. I. Mechanisms for endocrine-disrupting chemicals with estrogenic activity. *Environ Health Perspect*, 111, 904–1006, 2003.
3. Welshons WV et al., Large effects from small exposures. III. Endocrine mechanisms mediating effects of bisphenol A at levels of human exposure. *Endocrinology*, 147, S56–S69, 2006.
4. Grun F, Blumberg B, Perturbed nuclear receptor signaling by environmental obesogens as emerging factors in the obesity crisis. *Rev Endocr Metab Disord*, 8, 161–171, 2007.
5. Stahlhut RW et al., Concentrations of urinary phthalate metabolites are associated with increased waist circumference and insulin resistance in adult U.S. males. *Environ Health Perspect*, 115, 876–882, 2007.
6. Lang IA et al., Association of urinary bisphenol A concentration with medical disorders and laboratory abnormalities in adults. *JAMA*, 300, 1303–1310, 2008.
7. Heindel JJ, vom Saal FS, Overview of obesity and the role of developmental nutrition and environmental chemical exposures. *Mol Cell Endocrinol*, 304, 90–96, 2009.
8. Alonso-Magdalena P et al., Bisphenol A exposure during pregnancy disrupts glucose homeostasis in mothers and adult male offspring. *Environ Health Perspect*, 118, 1243–1250, 2010.
9. Watson CS et al., Nongenomic signaling pathways of estrogen toxicity. *Toxicol Sci*, 115, 1–11, 2010.
10. Shioda T et al., Importance of dosage standardization for interpreting transcriptomal signature profiles: Evidence from studies of xenoestrogens. *Proc Natl Acad Sci*, 103, 12033–12038, 2006.
11. Blumberg B, Obesogens, stem cells and the maternal programming of obesity. *J Develop Origins Health Disease*, 2, 3–8, 2011.

12. Choudhuri S et al., Molecular targets of epigenetic regulation and effectors of environmental influences. *Toxicol Appl Pharmacol*, 245, 378–393, 2010.

13. Weinhold B, Epigenetics: The science of change. *Environ Health Perspect*, 114, A160–A167, 2006.

14. Dolinoy DC et al., Maternal nutrient supplementation counteracts bisphenol A-induced DNA hypomethylation in early development. *Proc Natl Acad Sci*, 104, 13056–13061, 2007.

15. Cooke PS, Naaz A, The role of estrogens in adipocyte development and function. *Exp Biol Med*, 229, 1127–1135, 2004.

16. Newbold RR et al., Developmental exposure to endocrine disruptors and the obesity epidemic. *Reprod Toxicol*, 23, 290–296, 2007.

17. Howdeshell KL et al., Exposure to bisphenol A advances puberty. *Nature*, 401, 763–764, 1999.

18. Newbold RR et al., Developmental exposure to estrogenic compounds and obesity. *Birth Defects Res A Clin Mol Teratol*, 73, 478–480, 2005.

19. Heine PA et al., Increased adipose tissue in male and female estrogen receptor-alpha knockout mice. *Proc Natl Acad Sci*, 97, 12729–12734, 2000.

20. Jones ME et al., Aromatase-deficient (ArKO) mice have a phenotype of increased adiposity. *Proc Natl Acad Sci*, 97, 12735–12740, 2000.

21. Cooke PS et al., The role of estrogen and estrogen receptor-alpha in male adipose tissue. *Mol Cell Endocrinol*, 178, 147–154, 2001.

22. Jones ME et al., Aromatase-deficient (ArKO) mice accumulate excess adipose tissue. *J Steroid Biochem Mol Biol*, 79, 3–9, 2001.

23. Wild SH, Byrne CD, Evidence for fetal programming of obesity with a focus on putative mechanisms. *Nutr Res Rev*, 17, 153–162, 2004.

24. Yajnik CS, Fetal origins of adult disease: Where do we stand? *Int J Diab Dev Countries*, 21, 42–50, 2001.

25. Ogden CL et al., Prevalence of overweight and obesity in the United States, 1999–2004. *JAMA*, 295, 1549–1555, 2006.

26. Barker DJ, The developmental origins of adult disease. *J Am Coll Nutr*, 23, 588S–595S, 2004.

27. Oken E, Gillman MW, Fetal origins of obesity. *Obes Res*, 11, 496–506, 2003.

28. Baillie-Hamilton PF, Chemical toxins: A hypothesis to explain the global obesity epidemic. *J Altern Complement Med*, 8, 185–192, 2002.

29. Keith SW et al., Putative contributors to the secular increase in obesity: Exploring the roads less traveled. *Int J Obes (Lond)*, Online June 27, 2006.

30. Gluckman PD et al., Life-long echoes—A critical analysis of the developmental origins of adult disease model. *Biol Neonate*, 87, 127–139, 2005.

31. Stocker CJ et al., Fetal origins of insulin resistance and obesity. *Proc Nutr Soc*, 64, 143–151, 2005.

32. Adair LS, Cole TJ, Rapid child growth raises blood pressure in adolescent boys who were thin at birth. *Hypertension*, 41, 451–456, 2003.

33. Ruhlen RL et al., Low phytoestrogen levels in feed increase fetal serum estradiol resulting in the "fetal estrogenization syndrome" and obesity in CD-1 mice. *Environ Health Perspect*, 116, 322–328, 2008.

34. Somm E et al., Perinatal exposure to bisphenol a alters early adipogenesis in the rat. *Environ Health Perspect*, 117, 1549–1555, 2009.

35. Hager A et al., Body fat and adipose tissue cellularity in infants: A longitudinal study. *Metabolism*, 26, 607–614, 1977.

36. Gregoire FM, Adipocyte differentiation: From fibroblast to endocrine cell. *Exp Biol Med*, 226, 997–1002, 2001.

37. Ailhaud G et al., Cellular and molecular aspects of adipose tissue development. *Annu Rev Nutr*, 12, 207–233, 1992.

38. Johnson PR, Hirsch J, Cellularity of adipose depots in six strains of genetically obese mice. *J Lipid Res*, 13, 2–11, 1972.

39. Larsen TM et al., PPARgamma agonists in the treatment of type II diabetes: Is increased fatness commensurate with long-term efficacy? *Int J Obes Relat Metab Disord*, 27, 147–161, 2003.

40. Tong Q, Hotamisligil GS, Molecular mechanisms of adipocyte differentiation. *Rev Endocr Metab Disord*, 2, 349–355, 2001.

41. Gregoire FM et al., Understanding adipocyte differentiation. *Physiol Rev*, 78, 783–809, 1998.

42. Zhang JW et al., Role of CREB in transcriptional regulation of CCAAT/enhancer-binding protein beta gene during adipogenesis. *J Biol Chem*, 279, 4471–4478, 2004.

43. Krempler F et al., Leptin, peroxisome proliferator-activated receptor-gamma, and CCAAT/enhancer binding protein-alpha mRNA expression in adipose tissue of humans and their relation to cardiovascular risk factors. *Arterioscler Thromb Vasc Biol*, 20, 443–449, 2000.

44. Yamauchi T et al., The mechanisms by which both heterozygous peroxisome proliferator-activated receptor gamma (PPARgamma) deficiency and PPARgamma agonist improve insulin resistance. *J Biol Chem*, 276, 41245–41254, 2001.

45. Coleman RA, Lee DP, Enzymes of triacylglycerol synthesis and their regulation. *Prog Lipid Res*, 43, 134–176, 2004.

46. Chen HC et al., Increased insulin and leptin sensitivity in mice lacking acyl CoA:diacylglycerol acyltransferase 1. *J Clin Invest*, 109, 1049–1055, 2002.

47. Nativelle-Serpentini C et al., Aromatase activity modulation by lindane and bisphenol-A in human placental JEG-3 and transfected kidney E293 cells. *Toxicol In Vitro*, 17, 413–422, 2003.

48. Arase S et al., Endocrine disrupter bisphenol a increases in situ estrogen production in the mouse urogenital sinus. *Biol Reprod*, 84, 734–742, 2011.

49. Misso ML et al., Cellular and molecular characterization of the adipose phenotype of the aromatase-deficient mouse. *Endocrinology*, 144, 1474–1480, 2003.

50. Homma H et al., Estrogen suppresses transcription of lipoprotein lipase gene. Existence of a unique estrogen response element on the lipoprotein lipase promoter. *J Biol Chem*, 275, 11404–11411, 2000.

51. vom Saal FS, Sexual differentiation in litter-bearing mammals: Influence of sex of adjacent fetuses in utero. *J Anim Sci*, 67, 1824–1840, 1989.

52. Naaz A et al., Effect of ovariectomy on adipose tissue of mice in the absence of estrogen receptor alpha (ERalpha): A potential role for estrogen receptor beta (ERbeta). *Horm Metab Res*, 34, 758–763, 2002.

53. Joyner JM et al., Estrogen receptors in human preadipocytes. *Endocrine*, 15, 225–230, 2001.

54. Lea-Currie YR et al., Dehydroepiandrosterone and related steroids alter 3T3-L1 preadipocyte proliferation and differentiation. *Comp Biochem Physiol C Pharmacol Toxicol Endocrinol*, 123, 17–25, 1999.

55. Dieudonne MN et al., Opposite effects of androgens and estrogens on adipogenesis in rat preadipocytes: Evidence for sex and site-related specificities and possible involvement of insulin-like growth factor 1 receptor and peroxisome proliferator-activated receptor gamma2. *Endocrinology*, 141, 649–656, 2000.

56. Anderson LA et al., The effects of androgens and estrogens on preadipocyte proliferation in human adipose tissue: Influence of gender and site. *J Clin Endocrinol Metab*, 86, 5045–5051, 2001.

57. Cooper SC, Roncari DA, 17-beta-estradiol increases mitogenic activity of medium from cultured preadipocytes of massively obese persons. *J Clin Invest*, 83, 1925–1929, 1989.

58. Bailin PD et al., Public awareness drives market for safer alternatives: Bisphenol A market analysis report, 2008. http://www.iehn.org/publications.reports.bpa.php (accessed April 20, 2011).

59. Schonfelder G et al., Parent bisphenol A accumulation in human maternal-fetal-placental unit. *Environ Health Perspect*, 110, A703–A707, 2002.

60. Ikezuki Y et al., Determination of bisphenol A concentrations in human biological fluids reveals significant early prenatal exposure. *Human Reprod*, 17, 2839–2841, 2002.

61. Vandenberg LN et al., Human exposure to bisphenol A (BPA). *Reprod Toxicol*, 24, 139–177, 2007.

62. Vandenberg LN et al., Urinary, circulating, and tissue biomonitoring studies indicate widespread exposure to bisphenol A. *Environ Health Perspect*, 118, 1055–1070, 2010.

63. Zalko D et al., Biotransformations of bisphenol A in a mammalian model: Answers and new questions raised by low-dose metabolic fate studies in pregnant CD-1 mice. *Environ Health Perspect*, 111, 309–319, 2002.

64. Taylor JA et al., No effect of route of exposure (oral; subcutaneous injection) on plasma bisphenol A throughout 24 h after administration in neonatal female mice. *Reprod Toxicol*, 25, 169–176, 2008.

65. vom Saal FS, Hughes C, An extensive new literature concerning low-dose effects of bisphenol A shows the need for a new risk assessment. *Environ Health Perspect*, 113, 926–933, 2005.

66. Richter CA et al., In vivo effects of bisphenol A in laboratory rodent studies. *Reprod Toxicol*, 24, 199–224, 2007.

67. Akingbemi BT et al., Inhibition of testicular steroidogenesis by the xenoestrogen bisphenol A is associated with reduced pituitary luteinizing hormone secretion and decreased steroidogenic enzyme gene expression in rat Leydig cells. *Endocrinology*, 145, 592–603, 2004.

68. Markey CM et al., Mammalian development in a changing environment: Exposure to endocrine disruptors reveals the developmental plasticity of steroid-hormone target organs. *Evol Dev*, 5, 67–75, 2003.

69. Nikaido Y et al., Effects of maternal xenoestrogen exposure on development of the reproductive tract and mammary gland in female CD-1 mouse offspring. *Reprod Toxicol*, 18, 803–811, 2004.

70. Rubin BS et al., Perinatal exposure to low doses of bisphenol A affects body weight, patterns of estrous cyclicity, and plasma LH levels. *Environ Health Perspect*, 109, 657–680, 2001.

71. Takai Y et al., Preimplantation exposure to bisphenol A advances postnatal development. *Reprod Toxicol*, 15, 71–74, 2000.

72. Newbold RR et al., Developmental exposure to diethylstilbestrol (DES) alters uterine response to estrogens in prepubescent mice: Low versus high dose effects. *Reprod Toxicol*, 18, 399–406, 2004.

73. Rosen ED, MacDougald OA, Adipocyte differentiation from the inside out. *Nat Rev Mol Cell Biol*, 7, 885–896, 2006.

74. Masuno H et al., Bisphenol A in combination with insulin can accelerate the conversion of 3T3-L1 fibroblasts to adipocytes. *J Lipid Res*, 43, 676–684, 2002.

75. Sakurai K et al., Bisphenol A affects glucose transport in mouse 3T3-F442A adipocytes. *Br J Pharmacol*, 141, 209–214, 2004.

76. Deems RO et al., Expression of human GLUT4 in mice results in increased insulin action. *Diabetologia*, 37, 1097–1104, 1994.

77. Alonso-Magdalena P et al., The estrogenic effect of bisphenol A disrupts pancreatic beta-cell function in vivo and induces insulin resistance. *Environ Health Perspect*, 114, 106–112, 2006.

78. Budge H et al., Maternal nutritional programming of fetal adipose tissue development: Long-term consequences for later obesity. *Birth Defects Res C Embryo Today*, 75, 193–199, 2005.

79. Xi W et al., Effect of perinatal and postnatal bisphenol A exposure to the regulatory circuits at the hypothalamus-pituitary-gonadal axis of CD-1 mice. *Reprod Toxicol*, 39, 409–417, 2011.

80. Forsyth DS et al., Speciation of organotins in poly(vinyl chloride) products. *Food Addit Contam*, 10, 531–540, 1993.

81. Sadiki A, Williams DT, Speciation of organotin and organolead compounds in drinking water by gas chromatography—Atomic emission spectrometry. *Chemosphere*, 32, 1983–1992, 1996.

82. Smith MD et al., Poly(vinyl chloride) formulations: Acute toxicity to cultured human cell lines. *J Biomater Sci Polym Ed*, 7, 453–459, 1995.

83. Matthiessen P, Gibbs P, Critical appraisal of the evidence for tributyltin-mediated endocrine disruption in mollusks. *Environ Toxicol Chem*, 17, 37–43, 1998.

84. Saitoh M et al., Tributyltin or triphenyltin inhibits aromatase activity in the human granulosa-like tumor cell line KGN. *Biochem Biophys Res Commun*, 289, 198–204, 2001.

85. Grun F et al., Endocrine disrupting organotin compounds are potent inducers of adipogenesis in vertebrates. *Mol Endocrinol*, Online April 13, 2006.

86. Coe BL et al., A new 'crowded uterine horn' mouse model for examining the relationship between foetal growth and adult obesity. *Basic Clin Pharmacol Toxicol*, 102, 162–167, 2008.

6 Cigarette Smoking, Inflammation, and Obesity

Saibal K. Biswas, PhD, Ian L. Megson, PhD,
Catherine A. Shaw, PhD, and Irfan Rahman, PhD

CONTENTS

Obesity has already reached epidemic proportions in many countries, including the United States, the United Kingdom, and many upcoming economies. Latest estimates indicate that it now affects approximately 33% of adults worldwide [1–3]. Body mass index (BMI; the weight in kilograms divided by the square of the height in meters) is an indicator of obesity that is easy to calculate and is reasonably well correlated with direct anthropometric measures of body. A BMI greater than 28 is generally associated with a three- to fourfold increased risk of clinical conditions such as stroke, ischemic heart disease, or diabetes mellitus [1]. A central distribution of body fat (as determined by the ratio of waist circumference to hip circumference: 0.90 in women and 1.0 in men) is widely accepted to reflect the so-called visceral fat, which is associated with a higher risk than a more peripheral distribution and may be a better indicator of the risk than absolute fat mass or BMI. Childhood obesity increases the risk of subsequent morbidity, whether or not obesity persists into adulthood [1]. It is estimated that one in every three children born will develop diabetes associated with obesity [2,3]. Other than diabetes, obesity may also be associated with the development of cardiovascular diseases (CVDs); breast, colon, and prostate cancer; pulmonary conditions (asthma); sleep apnea; and osteoarticular disorders (rheumatoid arthritis and osteoporosis in women) [4–9]. These disorders are directly or indirectly exacerbated by tobacco smoke exposure, air pollution, and diesel exhaust, which all trigger inflammation.

ENERGY STORAGE, INTAKE, AND EXPENDITURE

Fat (or triglyceride) is the primary form in which potential chemical energy is stored in the body. The amount of triglyceride in adipose tissue is the cumulative sum of the differences between energy intake and energy expenditure. Although homeostatic mechanisms act to minimize the difference, imbalances over a long period can have a large-scale effect. The degree of control between energy intake and expenditure is achieved by coordinated effects mediated through endocrine and neural signals that arise from various tissues [10–14]. Such integration is central to the regulation of body fat stores (Figure 6.1). A large number of factors originating throughout the body relay afferent signals to a smaller number of functional centers in the central nervous system, which in turn signal the efferent pathways to regulate energy expenditure (e.g., through the sympathetic and parasympathetic nervous systems and thyroid hormones) and energy intake (through eating behavior) [15,16]. These factors can interact at many levels; for example, the effect of cholecystokinin on satiety is increased by estradiol and insulin and is dependent on parasympathetic afferent signals [17,18]. The release of insulin is increased by cholecystokinin and parasympathetic efferent activity and is inhibited by sympathetic efferent signals [19]. The redundancy of interactions within this system makes any pharmacological or surgical manipulation of a single component inadequate for long-term resolution of obesity. That body fat content can be regulated is evident from the responses of both lean and obese humans subjected to experimental manipulation of body weight, making it unlikely that behavior alone is the sole determinant of obesity. It has been observed that a decreased expenditure of energy and an increased propensity to store fat may precede the development of obesity, which suggests that the extra body fat in the obese person in some way corrects for low energy expenditure [16].

Current epidemiological studies on human obesity have shown that the regulation of energy balance is being acutely affected in a large number of subjects by environmental changes [20]. In general, increased energy intake and energy from fat is linked with obesity. However, decreased physical activity also plays a major role in weight gain, and susceptibility for gaining weight varies among individuals. Variations in basal metabolic rate (BMR) have also been associated with propensity to weight gain, which in turn may be linked to uncoupling proteins-2 and -3. However, *in vivo* studies are still required to establish the role of these proteins in the development of obesity. A wide array of hormones, cytokines, and neurotransmitters are involved in the regulation of energy intake, but their role in common polygenic obesity is still to be determined.

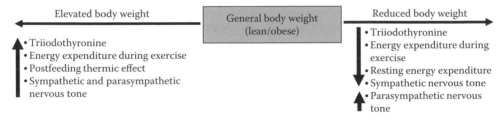

FIGURE 6.1 Metabolic alterations in adults due to weight gain or loss. Decreased body weight is associated with reduced energy expenditure during exercise, sympathetic nervous tones, and resting state energy expenditure. An almost opposite phenomenon is observed during increased weight gain.

Cigarette Smoking, Appetite, and Energy Expenditure

Smoking is a behavior that is maintained by physical addiction, psychological dependence, and habit and is associated with a wide variety of health problems relating to the cardiovascular, neurological, and pulmonary systems. Nicotine, the addictive component present in tobacco, has various mood-changing effects that contribute to and reinforce the highly controlled or compulsive pattern of drug use through smoking or via the use of nicotine gums and patches, or electronic cigarettes rich in nicotine. The pharmacological and biochemical effects of nicotine are powerful, with smokers reporting a mixture of relaxing, mood-lifting, and pleasurable effects. Smoking is also associated with decreased food intake and lower body weight particularly in chronic smokers. Nicotine is considered the major appetite-suppressing component of tobacco. Leptin and insulin are endogenous hormones that decrease appetite and increase energy expenditure by affecting the neuropeptide levels in the hypothalamus. Nicotine administration was found to reduce food intake and body weight. Acute (24 h) administration of nicotine lowered orexigenic neuropeptides expression, such as neuropeptide Y, agouti-related protein, and melanin-concentrating hormone. However, 3 days of nicotine treatment did not alter hypothalamic neuropeptides mRNA levels. Nicotine was not found to affect the intracellular signaling of leptin and insulin in the hypothalamus. These observations indicate that the acute anorectic effect of smoking may be explained in part by the decreased levels of orexigenic neuropeptides in the hypothalamus. The effect is not likely due to enhanced leptin or insulin signal transduction in the hypothalamus; however, chronic cigarette smoking may have differential effects on leptin and insulin signaling.

Studies on the influence of cigarette smoking on resting energy expenditure (REE) in normal-weight and obese smokers have indicated that REE increased in both obese and normal-weight smokers after smoking, but the increase was greater for normal-weight participants [21], suggesting the implications of smoking on obesity. However, the reliability of the observed alterations is lower for both normal-weight and obese smokers. Although smokers have lower mean BMI compared with nonsmokers, they have a more metabolically adverse fat distribution profile, with higher central adiposity [22]. The mechanism by which smoking affects fat distribution is not entirely clear. One hypothesis is that smoking has some kind of antiestrogenic effect. Another suggestion is that cigarette smoking may have an effect on the uptake and storage of triglyceride fatty acids via increasing the fat mass [23]. A precise explanation for the association may help to identify the mechanisms underlying the adverse health consequences of cigarette smoking and abdominal obesity. The strong negative correlation over time between smoking rates and obesity has led some to suggest that smoking cessation leads to weight gain [24].

Since one of the main effects of smoking is to decrease appetite, it may lure many individuals to use smoking as a means of losing body weight in spite of the health risks that smoking poses, such as chronic lung disease, chronic obstructive pulmonary disease (COPD)/emphysema, lung cancer, and CVDs. Nicotine has been reported to promote energy expenditure by increasing metabolic rate, decreasing metabolic efficiency, and decreasing caloric absorption [24]. Mice exposed to cigarette smoke experienced a decrease in appetite, leading to a weight loss on account of energy mobilization from adipose tissue [25]. Smoking is known to lead to decreased energy consumption and to promote the use of fat and overall energy expenditure, thus leading to a wasting effect on the body, an indicator of nutrient deficiencies [25]. Heavy smoking is associated with a greater susceptibility to obesity by affecting body fat distribution and visceral adiposity, the latter being an established risk factor for hyperglycemia (diabetes) and dyslipidemia (cardiovascular problems). The association between smoking and visceral adiposity may be partly explained by low physical activity including the lack of exercise and an unhealthy high fat containing-diet (mainly fast-food burgers, processed foods, fries, and fried snacks) that is frequently consumed by smokers [24]. Smoking also increases inflammation and oxidative stress leading to pancreatic beta-cell and endothelial cell dysfunction [26]. Smoking can lead to nutritional deficiency by causing inflammation in the digestion tract leading to pain, diarrhea, flatulence, acidity, increased gas formation, and impaired nutrient absorption [27]. Consistent smoke inhalation, whether second hand or direct, leads to peptic ulcers, liver disease, Crohn's disease, and heartburn. Smoking also disables the liver's ability to neutralize toxins, alcohol, and other drugs, eventually leading to hepatic damage and, ultimately, liver failure. Furthermore, smoking also affects the levels of vitamins and antioxidants in the body. Smoking decreases the levels of antioxidants, such as vitamins E and C, beta-carotene, selenium, and B-complex vitamins. Coupled with an already increased risk of a poorly balanced diet, smoking can lead to severe nutritional deficiency [28], associated with increased body mass/biometrics.

SMOKING AND HORMONAL MEDIATORS OF ENERGY HOMEOSTASIS

Cigarette smoke is an admixture of many potent oxidants, carcinogens/mutagens, and chemicals that are major risk factors for the development of various metabolic disorders. Mainstream cigarette smoke contains over 5000 chemical species, including high concentrations of oxidants/free radicals (10^{17}/puff) [29]. The aqueous phase of cigarette smoke condensate may undergo redox recycling (due to the presence of free iron) in the lungs of smokers [30]. The tar component of cigarette smoke contains high levels of relatively stable radicals (e.g., semiquinone radicals). The tar component effectively chelates metals and can bind iron (released from activated macrophages) to produce tar-semiquinone and tar-Fe^{2+} adducts, which can generate millimolar amounts of hydrogen peroxide (H_2O_2) over a prolonged period. Side-stream cigarette smoke contains more than 10^{15} reactive organic compounds per puff and contains carbon monoxide, ammonia, formaldehyde, N-nitrosamines, benzo(a)pyrene, benzene, isoprene, ethane, pentane, nicotine, aldehydes, acrolein, acetaldehyde, quinones, semiquinones, and other genotoxic and carcinogenic organic compounds.

Superoxide anion ($O_2^{\bullet-}$) and nitric oxide (NO) are the predominant free radicals of the gas phase of cigarette smoke. NO and $O_2^{\bullet-}$ quickly react to form more toxic peroxynitrite ($ONOO^-$). The semiquinone radicals in the tar component of cigarette smoke can reduce oxygen to produce so-called reactive oxygen species (ROS), including $O_2^{\bullet-}$, $^{\bullet}OH$, and H_2O_2 [31]. Oxidants present in cigarette smoke can stimulate alveolar macrophages to release a host of mediators, some of which are chemotactic and recruit neutrophils and other inflammatory cells into the lungs. Both neutrophils and macrophages can then generate ROS via the activation of the NADPH oxidase (now collectively known as NOX for NAD(P)H oxidase and DUOX for dual oxidase) complex system [32].

Cigarette smoke–derived oxidants (inhaled or endogenously produced by inflammatory cells) may affect many obesity-related hormones such as leptin, adiponectin, and resistin that are produced by the adipose tissue [32]. While leptin, a satiety hormone, regulates appetite and energy balance of the body, adiponectin suppresses atherogenesis and fibrotic diseases and might play a role as an anti-inflammatory hormone. Increased resistin, on the other hand, might cause insulin resistance and thus could link obesity with type 2 diabetes [32]. Ghrelin, produced in the stomach, is involved in the long-term regulation of energy metabolism and calorie intake. All of these hormones play an important role in energy homeostasis, glucose and lipid metabolism, cardiovascular function, and immunity, and they influence other organ systems, including the brain, liver, and skeletal muscle. Importantly, the functions of these enzymes are influenced by the cellular oxidant/antioxidant balance. In view of the local oxidative stress generated by adipocytes (discussed later) leading to activation of macrophages, this is still a further evidence to support a crucial role for oxidative stress in the complications related to obesity. Smoking, which is known to directly activate and recruit macrophages and other leukocytes in various tissues, can thus further exaggerate the effect of oxidative stress in obesity.

The adipocyte volume has been reported to be proportional to plasma insulin concentrations [18]. Insulin is transported to the central nervous system by a saturable transport system where it mediates reduction in food intake by inhibiting the expression of neuropeptide Y, enhancing the anorectic effects of cholecystokinin, and inhibiting neuronal norepinephrine reuptake [11,33]. It has been recently shown that insulin reduces food intake through an effect on leptin-mediated signaling. Cholecystokinin is a duodenal peptide secreted in the presence of food and is known to reduce food intake [14].

Obesity, Metabolism, and Energy Expenditure: Signaling Molecules

Leptin is synthesized in and secreted from adipose tissue and is a potential afferent signal of fat storage (Figure 6.2). In humans, the gene responsible for leptin expression is referred to as *LEP*. It is anorectic and increases energy expenditure, resulting in reduced body fat and restoration of insulin-sensitive glucose disposal in leptin-deficient (*ob/ob*) mice [34]. Plasma leptin concentrations have been reported to be directly correlated with body fat mass in obese human subjects [35]. Various hormones influence the expression of leptin in adipose tissue [35–37]. Leptin probably contributes to energy homeostasis in part by decreasing neuropeptide Y mRNA [34] or by blocking its action as an appetite stimulant; however, transgenic mice lacking the neuropeptide Y gene still respond to the anorexigenic effects of leptin, suggesting that it may also act via mechanisms that are independent of neuropeptide Y [34]. Neuropeptide Y is a potent central appetite stimulant that links afferent signals of the nutritional status of the organism from the endocrine, gastrointestinal, and central and peripheral nervous systems to effectors of energy intake and expenditure (Figure 6.2). Exogenous administration of neuropeptide Y has been reported to exert coordinated effects on energy intake and output and favor weight gain.

Ghrelin, a 28-amino-acid peptide preprohormone, was discovered as an agent that stimulates the release of growth hormone (GH) from the anterior pituitary. Studies established that ghrelin stimulates food intake in rodents, as well as in humans, and is strongly involved in the regulation of energy homeostasis. Ghrelin, along with several other hormones, has significant effects on appetite and energy balance [38]. Ghrelin increases adipose deposition by decreasing fat oxidation. Ghrelin has been shown to exhibit anticachectic action; hence, ghrelin may be used in treatment of cachexia caused by several cardiopulmonary diseases and cancer.

Adiponectin, also known as adipocyte complement-related protein (adipoQ), is an adipocyte-specific, secreted protein with roles in glucose and lipid homeostasis. Adiponectin is induced during adipocyte differentiation, and its secretion is stimulated by insulin. Administration of adiponectin leads to an insulin-independent decrease in plasma glucose. This is due to insulin-sensitizing effects involving adiponectin regulation of triglyceride metabolism (Figure 6.3). The role of adiponectin in lipid oxidation may involve the regulation of proteins associated with triglyceride metabolism, such as CD36, acyl-CoA oxidase, 5-activated protein kinase, and peroxisome proliferator–activated receptor-γ (PPAR-γ) [39]. Inhalation of cigarette smoke may be associated with abnormal triglyceride and cholesterol metabolism (increased accumulation of low-density lipoprotein [LDL] and decreased

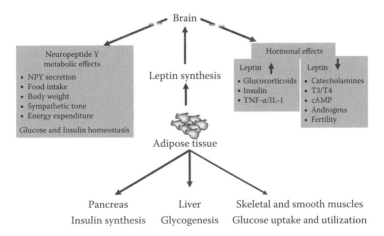

FIGURE 6.2 Effect of leptin on hypothalamus and peripheral organs such as liver, pancreas, and smooth muscles. Leptin released from the adipocytes triggers the brain to regulate a host of responses, such as food intake, fertility, insulin secretion, and sympathetic tones, and exerts peripheral responses on the liver, pancreas, and the smooth muscles.

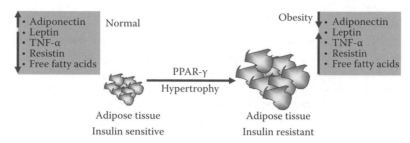

FIGURE 6.3   Adiponectin and related biochemical effects. Both cigarette and adipocytes lead to inflammation through PPAR-γ activation leading to obesity via elevation in resistin, free fatty acids, leptin, and TNF-α and decreasing adiponectin. The adipocytes in turn become resistant to insulin.

high-density lipoprotein [HDL]) and activation of PPAR-γ. A negative correlation between obesity and circulating adiponectin is shown, and adiponectin concentrations increase concomitantly with weight loss [40]. Patients with type 2 diabetes have low concentration of adiponectin which is associated with insulin resistance.

Sirtuins (SIRT: silent information regulator protein) are a family of nicotinamide adenine dinucleotide (NAD+)-dependent histone deacetylases conserved throughout evolution. In yeast, flies, and worms, Sir2 protein is related to increased longevity [41,42] due to caloric restriction [43–45]. Human sirtuins are of seven types (*SIRT1–7*) [46], of which SIRT1 and the yeast Sir2 have highest homology. SIRT1 modulates a wide variety of physiological processes ranging from cell protection against stress [43,47–50] and endocrine signaling specifically involved in glucose and fat metabolism [51–53]. SIRT1 represses transcription of PPAR-γ in adipose tissues, leading to inhibition of adipogenesis during fasting and activation of lipolysis [51]. This leads to loss of fat, considered to be an important effect of caloric restriction on longevity in mammals [51]. Although the effect of caloric restriction on extension of human lifespan is not clear, beneficial effects on cardiovascular risk factors have been well established [54,55]. SIRT1 level and activity are decreased in monocytes, epithelial and endothelial cells, and lungs of smokers and patients with COPD [56–58]. However, in the adipose tissue of various animals including humans, fasting leads to upregulation of SIRT1 [59–62]. It has, therefore, been hypothesized that therapeutic stimulation of SIRT1 may impart beneficial effects of caloric restriction in mammals [63,64] or in prevention of cardiopulmonary disorders. If reduction of body fat by activating SIRT1 with intact caloric intake could be achieved, this could lead to the development of novel prevention strategies for obesity and related disorders. Since in-depth studies of SIRT1 activation and its pleiotropic effect have not been carried out in humans, it is unclear as to the long-term outcome of such strategies [65–67]. Interestingly, SIRT1 has recently been shown to modulate CLOCK-gene expression [68,69], which may open new frontiers in obesity research since there is a link between smoking, dietary habits in particular late night eating, cellular metabolism, and the circadian clock/rhythm in humans. The idea that genetic variations in SIRT1 may influence the BMI and hence obesity has been put forth; however, studies pertaining to such hypothesis have yielded inconsistent results and need further investigations [70].

CIGARETTE SMOKE–MEDIATED OXIDATIVE STRESS, INFLAMMATION, AND OBESITY

Oxidative stress due to increased ROS or reactive nitrogen species (RNS) plays a critical role in the pathogenesis of various diseases and their complications. Activation of various inflammatory cells in response to smoking results in the release of a battery of cytokines and chemokines, including proinflammatory tumor necrosis factor-α (TNF-α) and interleukin (IL)-1β, both of which cause upregulation of adhesion molecules on the endothelium, increased permeability, and increased secretion of chemokines such as IL-8, macrophage inflammatory protein-2, or monocyte chemotactic protein-1 [71]. Cytokines and chemokines then act in concert to further promote the extravasation and accumulation/activation of leukocytes to produce ROS, such as superoxide anion and H_2O_2. Excessive release of ROS (oxidative stress/burden) can then lead to cellular and tissue damage associated with many chronic inflammatory diseases, such as atherosclerosis, asthma, and COPD. Chemokines released as a result of oxidative stress may in turn impinge on the fat cells and trigger a series of reactions leading to obesity or secondary complications of obesity. Growing evidence supports the notion that the condition of obesity may itself induce systemic oxidative stress, and increased oxidative stress in accumulated fat cells in turn may lead to dysregulation of adipocytokines and development of metabolic syndrome (e.g., increased circulating of bad lipid LDL). Increased oxidative stress in accumulated fat, therefore, is potentially an important target for the development of new therapies.

In studies involving obese mice, H_2O_2 production was found to be increased in adipose tissue, but not in other tissues. These results suggested that adipose tissue may be the major source of elevated plasma ROS in obese conditions (Figure 6.4). Oxidative stress affects both insulin secretion by pancreatic β-cells and glucose transport in muscle and adipose tissue. Increased oxidative stress in vascular walls is involved in the pathogenesis of hypertension and atherosclerosis. An association between smoking and increased risk of coronary heart disease was first reported in 1940 in an observational study by the Mayo Clinic [72]. Subsequently, numerous epidemiological studies have confirmed a strong and consistent association between cigarette smoking and morbidity and mortality associated with coronary heart disease [73]. In general, the relative risk of death due to coronary heart disease in smokers is two to four times greater than that in persons who have never smoked; thus, oxidative stress locally produced and disseminated to peripheral tissues via systemic circulation seems to be involved in the pathogenesis and outcome of these diseases. Furthermore, increased ROS release and the resultant lipid peroxidation end products in peripheral blood from accumulated fat in obesity

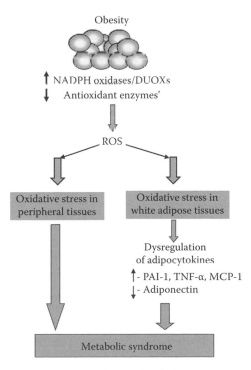

FIGURE 6.4 Oxidative stress in the adipocytes, followed by inflammatory response, can lead to the development of various metabolic alterations, such as diabetes and atherosclerosis.

may be involved in induction of insulin resistance in skeletal muscle and adipose tissue, impaired insulin secretion by β-cells, which are involved in pathogenesis of various vascular diseases, such as atherosclerosis and other cardiovascular disorders.

The other abundant source of $O_2^{\cdot-}$ and H_2O_2 is from the key phagocytes (i.e., neutrophils and macrophages), which have long been known to express a NOX that requires stimulation for assembly of its cytosolic components with the two subunits of the membrane flavocytochrome (gp91*phox* and p22*phox*) to generate high levels of $O_2^{\cdot-}$ upon activation of the cell [74]. The recent recognition that many cells express homologues of the catalytic subunit of the NOX, gp91*phox*, has raised questions about their mode of regulation to produce ROS either constitutively or in response to cytokines, growth factors, and calcium signals. Why, therefore, is oxidative stress only exhibited in accumulated fat and not more widespread in association with inflammatory cells? The answer to this question probably lies in the fact that mRNA expression levels of NOX subunits were increased only in white adipose tissues (WATs) and were associated with decreased mRNA expression levels of various antioxidant enzymes. A parallel increase in the expression of the transcription factor PC.1, which upregulates the transcription of the NOX gene [75], was also showed in adipose tissue of obese mice. Recently, it was reported that macrophages infiltrate the adipose tissues of obese individuals and are an important source of inflammatory cytokines, indicative of their activation in this setting [76,77]. Because activated macrophages are also known to produce ROS, it is possible that infiltrating macrophages are subject to augmentation of NOX and, consequently, increased ROS production in the adipose tissue of obese individuals. In this regard, a family of gp91phox homologous NOX proteins has been reported to be expressed in nonphagocytic cells, but not in macrophages [78]. Recent studies on adipocytes found that NOX4, a member of the NOX family, plays a role in the generation of H_2O_2 [79]. The expression of NOX4 was not detected in macrophages [80,81]. In contrast, expression of NOX4 in WAT, as well as gp91phox, and mRNA expression of NOX4 was significantly increased in WAT of obese mice. These results suggest that adipose NOX is elevated and contributes to ROS production in accumulated fat. In accumulated fat, therefore, elevated levels of fatty acids activate NOX and hence induce ROS production, which in turn upregulate mRNA expression of NOX, establishing a vicious cycle that augments oxidative stress in WAT and blood. It has also been reported that ROS increases the expression of monocyte chemotactic peptide-1 (MCP-1), a chemoattractant for monocytes and macrophages, in adipocytes. End-products of lipid peroxidation by ROS, such as F_2-isoprostanes, 4-hydroxy-2-nonenal, and malondialdehyde (MDA), are themselves potent chemoattractants [82]. Hence, it is possible that increased ROS production and MCP-1 secretion from accumulated fat may trigger macrophage recruitment and inflammation of adipose tissue in obesity. Thus, oxidative stress (triggered endogenously by cigarette smoking) in the adipocytes, followed by inflammatory response, can lead to the development of various metabolic alterations such as diabetes, cancer, and atherosclerosis (Figure 6.4).

The association between obesity and oxidative stress is now well established through large community-based cohort studies and validated biomarkers of lipid peroxidation such as F_2-isoprostanes, MDA, and 4-hydroxy-2-nonenal [83,84]. It is, however, not possible to determine from these sources whether obesity is a source of oxidative stress. It has been suggested that obesity is independently associated with oxidative stress [83]; the close association of obesity with other metabolic conditions leaves the possibility that oxidative stress and obesity may be related to other uninvestigated parameters. Therefore, further investigations of the relationships between obesity, inflammation, oxidative stress, and cardiopulmonary diseases [85] are required. In case obesity is established to be a state of increased oxidative stress, the potential for antioxidant therapy needs further investigations. For example, the use of statins (lipid-lowering drugs), which also work as antioxidants, alleviates cardiovascular problems associated with obesity [86–89]. There is an increasing evidence that prenatal exposure to cigarette smoke may lead to the development of a variety of diseases in adulthood, including type 2 diabetes, obesity, certain types of cancers, and respiratory disorders including asthma and bronchopulmonary dysplasia [90]. However, much remains to be established about gene–environment interactions in the prenatal stage: in particular, the mechanisms underlying cigarette smoke-induced immune imbalance (i.e., Th1/Th2), defects in stem cells, and epigenetic alterations (nuclear histone modifications and imprinting) and the link of asthma later in life are yet to be established. Accumulation of knowledge by addressing the aforementioned questions may lead to development of appropriate interventional strategies that will help to protect health not only at prenatal stage but also later in adulthood. This may relate to change in lifestyle (regular exercise; cessation of tobacco and its products; eating healthy food; and avoiding foods rich in fat, such as processed foods, pizzas, burgers, and chips).

ROLE OF iNOS IN OBESITY AND RELATION TO INFLAMMATION

NO free radical is synthesized by three different isoforms of NO synthase (NOS) and was originally discovered as an endothelium-derived relaxing factor (EDRF). Endothelial NOS (eNOS) and neuronal NOS (nNOS) are constitutively expressed and synthesize low levels of NO in response to a wide range of stimuli, including, in the case of eNOS, shear stress and insulin [91]. In contrast, inducible NOS (iNOS) is expressed when stimulated by inflammatory cytokines and can produce up to 1000-fold more NO than eNOS [92], which, while important for the immune response, can have detrimental effects on different cell types, including vascular smooth muscle cells (VSMCs) [93] and pancreatic β-cells [94].

Common vascular disease states including hypertension and atherosclerosis are associated with endothelial dysfunction, characterized by reduced bioactivity of NO [95]. Loss of the vasculoprotective effects of NO contributes to disease progression, but the mechanisms underlying endothelial dysfunction remain unclear. Increased $O_2^{\bullet-}$ production in animal models of vascular disease leads to reduced NO bioavailability and endothelial dysfunction. In human blood vessels, the NAD(P)H oxidase system is an important source of $O_2^{\bullet-}$ under pathological conditions and is functionally related to endothelial dysfunction. Furthermore, the C242T polymorphism in the NAD(P)H oxidase p22phox subunit is associated with significantly reduced $O_2^{\bullet-}$ production in patients carrying the 242T allele, suggesting a role for genetic variation in modulating vascular $O_2^{\bullet-}$ production. In vessels from patients with diabetes mellitus, endothelial dysfunction and NAD(P)H oxidase activity are significantly increased compared with matched nondiabetic vessels [95]. Furthermore, the vascular endothelium in diabetic vessels is a net source of $O_2^{\bullet-}$ rather than NO production, due to dysfunction of eNOS. This deficit is dependent on the eNOS cofactor, tetrahydrobiopterin, and is in part mediated by protein kinase C signaling.

These studies suggest an important role for both the NAD(P)H oxidases and eNOS in the increased vascular $O_2^{\bullet-}$ production and endothelial dysfunction in human vascular disease states. Obesity is associated with a chronic inflammatory response characterized by abnormal cytokines and chemokines production, increased acute phase reactants, and activation of inflammatory signaling pathways [96,97]. Recent studies have demonstrated that murine models of obesity are associated with infiltration of adipose tissue by macrophages and activation of several inflammatory genes [98]. The expression of iNOS may be one aspect of such inflammatory activation. Furthermore, iNOS expression is primarily regulated at transcriptional level, and, once transcribed, the enzyme may generate large amounts of NO over long periods of time. In other models of increased iNOS-derived NO (e.g., sepsis), excessive NO may contribute to increased basal bioactive NO and blunt classic, calcium-dependent vasodilatation (e.g., in response to acetylcholine) [98–100]. Thus, iNOS expression induced by cigarette smoke, oxidants, and inflammatory mediators could potentially contribute to several of the obesity-associated abnormalities discussed in this chapter.

Evidence of a significant increase rather than a reduction in basal NO in early stages of obesity has been found using several different approaches. Supporting these reports is the observation of an increased vasoconstrictor response to the nonselective NOS inhibitor L-NMMA, an effect of obesity that was lost in iNOS knockout (KO) mice. This was further supported by the effect of the specific iNOS inhibitor 1400 W to increase tone in the aorta of obese mice, whereas no effect was seen in lean mice. There was also an increase in the plasma nitrate and whole body NO production, which were reduced in iNOS KO mice. Furthermore, iNOS expression was found to be significantly increased in the aorta of obese mice. Earlier studies in vessels exposed to inflammatory cytokines rendered the mice septic using an injection of lipopolysaccharide/endotoxin [99], and iNOS gene transfer studies have all supported a role for iNOS-derived NO in causing vascular dysfunction during obesity [100].

A recent study showing that NO plays a role in energy balance offers potential mechanistic links with obesity and diabetes [101]: chronic administration of the NOS inhibitor, L-NAME, in mice led to a decrease in body weight gain, an effect that was more pronounced in mice on a high-fat diet. Concomitantly, L-NAME (an inhibitor of iNOS) also reversed the harmful effects of high-fat diet on hepatic triglyceride content, glucose tolerance, and *in vivo* insulin sensitivity. Such effects were attributed to the ability of L-NAME to increase energy dissipation by elevating the mRNA levels of uncoupling proteins-1 and -3 in muscles and brown adipose tissue, respectively. In addition, L-NAME also increased the expression of peroxisome proliferator–activated receptor-δ in muscles, a transcription factor central to oxidation of fats in muscles [102]. Since generation of NO in mitochondria by mitochondrial NOS decreases respiration and oxygen consumption [103], it appears that a decreased NO synthesis due to inhibition of NOS by L-NAME leads to enhanced fatty acid oxidation.

INFLAMMATION AND OBESITY

Advances in adipose tissue research over the past decade have led to a better understanding of the mechanisms linking obesity with metabolic syndrome and related complications [104]. Biomarkers of inflammation, such as leukocyte count, TNF-α, IL-6, and C-reactive protein (CRP), are all increased in obesity and insulin resistance; these markers are useful in predicting the development of type 2 diabetes and CVD. It is perhaps no coincidence that all the aforementioned biomarkers of inflammation are also hallmarks of smoking-induced oxidative stress. Thus, it is reasonable to surmise that many of the detrimental effects of smoking and obesity are mediated via a common pathway that is characterized by inflammation, which is triggered by oxidative stress. This interaction could explain the additive, if not synergistic, relationship between these factors in disease development and outcome.

Apart from serving as a storage depot for fat energy, adipose tissue also plays a role of an endocrine organ. Inflammatory cytokines, such as IL-6 and TNF-α, are expressed in human adipose tissue [105,106], and systemic increases in IL-6 concentrations are found to be correlated with increased adiposity. It has been reported that about one-third of the total circulating IL-6 originates from adipose tissue [85], which regulates the hepatic synthesis of the inflammatory acute phase protein, CRP [107]. Elevated serum CRP due to elevated IL-6 suggests an important role of inflammation in cardiovascular pathology due to obesity [108]. Increased CRP has also been found to be positively associated with increased BMI and waist-to-hip ratio in large community-based cohort studies [109,110].

Although it is now established that adipocytes are active participants in the generation of the inflammatory state in obesity, the initiating steps in the pathway are not fully ascertained. Adipocytes secrete several cytokines, including IL-6 and TNF-α, that promote inflammation. Obesity is also associated with an increased recruitment of macrophages in adipose tissue, which also induce an inflammatory response through the release of cytokines and chemokines. An in-depth understanding of the role of adipose tissue in the activation of inflammatory pathways may identify novel treatment strategies by reducing obesity-associated morbidity and mortality.

The aspect of inflammatory response in obesity is reviewed by Wellen et al. [111] in detail. It is clear that obesity promotes inflammatory response and insulin resistance [111]. This may be due to increased oxidative and endoplasmic reticulum (ER) stresses [112–114]. ROS-generating systems, such as mitochondrial electron transport chain, cytochrome 45- and its reductases, and xanthine/xanthine oxidase can all participate in this event in adipose cells/tissues.

Studies involving both cultured cells and whole animals have revealed that ER stress leads to activation of Janus kinase (JNK) and thus contributes to insulin resistance [104]. Interestingly, ER stress is also known to activate I-kappaB kinase (IKK, a cytosolic nuclear factor kappa-B, NF-κB, modulator) and thus may represent a common mechanism for the activation of these important signaling pathways involved in inflammation [115] particularly in endothelium [116]. Another mechanism that may play a role in the initiation of inflammation in obesity is oxidative stress. Increased delivery of glucose to adipose tissue may increase glucose uptake by endothelial cells in the fat pad, leading to excess production of ROS in mitochondria, which inflicts oxidative damage and activates inflammatory signaling cascades inside endothelial cells [116]. Endothelial injury in the adipose tissue is likely to attract inflammatory cells such as monocytes and cause platelet activation and further exacerbate the local inflammation. Hyperglycemia has earlier been reported to also stimulate ROS production in adipocytes, which leads to increased production of proinflammatory cytokines [117].

Since even moderate weight loss was found to be associated with decreased circulating levels of TNF-α, IL-6, and CRP [118], an idea has emerged that controlling the levels of these inflammatory proteins by reducing weight gain could be the effective prevention and treatment strategies for obesity. This idea is corroborated by a finding of significant decreases in urinary F_2-isoprostanes (8-epiPGF$_2$α) in obese men and women after only 3–4 weeks on weight loss programs and subjected to dietary modifications and increased physical activity in addition to smoking cessation [119]. However, long-term controlled studies establishing the beneficial effects of weight loss due to inflammation and oxidative stress, smoking cessation, in addition to other CVD risk factors, are still required.

FACTORS OVERLAPPING INFLAMMATION AND METABOLIC DISEASE

The first molecular link between inflammation and obesity—TNF-α—was established from the discovery that this inflammatory cytokine is overexpressed in the adipose tissues of rodent models of obesity [120]. TNF-α was found to be elevated in adipose tissue and muscle in obese humans [96,121] and other inflammatory genes are elevated in adipose tissue of obese animals [122]. Proatherogenic bioactive lipids activate lipid-targeted signaling pathways through fatty acid-binding proteins (FABPs) and nuclear receptors [111]. Inflammatory mediators and bioactive lipid mediators trigger several genes (TNF-α, IL-6, and matrix metalloproteinases [MMPs]) involved in obesity via fatty acid-binding protein (FABPs) and nuclear receptors, and adipocyte/macrophage FABaP2 (FABP4) and PPAR-γ in macrophages and adipocytes, and promoting insulin resistance [123–125]. It is, therefore, possible that several factors overlap inflammation and metabolic disease are important in obesity. Furthermore, it is conceivable that macrophage accumulation in adipose tissue may be a feature not only of obesity, but of other inflammatory conditions and insulin resistance as well.

OXIDATIVE/NITROSATIVE STRESS IN CARDIOVASCULAR DISEASE: IMPACT ON DISEASE PROGRESSION AND INFLUENCE OF OBESITY AND SMOKING AS RISK FACTORS

OXIDATIVE STRESS AND THE ENDOTHELIUM

The potential contribution of oxidative and nitrosative stress to the progression of CVD is well recognized, but highly complex. The monolayer of endothelial cells that lines all blood vessels is central to protection against CVDs, including hypertension and atherosclerosis. In healthy vessels, the endothelium secretes various antiatherogenic molecules, including the powerful vasodilator, NO, which helps to control vascular tone, maintains the integrity of the vessel wall, and resists the adhesion of leukocytes and platelets. It is now widely accepted that a critical early event in atheroma formation is endothelial cell injury and damage, resulting in endothelial dysfunction [126]. This can occur by several mechanisms: chemical injury can be caused by oxidative stress, including the oxidation of low-density lipoproteins (LDLs), resulting in the formation of damaging oxidized low-density lipoproteins (ox-LDLs), which can themselves cause further endothelial damage. Also, physical damage to the endothelium can occur from shear stress within a vessel; plaque tends to form in regions of low shear stress or at sites usually subjected to particularly turbulent blood flow, such as bifurcation points (aortic arch) in the arterial tree [127]. The consequences of an insult to the endothelium are several folds: first, the endothelium becomes dysfunctional, resulting in a decrease in the net production of NO by eNOS, promoting vasoconstriction and allowing the adhesion of circulating inflammatory cells. A decrease in the normal NO-producing capacity of the endothelium has been demonstrated in patients with risk factors for atherosclerosis, such as hypercholesterolemia, who have impaired endothelium-dependent vasodilatation of resistance vessels, which can be reversed by the delivery of exogenous NO [128]. Additionally, the insult to the endothelium triggers an inflammatory response. Recent findings show that shear stress–mediated angiogenic signaling is impaired by cigarette smoke exposure to human endothelial cells [129]. This is due to inhibition of eNOS by cigarette smoke–derived oxidants/aldehydes. Similarly, exposure of mice lacking the ApoE gene to cigarette smoke caused further lung injury and inflammation associated with endothelial dysfunction and COPD [130]. These studies highlight the impact of cigarette smoke–mediated oxidative stress in endothelial dysfunction, which occurs in obesity.

Oxidative Stress, Smoking, Hypertension, and Obesity

Hypertension, defined as chronically elevated blood pressure, is a complex clinical condition that is recognized as an important risk factor for coronary artery disease (CAD). Many studies have indicated that endothelial dysfunction is a feature of hypertension, but there is still some debate as to whether it is a cause or an effect. However, recent evidence supports the notion that increased angiotensin II–dependent ROS production from NAD(P)H oxidases, with an associated uncoupling of eNOS, leading to generation of further ROS and formation of highly cytotoxic peroxynitrite [132]. Taken together, these events result not only in the loss of the vasodilatory effects of NO, but also in the perpetuation of further endothelial damage induced by cigarette smoke containing reactive oxygen/carbonyl and nitrogen species [131], perhaps contributing to the predisposition of patients with hypertension to other vascular diseases.

Obesity, and particularly visceral obesity, is strongly associated with hypertension, mediated at least in part, through overactivity of the sympathetic nervous system, leading to an increase in peripheral resistance and sodium and water retention [132]. It is understood that increased circulating levels of leptin, free fatty acids, and perhaps insulin all act to increase sympathetic outflow from the hypothalamus, particularly when associated with low levels of adiponectin and ghrelin, which normally act to suppress sympathetic activity and are anti-inflammatory. An important impact of increased renal sympathetic drive is activation of the renin-angiotensin system, with the associated increase in oxidative stress and endothelial dysfunction [133], as discussed earlier. It is somewhat surprising and disappointing, therefore, that clinical trials of dietary antioxidants in hypertension have proved inconclusive, and it remains to be seen whether any more success will be achieved with phytochemicals in this arena (see later sections), given their potential for a combined antioxidant/anti-inflammatory effect.

Oxidative Stress, Lipid Peroxidation, and Inflammation in Atherogenesis

Atherosclerosis is characterized by the formation of lipid-rich plaques in the subendothelial space of conduit blood vessels [127,134–137] and is the process that underpins CAD, peripheral vascular disease, and some forms of stroke. The plaques consist of a necrotic core of lipid-laden inflammatory cells encapsulated by a fibrous, collagen-rich cap made up of VSMCs and extracellular matrix [138]. It is generally accepted that endothelial cell injury is a trigger for atherogenesis, leading to the expression of numerous inflammatory cytokines together with cell-surface adhesion molecules specific for monocytes. Adherent monocytes then translocate through the endothelial layer into the subendothelial space where they differentiate into macrophages that express scavenger receptors and secrete inflammatory cytokines. TNF-α, for example, is essentially produced by monocytes and macrophages in response to oxidative stress, and, in turn, it is the strongest known paracrine activator of monocytes and macrophages [139]. Upon stimulation, these cells also secrete a variety of products including IL-6, stimulating the liver to produce the acute phase reactant CRP [140]. TNF-α and CRP are both found in considerable quantities in atherosclerotic lesions, and they have also been associated with increased cardiovascular risk in numerous large population-based studies.

Besides instigating endothelial injury, oxidative stress is also an important mediator of lipid peroxidation, which is essential for the accumulation of LDL-derived lipids in macrophages that have infiltrated the blood vessel wall. Modification of LDL can occur by various means, including acetylation, exposure to MDA, or ROS-mediated peroxidation that leads to recognition by scavenger receptors and accumulation in macrophages [141]. Peroxynitrite ($ONOO^-$), formed by the rapid reaction of superoxide with NO, can also oxidize LDL [142–144], but might also have proatherogenic effects through modification of the protein, lipid, and antioxidant composition of LDL, most notably by depleting the antioxidant vitamin E content of the particle via the conversion of α-tocopherol to α-tocopherol quinone [141]. The oxidative/nitrosative status of an individual is, therefore, central to their risk of developing atheroma on a number of levels. It follows that both smoking and obesity predispose to increased ROS and encourage atherogenesis, and recent evidence suggests that the prevalence of ROS is likely to be enhanced in atheroma, not only through increased ROS generation but also through reduced synthesis of the endogenous antioxidant glutathione and concomitant depression of the activity of glutathione peroxidase [145].

In the case of obesity, oxidative stress acts in concert with other well-recognized risk factors that are usually associated with the obese condition—namely, hypertension, type 2 diabetes mellitus, and metabolic syndrome, which in turn are heavily linked to oxidative stress. The net effect of increased oxidant load are the raised levels of markers of oxidative stress [83], with an associated reduction in plasma total antioxidant status and superoxide dismutase (SOD) activity in blood [146]. Furthermore, there is now clear evidence that increased oxidative stress in accumulated fat is important in the development of metabolic syndrome on account of activation of NAD(P)H oxidase in adipocytes [147]. The importance of ROS in mediating many of the secondary pathologies that stem from obesity was further confirmed in this study by the benefit achieved through antioxidant treatment, with respect to dysregulation of the metabolic pathways relating to glucose and lipids, as well as the genes associated with adipocytokines.

These are encouraging findings with respect to phytochemicals, which might prove even more effective than conventional therapy (see later section on "Phytochemicals"). Hyperlipidemia is a critical risk factor for vascular disease that one might intuitively believe to be raised in obese individuals, but several studies do not necessarily show the expected correlation between BMI and either total cholesterol, LDL cholesterol, or serum triglyceride, particularly in humans. Indeed, although obesity is widely believed to be a risk factor for development of atherosclerosis [148,149], a body of evidence suggests that no correlation exists between obesity *per se* and plaque deposition in coronary arteries [150,151], although it clearly predisposes to other risk factors, most notably hypertension, insulin resistance, and diabetes [146,152]. Smoking, on the other hand, is a very well-recognized risk factor for vascular disease due to elevated levels of ox-LDL, an effect that is primarily mediated via its prooxidative [153,154] and proinflammatory effects [155].

IMPACT OF SMOKING AND OBESITY ON PLAQUE PROGRESSION AND RUPTURE, LEADING TO THROMBOTIC EVENTS

Atherosclerotic plaques evolve and grow as the ox-LDL accumulated in macrophage-derived foam cells causes further endothelial damage and is a chemoattractant for additional macrophage recruitment [156]; hence, a perpetual cycle of endothelial damage, monocyte recruitment, and accumulation of ox-LDL is established. Activated macrophages resident in the early lesion secrete numerous cytokines and growth factors, including platelet-derived growth factor (PDGF), basic fibroblast growth factor (bFGF), IL-1, TNF-α, and transforming growth factor-β (TGF-β) [127]. All of these factors induce VSMC hypertrophy and hyperplasia and promote secretion of extracellular matrix and connective tissue to form a mesh over the fatty streak. Eventually, calcification occurs and a fibrous cap forms over the top of the plaque, encapsulating the highly thrombogenic lipid core and maintaining a barrier between the plaque contents and the circulation [134–138]. Although atherosclerotic lesions can be widespread by middle age, the vast majority remain subclinical with only a small minority of plaques becoming symptomatic. The physical presence of a plaque within an arterial wall may impinge on the vessel lumen, causing partial occlusion of the vessel, which might be sufficient to cause substantial restriction of blood flow and tissue ischemia, resulting in chronic stable angina pectoris. A more serious situation arises if the fibrous cap is subject to mechanical breakdown or erosion such that it is considered to be unstable and liable to rupture, generating a thrombus and leading to more serious acute cardiovascular syndromes, such as unstable angina, myocardial infarction, and stroke [157]. The determinants of plaque vulnerability to rupture have yet to be fully identified, but a growing body of evidence is emerging that points to a critical role for both the thickness of the VSMC layer overlaying the core [158], and to unresolved inflammation within the plaque [135,159,160].

The crucial role of unresolved inflammation in the progression of atherosclerosis and ultimately to destabilization of the plaque is increasingly being identified as a potential target for therapeutic intervention. It is entirely possible that cigarette smoking and obesity, through their proinflammatory and proatherogenic effects, might exacerbate these important phases of plaque development, with potentially fatal consequences. Indeed, smoking is one of the most powerful risk factors for atherosclerotic disease, but the relationships between smoking and CVD result from multiple mechanisms that interact to contribute to atherosclerosis, vascular injury, thrombosis, and vascular dysfunction [161]. Several products of tobacco combustion, including nicotine, free radicals, and aromatic compounds, have been shown to cause release of catecholamines, endothelial injury, oxidation of LDL, increased plasma fibrinogen, and alteration of platelet activity (activation and its mean volume). All these agents are proatherogenic in nature [162].

Prospective cohort studies have consistently shown smoking to be one of the strongest risk factors for the development of peripheral vascular disease. The risk for progression of atherosclerotic peripheral vascular disease is also increased among patients who continue to smoke compared with those who quit [22,137]. The Atherosclerosis Risk in Community study showed a substantial increase in atherosclerosis progression in patients who smoked compared with those who had never smoked and an intermediate progression in former smokers. The progression of atherosclerosis attributable to smoking was more substantial than that due to other cardiovascular risk factors. The risk of progression of atherosclerosis was highest in smokers with obesity who had other risk factors, such as hypertension and diabetes mellitus, smoking being one of the strongest cardiovascular risk factors for atherosclerotic diseases [23]. Several studies have revealed increased plasma levels of TNF-α and of CRP in smokers as compared to nonsmokers [163,164], suggesting that part of the coronary risk associated with smoking may relate to increased inflammatory activity. However, the prevalence of CVD varies substantially among smoking individuals [165]; this could indicate that genetic factors are important determinants of the biological pathways linking smoking and obesity with CVD risk [166].

The effects of nicotine are much less important than the prothrombotic effects of other products of tobacco combustion, as there is no apparent dose–response relationship between nicotine and cardiovascular events [162]. Tobacco/cigarette smoke-derived nicotine and carbon monoxide produce acute cardiovascular consequences. These include altered myocardial performance, tachycardia, hypertension, and vasoconstriction [21]. Cigarette smoke, in view of its composition consisting of host of oxidants, causes redox signals that recruit and activate macrophages and other inflammatory cells. Persistent local or systemic oxidative stress, due to sustained smoking, leads to the expression of pro-inflammatory mediators and generation of lipid peroxides, which injure blood vessel walls by damaging endothelial cells, thus increasing permeability to lipids and other blood components. Among metabolic and biochemical changes induced by smoking, there is also is a tendency for increased serum cholesterol, reduced HDL, elevated plasma free fatty acids, elevated vasopressin, and a thrombogenic imbalance of prostacyclin and thromboxane A_2. In addition to rheologic and hematologic changes from increased erythrocytes, leukocytes, and fibrinogen, smokers have alterations in platelet aggregation and survival that cause thrombosis [21]. In fact, it has recently been shown that the CC polymorphism in the promoter region of the CD14 gene (CD14-159C/T) is associated with common carotid artery intima-media thickness in smokers, but not in nonsmokers [167]. Furthermore, smoking is known to reduce the activity of the endogenous fibrinolytic pathway that usually degrades thrombi in an effort to restore blood flow through an occluded vessel, while both smoking and obesity are prothrombotic through activation of platelets. Once again, one could envisage the potential benefits of phytochemicals, not only by preventing the inflammatory events that might predispose to plaque rupture, but also by reducing the propensity for thrombus formation.

PHYTOCHEMICAL MANAGEMENT OF OBESITY AND SMOKING-RELATED DISEASES ASSOCIATED WITH OXIDATIVE STRESS AND INFLAMMATION

Cigarette smoking induces oxidative stress and depletes antioxidants by elevation in oxidant levels, and a resultant depletion of cellular antioxidants is utilized to counter the effects of the oxidants. The downstream effect of smoke-dependent induction of oxidative stress leads to local generation of inflammatory cytokines, such as TNF-α, IL-1, IL-6, and IL-8. These cytokines in turn activate and recruit more inflammatory cells and may lead to systemic effects at various sites in the body. While oxidative injury to the lungs can result in lung cancers and COPD, inflammatory responses in the blood vessel may lead to various cardiovascular anomalies. In obese subjects, the risk of oxidative injury is heightened by the fact that the fatty stores by themselves behave as seats of inflammatory reactions and, as discussed earlier, may trigger oxidative stress and activation of local macrophages, thus leading to metabolic syndrome. This influence of obesity may augment consumption of the cellular antioxidant pools and further add to oxidative imbalance. Oxidatively modified molecules, especially lipids, act as triggers for expression of cell adhesion molecules in the vasculature. Circulating monocytes and platelets (smoking activates these cells) then adhere to the intimal surfaces and extravasate to the subintimal space, leading to atherogenesis; hence, antioxidant supplementation/therapies are logical, particularly via phytochemicals in addition to exercise, obesity, and cardiovascular managements via pharmacological means (use of lipid-lowering drugs) [168]. Such phytochemicals/polyphenols/bioactive botanicals include tomato-derived lycopene, broccoli-derived sulforaphane, garlic-derived allyl disulfides, turmeric-derived curcumin, red wine/grape-derived resveratrol, green tea-derived catechins, and berries-derived anthocyanins.

Plant-based diets have a lower caloric and increased nutrient density, which are important factors in curbing the obesity in the general population. Furthermore, phytochemicals have beneficial effects in protection against CVD and other cardiovascular risks caused by endothelial dysfunction and obesity [168,170,171]. Phytochemicals found in fruits and vegetables can affect the aforementioned processes by several mechanisms. Such mechanisms may involve regulation of cell proliferation and apoptosis [172], anti-inflammatory action [173], growth factors, such as insulin-like growth factor (IGF-1) [176], and carcinogenesis [177,178].

Overall, bioactive phytochemicals present in foods have been increasingly investigated for their potential health benefit effects and for prevention of chronic disorders such as cancer, CVD, and inflammatory and metabolic diseases including obesity. Polyphenols/phytochemicals are shown to modulate physiological and molecular pathways that are involved in energy metabolism, adiposity, and obesity. It may be noted, however, that bioactive phytochemicals have different beneficial effects when taken in whole fruits and vegetables (in food matrix) versus dietary supplementation. Furthermore, the effects are dependent on microbial flora of the gut. In the following section, we will focus on the beneficial effects of some polyphenols, such as resveratrol, catechins, anthocyanins, and curcumin, in controlling oxidative stress and inflammation associated with cardiovascular problems in obesity under oxidative stress induced by cigarette smoking.

RESVERATROL

Resveratrol is a widely studied polyphenol first identified in grape skins and has well-documented antioxidant and anti-inflammatory properties [179]. Resveratrol has been reported to have beneficial effects in several disease conditions, such as CVD, diabetes, cancer, and obesity [180–182]. One of the main mechanisms by which resveratrol exerts its beneficial effect on obesity is via the phosphorylation and activation of adenosine monophosphate (AMP)-activated protein kinase (AMPK), which upregulates fatty acid oxidation and increases uptake of glucose through translocation of Glut 4 [183]. In addition, by upregulating SIRT1, resveratrol increases PPAR-γ coactivator (PGC)-1α leading to mitochondrial biogenesis and oxidative phosphorylation, and thus leading to suppression of lipid accumulation [184,185]. In mice fed with atherogenic diet, resveratrol increases expression of SIRT1 leading to suppressed expression of PPAR-γ and accumulation of fat in liver [184]. In another study involving 3T3-L1 cells, treatment with resveratrol reduced PPAR-γ expression in part through ubiquitin-dependent proteasomal degradation [185]. Furthermore, treatment of isolated rat hepatocytes with resveratrol has been shown to inhibit fatty acid and triglyceride synthesis, thus contributing to its lipid-lowering effect [186]. Several studies in rodent models have indicated that administration of resveratrol can mimic the effects of caloric restriction, such as increase in longevity and motor functions, as well as prevention of cardiac and skeletal muscle dysfunction associated with aging [187]. Resveratrol also protects against liver damage by hepatotoxins through its antioxidant and anti-inflammatory properties [188].

In cell culture studies, resveratrol has been shown to enhance lipolytic activity in adipocytes by increasing the levels of cAMP [189] and inhibiting adipogenesis in isolated human adipocytes. When combined with genistein, the aforementioned effects of resveratrol have been shown to be potentiated [190,191]. These observations have been supported by studies on laboratory animals, wherein treatment with resveratrol significantly reduced fat depot size and total body fat in high-fat-fed and genetically obese rodents. In another study, mice fed with high-fat-atherogenic diet along with 125 mg resveratrol/kg diet exhibited less gain in body weight, accompanied by less fat and triglyceride accumulation, and had a lower liver weight compared to nonsupplemented mice [184]. Microarray analysis of genes in the liver subjected to treatment with resveratrol exhibited downregulation of genes involved in lipogenesis. Although various studies at molecular, cellular, and animal levels provide compelling evidences as to the ability of resveratrol in prevention of obesity through multiple mechanisms, in-depth epidemiological and clinical studies are still needed to establish whether the consumption of resveratrol will be effective in preventing obesity in humans.

CURCUMIN

Curcumin is one of the earliest identified and most studied polyphenol found in the spice turmeric; the perennial herb *Curcuma longa* has been in use since the second millennium BC [192].

Curcumin is a low-molecular-weight polyphenol belonging to the curcuminoid family of molecules and has been reported to have several beneficial biological properties, such as antioxidant, anti-inflammatory, anticancer, antiangiogenesis, chemopreventive, and chemotherapeutic properties [193]. Various studies involving cell and animal culture have explored the anti-inflammatory, antioxidant, and antiadiposity effects of curcumin. The antiadiposity effect of curcumin may underpin several mechanisms, such as modulation of energy metabolism, inflammation, and suppression of angiogenesis.

Curcumin suppresses angiogenesis and tumor growth through downregulation of vascular endothelial growth factor (VEGF), bFGF, and epidermal growth factor (EGF), as well as angiopoietin and hypoxia-inducible factors (HIFs)-1α [194,195]. Since angiogenesis is also required for adipogenesis, therefore, curcumin may prevent adipogenesis through suppression of angiogenesis within the adipose tissue [196]. Angiogenesis in the adipose tissue is mediated by adipose tissue secretion of several adipokines, such as leptin, adiponectin, resistin, visfatin, TNF-α, IL-6, IL-1, and VEGF [197]. Therefore, curcumin-dependent inhibition of angiogenesis in adipose tissue could be an important strategy for preventing adipogenesis and, hence, obesity. Curcumin also stimulates fatty acid oxidation by activating AMPK and downregulates acetyl-CoA carboxylase (ACC) activity through phosphorylation, which in turn downregulates the flow of acetyl-CoA to malonyl-CoA, leading to upregulation of carnitine palmitoyltransferase-1 (CPT-1) involved in the transfer of cytosolic long-chain fatty acyl-CoA into the mitochondria for oxidation [198]. Through activation of AMPK, curcumin also inhibits synthesis of glycerolipids by inhibiting glycerol-3-phosphate acyltransferase-1 (GPAT-1) activity, involved in esterification of fatty acids to glycerol to form storage forms of triglycerides [199].

Additional studies in animal models of obesity have revealed antiadipogenic effects of curcumin on body weight and fat, and energy metabolism. Administration of 2–10 g/kg curcumin for 2 weeks in rats was shown to reduce epididymal adipose tissue, attenuated liver fatty acid synthesis, and increased rat liver acetyl-CoA oxidase activity, the first enzyme involved in fatty acid oxidation [200]. Furthermore, curcumin also suppressed expression of PPAR-γ and C/EBPα in adipose tissue and thus suppressed adipogenesis and lipogenesis [200,201]. Adipose tissue growth and expansion was also suppressed by curcumin via suppression of differentiation of pre-adipocytes to adipocytes [202]. Most studies on curcumin have been focused on its antioxidant, anti-inflammatory, and anticarcinogenic properties; however, more studies are warranted on the antiobesity effects of curcumin.

Catechins

There are five major catechins in green tea, including catechin, epicatechin, epicatechin gallate, epigallocatechin, and epigallocatechin gallate (EGCG), of which EGCG comprises more than 40% of the total polyphenolic mixture of green tea catechins [203]. Various studies have reported the beneficial effects of consuming green tea, such as antioxidant and anti-inflammatory activities, anticancer and CVD, and obesity prevention properties.

EGCG elicits antiobesity effects through several different mechanisms, such as suppression of adipocyte differentiation and proliferation, inhibition of fat absorption from the intestine, and suppression of catechol-O-methyltransferase (COMT), an enzyme that inhibits fatty acid oxidation in brown adipose tissue [203]. The mechanism of action of green tea on fatty acid oxidation has been reviewed in detail elsewhere [204]. EGCG has been shown to inhibit adipocyte proliferation by decreasing phosphorylated ERK1/2, cdk2, and cyclin D1 proteins and cell growth arrest at Go/G1 [205] and by inducing apoptosis in mature adipocytes [206].

AMPK is the master switch involved in regulation of energy metabolism. Increased AMP:ATP ratio within the cell activates AMPK, which, therefore, acts as a sensor for cellular energy regulation [207]. AMP binding with AMPK allosterically activates AMPK by phosphorylation [208], which in turn downregulates anabolic pathways and enhances catabolic pathways through regulating the activity of several key enzymes of energy metabolism. AMPK inhibits the accumulation of fat by modulating downstream signaling components. EGCG increases both the expression and the phosphorylation of AMPK and phosphorylation downstream LKB1, leading to decreased esterification of fatty acids to triglyceride, hence increasing fatty acid oxidation [209]. EGCG and other catechins, thus, contributing to the reduction of adipogenesis and prevention of growth and expansion of adipose tissue through several mechanisms.

EGCG has been shown to decrease diet-induced adipogenesis and obesity by enhancing fat oxidation in mice [210]. Therefore, consumption of green tea may be regarded as an effective way for reducing body weight via increasing fatty acid oxidation and increasing energy expenditure. Although modulation of fatty acid oxidation is an important mechanism by which catechins influence adipogenesis, it must be noted that very high intake of catechins or EGCG may cause hepatotoxicity, inflammation, and necrotic damage of liver cells [211,212].

ANTHOCYANINS

Blueberries and blackberries are particularly the abundant source of phenolic compounds, such as hydroxycinnamic acids, flavonoids, and proanthocyanidines [213,214]. They are also rich in anthocyanins and contain more than 20 types of anthocyanins [215]. Several studies have reported that consumption of blueberries may provide health benefits, such as improvement in cognitive function [216], antioxidant effects [217], protection against inflammation [218] and endothelial dysfunction [213], and modulation of adiposity associated with obesity [214,215].

Administration of 2.9 mg/g purified anthocyanins to mice obtaining 60% calories from fat decreased their body and adipose tissue weight compared to high-fat-fed controls. On the contrary, mice fed with high-fat diet (45% calories from fat) and 10% freeze-dried extracts of whole blueberries resulted in the increase of body weight gain rather than the expected decrease [219]. Furthermore, administration of purified anthocyanins lowered serum triglyceride, cholesterol, and leptin levels. In contrast, liver lipid and triglyceride levels remained unaltered [220].

Bacterial transformation of blueberry juice increases the phenolic content and quadruples the antioxidant activity of blueberry juice. When administered to mice (40 mL/kg/day, for 3 weeks), the biotransformed blueberry juice was found to reduce body weight gain, abdominal fat pad size, and liver weights via its anorexic effect. However, chronic administration of this juice (80 mL/kg/day) in diabetic rats did not affect body weight gain, but was found to reduce blood glucose and insulin levels, and increase adiponectin levels [214]. Adiponectin has been shown to reverse insulin resistance and to lower muscle triglyceride levels by increasing influx and combustion of free fatty acids leading to decreased hepatic levels of triglycerides [221].

Diet-induced obesity is associated with adipocyte death within the adipocyte tissue. The dead adipocytes attract macrophages leading to release of proinflammatory cytokines like TNF-α, IL-6, and MCP-1 and hence cause inflammation, which further leads to development of insulin resistance [215,219,222]. Administration of 4% blueberry juice in obese mice leads to protection against adipocyte death and downregulation of TNF-α in macrophages. Furthermore, downregulation of CD11c in macrophages by blueberry juice leads to inhibition of macrophage infiltration [223]. Although contradicting and inconsistent results have been obtained by using different forms and concentrations of blueberry juice, the parameters affected by obesity, such as insulin sensitivity and inflammation were consistently found to be decreased by blueberry supplementation.

Obesity research has attracted a greater attention in recent years and has provided greater insights into neuroendocrine and hormonal control of hunger, satiety, and energy expenditure [224,225]. According to recent meta-analysis of genome-wide searches for susceptibility loci for obesity, at least 50 chromosomal segments have been identified that harbor alleles involved in adiposity or leanness [226]. It is suggested that genome-wide association studies in humans may give us greater insight on the mechanisms of triglyceride storage, an idea that is supported by the recent discovery of fat mass- and obesity-associated (FTO) gene [227]. Therefore, to identify and establish therapeutic targets for treatment, prevention and management of obesity still remains unclear, but personalized therapy may potentially be useful in the management of obesity and related complications.

CONCLUSIONS

Smoking, oxidative stress, inflammation, and obesity are intimately associated phenomena. While many sociopsychological factors influence both smoking and eating habits, the emerging physiological factors consequent to smoking and eating abuse lead to a variety of metabolic disorders including diabetes mellitus and can independently, or in conjunction with metabolic disorders, lead to CVDs including hypertension and atherosclerosis. Hormones synthesized by the adipocytes, such as leptin and adiponectin; hormones of the intestinal tract, such as cholecystokinin; and brain-related peptides, such as neuropeptide Y and ghrelin, undergo a complex interplay of regulatory cascades, which modulate hunger and cachexia, insulin secretion, and a wide variety of other metabolic effects. Interestingly, adipocytes laden with fats can themselves generate oxidants and free radicals, which in turn can initiate cytokine-dependent signals to activate and recruit macrophages and other inflammatory cells that may lead to the development of various metabolic disorders and more complex vascular diseases. Cigarette smoke, which itself consists of an array of oxidizing species, can elicit similar inflammatory responses and can either initiate obesity-dependent inflammatory processes or direct an obese condition to a particular disease; therefore, obesity–oxidative stress–cigarette smoking appears to be a multifactorial complication, and several focal points may be available for therapeutic targeting. Understanding the exact mechanism(s) involved in the etiopathogenesis of complications of obesity and smoking will reveal newer strategies in therapy for amelioration of such complications.

Phytochemicals from various plant/food sources may exert their antiobesity effects through one or a combination of several mechanisms, such as suppression of fat absorption, suppression of anabolic pathways, stimulation of catabolic pathways in adipose tissues, inhibition of angiogenesis in adipose tissues, inhibition of differentiation of preadipocytes to adipocytes, stimulation of apoptosis of mature adipocytes, and reduction of chronic inflammation and oxidatives stress associated with adiposity. Hence, phytochemicals serve as better, cost-effective, and less toxic long-term therapeutic alternatives for the prevention and management of obesity and associated cardiovascular pathologies.

ACKNOWLEDGMENT

We thank Dr. Jae-woong Hwang for formatting the references.

ABBREVIATIONS

ARDS	acute respiratory distress syndrome
BMI	body mass index
CAD	coronary artery disease
COPD	chronic obstructive pulmonary disease
CRP	C-reactive protein
EDRF	endothelium-derived relaxing factor
FABP	fatty acid–binding protein
IKK	I-kappa kinase
IL-1	interleukin 1
IL-6	interleukin 6
IL-8	interleukin 8
LDL	low-density lipoprotein

MCP-1   monocyte chemotactic peptide-1
MMP   matrix metalloproteinases
NO   nitric oxide
NOS   nitric oxide synthase
eNOS   endothelial NOS
iNOS   inducible NOS
nNOS   neuronal NOS
NOX   NADPH oxidases
PPAR-γ   peroxisome proliferator–activated receptor-γ
REE   resting energy expenditure
RNS   reactive nitrogen species
ROS   reactive oxygen species
TNF-α   tumor necrosis factor-α
WAT   white adipose tissue

REFERENCES

1. Van Itallie, T.B., Health implications of overweight and obesity in the United States, *Ann Intern Med*, 103, 983, 1985.
2. Mokdad, A.H. et al., The continuing increase of diabetes in the US, *Diabetes Care*, 24, 412, 2001.
3. Ogden, C.L. et al., Prevalence of overweight and obesity in the United States, 1999–2004, *JAMA*, 295, 1549, 2006.
4. Wiseman, M., The second World Cancer Research Fund/American Institute for Cancer Research expert report. Food, nutrition, physical activity, and the prevention of cancer: A global perspective, *Proc Nutr Soc*, 67, 253, 2008.
5. Calle, E.E. et al., Overweight, obesity, and mortality from cancer in a prospectively studied cohort of U.S. adults, *N Engl J Med*, 348, 1625, 2003.
6. Bronson, R. et al., Biomarkers as early predictors of long-term health status and human immune function, *Nutr Rev*, 57, S7, 1999.
7. Kannel, W.B. et al., Regional obesity and risk of cardiovascular disease; the Framingham Study, *J Clin Epidemiol*, 44, 183, 1991.
8. Kenchaiah, S. et al., Obesity and the risk of heart failure, *N Engl J Med*, 347, 305, 2002.
9. Field, A.E. et al., Impact of overweight on the risk of developing common chronic diseases during a 10-year period, *Arch Intern Med*, 161, 1581, 2001.
10. Flier, J.S., The adipocyte: Storage depot or node on the energy information superhighway? *Cell*, 80, 15, 1995.
11. Figlewicz, D.P. et al., Endocrine regulation of food intake and body weight, *J Lab Clin Med*, 127, 328, 1996.
12. Rohner-Jeanrenaud, F., A neuroendocrine reappraisal of the dual-centre hypothesis: Its implications for obesity and insulin resistance, *Int J Obes Relat Metab Disord*, 19, 517, 1995.
13. Friedman, M.I. et al., Integrated metabolic control of food intake, *Brain Res Bull*, 17, 855, 1986.
14. Geary, N., Role of gut peptides in meal regulation, in: *Obesity: Advances in Understanding and Treatment*, Weston, L.A. and Savage, L.M. (eds.), International Business Communications, Southborough, MA, pp. 2.1.1–3.2.34, 1996.
15. Leibel, R.L. et al., Metabolic and hemodynamic responses to endogenous and exogenous catecholamines in formerly obese subjects, *Am J Physiol*, 260, R785, 1991.
16. Arone, L.J. et al., Autonomic nervous system activity in weight gain and weight loss, *Am J Physiol*, 269, R222, 1995.
17. Butera, P.C. et al., Modulation of the satiety effect of cholecystokinin by estradiol, *Physiol Behav*, 53, 1235, 1993.
18. Woods, S.C. et al., The evaluation of insulin as a metabolic signal influencing behavior via the brain, *Neurosci Biobehav Rev*, 20, 139, 1996.
19. Bray, G.A., Nutrient intake is modulated by peripheral peptide administration, *Obes Res*, 3 Suppl 4, 569S, 1995.
20. Webber, J., Energy balance in obesity, *Proc Nutr Soc*, 62, 539, 2003.
21. Krupski, W.C., The peripheral vascular consequences of smoking, *Ann Vasc Surg*, 5, 291, 1991.

22. Howard, G. et al., Cigarette smoking and progression of atherosclerosis: The Atherosclerosis Risk in Communities (ARIC) Study, *JAMA*, 279, 119, 1998.
23. Gensini, G.F. et al., Classical risk factors and emerging elements in the risk profile for coronary artery disease, *Eur Heart J*, 19 Suppl A, A53, 1998.
24. Chiolero, A. et al., Consequences of smoking for body weight, body fat distribution, and insulin resistance, *Am J Clin Nutr*, 87, 801, 2008.
25. Chen, H. et al., Effect of short-term cigarette smoke exposure on body weight, appetite and brain neuropeptide Y in mice, *Neuropsychopharmacology*, 30, 713, 2005.
26. Ding, E.L. et al., Smoking and type 2 diabetes: Underrecognized risks and disease burden, *JAMA*, 298, 2675, 2007.
27. National Digestive Diseases Information Clearinghouse, Smoking and your digestive system, http://digestive.niddk,nih.gov/ddiseases/pubs/smoking/ (November 7, 2009).
28. Preston, A.M., Cigarette smoking-nutritional implications, *Prog Food Nutr Sci*, 15, 183, 1991.
29. Church, D.F. et al., Free-radical chemistry of cigarette smoke and its toxicological implications, *Environ Health Perspect*, 64, 111, 1985.
30. Zang, L.Y. et al., Detection of free radicals in aqueous extracts of cigarette tar by electron spin resonance, *Free Radic Biol Med*, 19, 161, 1995.
31. Pryor, W.A. et al., Oxidants in cigarette smoke. Radicals, hydrogen peroxide, peroxynitrate, and peroxynitrite, *Ann N Y Acad Sci*, 686, 12, 1993.
32. Meier, U. et al., Endocrine regulation of energy metabolism: Review of pathobiochemical and clinical chemical aspects of leptin, ghrelin, adiponectin, and resistin, *Clin Chem*, 50, 1511, 2004.
33. Schwartz, M.W. et al., Insulin in the brain: A hormonal regulator of energy balance, *Endocr Rev*, 13, 387, 1992.
34. Schwartz, M.W. et al., Specificity of leptin action on elevated blood glucose levels and hypothalamic neuropeptide Y gene expression in ob/ob mice, *Diabetes*, 45, 531, 1996.
35. Rosenbaum, M. et al., Effects of gender, body composition, and menopause on plasma concentrations of leptin, *J Clin Endocrinol Metab*, 81, 3424, 1996.
36. Kolaczynski, J.W. et al., Acute and chronic effects of insulin on leptin production in humans: Studies in vivo and in vitro, *Diabetes*, 45, 699, 1996.
37. Rentsch, J. et al., Regulation of ob gene mRNA levels in cultured adipocytes, *FEBS Lett*, 379, 55, 1996.
38. Hosoda, H. et al., Structural divergence of human ghrelin. Identification of multiple ghrelin-derived molecules produced by post-translational processing, *J Biol Chem*, 278, 64, 2003.
39. Tomas, E. et al., Enhanced muscle fat oxidation and glucose transport by ACRP30 globular domain: Acetyl-CoA carboxylase inhibition and AMP-activated protein kinase activation, *Proc Natl Acad Sci USA*, 99, 16309, 2002.
40. Faraj, M. et al., Plasma acylation-stimulating protein, adiponectin, leptin, and ghrelin before and after weight loss induced by gastric bypass surgery in morbidly obese subjects, *J Clin Endocrinol Metab*, 88, 1594, 2003.
41. Sinclair, D.A. et al., Extrachromosomal rDNA circles—A cause of aging in yeast, *Cell*, 91, 1033, 1997.
42. Blander, G. et al., The Sir2 family of protein deacetylases, *Annu Rev Biochem*, 73, 417, 2004.
43. Lin, S.J. et al., Requirement of NAD and SIR2 for life-span extension by calorie restriction in *Saccharomyces cerevisiae*, *Science*, 289, 2126, 2000.
44. Rogina, B. et al., Sir2 mediates longevity in the fly through a pathway related to calorie restriction, *Proc Natl Acad Sci USA*, 101, 15998, 2004.
45. Wang, Y. et al., Overlapping and distinct functions for a *Caenorhabditis elegans* SIR2 and DAF-16/FOXO, *Mech Ageing Dev*, 127, 48, 2006.
46. Frye, R.A., Phylogenetic classification of prokaryotic and eukaryotic Sir2-like proteins, *Biochem Biophys Res Commun*, 273, 793, 2000.
47. Luo, J. et al., Negative control of p53 by Sir2alpha promotes cell survival under stress, *Cell*, 107, 137, 2001.
48. Brunet, A. et al., Stress-dependent regulation of FOXO transcription factors by the SIRT1 deacetylase, *Science*, 303, 2011, 2004.
49. Araki, T. et al., Increased nuclear NAD biosynthesis and SIRT1 activation prevent axonal degeneration, *Science*, 305, 1010, 2004.
50. Alcendor, R.R. et al., Silent information regulator 2alpha, a longevity factor and class III histone deacetylase, is an essential endogenous apoptosis inhibitor in cardiac myocytes, *Circ Res*, 95, 971, 2004.
51. Picard, F. et al., Sirt1 promotes fat mobilization in white adipocytes by repressing PPAR-gamma, *Nature*, 429, 771, 2004.

52. Rodgers, J.T. et al., Nutrient control of glucose homeostasis through a complex of PGC-1alpha and SIRT1, *Nature*, 434, 113, 2005.

53. Frescas, D. et al., Nuclear trapping of the forkhead transcription factor FoxO1 via Sirt-dependent deacetylation promotes expression of glucogenetic genes, *J Biol Chem*, 280, 20589, 2005.

54. Larson-Meyer, D.E. et al., Effect of calorie restriction with or without exercise on insulin sensitivity, beta-cell function, fat cell size, and ectopic lipid in overweight subjects, *Diabetes Care*, 29, 1337, 2006.

55. Lefevre, M. et al., Caloric restriction alone and with exercise improves CVD risk in healthy non-obese individuals, *Atherosclerosis*, 203, 206, 2009.

56. Yang, S.R. et al., Sirtuin regulates cigarette smoke-induced proinflammatory mediator release via RelA/p65 NF-kappaB in macrophages in vitro and in rat lungs in vivo: Implications for chronic inflammation and aging, *Am J Physiol Lung Cell Mol Physiol*, 292, L567, 2007.

57. Rajendrasozhan, S. et al., SIRT1, an antiinflammatory and antiaging protein, is decreased in lungs of patients with chronic obstructive pulmonary disease, *Am J Respir Crit Care Med*, 177, 861, 2008.

58. Arunachalam, G. et al., SIRT1 regulates oxidant- and cigarette smoke-induced eNOS acetylation in endothelial cells: Role of resveratrol, *Biochem Biophys Res Commun*, 393, 66, 2010.

59. Cohen, H.Y. et al., Calorie restriction promotes mammalian cell survival by inducing the SIRT1 deacetylase, *Science*, 305, 390, 2004.

60. Kanfi, Y. et al., Regulation of SIRT1 protein levels by nutrient availability, *FEBS Lett*, 582, 2417, 2008.

61. Pedersen, S.B. et al., Low Sirt1 expression, which is upregulated by fasting, in human adipose tissue from obese women, *Int J Obes (Lond)*, 32, 1250, 2008.

62. Schug, T.T. et al., Sirtuin 1 in lipid metabolism and obesity, *Ann Med*, 43, 198, 2011.

63. Baur, J.A. et al., Resveratrol improves health and survival of mice on a high-calorie diet, *Nature*, 444, 337, 2006.

64. Lagouge, M. et al., Resveratrol improves mitochondrial function and protects against metabolic disease by activating SIRT1 and PGC-1alpha, *Cell*, 127, 1109, 2006.

65. Yang, T. et al., SIRT1 and endocrine signaling, *Trends Endocrinol Metab*, 17, 186, 2006.

66. Heltweg, B. et al., Antitumor activity of a small-molecule inhibitor of human silent information regulator 2 enzymes, *Cancer Res*, 66, 4368, 2006.

67. Chen, D. et al., Tissue-specific regulation of SIRT1 by calorie restriction, *Genes Dev*, 22, 1753, 2008.

68. Nakahata, Y. et al., The NAD+-dependent deacetylase SIRT1 modulates CLOCK-mediated chromatin remodeling and circadian control, *Cell*, 134, 329, 2008.

69. Asher, G. et al., SIRT1 regulates circadian clock gene expression through PER2 deacetylation, *Cell*, 134, 317, 2008.

70. Zillikens, M.C. et al., SIRT1 genetic variation is related to BMI and risk of obesity, *Diabetes*, 58, 2828, 2009.

71. Rahman, I. et al., Glutathione, stress responses, and redox signaling in lung inflammation, *Antioxid Redox Signal*, 7, 42, 2005.

72. English, J.P. et al., Tobacco and coronary diseases, *JAMA*, 115, 1327, 1940.

73. Willett, W.C. et al., Relative and absolute excess risks of coronary heart disease among women who smoke cigarettes, *N Engl J Med*, 317, 1303, 1987.

74. Babior, B.M., NADPH oxidase, *Curr Opin Immunol*, 16, 42, 2004.

75. Jackson, R.S. et al., Obesity and impaired prohormone processing associated with mutations in the human prohormone convertase 1 gene, *Nat Genet*, 16, 303, 1997.

76. Weisberg, S.P. et al., Obesity is associated with macrophage accumulation in adipose tissue, *J Clin Invest*, 112, 1796, 2003.

77. Xu, H. et al., Chronic inflammation in fat plays a crucial role in the development of obesity-related insulin resistance, *J Clin Invest*, 112, 1821, 2003.

78. Shiose, A. et al., A novel superoxide-producing NAD(P)H oxidase in kidney, *J Biol Chem*, 276, 1417, 2001.

79. Mahadev, K. et al., The NAD(P)H oxidase homolog Nox4 modulates insulin-stimulated generation of H_2O_2 and plays an integral role in insulin signal transduction, *Mol Cell Biol*, 24, 1844, 2004.

80. Yang, S. et al., Expression of Nox4 in osteoclasts, *J Cell Biochem*, 92, 238, 2004.

81. Sorescu, D. et al., Superoxide production and expression of nox family proteins in human atherosclerosis, *Circulation*, 105, 1429, 2002.

82. Curzio, M. et al., Possible role of aldehydic lipid peroxidation products as chemoattractants, *Int J Tissue React*, 9, 295, 1987.

83. Keaney, J.F. Jr. et al., Obesity and systemic oxidative stress: Clinical correlates of oxidative stress in the Framingham Study, *Arterioscler Thromb Vasc Biol*, 23, 434, 2003.

84. Dorjgochoo, T. et al., Obesity, age, and oxidative stress in middle-aged and older women, *Antioxid Redox Signal*, 14, 2453, 2011.

85. Yudkin, J.S. et al., Inflammation, obesity, stress and coronary heart disease: Is interleukin-6 the link? *Atherosclerosis*, 148, 209, 2000.

86. Knight, S.F. et al., Simvastatin and tempol protect against endothelial dysfunction and renal injury in a model of obesity and hypertension, *Am J Physiol Renal Physiol*, 298, F86, 2010.

87. Verreth, W. et al., Rosuvastatin restores superoxide dismutase expression and inhibits accumulation of oxidized LDL in the aortic arch of obese dyslipidemic mice, *Br J Pharmacol*, 151, 347, 2007.

88. Chinen, I. et al., Vascular lipotoxicity: Endothelial dysfunction via fatty-acid-induced reactive oxygen species overproduction in obese Zucker diabetic fatty rats, *Endocrinology*, 148, 160, 2007.

89. Higdon, J.V. et al., Obesity and oxidative stress: A direct link to CVD? *Arterioscler Thromb Vasc Biol*, 23, 365, 2003.

90. Doherty, S.P. et al., Early life insult from cigarette smoke may be predictive of chronic diseases later in life, *Biomarkers*, 14 Suppl 1, 97, 2009.

91. Michel, T. et al., Nitric oxide synthases: Which, where, how, and why? *J Clin Invest*, 100, 2146, 1997.

92. Nathan, C., Inducible nitric oxide synthase: What difference does it make? *J Clin Invest*, 100, 2417, 1997.

93. Iwashina, M. et al., Transfection of inducible nitric oxide synthase gene causes apoptosis in vascular smooth muscle cells, *Circulation*, 98, 1212, 1998.

94. Shimabukuro, M. et al., Role of nitric oxide in obesity-induced beta cell disease, *J Clin Invest*, 100, 290, 1997.

95. Channon, K.M. et al., Mechanisms of superoxide production in human blood vessels: Relationship to endothelial dysfunction, clinical and genetic risk factors, *J Physiol Pharmacol*, 53, 515, 2002.

96. Hotamisligil, G.S. et al., Increased adipose tissue expression of tumor necrosis factor-alpha in human obesity and insulin resistance, *J Clin Invest*, 95, 2409, 1995.

97. Mazurek, T. et al., Human epicardial adipose tissue is a source of inflammatory mediators, *Circulation*, 108, 2460, 2003.

98. Kessler, P. et al., Inhibition of inducible nitric oxide synthase restores endothelium-dependent relaxations in proinflammatory mediator-induced blood vessels, *Arterioscler Thromb Vasc Biol*, 17, 1746, 1997.

99. Chauhan, S.D. et al., Protection against lipopolysaccharide-induced endothelial dysfunction in resistance and conduit vasculature of iNOS knockout mice, *FASEB J*, 17, 773, 2003.

100. Gunnett, C.A. et al., NO-dependent vasorelaxation is impaired after gene transfer of inducible NO synthase, *Arterioscler Thromb Vasc Biol*, 21, 1281, 2001.

101. Tsuchiya, K. et al., Chronic blockade of nitric oxide synthesis reduces adiposity and improves insulin resistance in high fat-induced obese mice, *Endocrinology*, 148, 4548, 2007.

102. Barish, G.D. et al., PPAR delta: A dagger in the heart of the metabolic syndrome, *J Clin Invest*, 116, 590, 2006.

103. Giulivi, C. et al., Nitric oxide regulation of mitochondrial oxygen consumption I. Cellular physiology, *Am J Physiol Cell Physiol*, 291, C1225, 2006.

104. Lee, Y.H. et al., The evolving role of inflammation in obesity and the metabolic syndrome, *Curr Diab Rep*, 5, 70, 2005.

105. Eckel, R.H. et al., Report of the National Heart, Lung, and Blood Institute-National Institute of Diabetes and Digestive and Kidney Diseases Working Group on the pathophysiology of obesity-associated cardiovascular disease, *Circulation*, 105, 2923, 2002.

106. Mohamed-Ali, V. et al., Subcutaneous adipose tissue releases interleukin-6, but not tumor necrosis factor-alpha, in vivo, *J Clin Endocrinol Metab*, 82, 4196, 1997.

107. Heinrich, P.C. et al., Interleukin-6 and the acute phase response, *Biochem J*, 265, 621, 1990.

108. de Ferranti, S. et al., C-reactive protein and cardiovascular disease: A review of risk prediction and interventions, *Clin Chim Acta*, 317, 1, 2002.

109. Visser, M. et al., Elevated C-reactive protein levels in overweight and obese adults, *JAMA*, 282, 2131, 1999.

110. Festa, A. et al., The relation of body fat mass and distribution to markers of chronic inflammation, *Int J Obes Relat Metab Disord*, 25, 1407, 2001.

111. Wellen, K.E. et al., Inflammation, stress, and diabetes, *J Clin Invest*, 115, 1111, 2005.

112. Ozcan, U. et al., Endoplasmic reticulum stress links obesity, insulin action, and type 2 diabetes, *Science*, 306, 457, 2004.

113. Nakatani, Y. et al., Involvement of endoplasmic reticulum stress in insulin resistance and diabetes, *J Biol Chem*, 280, 847, 2005.

114. Ozawa, K. et al., The endoplasmic reticulum chaperone improves insulin resistance in type 2 diabetes, *Diabetes*, 54, 657, 2005.
115. Hung, J.H. et al., Endoplasmic reticulum stress stimulates the expression of cyclooxygenase-2 through activation of NF-kappaB and pp38 mitogen-activated protein kinase, *J Biol Chem*, 279, 46384, 2004.
116. Brownlee, M., Biochemistry and molecular cell biology of diabetic complications, *Nature*, 414, 813, 2001.
117. Lin, Y. et al., The hyperglycemia-induced inflammatory response in adipocytes: The role of reactive oxygen species, *J Biol Chem*, 280, 4617, 2005.
118. Ziccardi, P. et al., Reduction of inflammatory cytokine concentrations and improvement of endothelial functions in obese women after weight loss over one year, *Circulation*, 105, 804, 2002.
119. Roberts, C.K. et al., Effect of diet and exercise intervention on blood pressure, insulin, oxidative stress, and nitric oxide availability, *Circulation*, 106, 2530, 2002.
120. Sethi, J.K. et al., The role of TNF alpha in adipocyte metabolism, *Semin Cell Dev Biol*, 10, 19, 1999.
121. Kern, P.A. et al., The expression of tumor necrosis factor in human adipose tissue. Regulation by obesity, weight loss, and relationship to lipoprotein lipase, *J Clin Invest*, 95, 2111, 1995.
122. Soukas, A. et al., Leptin-specific patterns of gene expression in white adipose tissue, *Genes Dev*, 14, 963, 2000.
123. Makowski, L. et al., Lack of macrophage fatty-acid-binding protein aP2 protects mice deficient in apolipoprotein E against atherosclerosis, *Nat Med*, 7, 699, 2001.
124. Tontonoz, P. et al., PPARgamma promotes monocyte/macrophage differentiation and uptake of oxidized LDL, *Cell*, 93, 241, 1998.
125. Cousin, B. et al., A role for preadipocytes as macrophage-like cells, *FASEB J*, 13, 305, 1999.
126. Le Brocq, M. et al., Endothelial dysfunction: From molecular mechanisms to measurement, clinical implications, and therapeutic opportunities, *Antioxid Redox Signal*, 10, 1631, 2008.
127. Ross, R., Atherosclerosis—An inflammatory disease, *N Engl J Med*, 340, 115, 1999.
128. Chowienczyk, P.J. et al., Impaired endothelium-dependent vasodilation of forearm resistance vessels in hypercholesterolaemia, *Lancet*, 340, 1430, 1992.
129. Edirisinghe, I. et al., Cigarette-smoke-induced oxidative/nitrosative stress impairs VEGF- and fluid-shear-stress-mediated signaling in endothelial cells, *Antioxid Redox Signal*, 12, 1355, 2010.
130. Arunachalam, G. et al., Emphysema is associated with increased inflammation in lungs of atherosclerosis-prone mice by cigarette smoke: Implications in comorbidities of COPD, *J Inflamm (Lond)*, 7, 34, 2010.
131. Escobales, N. et al., Oxidative-nitrosative stress in hypertension, *Curr Vasc Pharmacol*, 3, 231, 2005.
132. Rahmouni, K. et al., Obesity-associated hypertension: New insights into mechanisms, *Hypertension*, 45, 9, 2005.
133. Vigili de Kreutzenberg, S. et al., Visceral obesity is characterized by impaired nitric oxide-independent vasodilation, *Eur Heart J*, 24, 1210, 2003.
134. Badimon, J.J. et al., Coronary atherosclerosis. A multifactorial disease, *Circulation*, 87, II3, 1993.
135. Libby, P., Inflammation in atherosclerosis, *Nature*, 420, 868, 2002.
136. Ludewig, B. et al., Arterial inflammation and atherosclerosis, *Trends Cardiovasc Med*, 12, 154, 2002.
137. Ross, R., The pathogenesis of atherosclerosis: A perspective for the 1990s, *Nature*, 362, 801, 1993.
138. Davies, M.J., The composition of coronary-artery plaques, *N Engl J Med*, 336, 1312, 1997.
139. Schreyer, S.A. et al., Accelerated atherosclerosis in mice lacking tumor necrosis factor receptor p55, *J Biol Chem*, 271, 26174, 1996.
140. Rader, D.J., Inflammatory markers of coronary risk, *N Engl J Med*, 343, 1179, 2000.
141. Graham, A. et al., Peroxynitrite modification of low-density lipoprotein leads to recognition by the macrophage scavenger receptor, *FEBS Lett*, 330, 181, 1993.
142. Darley-Usmar, V.M. et al., The simultaneous generation of superoxide and nitric oxide can initiate lipid peroxidation in human low density lipoprotein, *Free Radic Res Commun*, 17, 9, 1992.
143. Hogg, N. et al., Peroxynitrite and atherosclerosis, *Biochem Soc Trans*, 21, 358, 1993.
144. Radi, R. et al., Peroxynitrite-induced membrane lipid peroxidation: The cytotoxic potential of superoxide and nitric oxide, *Arch Biochem Biophys*, 288, 481, 1991.
145. Biswas, S.K. et al., Depressed glutathione synthesis precedes oxidative stress and atherogenesis in Apo-E(-/-) mice, *Biochem Biophys Res Commun*, 338, 1368, 2005.
146. Beltowski, J. et al., The effect of dietary-induced obesity on lipid peroxidation, antioxidant enzymes and total plasma antioxidant capacity, *J Physiol Pharmacol*, 51, 883, 2000.
147. Furukawa, S. et al., Increased oxidative stress in obesity and its impact on metabolic syndrome, *J Clin Invest*, 114, 1752, 2004.

148. Steinberger, J. et al., Obesity, insulin resistance, diabetes, and cardiovascular risk in children: An American Heart Association scientific statement from the Atherosclerosis, Hypertension, and Obesity in the Young Committee (Council on Cardiovascular Disease in the Young) and the Diabetes Committee (Council on Nutrition, Physical Activity, and Metabolism), *Circulation*, 107, 1448, 2003.

149. Hubert, H.B. et al., Obesity as an independent risk factor for cardiovascular disease: A 26-year follow-up of participants in the Framingham Heart Study, *Circulation*, 67, 968, 1983.

150. Auer, J. et al., Obesity, body fat and coronary atherosclerosis, *Int J Cardiol*, 98, 227, 2005.

151. Patel, Y.C. et al., Obesity, smoking and atherosclerosis. A study of interassociations, *Atherosclerosis*, 36, 481, 1980.

152. Sharma, A.M. et al., Obesity, hypertension and insulin resistance, *Acta Diabetol*, 42 Suppl 1, S3, 2005.

153. Lee, H.C. et al., Concurrent increase of oxidative DNA damage and lipid peroxidation together with mitochondrial DNA mutation in human lung tissues during aging—Smoking enhances oxidative stress on the aged tissues, *Arch Biochem Biophys*, 362, 309, 1999.

154. Burke, A. et al., Oxidative stress and smoking-induced vascular injury, *Prog Cardiovasc Dis*, 46, 79, 2003.

155. Olszanecka-Glinianowicz, M. et al., Serum concentrations of nitric oxide, tumor necrosis factor (TNF)-alpha and TNF soluble receptors in women with overweight and obesity, *Metabolism*, 53, 1268, 2004.

156. Simon, B.C. et al., Oxidized low density lipoproteins cause contraction and inhibit endothelium-dependent relaxation in the pig coronary artery, *J Clin Invest*, 86, 75, 1990.

157. Mitra, A.K. et al., "Vulnerable plaques"—Ticking of the time bomb, *Can J Physiol Pharmacol*, 82, 860, 2004.

158. Leskinen, M.J. et al., Regulation of smooth muscle cell growth, function and death in vitro by activated mast cells—A potential mechanism for the weakening and rupture of atherosclerotic plaques, *Biochem Pharmacol*, 66, 1493, 2003.

159. Lombardo, A. et al., Inflammation as a possible link between coronary and carotid plaque instability, *Circulation*, 109, 3158, 2004.

160. Robbins, M. et al., Inflammation in acute coronary syndromes, *Cleve Clin J Med*, 69 Suppl 2, SII130, 2002.

161. Villablanca, A.C. et al., Smoking and cardiovascular disease, *Clin Chest Med*, 21, 159, 2000.

162. Powell, J.T., Vascular damage from smoking: Disease mechanisms at the arterial wall, *Vasc Med*, 3, 21, 1998.

163. Tappia, P.S. et al., Cigarette smoking influences cytokine production and antioxidant defences, *Clin Sci (Lond)*, 88, 485, 1995.

164. de Maat, M.P. et al., Association of plasma fibrinogen levels with coronary artery disease, smoking and inflammatory markers, *Atherosclerosis*, 121, 185, 1996.

165. Sonmez, K. et al., Distribution of risk factors and prophylactic drug usage in Turkish patients with angiographically established coronary artery disease, *J Cardiovasc Risk*, 9, 199, 2002.

166. Talmud, P.J. et al., Analysis of gene-environment interaction in coronary artery disease: Lipoprotein lipase and smoking as examples, *Ital Heart J*, 3, 6, 2002.

167. Gander, M.L. et al., Effect of the G-308A polymorphism of the tumor necrosis factor (TNF)-alpha gene promoter site on plasma levels of TNF-alpha and C-reactive protein in smokers: A cross-sectional study, *BMC Cardiovasc Disord*, 4, 17, 2004.

168. Heber, D., Vegetables, fruits and phytoestrogens in the prevention of diseases, *J Postgrad Med*, 50, 145, 2004.

169. Witztum, J.L. et al., Oxidized phospholipids and isoprostanes in atherosclerosis, *Curr Opin Lipidol*, 9, 441, 1998.

170. Sánchez-Moreno, C. et al., Study of low-density lipoprotein oxidizability indexes to measure the antioxidant activity of dietary polyphenols, *Nutr Res*, 20, 941, 2000.

171. Ridker, P.M. et al., Comparison of C-reactive protein and low-density lipoprotein cholesterol levels in the prediction of first cardiovascular events, *N Engl J Med*, 347, 1557, 2002.

172. Pool-Zobel, B.L. et al., Mechanisms by which vegetable consumption reduces genetic damage in humans, *Cancer Epidemiol Biomarkers Prev*, 7, 891, 1998.

173. Ohashi, Y. et al., Prevention of intrahepatic metastasis by curcumin in an orthotopic implantation model, *Oncology*, 65, 250, 2003.

174. Minorsky, P.V., Lycopene and human health, *Plant Physiol*, 130, 1077, 2002.

175. Obermuller-Jevic, U.C. et al., Lycopene inhibits the growth of normal human prostate epithelial cells in vitro, *J Nutr*, 133, 3356, 2003.

176. Karas, M. et al., Lycopene interferes with cell cycle progression and insulin-like growth factor I signaling in mammary cancer cells, *Nutr Cancer*, 36, 101, 2000.
177. Giovannucci, E. et al., Intake of carotenoids and retinol in relation to risk of prostate cancer, *J Natl Cancer Inst*, 87, 1767, 1995.
178. Kucuk, O. et al., Lycopene supplementation in men with prostate cancer (Pca) reduced grade and volume of preneoplasia (PIN) and tumor, decreases serum prostate specific antigen (PSA) and modulates biomarkers of growth and differentiation, *International Carotenoid Meeting*, Cairns, Australia, 1999.
179. Burns, J. et al., Plant foods and herbal sources of resveratrol, *J Agric Food Chem*, 50, 3337, 2002.
180. Hung, L.M. et al., Cardioprotective effect of resveratrol, a natural antioxidant derived from grapes, *Cardiovasc Res*, 47, 549, 2000.
181. Atten, M.J. et al., Resveratrol regulates cellular PKC alpha and delta to inhibit growth and induce apoptosis in gastric cancer cells, *Invest New Drugs*, 23, 111, 2005.
182. van der Spuy, W.J. et al., Is the use of resveratrol in the treatment and prevention of obesity premature? *Nutr Res Rev*, 22, 111, 2009.
183. Zang, M. et al., Polyphenols stimulate AMP-activated protein kinase, lower lipids, and inhibit accelerated atherosclerosis in diabetic LDL receptor-deficient mice, *Diabetes*, 55, 2180, 2006.
184. Ahn, J. et al., Dietary resveratrol alters lipid metabolism-related gene expression of mice on an atherogenic diet, *J Hepatol*, 49, 1019, 2008.
185. Floyd, Z.E. et al., Modulation of peroxisome proliferator-activated receptor gamma stability and transcriptional activity in adipocytes by resveratrol, *Metabolism*, 57, S32, 2008.
186. Gnoni, G.V. et al., Resveratrol inhibits fatty acid and triacylglycerol synthesis in rat hepatocytes, *Eur J Clin Invest*, 39, 211, 2009.
187. Barger, J.L. et al., A low dose of dietary resveratrol partially mimics caloric restriction and retards aging parameters in mice, *PLoS One*, 3, e2264, 2008.
188. Bishayee, A. et al., Resveratrol and liver disease: From bench to bedside and community, *Liver Int*, 30, 1103, 2010.
189. Szkudelska, K. et al., Resveratrol, a naturally occurring diphenolic compound, affects lipogenesis, lipolysis and the antilipolytic action of insulin in isolated rat adipocytes, *J Steroid Biochem Mol Biol*, 113, 17, 2009.
190. Rayalam, S. et al., Resveratrol induces apoptosis and inhibits adipogenesis in 3T3-L1 adipocytes, *Phytother Res*, 22, 1367, 2008.
191. Park, H.J. et al., Combined effects of genistein, quercetin, and resveratrol in human and 3T3-L1 adipocytes, *J Med Food*, 11, 773, 2008.
192. Sharma, R.A. et al., Curcumin: The story so far, *Eur J Cancer*, 41, 1955, 2005.
193. Strimpakos, A.S. et al., Curcumin: Preventive and therapeutic properties in laboratory studies and clinical trials, *Antioxid Redox Signal*, 10, 511, 2008.
194. Bae, M.K. et al., Curcumin inhibits hypoxia-induced angiogenesis via down-regulation of HIF-1, *Oncol Rep*, 15, 1557, 2006.
195. Gururaj, A.E. et al., Molecular mechanisms of anti-angiogenic effect of curcumin, *Biochem Biophys Res Commun*, 297, 934, 2002.
196. Rupnick, M.A. et al., Adipose tissue mass can be regulated through the vasculature, *Proc Natl Acad Sci USA*, 99, 10730, 2002.
197. Tilg, H. et al., Adipocytokines: Mediators linking adipose tissue, inflammation and immunity, *Nat Rev Immunol*, 6, 772, 2006.
198. Ruderman, N.B. et al., AMPK as a metabolic switch in rat muscle, liver and adipose tissue after exercise, *Acta Physiol Scand*, 178, 435, 2003.
199. Ejaz, A. et al., Curcumin inhibits adipogenesis in 3T3-L1 adipocytes and angiogenesis and obesity in C57/BL mice, *J Nutr*, 139, 919, 2009.
200. Asai, A. et al., Dietary curcuminoids prevent high-fat diet-induced lipid accumulation in rat liver and epididymal adipose tissue, *J Nutr*, 131, 2932, 2001.
201. Wu, Z. et al., Conditional ectopic expression of C/EBP beta in NIH-3T3 cells induces PPAR gamma and stimulates adipogenesis, *Genes Dev*, 9, 2350, 1995.
202. Gurnell, M., Peroxisome proliferator-activated receptor gamma and the regulation of adipocyte function: Lessons from human genetic studies, *Best Pract Res Clin Endocrinol Metab*, 19, 501, 2005.
203. Meydani, M. et al., Dietary polyphenols and obesity, *Nutrients*, 2, 737, 2010.
204. Hursel, R. et al., Thermogenic ingredients and body weight regulation, *Int J Obes (Lond)*, 34, 659, 2010.
205. Lin, J.K. et al., Mechanisms of hypolipidemic and anti-obesity effects of tea and tea polyphenols, *Mol Nutr Food Res*, 50, 211, 2006.

206. Lin, J. et al., Green tea polyphenol epigallocatechin gallate inhibits adipogenesis and induces apoptosis in 3T3-L1 adipocytes, *Obes Res*, 13, 982, 2005.
207. Carling, D., AMP-activated protein kinase: Balancing the scales, *Biochimie*, 87, 87, 2005.
208. Ruderman, N.B. et al., Malonyl-CoA, fuel sensing, and insulin resistance, *Am J Physiol*, 276, E1, 1999.
209. Murase, T. et al., Catechin-induced activation of the LKB1/AMP-activated protein kinase pathway, *Biochem Pharmacol*, 78, 78, 2009.
210. Klaus, S. et al., Epigallocatechin gallate attenuates diet-induced obesity in mice by decreasing energy absorption and increasing fat oxidation, *Int J Obes (Lond)*, 29, 615, 2005.
211. Mazzanti, G. et al., Hepatotoxicity from green tea: A review of the literature and two unpublished cases, *Eur J Clin Pharmacol*, 65, 331, 2009.
212. Lambert, J.D. et al., Hepatotoxicity of high oral dose (-)-epigallocatechin-3-gallate in mice, *Food Chem Toxicol*, 48, 409, 2010.
213. Agouni, A. et al., Red wine polyphenols prevent metabolic and cardiovascular alterations associated with obesity in Zucker fatty rats (Fa/Fa), *PLoS One*, 4, e5557, 2009.
214. DeFuria, J. et al., Dietary blueberry attenuates whole-body insulin resistance in high fat-fed mice by reducing adipocyte death and its inflammatory sequelae, *J Nutr*, 139, 1510, 2009.
215. Strissel, K.J. et al., Adipocyte death, adipose tissue remodeling, and obesity complications, *Diabetes*, 56, 2910, 2007.
216. Joseph, J.A. et al., Reversals of age-related declines in neuronal signal transduction, cognitive, and motor behavioral deficits with blueberry, spinach, or strawberry dietary supplementation, *J Neurosci*, 19, 8114, 1999.
217. Youdim, K.A. et al., Polyphenolics enhance red blood cell resistance to oxidative stress: In vitro and in vivo, *Biochim Biophys Acta*, 1523, 117, 2000.
218. Lau, F.C. et al., Inhibitory effects of blueberry extract on the production of inflammatory mediators in lipopolysaccharide-activated BV2 microglia, *J Neurosci Res*, 85, 1010, 2007.
219. Cinti, S. et al., Adipocyte death defines macrophage localization and function in adipose tissue of obese mice and humans, *J Lipid Res*, 46, 2347, 2005.
220. Lumeng, C.N. et al., Obesity induces a phenotypic switch in adipose tissue macrophage polarization, *J Clin Invest*, 117, 175, 2007.
221. Prior, R.L. et al., Whole berries versus berry anthocyanins: Interactions with dietary fat levels in the C57BL/6J mouse model of obesity, *J Agric Food Chem*, 56, 647, 2008.
222. Cottart, C.H. et al., Resveratrol bioavailability and toxicity in humans, *Mol Nutr Food Res*, 54, 7, 2010.
223. Prior, R.L. et al., Purified berry anthocyanins but not whole berries normalize lipid parameters in mice fed an obesogenic high fat diet, *Mol Nutr Food Res*, 53, 1406, 2009.
224. Joost, H.G. et al., NO to obesity: Does nitric oxide regulate fat oxidation and insulin sensitivity?, *Endocrinology*, 148, 4545, 2007.
225. Coll, A.P. et al., The hormonal control of food intake, *Cell*, 129, 251, 2007.
226. Wuschke, S. et al., A meta-analysis of quantitative trait loci associated with body weight and adiposity in mice, *Int J Obes (Lond)*, 31, 829, 2007.
227. Frayling, T.M. et al., A common variant in the FTO gene is associated with body mass index and predisposes to childhood and adult obesity, *Science*, 316, 889, 2007.

7 Role of Neurotransmitters in Obesity Regulation

Sunny E. Ohia, PhD, Catherine A. Opere, PhD, Madhura Kulkarni, MPharm, and Ya Fatou Njie-Mbye, PhD

CONTENTS

INTRODUCTION

The main goal of this chapter is to provide a comprehensive review of neurotransmitters, neuropeptides, and other chemicals that have been reported to be involved in obesity regulation based on data obtained from animal and human studies. These substances affect obesity via several mechanisms: a decrease in food intake through satiety and nonsatiety pathways or an effect on energy expenditure through hyperactivity and thermogenesis. An induction of weight loss is a resultant action of the ingestion of compounds that mimic or alter the action of neurotransmitters and neuropeptides, as described in this chapter. The neurotransmitters discussed in this chapter include 5-hydroxytryptamine (5-HT) or serotonin; the catecholamines norepinephrine (NE) and dopamine (DA); and histamine. For neuropeptides, the focus is on neuropeptide Y (NPY), galanin, corticotropin-releasing factor (CRF), orexin, and melanocortin (MC). For both neurotransmitters and neuropeptides, an additional review of pharmacological receptors associated with their actions is provided. For brevity, only in highly relevant cases is a discussion of signal transduction pathways for neurotransmitters and neuropeptides included. We also discuss the role of other chemicals such as endocannabinoids and their respective receptors in the regulation of obesity. The reader is also provided with a bibliography of critical references for more information about the neurotransmitters and neuropeptides discussed in this chapter.

NEUROTRANSMITTERS AND RELEVANT PHARMACOLOGICAL RECEPTORS

5-Hydroxytryptamine

In addition to its well-known actions on the gastrointestinal tract and cardiovascular system, 5-HT (serotonin) plays an important role as a neurotransmitter in the central nervous system (CNS). 5-HT is biosynthesized from the essential amino acid tryptophan by two enzymes: tryptophan hydroxylase and aromatic L-amino acid decarboxylase. Dietary tryptophan is converted into 5-hydroxytryptophan (5-HTP) by tryptophan hydroxylase. At the nerve terminal, 5-HTP is rapidly converted into 5-HT by the enzyme L-amino acid decarboxylase. Newly synthesized 5-HT is stored in vesicles at serotonergic neurons and is released by exocytosis following a nerve action potential. In the nervous system, the effect of released 5-HT is terminated by a reuptake process into neurons by a specific transporter. The localization of 5-HT transporters on membranes of serotonergic axon terminals facilitates the reuptake process. It is pertinent to note that the 5-HT transporter plays an important role in the action of this neurotransmitter in the regulation of obesity. Drugs that inhibit the activity of this transporter (such as d-norfenfluramine and fluoxetine) increase the concentration of 5-HT at synaptic sites and have been reported to have a suppressive action on food intake.

Further evidence for the role of 5-HT in the regulation of feeding behavior is derived from both animal and human studies. For example, when 5-HT or its precursors, tryptophan and 5-HTP, are administered to experimental animals, a significant decrease in food intake, eating rate, and meal size results. Baseline levels of 5-HT and its metabolite, 5-hydroxyindoleacetic acid, are lower in the hypothalamus of obese Zucker rats when compared to their lean counterparts. Similarly, in obese humans, plasma concentrations of the tryptophan and brain 5-HT levels are low, indicating a role for this monoamine in the individual's ability to control caloric intake.

In general, compounds that increase the concentration of 5-HT (whether through inhibition of the transporter or via direct administration into the brain or periphery) have been shown to have a preferential suppressant action on carbohydrate and fat consumption with little or no effect on protein ingestion. In addition to well-known selective serotonin reuptake inhibitors (SSRIs) such as fluoxetine and fenfluramine, hydroxycitric acid has been reported to initiate its antiobesity action through an action on 5-HT metabolic pathway. Hydroxycitric acid increased brain concentrations of 5-HT in experimental animals and plasma 5-HT levels in humans. Although 5-HT appears to possess a selective action on carbohydrate and fat ingestion in animal studies, it is unclear whether these findings are relevant to humans. Be that as it may, an increase in 5-HT concentrations at synaptic and other sites produces a general inhibitory action on the pattern of food intake by modulating hunger and satiety.

The pharmacological actions of 5-HT are mediated by specific receptors of seven different families (5-HT_1–5-HT_7). Of all the 5-HT receptors described, 5-HT_{1A}, 5-HT_{1B}, 5-HT_{2C}, and, more recently, 5-HT_{2B} and 5-HT_6 receptor subtypes have been implicated in the regulation of feeding behavior. For example, activation of 5-HT_{1A} receptors can lead to increased food intake, whereas stimulation of 5-HT_{1B} and 5-HT_{2C} receptors will cause a decrease in food consumption. 5-HT_{1A} receptors are localized on nerve terminals; both 5-HT_{1B} and 5-HT_{2C} receptors are found on postsynaptic sites. Evidence linking the action on 5-HT on food intake and feeding behavior with specific receptor subtypes was based on animal studies in which selective antagonists of 5-HT_{1B} and 5-HT_{2C} receptors were found to block the anorectic actions of serotonergic drugs such as fenfluramine and fluoxetine. Further evidence is derived from studies using knockout mice that possess no functional 5-HT_{2C} receptors. 5-HT_{2C} receptor knockout mice demonstrate marked hyperphagia and late-onset obesity and exhibit metabolic hormone changes such as hyperleptinemia and hyperinsulinemia. Likewise, 5-HT_{1B} receptor knockout mice gained more weight than corresponding wild type, indicating a higher degree of food intake. The observations made in the knockout mice provide strong evidence that these genetically altered obese animals possess a deficient endogenous 5-HT satiety system. Animals deprived of food demonstrate intense food-seeking behavior and increased food intake when food is provided, a response that is linked to turnover of 5-HT and a differential expression of 5-HT_{2C} receptor subtypes in the hypothalamus.

In summary, studies on food intake and feeding behavior confirm a significant role for 5-HT (and its possible action on 5-HT_{1B} and 5-HT_{2C} receptors) in mediation of the hypophagic response induced by this monoamine. Attention is now being focused on producing receptor-selective 5-HT_{1B} and 5-HT_{2C} agonists that can serve as novel molecules for the treatment of obesity. Indeed, weight loss induced by fenfluramine is now ascribed to a direct stimulant action of its desmethyl metabolite, norfenfluramine on 5-HT_{2C} receptors. Recent findings have implicated 5-HT_{2B} receptors in the anorectic properties of dexfenfluramine (active d-enantiomer of fenfluramine). However, this receptor has been strongly associated with the cardiopulmonary adverse effects of dexfenfluramine. The effectiveness of 5-HT_{2C} receptor agonists in regulating appetite and food intake in humans shows significant promise for the serotonergic system in the development of new antiobesity drugs. 5-HT_{2C} receptor agonism increases anorexigenic proopiomelanocortin (POMC) production in the arcuate nucleus (ARC) area in the hypothalamus. A new generation of 5-HT_{2C} receptor-selective agonist, lorcaserin (ADP356), has been developed. Lorcaserin is believed to reduce food intake predominantly by influencing hypothalamic pathways involved in appetite. The drug completed phase III clinical trial; however, toxicology data in rodents presented to the FDA demonstrated a significant number of neoplasms in mammary and brain tissue of rats treated with lorcaserin for 2 years, and, hence, the FDA advisory panel recommended that lorcaserin should not be approved for the long-term treatment of obesity.

In addition to the 5-HT-receptors mentioned earlier, one of the recent additions to serotonin receptor family, 5-HT_6, has been implicated in the regulation of food intake. The 5-HT_6 receptor is expressed within the CNS with high levels in cortical and limbic regions. 5-HT_6 receptor antagonists such as PRX-07034 and BVT74316 have been shown to potently reduce food intake and bodyweight gain in rodent models and have recently entered clinical trials. However, the role of the 5-HT_6 receptor in the expression of appetite remains to be determined.

The ability of 5-HT to cause hypophagia may involve the interaction of this monoamine with other neurotransmitter and neuropeptide pathways; for example, NPY-induced hyperphagia can be blocked by fenfluramine. Treatment of animals with 5-HT (mainly through 5-HT_{1B} receptor agonism) has been reported to decrease hypothalamic NPY concentrations. Anorectic 5-HT drugs such as fenfluramine activate POMC neurons in the ARC, thus indicating a role for downstream MC pathways in the regulation of food intake and body weight. Orexin can stimulate 5-HT release in the hypothalamus, suggesting that serotonergic pathways are involved in the anorectic action of this neuropeptide. Thus, net result of increased CNS serotoninergic activity is an increase in anorexigenic and catabolic effects, a decrease in orexigenic and anabolic effects, and therefore weight loss.

It is clear from the discussion mentioned earlier that, as a neurotransmitter, 5-HT plays a crucial role in satiety response and may serve as a template for future antiobesity therapy. Compounds that increase its concentrations at synaptic sites or activate 5-HT_{1B} or 5-HT_{2C} receptors will continue to represent compelling therapeutic targets in the quest to develop highly selective pharmacological entities for the regulation of food intake and feeding behavior.

CATECHOLAMINES

Of the three major catecholamines, DA and NE have been linked to the regulation of appetite and feeding behavior. DA, an immediate precursor of NE and epinephrine, is a neurotransmitter in the CNS. It is synthesized from the amino acid tyrosine by two enzymes: tyrosine hydroxylase and aromatic L-amino acid decarboxylase. Tyrosine is converted to dihydroxyphenylalanine (DOPA) by tyrosine hydroxylase, which is subsequently metabolized to DA by aromatic L-amino acid decarboxylase. DA is presumed to be one of the target neurotransmitters linking genetic and environmental factors that contribute to obesity. It has a site-specific action on the regulation of food intake. The reinforcing action of DA on food intake is associated with the release of this neurotransmitter in the brain nucleus accumbens. The basal regulation of food intake, duration of meal consumption, is ascribed to DA release in the hypothalamus. DA acting on two regions of hypothalamus, the lateral hypothalamus and the ventromedial hypothalamus, appears to have opposing effects on food intake. For example, DA levels in lateral hypothalamus increase immediately in response to feeding, remain elevated during meal consumption, and normalize after meal termination. On the contrary, DA levels in hypothalamic ventromedial hypothalamus decrease after food intake and increase during fasting. Thus, hypothalamic DA is required to initiate each meal and is also responsible for the number of meals and duration of feeding. DA neurons originating in the midbrain (ventral tegmental area) that innervate nucleus accumbens are essential for motivation of food and food-related reward, whereas mesocortical DA is associated with emotional responses to feeding. Furthermore, DA neurons originating in the substantia nigra and projecting to the caudate putamen may be linked with sensory-motor aspects of feeding. Further support for the role of DA in the regulation of food intake has been demonstrated in DA knockout mice that do not express tyrosine hydroxylase activity. Although these animals do not lack the motor capabilities for feeding, they cannot initiate the feeding process. Thus, evidence from biomedical literature supports the fact that DA is essential for feeding.

DA exerts its pharmacological actions via activity on five receptor subtypes classified into D_1-like (D_1 and D_5) and D_2-like (D_2, D_3, and D_4) families. Both subtypes of DA receptors are found on hypothalamic neurons, thus supporting their role in the regulation of feeding behavior. Data from studies in animals show that chronic activation of D_1 and D_2 receptors results in a decrease in food consumption with concomitant body weight reduction. In humans, there is evidence that striatal D_2 receptor activity is significantly lower in obese individuals than in controls, a finding that was hypothesized to be due to the action of DA on motivation and reward circuits. In general, an effect of DA on D_1 receptors is presumed to be regulation of satiety signals, thus leading to a decrease in meal size and duration of feeding. Activation of D_2 receptors leads to a reduction in the rate of feeding. Drugs that activate or block DA receptors can affect appetite and feeding behavior; for example, the D_1/D_2 receptor agonist apomorphine has been shown to decrease both the rate and duration of feeding. On the other hand, behavioral studies in animals have revealed that antagonists of D_2 receptors can increase meal size and the duration of feeding. In humans, patients treated with antipsychotics that block D_2 receptors show an increase in body weight as a side effect. Clearly, both DA receptors play a very important role in the regulation of appetite and feeding behavior in both animals and humans. Moreover, neuropeptides like orexin, NPY, and MC system are known to interact with DA.

NE is a neurotransmitter that is released from sympathetic nerves. It is a metabolic product of the action of DA β-hydroxylase on DA. Compounds that produce effects that resemble sympathetic nerve stimulation (i.e., sympathomimetics) such as amphetamine, phentermine, and sibutramine have been employed as antiobesity drugs. The mechanism of action of these antiobesity compounds is complex with a diverse activity spectrum, such as a reduction in food intake or increase in energy expenditure (through hyperactivity and thermogenesis). Amphetamine was the first compound mimicking the action of sympathetic nerve stimulation that was employed for the treatment of obesity. Amphetamine reduces hunger, food intake, and the number of meals while increasing feeding latency and feeding rate. Due to its deleterious side effect on the cardiovascular system and high rate of abuse potential, this drug is no longer in use for the treatment of obesity. Sibutramine, a potent inhibitor of NE and serotonin reuptake, has antiobesity actions through an inhibitory action on food intake. This drug is indefinitely suspended from August 2010 based on several reports on cardiovascular complications such as increased heart rate, heart attack, and stroke. European Union drug regulatory agency cited that "drug's benefit do not outweigh the risk."

NE exerts its physiological and pharmacological actions via activation of three major receptor classes: α_1-, α_2-, and β-adrenoceptors. All three receptor classes have been implicated in the regulation of appetite and feeding behavior. In the brain, α_1- and α_2-adrenoceptors present in the paraventricular hypothalamus have been linked to the regulation of feeding behavior. In animal studies, stimulation of α_1-adrenoceptors suppresses food intake, whereas activation of α_2-adrenoceptors increases food intake. It appears that the observed antiobesity action of sympathomimetics could be related to the degree to which they act on α_1- and α_2-adrenoceptors; for example, sibutramine is presumed to decrease appetite via an inhibitory action on α_2-adrenoceptors. α-Adrenoceptors mediate glucose homeostasis through an effect on insulin and glucagon secretion, liver glucose production, and glucose uptake into muscle. Production of heat by the body (thermogenesis) can increase energy expenditure leading to weight loss. The adipose tissue serves both as a depot for fat storage and also as a dynamic endocrine organ involved in the control of energy balance. β_3-Adrenoceptors present in adipose tissue are involved in catecholamine-stimulated lipolysis and thermogenesis. The discovery that mutation of a gene encoding β_3-adrenoceptors at Trp 64/Arg is linked with the propensity to gain weight coupled with the observation that these receptors mediate thermogenesis in adipose tissue led to the search for antiobesity drugs that act via this pathway. It remains to be determined whether β_3-adrenoceptors present on adipose tissues may serve as a useful target for the treatment of obesity.

HISTAMINE

Histamine is a neurotransmitter in the CNS that has also been linked to the regulation of feeding behavior. Apart from the CNS, histamine is found in abundance in mast cells especially in skin, lungs, and the gastrointestinal tract. In the brain, histamine is synthesized in tuberomammillary nucleus hypothalamic neurons from the amino acid histidine. Histidine is decarboxylated to form histamine, a reaction that is catalyzed by the enzyme L-histidine decarboxylase. Unlike the catecholamines whose effect is terminated by reuptake mechanisms in synapses, histamine diffuses from synapses, where its action is terminated by degradative enzymes. Nerves containing histamine project throughout the brain to areas such as the thalamus and cerebral cortex. In animal studies, histamine has been shown to suppress food intake, and there is evidence that this neurotransmitter may regulate body weight and adiposity by an action on peripheral energy metabolism. Histamine-containing neurons have been linked to the rate of feeding and intake volume of meals. Histamine produces its pharmacological actions via effects on four different receptor subtypes: H_1, H_2, H_3, and H_4. Of these receptor subtypes, both H_1 and H_3 receptors have been associated with the regulation of appetite and feeding behavior. In animal studies, injection of H_1-receptor agonists or peripheral administration of the histamine precursor histidine suppressed food intake in rats and mice. Furthermore, H_1-receptor-deficient mice demonstrated an increase in food intake when compared to their normal counterparts. Similarly, histidine decarboxylase deficient mice also showed a marked increase in obesity. Taken together, data from animal studies reveal a role for H_1 receptors and histidine decarboxylase in the regulation of food intake and feeding behavior.

Administration of the H_3 receptor antagonist, thioperamide, into the brain has been reported to suppress food intake in rats. Presumably, by blocking inhibitory H_3 receptors present on histamine-containing nerve terminals, thioperamide indirectly causes an increase in the release and availability of this amine, leading to enhanced stimulation of postsynaptic H_1 receptors and the suppression of food intake. Based on this observation, several new compounds with antagonistic activity at H_3 receptors have been developed by pharmaceutical companies for potential use as antiobesity drugs. In spite of the evidence from preclinical studies that implicates histamine in the regulation of food intake, it remains to be determined whether compounds that interact with H_1 and H_3 receptors will be of therapeutic importance in the treatment of obesity in humans.

NEUROPEPTIDES AND RELEVANT PHARMACOLOGICAL RECEPTORS

NEUROPEPTIDE Y

NPY, a 36-amino-acid neurotransmitter that was discovered in 1982, is one of the most abundant and widely distributed neuropeptides in mammalian CNS. It belongs to a family of pancreatic polypeptides with similar structural homology known as the NPY family. Other members of this family include peptide YY, pancreatic polypeptide, and polypeptide Y. NPY, which is also one of the most studied neuropeptides, is highly conserved across species from *Drosophila* to humans. Biosynthesis of NPY involves posttranslational enzymatic cleavage of the 98-amino-acid preproNPY to the 69-amino-acid prohormone proNPY, which is further cleaved to NPY by the prohormone convertases (PC)1/3 and PC2. It is often colocalized and coreleased with NE neurotransmitter in both central and autonomic nervous system, where it is believed to modulate catecholamine release and activity. In addition to its regulatory role in the cardiovascular, reproductive, bone mass, and psychomotor systems, among others, NPY is a potent orexigenic neuropeptide that plays a central role in the regulation of appetite in the CNS. In the CNS, NPY is most abundant in the hypothalamic nuclei such as the ARC and paraventricular nucleus (PVN), both key areas in the regulation of feeding. Indeed, several studies have shown that injection of NPY into the PVN stimulates hyperphagia, reduced energy expenditure, and the induction of obesity in the long run.

NPY mediates its pharmacological actions by activating six G_i/G_o-protein-coupled NPY receptor subtypes (Y1 to Y6), all of which have been shown to be expressed in both CNS and peripheral tissues. Three of these receptor subtypes (Y1, Y2, and Y5) have been implicated in regulation of food intake; for example, evidence suggests that Y1 receptors are involved in selective stimulation of carbohydrate intake and meal size. Recent studies have shown that Y1 receptors are also involved in regulating bone homeostasis (Y1 receptor expression has been found on osteoblastic and bone marrow stromal cells) along with controlling body weight, thus adding another dimension to the potential use of Y1 receptor as an antiobesity medicine. Additionally, recent studies have revealed that antagonizing the peripheral Y1 receptors by increasing fat oxidation and energy expenditure is more beneficial in treating obesity. Because central Y1 receptors mediate central functions such as control of anxiety and emotionality, targeting peripheral as opposed to central Y1 receptors would provide an additional benefit of minimizing potential central side effects. Thus, it will be of great interest to develop compounds that antagonize Y1 receptors in peripheral tissues and confer beneficial effects on the bone mass, thereby providing new dimensions for treatment of obesity. Several studies utilizing receptor NPY agonists and receptor subtype antagonists have demonstrated that both Y1 and Y5 receptors independently and synergistically interact with each other to mediate NPY hyperphagic response. In contrast, the Y2 receptor subtype, which is located presynaptically (with postsynaptic expression in some brain regions) on neurons, suppresses carbohydrate intake. Lately, it was shown that variation in the 5′ region of the Y2 receptor gene is associated with obesity in Caucasian Danish subjects. Other studies report that Y2 receptors have no effect in satiated animals but suppress food intake in fasted animals. It appears that, under fasted conditions, Y2 receptor activity attenuates the release of PVN NPY and eliminates tonic inhibition of γ-aminobutyric acid (GABA) on POMC neurons, thereby stimulating release of α-melanocyte-stimulating hormone (α-MSH) with the net effect of decreased food intake. It has been hypothesized that, in satiated animals, the Y2-sensitive NPY and GABA are rendered inactive, while the activity of α-MSH and POMC neurons predominates to reduce food intake. Recently, a Y2 receptor agonist, Pyy3–36, was reported to reduce body weight in animals and humans. However, its short half-life (less than 20 min) minimized its potential application in treatment of obesity. A modified version of this peptide with greater stability and longer lasting effects needs to be developed.

In general, Y2 receptors regulate transport, synthesis, and release of NPY and other central mediators, in addition to playing a significant role in the NPY-mediated effects of leptin. Although the central orexigenic effect of NPY has been established in several studies, the use of transgenic mice has surprisingly revealed that neither overexpression nor deletion of NPY receptors interferes with normal weight and appetite. It appears that, although NPY is central to the regulation of food intake and energy balance, the body can adjust other orexigenic and anorexigenic signals to compensate for its receptor deletion or overexpression. The normal transgenic phenotype of both transgenic models thus reflects the rich functional redundancy of the system regulating food intake and energy balance. Based on studies utilizing transgenic models, it is not surprising that a Y5 antagonist was unsuccessful in clinical trials with human subjects. Although these observations suggest that NPY is not involved in morbid obesity, NPY analogs may still find clinical application as appetite suppressants and antiobesity drugs. In a recent development, the Y5 receptor antagonist, velneperit (S-2367), was successful in phase II clinical trials. In addition to being well tolerated in humans, this drug caused significant reduction in waist circumference and improved serum lipid profile in humans. Thus, NPY analogs provide an additional therapeutic target for treatment of obesity.

GALANIN

Galanin is a 29-amino-acid (30 in humans) peptide that is widely expressed in mammalian central nervous, peripheral nervous, and endocrine systems. It was originally identified in porcine intestines in 1983. It is colocalized with and regulates the release of several neurotransmitters and has been implicated in high-order physiological functions such as learning and memory, nociception, epileptic activity, spinal reflexes, sexual activity, mood changes, and food intake. The pharmacological effects of galanin are mediated through three G-protein-coupled receptors: GalR1, GalR2, and GalR3. It is unclear which of these receptors mediate the effects of galanin on the regulation of food intake. Injection of galanin into the brain stem stimulates food consumption. On the other hand, administration of galanin antagonists such as M40 decreases food intake. Evidence suggests that in the PVN of the hypothalamus, endogenous galanin selectively stimulates the intake of lipids and alcohol, and its production is stimulated by the same dietary components. Interestingly, consumption of a high-carbohydrate diet does not regulate endogenous galanin levels. Transgenic mice overexpressing galanin mRNA in hypothalamus exhibit a higher preference for a lipid diet. It is therefore conceivable that a potent galanin antagonist may have potential clinical application as an antiobesity drug.

CORTICOTROPIN-RELEASING FACTOR

CRF, also known as corticotropin-releasing hormone (CRH), is a 41-amino-acid neuropeptide that belongs to the CRH family of peptides. Other members of this family include urocortins I, II, and III. In addition to being one of the major physiologic secretagogues of adrenocorticotropic hormone (ACTH), CRF regulates the hypothalamic–pituitary axis; autonomic and behavioral responses to stress; cardiovascular, inflammatory, and gastrointestinal function; and food intake. CRF is synthesized by hypothalamic paraventricular neurons and is distributed throughout the brain and spinal cord. Biosynthesis of CRF involves cleavage of flanking amino acid base pairs from a 191-amino-acid precursor. CRF activates two seven-transmembrane-domain-spanning G-protein coupled receptors: CRF type 1 (CRF1) and CRF type 2 (CRF2). CRF1, which exhibits a higher affinity for CRF, is expressed in cortical, hypothalamic, limbic, cerebellar, and pituitary regions of the brain and in the gastrointestinal tract. In contrast, CRF2 exhibits a lower affinity for CRF and is distributed mainly in peripheral systems such as the gut and in more limited areas of brain compared to CRF1. Both receptors are positively coupled to adenylyl cyclase enzyme. In humans, CRF2(a) is localized in hypothalamic areas that control appetite such as the PVN, in the gastrointestinal tract, and on vagal afferent nerves, suggesting this receptor plays a role in the regulation of food intake.

Chronic intracerebroventricular (i.c.v.) administration of exogenous CRF in rats elicits a potent anorexic effect via stimulation of synthesis and secretion of POMC-related peptides, subsequently suppressing food intake and decreasing body weight. The discovery of endogenous-selective CRF2 receptor agonists (type 2 urocortins Ucn-II and Ucn-III) and the synthesis of more selective ligands continue to delineate the functional significance of the CRF systems in brain and gut. Using some of the newly found ligands, it has been shown that agonists with higher affinity for CRF2 exhibit a high potency of hypophagic response. For example, Ucn-I, which has a higher affinity for CRF2, is more potent at suppressing food intake and less potent at modulating stress compared with CRF1, which has a moderate affinity for this receptor subtype. In contrast, the selective CRF2 receptor antagonist antisauvagine-30 attenuates CRF-induced anorexia, unlike the CRF1 receptor antagonist counterpart. In support of this premise, deletion, reduction, or inhibition of CRF2 receptor subtype attenuates hypophagic effect caused by i.c.v. injection of Ucn-I and CRF. Other studies indicate that, in rats, CRF1 receptors mediate abbreviated, short-onset anorexia while CRF2 elicits delayed-onset anorexia. Furthermore, activation of both CRF1 and CRF2 receptor subtypes using nonselective agonists provokes both prolonged and short-onset anorexia. Clearly, the exact mechanisms by which the CRF receptor system regulates appetite suppression remain to be fully elucidated. It is conceivable that CRF antagonists may find therapeutic application in the treatment of overweight, obesity, and associated morbidities.

OREXINS

Orexins (previously known as hypocretins) A and B are neuropeptides that were initially identified in rat hypothalamus in 1998. These novel neuropeptides have been shown to be involved in the regulation of food intake, in addition to sleep/wakefulness and energy homeostasis. Several studies have now linked orexin to reward-based eating (consumption beyond homeostatic needs); hence, dysfunction of the orexin system may be a contributing factor in the overeating associated with obesity. Orexin A (33-amino-acid residues) and orexin B (28-amino-acid residues) are proteolytically derived from 130 to 131 preproorexin. Orexins interact with two seven-transmembrane-domain-spanning G-protein-coupled receptors: orexin receptor 1 (OX1R), which selectively binds orexin A, and orexin receptor 2 (OX2R), which has the same affinity for both orexin A and B. Originally localized in the lateral and posterior hypothalamus, orexin neurons project diffusely into brain regions, including areas involved in the regulation of energy homeostasis such as the ARC, paraventricular hypothalamus, and ventromedial hypothalamus. Interestingly, these hypothalamic regions also express orexin receptors, suggesting involvement of the orexin system in the regulation of food intake. In the lateral hypothalamus, orexin neurons are coexpressed with the hyperphagic endogenous opioid, dynorphin. Recent evidence demonstrates that orexin shows protective effect against the development of peripheral insulin resistance induced by high-fat diet in mice. Both orexins and their receptors are now known to be expressed in the gastrointestinal system as well. In rats, SB-334867, a selective OX1R antagonist, blocks orexin-A-induced gastric acid secretions.

Administration of orexin A elicits an OX1R-receptor-sensitive hyperphagic response that is less potent than that of NPY but comparable to that of melanin-concentration hormone (MCH). In rodents, acute administration of orexin A induces a transient orexigenic effect that is preceded by anorexia with no net increase in food intake over a 24-h period. It is therefore not surprising that chronic administration of orexin A does not induce obesity, unlike the orexigenic neuropeptides, NPY, and agouti-related protein (AGRP). OXR1 antagonist such as SB-334867 not only reverses orexin-A-induced hyperphagia but may also induce satiety when administered alone. However, SB-334867 has off-target effects that do not make it an ideal drug for treatment of obesity. Interestingly, orexin-A-induced feeding can also be blocked by nonselective opioid antagonist and partially reversed by NPY Y1 receptor antagonist, suggesting that control of food intake involves an integration of various pathways. The hyperphagic effect of orexin A is supported by the observation that mice lacking preproorexin are hypophagic with normal body weight. Hypophagia is also observed in the selective deletion of orexin neurons using ataxin-3 in mice. Ataxin-3-treated mice develop late-onset obesity, an effect that can be ascribed to an orexin-induced increase in thermogenesis. In contrast, orexin B induces little or no hyperphagic response and promotes grooming and searching activities. Although these observations indicate that orexin system does play the main regulatory role in food intake, ORX1R antagonists have the potential to reduce food intake and reduce body weight. A new dual orexin receptor antagonist, ACT-078573, selectively and reversibly blocks both ORX1R and ORX2R in nanomolar concentrations. This drug is effective for promoting sleep and has entered phase III clinical trials for treating insomnia patients. To date there is no report of selective ORX1R antagonist entering in clinical development.

MELANOCORTIN

The MC system consists of a group of four peptides: α-, β-, γ-MSHs, and ACTH, which are derived from posttranslational cleavage of the precursor molecule, POMC. Other members of the system include two endogenous antagonists (agouti and AGRP) and five MC receptor subtypes (MC1R–MC5R). Although the behavioral effects of ACTH and α-MSH have been known since 1955, it was not until the 1980s that the regulatory effect of MC peptides on food intake was illustrated. So far, two receptor subtypes, MC4R and, to a lesser extent, MC3R (also known as the central receptors), have been implicated in the regulation of food intake. MC3R is highly expressed in hypothalamic nuclei that control feeding such as ventromedial hypothalamus, ARC, lateral hypothalamus, and preoptic nucleus. MC4R is more widely expressed in multiple parts of the brain, including hypothalamic dorsal medial nucleus and PVN, which receive projections from ARC. Interestingly, MC3R and MC4R receptors are activated by all of the four MC peptides, with α-MSH exhibiting the highest selectivity for MC3R. The functional loss of MC4R is the most common genetic cause of human obesity. Increased body mass index, adipose mass, early-onset obesity, and risk to develop obesity are associated with single nucleotide polymorphism in MC4R or genetic variances near MC4R. In general, MC peptides suppress food intake and reverse positive energy balance, while MCR antagonists increase food intake and body weight. For example, the endogenous antagonists, agouti and AGRP, are competitive antagonists at MC4R that elicit a hyperphagic response. Similarly, synthetic-selective MC4R inhibitors such as HS024, HS028, and SHU9119 induce hyperphagia in both normal and satiated mice. Targeted gene deletion of central MC receptors (MC4R and MC3R) and precursor molecules (POMCs) can result in obese mice. Mice deficient in MC4R are hyperphagic and exhibit obese phenotype.

Additionally, evidence suggests that the MC system interacts with other systems to regulate food intake. For instance, in mice, centrally administered MCR agonists attenuate fasting or NPY-induced hyperphagia. On the other hand, NPY1 receptor inhibitors attenuate hyperphagia induced by selective MC4R antagonists. MC4R antagonists also attenuate the effects of leptin on food intake and body weight, suggesting the involvement of the MC system in the effects of leptin. In support of this hypothesis, leptin has been reported to stimulate hypothalamic POMC mRNA. Furthermore, administration of peripheral and central leptin to obese MC4R knockout mice does not alter food intake, thus implicating MC4R in the regulation of food intake by leptin. In addition to NPY and leptin, MC system appears to be regulated by serotonin via 5-HT$_{1B}$ and 5-HT$_{2C}$ receptors. 5-HT through its action on 5-HT$_{1B}$ receptor inhibits ARP neurons and decreases an inhibitory effect of ARP on POMC neurons. Furthermore, direct action of 5-HT on POMC is mediated through 5-HT$_{2C}$ receptor. 5-HT$_{2C}$ receptor is colocalized with POMC in the ARC, which directly regulates central MC system. Thus, 5-HT interacts with MC system, with both systems being effective in decreasing food intake. To date, no weight loss therapies target the MC system, but drug discovery efforts are being made in this direction. Indeed, 15 patent applications for MC4R ligand as potential antiobesity medicine were filed in the United States in 2008 alone. The effects of individual MC peptides on food intake are summarized as follows:

α-MSH

α-MSH is a 13-amino-acid MC receptor agonist that appears to be the primary endogenous agonist for central MC receptors mediating suppression of food intake. It is expressed in both central (highest levels in the hypothalamus) and peripheral tissues. Central administration of α-MSH has been shown to induce suppression of food intake in experimental animals such as rat. Injection of α-MSH into the ventricles of fasted rats has been shown to attenuate food intake. It also reverses NPY-mediated or dark-phase-mediated feeding following administration into the PVN. In addition to its central effects, α-MSH exhibits peripheral effects on weight gain. For example, it elicits weight loss in POMC-deficient and diet-induced obese mice. Taken together, these data suggest that α-MSH plays a vital role in MC-mediated inhibition of food intake.

β-MSH

β-MSH is a 22-amino-acid peptide derived from the C-terminus fragment of POMC that exhibits a higher affinity for MC4R than α-MSH or γ-MSH in humans and rats. Findings regarding its effect on the regulation of food intake are conflicting. Whereas it has been reported to be equivalent to α-MSH in attenuating food intake in rats fasted for 24 h, other studies indicate it failed to reduce the food intake of rats fasted for 48 h. Evidence from other studies suggests a dose-dependent attenuation of food intake in freely feeding rats after i.c.v. administration of β-MSH. Although some data suggest that β-MSH is involved in the regulation of food intake, the exact nature of its involvement remains to be fully elucidated.

ACTH

ACTH is a 39-amino-acid peptide formed by action of PC1 on POMC in anterior pituitary corticotrophs. It plays a significant role in regulation of appetite. Cleavage of ACTH by PC2 yields α-MSH. Other fragments of ACTH include ACTH(1–16), ACTH(4–16), and ACTH(7–16). Interestingly, ACTH is the only endogenous MC that activates all five MCRs. The anorectic effects of ACTH are mediated by ACTH(1–24), whose activity is protected by ACTH(25–39). Central administration of ACTH(1–24) attenuates feeding in both fasted and freely feeding rat. Furthermore, ACTH(1–24) was found to inhibit hyperphagic effect of intraperitoneally administered kappa opiate agonists. Neither adrenalectomy nor subcutaneous administration (dose up to 200 µg/kg in rats) of ACTH(1–24) was found to suppress food intake, suggesting that the anorectic effects ACTH are not linked to adrenal steroids nor are they mediated by interaction with peripheral feeding regulatory pathways but via sites in the CNS.

In summary, evidence from studies using experimental animals clearly demonstrates a role for several neuropeptides in the regulation of appetite and feeding behavior. The wide array of neuropeptides involved offers great potential for the identification of several classes of these agents that could ultimately be employed in the treatment of obesity in humans.

OTHER CHEMICALS AND RELEVANT PHARMACOLOGICAL RECEPTORS

ENDOCANNABINOIDS

It is well known that the cannabis plant (*Cannabis sativa*) and its extract have an appetite-stimulating action due to the presence of the psychoactive compound Δ^9-tetrahydrocannabinol (THC). The discovery of endogenous ligands for plant-derived cannabinoids (endocannabinoids) has led to the description of a physiological basis for the efficacy of these compounds in experimental animals and humans. Endocannabinoids are derived from arachidonic acid, and they include substances such as anandamide and 2-arachidonoylglycerol (2-AG). In low doses, centrally or systemically administered THC has been shown to stimulate feeding in a variety of animal models. In high doses, THC can decrease feeding due to its potent sedative actions. In humans, THC has also been reported to increase food intake, a factor that has been found to be beneficial in the treatment of conditions involving appetite loss such as AIDS and cancer. It is important to note that the hyperphagic effects of THC can be mimicked by endocannabinoids, anandamide, and 2-AG. Endocannabinoids have been linked with physiological process involved in the regulation of feeding behavior. Increased concentrations of anandamide and 2-AG have been found in the nucleus accumbens during fasting. A decline in the 2-AG level was found during the feeding state, suggesting that the endocannabinoids play an important role in the motivation to obtain food.

Both exogenous cannabinoids and endocannabinoids increase food intake and promote weight gain by stimulating two subtypes of receptors: CB1 and CB2. CB1 receptors are found in the CNS and some peripheral tissues, whereas CB2 receptors are localized in peripheral immune cells. CB1 receptors are linked to the regulation of appetite and feeding behavior. Evidence suggests that pharmacological blockade of CB1 receptors with drugs such as rimonabant (SR141716) produces a reduction of food intake and body weight. Indeed, CB1-gene-deficient mice are found to be lean and resistant to diet-induced obesity. However, rimonabant was withdrawn recently because of its substantial CNS side effects including depression and anxiety. Due to psychiatric disturbance associated with targeting CB1 receptor in the brain, development of antiobesity drugs targeting this receptor in the brain has been suspended and/or terminated globally. Attention is now focused on developing peripherally restricted CB1 receptor antagonists that are unable to cross blood-brain barrier. Such antagonists are thought to not only eliminate any CNS adverse effects observed with rimonabant, but also maintain therapeutic benefits in metabolic syndrome, including type 2 diabetes mellitus and nonalcoholic fatty liver diseases. An example of a compound that meets that criterion, URB447, was recently discovered. URB447 has been identified as a mixed CB1 antagonist/CB2 agonist with anorectic actions and devoid of CNS effects, making it a potential drug candidate for treatment of obesity.

In summary, it appears that endocannabinoids, acting on brain CB1 receptors, can stimulate appetite and feeding behavior in both experimental animals and humans. The discovery of the link between endocannabinoids and their potential to regulate feeding behavior provides immense opportunities for the treatment of diseases or conditions that require either an increase or decrease in appetite.

SUMMARY AND CONCLUSIONS

A wide variety of neurotransmitters and neuropeptides are involved in the regulation of appetite and feeding behavior in both experimental animals and humans. Receptors for classical neurotransmitters (5-HT, NE, and histamine) are well known and appear to be ready targets for development of compounds with therapeutic potential as antiobesity drugs. The neuropeptides NPY, galanin, CRF, orexin, and MC are a diverse group with potential to interact with classical neurotransmitters in the pathways involved in appetite and food regulation. The discovery of endocannabinoids and their receptors has revealed additional targets for the manipulation of pathways that control food intake in experimental animals and humans. In conclusion, concerted efforts need to be focused on the effects of neurotransmitters and neuropeptides that are important in the regulation of food intake and energy metabolism in humans. It may well be that formulations that contain more than one neurotransmitter or neuropeptide could produce the optimum action in terms of controlling food intake and energy metabolism.

BIBLIOGRAPHY

Bays, H.E., Current and investigational antiobesity agents and obesity therapeutic treatment targets, *Obesity Res.*, 12(8), 1197–1211, 2004.

Bays, H.E., Lorcaserin and adiposopathy: 5-HT2c agonism as a treatment for 'sick fat' and metabolic disease, *Expert Rev. Cardiovasc. Ther.*, 7(11), 1429–1445, 2009.

Bello, N.T. and Liang, N.C., The use of serotonergic drugs to treat obesity—Is there any hope?, *Drug Des. Devel. Ther.*, 5, 95–109, 2011.

Bermudez, F.J., Viveros, M.P., McPartland, J.M., and Rodriguez, F., The endocannabinoid system, eating behavior and energy homeostasis: The end or a new beginning? *Pharmacol. Biochem. Behav.*, 95(4), 375–382, 2010.

Cason, A.M., Smith, R.J., Tahsili, P. et al., Role of orexin/hypocretin in reward-seeking and addiction: Implications for obesity, *Physiol. Behav.*, 100(5), 419–428, 2010.

Cerulli, J., Lomaestro, B.M., and Malone, M., Update on the pharmacotherapy of obesity, *Ann. Pharmacother.*, 32, 88–102, 1998.

Choi, D.L., Davis, J.F., Fitzgerald, M.E., and Benoit, S.C., The role of orexin-A in food motivation, reward-based feeding behavior and food-induced neuronal activation in rats, *Neuroscience*, 167(1), 11–20, 2010.

Feletou, M. and Levens, N.R., Neuropeptide Y2 receptors as drug targets for the central regulation of body weight, *Curr. Opin. Invest. Drugs*, 6(10), 1002–1011, 2005.

Halford J.C.G., Pharmacology of appetite suppression: Implication for the treatment of obesity, *Curr. Drug Targets*, 2, 353–370, 2001.

Halford, J.C.G., Harrold, J.A., Lawton, C.L., and Blundell, J.E., Serotonin (5-HT) drugs: Effects on appetite expression and use for the treatment of obesity, *Curr. Drug Targets,* 6, 201–213, 2005.

Halford, J.C., Harrold, J.A., Boyland, E.J., Lawton, C.L., and Blundell, J.E., Serotonergic drugs: Effects on appetite expression and use for the treatment of obesity, *Drugs,* 67(1), 27–55, 2007.

Haynes, A.C., Jackson, B., Overend, P. et al., Effects of single and chronic intracerebroventricular administration of the orexins on feeding in the rat, *Peptides,* 20, 1099–1105, 1999.

Irani, B.G. and Haskell-Luevano, C., Feeding effects of melanocortin ligands—A historical perspective, *Peptides,* 26, 1788–1799, 2005.

King, P.J., The hypothalamus and obesity, *Curr. Drug Targets,* 6, 225–240, 2005.

Kirkham, T.C., Endocannabinoids in the regulation of appetite and body weight, *Behav. Pharmacol.,* 16, 297–313, 2005.

Marston, O.J., Garfield, A.S., and Heisler, L.K., Role of central serotonin and melanocortin systems in the control of energy balance, *Eur. J. Pharmacol.,* 660(1), 70–79, 2011.

Masaki, T. and Yoshimatsu, H., Molecular mechanisms of neuronal histamine and its receptors in obesity, *Curr. Mol. Pharmacol.,* 2(3), 249–252, 2009.

Mastorakos, G. and Zapanti E., The hypothalamic-pituitary-adrenal axis in the neuroendocrine regulation of food intake and obesity: The role of corticotropin releasing hormone, *Nutr. Neurosci.,* 7(5–6), 271–280, 2004.

Masuo, K., Roles of beta2- and beta3-adrenoceptor polymorphisms in hypertension and metabolic syndrome, *Int. J. Hypertens.,* 2010, 832821, 2010.

Mul, J.D., Van, B.R., Bergen, D.J. et al., Melanocortin receptor 4 deficiency affects body weight regulation, grooming behavior, and substrate preference in the rat, *Obesity,* 2011. Epub ahead of print.

Schaub, J.W., Bruce, E.B., and Haskell, L.C., Drugs, exercise, and the melanocortin-4 receptor- different means, same ends: Treating obesity, *Adv. Exp. Med. Biol.,* 681, 49–60, 2010.

Souza, C.J. and Burkey, B.F., Beta$_3$-adrenoceptor agonists as anti-diabetic and anti-obesity drugs in humans, *Curr. Pharmaceut. Des.,* 7, 1433–1449, 2001.

Tsujino, N. and Sakurai, T., Orexin/hypocretin: A neuropeptide at the interface of sleep, energy homeostasis, and reward system, *Pharmacol. Rev.,* 61(2), 162–176, 2009.

Tsuneki, H., Wada, T., and Sasaoka, T., Role of orexin in the regulation of glucose homeostasis, *Acta. Physiol. (Oxf.),* 198(3), 335–348, 2010.

Vucetic, Z. and Reyes, T.M., Central dopaminergic circuitry controlling food intake and reward: Implications for the regulation of obesity, *Wiley Interdiscip. Rev. Syst. Biol. Med.,* 2(5), 577–593, 2010.

Wang, G.J., Volkow, N.D., and Fowler, J.S., The role of dopamine in motivation for food in humans: Implications for obesity, *Expert Opin. Ther. Targets,* 6(5), 601–609, 2002.

Wu, Y.K., Yeh, C.F., Ly, T.W., and Hung, M.S., New perspective of cannabinoid 1 receptor antagonists: Approaches toward peripheral cannabinoid 1 blockers without crossing the blood-brain barrier, *Curr. Top. Med. Chem.,* 2011. Epub ahead of print.

Xu, Y.-L., Jackson, V.R., and Civelli, O., Orphan G protein-coupled receptors and obesity, *Eur. J. Pharmacol.,* 500, 243–253, 2004.

Xu, Z.Q.D., Zheng, K., and Hokfelt, T., Electrophysiological studies of galanin effects in brain—Progress during the last six years, *Neuropeptides,* 39, 269–275, 2005.

Zhang, L., Bijker, M.S., and Herzog, H., The neuropeptide Y system: Pathophysiological and therapeutic implications in obesity and cancer, *Pharmacol. Ther.,* 2011. Epub ahead of print.

8 Neurobiology of Obesity

Nina Eikelis, PhD

CONTENTS

INTRODUCTION

Food is a necessity of life, like sleep. It is also one of the pleasures of life. We may eat when we are not hungry, just because it tastes, looks, or smells good! In fact, a lot of people will eat much more than their body actually needs for fuel. Not surprisingly, the obesity epidemic is sweeping the world. These people go to extreme measures in hopes of getting a control over their body weight.

But why is it so difficult to control our body weight? In recent years, there has been a remarkable progress in the understanding of the molecular basis of obesity. Mammalian energy balance is controlled by complex networks between brain structures such as the hypothalamus, brainstem, and higher brain centers and in the periphery—the stomach, gut, liver, thyroid, and adipose tissue. Advances in molecular techniques have resulted in major advances being made in the understanding of hypothalamic circuits involved in body-weight regulation. In 1994, scientists discovered a gene (*ob* gene), a mutation of which causes severe obesity in a strain of laboratory mice. This gene encodes a hormone leptin, which is mainly secreted by fat cells and acts within the hypothalamus to reduce appetite and increase energy expenditure. When mice are injected with leptin, they lose weight dramatically. Overweight people have elevated leptin levels due to increased adipose tissue mass. However, they seem to be leptin resistant when it comes to its anorexigenic effects; despite high levels of leptin, they continue to overeat. Several mechanisms have been suggested to explain leptin resistance in humans, such as impaired leptin transport in the brain, where it informs the central nervous system (CNS) about the state of body fat, defects in leptin receptor, or altered leptin downstream signaling.

OBESITY EPIDEMIC

The Western world is experiencing an epidemic. While people should be aware of this epidemic, as the evidence is literally under their noses, the rise in obesity prevalence continues to sweep the world unabated. Globally, there are more than 1 billion overweight adults, and at least 300 million of these are obese. Often coexisting in developing countries with undernutrition, obesity is a multidimensional condition affecting virtually all ages and socioeconomic groups. Alarmingly, this trend is even greater in young children, suggesting that this problem will escalate in the foreseeable future.

Why is this happening? A decade or two ago, it was common to blame the individual for being overweight. And while there is no doubt that the rising epidemic reflects the changes in lifestyle due to a simultaneous decrease in activity and increase in caloric intake to great extent, today, however, a different approach is taken to the problem of weight control, with strong and complex factors involved in the tendency to increase body weight. Twin and adoption studies, as well as experimental models of obesity now indicate that obesity results from both genetic and environmental factors.

The health, economic, and psychosocial consequences of obesity are substantial. The health consequences of obesity range from a number of nonfatal complaints that impact on the quality of life, such as skin problems, particularly infectious in flexural creases, respiratory difficulties, and infertility, to complaints that lead to an increased risk of premature death including diabetes, gallbladder disease, and cardiovascular problems (hypertension, stroke, and heart disease). For example, hypertension and diabetes are between two and six times more prevalent among heavier people.

From a social perspective, being overweight may have deleterious effects on people's self-esteem, social and economic characteristics, and physical health. In our culture, being thin means more than just good health; it symbolizes self-control, hard work, ambition, and success in life. Positive attributes are given to thin people, whereas those with less than perfect bodies are often blamed and thought to be lazy and self-indulgent.

REGULATION OF BODY WEIGHT

The regulation of body weight may be considered a homeostatic process, directed at conserving energy balance, seeking food in times of need, and storing energy in times of plenty. However, the homeostatic system in humans is strongly biased toward weight gain and storage of fat, with only a few mechanisms that encourage weight loss. This biased homeostatic system is probably due to little evolutionary pressure to decrease food intake once energy stores are full [1].

Regulation of body weight in humans involves genetic, environmental, and psychosocial factors through physiological regulators of food intake and energy expenditure [2]. Most animals, including humans, can maintain constant body weight over prolonged periods of time. This means that energy intake (derived from ingested foods) must equal energy expenditure over a long term to maintain a stable body weight. While the equation seems pretty straightforward, regulation of body weight is a far more complex interplay of energy intake and expenditure, satiety factors, and other controls of appetite.

Food intake elicits sensory inputs, nutrient, and gastrointestinal signals mediated by distension of the stomach or local hormones, which together modulate appetite. The mechanisms involve different neurotransmitters such as norepinephrine, dopamine, serotonin, orexins, melanocortins, and neuropeptide Y (NPY) just to name a few [3]. All these signals produce neural and humoral outputs that cause appropriate adjustments in nutrient intake and metabolism [4].

Many of the hormones that are involved in the regulation of body weight via appetite and satiety are released from the gastrointestinal tract after a meal. Some of these are cholecystokinin (CCK), glucagon, and gastrin-releasing peptide, which act by reducing food intake after a meal. Nutrients such as glucose and fatty acids provide another signal that regulates food intake. Long-term regulators of food intake include insulin, ghrelin, corticosteroids, and leptin.

In addition to appetite, thermogenesis is another mechanism involved in body-weight regulation. Several prospective studies have shown that a relatively low energy expenditure predicts body-weight gain [5–7]. Results from most overfeeding studies indicate that short-term diet-induced weight gain is associated with an increase in energy expenditure [8,9]. Similarly, underfeeding is accompanied by a decrease in energy expenditure beyond the predicted values [10–12]. Such overcompensatory metabolic changes are presumably acting to oppose any further weight gain.

It is currently assumed that the major factors involved in obesity include the genetic background of an individual and his or her dietary and physical activity habits. The role of inheritance in human obesity has been extensively studied over the last decade, with adoption and twin studies showing that obesity has a genetic component. More recently, the studies have shown that both body fat mass and the partitioning between the central and peripheral fat depots are influenced by genetics [13]. It is likely therefore that genes involved in weight gain increase the susceptibility of an individual to develop obesity when exposed to the environment that favors positive energy balance.

The discovery and cloning of specific genes involved in fat accumulation have led to a renewed interest in genetic factors responsible for the development of human obesity. The relatively recent isolation of the *ob* gene, which encodes leptin, has attracted particular attention. Other genetic mutations that lead to the excessive accumulation of fat in animal models have also been identified, and some of them involve the leptin receptor, melanocortin-4 receptor, and proopiomelanocortin (POMC).

Body weight is regulated by the CNS, which can sense the body's metabolic status from a wide range of humoral and neural signals. The integration of the signals takes place largely, but not solely, in the hypothalamus. The hypothalamus is the structure that is generally considered to be the most sensitive to manipulations that modulate appetite and eating behaviors. Hypothalamic amines, hormones, and neurotransmitters participate in a complex network of systems that influence eating behavior and the metabolism of specific nutrients. Stimulation of some systems results in an increase in food consumption, while stimulation of other systems results in a reduction in food intake and storage. Therefore, it is likely that disturbances in one or many of these systems may underlie body-weight changes.

LEPTIN

ob Gene

The *ob* gene was first discovered in adipose tissue of the obese mouse through positional cloning [14]. The full coding sequence contains 167 amino acids and represents a 21-amino-acid signal peptide and 146-amino-acid circulating bioactive hormone [14]. In both human and mouse, the leptin gene is composed of three exons and two introns. Interestingly, the leptin peptide has structural similarities to members of the cytokine family [15].

In mammals, leptin is predominantly produced in adipose tissue and secreted into the bloodstream. However, nonadipocyte leptin production has also been documented in the stomach [16], placenta [17], and brain [18,19]. Nonadipose sources of leptin production may perhaps suggest a far more complex role for leptin than originally thought.

Leptin Protein

The *ob* gene codes for a protein secreted by fat cells. This protein is hypothesized to regulate fat storage by signaling the brain to suppress appetite when the body's fat stores are full. When mutated in mice, the *ob* gene is no longer able to express leptin and therefore can no longer deliver its appetite-suppressing message. The mice consequently develop a syndrome that resembles extreme obesity and type II diabetes in humans.

Human leptin is 84% homologous to mouse and 83% homologous to rat leptin. Leptin consists of four antiparallel α-helices (A, B, C, and D), connected by two long crossover links (AB and CD) and one short loop (BC), arranged in a left-handed twisted helical bundle. The four-helix bundle is folded as packing of antiparallel helix pairs A and D against B and C, and a disulfide bond between the C-terminus of the protein and the beginning of the CD loop is important for stability and biological activity [20].

Leptin Receptors

While leptin is predominantly produced by adipocytes, leptin receptors are located in many tissues. The leptin receptor is encoded by the diabetes (*db*) gene. Tartaglia et al. [21] were the first to isolate and describe the leptin receptor (Ob-R) in a mouse. To date, at least six leptin receptor isoforms have been described [22]. Alternative gene splicing explains the number of leptin receptors. All isoforms share the same extracellular domain; however, only one of them, the long form, has all the intracellular motifs required for signal transduction via the JAK-STAT pathway (Figure 8.1).

Based on sequence homology, the OB-R belongs to the class I cytokine receptor family, which includes receptors for interleukin-6, leukocyte inhibitory factor, and granulocyte-colony-stimulating factor [23]. Leptin-OB-Rb complex formation leads to the induction of tyrosine phosphorylation through its association with JAK2 (Figure 8.1). The activated JAK2 phosphorylates a distal tyrosine (Tyr-1138) on the receptor, similar to STATs proteins. Although leptin can activate STAT1, STAT3, STAT5, and STAT6, it only activates STAT3 in the rodent hypothalamus.

Mutations in the functional leptin receptor result in an obese phenotype identical to that of *ob* mice. In fatty Zucker rats, a point mutation in the extracellular domain inhibits signal transduction. On the other hand, *db/db* mice predominantly express the short form of leptin receptor, which leaves these mice with a nonsignaling leptin receptor system.

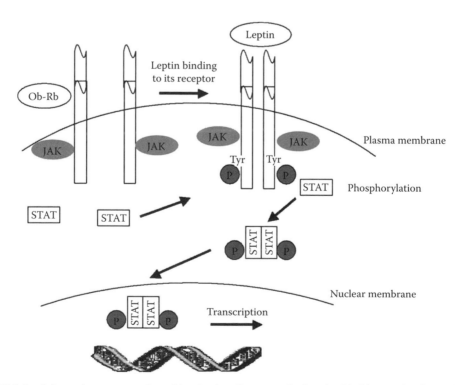

FIGURE 8.1 Schematic representation of leptin signaling cascade. Leptin-Ob-Rb complex formation leads to the induction of tyrosine phosphorylation through its association with JAK2, which leads to the activation of STAT proteins.

Ob-Rb is highly expressed in the hypothalamus. Experimental studies have identified the hypothalamic arcuate nucleus (ARC), DMH, PVN, VMH, and lateral hypothalamic nucleus as principle sites of leptin receptor expression in the CNS [24,25]. Each of these nuclei is important in regulating body weight.

A soluble form of leptin receptor consisting of an extracellular domain only also exists. It binds leptin with an affinity similar to that of membrane receptors. Results from animal experiments have demonstrated that the soluble form of leptin receptor may modulate leptin levels in plasma by delaying its clearance, and it may determine the amount of free versus bound leptin [26]. In obese subjects, a considerable greater proportion of leptin circulates in the free form compared to lean individuals, and the amount of free leptin increases with the increasing body mass index (BMI), suggesting that the soluble form of this receptor is saturated in the state of obesity [27]. In addition, short-term fasting results in a decrease of total leptin levels, which is mostly attributable to the decrease in free leptin.

Mutations in *db* gene are extremely rare in humans. The first case of leptin receptor mutation was first described by Clement [22]. In these patients, a single G-A substitution in the splice donor site of exon 16 resulted in a nonfunctional leptin receptor lacking both transmembrane and intracellular domain. As a result of that mutation, the truncated leptin receptor is unable to activate STAT signal transduction pathway. Similar to the *ob* gene mutation in humans, human *db* mutation results in hyperphagia and early onset obesity, with BMI reaching as high as 70 kg/m^2.

Transport of Leptin into the CNS

Leptin is primarily secreted by adipocytes, circulates in blood, in part while linked to binding proteins, and exerts its effects in specific regions of the brain. The delivery of leptin into the brain represents a crucial step toward the regulation of body weight and energy balance. How leptin gains access to specific regions in the brain is still a controversial issue. Different studies have demonstrated the presence of leptin receptors in the brain capillaries as well as binding of leptin to human and mouse brain capillaries [28,29]. Potentially, the presence of leptin receptors in the brain capillaries would allow leptin access through the capillary wall to specific regions (such as hypothalamic nuclei) in order to exert its effects.

In rodents, leptin enters the brain via saturable transport mechanisms across the blood-brain barrier. Results from the previous studies demonstrated that brain microvessels express the short form of the leptin receptor (Ob-Ra) at a high rate. It has been suggested that the same short form of leptin receptor, which is highly expressed in the choroid plexus (the site of CSF production), mediates blood-to-CSF leptin transport. In fact, the experiments conducted by Hileman and coworkers [30] on Madin-Darby Canine Kidney showed that the short form of leptin receptor is capable of mediating transcellular transport of leptin. These data further suggest that the short form of the leptin receptor expressed at the blood-brain barrier is capable of transporting leptin from the circulation into the brain. It is also of interest to note that the receptor is preferentially expressed on the apical membrane, which faces the bloodstream. Therefore, the Ob-Ra is well positioned to mediate the transport of leptin from the circulation into the brain. Once in the brain, leptin can reach the neurons containing the long-form signaling leptin receptor (Ob-Rb) to activate the signal transduction pathway [30]. These data are supportive of the concept that Ob-Ra mediates passage of leptin across the cerebral microvessels that constitute the blood-brain barrier. Furthermore, deficits in Ob-Ra function at this site could result in leptin resistance. On the other hand, leptin is present in the CSF of Koletsky rats, which lack leptin receptors altogether, thereby suggesting that leptin receptors are perhaps not essential for leptin receptor transport into CSF. In addition, recent evidence from our laboratory also suggests that leptin is actually synthesized by the human brain itself, as evident from the net leptin efflux into the internal jugular vein [19,31,32] as well as leptin mRNA expression in the human cadaver hypothalami [33,34].

Human obesity is characterized by a state of leptin resistance, which is likely caused by a combination of resistance at the receptor and postreceptor levels as well as reduced transport of circulating leptin across the blood-brain barrier. A few lines of evidence have suggested impaired leptin transport across the blood-brain barrier. For example, it has been demonstrated that obese humans have a reduced CSF-to-serum ratio for leptin. Experimental evidence also supports the idea of impaired leptin transport across the brain in obesity in showing that some obese animal models that no longer respond to peripherally administered leptin can still respond to leptin given centrally.

Leptin and Eating Disorders

Since eating disorders such as anorexia nervosa and bulimia nervosa are characterized by abnormal eating behaviors, dysregulation of endogenous endocrine axes, alterations of reproductive and immune functions, and increased physical activity, extensive research has been carried out in the last decade in order to ascertain a role of leptin in the pathophysiology of eating disorders.

It has been reported that plasma leptin levels are dramatically reduced in underweight anorectic patients as compared to healthy age-matched people [35]. However, although markedly reduced, circulating leptin is significantly and positively correlated with the person's BMI, indicating that even at an extremely low body weight and fat, circulating leptin still functions as a signal of energy stores. Longitudinal studies have shown that in anorexia nervosa patients undergoing refeeding during recovery, circulating leptin levels increase progressively and reach values disproportionately higher than compared to stable weight healthy people [35]. It has even been suggested that hyperleptinemia in these patients during refeeding treatment may be one of the factors in patient's difficulties of reaching and maintaining the target weight. In fact, it has been demonstrated that in patients undergoing refeeding treatment, a too rapid weight gain, followed by hyperleptinemia, is associated with poor prognosis [36].

In normal weight patients with bulimia nervosa, plasma leptin levels have been reported to be increased, decreased, or normal [37–39]. The reason for such a discrepancy among the results may be due to the heterogeneous composition of the patient groups. It seems that a group of bulimic patients hyposecreted leptin despite the body weight being similar to otherwise healthy people [37]. Therefore, even if body weight is a major determinant of circulating leptin levels, other factors are likely to be involved in suppressing leptin production in these patients. It has been proposed that the chronicity and severity of the illness could be determinants of the leptin hyposecretion [37]. While leptin does not seem to be directly involved in the pathogenesis of eating disorders, derangements in its physiology may contribute to some clinical alterations occurring in the course of these disorders.

Mechanisms of Leptin Action in the Brain

The brain has been hypothesized to be the primary site of leptin action, as peripherally administered leptin has been shown to rapidly induce the hypothalamic signal transduction pathway. *In situ* hybridization studies have shown that the Ob-Rb is predominantly expressed in hypothalamic nuclei such as the ARC, the dorsomedial nucleus of the hypothalamus (DMH), the paraventricular nucleus (PVN), the ventromedial nucleus of the hypothalamus (VMH), and the lateral hypothalamus (LH). Early experimental work demonstrated that destruction of the PVN and VMH produced hyperphagia and obesity, while lesions to the LH caused anorexia.

Leptin-sensitive neurons in the hypothalamus are known to express neuropeptides and neurotransmitters involved in the central regulation of appetite. The long-form leptin receptor has been shown to be coexpressed with NPY, agouti-related peptide (AgRP), POMC, and cocaine- and amphetamine-regulated transcript (CART) in the ARC. Therefore, leptin-sensitive neurons in the ARC may influence other peptides involved in the regulation of appetite. In addition, leptin is known to modulate the effects of the orexigenic peptides in the brain by inhibiting their synthesis such as in the case of NPY [40,41].

Leptin Resistance in Obesity

The observation that high leptin levels in overweight and obese individuals fail to induce weight loss has given rise to the notion of "leptin resistance." While the mechanisms underlying leptin resistance are still the matter of considerable research, a number of biological processes hypothesized to be involved include leptin binding to blood-borne proteins (one of which is the soluble leptin receptor), active and/or passive transport of leptin into the brain, leptin receptor expression levels, and alterations of leptin receptor second messenger responsiveness [22].

The failure of leptin to reach its target in the brain, in particular the hypothalamus, has received much attention. Experimental studies provided some evidence of leptin-impaired transport across the blood-brain barrier in animal models of diet-induced obesity [42]. Moreover, in some animal models, the delivery of leptin into the CNS seems to be a crucial step toward the regulation of food intake and energy balance. Different studies have shown the presence of specific leptin receptors in the brain capillaries as well as binding of leptin to brain capillaries [28,43]. Therefore, the presence of the leptin receptors on endothelial cells would suggest that leptin can gain access to the specific hypothalamic nuclei to initiate the signaling cascade. Leptin has also been shown to be transported by a saturable transport system, the activity of which is impaired in obesity [44].

When first discovered, leptin was thought to be secreted exclusively by adipocytes into the bloodstream [14]. Later evidence, however, suggests that adipose tissue may not be the only site of leptin production with demonstration of leptin gene expression in other tissues, such as stomach [16], placenta [45], and skeletal muscles [46]. The results of previous studies from our laboratory demonstrated a net efflux of leptin from the brain into the internal jugular veins [19,32]. This observation suggests that perhaps the brain itself produces leptin that is subsequently released into the circulation and contributes to total leptin plasma pool [32]. In fact, leptin mRNA expression has been shown in the rat pituitary and the brain [18].

Another possible mechanism in leptin resistance could involve defects in the leptin receptor. There are a few isoforms of the leptin receptor that are spliced abnormally and therefore do not result in the appropriate signal transduction. The mutation of the *db* gene generates a truncated version of the leptin receptor, lacking most of the intracellular domain. In *fa/fa* Zucker rats, there is a missense mutation in the leptin receptor. This mutation causes obesity, despite the fact that the expression of the leptin gene is significantly augmented. Therefore, these examples demonstrate that the defects in the leptin receptor may result in leptin resistance.

There has been an extensive search in the human hypothalamic leptin receptors for possible variations that would explain the leptin resistance in human obesity. The full-length functional receptor, Ob-Rb, identified by Tartaglia was found to be expressed in the human hypothalamus. In addition, no abnormal splicing of the human leptin receptor was observed, together with the demonstration that there was no difference between the leptin receptor mRNA expression between lean and obese individuals. Some sequence variations have been detected in the human leptin receptor, with most variation being the single-base substitutions that did not result in the change of the amino acid. There was a single-base substitution detected in the leptin receptor gene that results in the change of the amino acid from glutamine to arginine. However, this substitution was detected in both lean and obese individuals, therefore making this polymorphism unlikely to underlie the basis for leptin resistance in humans. There are a few mutations in the human leptin receptor gene that result in the truncated receptor unable to activate the signal transduction pathway. These mutations result in the early onset obesity, highlighting the importance of leptin in body-weight regulation in humans. However, mutations in the leptin receptor gene are very rare in humans.

We have examined full-length leptin receptor expression (Ob-Rb) in the human hypothalamus in males and females across a broad range of BMI (Figure 8.2). However, we have not found any relation between the level of its expression and adiposity, suggesting that other factors must operate that regulate Ob-Rb levels. So, it would seem that leptin resistance cannot be simply explained on the basis of mutations in the leptin receptor.

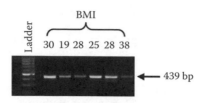

FIGURE 8.2   Leptin receptor (Ob-Rb) expression in the human hypothalamus of six donors of different BMI. No association was found between adiposity and Ob-Rb expression.

Since most cases of human obesity are not associated with inappropriate leptin levels or mutated leptin receptor, a defect could lie in the signaling cascade. SOCS-3 (suppressor of cytokine signaling 3) has been demonstrated to play a role in leptin resistance [47]. SOCS proteins are negative regulators of the JAK/STAT signaling pathways. It has been shown experimentally that injection of leptin stimulates the production of SOCS-3. The signaling cascade induced by leptin binding to its receptor is blocked due to SOCS-3 binding to leptin.

Although several biological mechanisms that may participate in leptin resistance have been identified, it still remains to be determined the sequence of events that initiate this state and as well as treatment possibilities.

Leptin Signaling Pathways

It is clear that leptin and its receptors are only one of many maybe important determinants in the control of body weight and the pathogenesis of obesity (Table 8.1). It has been proposed that two classes of neurons account for leptin's actions in the CNS, namely, NPY- and POMC-containing neurons (Figure 8.3).

TABLE 8.1

Neuropeptide Systems Involved in the Control of Food Intake

Orexigenic (Increase Energy Intake)	Anorexigenic (Decrease Energy Intake)
AgRP	Leptin
NPY	α-MSH
Melanin-concentrating hormone	CCK
Ghrelin	Corticotrophin-releasing factor
Orexin	Glucagon
Opioid	Neurotensin

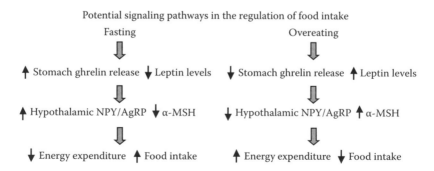

FIGURE 8.3   Schematic representation of the potential signaling pathways in the regulation of food intake.

Role of NPY in the Control of Food Intake

NPY, a 36-amino-acid protein, is synthesized as a long precursor molecule with the active portion at the amino end of the polypeptide. It is expressed in many areas of the brain acting as a transmitter in the nervous system. It selectively binds to Y1 and Y5 receptors in the hypothalamus and is a potent stimulator of feeding. Most attention given to NPY's role in feeding behavior has focused on its central action in the hypothalamus, where a single injection of NPY stimulates overeating, and its repeated administration results in obesity.

NPY seems to be a partner of leptin in the regulation of body fat by participation in the energy balance and neuroendocrine signaling. Leptin appears to inhibit feeding partly by suppressing the synthesis of NPY. Not surprisingly, leptin deficiency results in the elevation of the central NPY levels.

In order to examine the role that NPY plays in feeding behavior, scientists have examined NPY gene knockout mutants. Since knockout NPY mutant mice birth rates follow mathematical probability calculations, and these mice have normal lives and fertility, it can be concluded that NPY presence is not vital to maintain a seemingly normal feeding and body-weight regulation. Although NPY is clearly involved in the control of feeding behavior, leptin effects on body weight are only partly mediated by its effects on NPY expression. No doubt there are other overlapping systems in the control of food intake and energy homeostasis.

Central Melanocortin System in the Regulation of Food Intake

One of the central systems activated by leptin is the melanocortin system. The melanocortin system refers to a family of peptide hormones and hormone receptors that controls a number of functions in our bodies such as energy metabolism, sexual functions, and skin pigmentation. Bioactive peptides, generated from the prohormone called POMC, are key regulators of appetite control and energy homeostasis. It is therefore important to understand many aspects of POMC gene regulation particularly in the brain, as pharmacological manipulations of POMC expression/processing could be a potential strategy to combat obesity.

Proteolytic processing of POMC results in a number of different hormones and neuropeptides that are mainly divided into two classes: melanocortins and endorphins. Melanocortin peptides include adrenocorticotrophin and α-, β-, and γ-melanocyte-stimulating hormones (MSH) that exert their effects via G-protein-coupled melanocortin receptors, MC-1 through to MC-5.

Agouti-related protein (AgRP) is a naturally occurring antagonist of melanocortin action. It is a neuropeptide expressed in the ARC of the hypothalamus that increases appetite and decreases metabolism. It is one of the most potent and long-lasting of appetite stimulators. AgRP levels are elevated in obese males [48]. AgRP is an endogenous antagonist at the MC3-R and MC4-R, whereas POMC products, such as α-MSH, act as agonists [49].

Leptin has been shown to activate AgRP-containing neurons and POMC-/CART-containing neurons in the hypothalamus via activation of the long-form leptin receptor coexpressed in these neurons. Central infusion of leptin stimulates expression of the POMC gene while reducing the expression of the AgRP gene in the ARC of the hypothalamus. Not surprisingly, animals either deficient in leptin or leptin-signaling pathways have increased levels of AgRP but reduced POMC levels.

The melanocortin system plays a key role in the central control of appetite and energy expenditure, which is highlighted by the studies showing that mice deficient in MC-4 receptors, as well as mice with increased levels of AgRP, are obese. In humans, mutations in the α-MSH gene also lead to obesity. Abnormalities in the melanocortin system produce obesity through changes in appetite and food intake. Moreover, melanocortin agonists have been shown to suppress appetite. Animals and humans with defects in the central melanocortin system display a characteristic melanocortin obesity phenotype typified by increased adiposity, hyperphagia, metabolic defects, and increased linear growth.

GHRELIN EFFECTS IN THE HYPOTHALAMUS

The hormone ghrelin is expressed mainly in the stomach. It was initially discovered as the endogenous ligand of the growth hormone secretagogue receptor type 1a [50]. Now it is also known to participate in the regulation of energy homeostasis. It is the only known systemic signal to date to promote a positive energy balance by stimulating food intake and decreasing fat oxidation [51]. During fasting, ghrelin levels are increased; however, they fall after meals. As such, this hormone plays a critical role in signaling the brain when we are hungry or full and has become an important focus of obesity research.

In both rodents and humans, ghrelin acts to increase hunger through its actions on the hypothalamic feeding centers. It has been shown that ghrelin-dependent food intake is at least partially mediated by its action in the ARC nucleus [52]. The neurons of the ARC are also known to express NPY and AgRP. In fact, it has been demonstrated that ghrelin increases the expression of these two orexigenic peptides [52], which perhaps suggest indirect actions of ghrelin on food intake via the NPY/AgRP signaling pathway.

There is some evidence that ghrelin administration in humans leads to reported sensations of hunger. Ghrelin administration in the experimental setting leads to increased AgRP and NPY mRNA levels in the ARC of the hypothalamus [52]. This perhaps indicates that AgRP/NPY neurons are the primary target of ghrelin's orexigenic effects in the hypothalamus.

In a recent elegant study, Theander-Carrillo et al. reported that apart from ghrelin's stimulation of appetite, it also has effect on adipocyte metabolism [53]. In white adipocytes, ghrelin caused glucose and triglyceride uptake, increased lipogenesis, and inhibited lipid oxidation, while in brown adipose tissue, ghrelin inhibited the expression of uncoupling proteins, which usually contribute to energy expenditure [53].

Ghrelin can also regulate feeding by inhibition of leptin. Leptin receptors are found in the hypothalamus, including the ARC, and hypothalamic NPY-positive neurons are the target of leptin action. Leptin suppresses arcuate NPY mRNA expression, and ghrelin can reverse leptin-induced downregulation of NPY expression, thereby inhibiting leptin effects. Therefore, it would seem that leptin and ghrelin share the hypothalamic NPY/AgRP signaling pathway.

CONCLUSIONS

Nothing seems simpler or more natural than eating. Yet, every article on feeding behavior emphasizes how complex it is! Feeding behavior has intrigued scientists for centuries; however, it was not until the late 1990s that the most amazing discoveries were made. The discovery of the fat-derived peptide, leptin, sets in motion an intense research effort to better understand the genetic, hormonal, and neurochemical basis of obesity. No other hormone has drawn more attention than leptin in the studies on the control of body weight and appetite. Several neuropeptides and transmitters have been identified and shown to be the mediators of leptin's central actions with POMC and NPY having opposing effects. It is unlikely that leptin has evolved to prevent obesity because high circulating leptin does not prevent the development of obesity.

REFERENCES

1. Wilding, J.P., Neuropeptides and appetite control, *Diabet Med*, 19, 619–627, 2002.
2. Jebb, S.A., Aetiology of obesity, *Br Med Bull*, 53, 264–285, 1997.
3. Bessesen, D.H. and Faggioni, R., Recently identified peptides involved in the regulation of body weight, *Semin Oncol*, 25, 28–32, 1998.
4. Bray, G.A., Treatment for obesity: A nutrient balance/nutrient partition approach, *Nutr Rev*, 49, 33–45, 1991.
5. Roberts, S.B. et al., Energy expenditure and intake in infants born to lean and overweight mothers, *N Engl J Med*, 318, 461–466, 1988.

6. Griffiths, M. et al., Metabolic rate and physical development in children at risk of obesity, *Lancet*, 336, 76–78, 1990.

7. Ravussin, E. et al., Reduced rate of energy expenditure as a risk factor for body-weight gain, *N Engl J Med*, 318, 467–472, 1988.

8. Tremblay, A. et al., Overfeeding and energy expenditure in humans, *Am J Clin Nutr*, 56, 857–62, 1992.

9. Norgan, N.G. and Durnin, J.V., The effect of 6 weeks of overfeeding on the body weight, body composition, and energy metabolism of young men, *Am J Clin Nutr*, 33, 978–988, 1980.

10. Leibel, R.L., Rosenbaum, M., and Hirsch, J., Changes in energy expenditure resulting from altered body weight, *N Engl J Med*, 332, 621–628, 1995.

11. Mansell, P.I. and MacDonald, I.A., The effect of underfeeding on the physiological response to food ingestion in normal weight women, *Br J Nutr*, 60, 39–48, 1988.

12. Bessard, T., Schutz, Y., and Jequier, E., Energy expenditure and postprandial thermogenesis in obese women before and after weight loss, *Am J Clin Nutr*, 38, 680–693, 1983.

13. Perusse, L. et al., Familial aggregation of abdominal visceral fat level: Results from the Quebec family study, *Metabolism*, 45, 378–382, 1996.

14. Zhang, Y. et al., Positional cloning of the mouse obese gene and its human homologue, *Nature*, 372, 425–432, 1994.

15. Fruhbeck, G., A heliocentric view of leptin, *Proc Nutr Soc*, 60, 301–318, 2001.

16. Bado, A. et al., The stomach is a source of leptin, *Nature*, 394, 790–793, 1998.

17. Hassink, S.G. et al., Placental leptin: An important new growth factor in intrauterine and neonatal development?, *Pediatrics*, 100, E1, 1997.

18. Morash, B. et al., Leptin gene expression in the brain and pituitary gland, *Endocrinology*, 140, 5995–5998, 1999.

19. Wiesner, G. et al., Leptin is released from the human brain: Influence of adiposity and gender, *J Clin Endocrinol Metab*, 84, 2270–2274, 1999.

20. Zhang, F. et al., Crystal structure of the obese protein leptin-E100, *Nature*, 387, 206–209, 1997.

21. Tartaglia, L.A. et al., Identification and expression cloning of a leptin receptor, OB-R, *Cell*, 83, 1263–1271, 1995.

22. Ahima, R.S. and Flier, J.S., Leptin, *Annu Rev Physiol*, 62, 413–437, 2000.

23. Ishida-Takahashi, R. et al., Rapid inhibition of leptin signaling by glucocorticoids in vitro and in vivo, *J Biol Chem*, 279, 19658–19664, 2004.

24. Mercer, J.G. et al., Localization of leptin receptor mRNA and the long form splice variant (Ob-Rb) in mouse hypothalamus and adjacent brain regions by in situ hybridization, *FEBS Lett*, 387, 113–116, 1996.

25. Fei, H. et al., Anatomic localization of alternatively spliced leptin receptors (Ob-R) in mouse brain and other tissues, *Proc Natl Acad Sci USA*, 94, 7001–7005, 1997.

26. Huang, L., Wang, Z., and Li, C., Modulation of circulating leptin levels by its soluble receptor, *J Biol Chem*, 276, 6343–6349, 2001.

27. Sinha, M.K. et al., Evidence of free and bound leptin in human circulation. Studies in lean and obese subjects and during short-term fasting, *J Clin Invest*, 98, 1277–1282, 1996.

28. Bjorbaek, C. et al., Expression of leptin receptor isoforms in rat brain microvessels, *Endocrinology*, 139, 3485–3491, 1998.

29. Golden, P.L., Maccagnan, T.J., and Pardridge, W.M., Human blood-brain barrier leptin receptor. Binding and endocytosis in isolated human brain microvessels, *J Clin Invest*, 99, 14–18, 1997.

30. Hileman, S.M. et al., Transcellular transport of leptin by the short leptin receptor isoform ObRa in Madin-Darby Canine Kidney cells, *Endocrinology*, 141, 1955–1961, 2000.

31. Esler, M. et al., Leptin in human plasma is derived in part from the brain, and cleared by the kidneys, *Lancet*, 351, 879, 1998.

32. Eikelis, N. et al., Extra-adipocyte leptin release in human obesity and its relation to sympathoadrenal function, *Am J Physiol Endocrinol Metab*, 286 (5), E744–E752, 2004.

33. Eikelis, N. et al., Reduced brain leptin in patients with major depressive disorder and in suicide victims, *Mol Psychiatry*, 11 (9), 800–801, 2006.

34. Eikelis, N. and Esler, M., The neurobiology of human obesity, *Exp Physiol*, 90, 673–682, 2005.

35. Hebebrand, J. et al., Leptin levels in patients with anorexia nervosa are reduced in the acute stage and elevated upon short-term weight restoration, *Mol Psychiatry*, 2, 330–334, 1997.

36. Remschmidt, H., Schmidt, M.H., and Gutenbrunner, C., Prediction of long-term outcome in anorectic patients from longitudinal weight measurements during inpatient treatment: A cross validation study, in *Child and Youth Psychiatry: Europen Perspectives*. Vol 1. *Anorexiaa Nervosa*. Hogrefe & Huber Publishers, Toronto, Canada, 1990, pp. 150–167.

37. Monteleone, P. et al., Leptin secretion is related to chronicity and severity of the illness in bulimia nervosa, *Psychosom Med*, 64, 874–879, 2002.
38. Monteleone, P. et al., Opposite modifications in circulating leptin and soluble leptin receptor across the eating disorder spectrum, *Mol Psychiatry*, 7, 641–646, 2002.
39. Jimerson, D.C. et al., Decreased serum leptin in bulimia nervosa, *J Clin Endocrinol Metab*, 85, 4511–4514, 2000.
40. Erickson, J.C., Hollopeter, G., and Palmiter, R.D., Attenuation of the obesity syndrome of ob/ob mice by the loss of neuropeptide Y, *Science*, 274, 1704–1707, 1996.
41. Cusin, I. et al., The weight-reducing effect of an intracerebroventricular bolus injection of leptin in genetically obese fa/fa rats. Reduced sensitivity compared with lean animals, *Diabetes*, 45, 1446–1450, 1996.
42. Banks, W.A. and Farrell, C.L., Impaired transport of leptin across the blood-brain barrier in obesity is acquired and reversible, *Am J Physiol Endocrinol Metab*, 285, E10–5, 2003.
43. Banks, W.A. et al., Leptin enters the brain by a saturable system independent of insulin, *Peptides*, 17, 305–311, 1996.
44. Banks, W.A., The many lives of leptin, *Peptides*, 25, 331–338, 2004.
45. Hoggard, N. et al., Leptin and leptin receptor mRNA and protein expression in the murine fetus and placenta, *Proc Natl Acad Sci USA*, 94, 11073–11078, 1997.
46. Wang, J. et al., A nutrient-sensing pathway regulates leptin gene expression in muscle and fat, *Nature*, 393, 684–688, 1998.
47. Bjorbaek, C. et al., The role of SOCS-3 in leptin signaling and leptin resistance, *J Biol Chem*, 274, 30059–30065, 1999.
48. Katsuki, A. et al., Plasma levels of agouti-related protein are increased in obese men, *J Clin Endocrinol Metab*, 86, 1921–1924, 2001.
49. Ollmann, M.M. et al., Antagonism of central melanocortin receptors in vitro and in vivo by agouti-related protein, *Science*, 278, 135–138, 1997.
50. Kojima, M. et al., Ghrelin is a growth-hormone-releasing acylated peptide from stomach, *Nature*, 402, 656–660, 1999.
51. Tschop, M., Smiley, D.L., and Heiman, M.L., Ghrelin induces adiposity in rodents, *Nature*, 407, 908–913, 2000.
52. Kamegai, J. et al., Chronic central infusion of ghrelin increases hypothalamic neuropeptide Y and Agouti-related protein mRNA levels and body weight in rats, *Diabetes*, 50, 2438–2443, 2001.
53. Theander-Carrillo, C. et al., Ghrelin action in the brain controls adipocyte metabolism, *J Clin Invest*, 116 (7), 1983–1993, 2006.

9 Leptin as a Vasoactive Adipokine

Link between Metabolism and Vasculature

Anne Bouloumié, PhD, Cyrile Anne Curat, PhD,
Alexandra Miranville, PhD, Karine Lolmède, PhD,
and Coralie Sengenès, PhD

CONTENTS

In the past years, the discovery of leptin has open new perspectives and brought new concepts in understanding the regulation of the body weight. With the recognition of its important endocrine activity, the adipose tissue has acquired a central role not only in the regulation of energy homeostasis but also in the immune function and reproductive capacity. Obesity is frequently clustered with a number of cardiovascular risk factors such as insulin resistance, diabetes mellitus, hyperlipidemia, and arterial hypertension, commonly referred to as the metabolic syndrome. Although each component of the metabolic syndrome may contribute to the increased risk of cardiovascular disease observed in obesity, the adipose tissue may also *directly* influence the pathogenesis of hypertension and atherosclerosis by the secretion of adipocytokines and more particularly leptin.

Leptin is an adipocyte-derived hormone [1–3] that exhibits structural similarities with the cytokine family. Other tissues also express leptin, although at lower levels, including placenta, ovaries, skeletal muscle, stomach, pituitary, and liver [4]. Leptin gene expression in adipocyte is regulated in the context of hormonal and nutritional status (Table 9.1) (for review [5]).

CENTRAL EFFECTS OF LEPTIN

The interest in leptin focused initially on appetite and body weight regulation (Figure 9.1).

TABLE 9.1

Regulation of Leptin Expression

Upregulation	Downregulation
Refeeding	Fasting/dieting
Insulin/glucose	β-Adrenoceptor agonists
Estrogens	Androgens
Glucocorticoids	PPARγ agonists (thiazolidinediones)
TNFα/IL-1	Cigarette smoking
Acute inflammation	

Source: Margetic, S. et al., *Int. J. Obes. Relat. Metab. Disord.*, 26(11), 1407, 2002.

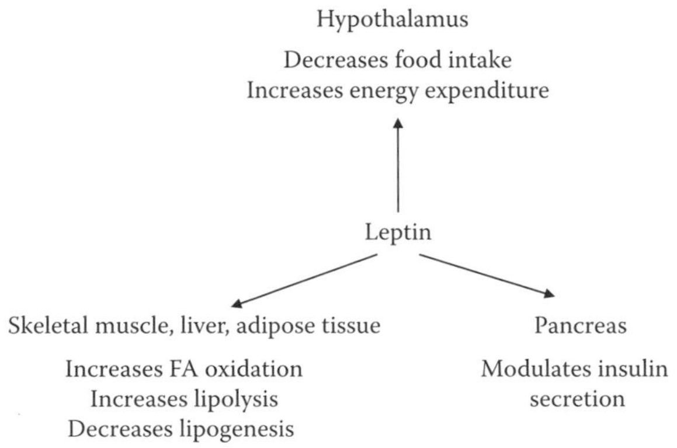

Hypothalamus

Decreases food intake
Increases energy expenditure

↑

Leptin

Skeletal muscle, liver, adipose tissue   Pancreas

Increases FA oxidation   Modulates insulin
Increases lipolysis   secretion
Decreases lipogenesis

FIGURE 9.1   Central and peripheral effect of leptin on energy homeostasis.

ENERGY HOMEOSTASIS

Leptin acts as an afferent satiety signal influencing the central regulation of food intake and energy expenditure via central leptin receptors. Fasting and dieting induces a fall in leptin, signal for the brain to initiate adaptive responses, such as suppression of reproductive and thyroid function and stimulation of the hypothalamic–pituitary–adrenal axis.

Two genetic obese animal models, the ob/ob and db/db mouse, have been extensively investigated, the former being defective in leptin synthesis, the latter in leptin receptor function. Several isoforms (a–f) of the leptin receptor (Ob-R) exist as a result of alternative mRNA splicing [6]. Db/db mice lack the long isoform of the Ob-R (Ob-Rb) that has a cytoplasmic domain required for activation of signal transducers and activators of transcription (STAT) but still express the four other isoforms of the leptin receptor (the short isoforms Ob-Ra, Ob-Rc, Ob-Rd, Ob-Re). The short isoforms exhibit abbreviated intracellular amino acid sequences and have little intracellular signaling capacity [6]. Their physiological role is less clear. The short isoforms Ob-Ra and Ob-Rc seem to be important for blood–brain barrier function as leptin transport system [7], whereas the circulating Ob-Re isoform might play a role in preventing the hormone from degradation and clearance. The long-form leptin receptor belongs to the cytokine-receptor superfamily coupled to the janus kinase (JAK)/STAT pathway. This pathway is essential for the regulation of energy homeostasis by leptin but not for the leptin-dependent control of reproductive function and glucose homeostasis [8]. Activation of the phosphoinositol-3 kinase–dependent pathways [9] as well as inhibition of AMP-activated protein kinase (AMPK)-dependent pathways [10] are also involved in the control of appetite and weight loss by leptin.

Although single cases of leptin deficiency in humans have been reported, most obese subjects as well as animals with diet-induced obesity are characterized by elevated systemic leptin concentrations. Those observations have led to the concept of a hypothalamic leptin-resistant state associated with obesity concerning the action of leptin on body weight and appetite [11]. Suppressor of cytokine signaling (SOCS) proteins have emerged recently as potential mechanism of leptin resistance. In the hypothalamus, SOCS-3 is thought to contribute to the physiological negative feedback of the leptin signaling by its inhibition of JAK activity once activated by STAT-3 [12]. SOCS-3 haploinsufficiency or brain SOCS-3 deficiency increases leptin sensitivity and protects mice against development of high-fat diet-induced obesity [13,14]. Thus, SOCS-3 appears to be an important mechanism of leptin resistance, suggesting that targeting SOCS-3 may be an interesting therapeutic approach for the treatment of obesity and associated diseases. Protein tyrosine phosphatase 1b (PTP1b) is another negative regulator of leptin signaling that might contribute to leptin resistance. Mice lacking PTP1b exhibit enhanced leptin sensitivity and are protected from diet-induced obesity [15,16]. Inhibition of this pathway is also considered as a potential target for antiobesity drug.

BLOOD PRESSURE

Besides its effect on appetite and energy homeostasis, leptin exerts a control on blood pressure. A positive correlation is found between mean blood pressure and leptin serum levels in lean subjects with essential hypertension [17]. Leptin acts in the hypothalamus to increase blood pressure through activation of the sympathetic nervous system [18]. Administration of leptin to the ob/ob mice increases arterial pressure despite reduction in food intake and body weight, as well as urinary catecholamine. Since blood pressure was normalized after acute alpha adrenergic or ganglionic blockade, it appears that leptin exerts a sympathetically mediated pressor response [19]. Long-term sympathoactivation could raise arterial pressure by causing peripheral vasoconstriction and by increasing renal tubular sodium reabsorption (Figure 9.2). Leptin was shown to increase sympathetic activity to the kidney and extremities [20], and in human, obesity is associated with increased sympathetic activity to the kidney [21]. Leptin may thus represent a link between excess adiposity and increased cardiovascular sympathetic activity in human obesity, leading to hypertension [22].

The observation that in the agouti mice, a genetic-induced obesity rodent model characterized by a resistance to the anorexic and weight-reducing effect of leptin, the renal sympathoactivation of leptin is preserved [23], has led to the concept of a selective hypothalamic leptin resistance. The mechanisms underlying the selective hypothalamic leptin resistance are not well defined. Several hypotheses are suggested. In diet-induced obese mice, the inability of leptin to activate leptin-signaling pathways such as STAT3 proteins has been shown to be restricted to the arcuate nucleus where a specific upregulation of SOCS-3 was found [24]. Since leptin-induced increase in renal sympathetic activity and blood pressure are mediated by the ventromedial and dorsomedial hypothalamus [25], it is suggested that the leptin resistance associated with obesity is restricted

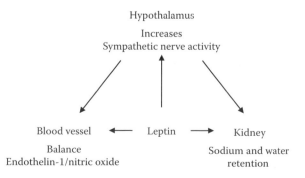

FIGURE 9.2 Central and peripheral effect of leptin on blood pressure.

to specific hypothalamic area such as the arcuate nucleus. The selectivity in leptin resistance may also relate to the divergent signaling pathways downstream from the leptin receptor depending on the physiological processes [26].

PERIPHERAL EFFECTS OF LEPTIN

The signaling form of the leptin receptor, initially described to be expressed only in the hypothalamus, is also found in peripheral tissues.

FATTY ACID METABOLISM

Ob-Rb is expressed on the major tissues involved in the regulation of glucose and fatty acid (FA) metabolism, pancreas, adipose tissue, muscle, and liver (Figure 9.1). The presence of Ob-Rb in pancreatic islets [27] indicates that leptin can regulate directly the secretion of insulin in rodents, although inconsistent results are reported [28,29]. In the other metabolically active tissues, the clear effect of leptin is the promotion of energy dissipation through stimulation of FA oxidation and the prevention of ectopic lipid deposition [30]. In adipocytes, leptin directly decreases lipogenesis [31], increases the enzymes involved in FA oxidation, and stimulates a novel form of lipolysis in which glycerol is released without a proportional release of free FA [32]. In liver and muscle, leptin also inhibits lipogenesis and stimulates FA oxidation [33]. The mechanism underlying these actions of leptin may be via binding to its receptor with succeeding activation of the JAK/STAT pathway, by direct stimulation of the AMPK [34] which will phosphorylate and thereby inhibit acetyl-CoA carboxylase activity and lipogenesis, as well as the inhibition of the expression of sterol response element binding protein-1c (SREBP-1c) [35].

The lack of adipose tissue and thus no leptin as observed in lipodystrophy or incorrect leptin action is associated with ectopic fat deposition in liver, pancreas, and muscle [33]. Administration of leptin to lipodystrophic patients [36] or to rodent models of leptin deficiency [37] reverses many lipotoxic effects, in part due to the direct effects of leptin on lipid metabolism. However, the impact of hyperleptinemia in the peripheral regulation of metabolic fluxes under the background of insulin resistance remains to be determined in obese people.

VASCULAR WALL HOMEOSTASIS

The blood vessel wall is composed of three different layers: intima, media, and adventitia. The intima is a monolayer of endothelial cells, which separates circulating blood from the underlying media. The media consist of concentric layers of smooth muscle cells and elastic lamella. The outer layer of the vessel, the tunica adventitia, is formed of collagen and elastic fibers, fibroblasts, and vasa vasorum. With the discovery of nitric oxide as an endothelium-derived relaxing factor in the 1980s, the endothelial layer has acquired the status of a paracrine tissue, the integrity of which is necessary for vascular homeostasis. Through its production of contractile and relaxant factors, the endothelium regulates not only the medial function but also a wide range of proatherogenic and inflammatory processes such as the platelet activation and aggregation, the proliferation and migration of the smooth muscle cells, as well as the infiltration of inflammatory cells within the vessel wall [38]. Endothelial dysfunction mainly characterized by an impaired NO production and/or bioavailability is observed in obesity [39] and is considered as one of the primary events in the genesis of cardiovascular diseases. Although mechanisms linking obesity with endothelial dysfunction have not yet been fully clarified, several observations suggest that hyperleptinemia might contribute to endothelial dysfunction. Indeed, in obese women, leptin was positively correlated with plasma levels of soluble thrombomodulin (sTM) and vascular cell adhesion molecule (VCAM-1), two markers of endothelial activation [40]. This relationship was independent of BMI, waist-to-hip ratio (WHR), C-reactive protein, and insulin sensitivity. Many blood vessels are surrounded by adipose tissue in variable amounts. Several works [41,42] support the hypothesis of

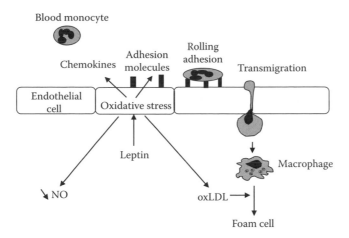

FIGURE 9.3 Hyperleptinemia and endothelial dysfunction.

a paracrine role of white adipose tissue in the regulation of vascular function. Increasing reports suggest that the periadventitial adipose tissue has a pathophysiological role in the vascular dysfunction associated with obesity [43–45] (Figure 9.3).

We and others have described the expression of the Ob-Rb in human endothelial cells [46,47]. Later on, the presence of Ob-Rb was also found in smooth muscle cells [48] as well as in platelets [49] and inflammatory cells [50].

Vascular Tone

Vascular tone is regulated through the actions of locally produced factors. NO is a critical modulator of blood flow and is released by the endothelium in response to shear stress, thereby playing an important role in flow-mediated vasodilation. Endothelial release of NO opposes the vasoconstrictor effects of norepinephrine, endothelin-1, and angiotensin II. Endothelin-1 is one of the most potent vasoconstrictor factors produced in the arterial wall. Vascular tone in health reflects the balance of these opposing factors. Several observations suggest that hyperleptinemia may contribute to the alteration of the endothelial-dependent dilation in obese. For example, plasma leptin correlates inversely with the extent of NO-dependent coronary vasodilation in healthy obese male [51], and obese-related concentrations of leptin infused to anesthetized dogs induce an impairment of the acetylcholine-induced dilations of the coronary arteries suggesting that hyperleptinemia produces significant coronary endothelial dysfunction [52]. However, on the contrary, no relationship between plasma leptin and flow-mediated dilatation of the brachial artery was found in healthy adolescents [53] and in normolipidemic healthy obese women [54]. Those observations suggest that the hyperleptinemia-dependent effect on the vascular tone is dependent on the vascular bed location.

Nitric Oxide Production

Direct vasodilatory actions of leptin have been inconsistently reported. It appears that any direct effects of leptin on the endothelial-dependent production of NO may be restricted to some vascular beds and that they are generally insufficient to oppose to the sympathetically mediated vasoconstriction [55,56]. Fruhbeck described that acute administration of leptin increases endothelial NO release and decreases blood pressure in anesthetized Wistar rats [57]. Such an effect is only observed in sympathectomized rats, suggesting that leptin-dependent activation of the sympathetic nervous system offsets the vasodilatory effect of leptin [58]. The mechanism by which leptin induces NO production in some vascular beds is in part related to the activation of the Akt-endothelial nitric-oxide synthase phosphorylation pathway [59].

Endothelin-1 Production

Leptin at high concentrations upregulates endothelin-1 production *in vitro* in the human umbilical vein endothelial cells (HUVECs) [60]. Since endothelin-1 not only exerts potent direct vasoconstrictory effect but also may itself reduce bioavailable NO, increased vascular production of endothelin-1 has been suggested as a potential mechanism for endothelial dysfunction associated with obesity [39,61]. In favor with such an hypothesis, blockade of the endothelin A (ETA) receptors induces significant vasodilation in overweight and obese patients but not in lean hypertensive subjects [62].

Vascular Wall Remodeling

After the first demonstration in the West of Scotland Coronary Prevention Study (WOSCOPS) that hyperleptinemia is an independent risk factor for coronary heart disease [63], recent studies have confirmed a role for increased leptin concentration in cardiovascular disease [64–66]. Reilly et al. reported an association between plasma leptin levels and the degree of coronary artery calcification in type 2 diabetic patients after controlling for traditional indices such as obesity and C-reactive protein [67]. Leptin levels are increased in nondiabetic patients with restenosis after stenting, whereas no differences were demonstrated in patients without restenosis and in control subjects [68]. Finally, leptin impairs the vascular compliance [53]. An increase in vascular stiffness has long-term adverse effects on the cardiovascular system by increasing impedance to blood flow and thereby increasing cardiovascular work and contributing to the development of left ventricular hypertrophy [69]. In animal models, neointimal formation after endovascular arterial injury is markedly attenuated in db/db mice [70], whereas it is promoted by leptin in normal strains [71]. The pathobiology of restenosis in stented arteries is linked to neointimal hyperplasia. Atherosclerotic lesions are the result of an excessive proliferative and inflammatory response that involves several cellular events, including smooth muscle cell migration and proliferation, inflammatory cell infiltration, neovascularization, production of extracellular matrix, and accumulation of lipids [72]. Leptin signaling has been implicated in the promotion of atherosclerosis [73]. Indeed, *in vivo*, the expression of leptin receptors is increased in atherosclerotic lesions [74,75], and leptin signaling promotes atherosclerosis in mice models [76,77]. *In vitro* proatherogenic effects of leptin include endothelial cell activation, migration, and proliferation; smooth muscle cell proliferation, migration, hypertrophy, and calcification; activation of monocytes; and modulation of the immune response, as well as platelet aggregation.

Leptin and Endothelial Cells

Neovascularization within the plaque is known to be essential in the atheromatous plaque formation [78,79]. Atherosclerotic aortic plaques demonstrated marked increase in Ob-Rb immunoreactivity, predominantly in foam cells, vascular smooth muscle cells, and the vascular endothelial lining of intimal neovessels [80]. We [46] and others [47] showed that leptin increases *in vitro* the proliferation and the migration of endothelial cells and promotes the formation of new blood vessels *in vivo* on various angiogenic models. Such a proangiogenic effect of leptin has been suggested to participate to the growth of the fat mass itself since the development of the adipose tissue is dependent not only on its own vasculature [81] but also in the progression of the atheromatous plaques [80] and the neointimal hyperplasia after endothelial damage.

Endothelial cells play an important role in the initiation and maintenance of inflammatory processes and acute tissue injuries. Indeed, the activation of the endothelial cell surface leads to the expression of several adhesion molecules as well as chemokines that promote the adhesion and transmigration of circulatory inflammatory cells into the vascular wall (Figure 9.2). The adhesion of blood-borne monocytes and migration through the endothelial surface are prerequisites for the monocyte-macrophage conversion. We have recently demonstrated that *in vitro* leptin at high concentration promotes the adhesion as well as the transmigration of human blood monocytes through the endothelial cell layer [82]. Moreover, we [83] and others have shown that leptin leads to the increased endothelial expression of the monocyte-chemoattractant protein-1 (MCP-1). Furthermore, this effect is dependent on the leptin-induced production of reactive oxygen species [83,84]. It is thus tempting to speculate that the intracellular accumulation of oxidant radicals stimulated by high leptin concentrations and the consecutive expression of MCP-1 in endothelial cells might play a key role in the infiltration of inflammatory cells within the vessel wall. In addition, chronic endothelial oxidative stress under hyperleptinemia, as in human obesity, might be involved in the genesis of endothelial dysfunction linked to atherosclerosis through a direct interaction with NO to form a more harmful oxygen radical compound, the peroxynitrite, thus leading to a decreased NO bioavailability (Figure 9.2).

Leptin and Smooth Muscle Cells

High leptin concentrations stimulate the proliferation and migration of smooth muscle cells [85] as well as smooth muscle cell hypertrophy through the p38 MAP kinase pathway [86]. Moreover, leptin at obese-relevant concentration promotes accumulation of reactive oxygen species in human smooth muscle cells [87]. Finally, Parhami et al. [75] demonstrated that leptin enhances the calcification of vascular cells.

Leptin and Inflammation

Inflammatory reaction in the vascular wall plays an important role in the development of atherosclerosis and in plaque destabilization and rupture. Consequently, systemic markers of inflammation, in particular CRP, are independent risk factors of cardiovascular events [88]. CRP exerts many proatherogenic effects including impairment of endothelial NO production, activation of vascular smooth muscle cells, and stimulation of monocyte adhesion to endothelial surface [89]. Leptin exerts strong proinflammatory and immunostimulatory effects [90]. Leptin, *per se*, acts on monocytes/macrophages by inducing their release of proinflammatory cytokines and oxygen radicals and eicosanoids [91–93]. Leptin also affects natural killer (NK) cell development and activation both *in vitro* and *in vivo* [94]. Moreover, leptin has been demonstrated to also modulate adaptive immune response [95]. In addition, inflammatory stimuli have previously been shown to induce elevated systemic leptin concentrations [96], proposing that leptin induction is part of the ubiquitous acute phase reaction. In agreement, plasma leptin has been demonstrated to correlate with acute phase reactants, such as CRP both in normal weight and in obese subjects [97–99]. Taken together, these data suggest that leptin might contribute to proinflammatory state associated with obesity.

Leptin and Platelets

Human obesity is associated with an elevated risk for arterial and venous thrombosis [100], and hyperleptinemia has been suggested to play a role in the development of atherothrombotic disease in obesity [101,102]. Platelets express the leptin receptor, and leptin potentiates platelet aggregation through leptin receptor–dependent mechanism [49,103]. Leptin deficient ob/ob mice have delayed and unstable thrombus formation after arterial injury, and leptin normalizes this phenotype [104], whereas inhibition of endogenous leptin protects mice from arterial and venous thrombosis [105].

CONCLUSION

Leptin is now well recognized as adipose tissue originating signal that informs the hypothalamus about the amount of energy storage to modulate in adequacy the metabolic fluxes, energy intake and expenditure, as well as the reproductive capacity and the immune function. The leptin-dependent regulation of the vascular tone according to the vessel bed location plays certainly in addition an important role in the efficiency of the oxygen and nutrients delivery to tissues and the subsequent effectiveness of metabolic activities. Such effects are reminiscent to those of insulin on the vascular reactivity [106]. Despite this acute action of leptin, the majority of studies performed to date indicate that chronic hyperleptinemia is atherogenic. Although it is not clear whether hyperleptinemia is associated with the development of a peripheral leptin resistance, high concentrations of leptin are known to increase oxidative stress in endothelial cells. The long-term consequences of oxidative stress may include reductions in NO bioavailability and an increase in the expression of adhesion molecules and chemokines that mediate vascular inflammation and atherogenesis. Furthermore, the associated metabolic changes that occur in insulin-resistance state (e.g., increased levels of plasma FA) associated with obesity are also known to impair endothelial function. Thus, hyperlepti-nemia together with insulin resistance might exert powerful detrimental effects on the vascular wall leading to the genesis of vascular pathologies associated with obesity [107,108].

REFERENCES

1. Campfield, L. A.; Smith, F. J.; Guisez, Y.; Devos, R.; Burn, P. *Science* 1995, *269*(5223), 546–549.
2. Halaas, J. L.; Gajiwala, K. S.; Maffei, M.; Cohen, S. L.; Chait, B. T.; Rabinowitz, D.; Lallone, R. L.; Burley, S. K.; Friedman, J. M. *Science* 1995, *269*(5223), 543–546.
3. Pelleymounter, M. A.; Cullen, M. J.; Baker, M. B.; Hecht, R.; Winters, D.; Boone, T.; Collins, F. *Science* 1995, *269*(5223), 540–543.
4. Muoio, D. M.; Lynis, D. G. *Best Pract Res Clin Endocrinol Metab* 2002, *16*(4), 653–666.
5. Margetic, S.; Gazzola, C.; Pegg, G. G.; Hill, R. A. *Int J Obes Relat Metab Disord* 2002, *26*(11), 1407–1433.
6. Bjorbaek, C.; Uotani, S.; da Silva, B.; Flier, J. S. *J Biol Chem* 1997, *272*(51), 32686–32695.
7. Hileman, S. M.; Pierroz, D. D.; Masuzaki, H.; Bjorbaek, C.; El Haschimi, K.; Banks, W. A.; Flier, J. S. *Endocrinology* 2002, *143*(3), 775–783.
8. Bates, S. H.; Stearns, W. H.; Dundon, T. A.; Schubert, M.; Tso, A. W.; Wang, Y.; Banks, A. S.; Lavery, H. J.; Haq, A. K.; Maratos-Flier, E.; Neel, B. G.; Schwartz, M. W.; Myers, M. G., Jr. *Nature* 2003, *421*(6925), 856–859.
9. Rahmouni, K.; Haynes, W. G.; Morgan, D. A.; Mark, A. L. *Hypertension* 2003, *41*(3 Pt 2), 763–767.
10. Minokoshi, Y.; Alquier, T.; Furukawa, N.; Kim, Y. B.; Lee, A.; Xue, B.; Mu, J.; Foufelle, F.; Ferre, P.; Birnbaum, M. J.; Stuck, B. J.; Kahn, B. B. *Nature* 2004, *428*(6982), 569–574.
11. Considine, R. V.; Sinha, M. K.; Heiman, M. L.; Kriauciunas, A.; Stephens, T. W.; Nyce, M. R.; Ohannesian, J. P.; Marco, C. C.; McKee, L. J.; Bauer, T. L. *N Engl J Med* 1996, *334*(5), 292–295.
12. Flier, J. S. *Cell* 2004, *116*(2), 337–350.
13. Howard, J. K.; Cave, B. J.; Oksanen, L. J.; Tzameli, I.; Bjorbaek, C.; Flier, J. S. *Nat Med* 2004, *10*(7), 734–738.
14. Mori, H.; Hanada, R.; Hanada, T.; Aki, D.; Mashima, R.; Nishinakamura, H.; Torisu, T.; Chien, K. R.; Yasukawa, H.; Yoshimura, A. *Nat Med* 2004, *10*(7), 739–743.
15. Zabolotny, J. M.; Bence-Hanulec, K. K.; Stricker-Krongrad, A.; Haj, F.; Wang, Y.; Minokoshi, Y.; Kim, Y. B.; Elmquist, J. K.; Tartaglia, L. A.; Kahn, B. B.; Neel, B. G. *Dev Cell* 2002, *2*(4), 489–495.
16. Cheng, A.; Uetani, N.; Simoncic, P. D.; Chaubey, V. P.; Lee-Loy, A.; McGlade, C. J.; Kennedy, B. P.; Tremblay, M. L. *Dev Cell* 2002, *2*(4), 497–503.
17. Agata, J.; Masuda, A.; Takada, M.; Higashiura, K.; Murakami, H.; Miyazaki, Y.; Shimamoto, K. *Am J Hypertens* 1997, *10*(10 Pt 1), 1171–1174.
18. Carlyle, M.; Jones, O. B.; Kuo, J. J.; Hall, J. E. *Hypertension* 2002, *39*(2 Pt 2), 496–501.
19. Aizawa-Abe, M.; Ogawa, Y.; Masuzaki, H.; Ebihara, K.; Satoh, N.; Iwai, H.; Matsuoka, N.; Hayashi, T.; Hosoda, K.; Inoue, G.; Yoshimasa, Y.; Nakao, K. *J Clin Invest* 2000, *105*(9), 1243–1252.
20. Haynes, W. G.; Morgan, D. A.; Walsh, S. A.; Mark, A. L.; Sivitz, W. I. *J Clin Invest* 1997, *100*(2), 270–278.
21. Vaz, M.; Jennings, G.; Turner, A.; Cox, H.; Lambert, G.; Esler, M. *Circulation* 1997, *96*(10), 3423–3429.
22. Eikelis, N.; Schlaich, M.; Aggarwal, A.; Kaye, D.; Esler, M. *Hypertension* 2003, *41*(5), 1072–1079.
23. Rahmouni, K.; Haynes, W. G.; Morgan, D. A.; Mark, A. L. *Hypertension* 2002, *39*(2 Pt 2), 486–490.
24. Munzberg, H.; Flier, J. S.; Bjorbaek, C. *Endocrinology* 2004, *145*(11), 4880–4889.
25. Marsh, A. J.; Fontes, M. A.; Killinger, S.; Pawlak, D. B.; Polson, J. W.; Dampney, R. A. *Hypertension* 2003, *42*(4), 488–493.
26. Rahmouni, K.; Correia, M. L.; Haynes, W. G.; Mark, A. L. *Hypertension* 2005, *45*(1), 9–14.
27. Emilsson, V.; Liu, Y. L.; Cawthorne, M. A.; Morton, N. M.; Davenport, M. *Diabetes* 1997, *46*(2), 313–316.
28. Tanizawa, Y.; Okuya, S.; Ishihara, H.; Asano, T.; Yada, T.; Oka, Y. *Endocrinology* 1997, *138*(10), 4513–4516.

29. Kieffer, T. J.; Heller, R. S.; Leech, C. A.; Holz, G. G.; Habener, J. F. *Diabetes* 1997, *46*(6), 1087–1093.

30. Ceddia, R. B.; Somwar, R.; Maida, A.; Fang, X.; Bikopoulos, G.; Sweeney, G. *Diabetologia* 2005, *48*(1), 132–139.

31. Bai, Y.; Zhang, S.; Kim, K. S.; Lee, J. K.; Kim, K. H. *J Biol Chem* 1996, *271*(24), 13939–13942.

32. Wang, M. Y.; Lee, Y.; Unger, R. H. *J Biol Chem* 1999, *274*(25), 17541–17544.

33. Unger, R. H.; Orci, L. *Biochim Biophys Acta* 2002, *1585*(2–3), 202–212.

34. Minokoshi, Y.; Kim, Y. B.; Peroni, O. D.; Fryer, L. G.; Muller, C.; Carling, D.; Kahn, B. B. *Nature* 2002, *415*(6869), 339–343.

35. Muller-Wieland, D.; Kotzka, J. *Ann N Y Acad Sci* 2002, *967*, 19–27.

36. Oral, E. A.; Simha, V.; Ruiz, E.; Andewelt, A.; Premkumar, A.; Snell, P.; Wagner, A. J.; DePaoli, A. M.; Reitman, M. L.; Taylor, S. I.; Gorden, P.; Garg, A. *N Engl J Med* 2002, *346*(8), 570–578.

37. Shimomura, I.; Hammer, R. E.; Ikemoto, S.; Brown, M. S.; Goldstein, J. L. *Nature* 1999, *401*(6748), 73–76.

38. Weber, C. *J Mol Med* 2003, *81*(1), 4–19.

39. Mather, K. J.; Lteif, A.; Steinberg, H. O.; Baron, A. D. *Diabetes* 2004, *53*(8), 2060–2066.

40. Porreca, E.; Di Febbo, C.; Fusco, L.; Moretta, V.; Di Nisio, M.; Cuccurullo, F. *Atherosclerosis* 2004, *172*(1), 175–180.

41. Verlohren, S.; Dubrovska, G.; Tsang, S. Y.; Essin, K.; Luft, F. C.; Huang, Y.; Gollasch, M. *Hypertension* 2004, *44*(3), 271–276.

42. Lohn, M.; Dubrovska, G.; Lauterbach, B.; Luft, F. C.; Gollasch, M.; Sharma, A. M. *FASEB J.* 2002, *16*(9), 1057–1063.

43. Yudkin, J. S.; Eringa, E.; Stehouwer, C. D. *Lancet* 2005, *365*(9473), 1817–1820.

44. Henrichot, E.; Juge-Aubry, C. E.; Pernin, A.; Pache, J. C.; Velebit, V.; Dayer, J. M.; Meda, P.; Chizzolini, C.; Meier, C. A. *Arterioscler Thromb Vasc Biol* 2005, *25*(12), 2594–2599.

45. Galvez, B.; de Castro, J.; Herold, D.; Dubrovska, G.; Arribas, S.; Gonzalez, M. C.; Aranguez, I.; Luft, F. C.; Ramos, M. P.; Gollasch, M.; Fernandez Alfonso, M. S. *Arterioscler Thromb Vasc Biol* 2006, *26*(6), 1297–1302.

46. Bouloumie, A.; Drexler, H. C.; Lafontan, M.; Busse, R. *Circ Res* 1998, *83*(10), 1059–1066.

47. Sierra-Honigmann, M. R.; Nath, A. K.; Murakami, C.; Garcia-Cardena, G.; Papapetropoulos, A.; Sessa, W. C.; Madge, L. A.; Schechner, J. S.; Schwabb, M. B.; Polverini, P. J.; Flores-Riveros, J. R. *Science* 1998, *281*(5383), 1683–1686.

48. Fortuno, A.; Rodriguez, A.; Gomez-Ambrosi, J.; Muniz, P.; Salvador, J.; Diez, J.; Fruhbeck, G. *Endocrinology* 2002, *143*(9), 3555–3560.

49. Nakata, M.; Yada, T.; Soejima, N.; Maruyama, I. *Diabetes* 1999, *48*(2), 426–429

50. Gainsford, T.; Willson, T. A.; Metcalf, D.; Handman, E.; McFarlane, C.; Ng, A.; Nicola, N. A.; Alexander, W. S.; Hilton, D. J. *Proc Natl Acad Sci USA* 1996, *93*(25), 14564–14568.

51. Sundell, J.; Huupponen, R.; Raitakari, O. T.; Nuutila, P.; Knuuti, J. *Obes Res* 2003, *11*(6), 776–782.

52. Knudson, J. D.; Dincer, U. D.; Zhang, C.; Swafford, A. N. Jr.; Koshida, R.; Picchi, A.; Focardi, M.; Dick, G. M.; Tune, J. D. *Am J Physiol Heart Circ Physiol* 2005, *289*(1), H48–H56

53. Singhal, A.; Farooqi, I. S.; Cole, T. J.; O'Rahilly, S.; Fewtrell, M.; Kattenhorn, M.; Lucas, A.; Deanfield, J. *Circulation* 2002, *106*(15), 1919–1924.

54. Oflaz, H.; Ozbey, N.; Mantar, F.; Genchellac, H.; Mercanoglu, F.; Sencer, E.; Molvalilar, S.; Orhan, Y. *Diabetes Nutr Metab* 2003, *16*(3), 176–181.

55. Gardiner, S. M.; Kemp, P. A.; March, J. E.; Bennett, T. *Br J Pharmacol* 2000, *130*(4), 805–810.

56. Mitchell, J. L.; Morgan, D. A.; Correia, M. L.; Mark, A. L.; Sivitz, W. I.; Haynes, W. G. *Hypertension* 2001, *38*(5), 1081–1086.

57. Fruhbeck, G. *Diabetes* 1999, *48*(4), 903–908.

58. Lembo, G.; Vecchione, C.; Fratta, L.; Marino, G.; Trimarco, V.; d'Amati, G.; Trimarco, B. *Diabetes* 2000, *49*(2), 293–297.

59. Vecchione, C.; Maffei, A.; Colella, S.; Aretini, A.; Poulet, R.; Frati, G.; Gentile, M. T.; Fratta, L.; Trimarco, V.; Trimarco, B.; Lembo, G. *Diabetes* 2002, *51*(1), 168–173.

60. Quehenberger, P.; Exner, M.; Sunder-Plassmann, R.; Ruzicka, K.; Bieglmayer, C.; Endler, G.; Muellner, C.; Speiser, W.; Wagner, O. *Circ Res* 2002, *90*(6), 711–718.

61. Mather, K. J.; Mirzamohammadi, B.; Lteif, A.; Steinberg, H. O.; Baron, A. D. *Diabetes* 2002, *51*(12), 3517–3523.

62. Cardillo, C.; Campia, U.; Iantorno, M.; Panza, J. A. *Hypertension* 2004, *43*(1), 36–40.

63. Wallace, A. M.; McMahon, A. D.; Packard, C. J.; Kelly, A.; Shepherd, J.; Gaw, A.; Sattar, N. *Circulation* 2001, *104*(25), 3052–3056.

64. Schulze, P. C.; Kratzsch, J.; Linke, A.; Schoene, N.; Adams, V.; Gielen, S.; Erbs, S.; Moebius-Winkler, S.; Schuler, G. *Eur J Heart Fail* 2003, *5*(1), 33–40.

65. Wolk, R.; Johnson, B. D.; Somers, V. K. *J Am Coll Cardiol* 2003, *42*(9), 1644–1649.

66. Ren, J. *J Endocrinol* 2004, *181*(1), 1–10.

67. Reilly, M. P.; Iqbal, N.; Schutta, M.; Wolfe, M. L.; Scally, M.; Localio, A. R.; Rader, D. J.; Kimmel, S. E. *J Clin Endocrinol Metab* 2004, *89*(8), 3872–3878.

68. Piatti, P.; Di Mario, C.; Monti, L. D.; Fragasso, G.; Sgura, F.; Caumo, A.; Setola, E.; Lucotti, P.; Galluccio, E.; Ronchi, C.; Origgi, A.; Zavaroni, I.; Margonato, A.; Colombo, A. *Circulation* 2003, *108*(17), 2074–2081.

69. Cooke, J. P.; Oka, R. K. *Circulation* 2002, *106*(15), 1904–1905.

70. Stephenson, K.; Tunstead, J.; Tsai, A.; Gordon, R.; Henderson, S.; Dansky, H. M. *Arterioscler Thromb Vasc Biol* 2003, *23*(11), 2027–2033.

71. Schafer, K.; Halle, M.; Goeschen, C.; Dellas, C.; Pynn, M.; Loskutoff, D. J.; Konstantinides, S. *Arterioscler Thromb Vasc Biol* 2004, *24*(1), 112–117.

72. Ross, R. *Nature* 1993, *362*(6423), 801–809.

73. Wolk, R.; Berger, P.; Lennon, R. J.; Brilakis, E. S.; Johnson, B. D.; Somers, V. K. *J Am Coll Cardiol* 2004, *44*(9), 1819–1824.

74. Kang, S. M.; Kwon, H. M.; Hong, B. K.; Kim, D.; Kim, I. J.; Choi, E. Y.; Jang, Y.; Kim, H. S.; Kim, M. S.; Kwon, H. C. *Yonsei Med J* 2000, *41*(1), 68–75.

75. Parhami, F.; Tintut, Y.; Ballard, A.; Fogelman, A. M.; Demer, L. L. *Circ Res* 2001, *88*(9), 954–960.

76. Hasty, A. H.; Shimano, H.; Osuga, J.; Namatame, I.; Takahashi, A.; Yahagi, N.; Perrey, S.; Iizuka, Y.; Tamura, Y.; Amemiya-Kudo, M.; Yoshikawa, T.; Okazaki, H.; Ohashi, K.; Harada, K.; Matsuzaka, T.; Sone, H.; Gotoda, T.; Nagai, R.; Ishibashi, S.; Yamada, N. *J Biol Chem* 2001, *276*(40), 37402–37408.

77. Bodary, P. F.; Gu, S.; Shen, Y.; Hasty, A. H.; Buckler, J. M.; Eitzman, D. T. *Arterioscler Thromb Vasc Biol* 2005, *25*(8), e119–e122.

78. Kahlon, R.; Shapero, J.; Gotlieb, A. I. *Can J Cardiol* 1992, *8*(1), 60–64.

79. O'Brien, E. R.; Garvin, M. R.; Dev, R.; Stewart, D. K.; Hinohara, T.; Simpson, J. B.; Schwartz, S. M. *Am J Pathol* 1994, *145*(4), 883–894.

80. Park, H. Y.; Kwon, H. M.; Lim, H. J.; Hong, B. K.; Lee, J. Y.; Park, B. E.; Jang, Y.; Cho, S. Y.; Kim, H. S. *Exp Mol Med* 2001, *33*(2), 95–102.

81. Rupnick, M. A.; Panigrahy, D.; Zhang, C. Y.; Dallabrida, S. M.; Lowell, B. B.; Langer, R.; Folkman, M. J. *Proc Natl Acad Sci USA* 2002, *99*(16), 10730–10735.

82. Curat, C. A.; Miranville, A.; Sengenes, C.; Diehl, M.; Tonus, C.; Busse, R.; Bouloumie, A. *Diabetes* 2004, *53*(5), 1285–1292.

83. Bouloumie, A.; Marumo, T.; Lafontan, M.; Busse, R. *FASEB J* 1999, *13*(10), 1231–1238.

84. Yamagishi, S. I.; Edelstein, D.; Du, X. L.; Kaneda, Y.; Guzman, M.; Brownlee, M. *J Biol Chem* 2001, *276*(27), 25096–25100.

85. Oda, A.; Taniguchi, T.; Yokoyama, M. *Kobe J Med Sci* 2001, *47*(3), 141–150.

86. Shin, H. J.; Oh, J.; Kang, S. M.; Lee, J. H.; Shin, M. J.; Hwang, K. C.; Jang, Y.; Chung, J. H. *Biochem Biophys Res Commun* 2005, *329*(1), 18–24.

87. Li, L.; Mamputu, J. C.; Wiernsperger, N.; Renier, G. *Diabetes* 2005, *54*(7), 2227–2234.

88. Lind, L. *Atherosclerosis* 2003, *169*(2), 203–214.

89. Venugopal, S. K.; Devaraj, S.; Jialal, I. *Curr Opin Nephrol Hypertens* 2005, *14*(1), 33–37.

90. Otero, M.; Lago, R.; Lago, F.; Casanueva, F. F.; Dieguez, C.; Gomez-Reino, J. J.; Gualillo, O. *FEBS Lett* 2005, *579*(2), 295–301.

91. Mancuso, P.; Canetti, C.; Gottschalk, A.; Tithof, P. K.; Peters-Golden, M. *Am J Physiol Lung Cell Mol Physiol* 2004, *287*(3), L497–L502.

92. Zarkesh-Esfahani, H.; Pockley, G.; Metcalfe, R. A.; Bidlingmaier, M.; Wu, Z.; Ajami, A.; Weetman, A. P.; Strasburger, C. J.; Ross, R. J. *J Immunol* 2001, *167*(8), 4593–4599.

93. Raso, G. M.; Pacilio, M.; Esposito, E.; Coppola, A.; Di Carlo, R.; Meli, R. *Br J Pharmacol* 2002, *137*(6), 799–804.

94. Zhao, Y.; Sun, R.; You, L.; Gao, C.; Tian, Z. *Biochem Biophys Res Commun* 2003, *300*(2), 247–252.

95. La Cava, A.; Matarese, G. *Nat Rev Immunol* 2004, *4*(5), 371–379.

96. Faggioni, R.; Feingold, K. R.; Grunfeld, C. *FASEB J* 2001, *15*(14), 2565–2571.

97. Shamsuzzaman, A. S.; Winnicki, M.; Wolk, R.; Svatikova, A.; Phillips, B. G.; Davison, D. E.; Berger, P. B.; Somers, V. K. *Circulation* 2004, *109*(18), 2181–2185.

98. van Dielen, F. M.; van't Veer, C.; Schols, A. M.; Soeters, P. B.; Buurman, W. A.; Greve, J. W. *Int J Obes Relat Metab Disord* 2001, *25*(12), 1759–1766.

99. Kazumi, T.; Kawaguchi, A.; Hirano, T.; Yoshino, G. *Metabolism* 2003, *52*(9), 1113–1116.
100. Korner, J.; Aronne, L. J. *J Clin Invest* 2003, *111*(5), 565–570.
101. Konstantinides, S.; Schafer, K.; Koschnick, S.; Loskutoff, D. J. *J Clin Invest* 2001, *108*(10), 1533–1540.
102. Konstantinides, S.; Schafer, K.; Loskutoff, D. J. *Ann NY Acad Sci* 2001, *947*, 134–141.
103. Corsonello, A.; Perticone, F.; Malara, A.; De Domenico, D.; Loddo, S.; Buemi, M.; Ientile, R.; Corica, F. *Int J Obes Relat Metab Disord* 2003, *27*(5), 566–573.
104. Bodary, P. F.; Westrick, R. J.; Wickenheiser, K. J.; Shen, Y.; Eitzman, D. T. *JAMA* 2002, *287*(13), 1706–1709.
105. Konstantinides, S.; Schafer, K.; Neels, J. G.; Dellas, C.; Loskutoff, D. J. *Arterioscler Thromb Vasc Biol* 2004, *24*(11), 2196–2201.
106. Ritchie, S. A.; Ewart, M. A.; Perry, C. G.; Connell, J. M.; Salt, I. P. *Clin Sci (Lond)* 2004, *107*(6), 519–532.
107. Piatti, P.; Monti, L. D. *Curr Opin Pharmacol* 2005, *5*(2), 160–164.
108. Werner, N.; Nickenig, G. *Arterioscler Thromb Vasc Biol* 2004, *24*(1), 7–9.

10 Leptin-Induced Inflammation
A Link between Obesity and Cancer

Na-Young Song, PhD and Young-Joon Surh, PhD

CONTENTS

INTRODUCTION

It is well known that chronic inflammation is closely related to several malignancies. Once cells are activated by inflammatory stimuli, both reactive oxygen/nitrogen species (ROS/RNS) are massively generated, which cause irreversible DNA damage (Kundu and Surh 2008). Thus, chronic inflammation itself can act as an initiator of the multistage carcinogenesis. Furthermore, proinflammatory cytokines and chemokines released from the inflamed cells can overactivate various cellular signaling molecules, such as nuclear factor κB (NF-κB) and hypoxia-inducible factor-1 α (HIF-1α), leading to promotion and progression of cancer as well as profound inflammation (Cramer and Johnson 2003; Cramer et al. 2003; Frede et al. 2005; Karin and Greten 2005). This vicious cycle of chronic inflammation might accelerate carcinogenesis.

Obesity represents a chronic mild inflammatory state as well (Baker et al. 2011). Circulating levels of proinflammatory mediators, such as tumor necrosis factor α (TNF-α), interleukin (IL)-6, and C-reactive protein (CRP), are significantly increased in obese subjects compared with normal lean individuals (Hotamisligil 1999; Das 2001; Browning et al. 2008). Systemic inflammation in obese people may enhance the risk of cancer (Cleary and Maihle 1997; Calle et al. 2003; von Hafe et al. 2004; Silha et al. 2005; Frezza et al. 2006), but the underlying molecular mechanisms are not clarified yet.

Obesity is defined as an accumulation of excess body fat, particularly white adipose tissue (WAT) which can exert endocrine functions by releasing various adipokines (Trayhurn 2007). Adipokines include cytokines, such as IL-6, IL-10, TNF-α, and transforming growth factor β (TGF-β); chemokines including plasminogen activator inhibitor-1 (PAI-1) and haptoglobin; and adipose-derived hormones (e.g., leptin, adiponectin, and resistin) (Trayhurn and Wood 2005). Since leptin and adiponectin are produced predominantly by WAT, these substances are referred to as the most representative adipokines (Fain et al. 2004). Whereas adiponectin has an anti-inflammatory effect, leptin can stimulate proinflammatory signals (Stofkova 2009). A ratio of leptin to adiponectin is remarkably elevated in obesity, which can account for chronic inflammation in obese people (van Kruijsdijk et al. 2009; Labruna et al. 2011). In this respect, leptin is suggested as a linker molecule between obesity and cancer. Here we highlight the role of leptin in obesity-induced carcinogenesis, particularly in the context of inflammation.

LEPTIN AND INFLAMMATION

OBESITY, LEPTIN, AND INFLAMMATION

Leptin, a product of *ob* gene, has been identified as an anorexic hormone. When leptin binds to its receptor (Ob-R) in the hypothalamus of the brain, it can inhibit an appetite and consequently regulate body weight (Maffei et al. 1995; Hakansson et al. 1998). Leptin-deficient *ob/ob* mice show increased food intake and subsequently manifest an obese phenotype, and these effects were mitigated by replenishment with leptin (Halaas et al. 1995; Weigle et al. 1995). However, human obesity is rarely associated with leptin deficiency. Unexpectedly, obese subjects exhibit an extremely higher plasma level of leptin due to leptin resistance, a status that the hypothalamic leptin receptor fails to respond to leptin, resulting in increased production of leptin as a compensation (Considine et al. 1996; Myers et al. 2010).

Leptin signaling is primarily mediated by its receptor Ob-R that recruits Janus kinase 2 (JAK2) (Fruhbeck 2006). When leptin interacts with Ob-R, JAK2 undergoes autophosphorylation, leading to subsequent phosphorylation of downstream signaling molecules, such as mitogen-activated protein kinases (MAPKs) and signal transducer and activator of transcription pathway 3 (STAT3) (Banks et al. 2000; Hegyi et al. 2004). Elevated circulating leptin targets not only hypothalamus but also peripheral organs expressing Ob-R, such as liver, heart, prostate, ovaries, and intestine (Margetic et al. 2002). Thus, leptin evokes peripheral effects by activating the JAK2-STAT3 and MAPK pathways as illustrated in Figure 10.1. These include insulin regulation in the liver and reproduction in the ovary (Margetic et al. 2002). In addition to these organ-specific peripheral actions, leptin stimulates the inflammatory response which does not appear to be limited to a specific organ, but rather represents a systemic phenomenon. Increased amounts of plasma leptin correlated with elevated levels of circulating inflammatory markers including TNF-α, CRP, PAI-1, and IL-6 in obese individuals (Corica et al. 1999). Furthermore, leptin enhances biosynthesis of proinflammatory mediators in various cell lines (Raso et al. 2002; Dreyer et al. 2003; Lappas et al. 2005; Vuolteenaho et al. 2009). Immunomodulatory effects of leptin might be achieved via two different mechanisms: first, leptin directly activates immune cells, resulting in production of proinflammatory mediators able to affect peripheral tissues, and second, leptin activates the proinflammatory signaling pathways, including those mediated by NF-κB, in peripheral tissues (Figure 10.1). Both mechanisms will be discussed more in detail in the following sections. Thus, leptin is thought to be responsible for chronic inflammation in obesity.

Leptin-induced inflammation in obesity could be sustained by obesity-induced hypoxia. Obese mice show increased levels of hypoxic markers as well as HIF-1α in WAT (Hosogai et al. 2007; He et al. 2011). The adipose hypoxia stimulates the secretion of the proinflammatory mediators, such as TNF-α, IL-1, and IL-6 in the adipocytes, leading to a profound inflammatory state (Ye et al. 2007). Moreover, leptin expression is upregulated in human preadipocytes under hypoxic conditions (Wang et al. 2008). Leptin may also induce transcriptional activation of HIF-1α, suggesting the existence of a positive feedback loop among leptin, hypoxia, and inflammation (Gonzalez-Perez et al. 2010). Table 10.1 summarizes the proinflammatory signaling stimulated or mediated by leptin.

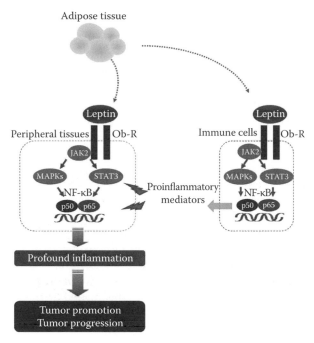

FIGURE 10.1 Leptin stimulates proinflammatory responses, leading to tumor promotion and progression: a possible link between obesity and cancer. The obese protein leptin, produced by the WAT, induces the production of the proinflammatory mediators from various immune cells. Once secreted, these substances can circulate in the peripheries and activate the NF-κB signaling in a paracrine manner. In addition, leptin directly affects the peripheral tissues, leading to NF-κB-dependent cellular events. As a consequence, leptin may develop the microenvironment favorable to tumor promotion and progression.

TABLE 10.1
Leptin-Induced Proinflammatory Signaling

Animal/Cell Type	Effects	Reference
Eosinophils	↑ Secretion of IL-6 and IL-8	Wong et al. (2007)
Human PBMCs	↑ Release of TNF-α, IL-6, and INF-γ	Zarkesh-Esfahani et al. (2001)
T lymphocytes	↑ Th1 cytokine production	Lord et al. (1998)
	↓ Th2 responses	
Murine macrophage	↑ Production of NO and PGE$_2$	Raso et al. (2002)
Monocytes	↑ NF-κB-dependent release of IL-1	Dreyer et al. (2003)
Human placenta	↑ NF-κB-dependent release of IL-1β, IL-6, and TNF-α	Lappas et al. (2005)
Wistar rats	↑ Severity of TNBS-induced colitis	Barbier et al. (2001)
Human osteoarthritis cartilage	↑ Production of NO and PGE$_2$	Vuolteenaho et al. (2009)
C6 glioma cells	↑ Degradation of IκB-α	Mattace Raso et al. (2006)
	↑ NO production	
ob/ob and *db/db* mice	Restoration of the decreased phagocytic function of macrophages	Loffreda et al. (1998)
ob/ob mice	↑ Susceptibility to DSS-induced colitis	Siegmund et al. (2002)
Wistar rats	↑ Severity of TNBS-induced colitis	Barbier et al. (2001)

Leptin Activates the Inflammatory Responses in the Immune Cells

Leptin has been reported to regulate inflammatory responses in various immune cells. Thus, leptin stimulates secretion of proinflammatory cytokines IL-6 and IL-8 from eosinophils and expression of adhesion molecules on the surface of eosinophils which facilitates chemokinesis in these cells (Wong et al. 2007). Leptin also induces the release of TNF-α, IL-6, and INF-γ in human peripheral blood mononuclear cells (PBMCs) (Zarkesh-Esfahani et al. 2001). In addition to cytokine release, leptin increases production of nitric oxide (NO) and prostaglandin E_2 (PGE$_2$), resulting from overexpression of inducible NO synthase and cyclooxygenase-2, respectively. Moreover, leptin modulates cellular immune responses by increasing Th1 cytokine production and concomitantly decreasing Th2 responses (Lord et al. 1998).

Leptin signaling is impaired in genetically leptin-deficient *ob/ob* and leptin receptor-deficient *db/db* mice (Halaas et al. 1995; Chen et al. 1996). Phagocytosis and expression of proinflammatory cytokines are decreased in leptin signaling-defective *ob/ob* and *db/db* mice compared with control mice (Loffreda et al. 1998). Leptin replacement restores the phagocytic function of macrophages in *ob/ob* mice that still have the intact Ob-R, but not in *db/db* mice, suggesting that leptin plays a crucial role in the proinflammatory immune responses (Loffreda et al. 1998). Consistent with *in vitro* data, leptin is involved in the cell-mediated immunity *in vivo*. While Th1 responses are predominant under leptin-elevated conditions such as rheumatoid arthritis, leptin-deficient *ob/ob* mice shift the Th1/Th2 balance favorable to Th2, leading to amelioration of rheumatoid arthritis (Busso et al. 2002).

Leptin Stimulates the Proinflammatory Signaling Pathways in Peripheries

Leptin is supposed to play an important role in the inflammation in peripheral tissues expressing Ob-R, including colon, liver, and placenta (Hoggard et al. 1997; Masuzaki et al. 1997; Cohen et al. 2005; Hansen et al. 2008). Dextran sulfate sodium (DSS) and trinitrobenzene sulfonic acid (TNBS) are prototypic inducers of colitis. DSS-fed *ob/ob* mice showed less severe colitis compared with control mice in terms of stool consistency, bleeding, and cytokine release, and these effects were reverted by leptin replacement (Siegmund et al. 2002). A plasma leptin concentration was increased in the TNBS-induced colitis model, and exogenous leptin injection exacerbated the inflammatory injuries in the colonic mucosa (Barbier et al. 2001). Moreover, leptin receptor-deficient *db/db* mice were resistant to concanavalin A–induced hepatitis (Gove et al. 2009). Treatment with leptin also stimulated NF-κB-dependent release of proinflammatory cytokines, such as IL-1β, IL-6, and TNF-α, in human placental tissues (Lappas et al. 2005).

NF-κB Might Bridge Leptin-Induced Inflammation and Cancer

It is well known that the transcription factor NF-κB is a key player in inflammation-associated carcinogenesis. Uncontrolled activation of NF-κB induces continuous expression of genes encoding proteins with proinflammatory, antiapoptotic, and proangiogenic functions, consequently facilitating tumorigenesis (Karin and Greten 2005; Kundu and Surh 2008). Several *in vitro* studies have shown that leptin activates NF-κB through phosphorylation of MAPKs and/or degradation of IκB-α, a negative regulator of NF-κB (Lappas et al. 2005; Mattace Raso et al. 2006). Besides directly activating NF-κB, leptin can provoke NF-κB activation in nearby cells in a rather indirect manner. As illustrated in Figure 10.1, leptin induces the release of the proinflammatory mediators, such as IL-1, IL-6, and TNF-α, from the immune cells which can stimulate the NF-κB signaling in a paracrine fashion. Thus, obese protein leptin might stimulate proinflammatory responses via direct and/or indirect activation of NF-κB, contributing to carcinogenesis.

LEPTIN AND CARCINOGENESIS

ELEVATED EXPRESSION LEVELS OF LEPTIN AND ITS RECEPTOR IN TUMORS

Several clinical studies report that leptin and its receptor Ob-R are overexpressed in tumors. Human breast and gastric carcinomas exhibit significant expression of Ob-R compared with normal surrounding tissues (Ishikawa et al. 2004, 2006). Overexpression of Ob-R is a predictable marker of poor prognosis in breast and ovarian cancers (Ishikawa et al. 2004; Uddin et al. 2009). Leptin expression is also elevated in human colorectal cancer, hepatocellular carcinoma, gastric cancer, and endometrial cancer (Wang et al. 2004; Koda et al. 2007a,b). Increased leptin expression correlates with severe clinicopathological features and unfavorable outcome in gastric cancer (Zhao et al. 2007). Moreover, a high circulating level of leptin is closely associated with an increased risk of breast, colon, and prostate cancer (Hsing et al. 2001; Stattin et al. 2001, 2003; Chia et al. 2007; Wu et al. 2009). In case of colon cancer, however, elevated leptin is not linked to an increased cancer risk in women (Stattin et al. 2003; Chia et al. 2007). An enhanced circulating level of leptin is unlikely to affect the tumor growth in women, due to their relatively high plasma levels of leptin even under normal healthy conditions, compared to men. Moreover, a plasma concentration of estrogen needs to be considered as another factor that can influence the colon tumorigenesis in women.

Although it is still uncertain whether increased expression of leptin and Ob-R in several tumors is a cause or a result of obesity-associated cancer, it is quite obvious that leptin regulates growth and locomotion of cancer cells through Ob-R, based on the results from abundant *in vivo* and *in vitro* studies. Thus, leptin might accelerate tumorigenesis in the promotion and progression stages, even though leptin itself is not likely to be a tumor initiator.

LEPTIN PROMOTES TUMORIGENESIS

Leptin can stimulate proliferation of assorted types of cancer cells. Treatment with 50–500 ng/mL of leptin markedly promotes cell growth in various cancer cell lines, including those of breast, endometrium, colon, prostate, esophagus, bile duct, liver, and melanocyte (Hu et al. 2002; Okumura et al. 2002; Somasundar et al. 2004; Yin et al. 2004; Ogunwobi et al. 2006; Sharma et al. 2006; Chen et al. 2007; Ogunwobi and Beales 2007; Fava et al. 2008; Brandon et al. 2009). Leptin induced cancer cell proliferation might be mainly mediated by Ob-R-bound JAK2. AG490, a pharmacological inhibitor of JAK2, abrogated leptin-induced cell growth in hepatocarcinoma, endometrium cancer, and breast cancer (Yin et al. 2004; Sharma et al. 2006; Chen et al. 2007). Phosphotidylinositol 3-kinase (PI3K) and MAPKs seem to be downstream effectors of JAK2 in leptin-induced cancer cell proliferation. Leptin acts as a growth factor not only in breast cancer cells but also in normal mammary epithelial cells, suggesting that leptin-induced proliferation is not a cancer-specific event (Hu et al. 2002). However, Ob-R is frequently overexpressed in cancer cells compared with normal counterparts, which might limit the uncontrolled proliferative action of leptin in cancerous cells.

Leptin promotes cancer growth *in vivo* as well (Table 10.2). When nude mice bearing MCF-7 human breast cancer cells were exposed to exogenous human recombinant leptin, estrogen-induced tumor growth was potentiated (Mauro et al. 2007). It has been reported that leptin is a potent promoter of azoxymethane (AOM)-induced mouse colorectal carcinogenesis (Endo et al. 2011). According to this study, Ob-R-deficient *db/db* mice are less prone to AOM-induced colorectal cancer, which suggests that the leptin signaling plays an important role in promoting proliferation of epithelial cells in colonic mucosa (Endo et al. 2011). In line with this notion, a leptin receptor antagonist reduced mammary tumor growth in a xenograft model (Gonzalez et al. 2006). Interestingly, the growth of implanted tumor was suppressed in mice housed under leptin-reducing conditions, such as enriched environment (Cao et al. 2010).

TABLE 10.2
Leptin-Induced Carcinogenesis

Animal Strain/Species	Route of Administration	Effects	Reference
Nude mice bearing MCF-7 cells	Intraperitoneal injection of 230 μg/kg leptin	↑ Estrogen-induced tumor growth	Mauro et al. (2007)
BALB/c mice bearing mouse 4T1 cells	Local injection of a leptin receptor antagonist into the mammary fat pad	↓ Mammary tumor growth	Gonzalez et al. (2006)
db/db mice	Intraperitoneal injection of 10 mg/kg AOM	↓ Colon tumor sizes ↓ Colon tumor multiplicity	Endo et al. (2011)
C57BL/6J mice	Intraperitoneal injection of 2 μg recombinant leptin everyday for 15 weeks after initial AOM injection	↑ Colon tumor sizes	Endo et al. (2011)
Rats	Implantation of leptin-containing disk on the dorsal thorax	↑ The number of blood vessels	Anagnostoulis et al. (2008)

LEPTIN INDUCES TUMOR PROGRESSION

Leptin is also involved in cancer progression including angiogenesis and metastasis that are essential for prolonged survival of tumors. The number of blood vessels was found to be increased in leptin-containing disk implanted on the dorsal thorax of rats, indicative of an angiogenic effect of leptin (Anagnostoulis et al. 2008). Leptin-induced angiogenesis might be mediated by vascular endothelial growth factor (VEGF), a major angiogenic factor, based on the observations that leptin upregulates VEGF expression in several cancer cell lines (Carino et al. 2008; Gonzalez-Perez et al. 2010; Zhou et al. 2011). Moreover, expression levels of leptin and Ob-R are positively correlated with a degree of vascularization in hepatocellular carcinoma tissues (Ribatti et al. 2008). Leptin-induced angiogenesis in cancer cells can develop the microenvironment to overcome shortage of oxygen and nutrients, favorable to cancer cell survival.

In addition to stimulating angiogenesis, leptin induces invasion and migration in various types of cancer cells (Saxena et al. 2007, 2008; Jaffe and Schwartz 2008; McMurtry et al. 2009; Yang et al. 2009; Yeh et al. 2009; Ratke et al. 2010). Increased motility and invasiveness are likely due to leptin-induced upregulation of certain molecules related to cellular locomotion, such as integrins, cadherins, RhoA, and matrix metalloproteinases (MMPs) (Attoub et al. 2000; Park et al. 2001; Mauro et al. 2007; Nath et al. 2008; Yeh et al. 2009; Huang et al. 2011). Moreover, leptin promotes epithelial to mesenchymal transition, a primary feature of metastatic cancer (Nath et al. 2008).

Leptin-induced tumor progression seems to be regulated by NF-κB. Pharmacological inhibitors of NF-κB, such as pyrrolidine dithiocarbamate and tosylphenylalanine chloromethyl ketone, abrogated leptin-induced upregulation of VEGF, MMPs, and integrins (Yeh et al. 2009; Gonzalez-Perez et al. 2010; Huang et al. 2011). Thus, the obese protein leptin may stimulate inflammation-associated oncogenic events via NF-κB activation, providing the molecular basis of obesity-induced carcinogenesis.

CONCLUDING REMARKS

Obesity is a prime etiologic factor for various types of tumors (Cleary and Maihle 1997; Calle et al. 2003; von Hafe et al. 2004; Silha et al. 2005; Frezza et al. 2006). Adipose tissue mass is increased in obesity, leading to substantial elevation of adipokines (Trayhurn 2007). Among the adipokines, leptin might play a most prominent role in obesity-induced inflammation and carcinogenesis. An elevated serum level of leptin has been associated with inflammation and an increased cancer risk in several clinical studies (Corica et al. 1999; Wang et al. 2004; Koda et al. 2007a,b).

Although multiple lines of evidence support the carcinogenic functions of leptin, controversies still remain. It has been reported that correlation between the serum leptin level and the risk of prostate cancer is not statistically significant (Hsing et al. 2001). In the case of colon cancer, there was no significant difference observed in the number of AOM-induced aberrant crypt foci (ACF) between *ob/ob* and *db/db* mice (Ealey et al. 2008). According to their presumption, *db/db* mice are expected to develop more ACF compared with *ob/ob* mice if leptin is a tumor promoter, due to hyperleptinemia and existence of a functional short-form Ob-R in long-form Ob-R-defective *db/db* mice. Moreover, leptin failed to promote the tumor growth in the xenograft model and colon tumorigenesis in Apc$^{Min/+}$ mice, although it stimulated the proliferation of colon cancer cells (Aparicio et al. 2005).

In spite of the contradictory observations, the role of leptin as a tumor promoter is complemented with multiple lines of convincing evidence. First, *db/db* mice have a nonfunctional long-form Ob-R unable to mediate cell proliferation via JAK2 activation, which may explain no difference in ACF formation between *ob/ob* and *db/db* mice (Ghilardi and Skoda 1997). Compared to *ob/ob* and *db/db* mice, KK-A^y mice are thought to be a more reliable for leptin-induced carcinogenesis, as the latter mice elicit an obese phenotype concomitantly with hyperleptinemia and expression of the intact leptin receptor (Gohda et al. 2006). KK-A^y mice are more susceptible to a AOM-induced tumor development as well as angiogenesis compared with normal lean C57BL/6J mice, providing solid evidence for the oncogenic role of leptin in obesity-induced carcinogenesis (Teraoka et al. 2011). In addition, leptin stimulates tumor growth in AOM-initiated and leptin-promoted colon cancer model (Endo et al. 2011).

As summarized in Figure 10.1, leptin stimulates proinflammatory responses in immune cells, resulting in secretion of various proinflammatory cytokines. Released cytokines influence other peripheral and tumor tissues in a paracrine manner. Moreover, leptin can directly affect both peripheral and tumor tissues, creating tumor-favorable microenvironment mainly via NF-κB activation. In conclusion, the obese protein leptin is a missing link bridging obesity and cancer. Hence, obesity-induced carcinogenesis might be predicted by monitoring the serum leptin level and prevented by improving leptin resistance. Further investigation is required to clarify the effect of leptin on obesity-associated carcinogenesis and to elucidate the underlying mechanisms.

ACKNOWLEDGMENT

This work was supported by the National Center of Efficacy Evaluation for the Development of Health Products Targeting Digestive Disorders (NCEED) grant (A102063) from the Ministry of Health and Welfare, Republic of Korea.

REFERENCES

Anagnostoulis, S., A. J. Karayiannakis, M. Lambropoulou, A. Efthimiadou, A. Polychronidis, and C. Simopoulos. 2008. Human leptin induces angiogenesis in vivo. *Cytokine* 42 (3):353–357.

Aparicio, T., L. Kotelevets, A. Tsocas, J. P. Laigneau, I. Sobhani, E. Chastre, and T. Lehy. 2005. Leptin stimulates the proliferation of human colon cancer cells in vitro but does not promote the growth of colon cancer xenografts in nude mice or intestinal tumorigenesis in Apc$^{Min/+}$ mice. *Gut* 54 (8):1136–1145.

Attoub, S., V. Noe, L. Pirola, E. Bruyneel, E. Chastre, M. Mareel, M. P. Wymann, and C. Gespach. 2000. Leptin promotes invasiveness of kidney and colonic epithelial cells via phosphoinositide 3-kinase-, rho-, and rac-dependent signaling pathways. *FASEB J* 14 (14):2329–2338.

Baker, R. G., M. S. Hayden, and S. Ghosh. 2011. NF-κB, inflammation, and metabolic disease. *Cell Metab* 13 (1):11–22.

Banks, A. S., S. M. Davis, S. H. Bates, and M. G. Myers Jr. 2000. Activation of downstream signals by the long form of the leptin receptor. *J Biol Chem* 275 (19):14563–14572.

Barbier, M., S. Attoub, M. Joubert, A. Bado, C. Laboisse, C. Cherbut, and J. P. Galmiche. 2001. Proinflammatory role of leptin in experimental colitis in rats benefit of cholecystokinin-B antagonist and β3-agonist. *Life Sci* 69 (5):567–580.

Brandon, E. L., J. W. Gu, L. Cantwell, Z. He, G. Wallace, and J. E. Hall. 2009. Obesity promotes melanoma tumor growth: Role of leptin. *Cancer Biol Ther* 8 (19):1871–1879.

Browning, L. M., J. D. Krebs, E. C. Magee, G. Fruhbeck, and S. A. Jebb. 2008. Circulating markers of inflammation and their link to indices of adiposity. *Obes Facts* 1 (5):259–265.

Busso, N., A. So, V. Chobaz-Peclat, C. Morard, E. Martinez-Soria, D. Talabot-Ayer, and C. Gabay. 2002. Leptin signaling deficiency impairs humoral and cellular immune responses and attenuates experimental arthritis. *J Immunol* 168 (2):875–882.

Calle, E. E., C. Rodriguez, K. Walker-Thurmond, and M. J. Thun. 2003. Overweight, obesity, and mortality from cancer in a prospectively studied cohort of U.S. adults. *N Engl J Med* 348 (17):1625–1638.

Cao, L., X. Liu, E. J. Lin, C. Wang, E. Y. Choi, V. Riban, B. Lin, and M. J. During. 2010. Environmental and genetic activation of a brain-adipocyte BDNF/leptin axis causes cancer remission and inhibition. *Cell* 142 (1):52–64.

Carino, C., A. B. Olawaiye, S. Cherfils, T. Serikawa, M. P. Lynch, B. R. Rueda, and R. R. Gonzalez. 2008. Leptin regulation of proangiogenic molecules in benign and cancerous endometrial cells. *Int J Cancer* 123 (12):2782–2790.

Chen, C., Y. C. Chang, C. L. Liu, T. P. Liu, K. J. Chang, and I. C. Guo. 2007. Leptin induces proliferation and anti-apoptosis in human hepatocarcinoma cells by up-regulating cyclin D1 and down-regulating Bax via a Janus kinase 2-linked pathway. *Endocr Relat Cancer* 14 (2):513–529.

Chen, H., O. Charlat, L. A. Tartaglia, E. A. Woolf, X. Weng, S. J. Ellis, N. D. Lakey, J. Culpepper, K. J. Moore, R. E. Breitbart, G. M. Duyk, R. I. Tepper, and J. P. Morgenstern. 1996. Evidence that the diabetes gene encodes the leptin receptor: Identification of a mutation in the leptin receptor gene in *db/db* mice. *Cell* 84 (3):491–495.

Chia, V. M., P. A. Newcomb, J. W. Lampe, E. White, M. T. Mandelson, A. McTiernan, and J. D. Potter. 2007. Leptin concentrations, leptin receptor polymorphisms, and colorectal adenoma risk. *Cancer Epidemiol Biomarkers Prev* 16 (12):2697–2703.

Cleary, M. P. and N. J. Maihle. 1997. The role of body mass index in the relative risk of developing premenopausal versus postmenopausal breast cancer. *Proc Soc Exp Biol Med* 216 (1):28–43.

Cohen, P., G. Yang, X. Yu, A. A. Soukas, C. S. Wolfish, J. M. Friedman, and C. Li. 2005. Induction of leptin receptor expression in the liver by leptin and food deprivation. *J Biol Chem* 280 (11):10034–10039.

Considine, R. V., M. K. Sinha, M. L. Heiman, A. Kriauciunas, T. W. Stephens, M. R. Nyce, J. P. Ohannesian, C. C. Marco, L. J. McKee, T. L. Bauer et al. 1996. Serum immunoreactive-leptin concentrations in normal-weight and obese humans. *N Engl J Med* 334 (5):292–295.

Corica, F., A. Allegra, A. Corsonello, M. Buemi, G. Calapai, A. Ruello, V. Nicita Mauro, and D. Ceruso. 1999. Relationship between plasma leptin levels and the tumor necrosis factor-α system in obese subjects. *Int J Obes Relat Metab Disord* 23 (4):355–360.

Cramer, T. and R. S. Johnson. 2003. A novel role for the hypoxia inducible transcription factor HIF-1α: Critical regulation of inflammatory cell function. *Cell Cycle* 2 (3):192–193.

Cramer, T., Y. Yamanishi, B. E. Clausen, I. Forster, R. Pawlinski, N. Mackman, V. H. Haase, R. Jaenisch, M. Corr, V. Nizet, G. S. Firestein, H. P. Gerber, N. Ferrara, and R. S. Johnson. 2003. HIF-1α is essential for myeloid cell-mediated inflammation. *Cell* 112 (5):645–657.

Das, U. N. 2001. Is obesity an inflammatory condition? *Nutrition* 17 (11–12):953–966.

Dreyer, M. G., C. E. Juge-Aubry, C. Gabay, U. Lang, F. Rohner-Jeanrenaud, J. M. Dayer, and C. A. Meier. 2003. Leptin activates the promoter of the interleukin-1 receptor antagonist through p42/44 mitogen-activated protein kinase and a composite nuclear factor κB/PU.1 binding site. *Biochem J* 370 (Pt 2):591–599.

Ealey, K. N., S. Lu, and M. C. Archer. 2008. Development of aberrant crypt foci in the colons of *ob/ob* and *db/db* mice: Evidence that leptin is not a promoter. *Mol Carcinog* 47 (9):667–677.

Endo, H., K. Hosono, T. Uchiyama, E. Sakai, M. Sugiyama, H. Takahashi, N. Nakajima, K. Wada, K. Takeda, H. Nakagama, and A. Nakajima. 2011. Leptin acts as a growth factor for colorectal tumours at stages subsequent to tumour initiation in murine colon carcinogenesis. *Gut* 60 (11):1363–1371.

Fain, J. N., A. K. Madan, M. L. Hiler, P. Cheema, and S. W. Bahouth. 2004. Comparison of the release of adipokines by adipose tissue, adipose tissue matrix, and adipocytes from visceral and subcutaneous abdominal adipose tissues of obese humans. *Endocrinology* 145 (5):2273–2282.

Fava, G., G. Alpini, C. Rychlicki, S. Saccomanno, S. DeMorrow, L. Trozzi, C. Candelaresi, J. Venter, A. Di Sario, M. Marzioni, I. Bearzi, S. Glaser, D. Alvaro, L. Marucci, H. Francis, G. Svegliati-Baroni, and A. Benedetti. 2008. Leptin enhances cholangiocarcinoma cell growth. *Cancer Res* 68 (16):6752–6761.

Frede, S., P. Freitag, T. Otto, C. Heilmaier, and J. Fandrey. 2005. The proinflammatory cytokine interleukin 1β and hypoxia cooperatively induce the expression of adrenomedullin in ovarian carcinoma cells through hypoxia inducible factor 1 activation. *Cancer Res* 65 (11):4690–4697.

Frezza, E. E., M. S. Wachtel, and M. Chiriva-Internati. 2006. Influence of obesity on the risk of developing colon cancer. *Gut* 55 (2):285–291.

Fruhbeck, G. 2006. Intracellular signalling pathways activated by leptin. *Biochem J* 393 (Pt 1):7–20.

Ghilardi, N. and R. C. Skoda. 1997. The leptin receptor activates janus kinase 2 and signals for proliferation in a factor-dependent cell line. *Mol Endocrinol* 11 (4):393–399.

Gohda, T., M. Tanimoto, S. Kaneko, T. Shibata, K. Funabiki, S. Horikoshi, and Y. Tomino. 2006. Minor gene effect of leptin receptor variant on the body weight in KK/Ta mice. *Diabetes Obes Metab* 8 (5):581–584.

Gonzalez, R. R., S. Cherfils, M. Escobar, J. H. Yoo, C. Carino, A. K. Styer, B. T. Sullivan, H. Sakamoto, A. Olawaiye, T. Serikawa, M. P. Lynch, and B. R. Rueda. 2006. Leptin signaling promotes the growth of mammary tumors and increases the expression of vascular endothelial growth factor (VEGF) and its receptor type two (VEGF-R2). *J Biol Chem* 281 (36):26320–26328.

Gonzalez-Perez, R. R., Y. Xu, S. Guo, A. Watters, W. Zhou, and S. J. Leibovich. 2010. Leptin upregulates VEGF in breast cancer via canonic and non-canonical signalling pathways and NF-κB/HIF-1α activation. *Cell Signal* 22 (9):1350–1362.

Gove, M. E., D. H. Rhodes, M. Pini, J. W. van Baal, J. A. Sennello, R. Fayad, R. J. Cabay, M. G. Myers Jr., and G. Fantuzzi. 2009. Role of leptin receptor-induced STAT3 signaling in modulation of intestinal and hepatic inflammation in mice. *J Leukoc Biol* 85 (3):491–496.

Hakansson, M. L., H. Brown, N. Ghilardi, R. C. Skoda, and B. Meister. 1998. Leptin receptor immunoreactivity in chemically defined target neurons of the hypothalamus. *J Neurosci* 18 (1):559–572.

Halaas, J. L., K. S. Gajiwala, M. Maffei, S. L. Cohen, B. T. Chait, D. Rabinowitz, R. L. Lallone, S. K. Burley, and J. M. Friedman. 1995. Weight-reducing effects of the plasma protein encoded by the *obese* gene. *Science* 269 (5223):543–546.

Hansen, G. H., L. L. Niels-Christiansen, and E. M. Danielsen. 2008. Leptin and the obesity receptor (OB-R) in the small intestine and colon: A colocalization study. *J Histochem Cytochem* 56 (7):677–685.

He, Q., Z. Gao, J. Yin, J. Zhang, Z. Yun, and J. Ye. 2011. Regulation of HIF-1α activity in adipose tissue by obesity-associated factors: Adipogenesis, insulin, and hypoxia. *Am J Physiol Endocrinol Metab* 300 (5):E877–E885.

Hegyi, K., K. Fulop, K. Kovacs, S. Toth, and A. Falus. 2004. Leptin-induced signal transduction pathways. *Cell Biol Int* 28 (3):159–169.

Hoggard, N., L. Hunter, J. S. Duncan, L. M. Williams, P. Trayhurn, and J. G. Mercer. 1997. Leptin and leptin receptor mRNA and protein expression in the murine fetus and placenta. *Proc Natl Acad Sci U S A* 94 (20):11073–11078.

Hosogai, N., A. Fukuhara, K. Oshima, Y. Miyata, S. Tanaka, K. Segawa, S. Furukawa, Y. Tochino, R. Komuro, M. Matsuda, and I. Shimomura. 2007. Adipose tissue hypoxia in obesity and its impact on adipocytokine dysregulation. *Diabetes* 56 (4):901–911.

Hotamisligil, G. S. 1999. The role of TNFα and TNF receptors in obesity and insulin resistance. *J Intern Med* 245 (6):621–625.

Hsing, A. W., S. Chua Jr., Y. T. Gao, E. Gentzschein, L. Chang, J. Deng, and F. Z. Stanczyk. 2001. Prostate cancer risk and serum levels of insulin and leptin: A population-based study. *J Natl Cancer Inst* 93 (10):783–789.

Hu, X., S. C. Juneja, N. J. Maihle, and M. P. Cleary. 2002. Leptin—A growth factor in normal and malignant breast cells and for normal mammary gland development. *J Natl Cancer Inst* 94 (22):1704–1711.

Huang, C. Y., H. S. Yu, T. Y. Lai, Y. L. Yeh, C. C. Su, H. H. Hsu, F. J. Tsai, C. H. Tsai, H. C. Wu, and C. H. Tang. 2011. Leptin increases motility and integrin up-regulation in human prostate cancer cells. *J Cell Physiol* 226 (5):1274–1282.

Ishikawa, M., J. Kitayama, and H. Nagawa. 2004. Enhanced expression of leptin and leptin receptor (OB-R) in human breast cancer. *Clin Cancer Res* 10 (13):4325–4331.

Ishikawa, M., J. Kitayama, and H. Nagawa. 2006. Expression pattern of leptin and leptin receptor (OB-R) in human gastric cancer. *World J Gastroenterol* 12 (34):5517–5522.

Jaffe, T. and B. Schwartz. 2008. Leptin promotes motility and invasiveness in human colon cancer cells by activating multiple signal-transduction pathways. *Int J Cancer* 123 (11):2543–2556.

Karin, M. and F. R. Greten. 2005. NF-κB: Linking inflammation and immunity to cancer development and progression. *Nat Rev Immunol* 5 (10):749–759.

Koda, M., M. Sulkowska, L. Kanczuga-Koda, E. Surmacz, and S. Sulkowski. 2007a. Overexpression of the obesity hormone leptin in human colorectal cancer. *J Clin Pathol* 60 (8):902–906.

Koda, M., M. Sulkowska, A. Wincewicz, L. Kanczuga-Koda, B. Musiatowicz, M. Szymanska, and S. Sulkowski. 2007b. Expression of leptin, leptin receptor, and hypoxia-inducible factor 1α in human endometrial cancer. *Ann N Y Acad Sci* 1095:90–98.

Kundu, J. K. and Y. J. Surh. 2008. Inflammation: Gearing the journey to cancer. *Mutat Res* 659 (1–2):15–30.

Labruna, G., F. Pasanisi, C. Nardelli, R. Caso, D. F. Vitale, F. Contaldo, and L. Sacchetti. 2011. High leptin/ adiponectin ratio and serum triglycerides are associated with an "at-risk" phenotype in young severely obese patients. *Obesity (Silver Spring)* 19 (7):1492–1496.

Lappas, M., M. Permezel, and G. E. Rice. 2005. Leptin and adiponectin stimulate the release of proinflammatory cytokines and prostaglandins from human placenta and maternal adipose tissue via nuclear factor-κB, peroxisomal proliferator-activated receptor-γ and extracellularly regulated kinase 1/2. *Endocrinology* 146 (8):3334–3342.

Loffreda, S., S. Q. Yang, H. Z. Lin, C. L. Karp, M. L. Brengman, D. J. Wang, A. S. Klein, G. B. Bulkley, C. Bao, P. W. Noble, M. D. Lane, and A. M. Diehl. 1998. Leptin regulates proinflammatory immune responses. *FASEB J* 12 (1):57–65.

Lord, G. M., G. Matarese, J. K. Howard, R. J. Baker, S. R. Bloom, and R. I. Lechler. 1998. Leptin modulates the T-cell immune response and reverses starvation-induced immunosuppression. *Nature* 394 (6696):897–901.

Maffei, M., J. Halaas, E. Ravussin, R. E. Pratley, G. H. Lee, Y. Zhang, H. Fei, S. Kim, R. Lallone, S. Ranganathan et al. 1995. Leptin levels in human and rodent: Measurement of plasma leptin and ob RNA in obese and weight-reduced subjects. *Nat Med* 1 (11):1155–1161.

Margetic, S., C. Gazzola, G. G. Pegg, and R. A. Hill. 2002. Leptin: A review of its peripheral actions and interactions. *Int J Obes Relat Metab Disord* 26 (11):1407–1433.

Masuzaki, H., Y. Ogawa, N. Sagawa, K. Hosoda, T. Matsumoto, H. Mise, H. Nishimura, Y. Yoshimasa, I. Tanaka, T. Mori, and K. Nakao. 1997. Nonadipose tissue production of leptin: Leptin as a novel placenta-derived hormone in humans. *Nat Med* 3 (9):1029–1033.

Mattace Raso, G., E. Esposito, A. Iacono, M. Pacilio, A. Coppola, G. Bianco, S. Diano, R. Di Carlo, and R. Meli. 2006. Leptin induces nitric oxide synthase type II in C6 glioma cells. Role for nuclear factor-κB in hormone effect. *Neurosci Lett* 396 (2):121–126.

Mauro, L., S. Catalano, G. Bossi, M. Pellegrino, I. Barone, S. Morales, C. Giordano, V. Bartella, I. Casaburi, and S. Ando. 2007. Evidences that leptin up-regulates E-cadherin expression in breast cancer: Effects on tumor growth and progression. *Cancer Res* 67 (7):3412–3421.

McMurtry, V., A. M. Simeone, R. Nieves-Alicea, and A. M. Tari. 2009. Leptin utilizes Jun N-terminal kinases to stimulate the invasion of MCF-7 breast cancer cells. *Clin Exp Metastasis* 26 (3):197–204.

Myers, M. G. Jr., R. L. Leibel, R. J. Seeley, and M. W. Schwartz. 2010. Obesity and leptin resistance: Distinguishing cause from effect. *Trends Endocrinol Metab* 21 (11):643–651.

Nath, A. K., R. M. Brown, M. Michaud, M. R. Sierra-Honigmann, M. Snyder, and J. A. Madri. 2008. Leptin affects endocardial cushion formation by modulating EMT and migration via Akt signaling cascades. *J Cell Biol* 181 (2):367–380.

Ogunwobi, O. O. and I. L. Beales. 2007. The anti-apoptotic and growth stimulatory actions of leptin in human colon cancer cells involves activation of JNK mitogen activated protein kinase, JAK2 and PI3-kinase/ Akt. *Int J Colorectal Dis* 22 (4):401–409.

Ogunwobi, O., G. Mutungi, and I. L. Beales. 2006. Leptin stimulates proliferation and inhibits apoptosis in Barrett's esophageal adenocarcinoma cells by cyclooxygenase-2-dependent, prostaglandin-E_2-mediated transactivation of the epidermal growth factor receptor and c-Jun NH2-terminal kinase activation. *Endocrinology* 147 (9):4505–4516.

Okumura, M., M. Yamamoto, H. Sakuma, T. Kojima, T. Maruyama, M. Jamali, D. R. Cooper, and K. Yasuda. 2002. Leptin and high glucose stimulate cell proliferation in MCF-7 human breast cancer cells: Reciprocal involvement of PKC-α and PPAR expression. *Biochim Biophys Acta* 1592 (2):107–116.

Park, H. Y., H. M. Kwon, H. J. Lim, B. K. Hong, J. Y. Lee, B. E. Park, Y. Jang, S. Y. Cho, and H. S. Kim. 2001. Potential role of leptin in angiogenesis: Leptin induces endothelial cell proliferation and expression of matrix metalloproteinases in vivo and in vitro. *Exp Mol Med* 33 (2):95–102.

Raso, G. M., M. Pacilio, E. Esposito, A. Coppola, R. Di Carlo, and R. Meli. 2002. Leptin potentiates IFN-γ-induced expression of nitric oxide synthase and cyclo-oxygenase-2 in murine macrophage J774A.1. *Br J Pharmacol* 137 (6):799–804.

Ratke, J., F. Entschladen, B. Niggemann, K. S. Zanker, and K. Lang. 2010. Leptin stimulates the migration of colon carcinoma cells by multiple signaling pathways. *Endocr Relat Cancer* 17 (1):179–189.

Ribatti, D., A. S. Belloni, B. Nico, M. Di Comite, E. Crivellato, and A. Vacca. 2008. Leptin-leptin receptor are involved in angiogenesis in human hepatocellular carcinoma. *Peptides* 29 (9):1596–1602.

Saxena, N. K., D. Sharma, X. Ding, S. Lin, F. Marra, D. Merlin, and F. A. Anania. 2007. Concomitant activation of the JAK/STAT, PI3K/AKT, and ERK signaling is involved in leptin-mediated promotion of invasion and migration of hepatocellular carcinoma cells. *Cancer Res* 67 (6):2497–2507.

Saxena, N. K., L. Taliaferro-Smith, B. B. Knight, D. Merlin, F. A. Anania, R. M. O'Regan, and D. Sharma. 2008. Bidirectional crosstalk between leptin and insulin-like growth factor-I signaling promotes invasion and migration of breast cancer cells via transactivation of epidermal growth factor receptor. *Cancer Res* 68 (23):9712–9722.

Sharma, D., N. K. Saxena, P. M. Vertino, and F. A. Anania. 2006. Leptin promotes the proliferative response and invasiveness in human endometrial cancer cells by activating multiple signal-transduction pathways. *Endocr Relat Cancer* 13 (2):629–640.

Siegmund, B., H. A. Lehr, and G. Fantuzzi. 2002. Leptin: A pivotal mediator of intestinal inflammation in mice. *Gastroenterology* 122 (7):2011–2025.

Silha, J. V., M. Krsek, P. Sucharda, and L. J. Murphy. 2005. Angiogenic factors are elevated in overweight and obese individuals. *Int J Obes (Lond)* 29 (11):1308–1314.

Somasundar, P., K. A. Frankenberry, H. Skinner, G. Vedula, D. W. McFadden, D. Riggs, B. Jackson, R. Vangilder, S. M. Hileman, and L. C. Vona-Davis. 2004. Prostate cancer cell proliferation is influenced by leptin. *J Surg Res* 118 (1):71–82.

Stattin, P., R. Palmqvist, S. Soderberg, C. Biessy, B. Ardnor, G. Hallmans, R. Kaaks, and T. Olsson. 2003. Plasma leptin and colorectal cancer risk: A prospective study in Northern Sweden. *Oncol Rep* 10 (6):2015–2021.

Stattin, P., S. Soderberg, G. Hallmans, A. Bylund, R. Kaaks, U. H. Stenman, A. Bergh, and T. Olsson. 2001. Leptin is associated with increased prostate cancer risk: A nested case-referent study. *J Clin Endocrinol Metab* 86 (3):1341–1345.

Stofkova, A. 2009. Leptin and adiponectin: From energy and metabolic dysbalance to inflammation and auto-immunity. *Endocr Regul* 43 (4):157–168.

Teraoka, N., M. Mutoh, S. Takasu, T. Ueno, K. Nakano, M. Takahashi, T. Imai, S. Masuda, T. Sugimura, and K. Wakabayashi. 2011. High susceptibility to azoxymethane-induced colorectal carcinogenesis in obese KK-A^y mice. *Int J Cancer* 129 (3):528–535.

Trayhurn, P. 2007. Adipocyte biology. *Obes Rev* 8 Suppl 1:41–44.

Trayhurn, P. and I. S. Wood. 2005. Signalling role of adipose tissue: Adipokines and inflammation in obesity. *Biochem Soc Trans* 33 (Pt 5):1078–1081.

Uddin, S., R. Bu, M. Ahmed, J. Abubaker, F. Al-Dayel, P. Bavi, and K. S. Al-Kuraya. 2009. Overexpression of leptin receptor predicts an unfavorable outcome in Middle Eastern ovarian cancer. *Mol Cancer* 8:74.

van Kruijsdijk, R. C., E. van der Wall, and F. L. Visseren. 2009. Obesity and cancer: The role of dysfunctional adipose tissue. *Cancer Epidemiol Biomarkers Prev* 18 (10):2569–2578.

von Hafe, P., F. Pina, A. Perez, M. Tavares, and H. Barros. 2004. Visceral fat accumulation as a risk factor for prostate cancer. *Obes Res* 12 (12):1930–1935.

Vuolteenaho, K., A. Koskinen, M. Kukkonen, R. Nieminen, U. Paivarinta, T. Moilanen, and E. Moilanen. 2009. Leptin enhances synthesis of proinflammatory mediators in human osteoarthritic cartilage—Mediator role of NO in leptin-induced PGE$_2$, IL-6, and IL-8 production. *Mediators Inflamm* 2009:345838.

Wang, B., I. S. Wood, and P. Trayhurn. 2008. Hypoxia induces leptin gene expression and secretion in human preadipocytes: Differential effects of hypoxia on adipokine expression by preadipocytes. *J Endocrinol* 198 (1):127–134.

Wang, X. J., S. L. Yuan, Q. Lu, Y. R. Lu, J. Zhang, Y. Liu, and W. D. Wang. 2004. Potential involvement of leptin in carcinogenesis of hepatocellular carcinoma. *World J Gastroenterol* 10 (17):2478–2481.

Weigle, D. S., T. R. Bukowski, D. C. Foster, S. Holderman, J. M. Kramer, G. Lasser, C. E. Lofton-Day, D. E. Prunkard, C. Raymond, and J. L. Kuijper. 1995. Recombinant ob protein reduces feeding and body weight in the *ob/ob* mouse. *J Clin Invest* 96 (4):2065–2070.

Wong, C. K., P. F. Cheung, and C. W. Lam. 2007. Leptin-mediated cytokine release and migration of eosinophils: Implications for immunopathophysiology of allergic inflammation. *Eur J Immunol* 37 (8):2337–2348.

Wu, M. H., Y. C. Chou, W. Y. Chou, G. C. Hsu, C. H. Chu, C. P. Yu, J. C. Yu, and C. A. Sun. 2009. Circulating levels of leptin, adiposity and breast cancer risk. *Br J Cancer* 100 (4):578–582.

Yang, S. N., H. T. Chen, H. K. Tsou, C. Y. Huang, W. H. Yang, C. M. Su, Y. C. Fong, W. P. Tseng, and C. H. Tang. 2009. Leptin enhances cell migration in human chondrosarcoma cells through OBRl leptin receptor. *Carcinogenesis* 30 (4):566–574.

Ye, J., Z. Gao, J. Yin, and Q. He. 2007. Hypoxia is a potential risk factor for chronic inflammation and adi-ponectin reduction in adipose tissue of *ob/ob* and dietary obese mice. *Am J Physiol Endocrinol Metab* 293 (4):E1118–E1128.

Yeh, W. L., D. Y. Lu, M. J. Lee, and W. M. Fu. 2009. Leptin induces migration and invasion of glioma cells through MMP-13 production. *Glia* 57 (4):454–464.

Yin, N., D. Wang, H. Zhang, X. Yi, X. Sun, B. Shi, H. Wu, G. Wu, X. Wang, and Y. Shang. 2004. Molecular mechanisms involved in the growth stimulation of breast cancer cells by leptin. *Cancer Res* 64 (16):5870–5875.

Zarkesh-Esfahani, H., G. Pockley, R. A. Metcalfe, M. Bidlingmaier, Z. Wu, A. Ajami, A. P. Weetman, C. J. Strasburger, and R. J. Ross. 2001. High-dose leptin activates human leukocytes via receptor expression on monocytes. *J Immunol* 167 (8):4593–4599.

Zhao, X., K. Huang, Z. Zhu, S. Chen, and R. Hu. 2007. Correlation between expression of leptin and clinicopathological features and prognosis in patients with gastric cancer. *J Gastroenterol Hepatol* 22 (8):1317–1321.

Zhou, W., S. Guo, and R. R. Gonzalez-Perez. 2011. Leptin pro-angiogenic signature in breast cancer is linked to IL-1 signalling. *Br J Cancer* 104 (1):128–137.

11 Overview of Ghrelin, Appetite, and Energy Balance*

Rafael Fernández-Fernández, PhD
and Manuel Tena-Sempere, MD, PhD

CONTENTS

INTRODUCTION

Homeostatic control of energy balance is a key biological function essential for the survival of individuals and species. Maintenance of the energy status of an organism critically relies on the dynamic balance between energy expenditure and food intake. In this equation, expression of appetite (defined as the motivational drive toward an energy source) appears as a pivotal, highly regulated phenomenon, based on the complex physiological interaction of afferent signals (which promote or inhibit appetite) and effector mechanisms (which restrain or get into motion the drive toward food intake). Among the former, multiple peripheral factors, arising mostly from the adipose tissue, the pancreas, and the gastrointestinal tract, have been identified in the last decades as powerful regulators of central circuits at the hypothalamus, as well as in the brain stem and limbic system. At those sites, such factors actively modulate neuropeptide release and, thereby, participate in the control of food intake and energy expenditure.[1,2]

In this context, leptin is probably the most illustrative paradigm of peripheral regulator of energy balance. Leptin was originally identified in 1994 as a secreted hormone, primarily produced in the white adipose tissue, displaying a very potent satiating activity. Interestingly, circulating leptin levels were demonstrated to directly correlate with the amount of adiposity. Therefore, leptin appeared to serve an essential function in signaling the amount of body energy stores to the hypothalamic centers controlling food intake, thus contributing to body weight homeostasis.[3,4] Indeed, a wealth of experimental and epidemiological evidence, gathered in the last decade, has fully confirmed the crucial role of leptin in the control of metabolism and energy balance. Moreover, identification of

---

* *Grant support*: The work from the authors' laboratory described herein was funded by grants BFI 2000-0419-CO3-03 and BFI 2002-00176 from DGESIC (Ministerio de Ciencia y Tecnología, Spain), funds from Instituto de Salud Carlos III (Red de Centros RCMN C03/08 and Project PI042082), and EU research contract EDEN QLK4-CT-2002-00603.

leptin in the mid-1990s, coinciding with the exponential increase in the prevalence of obesity and other weight disorders, boosted an extraordinary activity, in terms of basic and clinical research, aimed at identifying the molecular and physiological basis for the dynamic regulation of body weight. This research activity has not only helped to characterize the physiology of leptin but has also significantly contributed to enlarge our knowledge on the molecules and networks involved in the dynamic control of food intake. One of these molecules turned out to be the gut-derived hormone, ghrelin.

DISCOVERY OF GHRELIN

The gastric hormone ghrelin was originally identified by the group of Kangawa in late 1999 (at the National Cardiovascular Center Research Institute, Osaka, Japan) during their search for an endogenous ligand of the growth hormone (GH) secretagogue receptor (GHS-R).[5,6] Cloning of ghrelin was the endpoint of a long search for the endogenous counterpart of a large family of peptidyl and nonpeptidyl synthetic compounds, globally termed GHSs, with ability to elicit GH release *in vivo* and *in vitro* in a wide spectrum of species, including humans.[7,8] Synthesis of the first GHSs dates back to the late 1970s, when Bowers and coworkers reported that some synthetic peptide analogues of met-enkephalin, although devoid of any opioid activity, specifically induced GH secretion.[9] Although early GHSs showed very weak activity, further development of many peptide- and nonpeptide-related molecules led to the generation of much more potent GH secretagogues. Thus, GHRP-6 was the first hexapeptide shown to actively release GH *in vivo*,[10] and it is still considered as golden standard for peptidergic GHSs. Among nonpeptidyl members of the family, MK-0677 is probably the most representative GHS, showing a potent GH-releasing effect even after oral administration.[11]

A major breakthrough in the course of identification of ghrelin was the cloning in 1996 of the GHS-R, distinct from that of the major elicitor of GH release, the GH-releasing hormone receptor (GHRH-R).[12] This provided a conclusive evidence for the existence of the natural counterpart of GHSs: the endogenous ligand of GHS-R. Moreover, discovery of GHS-R allowed the implementation of routines for identification of its ligand, using an orphan receptor strategy. Given the prominent expression of GHS-R reported at the pituitary and hypothalamus (among other central areas), its potential ligand was expected to exist also in the brain.[13] However, the weak activation of GHS-R reporter systems by brain extracts suggested that such ligand might only be present at low levels at this site. Instead, a very prominent expression of this molecule was finally demonstrated by Kojima and coworkers in rat stomach extracts.[5] This molecule turned out to be a 28-amino-acid peptide, highly conserved between rat and human species, harboring an essential *n*-octanoyl modification at Ser3. This molecule was named *ghrelin*, from Proto-Indo-European root *ghre*, which means growth, and the suffix *relin*, for its reported GH-releasing activity.[5]

STRUCTURE OF GHRELIN AND ITS FUNCTIONAL RECEPTOR, THE GHS-R

The functional ghrelin peptide results from the cleavage of a precursor form, the preproghrelin, which is composed of 117 amino acids. In the human and rat, the mature ghrelin peptide consists of 28 amino acids, with divergence in two residues only.[5] Even in nonmammalian species, such as chicken, the sequence homology is rather high, with 54% identity with human ghrelin.[14] In the rat, a second form of the peptide, termed des-Gln(14)-ghrelin, has been described. Its biological activity and sequence are identical to ghrelin, except for the lack of one glutamine in position 14.[15] However, this variant is present only in low amounts in the stomach, indicating that 28-amino-acid ghrelin is the main active form of the molecule.[16] Interestingly, while no obvious structural homology between ghrelin and peptidyl GHSs was found, the gastric peptide motilin was shown to share 36% structural homology with ghrelin.[17] In fact, after the discovery of ghrelin, Tomasetto et al. reported the identification of a gastric peptide called motilin-related peptide (MTLRP),[18] whose amino acid sequence was identical to preproghrelin, except for the lack of Ser26.[18] In terms of structure–function relationship, the N-terminal seven-amino-acid stretch of ghrelin is very well conserved across vertebrate species,[19] suggesting that this region is relevant for its biological functions.

Another highly conserved (and rather unique) feature of ghrelin molecule is the addition of an *n*-octanoyl group at Ser3, which appears essential for most of its biological activities.[5] Such a post-translational modification (acylation) is the first reported in a secreted protein,[20] yet acyl modifications had been previously observed in G proteins and membrane-bound receptors. The enzymatic system responsible for acylation of ghrelin was identified in 2009, and was named GOAT, which stands for Ghrelin O-Acyltransferase.[21] The biological roles, if any, of unacylated ghrelin (whose concentration in plasma largely exceeds that of mature ghrelin) have remained largely neglected. Nonetheless, compelling evidence has been recently presented demonstrating that des-acyl ghrelin is not merely an inert form of the molecule.[22,23]

The biological actions of ghrelin are mostly conducted through interaction with its specific cell surface receptor, namely, the GHS-R. The cognate ghrelin receptor belongs to the large family of G-protein-coupled, seven-transmembrane domain receptors.[12,24] This receptor is highly expressed at central neuroendocrine tissues such as the pituitary and hypothalamus.[13] Two GHS-R subtypes, generated by alternative splicing of a single gene, have been described: the full-length type 1a receptor and the truncated GHS-R type 1b.[12,24] The GHS-R1a is the functionally active, signal-transducing form of the receptor. In contrast, the GHS-R1b lacks the transmembrane domains 6 and 7, and it is apparently devoid of high-affinity ligand binding and signal transduction capacity.[27] Thus, its functional role, if any, remains unclear. In addition, evidence for GHS-R1a-independent biological actions of ghrelin, as well as of synthetic GHSs, has been presented recently.[22,24] These seem to include (at least some of) the potential weight-gain-promoting effects of ghrelin.[25] However, the search of ghrelin receptor(s) other than GHS-R has not yet provided conclusive evidence.

DISTRIBUTION AND BIOLOGICAL FUNCTIONS OF GHRELIN: AN OVERVIEW

Despite its identification in the context of GH control (see "Discovery of ghrelin" section), in recent years, it has become evident that the biological actions of ghrelin are much wider than those originally anticipated. Indeed, a striking feature of ghrelin is its widespread pattern of distribution.[22,23] Thus, while the peptide was initially isolated from the stomach (which is undoubtedly the major source of circulating ghrelin), ghrelin expression has also been demonstrated in an array of tissues and cell types including small intestine, pancreas, lymphocytes, placenta, kidney, lung, pituitary, brain, and the gonads.[22,23,26,27] Overall, such a ubiquitous pattern of expression strongly suggests that, in addition to systemic actions of the gut-derived peptide, locally produced ghrelin might be provided with paracrine/autocrine regulatory effects in different tissues, whose physiological relevance awaits to be completely defined.

In terms of endocrine function, the first biological effect assigned to ghrelin was the ability to elicit GH secretion, as predicted by its capacity to activate GHS-R1a in cell reporter systems. This GH secretagogue action is conducted at both the pituitary and the hypothalamus, where ghrelin has been proven to regulate GHRH and somatostatin systems.[28] Yet, the importance of gut-derived ghrelin in the control of GH secretion remains controversial. In addition, a wealth of data have now demonstrated that ghrelin may serve additional central neuroendocrine functions, such as modulation of lactotropic, corticotropic, and gonadotropic axes.[26,27] Indeed, ghrelin has been proposed as putative neuroendocrine integrator linking the function of several endocrine systems essential for survival. These likely include the neuroendocrine networks responsible for the control of body weight and energy balance, as revised in detail in "Ghrelin and the control of appetite: major effects and mechanisms of action" section.

Finally, besides the endocrine actions of ghrelin summarized earlier, solid evidence has been presented recently showing that ghrelin is involved also in the regulation of quite diverse peripheral nonendocrine functions. These include regulation of gastric motility and acid secretion, different effects upon the cardiovascular system, modulation of glucose metabolism and pancreatic insulin secretion, as well as control of adipogenesis and cell proliferation. Detailed description of these functional properties of ghrelin exceeds the goals of this chapter and has been recently provided elsewhere.[20,22,23]

GHRELIN AND THE CONTROL OF APPETITE: MAJOR EFFECTS AND MECHANISMS OF ACTION

Undoubtedly, one of the facets of ghrelin physiology that has attracted more attention is that related to its ability to promote food intake. Retrospectively considered, the fact that ghrelin was able to enhance body weight should not be considered totally unexpected, given previous reports on the ability of GHSs to stimulate food intake. Nonetheless, these effects of GHSs had remained largely neglected.[22] Thus, demonstration in 2000 that administration of ghrelin efficiently induced body weight gain[29] opened a new dimension of ghrelin biology, focused in the characterization of the effects and mechanisms of action of this gut-derived hormone in the control of appetite and energy balance.

There is undisputed evidence indicating that administration of ghrelin to rodents stimulates food intake,[29] an effect that is far more potent after intracerebral delivery of the peptide, which suggests a primary central site of action. The relevance of central vs. peripheral ghrelin in the control of food intake remains controversial, mainly due to conflictive data on the expression of only minute amounts of ghrelin at the hypothalamus. Nonetheless, the importance of ghrelin/GHS-R signaling in the homeostatic control of body weight is supported by the observed decrease in food intake after antisense disruption of GHS-R at the hypothalamus,[30] and the effects of centrally and peripherally injected ghrelin in body weight.[22] Although the potency of systemically derived ghrelin in terms of food intake induction is somewhat modest, the latter is a rather unusual feature, as virtually all the orexigens known to date are only effective when acting centrally. This has led to the conclusion that ghrelin is the most important, if not the only one, appetite stimulant in the bloodstream,[31] which may serve important roles as meal-initiating signal, as well as in the long-term regulation of body weight in combination with leptin (see "Regulation of ghrelin levels and interaction with leptin system" section).

The central circuitries whereby ghrelin conducts its modulatory actions upon food intake have been exhaustively explored in the last years. Assuming a bipartite model of food intake control at the hypothalamus, with neuropeptide Y(NPY)/Agouti-related peptide (AGRP) neurons as major orexigenic effectors, and proopiomelanocortin (POMC)/cocaine-amphetamine-regulated transcript (CART) neurons as major anorexigenic effectors, ghrelin has been demonstrated to modulate expression of some (if not all) of the elements of this network. Thus, ghrelin appears to enhance AGRP and NPY after acute and chronic administration, action that might contribute to the observed short- and long-term effects of ghrelin on body weight gain.[22] In addition, ghrelin has been shown to target POMC and CART neurons at the hypothalamus. Moreover, orexins and other neuropeptides with roles in the central control of appetite are apparently modulated by ghrelin. This complex mode of action of ghrelin upon the hypothalamic centers controlling energy balance and food intake is schematically depicted in Figure 11.1. In addition, it has been shown that central effects of ghrelin on food intake are mediated by hypothalamic fatty acid metabolism and AMP-activated protein kinase (AMPK).[32]

Notwithstanding, some of the reported effects of ghrelin on food intake might not derive from direct central actions of the gut-derived peptide, but rather might be mediated by peripheral activation of afferent activity of the vagal nerve.[33] Indeed, blockade of gastric vagal inputs has been shown to blunt ghrelin effects in terms of food intake and hypothalamic NPY expression,[34] and vagal resection associated to gastroplastic surgery has been implicated in the lowering of ghrelin levels following some of these surgical procedures,[35] yet the latter is still a matter of debate. Additional contributors to the observed effects of ghrelin upon body weight are likely its direct actions upon the adipose tissue, where it mostly promotes adipogenesis and antagonizes lipolysis, and its ability to reduce cellular fat utilization and to decrease locomotor activity. These, together with its potent orexigenic action, drive the energy equation toward a state of positive energy balance.[22]

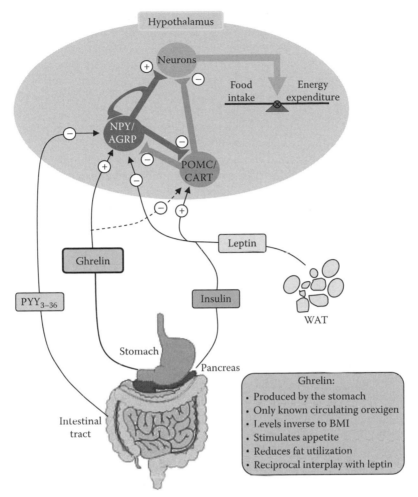

FIGURE 11.1 Diagrammatic presentation of the major biological actions of ghrelin in the control of appetite. Produced by the stomach under the regulation of metabolic cues (putative regulators: preprandial state, caloric meal intake, BMI, leptin, insulin), ghrelin mostly operates at central levels by modulating the function of leptin-responsive circuits, such as NPY/AGRP neurons. Other hypothalamic targets of ghrelin (such as PMOC/CART neurons) have also been suggested. In addition, some of the orexigenic actions of ghrelin might be mediated by the hypothalamic AMPK or conducted via modulation of vagal afferents (*not shown*). Importantly, the function of ghrelin in the control of appetite and energy balance is counterbalanced by the concerted action of a set of peripheral signals, of adipose (leptin and other adipocytokines), pancreatic (insulin), and gastrointestinal (PYY$_{3-36}$ and other gut-hormone) origin. Among these, the most prominent functional opponent for ghrelin actions appears to be leptin, which dynamically interplays with ghrelin in the long-term control of energy homeostasis.

REGULATION OF GHRELIN LEVELS AND INTERACTION WITH LEPTIN SYSTEM

While the pharmacological evidence for the appetite promoting effects of ghrelin was unquestioned, its physiological relevance in the dynamic regulation of body weight and energy homeostasis was initially the subject of an intense debate. Several observations seemed to cast doubts on the importance of ghrelin in this function, including (1) the low to negligible expression of ghrelin at the hypothalamus, (2) the limited passage of circulating ghrelin through the blood-brain barrier, and (3) the modest orexigenic effects of ghrelin after its systemic administration.[22] In addition, initial studies on mouse models of genetic inactivation of ghrelin and its functional receptor evidenced rather mild metabolic phenotypes, without a clear-cut effect of the absence of ghrelin signaling upon body weight.[36,37] Nonetheless, recent experimental observations appeared to dissipate those concerns, as expression of ghrelin has been demonstrated in discrete neuronal populations at the hypothalamus,[38] ghrelin or GHSs have been proven to act at hypothalamic regions (such as certain areas of the arcuate nucleus) where the permeability of the blood-brain barrier is significantly enhanced,[22] and, albeit less potent, consistent orexigenic responses to peripheral ghrelin delivery have been obtained in different experimental models, in contrast to other well-known orexigens devoid of systemic activity.[22] Moreover, detailed metabolic analyses of GHS-R knockout animals have shown that mice lacking ghrelin signaling are resistant to develop diet-induced obesity.[39]

One of the hallmarks of gut-derived ghrelin is that its circulating levels appear to be regulated by a number of metabolic factors. Strikingly, ghrelin concentrations have been reported to increase pre-prandially, thus suggesting a role in meal initiation.[40] Moreover, circulating ghrelin levels decrease after meal intake, the magnitude of such a drop being proportional to the ingested caloric load.[41] In addition, ghrelin concentrations seem to be inversely correlated with the body mass index (BMI), and ghrelin levels have been reported to increase in fasting conditions or persistent undernutrition, in a wide array of species.[22] Taken together, these observations support the contention that ghrelin may play complementary roles in the short-term regulation of premeal hunger and the duration of episodes of ingestion, as well as in the long-term control of energy homeostasis, acting as signal for energy insufficiency.[42] In keeping with the proposed metabolic control of ghrelin, as ultimate afferent signaling energy deficit, changes in glucose homeostasis, insulin, and leptin have been demonstrated, among others, as putative regulators of ghrelin secretion.[22]

From a homeostatic perspective, the functions and regulation of ghrelin cannot be independently considered but rather integrated in the context of a complex network of peripheral modulators of energy balance and food intake. Within this system, ghrelin possesses quite unique features, as it is the only known circulating orexigen, and may serve both short- and long-term regulatory functions.[22,23] The major functional "opponent" of ghrelin appears to be leptin.[42] Indeed, leptin and ghrelin show remarkable opposite characteristics in terms of their effects on food intake and energy balance, as well as in their correlation with the nutritional state and BMI. Thus, while excess of body weight/adiposity is associated with elevated leptin levels, situations of negative energy balance/low BMI are generally linked to persistently elevated ghrelin levels. This inverse relationship has led to the proposal that leptin (as signal for energy abundance) and ghrelin (as signal for energy insufficiency) are the two major peripheral players in the maintenance of appropriate food intake and energy stores.[42] The neuro-endocrine substrate for such a reciprocal interaction appears to involve the convergent actions of these hormones onto similar central pathways,[42] as ghrelin has been shown to regulate leptin-responsive neurons in specific hypothalamic areas.[22,42] Additional levels of interplay between leptin and ghrelin are found at the periphery, where leptin has been suggested to modulate ghrelin expression.[22] Overall, while probably being a partial simplification of a complex regulatory system, this *yin-yang* model of regulation of appetite and energy homeostasis by orexigenic (ghrelin) and anorexigenic (leptin) signals is tremendously illustrative of the basic mechanisms governing energy homeostasis, whose deregulation may lead/contribute to alterations in body weight such as obesity, anorexia, or cachexia.[42] Obviously, other peripheral factors, such as insulin and other gastrointestinal hormones (e.g., PYY_{3-36}) and adipocytokines, likely contribute, together with ghrelin and leptin, to the dynamic control of appetite, metabolism, and energy balance, as schematically presented in Figure 11.1.

GHRELIN AS NEUROENDOCRINE INTEGRATOR LINKING ENERGY STATUS AND OTHER KEY FUNCTIONS

The pleiotropic nature of ghrelin, and the diversity of its biological functions, clearly demonstrates that ghrelin is much more than a "simple" regulator of appetite. Instead, ghrelin appears to play a fundamental role in several key endocrine and nonendocrine systems, suggesting that ghrelin is an important member of the survival kit of nature.[42] Interestingly, the concurrent actions of ghrelin upon different neuroendocrine axes make it a suitable candidate for the integrated control of energy balance and other essential endocrine functions, such as growth and reproduction. The former has been assumed on the basis of the ability of ghrelin to elicit GH secretion, yet its physiological relevance remains to be fully defined. Indeed, from a teleological point of view, the proposed role of ghrelin as a signal for energy insufficiency is difficult to reconcile with a supposed action of this molecule as major elicitor of GH secretion and growth.

In contrast, although the potential link between ghrelin and reproduction has received limited attention to date, some fragmentary data strongly suggest that ghrelin may operate as putative modulator (mostly inhibitor) of the reproductive axis in different mammalian species, including primates, sheep, and rats.[26,27,43] As evidence for the reproductive "facet" of ghrelin, its expression has been demonstrated in human and rodent placenta, and ghrelin has been reported to inhibit early embryo development *in vitro* and pregnancy outcome *in vivo*.[26,27] In addition, ghrelin has been shown to suppress luteinizing hormone (LH) secretion *in vivo* and to decrease LH responsiveness to gonadotropin-releasing hormone (GnRH) *in vitro*. Moreover, repeated administration of ghrelin induced a partial delay in the timing of puberty in male rats.[44,45] Finally, transcripts of ghrelin and its cognate receptor have also been identified in rat and human gonads, and ghrelin has been reported to inhibit stimulated testicular testosterone secretion.[26,27] Given its proposed role as peripheral signal for energy insufficiency,[42] the data mentioned earlier suggest that ghrelin exerts a negative influence on the gonadotropic axis, contributing to the complex neuroendocrine network linking energy status and fertility. From a general perspective, ghrelin appears to operate as neuroendocrine integrator involved in the coordinated control of several functions essential for the survival of organisms and/or species, such as food intake and energy homeostasis, growth, and reproduction.

MAJOR CONCLUSIONS AND FUTURE PERSPECTIVES

Despite the astonishing amount of studies published on ghrelin during the last 5 years (more than 3400 scientific papers and reviews registered in PubMed database), there are still controversies and open questions regarding ghrelin physiology that await to be elucidated, as exhaustively revised recently elsewhere.[31] In the context of appetite control, a key issue to be defined is the contribution of central vs. peripheral ghrelin in the control of food intake and the relevance of centrally produced ghrelin, if any, in the neuronal networks involved in such function. Other important aspects to be fully characterized are the mechanisms (neuronal targets and central effectors) whereby ghrelin conducts its orexigenic actions, and whether some of the body weight-gain-promoting effects of ghrelin might be mediated via GHS-R1a-independent mechanisms, as recently suggested by pharmacological studies.[25] From a metabolic perspective, the reciprocal interplay between leptin and ghrelin, and more importantly, between ghrelin and insulin, remains to be fully clarified, as conflictive data on the ability of ghrelin to modulate insulin secretion have been presented.[31] Finally, a contentious issue is whether unacylated ghrelin is provided with specific or common physiologic functions. In this sense, original reports firmly demonstrated that octanoylation of ghrelin at Ser3 is mandatory for GHS-R1a binding and stimulation of GH secretion.[5,6] While this contention remains undisputed, a wealth of data presented in the last years strongly suggest that unacylated ghrelin is not merely an inert form of the molecule. In contrast, several nonendocrine actions of octanoylated ghrelin can be mimicked by its des-acyl counterpart,[22,23] including cardiovascular, adipogenic, and (anti)proliferative effects. More important for the purpose of this chapter, evidence for central and/or peripheral neuroendocrine and metabolic effects of ghrelin independent of GHS-R1a has also been recently reported.[25,45,46] These included demonstration of the ability of des-acyl ghrelin to modulate hypothalamic expression of neuropeptides relevant for food intake control, such as CART, and to induce significant decreases in body weight and food intake in mice. These observations suggest that in rodents unacylated ghrelin might operate as counterbalance signal for ghrelin in some of its metabolic responses, in line with recent reports in humans.[47]

In summary, ghrelin has emerged during the last decade as a key metabolic regulator playing an essential role in the control of food intake and energy balance. Among other unique features, ghrelin appears as the only known circulating orexigenic factor, whose serum profile (with preprandial elevation and postprandial decrease) is highly suggestive of a major function of ghrelin as premeal hunger signal. In addition, circulating ghrelin levels seem to be negatively correlated with BMI, leading to the hypothesis that ghrelin operates as peripheral signal for energy insufficiency. Indeed, on the basis of their biological properties and their reciprocal fluctuation, leptin and ghrelin have been proposed as the most prominent antagonic afferents of a dynamic (*yin-yang*) regulatory system, which allows precise tuning of the long-term control of body weight and energy balance. Importantly, the biological roles of ghrelin clearly exceed those related with its metabolic facet, as ghrelin has been involved in a wide diversity of functions, from cell proliferation to reproduction. Complete elucidation of ghrelin biology promises to be an active field in endocrine research in the coming years.

ACKNOWLEDGMENTS

The authors are indebted to C. Dieguez, E. Aguilar, L. Pinilla, and other members of the research team at the Physiology Section of the University of Córdoba, for continuous collaboration and support in their studies on neuroendocrine aspects of ghrelin physiology, as well as for helpful discussions during preparation of this chapter.

REFERENCES

1. Kalra, S.P. et al., Interacting appetite-regulating pathways in the hypothalamic regulation of body weight, *Endocr. Rev.*, 20, 68, 1999.
2. Small, C.J. and Bloom, S.R., Gut hormones and the control of appetite, *Trends Endocrinol. Metab.*, 15, 259, 2004.
3. Casanueva, F.F. and Dieguez, C., Neuroendocrine regulation and actions of leptin, *Front. Neuroendocrinol.*, 20, 317, 1999.
4. Ahima, R.S. et al., Leptin regulation of neuroendocrine systems, *Front. Neuroendocrinol.*, 21, 263, 2000.
5. Kojima, M. et al., Ghrelin is a growth-hormone-releasing acylated peptide from stomach, *Nature*, 402, 656, 1999.
6. Kojima, M. et al., Ghrelin: Discovery of the natural endogenous ligand for the growth hormone secretagogue receptor, *Trends Endocrinol. Metab.*, 12, 118, 2001.
7. Casanueva, F.F. and Dieguez, C., Growth hormone secretagogues physiological role and clinical utilities, *Trends Endocrinol. Metab.*, 10, 30, 1999.
8. Smith, R.G. et al., Peptidomimetic regulation of growth hormone secretion, *Endocr. Rev.*, 18, 621, 1997.
9. Bowers, C.Y., Growth hormone-releasing peptide (GHRP), *Cell Mol. Life Sci.*, 54, 1316, 1998.
10. Camanni, F., Ghigo, E., and Arvat, E., Growth hormone-releasing peptides and their analogs, *Front. Neuroendocrinol.*, 19, 47, 1998.
11. Patchett, A.A. et al., Design and biological activities of L-163,191 (MK-0677): A potent, orally active growth hormone secretagogue, *Proc. Natl. Acad. Sci. USA*, 92, 7001, 1995.
12. Howard, A.D. et al., A receptor in pituitary and hypothalamus that functions in growth hormone release, *Science*, 273, 974, 1996.
13. Guan, X.M. et al., Distribution of mRNA encoding the growth hormone secretagogue receptor in brain and peripheral tissues, *Brain Res. Mol. Brain Res.*, 48, 23, 1997.
14. Kaiya, H. et al., Chicken ghrelin: Purification, cDNA cloning, and biological activity, *Endocrinology*, 143, 3454, 2002.
15. Hosada, H. et al., Purification and characterization of rat des-Gln 14-Ghrelin, a second endogenous ligand for the growth hormone secretagogue receptor, *J. Biol. Chem.*, 275, 21995, 2000.
16. Hosada, H. et al., Ghrelin and des-acyl ghrelin: Two major forms of rat ghrelin peptide in gastrointestinal tissue, *Biochem. Biophys. Res. Commun.*, 279, 909, 2000.
17. Folwaczny, C., Chang, J.K., and Tschop, M., Ghrelin and motilin: Two sides of one coin? *Eur. J. Endocrinol.*, 144, R1, 2001.
18. Tomasetto, C. et al., Identification and characterization of a novel gastric peptide hormone: The motilin-related peptide, *Gastroenterology*, 119, 395, 2000.

19. Kojima, M. and Kangawa, K., Ghrelin: Structure and function, *Physiol. Rev.*, 85, 495, 2005.
20. Gualillo, O. et al., Ghrelin, a widespread hormone: Insights into molecular and cellular regulation of its expression and mechanism of action, *FEBS Lett.*, 552, 105, 2003.
21. Yang, J., Brown, M.S., Liang, G., Grishin, N.V., and Goldstein, J.L., Identification of the acyltransferase that octanoylates ghrelin, an appetite-stimulating peptide hormone, *Cell*, 132(3), 387–396, February 8, 2008.
22. van der Lely, A.J. et al., Biological, physiological, pathophysiological, and pharmacological aspects of ghrelin, *Endocr. Rev.*, 25, 426, 2004.
23. Korbonits, M. et al., Ghrelin—A hormone with multiple functions, *Front. Neuroendocrinol.*, 25, 27, 2004.
24. McKee, K.K. et al., Molecular analysis of rat pituitary and hypothalamic growth hormone secretagogue receptors, *Mol. Endocrinol.*, 11, 415, 1997.
25. Halem, H.A. et al., A novel growth hormone secretagogue-1a receptor antagonist that blocks ghrelin-induced growth hormone secretion but induces increased body weight gain, *Neuroendocrinology*, 81, 339, 2005.
26. Barreiro, M.L. and Tena-Sempere, M., Ghrelin and reproduction: A novel signal linking energy status and fertility? *Mol. Cell. Endocrinol.*, 226, 1, 2004.
27. Tena-Sempere, M., Exploring the role of ghrelin as novel regulator of gonadal function, *Growth Horm. IGF Res.*, 15, 83, 2005.
28. Seoane, L.M. et al., Agouti-related peptide, neuropeptide Y, and somatostatin-producing neurons are targets for ghrelin actions in the rat hypothalamus, *Endocrinology*, 144, 544, 2003.
29. Tschop, M. et al., Ghrelin induces adiposity in rodents, *Nature*, 407, 908, 2000.
30. Shuto, Y. et al., Hypothalamic growth hormone secretagogue receptor regulates growth hormone secretion, feeding, and adiposity, *J. Clin. Invest.*, 109, 1429, 2002.
31. Cummings, D.E., Foster-Schubert, K.E., and Overduin, J., Ghrelin and energy balance: Focus on current controversies, *Curr. Drug Targets*, 6, 153, 2005.
32. López, M. et al., Hypothalamic fatty acid metabolism mediates the orexigenic action of ghrelin, *Cell Metab.*, 7(5), 389–399, May 2008.
33. Asakawa, A. et al., Ghrelin is an appetite-stimulatory signal from stomach with structural resemblance to motilin, *Gastroenterology*, 120, 337, 2001.
34. Date, Y. et al., The role of the gastric afferent vagal nerve in ghrelin-induced feeding and growth hormone secretion in rats, *Gastroenterology*, 123, 1120, 2002.
35. Cummings, D.E. et al., Gastric bypass for obesity: Mechanisms of weight loss and diabetes resolution, *J. Clin. Endocrinol. Metab.*, 89, 2608, 2004.
36. Sun, Y., Ahmed, S., and Smith, R.G., Deletion of ghrelin impairs neither growth nor appetite, *Mol. Cell. Biol.*, 23, 7973, 2003.
37. Sun, Y. et al., Ghrelin stimulation of growth hormone release and appetite is mediated through the growth hormone secretagogue receptor, *Proc. Natl. Acad. Sci. USA*, 101, 4679, 2004.
38. Crowley, M.A. et al., The distribution and mechanisms of action of ghrelin in the CNS demonstrates a novel hypothalamic circuit regulating energy homeostasis, *Neuron*, 37, 649, 2003.
39. Zigman, J.M. et al., Mice lacking ghrelin receptors resist the development of diet-induced obesity, *J. Clin. Invest.*, 115, 3564, 2005.
40. Cummings, D.E. et al., A preprandial rise in plasma ghrelin levels suggests a role in meal initiation in humans, *Diabetes*, 50, 1714, 2001.
41. Callahan, H.S. et al., Postprandial suppression of plasma ghrelin levels is proportional to ingested caloric load but does not predict intermeal interval in humans, *J. Clin. Endocrinol. Metab.*, 89, 1319, 2004.
42. Zigman, J.M. and Elmquist, J.K., From anorexia to obesity—The yin and yang of body weight control, *Endocrinology*, 144, 3749, 2003.
43. Iqbal, J. et al., Effects of central infusion of ghrelin on food intake and plasma levels of growth hormone, luteinizing hormone, prolactin, and cortisol secretion in sheep, *Endocrinology*, 147, 510, 2006.
44. Fernandez-Fernandez, R. et al., Effects of chronic hyperghrelinemia on puberty onset and pregnancy outcome in the rat, *Endocrinology*, 146, 3018, 2005.
45. Martini, A.C. et al., Comparative analysis of the effects of ghrelin and un-acylated ghrelin upon luteinizing hormone secretion in male rats, *Endocrinology*, doi10.1210/en.2005.1422.
46. Asakawa, A. et al., Stomach regulates energy balance via acylated ghrelin and desacyl ghrelin, *Gut*, 54, 18, 2005.
47. Broglio, F. et al., Non-acylated ghrelin counteracts the metabolic but not the neuroendocrine response to acylated ghrelin in humans, *J. Clin. Endocrinol. Metab.*, 89, 3062, 2004.

12 Molecular Genetics of Obesity Syndrome
Role of DNA Methylation

Rama S. Dwivedi, PhD, Maria R. Wing, PhD, and Dominic S. Raj, MD

CONTENTS

INTRODUCTION

The prevalence of obesity in developed and industrialized countries has reached alarming levels. According to the World Health Organization (WHO 2009) there were 1 billion adults over-weight (BMI > 25.0), and about 300 million obese (BMI > 30) in 2005. Based on the data from 2007–2008 National Health and Nutrition Examination Survey, the percentage of overweight children between the ages 6 and 11 increased from 6.5% to 19.6% compared with 1976–1980. In 2001, nearly 58 million Americans were overweight; among them, 40 million people were obese, and 300,000 die each year due to obesity-related disorders (Allison et al. 1999). These numbers have since increased, and between 2005 and 2006, the National Health and Nutrition Examination Survey reported that an estimated 32.7% of U.S. adults 20 years and older were overweight, 34.3% were obese, and 5.9% were extremely obese.

A great economic and financial stress has been placed on the society as obesity-related disorders such as type 2 diabetes, osteoporosis, hypertension, heart and liver disease, postmenopausal breast cancer, colon cancer, and endometrial cancer have increased dramatically. Annual medical costs to treat these diseases are expected to exceed $100 billion in the United States, thus making obesity a major public health concern (Correia and Haynes 2005). According to projections calculated from the National Health and Nutrition Survey, if the increase in obesity continues at present rates, 86% of Americans will be overweight, and 51% will be obese by the year 2030. In addition, health-care costs due to obesity are estimated to double every decade, reaching $860–957 billion by the year 2030 (Wang et al. 2008). One of the national public health goals for the year 2010 was to reduce the incidence of obesity among adults to less than 15%. According to the Center for Disease Control and Prevention, every state in the United States failed to meet this *Healthy People 2010* objective, with rates of obesity increasing by 1.1% in U.S. adults since 2007 (CDC 2009).

These statistics are startling and illustrate the importance of interventions to slow the obesity epidemic. Many factors influence an individual's predisposition to weight gain and obesity, including genetics, environment, and lifestyle. Researchers have identified several genetic variants in important genes that are associated with obesity, but there are potentially many more that have not been identified. In addition, identifying epigenetic modifications may be equally important, since these changes are potentially reversible. The focus of this chapter is to describe the putative role of DNA methylation in regulating and altering the function of obesity-related genes, which may hopefully lead to treatments and prevention of obesity.

MOLECULAR GENETICS OF OBESITY

Update of the human obesity gene map in 2005 revealed that about 425 genes or biomarkers were directly or indirectly linked with the onset of human obesity (Snyder et al. 2004; Perusse et al. 2005). Some genes, such as those that regulate expression of uncoupling proteins, leptin, leptin receptors, adrenergic receptors, peroxisome proliferator–activated receptors (PPARs), and fatty-acid-binding proteins, may modulate the control of energy metabolism and may be affected by dietary composition and physical activity. Specific genes like pro-opiomelanocortin are involved in controlling food intake, while others such as PPARs regulate adipogenesis affecting body weight and fat deposition in individuals who are carriers of defective gene mutations and/or polymorphisms. Variations in adrenergic receptors and the leptin receptor have been shown to be positively correlated with increased weight gain (Snyder et al. 2004; Perusse et al. 2005).

The genetic basis of obesity was significantly advanced by the discovery of the leptin gene in the obese mouse model in 1994 (Zhang et al. 1994). Since then, autosomal recessive mutations in the genes for leptin (Issad et al. 1998; Strobel et al. 1998), leptin and melanocortin-4 receptors (Clement et al. 1998; Govaerts et al. 2005), prohormone, convertase-1 (Jackson et al. 1997), and pro-opiomelanocortin (Krude et al. 1998) have been linked to the onset of obesity in humans. Deletion of a single guanine nucleotide in the leptin gene in children was associated with increased weight gain, which was reversed by administration of recombinant leptin causing a significant loss of weight and adipose tissue mass (Strobel et al. 1998). A truncated leptin receptor lacking both the transmembrane and the intracellular domain was present in the children of a family with a mutation in the human leptin receptor gene and was associated with obesity and pituitary dysfunction. Thus, a genetic defect in leptin and/or leptin receptors may be one of the factors contributing to the impaired regulation of body weight in obese children (Paracchini et al. 2005). However, a correlation with leptin gene and association with leptin receptor variants and common obesity has been inconsistent (Duarte et al. 2007; Marti et al. 2009).

There are many candidate genes found to be altered in Mendelian or rare obesity syndromes, such as leptin, pro-opiomelanocortin, melanocortin-4 receptor, and Bardet–Biedel syndrome loci (Jacobson et al. 2002). An established association between monogenic forms of obesity and mutations in the melanocortin-4 receptor, accounting for about 4% of early-onset obesity, has been reported (Hirschhorn and Altshuler 2002). However, mutations in the melanocortin-4 receptor do not seem to play a prominent role in the late-onset more common type of obesity, with mutations only present in 1%–2% of obese adults (Hinney et al. 2010). Mutations in the leptin gene lead to severe early-onset obesity. Although treatment with leptin successfully reverses the progression of early-onset obesity, it has not proven to be effective in treating this syndrome (Farooqi et al. 2002). Ultimately, identification of the rare mutations in candidate genes may facilitate in identifying the pathways that can lead to severe obesity.

Genetic defects in the prohormone convertase-1 that is involved in the posttranslational processing and sorting of prohormones and neuropeptides have been implicated in neuroendocrine control of energy balance in obese children (Jackson et al. 1997). Genetic mutations associated with additional manifestations of the obesity syndrome such as adrenal insufficiency, red hair (pro-opiomelanocortin), impaired fertility (prohormone convertase-1, leptin, and leptin receptor), and impaired immunity (leptin gene) have been suggested as causative factors (Krude et al. 1998). A defect in pro-opiomelanocortin protein due to impaired synthesis of melanocortin peptides, adrenocorticotrophin, melanocyte-stimulating hormones (MSH), α, β, γ, and opioid receptor ligand β-endorphin results in early-onset obesity due to increased food intake and/or reduced energy utilization.

Another important monogenic form of obesity is due to mutations in the PPAR gamma-2 (PPARγ-2) gene (Ristow et al. 1998). More than 30 rare mutations have been identified worldwide that occur very infrequently in association with obesity. The melanocortin-4 gene, which can be detected in 2%–4% of all extremely obese children, has also been linked to the onset of obesity (Hinney et al. 1999; Sina et al. 1999). Children with melanocortin-4 gene mutations have been found to eat more meals than controls without mutations (Vaisse et al. 2000; Farooqi et al. 2002; Govaerts et al. 2005). Experimental studies using melanocortin-4 gene knockout mice have demonstrated a significant increment in food uptake when compared with controls leading to the development of obesity (Huszar et al. 1997). These findings support earlier observations made by Farooqi et al. (2002) in regard to the additional meals being taken by obese children.

Polymorphisms in the sterol regulatory element-binding transcription factor 1 gene have been suggested to predispose diabetic patients to obesity (Eberle et al. 2004). Analysis of the human melanin-concentrating hormone receptor-1 gene has identified 11 infrequent variations and two single-nucleotide polymorphisms, or SNPs, in its coding sequence and 18 SNPs (eight novel) in the flanking sequence of this gene in subjects with juvenile-onset obesity syndrome (Wermter et al. 2005). The mitogen-activated protein kinases (ERK, p38 and JNK, MAPKs) have also been proposed to play an important role in the differentiation of preadipocyte cell lines to adipocytes with a consequent effect on obesity (Bost et al. 2005). Recent studies with obese and type 2 diabetic (db/db) mice suggest that osteopontin may also be a factor in the etiology of obesity syndrome (Sahai et al. 2004a,b). These findings indicate that upregulation of osteopontin signaling in obese mice potentiates the development of hepatic fibrosis and nonalcoholic steatohepatitis (Sahai et al. 2004b; Bost et al. 2005). While heredity and environmental factors play a critical role in the development of obesity and related disorders, at this stage, their respective roles and significance remain unresolved.

CLINICAL SYNDROMES OF OBESITY

A number of clinical syndromes such as the Prader–Willi syndrome (PWS) with endocrine disorders, acanthosis nigricans characterized by thickening and pigmentation of skin folds, Blount's disease associated with orthopedic anomalies, sleep disorders, neurological (pseudotumor cerebri) and cardiovascular problems, and polycystic ovary syndrome are associated with obesity.

PRADER–WILLI SYNDROME: A CLINICAL DESCRIPTION

The PWS is a common syndrome associated with human obesity. It was first described in 1956, although specific diagnostic criteria were not established until 1993 (Holm et al. 1993). The main clinical characteristics of this syndrome are hypotonia during the neonatal period and failure to thrive due to feeble sucking reflex and low energy intake. In males, bilateral cryptorchidism associated with profound hypotonia may draw attention to the diagnosis. Hypoplasia of the external genitalia (labia minora and clitoris) also occurs in females but may be difficult to recognize. Limited hip and knee extension may be detected during routine newborn examination for congenital dislocation of the hip. Hands are frequently delicate with a puffy appearance. Orthopedic problems, for example, scoliosis, are common, as a consequence of both the syndrome itself and the presence of gross obesity (Holm et al. 1993).

Gastrointestinal symptoms such as hyperphagia, a continuous hunger apparently without normal sensation of satiety, vomiting, and rectal bleeding may occur. The insatiable hunger has been attributed to anomalies in the development of the parvocellular oxytocin (OXT) neurons of the hypothalamic paraventricular nucleus (Swaab et al. 1995). Hyperphagia is commonly associated with aggressive and self-abusive behavior, theft of food, poor social relationships, and mental retardation.

Obesity has been identified as one of the major contributing factors for the morbidity and mortality associated with the PWS. Development of noninsulin-dependent diabetes mellitus and impaired cardiac and pulmonary function, leading to severe disability and early death, has also been described.

ROLE OF DNA METHYLATION

Robinson et al. (1993) reported that the PWS may be associated with deletion of the q11–q13 fragment of paternal chromosome 15 or the presence of uniparental disomy, that is, two complete chromosomes 15 of maternal origin. A third type of genetic or epigenetic alteration involving impairment of the imprinting center due to changes in methylation patterns has also been proposed. DNA methylation is the covalent modification of DNA that is associated with the regulation of gene expression during development, genomic imprinting, X-chromosome inactivation, and silencing of functional genes (Feinberg and Vogelstein 1983; Feinberg et al. 2002). The PWS is a neurodevelopmental disorder that arises from lack of expression of paternally inherited genes known to be imprinted and located in the chromosome 15q11–q13 region. This is considered the most common syndrome causing life-threatening obesity with an incidence estimated to be 1 in 10,000–20,000 individuals. Approximately 99% of patients have an abnormality in the parent-specific methylation imprint within the PWS imprinting center at chromosome 15q11.2–q12. Among these subjects, 70% have a paternal deletion, 25% have a maternal uniparental disomy, and less than 5% have a mutation in the imprinting center.

A *de novo* paternally derived chromosome 15q11–q13 deletion is the cause of the PWS in about 70% of patients, and maternal disomy 15 accounts for about 25% of cases. The remaining cases result from genomic imprinting defects (microdeletions or epimutations) of the imprinting center in the 15q11–q13 region or from chromosome 15 translocations (Shao et al. 2005). A deficiency of methyl-(CpG)-binding protein 2 in the PWS causes an epimutation at the maternal small nuclear ribonucleoprotein polypeptide N promoter allele. This results in an open chromatin structure that is associated with increased histone H3 acetylation, H3(K4) methylation, and decreased H3(K9) methylation (Makedonski et al. 2005). Methylation-specific PCR and real-time PCR analyses in a young woman with the PWS due to a mosaic imprinting defect demonstrated that approximately 50% of a patient's blood cells had an imprinting defect, whereas 50% of the cells were normal (Wey et al. 2005).

Imprinting of the 2 Mb PWS and Angelman syndrome (AS) domain in human chromosome 15q11–q13 and its mouse orthologue in mouse chromosome-7c was believed to be regulated by a regional imprinting control center. However, the mechanism by which this occurs remains unclear. The entire 2 Mb domain contains numerous paternally expressed genes and at least two maternally expressed genes.

A breakthrough in understanding regulation of the imprinting control mechanism was achieved by studying the PWS and AS in families with imprinting mutations caused by microdeletions of two sequences: a 4.3 kb sequence (PWS–SRO) that includes the small nuclear ribonucleoprotein polypeptide N promoter/exon1 and an 880 bp sequence (AS–SRO) located 35 kb upstream to the transcription start site. Deletion of the latter (AS–SRO) sequence was implicated in AS and the former (PWS–SRO) sequence in the PWS. These sequences, although separated by a 35 kb intervening sequence, are able to communicate and constitute an imprinting center that regulates imprinting of the entire 2 Mb domain. In view of the altered methylation patterns in the PWS imprinting center, it is currently being diagnosed by identification of an abnormal DNA methylation patterns in the small nuclear ribonucleoprotein polypeptide N gene (Chen et al. 2004).

COMMON OBESITY AND DNA METHYLATION

The introduction of genome-wide association studies, or GWAS, leads to a hypothesis freeway to identify genes, independent of function, associated with more common forms of obesity. This method allows for millions of SNPs across the entire genome to be typed at one time. It has been a successful approach, identifying at least 30 loci associated with obesity and obesity measures to date (Speliotes et al. 2010). These studies have identified genes involved in overall obesity that regulate energy balance in the brain (Thorleifsson et al. 2009; Willer et al. 2009; Speliotes et al. 2010), as well as genes associated with fat distribution phenotypes such as waist-to-hip ratio, which are involved in adipogenesis development and function in adipose tissue (Lindgren et al. 2009; Heid et al. 2010). Although there have been several loci identified from variants associated with obesity and adiposity measures such as BMI, GWAS require large sample sizes in order to have enough power to detect common variation with small effects.

The most successful candidate so far has been the fat mass- and obesity-associated gene, or *FTO* (Dina et al. 2007; Frayling et al. 2007; Scuteri et al. 2007). Intron 1 variants have been associated with increased fat mass in children and adults, with individuals with two risk alleles being 3 kg heavier than individuals without the risk alleles (Frayling et al. 2007). Risk variants have also shown association with increased energy intake (Sonestedt et al. 2009) and decreased satiety (den Hoed et al. 2009). *FTO* is a 2-oxyglutarate-dependent nucleic acid demethylase (Gerken et al. 2007; Sanchez-Pulido and Andrade-Navarro 2007) with high expression levels in the brain (Fredriksson et al. 2008). Knockout mice have reduced adipose tissue and lean body mass, increased energy expenditure, increased food intake, and die before 4 weeks of age (Fischer et al. 2009). Another group created a dominant point mutation (I367F) in the *FTO* gene that more closely resembles the human phenotype (Church et al. 2009). This mutation leads to a decrease in *FTO* function, leading to reduced fat mass, upregulation of fat and carbohydrate metabolism genes, and increased energy expenditure. Studies to date illustrate that *FTO* plays a vital role in regulating key signals in the energy sensing centers of the brain through the maintenance of appetite and energy intake.

A recent study investigated genotype and epigenetic interactions by measuring overall methylation patterns of known type 2 diabetes loci. Of all the genes tested, the obesity risk allele for an SNP in *FTO* was the only one significantly associated with increased methylation (Bell et al. 2010). This increase in methylation was affected by the phase of CpG-creating SNPs that were in high linkage disequilibrium with the *FTO* risk allele. This study illustrates the significance of looking at linkage disequilibrium patterns and haplotypes when studying epigenetic and genotype interactions.

Other studies have investigated other epigenetic changes that may lead to obesity. These epigenetic changes are heritable and cause changes in gene function without changing the sequence of DNA. Disease can occur when normal methylation patters are disrupted, which can cause upregulation or downregulation of important genes. An example of this was shown in H3K9-specific lysine-specific demethylase 3A knockout mice. Mice without this gene show dysregulation of the expression of metabolic genes, such as the PPAR α (a gene involved in fatty acid metabolism) and uncoupling protein 1, which cause these mice to develop hyperlipidemia and obesity (Tateishi et al. 2009). In knockout mice, the expression of PPAR α is decreased by 50% in myocytes when compared to wild-type mice. Another study found that mice lacking the protein *N*-arginine methyltransferase 2 show decreased methylation of hypothalamic STAT3, which regulates leptin signaling and results in a lean phenotype, identifying this gene as a potential therapeutic target for obesity in the future (Iwasaki et al. 2010).

Recently, potential genes involved in obesity epigenetics were identified using a bioinformatic analysis identified genes involved with obesity that have been shown to undergo methylation changes in their promoters (Campion et al. 2009). This included genes functioning in adipogenesis (PPARγ), inflammation (suppressor of cytokine signaling 3), insulin resistance (tumor necrosis factor alpha), and fat metabolism (lipoprotein lipase).

Imprinting studies also have identified loci such as GNAS, which transcribes several different gene products and has both maternally and paternally imprinted genes (Weinstein et al. 2010). The G-protein α-subunit is essential in signaling pathways such as those involved in lipogenesis and in the activation of transcription factors. Mutations in the maternally imprinted genes lead to obesity in mice and humans through G-protein α-subunit deficiency, while mutations in paternally imprinted genes cause mice to be severely lean due to the lack of the G-protein α-subunit isoform XLα-subunit.

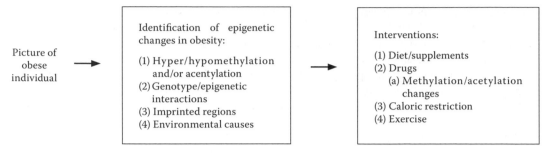

FIGURE 12.1   The future of obesity epigenetics.

Other genes showing genomic imprinting in obesity include preadipocyte factor 1/delta, *Drosophila* homolog-like 1, and paternally expressed gene 1/mesoderm-specific transcript, which are involved in adipocyte differentiation and function. Follow-up of these potential targets along with identification of new epigenetic modifications present in obesity will aid in our understanding of the obesity epidemic.

CONCLUSIONS

New molecular and genetic tools are becoming available that should expedite the identification of candidate obesity genes. Since the complete sequence of the human genome and other species are now available, they may be used to study the imprinting center and its critical sites for methylation-mediated mutations in candidate obesity genes. Information about methylation-based functional and transcriptional activation/inactivation of candidate genes involved in early-onset obesity may be useful in the development of antiobesity drugs. Although GWAS have identified several genes associated with common obesity, the variants have small effect sizes. Next generation sequencing should aid in the identification of rare variants, hopefully with larger effects on weight gain and obesity. This will identify potential targets for interventions, such as diet changes, supplements, or drugs that cause changes in methylation or acetylation patterns (Figure 12.1).

REFERENCES

Allison, D. B., K. R. Fontaine, J. E. Manson et al. 1999. Annual deaths attributable to obesity in the United States. *JAMA* 282 (16):1530–1538.

Bell, C. G., S. Finer, C. M. Lindgren et al. 2010. Integrated genetic and epigenetic analysis identifies haplotype-specific methylation in the FTO type 2 diabetes and obesity susceptibility locus. *PLoS One* 5 (11):e14040.

Bost, F., M. Aouadi, L. Caron et al. 2005. The role of MAPKs in adipocyte differentiation and obesity. *Biochimie* 87 (1):51–56.

Campion, J., F. I. Milagro, and J. A. Martinez. 2009. Individuality and epigenetics in obesity. *Obes Rev* 10 (4):383–392.

CDC. 2009. Vital signs: State-specific obesity prevalence among adults—United States. *MMWR Morb Mortal Wkly Rep* 59 (30):951–955.

Chen, C. J., M. L. Hsu, Y. S. Yuh et al. 2004. Early diagnosis of Prader-Willi syndrome in a newborn. *Acta Paediatr Taiwan* 45 (2):108–110.

Church, C., S. Lee, E. A. Bagg et al. 2009. A mouse model for the metabolic effects of the human fat mass and obesity associated FTO gene. *PLoS Genet* 5 (8):e1000599.

Clement, K., C. Vaisse, N. Lahlou et al. 1998. A mutation in the human leptin receptor gene causes obesity and pituitary dysfunction. *Nature* 392 (6674):398–401.

Correia, M. L. and W. G. Haynes. 2005. Emerging drugs for obesity: Linking novel biological mechanisms to pharmaceutical pipelines. *Expert Opin Emerg Drugs* 10 (3):643–660.

den Hoed, M., M. S. Westerterp-Plantenga, F. G. Bouwman et al. 2009. Postprandial responses in hunger and satiety are associated with the rs9939609 single nucleotide polymorphism in FTO. *Am J Clin Nutr* 90 (5):1426–1432.

Dina, C., D. Meyre, S. Gallina et al. 2007. Variation in FTO contributes to childhood obesity and severe adult obesity. *Nat Genet* 39 (6):724–726.

Duarte, S. F., E. A. Francischetti, V. A. Genelhu et al. 2007. LEPR p.Q223R, beta3-AR p.W64R and LEP c.-2548G>A gene variants in obese Brazilian subjects. *Genet Mol Res* 6 (4):1035–1043.

Eberle, D., K. Clement, D. Meyre et al. 2004. SREBF-1 gene polymorphisms are associated with obesity and type 2 diabetes in French obese and diabetic cohorts. *Diabetes* 53 (8):2153–2157.

Farooqi, I. S., G. Matarese, G. M. Lord et al. 2002. Beneficial effects of leptin on obesity, T cell hyporesponsiveness, and neuroendocrine/metabolic dysfunction of human congenital leptin deficiency. *J Clin Invest* 110 (8):1093–1103.

Feinberg, A. P., H. Cui, and R. Ohlsson. 2002. DNA methylation and genomic imprinting: Insights from cancer into epigenetic mechanisms. *Semin Cancer Biol* 12 (5):389–398.

Feinberg, A. P. and B. Vogelstein. 1983. Hypomethylation distinguishes genes of some human cancers from their normal counterparts. *Nature* 301:89–92.

Fischer, J., L. Koch, C. Emmerling et al. 2009. Inactivation of the Fto gene protects from obesity. *Nature* 458 (7240):894–898.

Frayling, T. M., N. J. Timpson, M. N. Weedon et al. 2007. A common variant in the FTO gene is associated with body mass index and predisposes to childhood and adult obesity. *Science* 316 (5826):889–894.

Fredriksson, R., M. Hagglund, P. K. Olszewski et al. 2008. The obesity gene, FTO, is of ancient origin, up-regulated during food deprivation and expressed in neurons of feeding-related nuclei of the brain. *Endocrinology* 149 (5):2062–2071.

Gerken, T., C. A. Girard, Y. C. Tung et al. 2007. The obesity-associated FTO gene encodes a 2-oxoglutarate-dependent nucleic acid demethylase. *Science* 318 (5855):1469–1472.

Govaerts, C., S. Srinivasan, A. Shapiro et al. 2005. Obesity-associated mutations in the melanocortin 4 receptor provide novel insights into its function. *Peptides* 26 (10):1909–1919.

Heid, I. M., A. U. Jackson, J. C. Randall et al. 2010. Meta-analysis identifies 13 new loci associated with waist-hip ratio and reveals sexual dimorphism in the genetic basis of fat distribution. *Nat Genet* 42 (11):949–960.

Hinney, A., A. Schmidt, K. Nottebom et al. 1999. Several mutations in the melanocortin-4 receptor gene including a nonsense and a frameshift mutation associated with dominantly inherited obesity in humans. *J Clin Endocrinol Metab* 84 (4):1483–1486.

Hinney, A., C. I. Vogel, and J. Hebebrand. 2010. From monogenic to polygenic obesity: Recent advances. *Eur Child Adolesc Psychiatry* 19 (3):297–310.

Hirschhorn, J. N. and D. Altshuler. 2002. Once and again—Issues surrounding replication in genetic association studies. *J Clin Endocrinol Metab* 87 (10):4438–4441.

Holm, V. A., S. B. Cassidy, M. G. Butler et al. 1993. Prader-Willi syndrome: Consensus diagnostic criteria. *Pediatrics* 91 (2):398–402.

Huszar, D., C. A. Lynch, V. Fairchild-Huntress et al. 1997. Targeted disruption of the melanocortin-4 receptor results in obesity in mice. *Cell* 88 (1):131–141.

Issad, T., A. Strobel, L. Camoin et al. 1998. [Leptin and puberty in humans: Hypothesis of the critical adipose mass revisited]. *Diabetes Metab* 24 (4):376–378.

Iwasaki, H., J. C. Kovacic, M. Olive et al. 2010. Disruption of protein arginine N-methyltransferase 2 regulates leptin signaling and produces leanness in vivo through loss of STAT3 methylation. *Circ Res* 107 (8):992–1001.

Jackson, R. S., J. W. Creemers, S. Ohagi et al. 1997. Obesity and impaired prohormone processing associated with mutations in the human prohormone convertase 1 gene. *Nat Genet* 16 (3):303–306.

Jacobson, P., O. Ukkola, T. Rankinen et al. 2002. Melanocortin 4 receptor sequence variations are seldom a cause of human obesity: The Swedish Obese Subjects, the HERITAGE Family Study, and a Memphis cohort. *J Clin Endocrinol Metab* 87 (10):4442–4446.

Krude, H., H. Biebermann, W. Luck et al. 1998. Severe early-onset obesity, adrenal insufficiency and red hair pigmentation caused by POMC mutations in humans. *Nat Genet* 19 (2):155–157.

Lindgren, C. M., I. M. Heid, J. C. Randall et al. 2009. Genome-wide association scan meta-analysis identifies three loci influencing adiposity and fat distribution. *PLoS Genet* 5 (6):e1000508.

Makedonski, K., L. Abuhatzira, Y. Kaufman et al. 2005. MeCP2 deficiency in Rett syndrome causes epigenetic aberrations at the PWS/AS imprinting center that affects UBE3A expression. *Hum Mol Genet* 14 (8):1049–1058.

Marti, A., J. L. Santos, M. Gratacos et al. 2009. Association between leptin receptor (LEPR) and brain-derived neurotrophic factor (BDNF) gene variants and obesity: A case-control study. *Nutr Neurosci* 12 (4):183–188.

Paracchini, V., P. Pedotti, and E. Taioli. 2005. Genetics of leptin and obesity: A HuGE review. *Am J Epidemiol* 162 (2):101–114.

Perusse, L., T. Rankinen, A. Zuberi et al. 2005. The human obesity gene map: The 2004 update. *Obes Res* 13 (3):381–490.

Ristow, M., D. Muller-Wieland, A. Pfeiffer et al. 1998. Obesity associated with a mutation in a genetic regulator of adipocyte differentiation. *N Engl J Med* 339 (14):953–959.

Robinson, W. P., R. Spiegel, and A. A. Schinzel. 1993. Deletion breakpoints associated with the Prader-Willi and Angelman syndromes (15q11–q13) are not sites of high homologous recombination. *Hum Genet* 91 (2):181–184.

Sahai, A., P. Malladi, H. Melin-Aldana et al. 2004a. Upregulation of osteopontin expression is involved in the development of nonalcoholic steatohepatitis in a dietary murine model. *Am J Physiol Gastrointest Liver Physiol* 287 (1):G264–G273.

Sahai, A., P. Malladi, X. Pan et al. 2004b. Obese and diabetic db/db mice develop marked liver fibrosis in a model of nonalcoholic steatohepatitis: Role of short-form leptin receptors and osteopontin. *Am J Physiol Gastrointest Liver Physiol* 287 (5):G1035–G1043.

Sanchez-Pulido, L. and M. A. Andrade-Navarro. 2007. The FTO (fat mass and obesity associated) gene codes for a novel member of the non-heme dioxygenase superfamily. *BMC Biochem* 8:23.

Scuteri, A., S. Sanna, W. M. Chen et al. 2007. Genome-wide association scan shows genetic variants in the FTO gene are associated with obesity-related traits. *PLoS Genet* 3 (7):e115.

Shao, J., L. Qiao, R. C. Janssen et al. 2005. Chronic hyperglycemia enhances PEPCK gene expression and hepatocellular glucose production via elevated liver activating protein/liver inhibitory protein ratio. *Diabetes* 54 (4):976–984.

Sina, M., A. Hinney, A. Ziegler et al. 1999. Phenotypes in three pedigrees with autosomal dominant obesity caused by haploinsufficiency mutations in the melanocortin-4 receptor gene. *Am J Hum Genet* 65 (6):1501–1507.

Snyder, E. E., B. Walts, L. Perusse et al. 2004. The human obesity gene map: The 2003 update. *Obes Res* 12 (3):369–439.

Sonestedt, E., C. Roos, B. Gullberg et al. 2009. Fat and carbohydrate intake modify the association between genetic variation in the FTO genotype and obesity. *Am J Clin Nutr* 90 (5):1418–1425.

Speliotes, E. K., C. J. Willer, S. I. Berndt et al. 2010. Association analyses of 249,796 individuals reveal 18 new loci associated with body mass index. *Nat Genet* 42 (11):937–948.

Strobel, A., T. Issad, L. Camoin et al. 1998. A leptin missense mutation associated with hypogonadism and morbid obesity. *Nat Genet* 18 (3):213–215.

Swaab, D. F., J. S. Purba, and M. A. Hofman. 1995. Alterations in the hypothalamic paraventricular nucleus and its oxytocin neurons (putative satiety cells) in Prader-Willi syndrome: A study of five cases. *J Clin Endocrinol Metab* 80 (2):573–579.

Tateishi, K., Y. Okada, E. M. Kallin et al. 2009. Role of Jhdm2a in regulating metabolic gene expression and obesity resistance. *Nature* 458 (7239):757–761.

Thorleifsson, G., G. B. Walters, D. F. Gudbjartsson et al. 2009. Genome-wide association yields new sequence variants at seven loci that associate with measures of obesity. *Nat Genet* 41 (1):18–24.

Vaisse, C., K. Clement, E. Durand et al. 2000. Melanocortin-4 receptor mutations are a frequent and heterogeneous cause of morbid obesity. *J Clin Invest* 106 (2):253–262.

Wang, Y., M. A. Beydoun, L. Liang et al. 2008. Will all Americans become overweight or obese? Estimating the progression and cost of the US obesity epidemic. *Obesity (Silver Spring)* 16 (10):2323–2330.

Weinstein, L. S., T. Xie, A. Qasem et al. 2010. The role of GNAS and other imprinted genes in the development of obesity. *Int J Obes (Lond)* 34 (1):6–17.

Wermter, A. K., K. Reichwald, T. Buch et al. 2005. Mutation analysis of the MCHR1 gene in human obesity. *Eur J Endocrinol* 152 (6):851–862.

Wey, E., D. Bartholdi, M. Riegel et al. 2005. Mosaic imprinting defect in a patient with an almost typical expression of the Prader-Willi syndrome. *Eur J Hum Genet* 13 (3):273–277.

WHO. 2009. Global health risks: Mortality and burden of disease attributable to selected major risks. [Cited. Available from http://www.who.int/healthinfo/global_burden_disease/GlobalHealthRisks_report_full. pdf.]

Willer, C. J., E. K. Speliotes, R. J. Loos et al. 2009. Six new loci associated with body mass index highlight a neuronal influence on body weight regulation. *Nat Genet* 41 (1):25–34.

Zhang, Y., R. Proenca, M. Maffei et al. 1994. Positional cloning of the mouse obese gene and its human homologue. *Nature* 372 (6505):425–432.

13 Sleep and Obesity

Michelle A. Miller, PhD, MAcadMEd, FFPH
and Francesco P. Cappuccio, FRCP, FFPH, FAHA

CONTENTS

INTRODUCTION

A variety of cultural, social, psychological, behavioral, pathophysiological, and environmental factors influence an individual's sleep pattern and associated quantity and quality of sleep. Moreover, societal changes can influence these patterns. In the modern society, we have seen the introduction of longer working hours, more shift work, and 24/7 availability of commodities. These changes have been paralleled by secular trends of curtailed duration of sleep to fewer hours per day across westernized populations (Akerstedt and Nilsson 2003). This has led to increased reporting of fatigue, tiredness, and excessive daytime sleepiness (EDS) (Bliwise 1996). There is now a growing body of evidence to support an epidemiological link between quantity of sleep (short and long duration of sleep) and cardio-metabolic risk factors, including obesity (Cappuccio et al. 2008). The deleterious effects of sleep deprivation can be seen on a variety of systems within the body, with detectable changes in metabolic (Knutson et al. 2007; Spiegel et al. 2009), endocrine (Spiegel et al. 1999; Taheri et al. 2004), and immune pathways (Miller and Cappuccio 2007).

OVERWEIGHT AND OBESITY

An elevated body mass index (BMI) is a major risk factor for heart disease, stroke, type 2 diabetes, and other chronic diseases. Overweight individuals are defined as having a BMI of 25–30 kg/m², and as such 44% of men and 35% of women in the United Kingdom are overweight. In addition, 23% of men and 24% of women are obese (BMI >30 kg/m²). The International Obesity Task Force estimates that approximately 60% of the 350 million adults living in the EU may be overweight or obese. Obesity is especially common in Mediterranean countries. From Greece to Germany, the proportion of overweight or obese men is higher than in the United States even though the rates of obesity in the United States have doubled since 1980 (Flegal et al. 1998, 2002). Of great concern is the ever growing rate of obesity among children. Among the EU's 103 million children, the number of those overweight rises by 400,000 each year. The World Health Organization (WHO) estimates that if current trends continue, the number of overweight people globally will increase to 1.5 billion by 2015. The WHO estimates that over the next 10 years, cardiovascular disease (CVD)—primarily coronary heart disease (CHD) and stroke—will increase most notably in the regions of the Eastern Mediterranean and Africa, where CVD-related deaths are predicted to rise by over 25% (WHO 2006).

SLEEP AND OBESITY IN ADULTS AND IN CHILDREN AND ADOLESCENTS

The prevalence of obesity worldwide in both adults and children is increasing and is associated with an increased risk of morbidity and mortality as well as reduced life expectancy (Poirier et al. 2006). Obesity in childhood is a cause of psychosocial problems including low self-esteem and frequently continues into adulthood where it is a cause of major morbidity and mortality including CVD and type 2 diabetes. It is clear that obesity may have its effect on CVD through a number of different known and possibly as yet unknown mechanisms, and it has been proposed that sleep may have an effect on these mechanisms. Moreover, there has been a secular reduction in sleeping time. National surveys in the United States report that the average sleep duration in 2005 was around 6.8 h and that this represents a reduction in self-reported sleep duration of approximately 1.5 to 2 h over the past 50 years (National Sleep Foundation 2005). This sleep curtailment has been attributed to lifestyle changes.

There is a growing number of studies that report an association between duration of sleep (short as well as long) and ill-health, including relationships with self-reported well-being (Steptoe et al. 2006), all-cause (Ferrie et al. 2007; Cappuccio et al. 2010b) and cause-specific morbidity and mortality (Cappuccio et al. 2011), and with chronic conditions including type 2 diabetes (Cappuccio et al. 2010a), respiratory disorders (Somers et al. 2008), hypertension (Cappuccio et al. 2007), and obesity (Cappuccio et al. 2008). The implication of these studies is important especially with regard to the association between sleep and obesity in children (Taheri 2006; Currie and Cappuccio 2007; Patel and Hu 2008) as well as in adults (Cizza et al. 2005; Patel and Hu 2008; Stranges et al. 2008).

CROSS-SECTIONAL STUDIES

A recent systematic review and meta-analysis of cross-sectional studies in children and adults provides the global evidence in support of the presence of a relationship between short duration of sleep and obesity, providing a quantitative estimate of the risk (Cappuccio et al. 2008). The meta-analysis included a total of 36 population samples with 30,002 children and 604,509 adult participants from around the world. Age ranged from 2 to 102 years and included boys, girls, men, and women. The observed association was seen to be consistent across different populations and was observed in both children and adults. In children, the pooled odds ratio (OR) for short duration of sleep (≤10 h per night) and obesity was 1.89 (1.46–2.43; $P < 0.0001$), and in adults (short sleep defined as ≤5 h per night) the pooled OR was 1.55 (1.43–1.68; $P < 0.0001$). There was no evidence of publication bias.

A major limitation of this analysis is that the studies are cross-sectional and the results therefore cannot be used to determine temporal sequence, hence, causality. Furthermore, these studies do not give any indication as to whether an individual's sleeping habits may change with time and what consequence this may have. Moreover, all studies used sleep questionnaires to determine self-reported sleep duration within their populations, and a variety of different methods were used to determine obesity, particularly in children, making the various studies more difficult to reconcile. Likewise, there was considerable variation within the studies for the degree of adjustment for potential confounders.

Data from the recently published *Early Childhood Longitudinal Study-Kindergarten* (ECLS-K) also confirms that greater hours of sleep by children was associated with lower initial levels of BMI (Miller 2011).

PROSPECTIVE STUDIES

Adults

To date, many of the prospective studies in adults have failed to provide consistency in support of the view that short sleep duration predicts the future development of obesity (Bjorkelund et al. 2005; Gangwisch et al. 2005; Stranges et al. 2008; Lauderdale et al. 2009). It is possible that the observed relationships may be confounded by comorbidity, such as chronic mental illness, causing a decrease in the levels of physical activity and a reduction in sleep, etc. In a study of more than 5000 white male civil servants from the Whitehall II study, we demonstrated that both short and long sleep duration are cross-sectionally associated with an increase in BMI and an increased OR for obesity (Stranges et al. 2008). However, while these associations were highly significant, further prospective analysis failed to show any effect of sleep duration on BMI or any increase risk of obesity over the following 5 years (Stranges et al. 2008). One very large study ($n > 60,000$), carried out in women only, however, shows a small effect (HR 1.15 and 1.06 for those sleeping ≤ 5 h and ≤ 6 h per night, respectively) (Patel et al. 2006). Furthermore, the recent large prospective study by Watanabe and colleagues provides support for a relationship between sleep duration and weight gain in adults. They studied over 35,000 employees (31,477 men and 3,770 women) of a Japanese electrical power company. The results clearly demonstrate that in men who slept less than 5 h, there was an increased risk of obesity (OR) over a 1-year follow-up period (1.91 [1.36–2.67]) (Watanabe et al. 2010). Interestingly, although a cross-sectional association between obesity and sleep was observed in these women, there was no significant prospective association. This warrants further investigation but may in part be due to the relatively small percentage of women (~10%) in the cohort.

Recent data from the Helsinki Health study demonstrates that, in women but not men, short sleep duration is associated with major weight gain (OR 1.52; 95% confidence interval [CI]: 1.08, 2.14) during the 5–7 year follow-up period. This association persisted even after the adjustment for several covariates. Long sleep duration in women was also associated with major weight gain after adjusting for age (OR 1.35; 95% CI: 1.00–1.81). Similar associations were not observed in men, but it is of interest to note that 80% of the individuals in this study were women ($n = 5729$ vs. 1298 men) (Lyytikäinen et al. 2010). In the same cohort, it has also been shown that sleep problems (trouble falling asleep, waking up several times per night, and trouble staying asleep), which were assessed using the Jenkins sleep questionnaire, were associated with major weight gain during the 5–7 year follow-up, in women but not in men. The final component of the questionnaire that determines if individuals wake up after their usual amount of sleep, feeling tired or worn out was not associated with weight gain, and the observations persisted following adjustment for multiple confounders (Lyytikäinen et al. 2011). The study also found that occasional sleep problems were associated with weight gain (Lyytikäinen et al. 2011).

Children and Adolescents

Unlike in adults, in children and adolescents, the emerging prospective does support the view that short sleep predicts future obesity. In one such nationally representative U.S. study of over 2000 children and adolescents (aged 3–12 at baseline), the associations between sleep and the BMI were estimated. Following adjustment for baseline BMI, it was observed that children who slept less at the time of the first assessment had higher BMIs 5 years later and were more likely to be overweight (Snell et al. 2007). A more recent prospective study of 1916 preadolescent children also observed that children presenting a persistent short sleep trajectory between the ages of 2.5 and 10 years have an increased OR of being in the overweight BMI trajectory (OR = 1.55, 95% CI: 1.39, 1.71) or in the obese BMI trajectory (OR = 3.26, 95% CI: 3.20, 3.29) compared with the 11 h trajectory (Seegers et al. 2011). Further prospective data from the United States has recently reported on survey data of 1930 children aged from 0 to 13 years at baseline. It demonstrates that for children in the younger age range (0–4 years at baseline), short duration of nighttime sleep at baseline was strongly associated with increased risk of subsequent overweight or obesity (OR = 1.80; 95% CI: 1.16–2.80). For children in the older age range of 5–13 years, it was found that baseline sleep was not associated with subsequent weight status whereas their current sleep duration was associated with current weight (Bell and Zimmerman 2010). These results suggest that insufficient sleep, at least in young children, may be an important and modifiable risk factor for future obesity.

SLEEP, OBESITY, AND ETHNICITY

To date, the vast majority of sleep research has been performed in whites of European descent and to a lesser extent in African Americans, making generalization of the findings to other ethnic and racial groups difficult. As yet, very little sleep research has been done in other ethnic minority groups including U.S. Hispanics. A recent review (Loredo et al. 2010) suggests that, given the pattern of risk factors in Hispanics, it is likely that the prevalence of sleep disorders, including obstructive sleep apnea (OSA), which is characterized by the complete or partial collapse of the pharyngeal airway during sleep, will be high in these individuals. A recent study, in African Americans, not only supports the idea of an association between sleep quality and obesity but also suggests that perceived stress may modify the association. They found that there was an increased likelihood of obesity in the medium stress category, OR (95% CI): 1.09 (1.02–1.17) (Bidulescu et al. 2010). Unlike previous studies, a study carried out in 5877 Saudi students aged between 10 and 19 years used a cutoff of < or = 7 h to see if short sleep was related to obesity. While the study demonstrated that sleeping < or = 7 h significantly increased the risk of obesity, it is difficult to compare these findings with the previous studies in children where a more conservative cutoff of 10 h has normally been used (Bawazeer et al. 2009).

Racial/ethnic differences in early-life risk factors may also be important in the development of childhood obesity. A recent prospective study of 1343 white, 355 black, and 128 Hispanic mother–child pairs demonstrated that black and Hispanic children had a more rapid weight gain in infancy (OR: 2.01 for black, 1.75 for Hispanic). Moreover, black and Hispanic children were less likely to sleep at least 12 h/day in infancy (Taveras et al. 2010).

MECHANISMS

It is clear that there is increasing evidence to support a link between short sleep and the development of obesity. It is, however, still possible that obesity may lead to short sleep. Indeed, obese individuals are at increased risk of OSA, a condition that is associated with disturbed and short sleep. It is therefore conceivable that a bidirectional pathway may exist between sleep and obesity, and it is important to consider this when the mechanisms underlying these associations are considered (see Figure 13.1).

SLEEP, LEPTIN AND GHRELIN, AND OBESITY

It has been suggested that short sleep may lead to obesity through the activation of hormonal responses leading to an increase in appetite and caloric intake. In the first randomized crossover clinical trial of short-term sleep deprivation, Spiegel et al. demonstrated that sleep deprivation was

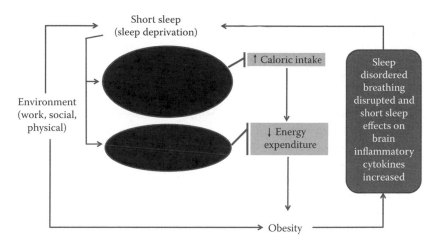

FIGURE 13.1   Bidirectional model of the association between sleep deprivation and obesity.

associated with decreased leptin and increased ghrelin levels (Spiegel et al. 2004). The individuals in this study were subjected to an extreme acute sleep deprivation (<4h per night) for 2 days and compared with 2 days with 10h of sleep. A constant glucose infusion provided the individuals with their caloric intake. Following sleep restriction, there was a decrease in leptin and increase in ghrelin, and the change in ghrelin to leptin ratio was associated with a positive change in hunger, suggesting that if the individuals had had access to food, they may have increased their food intake. If this mechanism was activated on a long-term basis, it could lead to the development of obesity.

Sleep, Orexigenic Neurons, and Obesity

Hypothalamic orexin neurons regulate arousal. Orexin A and orexin B (also referred to as hypocretin A and hypocretin B) have potent wake-promoting effects and stimulate food intake. The orexin system activates the appetite-promoting neuropeptide Y. In animal models, experimental sleep deprivation results in increased orexinergic activity. It is unclear if sleep deprivation under comfortable conditions in humans (e.g., TV watching) would have similar upregulating effects.

Sleep, Energy Transport, and Obesity

Studies on the effect of sleep deprivation on energy metabolism in humans come mainly from short-lived severe sleep deprivation experiments in young volunteers and as such cannot be extrapolated to longer-term effects of sustained sleep curtailment in the general population. In animal models, recent data suggests that acute sleep loss leads to changes in the circadian clock and altered metabolism, especially in relation to energy stores. However, energy stores were also altered in conditions of chronic sleep loss induced by mechanical stimuli, but not via light stimuli, suggesting that the changes in energy stores are caused by stress rather than sleep loss *per se* (Harbison and Sehgal 2009).

The results obtained from the Nurses Health study demonstrated that short sleep duration leads to an increase in weight with time. However, in this study, there was no evidence to suggest that this resulted from an increase in appetite. It has therefore been suggested that effects observed may be the result of changes in energy metabolism (Ayas et al. 2003). Three components constitute total energy expenditure (TEE). The first is the resting metabolic rate (RMR), which is the energy an individual expends at rest; the second is the thermic effect of meals (TEM), which is the energy used in the process of consuming and storing a meal; and the third component is the activity-related energy expenditure (AEE), which is the energy used in all volitional and nonvolitional activities

(Ayas et al. 2003). In a recent review, it has been suggested that individuals with sleep problems may have a reduction in their energy expenditure, but it is not yet clear whether this is true for all short sleepers (Knutson et al. 2007).

SLEEP AND LIPIDS

Findings from cross-sectional studies have demonstrated an association between short sleep and higher cholesterol in both men and women (Bjorvatn et al. 2007; Choi et al. 2008). Lower HDL concentrations were also observed in short-sleeping adult women with type 2 diabetes (Williams et al. 2007) and in adult Japanese women (Kaneita et al. 2008). A more recent follow-up study, conducted in the United States, indicates that short sleep durations in adolescent women (grades 7–12 at baseline) could be a significant risk factor for high cholesterol in young adulthood (ages 18–26) (Gangwisch et al. 2010).

SLEEP, CORTISOL, AND THE HYPOTHALAMIC–PITUITARY–ADRENAL AXIS

Studies indicate an association between obesity and EDS (Vgontzas and Kales 1999). Moreover, young adult studies indicate that sleep curtailment results in a constellation of metabolic and endocrine alterations, including increased evening concentrations of cortisol (Van Cauter and Knutson 2008). In a recent review, Vgontzas et al. suggested that it may be possible to subtype obese individuals according to whether they display an activation of proinflammatory cytokines with or without activation of the hypothalamic–pituitary–adrenal (HPA) axis (Vgontzas et al. 2008). Within obese individuals with or without sleep apnea, those who slept objectively better at night are paradoxically sleepier (objectively) during the day than those who slept worse. Further analysis suggests that those individuals who slept worse have an increased level of emotional stress. They propose that one obesity subtype is associated with emotional distress, poor sleep, fatigue, HPA axis "hyperactivity," and hypocytokinemia, while the other is associated with nondistress, better sleep but more sleepiness, HPA axis "normo- or hypoactivity," and hypercytokinemia. It is thought that by subtyping individuals in this way, it may lead to better treatment and prevention options.

SLEEP, INFLAMMATION, AND OBESITY

Activation of inflammatory pathways by short sleep has been implicated in the development of obesity. Obesity leads to a change in an individual's metabolic profile and an accumulation of adipose tissue (fat), which is composed of connective tissue and adipocytes. Adipose tissue is an important endocrine organ that produces inflammatory cytokines. Hence, an increase in adiposity may be associated with increased cytokine production. Indeed, a one unit higher BMI and a 0.01 unit greater waist-hip ratio (WHR) have been previously associated with a 2% increase in circulating sE-selectin level (Miller and Cappuccio 2006).

Adipose tissue also produces hormones such as resistin and leptin. Leptin plays a key role in regulating energy intake and expenditure. It has an important role in appetite regulation, and recent evidence suggests that it also has profound inflammatory effects. Although the underlying mechanisms are unclear, it has been proposed that leptin may bind to circulating hs-CRP, resulting in an attenuation of its physiological effects (Knutson et al. 2007). This is of interest as short-term sleep deprivation has been associated with an increase in hs-CRP (Meier-Ewert et al. 2004). To date, the potential impact of chronic sleep deprivation on the inflammatory system and immune responses has not been fully investigated. In a combined study of men and women, Taheri et al. failed to demonstrate any significant association between hs-CRP levels and sleep duration (Taheri et al. 2007). By contrast, in participants from the Cleveland family study, Patel et al. have demonstrated that increased habitual sleep duration, based on self-reported sleep questionnaire data, was associated with an increase in both hs-CRP ($P < 0.004$) and IL-6 ($P < 0.0003$). In the same study, however, sleep duration, as determined by polysomnography on the night prior to blood sampling, was inversely associated with TNF-α ($P < 0.02$) (Patel et al. 2009).

We have examined the relationship between markers of inflammation and sleep duration in over 4000 individuals from the Whitehall II study. We demonstrated marked gender differences in the observed relationships. In men, there was no association between hs-CRP and sleep. In women, however, there was a significant nonlinear association (Miller et al. 2009). In contrast to Patel et al., in our study, the level of hs-CRP was significantly higher in short sleepers (5 h or less) after multiple adjustments ($P = 0.04$) (interaction $P < 0.05$) (Patel et al. 2009), and while hs-CRP did appear to be higher in those women who slept more than 8 h as compared to those sleeping 7 h, the difference was not significant (Miller et al. 2009). This gender-specific observation is, however, consistent with the finding of Suarez et al. who demonstrated that indices of sleep disturbance were associated with higher fibrinogen and inflammatory biomarkers but only in women (Suarez 2008).

In the Whitehall II study, following multiple adjustments, there were no overall linear or nonlinear trends between sleep duration and IL-6. However, in women but not men (interaction $P < 0.05$), levels of IL-6 tended to be lower in individuals who slept 8 h (11% [95% CI: 4–17]) as compared to 7 h (Miller et al. 2009). This is in contrast to the Cleveland family study in which increasing sleep was associated with an increase in IL-6 (Patel et al. 2009).

The observed gender interactions in the relationship between sleep and inflammation may account for some of the observed differences in outcome between studies. Taheri et al. may have failed to find an association between sleep and markers of inflammation as the number of females in their study was much smaller, and a gender-adjusted analysis, as opposed to a sex-stratified analysis, was used (Taheri et al. 2007). Longitudinal studies are required to investigate fully possible temporal relationships between short sleep and markers of inflammation in both male and female individuals.

Other factors might be important in the relationship between sleep, obesity, and inflammation including ethnicity. In previous studies, we have demonstrated ethnic differences in inflammatory markers (Miller et al. 2003), and a recent study has demonstrated that the inflammatory responses to sleep loss appear to be mediated by both sex and ethnicity. The investigators studied 74 healthy adults (57% men, 63% African American, mean age 29.9 years) after two nights of baseline sleep (10 h time in bed) and then after five nights of sleep restriction (4 h time in bed) per night. A further control group received 10 h in bed throughout the whole study. The level of adiponectin was compared following the second night of baseline sleep and the fifth night of sleep restriction or control sleep. In Caucasian women, sleep restriction resulted in a decrease in adiponectin levels ($Z = -2.19$, $P = 0.028$). By contrast, adiponectin levels were increased among African American women ($Z = -2.73$, $P = 0.006$) following sleep restriction. No significant effects of sleep restriction on adiponectin levels were found among men in either ethnic group. A 2 × 2 between-group analysis of covariance on adiponectin change scores controlling for BMI confirmed significant interactions between sleep restriction and race/ethnicity ($P < 0.001$), as well as among sleep restriction, race/ethnicity, and sex ($P = 0.043$) (Simpson et al. 2010).

SLEEP, EATING PATTERNS, AND OBESITY

A recent study comparing the identified eating patterns among women with varying sleep duration demonstrated that the tendency to eat during conventional eating hours decreased with decreasing sleep duration and that there was an increase in snacking in short sleeping women. These behaviors were also associated with an increased intake of fat and sweets for energy and a decreased intake of fruit and vegetables (Kim et al. 2010). These eating patterns are all consistent with an increased risk of obesity. In children, it has also been observed that U.S. preschool-aged children ($n = 8550$) who were exposed to three household routines of regularly eating the evening meal as a family, obtaining adequate nighttime sleep, and having limited screen-viewing time had a lower prevalence of obesity (~40%) than those children who were not exposed to such routines (Anderson and Whitaker 2010). These findings suggest that having set routines in children may be a useful way to address the increasing rate of childhood obesity.

SLEEP AND WEIGHT LOSS

A recent study conducted in 10 healthy adults has suggested that insufficient sleep may undermine the body's ability to lose weight as fat (Nedeltcheva et al. 2010). The individuals studied were non-smoking individuals who reported sleeping 6.5–8.5 h per night and who had a BMI in the range of 25–32 kg/m^2. They were randomly assigned to sleep either 5.5 or 8.5 h each night in conjunction with moderate caloric restriction and were monitored in a closed clinical research environment. At the end of the treatment period, both sleep groups (5.5 and 8.5 h) had managed an equivalent weight loss of approx. 3 kg. However, interestingly further analysis revealed that while those individuals sleeping 8.5 h lost most of their weight as a result of a loss of fat mass, those sleeping 5.5 h loss mainly fat-free mass. There were also significant differences in fasting respiratory quotients between the two groups, suggesting that these individuals may have converted more body protein into glucose to support the more prolonged needs of a body that was awake longer. The results suggest that sleep restriction may reduce the ability of the body to lose fat mass and may be of importance for effective weight-loss regimes.

SLEEP EXTENSION AS A TREATMENT FOR OBESITY

The sleep–obesity hypothesis is complicated by the possible bidirectional causality pathway (Figure 13.1). A randomized clinical trial of the effect of sleep extension on obesity could represent a proof of concept (Cizza et al. 2010). In this study, the feasibility of increasing sleep duration to a healthy length (approximately 7(1/2) h) is being assessed along with measures to determine the effect of sleep extension on body weight. At the same time, the long-term effects of sleep extension on endocrine (leptin and ghrelin) and immune (cytokines) parameters, the prevalence of metabolic syndrome, body composition, psychomotor vigilance, mood, and quality of life will be examined. The investigators are recruiting 150 obese participants who usually sleep less than 6(1/2) h. They are stratified by age (above and below 35 years) and the presence or absence of metabolic syndrome. They are being randomized into an intervention or control group and are then being followed up. As of January 2010, it was reported that 109 participants had been randomized, 64 to the Intervention group and 45 to the Comparison group. Of these, 63 are African Americans and 83 are female. This will be a proof of concept study, which, if successful, may provide an alternative treatment option for obese patients. The major limitations of this trial are the relatively small number of participants and the fact that it is not possible to blind the study.

SLEEP AND LIFESTYLE INTERVENTION FOR THE TREATMENT OF OBESITY

One study that appears to be addressing the observed rise in obesity in young individuals is the Control, Evaluation, and Modification of Lifestyles in Obese Youth (CEMHaVi) program. It is a unique 2 year health-wellness program of physical activity and health education for obese youths. Results from the first year of study have indicated that a program of enjoyable physical activity in both young girls ($n = 14$ [13.4 ± 2.9 years]) and boys ($n = 12$ [12.3 ±–2.8 years]) resulted in a significant improvement in quality and quantity of sleep ($P < 0.05$) and obesity ($P < 0.05$). Academic performance also improved ($P < 0.001$) (Vanhelst et al. 2010).

SLEEP, OBESITY, AND OBSTRUCTIVE SLEEP APNEA

Evidence suggests that sleep-related breathing disorders, such as OSA, are contributing factors for the development of CVD. In OSA, during sleep there is a repetitive interruption of ventilation caused by collapse of the pharyngeal airway. An obstructive apnea is a ≥10 s pause in respiration associated with ongoing ventilatory effort. Obstructive hypopneas are decreases in—but not complete cessation of—ventilation, with an associate fall in oxygen saturation and/or arousal. A patient is diagnosed with OSA when they have an apnea–hypopnea index (AHI = number of apneas and hypopneas per hour of sleep) >5 and symptoms of EDS. Other signs and symptoms include disruptive snoring, obesity, and/or enlarged neck size and hypersomnolence (Guilleminault 1985). In particular, obesity appears to be a risk factor for OSA, and it has been proposed that the associated lack of sleep observed in OSA patients may also lead to the development of obesity thus potentiating a vicious cycle. Furthermore, it is important to note that the onset of CVD in the context of obesity and OSA begins early in childhood. The recognition of obesity and OSA in children should therefore be of paramount importance to clinicians (Bhattacharjee et al. 2011). Increased oxidative stress, insulin resistance, and low-grade inflammation are common both to obesity and OSA; this makes the determination of their relative roles in the development of CVD very challenging (Pack and Pien 2011). Many studies investigating OSA have tried to address this problem by matching for obesity in a case-controlled fashion, but many obesity studies have failed to rule out the presence of OSA. It is of interest to note that effective treatment for OSA using continuous positive airway pressure (CPAP) leads to reduction in cardiovascular events to the level seen in controls (Marin et al. 2005). Recent evidence also suggests that there may be a causal link between OSA and CVD and, in particular, hypertension that is independent of obesity (Budhiraja et al. 2010).

SUMMARY

While sustained sleep curtailment and ensuing EDS are undoubtedly cause for concern, the link to obesity has yet to be proven as a causal link. There is still a real possibility of reverse causality, and it is conceivable that there may be a bidirectional model for the association between short sleep and obesity (Figure 13.1). Societal pressure and changes in the physical environment may lead to a chronic curtailment of sleep leading to an increase in caloric intake and a reduction in energy expenditure and hence obesity. Alternatively, the same environmental pressures may lead to obesity, which may lead to a reduction in sleep as a result of an increase in sleep-disordered breathing and disruption in underlying metabolic and inflammatory processes. Notwithstanding this, the potential public health implications of a causal relationship between short duration of sleep and obesity have already been widely disseminated in the media. It is therefore of utmost importance that properly conducted prospective studies, in which weight, height, waist measurements, and adiposity are measured at baseline and again at subsequent data collection times together with more accurate objective measurement of sleep duration (including naps) and confounding factors or mediators, such as depression, are conducted in order to determine causality.

Finally, randomized controlled clinical trials of the effects of sleep on the development of weight gain and on effects of sleep extension on the reduction of body weight in obese people would be needed.

REFERENCES

Akerstedt, T. and Nilsson, P. M. 2003. Sleep as restitution: An introduction. *J. Intern. Med.*, 254 (1), 6–12.

Anderson, S. E. and Whitaker, R. C. 2010. Household routines and obesity in US preschool-aged children. *Pediatrics*, 125 (3), 420–428.

Ayas, N. T., White, D. P., Manson, J. E., Stampfer, M. J., Speizer, F. E., Malhotra, A., and Hu, F. B. 2003. A prospective study of sleep duration and coronary heart disease in women. *Arch. Intern. Med.*, 163 (2), 205–209.

Bawazeer, N. M., Al-Daghri, N. M., Valsamakis, G., Al-Rubeaan, K. A., Sabico, S. L., Huang, T. T., Mastorakos, G. P., and Kumar, S. 2009. Sleep duration and quality associated with obesity among Arab children. *Obesity* (Silver Spring), 17 (12), 2251–2253.

Bell, J. F. and Zimmerman, F. J. 2010. Shortened nighttime sleep duration in early life and subsequent childhood obesity. *Arch. Pediatr. Adolesc. Med.*, 164 (9), 840–845.

Bhattacharjee, R., Kim, J., Kheirandish-Gozal, L., and Gozal, D. 2011. Obesity and obstructive sleep apnea syndrome in children: A tale of inflammatory cascades. *Pediatr. Pulmonol.*, 46 (4), 313–323.

Bidulescu, A., Din-Dzietham, R., Coverson, D. L., Chen, Z., Meng, Y. X., Buxbaum, S. G., Gibbons, G. H., and Welch, V. L. 2010. Interaction of sleep quality and psychosocial stress on obesity in African Americans: The Cardiovascular Health Epidemiology Study (CHES). *BMC Public Health*, 10, 581.

Bjorkelund, C., Bondyr-Carlsson, D., Lapidus, L., Lissner, L., Mansson, J., Skoog, I., and Bengtsson, C. 2005. Sleep disturbances in midlife unrelated to 32-year diabetes incidence: The prospective population study of women in Gothenburg. *Diabetes Care*, 28 (11), 2739–2744.

Bjorvatn, B., Sagen, I. M., Øyane, N., Waage, S., Fetveit, A., Pallesen, S., and Ursin, R. 2007. The association between sleep duration, body mass index and metabolic measures in the Hordaland Health Study. *J. Sleep Res.*, 16 (1), 66–76.

Bliwise, D. L. 1996. Historical change in the report of daytime fatigue. *Sleep*, 19 (6), 462–464.

Budhiraja, R., Budhiraja, P., and Quan, S. F. 2010. Sleep-disordered breathing and cardiovascular disorders. *Respir. Care*, 55 (10), 1322–1332; discussion 1330–1332. [Review.]

Cappuccio, F. P., D'Elia, L., Strazzullo, P., and Miller, M. A. 2010a. Quantity and quality of sleep and incidence of type 2 diabetes: A systematic review and meta-analysis. *Diabetes Care*, 33 (2), 414–420.

Cappuccio, F. P., D'Elia, L., Strazzullo, P., and Miller, M. A. 2010b. Sleep duration and all-cause mortality: A systematic review and meta-analysis of prospective studies. *Sleep*, 33 (5), 585–592.

Cappuccio, F. P., D'Elia, L., Strazzullo, P., and Miller, M. A. 2011. Sleep duration predicts cardiovascular outcomes: A systematic review and meta-analysis of prospective studies. *Eur. Heart J.*, 32 (12), 1484–1492. [Epub ahead of print.]

Cappuccio, F. P., Stranges, S., Kandala, N.-B., Miller, M. A., Taggart, F. M., Kumari, M., Ferrie, J. E., Shipley, M. J., Brunner, E. J., and Marmot, G. 2007. Gender-specific associations of short sleep duration with prevalent and incident hypertension. The Whitehall II Study. *Hypertension*, 50 (4), 694–701.

Cappuccio, F. P., Taggart, F. M., Kandala, N.-B., Currie, A., Peile, E., Stranges, S., and Miller, M. A. 2008. Meta-analysis of short sleep duration and obesity in children, adolescents and adults. *Sleep*, 31 (5), 619–626.

Choi, K. M., Lee, J. S., Park, H. S., Baik, S. H., Choi, D. S., and Kim, S. M. 2008. Relationship between sleep duration and the metabolic syndrome: Korean National Health and Nutrition Survey 2001. *Int. J. Obes. (Lond.)*, 32 (7), 1091–1097. [Epub ahead of print.]

Cizza, G., Marincola, P., Mattingly, M., Williams, L., Mitler, M., Skarulis, M., and Csako, G. 2010. Treatment of obesity with extension of sleep duration: A randomized, prospective, controlled trial. *Clin. Trials*, 7 (3), 274–285.

Cizza, G., Skarulis, M., and Mignot, E. 2005. A link between short sleep and obesity: Building the evidence for causation. *Sleep*, 28 (10), 1217–1220.

Currie, A. and Cappuccio, F. P. 2007. Sleep in children and adolescents: A worrying scenario: Can we understand the sleep deprivation-obesity epidemic? *Nutr. Metab. Cardiovasc. Dis.*, 17 (3), 230–232.

Ferrie, J. E., Shipley, M. J., Cappuccio, F. P., Brunner, E., Miller, M. A., Kumari, M., and Marmot, M. G. 2007. A prospective study of change in sleep duration: Associations with mortality in the Whitehall II cohort. *Sleep*, 30 (12), 1659–1666.

Flegal, K., Carroll, M., Kuczmarski, F., and Johnson, C. 1998. Overweight and obesity in the United States: Prevalence and trends, 1960–1994. *Int. J. Obes. Relat. Metab. Disord.*, 22, 39–47.

Flegal, K., Carroll, M., Ogden, C., and Johnson, C. 2002. Prevalence and trends in obesity among US adults, 1999–2000. *JAMA*, 288, 1723–1727.

Gangwisch, J. E., Malaspina, D., Babiss, L. A. et al. 2010. Short sleep duration as a risk factor for hypercholesterolemia: Analyses of the National Longitudinal Study of Adolescent Health. *Sleep*, 33 (7), 956–961.

Gangwisch, J. E., Malaspina, D., Boden-Albala, B., and Heymsfield, S. B. 2005. Inadequate sleep as a risk factor for obesity: Analyses of the NHANES I. *Sleep*, 28 (10), 1289–1296.

Guilleminault, C. 1985. Obstructive sleep apnea. The clinical syndrome and historical perspective. *Med. Clin. North Am.*, 69 (6), 1187–1203.

Harbison, S. T. and Sehgal, A. 2009. Energy stores are not altered by long-term partial sleep deprivation in *Drosophila melanogaster*. *PLoS One*, 4 (7), e6211.

Kaneita, Y., Uchiyama, M., Yoshiike, N., and Ohida, T. 2008. Associations of usual sleep duration with serum lipid and lipoprotein levels. *Sleep*, 31 (5), 645–652.

Kim, S., Deroo, L. A., and Sandler, D. P. 2010. Eating patterns and nutritional characteristics associated with sleep duration. *Public Health Nutr.*, 14 (5), 1–7. [Epub ahead of print.]

Knutson, K. L., Spiegel, K., Penev, P., and Van Cauter, E. 2007. The metabolic consequences of sleep deprivation. *Sleep Med. Rev.*, 11 (3), 163–178.

Lauderdale, D. S., Knutson, K. L., Rathouz, P. J., Yan, L. L., Hulley, S. B., and Liu, K. 2009. Cross-sectional and longitudinal associations between objectively measured sleep duration and body mass index: The CARDIA Sleep Study. *Am. J. Epidemiol.*, 170 (7), 805–813.

Loredo, J. S., Soler, X., Bardwell, W., Ancoli-Israel, S., Dimsdale, J. E., and Palinkas, L. A. 2010. Sleep health in U.S. Hispanic population. *Sleep*, 33 (7), 962–967.

Lyytikäinen, P., Lallukka, T., Lahelma, E., and Rahkonen, O. 2011. Sleep problems and major weight gain: A follow-up study. *Int. J. Obes. (Lond.)*, 35, 109–114.

Lyytikäinen, P., Rahkonen, O., Lahelma, E., and Lallukka, T. 2010. Association of sleep duration with weight and weight gain: A prospective follow-up study. *J. Sleep Res.* doi: 10.1111/j.1365-2869.2010.00903.x. [Epub ahead of print.]

Marin, J. M., Carrizo, S. J., Vicente, E., and Agusti, A. G. 2005. Long-term cardiovascular outcomes in men with obstructive sleep apnoea-hypopnoea with or without treatment with continuous positive airway pressure: An observational study. *Lancet*, 365 (9464), 1046–1053.

Meier-Ewert, H. K., Ridker, P. M., Rifai, N. et al. 2004. Effect of sleep loss on C-reactive protein, an inflammatory marker of cardiovascular risk. *J. Am. Coll. Cardiol.*, 43 (4), 678–683.

Miller, D. P. 2011. Associations between the home and school environments and child body mass index. *Soc. Sci. Med.*, 72 (5), 677–684. [Epub ahead of print.]

Miller, M. A. and Cappuccio, F. P. 2006. Cellular adhesion molecules and their relationship with measures of obesity and metabolic syndrome in a multiethnic population. *Int. J. Obes. (Lond.)*, 30 (8), 1176–1182.

Miller, M. A. and Cappuccio, F. P. 2007. Inflammation, sleep, obesity and cardiovascular disease. *Curr. Vasc. Pharmacol.*, 5, 93–102.

Miller, M. A., Kandala, N.-B., Kivimaki, M. et al. 2009. Gender differences in the cross-sectional relationships between sleep duration and markers of inflammation: Whitehall II study. *Sleep*, 32 (7), 857–864.

Miller, M. A., Sagnella, G. A., Kerry, S. M., Strazzullo, P., Cook, D. G., and Cappuccio, F. P. 2003. Ethnic differences in circulating soluble adhesion molecules: The Wandsworth Heart and Stroke Study. *Clin. Sci. (Lond.)*, 104 (6), 591–598.

National Sleep Foundation 2005. Sleep in America Poll Washington, DC. http://www.sleepfoundation.org/article/sleep-america-polls/2005-adult-sleep-habits-and-styles (accessed February 10, 2011).

Nedeltcheva, A. V., Kilkus, J. M., Imperial, J., Schoeller, D. A., and Penev, P. D. 2010. Insufficient sleep undermines dietary efforts to reduce adiposity. *Ann. Intern. Med.*, 153, 435–441.

Pack, A. I. and Pien, G. W. 2011. Update on sleep and its disorders. *Ann. Rev. Med.*, 62, 447–460.

Patel, S. R. and Hu, F. B. 2008. Short sleep duration and weight gain: A systematic review. *Obesity* (Silver Spring), 16 (3), 643–653.

Patel, S. R., Malhotra, A., White, D. P., Gottlieb, D. J., and Hu, F. B. 2006. Association between reduced sleep and weight gain in women. *Am. J. Epidemiol.*, 164 (10), 947–954.

Patel, S. R., Zhu, X., Storfer-Isser, A., Mehra, R., Jenny, N. S., Tracy, R., and Redline, S. 2009. Sleep duration and biomarkers of inflammation. *Sleep*, 32 (2), 200–204.

Poirier, P., Giles, T. D., Bray, G. A., Hong, Y., Stern, J. S., Pi-Sunyer, F. X., and Eckel, R. H. 2006. Obesity and cardiovascular disease: Pathophysiology, evaluation, and effect of weight loss: An update of the 1997 American Heart Association Scientific Statement on Obesity and Heart Disease from the Obesity Committee of the Council on Nutrition, Physical Activity, and Metabolism. *Circulation*, 113 (6), 898–918.

Seegers, V., Petit, D., Falissard, B., Vitaro, F., Tremblay, R. E., Montplaisir, J., and Touchette, E. 2011. Short sleep duration and body mass index: A prospective longitudinal study in preadolescence. *Am. J. Epidemiol.*, 173 (6), 621–629. [Epub ahead of print.]

Simpson, N. S., Banks, S., Arroyo, S., and Dinges, D. F. 2010. Effects of sleep restriction on adiponectin levels in healthy men and women. *Physiol. Behav.*, 101 (5), 693–698.

Snell, E. K., Adam, E. K., and Duncan, G. J. 2007. Sleep and the body mass index and overweight status of children and adolescents. *Child Dev.*, 78 (1), 309–323.

Somers, V. K., White, D. P., Amin, R. et al. 2008. Sleep apnea and cardiovascular disease: An American Heart Association/American College of Cardiology Foundation Scientific Statement from the American Heart Association Council for High Blood Pressure Research Professional Education Committee, Council on Clinical Cardiology, Stroke Council, and Council on Cardiovascular Nursing. *J. Am. Coll. Cardiol.*, 52 (8), 686–717.

Spiegel, K., Leproult, R., and Van Cauter, E. 1999. Impact of sleep debt on metabolic and endocrine function. *Lancet*, 354 (9188), 1435–1439.

Spiegel, K., Tasali, E., Leproult, R., and Van Cauter, C. E. 2009. Effects of poor and short sleep on glucose metabolism and obesity risk. *Nat. Rev. Endocrinol.*, 5 (5), 253–261.

Spiegel, K., Tasali, E., Penev, P., and Van, C. E. 2004. Brief communication: Sleep curtailment in healthy young men is associated with decreased leptin levels, elevated ghrelin levels, and increased hunger and appetite. *Ann. Intern. Med.*, 141 (11), 846–850.

Steptoe, A., Peacey, V., and Wardle, J. 2006. Sleep duration and health in young adults. *Arch. Intern. Med.*, 166 (16), 1689–1692.

Stranges, S., Cappuccio, F. P., Kandala, N. B. et al. 2008. Cross-sectional versus prospective associations of sleep duration with changes in relative weight and body fat distribution: The Whitehall II Study. *Am. J. Epidemiol.*, 167 (3), 321–329.

Suarez, E. C. 2008. Self-reported symptoms of sleep disturbance and inflammation, coagulation, insulin resistance and psychosocial distress: Evidence for gender disparity. *Brain Behav. Immun.*, 22 (6), 960–968. [Epub ahead of print.]

Taheri, S. 2006. The link between short sleep duration and obesity: We should recommend more sleep to prevent obesity. *Arch. Dis. Child*, 91 (11), 881–884.

Taheri, S., Austin, D., Lin, L., Nieto, F. J., Young, T., and Mignot, E. 2007. Correlates of serum C-reactive protein (CRP)—No association with sleep duration or sleep disordered breathing. *Sleep*, 30 (8), 991–996.

Taheri, S., Lin, L., Austin, D., Young, T., and Mignot, E. 2004. Short sleep duration is associated with reduced leptin, elevated ghrelin, and increased body mass index. *PLoS Med.*, 1 (3), e62.

Taveras, E. M., Gillman, M. W., Kleinman, K., Rich-Edwards, J. W., and Rifas-Shiman, S. L. 2010. Racial/ethnic differences in early-life risk factors for childhood obesity. *Pediatrics*, 125 (4), 686–695. [Epub ahead of print.]

Van Cauter, E. and Knutson, K. L. 2008. Sleep and the epidemic of obesity in children and adults. *Eur. J. Endocrinol.*, 159 (Suppl 1), S59–S66.

Vanhelst, J., Marchand, F., Fardy, P. et al. 2010. The CEMHaVi program: Control, evaluation, and modification of lifestyles in obese youth. *J. Cardiopulm. Rehabil. Prev.*, 30 (3), 181–185.

Vgontzas, A. N., Bixler, E. O., Chrousos, G. P., and Pejovic, S. 2008. Obesity and sleep disturbances: Meaningful sub-typing of obesity. *Arch. Physiol. Biochem.*, 114 (4), 224–236.

Vgontzas, A. N. and Kales, A. 1999. Sleep and its disorders. *Annu. Rev. Med.*, 50, 387–400.

Watanabe, M., Kikuchi, H., Tanaka, K., and Takahashi, M. 2010. Association of short sleep duration with weight gain and obesity at 1-year follow-up: A large-scale prospective study. *Sleep*, 33 (2), 161–167.

WHO Europe 2006, WHO European Ministerial Conference on Counteracting Obesity. Diet and Physical Activity for Health EUR/06/5062700/9.

Williams, C. J., Hu, F. B., Patel, S. R., and Mantzoros, C. S. 2007. Sleep duration and snoring in relation to biomarkers of cardiovascular disease risk among women with type 2 diabetes. *Diabetes Care*, 30 (5), 1233–1240.

Part III

Obesity and Degenerative Diseases

14 Oxidative Stress Status in Humans with Metabolic Syndrome

C.-Y. Oliver Chen, PhD and
Jeffrey B. Blumberg, PhD, FASN, FACN, CNS

CONTENTS

INTRODUCTION

The concept of metabolic syndrome (MetS) was first introduced by Reaven as "syndrome X" [1]. Subsequently, the World Health Organization (WHO) [2] and the National Cholesterol Education Program Adult Treatment Panel (ATP III) [3,4] defined criteria of MetS with a specific focus on dyslipidemia, hyperglycemia, hypertension, and obesity as key signs—that is, a constellation of risk factors leading to cardiovascular disease (CVD) [4]. Using ATP III criteria, the

National Health and Nutrition Examination Survey (NHANES) II Mortality Study [5] indicated a nearly linear correlation between the number of these MetS components and mortality from CVD [5] and estimated a prevalence of MetS at 23.7%, or ~47,000,000 adults in the United States [6]. Although the precise etiology of MetS is unresolved and undoubtedly complex, abdominal obesity, insulin resistance, and physical inactivity are significant contributing risk factors and, thus, suggest a number of practical solutions for both prevention and treatment of the condition [7].

Reactive oxygen, nitrogen, and halide species (or free radicals) such as hydrogen peroxide, peroxynitrite, and hypochlorous acid, respectively, have been implicated in the etiology of CVD and type II diabetes [8]. Consistent with free radicals initiating or promoting the pathophysiology of these diseases, dietary antioxidants have been implicated in a reduction of their risk, although it is important to recognize that these compounds function importantly via mechanisms unrelated to their antioxidant properties [9,10]. These relationships have given rise to hypotheses that oxidative stress may be linked to early events in the development of CVD (as well as diabetes) via both independent mechanisms and dynamic interactions between the dyslipidemia, hyperglycemia, hypertension, and obesity of MetS. Examining antioxidant defenses and biomarkers of oxidative stress *in vivo* in human studies offers a robust approach to testing these hypotheses. These studies generally utilize determinations of (1) the modulation of antioxidant enzyme activity; (2) the concentration of antioxidants or measures of total antioxidant capacity; or (3) products of oxidatively modified lipids, protein, or DNA (Figure 14.1). However, these data must be interpreted with caution as they may not necessarily reflect a clinically significant or pathogenic event but instead indicate a temporary response of the antioxidant defense network. Assays for determining oxidation products of lipids, proteins, and DNA have been previously reviewed [11–16] and are beyond the scope of this chapter.

We consider here evidence from human studies suggesting a role of antioxidant defenses and oxidative stress in the etiology and/or progression of MetS and subsequent risk for CVD.

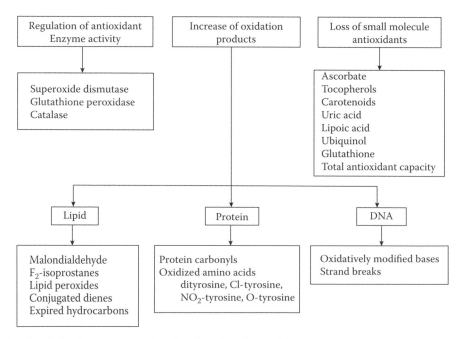

FIGURE 14.1 Oxidative stress sorted as functionality of antioxidants and products of oxidation. We consider here evidence from human studies suggesting a role of antioxidant defenses and oxidative stress in the etiology and/or progression of MS and subsequent risk for CVD.

INCREASES IN OXIDATION PRODUCTS IN PATIENTS WITH COMPONENTS OF METABOLIC SYNDROME

Oxidative stress is the disturbance in the oxidant–antioxidant balance in favor of the former and can be a consequence of diminished protection by antioxidant defenses or increased generation of free radicals, with both resulting in production of oxidation products (e.g., lipid peroxides) [16].

BIOMARKERS OF LIPID PEROXIDATION

OBESITY AND LIPID PEROXIDATION

Obesity, a key component of MetS [17–19], appears to be associated with increased generation of free radicals and lipid peroxidation reactions [20]. For example, in an observational study of 140 nondiabetic men and women (mean age, 59 years), body mass index (BMI in kg/m^2 even when units are not provided in the following) and waist circumference (WC in cm when units are not provided in the following) were directly associated with plasma thiobarbituric acid reactive substances (TBARS) and urinary 8-epi-prostaglandin-F2α (8-isoP), products of lipid peroxidation [21]. Analyses of 2828 subjects (mean age, 61 years; age is expressed in the following as a mean in years) from the Framingham cohort revealed a linear correlation between obesity and lipid peroxidation, as each 5 units of BMI was associated with a 9.9% increase in urinary 8-isoP after adjustment for creatinine [22]. Similarly, 8-isoP has also been associated in studies of age-matched men with adiposity, insulin resistance, and endothelial adhesion molecules [23,24]. Overweight/obesity in adolescents has become a serious public health issue because this group is at increased risk for development of metabolic diseases later in life. Analyses of 113 healthy peripubertal children (age, 12.9; 58 F) revealed that 55 obese children with age- and gender-adjusted BMI ≥95th percentile had significantly elevated plasma 8-isoP concentrations compared to 43 normal-weight children with BMI <85th percentile (99 ± 7 vs. 75 ± 4 pg/mL) [25]. Children born large and small for gestational age (LGA, SGA) are also at risk of metabolic dysfunction later in life. Urinary 8-isoP status in 31 obese LGA and SGA peripubertal children (age, 7.5) was ~1.5 fold larger than 15 obese children born appropriate for gestational age (age, 7.7) [26]. Although 8-isoP is the best validated measure of lipid peroxidation *in vivo*, it is worth noting that no difference was found when malondialdehyde (MDA), another biomarker of lipid peroxidation, was determined in a study with nine obese normotensive men (BMI, 32.6; age, 31) and age-matched controls [27]. Further, the type of obesity may dictate the magnitude of lipid peroxidation, as Davi et al. [28] found that urinary 8-isoP was higher in 24 android obese, nonsmoking women (BMI, 39; waist-to-hip ratio [WHR], 0.96; age, 45) than in 25 gynoid obese women (BMI, 33; WHR, 0.80; age, 40) but higher in all obese women when compared to 24 nonobese women (BMI, 22.5; age, 38).

HYPERGLYCEMIA AND LIPID PEROXIDATION

Hyperglycemia can increase the generation of free radicals via autoxidation events, polyol pathways, and Amadori reactions [9,29]; for example, an acute oral administration of 100 g glucose to eight healthy men (BMI, 22.4; age, 23) increased plasma MDA [30]. Consistent with this result, Facchini et al. [31] found that plasma lipid peroxides were significantly higher in 12 insulin-resistant healthy people (BMI, 25.9; age, 49) than in 12 insulin-sensitive individuals (BMI, 24.6; age, 47). Quantifying the relationship between obesity and lipid peroxidation, Keaney et al. [22] calculated that each 25 mg/dL increase in fasting glucose was associated with a 4.3% increase in urinary 8-isoP (adjusted for creatinine).

HYPERTENSION AND LIPID PEROXIDATION

Koska et al. [32] found increased MDA and lipofuscin concentrations in plasma of 11 men with essential hypertension (blood pressure [BP, in mmHg], 151/97; BMI, 28.6; age, 44.3) when compared to 10 normotensive men (BP, 119/79; BMI, 25.3; age, 44.4) at 0.85 vs. 1.3 ng/mL and 11.8 vs. 16.2 units, respectively. Further, the PREDMIED study in Spain assessed 1130 asymptomatic individuals at high risk for coronary heart disease (CHD), aged 55–80 years, BMI ≥25, and showed that lipid peroxidation, assessed by circulating oxidized low-density lipoprotein cholesterol (LDL), was associated with systolic and diastolic blood pressure ($r = 0.17$, $P < 0.05$; $r = 0.17$, $P < 0.01$, respectively) after taking into account the confounding factors of sex, age, glucose, LDL/high-density lipoprotein cholesterol (HDL) ratio, tobacco consumption, lipid-lowering agents, angiotensin-converting enzyme (ACE) inhibitors, and sodium and potassium intake [33]. Importantly, the magnitude of lipid peroxidation appears greater in people with two or more risk factors of MetS than in those with one or less. Konukoglu et al. [34] found that obesity and hypertension were associated with a greater oxidative stress status than with either obesity or hypertension alone as plasma TBARS ascended in order in 25 nonobese normotensives (BP, 95.5/75.4; BMI, 21.5; age, 54.5), 25 nonobese hypertensives (BP, 165.5/105.3; BMI, 23.5; age, 56.5), 35 obese normotensives (BP, 109.5/75.5; BMI, 32.5; age, 60.5), and 45 obese hypertensives (BP, 168.8/115.6; BMI, 33.8; age, 58.5) at 5.55, 6.85, 7.20, and 8.45 mol/L, respectively. When Stojiljkovic et al. [35] examined the relationship between lipid peroxidation and hypertension, obesity, and insulin resistance, they found increased urinary 8-isoP excretion in 10 obese hypertensives with insulin resistance (BMI, 31; BP, 131/88; age, 40) compared to 12 healthy normotensives without insulin resistance (BMI, 22; BP, 106/72; age, 38) at 5.0 vs. 3.3 ng/mg creatine, respectively. Using ATP III guidelines, Hansel et al. [36] found that plasma 8-isoP was 3.7-fold greater in 10 MetS patients (BMI, 31.1; WC, 102.3; BP, 148/85; age, 53.5) than in 11 healthy individuals (BMI, 23.4; WC, 81; BP, 127/80; age, 52.3) in a case control study. In contrast, also using ATP III criteria, Sjogren et al. [37] observed no difference in urinary 8-isoP between 22 men with MetS (BMI, 30.1; WC, 108; BP, 148/87) and healthy men (BMI, 24.2; WC, 92; BP, 120/75) or men with one or two MetS risk factors (BMI, 26.1; WC, 97; BP, 141/83) in a cross-sectional cohort of 289 men (aged 62–64 years). The absence of a correlation here between lipid peroxidation and MetS could be attributed to a lack of power with so few MetS patients in this population.

SUSCEPTIBILITY OF LOW-DENSITY LIPOPROTEIN TO OXIDATION

Oxidation of lipoproteins, especially LDL, has been implicated in the pathogenesis of atherosclerosis and CVD [38]. Thus, it is of interest to note that Myara et al. [39] found that the resistance of LDL to oxidation *in vitro* was negatively correlated with BMI ($r = -0.35$) in 75 obese patients (BMI, 30–50). However, as *in vitro* LDL oxidation assays may indicate only the oxidizability of LDL with a modest relationship to *in vivo* pathophysiology, some studies have evaluated circulating oxidized LDL (oxLDL) *in vivo*, although the origin of oxLDL in the circulation is unclear. Consistent with Myara et al. [39], Couillard et al. [24] found a positive correlation ($r = 0.52$) between oxLDL and WC in 56 sedentary men with abdominal obesity (WC, 102; BMI, 30.4; age, 40), and Kassi et al. [40] reported that 40 overweight postmenopausal women (BMI, 32.4) had an 82% greater oxLDL than 55 nonoverweight women (BMI, 23.5). Extending this relationship to glycemic status, Kopprasch et al. [41] found that oxLDL was higher in 113 subjects with impaired glucose tolerance (BMI, 28.0; age, 60) than in 376 with normal glucose tolerance (BMI, 26.4; age, 57). Similarly, Mizuno et al. [42] found higher oxLDL in 12 healthy, nonsmoking, insulin-resistant men (BMI, 24.5; age, 29.1) than in 24 insulin-sensitive men (BMI, 22.1; age, 28.7) at 146 vs. 101 IU/L, respectively. Examining the effect of oxLDL on the evolution of insulin resistance in a population-based observational study (Coronary Artery Risk Development in Young Adults) and its ancillary study (Young Adult Longitudinal Trends in Antioxidants) during 2000–2006,

Park et al. [43] found that the association between oxLDL and insulin resistance was independent of obesity. In contrast, Schwenke et al. [44] found no correlation between glucose intolerance and *in vitro* LDL susceptibility to oxidation in 352 men and postmenopausal women from the Insulin Resistance Atherosclerosis study.

Examining directly 1147 MetS patients (BMI, 29; WC, 102; BP, 139/72; age, 74) with their multiple risk factors for CVD according to ATP III criteria, Holvoet et al. [45] found elevated oxLDL in comparison to 1886 healthy subjects (BMI, 27; WC, 98; BP, 134/71; age, 74), independent of sex and ethnicity. From the Japan Obesity and Metabolic Syndrome (JOMETS) study, Kotani et al. [46] reported that serum concentration of serum amyloid A (SAA)-LDL, a product formed from the oxidative interaction between SAA and LDL, was 40% larger in 286 MetS patients (BMI, 31.6; BP, 143/85; WC, 101; age, 52.7) diagnosed according to the NCEP-ATP III criteria than obese outpatients (BMI, 30.3; BP, 131/79; WC, 97.2; age, 47.7). Employing WHO criteria, a similar correlation between increasing number of MetS criteria and oxLDL was reported in a cross-sectional study in Sweden among 391 nondiabetic men [47,48]; however, as with their inability to detect a difference using urinary 8-isoP, Sjogren et al. [37] found no difference in oxLDL concentrations between MetS and healthy men.

PRODUCTION OF PROTEIN OXIDATION

Nitrotyrosine (NT) can serve as a biomarker of peroxynitrite radical attack on proteins, although no studies have been conducted assessing MetS with NT [49–51]. Although Marfella et al. [52] found that acute hyperglycemia induced by glucose infusion increased plasma NT from 0.2 to 0.5 µmol/L in 20 healthy subjects (BMI, 24; age, 34), Bo et al. [53] found no difference in plasma NT between 96 healthy subjects (BMI, 22.9; WC, 85.9; BP, 126.9/80.5; age, 53.8) and 204 people with central obesity (BMI, 29.4; WC, 101.9; BP, 138.6/86.4; age, 55.3) in a cohort study. Plasma NT was found to be elevated in 40 type 2 diabetic patients (BMI, 26.2; age, 56.2) relative to 35 healthy subjects with a similar BMI (BMI, 25.9; age, 55.4) [50].

CHANGES OF ANTIOXIDANT DEFENSE MECHANISMS IN PATIENTS WITH COMPONENTS OF METABOLIC SYNDROME

SMALL MOLECULE ANTIOXIDANTS

Nonenzymatic, small-molecule dietary antioxidants include vitamins C and E, carotenoids, polyphenols, and other compounds. In addition to their presence in some foods, endogenous synthesis of α-lipoic acid, glutathione (GSH), uric acid, ubiquinols, and other compounds contributes to the body's antioxidant defense network. If the etiology or progression of MetS was associated with oxidative stress, then an increased utilization and requirement or lower concentrations in a vicious cycle with oxidative stress would be anticipated for these antioxidants. Serum antioxidant status has been associated in several studies with MetS [54–57]. Using data from the National Health and Examination Survey 2001–2006, Beydoun et al. [58] found that the prevalence of MetS was 32.0% among men and 29.5% among women aged 20–85. In this cohort, MetS was associated with lower serum carotenoid status, even after controlling for total cholesterol and triglycerides, than those without MetS. Among the carotenoids, β-carotene (both sexes), β-cryptoxanthin (men), and lutein plus zeaxanthin (women) were inversely related to MetS. Vitamin C exhibited a similar pattern with an inverse linear association with MetS and related conditions like insulin resistance and hyperuricemia. After controlling for serum lipids, vitamin E was observed not to have a significant relationship with MetS. As cross-sectional studies preclude inference about temporality of these associations, it is not clear whether the lower status of carotenoids and vitamin C is the result of oxidative stress caused by MetS or the direct outcome of lower fruit and vegetable intake that affects the pathogenesis of MetS.

OBESITY AND DIETARY ANTIOXIDANTS

The increases in lipid peroxidation associated with obesity suggest an increased utilization of anti-oxidant vitamins. Indeed, Myara et al. [39] found an inverse association between BMI and plasma vitamin E ($r = -0.53$) in a study of 75 nondiabetic, normotensive obese patients (age, 39.1). Botella-Carretero et al. [59] also found that both serum retinol and α-tocopherol correlated inversely with BMI ($r = -0.334$, $P = 0.002$ and $r = -0.299$, $P = 0.007$, respectively) in 80 patients with morbid obesity (BMI, 48.1; WC, 125; age, 40.1). In contrast, no such association was found by Visentin et al. [27] with plasma vitamins A, C, and E; β-carotene; or lycopene in nine obese, normotensive men (BMI, 32.6; age, 31) and nine nonobese men (BMI, 23.3). Menke et al. [60] reported that the plasma coenzyme Q10 and redox ratio (oxidized to total coenzyme Q10) were not different between 67 obese children and 50 age-matched, normal-weight children. However, these studies are of small size and also absent assessments of diet and oxidative stress, so it is not possible to determine whether the results are due to changes in antioxidant intake or utilization *in vivo*, free radical generation, or compensatory mechanisms in endogenous antioxidant synthesis.

INSULIN RESISTANCE AND DIETARY ANTIOXIDANTS

Inverse associations between insulin resistance and plasma vitamin E ($r = -0.21$) and β-carotene ($r = -0.2$) were observed among 103 Korean children by Konukoglu et al. [61]. Facchini et al. [31] also observed lower plasma α- and β-carotene, lutein, and α-tocopherol in 12 healthy insulin-resistant individuals (BMI, 25.9; age, 49) than in 12 insulin-sensitive individuals (BMI, 24.6; age, 47). Konukoglu et al. [61], however, found that erythrocyte GSH was not different between 18 middle-aged subjects with normal glucose tolerance and 15 with impaired glucose tolerance. To date, the evaluation of insulin resistance with assays purporting to measure total antioxidant capacity has not revealed any relationship between these parameters, even when other biomarkers of oxidative stress were affected [41] or when hyperglycemia or hyperinsulinemia was induced [62].

METABOLIC SYNDROME AND DIETARY ANTIOXIDANTS

Ford et al. [54] observed in 8808 adults from the NHANES III cohort that those with MetS had lower plasma retinyl esters, vitamins C and E, and carotenoids after adjustments for age, sex, race, education, smoking, physical activity, fruit and vegetable intake, and supplement use. Examining 374 Dutch men aged 40–80 years in a population-based, cross-sectional study, Sluijs et al. [57] found that there was a significant inverse association between total carotenoid intake and incidence of MetS. Men in the highest quartile of carotenoid intake (mean intake, 15.4 mg/day) had a 58% lower risk of MetS than those who were in the lowest quartile (59 mg/day) with the strongest associations for lycopene and β-carotene. Concerned by the growing prevalence of MetS among children [63], Molnar et al. [64] examined 15 children with MetS (BMI, 34.2; age, 13.4), 17 with obesity (BMI, 30.4; age, 14.4), and 16 healthy children (BMI, 20.7; age, 16.2) and also found significant reductions in plasma α-tocopherol, β-carotene, and total antioxidant capacity. Examining the associations between serum carotenoid concentrations and incidence of MetS in 1523 Australians aged 25 years and older, Coyne et al. [56] found that serum α- and β-carotene and the sum of five carotenoid concentrations (α- and β-carotene, β-cryptoxanthin, lutein, and lycopene) were significantly lower in people with MetS, diagnosed based on International Diabetes Federation 2005 criteria, than healthy people. In contrast, using ATP III criteria, Miles et al. [65] found that total plasma ubiquinol was higher in 134 MetS subjects (BMI, 33.2; age, 49.9) than in 178 healthy subjects (BMI, 26.5; age, 43). It may be possible, then, that MetS is associated with lower dietary antioxidant status due to increased utilization but higher endogenous antioxidant status due to induction of compensatory mechanisms and thus no readily apparent change in total antioxidant capacity.

ANTIOXIDANT ENZYMES

Antioxidant enzymes could be subject to compensatory regulation in MetS associated with oxidative stress. Ozata et al. [66] found that the activity of erythrocyte superoxide dismutase (SOD) and GSH peroxidase (GSHPx) was lower in 76 obese men (BMI, 36.6; mean age, 49.1) than in 24 healthy men (BMI, 21.2; mean age, 48.5). However, Visentin et al. [27] found no difference in the activity of erythrocyte SOD, GSHPx, or catalase in nine normotensive, obese men (BMI, 32.6; mean age, 31) vs. nine healthy men (BMI, 23.3; mean age, 31). Although neither of these studies suggests an upregulation of antioxidant enzymes with obesity, it should be noted that their populations were small and of different ages, factors that can affect this outcome [67]. Further, questions regarding compensatory mechanis-MetS might best include a longitudinal rather than a cross-sectional examination. Investigating the response of antioxidant enzymes to acute hyperglycemia, Koska et al. [30] induced an increase in erythrocyte GSHPx and SOD activity by administering 100g glucose to eight healthy males (BMI, 22.4; mean age, 23); however, the chronic hyperglycemia of 103 Korean children with insulin resistance was associated with an attenuated activity of erythrocyte catalase [68]. Interestingly, Pedro-Botet et al. [69] found that hypertension was also associated with lower activity of SOD and GSHPx when they compared 30 normolipidemic, untreated mild hypertensive patients with 164 age-matched, healthy subjects at 806 vs. 931 U/g Hb and 5491 vs. 6669 U/L, respectively; however, the influence of the combined constellation of MetS signs on antioxidant enzymes has yet to be determined.

PARAOXONASE

Paraoxonase-1 (PON-1) is an ester hydrolase bound to HDL that catalyzes the hydrolysis of a number of organic esters and protects LDL from oxidation. PON-1 activity is considerably lower in patients with diabetes, hypercholesterolemia, and myocardial infarction [70,71]. With regard to the critical MetS sign of obesity, Ferretti et al. [72] found that 12 obese women (BMI, 45.3; age, 38.2) had fourfold less PON-1 activity than 31 healthy controls (BMI, 20.1; age, 31.5) at 112.2 vs. 470.5 U/mg. Chen et al. [73] found that 32 patients with essential hypertension had a 23% lower PON-1 activity than 33 healthy people. Further, an inverse correlation ($r = -0.76$) was observed between PON-1 activity and LDL lipid peroxides. Employing WHO criteria, Garin et al. [74] observed that 139 MetS patients (BMI, 30; BP, 139/82; age, 62.1) had 22% lower serum PON-1 activity than 634 non-MetS patients (BMI, 26.6; BP, 130/79; age, 59.6), a decrement sufficient to attenuate the antioxidant protection of LDL by HDL [75]. Hashemi et al. [76] also reported that serum PON-1 activity was significantly lower by 24% in 106 Iranian MetS patients (BMI 29.2; WC, 99; BP, 126/81; age, 43.5), diagnosed using ATP III criteria, than 231 healthy subjects (BMI 23.8; WC, 82; BP, 114/74; age, 35.6). Using ATP III criteria, Senti et al. [77] found that the magnitude of attenuation of PON-1 activity was dependent on the number of MetS signs and related metabolic disturbances in a cohort of 713 men and 651 women aged 25–74 years. In contrast and also using ATP III criteria, Hansel et al. [36] found no difference in serum PON-1 activity between 10 MetS patients (age, 53.5) and 11 healthy, normolipidemic controls (age, 52.3), although they did observe that HDL from MetS patients had less resistance to LDL oxidation *in vitro*. Tabur et al. [78] also found no difference in PON-1 activity between 40 MetS patients (BMI, 40; WC, 75.1; BP, 98/65; age, 33.1) and 24 healthy controls (BMI, 23; WC, 75.1; BP, 146/95; age, 34.7). Results such as these are encouraging investigations exploring the therapeutic potential of PON-1 induction in patients with MetS.

CHANGES IN BIOMARKERS OF OXIDATIVE STRESS IN PATIENTS WITH COMPONENTS OF METABOLIC SYNDROME

The management goal for patients with MetS is reducing the risk of atherosclerosis and CVD [79]; thus, the initial treatment emphasis, before introducing pharmacotherapy, is on mitigating the modifiable lifestyle factors of obesity and physical inactivity [79–81]. Both lifestyle changes and medications may affect MetS and CVD risk via an impact on oxidative stress status.

PHYSICAL ACTIVITY, METABOLIC SYNDROME, AND OXIDATIVE STRESS STATUS

Regular exercise training in older adults is associated with significant reductions in several metabolic risk factors for CVD [82]. Similar exercise programs may contribute to the prevention of MetS, as Ekelund et al. [83] found that the level of energy expenditure in physical activity was inversely associated in a dose-dependent fashion with development of MetS signs over 5.6 years in a prospective study of 605 healthy adults (BMI, 26; age, 53.2). In a randomized clinical trial, Stewart et al. [84] provided 6 months of supervised exercise training (per the American College of Sports Medicine [85]) to 51 older adults (BMI, 29.4; BP, 140/77; age, 63), 22 who presented with MetS according to ATP III criteria. In addition to improvements in body composition and fitness, the subjects lost 2.2 kg body weight and reduced their BP by 5.3/3.7 mmHg. Importantly, no subjects developed MetS during the intervention period, and nine who presented with MetS were no longer so classified. Physical activity can also increase insulin sensitivity. For example, by subjecting 28 MetS patients (BMI, 32; age, 52) to a 40 min exercise program for 3 days a week over 8 weeks, Dumortier et al. [81] found that their insulin response improved twofold, and they also noted significant decreases in body weight (−2.6 kg), BMI (−0.96), and body fat (−1.55%). The benefits of regular exercise on reductions in metabolic risk factor may be ascribed to decreased oxidative stress and enhanced antioxidant defense among fit individuals. Examining 40 postmenopausal women (BMI, 25.6; age, 65.1), Pialoux et al. [86] reported that cardiorespiratory fitness, determined by maximum oxygen consumption in a graded exercise test, was associated to decreased plasma 8-oxo-deoxy-guanosine, a biomarker of DNA oxidation, and 8-isoP and increased glutathione peroxidase and catalase activities. Exercise programs can also impact measures of oxidative stress. For example, Vasankari et al. [87] found that a 10 month program of 3–5 h of walking per week decreased the ratio of LDL-conjugated dienes to LDL by 16% and enhanced the total antioxidant capacity of LDL by 13.5% in 104 sedentary volunteers (BMI, 29; age, 44). Exercise training can also significantly reduce measures of lipid peroxidation and inflammation *in vivo* in obese individuals [88]. For example, Roberts et al. [89] reported that 45–60 min of supervised aerobic exercise at 70%–85% maximum heart rate over 3 weeks decreased serum 8-isoP from 202.6 to 131.3 pg/mL in 31 obese, older men (BMI, 35.4; age, 63.3), including 15 presenting with MetS and all others with at least one MetS factor. At the end of the exercise program, the number of men with MetS according to WHO criteria decreased from 15 to 5.

HYPOCALORIC DIETS, METABOLIC SYNDROME, AND OXIDATIVE STRESS STATUS

Calorie reduction or restriction is an established approach to reducing body weight, and some studies indicate that success is associated with a reduction in measures of oxidative stress, as well. For example, Dandona et al. [90] found that a 1000 kcal/day diet regimen over 4 weeks induced a 12.3 kg loss of weight in nine obese patients (BMI, 40.7; age, 45.3) and concomitantly significant reductions in oxidative damage to lipids (1.68 vs. 1.47 μmol TBARS/L), proteins (1.39 vs. 1.17 μmol protein carbonyls/mg protein), and amino acids (o-tyrosine/phenylalanine, 0.42 vs. 0.36) with no changes in the status of α-tocopherol, β-carotene, or lycopene. Similarly, Davi et al. [28] found that a 1200 kcal/day diet consumed by 11 android obese women was associated with a significant 32% reduction in urinary 8-isoP; nine other women in this study who failed to comply with the diet and lost no weight showed no change in their urinary 8-isoP.

Although drug treatments specific for MetS signs are discussed later, gastrointestinal lipase inhibitors such as orlistat are described here as they are specifically indicated as adjuncts to hypocaloric, weight-loss diets [91]. Use of orlistat for 6 months in an obese population (BMI, 36.1; WC, 105; age, 49.7) not only reduced BMI and WC but also reduced plasma MDA from 2.0 vs. 0.89 μmol/L, the latter value being equivalent to nonobese controls, in direct association with BMI ($r = 0.36$) [92]. However, Samuelsson et al. [93] observed no change in plasma 8-isoP with orlistat and/or hypocaloric diets. As exercise can modulate antioxidant defenses [67], it is worth noting that the combination of orlistat with exercise and a low-calorie diet decreased serum MDA from 1.79 to 1.20 mg/L in a study of 12 obese subjects (BMI, 39.1; age, 37.3), while 11 subjects in the drug-plus-diet group (BMI, 37.9; age, 40) showed no such relationship [94]. However, results on oxidative stress from studies of orlistat are confounded by their action in decreasing the absorption of fat-soluble antioxidants such as carotenoids and tocopherols.

PHARMACOTHERAPY OF METABOLIC SYNDROME AND OXIDATIVE STRESS

Although the first line of treatment for MetS patients includes lifestyle modifications, pharmacotherapy is the second line of treatment and specifically targeted to each of its signs: dyslipidemia, hyperglycemia, and hypertension, as well as obesity (see earlier discussion of lipase inhibitors). With a growing appreciation of the putative role of oxidative stress, supplementation with dietary antioxidants is also being considered as another potential adjunct in the prevention and treatment of MetS.

ANTIHYPERGLYCEMIA THERAPY

Long-term therapy with thiazolidinediones improves insulin sensitivity and decreases the progression of carotid intima-media thickness [95]. Interestingly, treatment with repaglinide for 2 months in a randomized clinical trial significantly enhanced total serum antioxidant capacity and serum SOD activity in 46 type 2 diabetics (BMI, 27.7; age, 50.5), initial values of which were lower than age- and sex-matched controls [96]. Although the improvement in these antioxidant defenses may be attributed to improved glycemic control, it is worth noting that this class of drugs is composed of benzoic acid derivatives capable of directly scavenging free radicals. In an 8 week, randomized clinical trial with 15 obese patients, troglitazone was found to significantly reduce plasma TBARS as well as increase the resistance of LDL to oxidation *in vitro* without affecting vitamin E content [97].

ANTIHYPERTENSION THERAPY

The drugs employed to treat hypertension include thiazide diuretics, ACE inhibitors, angiotensin receptor blockers (ARBs), calcium channel blockers, and β-blockers, often in conjunction with dietary modifications such as reductions in total calorie and sodium intake [98,99]. Saez et al. [99] found that combined drug (ARBs or β-blockers) and diet treatments in 89 hypertensive patients (BMI, 29.5; BP 139/88; age, 46) were associated with significant decreases in MDA and increases in GSH as well as SOD, GSHPx, and catalase activity in blood; however, no significant correlation between BP reduction and these biomarkers of oxidative stress was found. In contrast, erythrocyte oxidized/reduced GSH was not altered by either ARB or calcium channel blocker regimens in a randomized trial of 49 nonsmoking, untreated hypertensives (BP, 151/96; BMI, 27; age, 52.5), although this ratio was significantly higher than that of the 32 placebo controls (BMI, 24.5; age, 51) [100]. A clinical trial of ARBs conducted in 12 MetS patients (BP, 145/85; BMI, 37; age, 45.2) similarly failed to find significant changes in biomarkers of oxidative stress, including plasma TBARS and urinary 8-isoP, after the intervention [101]. The hypothesis that an antioxidant supplement combined with antihypertensive therapy might improve clinical outcomes in MetS patients was tested by Sola et al. [102] in a trial with an ARB plus 300 mg/day α-lipoic acid. After 4 weeks of treatment in 15 MetS patients (BP, 135/85; BMI, 34; age, 48), the drug-plus-antioxidant combination reduced serum 8-isoP by 22%, the drug alone decreased it by 15%, and the antioxidant alone had no effect on 8-isoP; however, the antihypertensive efficacy of the first two groups was quite small and null for α-lipoic acid, despite some indication that it possesses some such activity [103].

DYSLIPIDEMIA THERAPY

Although atherogenic dyslipidemia is characterized by the abnormal profiles of many constituent lipids, LDL is the primary target of therapy, and statins are the principal class of therapeutic drugs [79,104]. Deedwania et al. [105] examined 2268 dyslipidemia patients and found that the 811 who met the ATP III criteria for MetS all benefited from statin treatment, albeit with some differences noted between individual agents. Importantly, all statins possess some antioxidant activity, providing them with at least a dual mechanism action in their use for patients with dyslipidemia as well as MetS and type 2 diabetes mellitus. For example, 3 months of atorvastatin therapy increased the *ex vivo* resistance of LDL to oxidation in 12 normocholesterolemic type 2 diabetic patients [106]. Similarly, 12 weeks of rosuvastatin therapy reduced oxLDL by 55% compared to placebo in a trial of 18 patients with familial combined hyperlipidemia (BMI, 28; age, 53.9) [107]. Further, Kural et al. [108] reported that a 10 week atorvastatin regimen enhanced total antioxidant capacity and serum PON activity by 7.6% and 23.6%, respectively, in 40 patients (age, 53.5) with dyslipidemia.

Studies of statins and oxidative stress are confounded by the inhibitory action of these drugs on 3-hydroxy-3-methylglutaryl coenzyme A, a critical step in the pathway not only for cholesterol but also for the synthesis of antioxidant ubiquinols such as coenzyme Q10. Significant reductions in the ubiquinol content of LDL and a greater oxidizability of LDL *ex vivo* were found in a trial of 28 men with primary hyperlipidemia and CHD (BMI, 27.1; BP, 147/88; age, 56) who received a 6 week treatment with lovastatin [109]. Similarly, atorvastatin has been found in clinical trials to reduce plasma ubiquinol concentrations [110]. Perhaps as a function of their lipid-lowering action, statins have also been reported to decrease vitamin E status [109]. Thus, in addition to supplementing patients taking statins with coenzyme Q10, some investigators have suggested including vitamin E supplements. For example, Manuel-Keenoy et al. [111] supplemented 11 type 1 diabetics receiving atorvastatin with 250 IU vitamin E daily for 6 months and found that their α-tocopherol status was markedly enhanced, while 11 patients receiving the drug alone showed a decrease in plasma concentrations of the vitamin. Consistent with these results, the TBARS content of LDL was reduced in the vitamin-E-supplemented group and elevated in the drug-only group. Importantly, several studies have revealed that the antioxidant potency of statins in LDL varies by individual compounds and is independent of their cholesterol-lowering potency (e.g., with atorvastatin and fluvastatin increasing resistance to oxidation but little such action by simvastatin, depending on the assay utilized) [112,113].

Statins have also been shown to beneficially affect biomarkers of oxidative stress other than LDL oxidizability. Among a group of 35 hypercholesterolemic patients (BMI, 29; age, 54), Shishehbor et al. [114] found a reduction in plasma measures of protein oxidation independent of improvements in lipid profiles (i.e., declines in chlorinated tyrosine, NT, and dityrosine by 30%, 25%, and 32%, respectively) following a 12 week atorvastatin regimen. However, as noted earlier, studies of statins in MetS patients are few, and those that address in a comprehensive way the impact of the therapy on antioxidant defenses and biomarkers of oxidative stress are even more limited.

ANTIOXIDANT SUPPLEMENTATION

A theoretical rationale for antioxidant supplementation in MetS can be proffered by examining the effect of these nutrients on each of the four individual components of the syndrome and their contribution to the generation of oxidative stress; however, as little direct evidence is available to test this hypothesis, further research in this area is warranted. For example, as noted earlier, hypertension increases oxidative stress as indicated by increases in plasma TBARS and urinary 8-isoP [32–34]. Conversely, Hajjar et al. [115] have shown in a randomized clinical trial that supplementation with 500–2000 mg/day vitamin C for 6 months reduced BP by 4.4/2.8 in 31 hypertensives (BP, 140–180/90–100). Also, Ward et al. [116] obtained a mean decrease of systolic BP 1.8 with 500 mg/day vitamin C in a trial of 69 treated hypertensives (systolic BP, 136.5;

BMI, 28.7; age, 62) already receiving antihypertensive therapies. The vitamin C supplement did not affect plasma levels of urinary 8-isoP or serum oxLDL.

Vitamin E has been well established as a chain-breaking antioxidant effective in reducing lipid peroxidation reactions. Brockes et al. [117] found that LDL in normotensive individuals had a greater resistance to oxidation *ex vivo* than in hypertensives, but after 400 IU/day vitamin E supplementation for 2 months in both groups, significant differences in this parameter were eliminated. Vitamin E has also been noted to increase insulin sensitivity via an inhibition of protein kinase C and activation of diacylglycerol kinase [118]. For example, in a randomized clinical trial, Barbagallo et al. [119] supplemented 24 hypertensive patients with normal blood glucose and insulin (BP, >140/90; BMI, 25.3; age, 47) with 600 mg/day vitamin E for 4 weeks and found significant increases in whole body glucose disposal and the ratio of plasma reduced to oxidized GSH. Investigating 41 overweight subjects (BMI, 32.3; age, 47) with normal glycemic status, Manning et al. [120] tested 800 IU/day vitamin E in a randomized clinical trial for 3 months and found significant reductions in fasting plasma insulin and lipid peroxides and an increase in insulin sensitivity compared to no change in any of these parameters among the 39 subjects (BMI, 33.2; age, 51) receiving placebo. The decrease in plasma insulin was significantly correlated with the increase in plasma vitamin E ($r = -0.235$). In contrast, McSorley et al. [121] found no effect of 800 IU/day vitamin E supplementation for 12 weeks on fasting plasma glucose or insulin sensitivity in 13 adult children of parents with type 2 diabetes with normal glucose tolerance (BMI, 24.8; age, 28) in a randomized, crossover trial. Results from Skrha et al. [122] suggested a deleterious effect of 600 mg/day vitamin E administered for 3 months when they observed a 7.3% reduction in insulin sensitivity in 11 obese subjects with type 2 diabetes (BMI, 31.6; age, 45).

Hildebrandt et al. [123] tested 600 mg/day N-acetylcysteine, a GSH prodrug, for 8 weeks in 11 obese subjects with impaired glucose tolerance (BMI, 35.7; age, 45.4) and observed increased plasma thiol status but further reduced glucose tolerance. Like the outcome of the study by Skrha et al. [122], these results suggest that some people may experience untoward results from an antioxidant intervention, and caution in future studies is advisable.

Dietary flavonoids possess an array of bioactivity, including antioxidation, anti-inflammation, and glucoregulation. A growing body of evidence suggests their consumption is associated to a reduction in CVD risk. Egert et al. [124] in a randomized, double-blinded, placebo-controlled crossover trial with overweight subjects (BMI, 30.6; WC, 104.3; BP, 130.3/82.6; age, 45.1) found that 150 mg/day quercetin, a flavonol, for 6 weeks significantly reduced systolic BP by 2.6 mmHg and plasma oxidized LDL concentrations by 14% as compared to placebo. Basu et al. [125] tested the effect of drinking four cups of green tea daily for 8 weeks on body weight, glucose, lipid profile, and biomarkers of oxidative stress in 35 obese subjects with MetS in a randomized, controlled prospective trial, and found the intervention decreased body weight by 2.5 kg, BMI by 1.9 kg/m², and plasma MDA as compared to water. These results suggest that, in addition to the essential vitamins C and E, phytochemical antioxidants such as the flavonoids and related polyphenols should be tested for their potential benefit to reduce the risk of MetS or treat selected signs of MetS.

Czernichow et al. [126] tested the effect of daily antioxidant supplementation (120 mg vitamin C, 30 mg vitamin E, 6 mg β-carotene, and 100 µg selenium and 20 mg zinc) for 7.5 years on the incidence of MetS in a French cohort of 5220 adults (age, 49.4). They found that there was no beneficial effect of this antioxidant supplement on the incidence of MetS in this generally well-nourished population. Given that serum antioxidant status has been found to be inadequate in MetS patient [54], this result suggests that the effect of an antioxidant intervention on the incidence of MetS in a population with poor diets should be examined.

CONCLUSION

Each component of the constellation of MetS signs—dyslipidemia, hyperglycemia, hypertension, and obesity—has been associated, though not unequivocally, with an elevation of oxidative stress status. Moreover, reductions in these conditions appear generally associated with attenuation of biomarkers of oxidative stress, although these inverse correlations are not always strong. Although hypotheses can readily be proffered regarding a vicious cycle of free radicals and pathology in the progression of these conditions and the potential for a beneficial impact of antioxidants in slowing the progress of MetS toward CVD, few direct data are available to support this approach as an adjunct to established lifestyle modifications and drug therapies for prevention or treatment. Nonetheless, the biological plausibility of these relationships clearly warrants further research in this area.

New research should consider variables that are particular to current approaches to MetS; for example, without careful planning, hypocaloric diets can readily be poor in antioxidant nutrients such as carotenoids and vitamin E, particularly when low-fat menus are stressed. Physical activity is to be encouraged, but it is important to recognize that intense exercise can generate free radicals and increase the requirement for antioxidant nutrients. While training regimens can upregulate some antioxidant enzymes, although perhaps not in older adults, this may not obviate the need for greater intake of antioxidant nutrients from food and supplements. Further, some of the drugs used to treat MetS interact with the antioxidant defense network (e.g., statins, which inhibit ubiquinol synthesis and reduce vitamin E status), again suggesting a value for supplementation. Of course, the potential for adverse drug–nutrient interactions, particularly with regard to dietary supplements, should always be considered. As it is always a challenge to design antioxidant interventions to alleviate oxidative stress, studies must be undertaken to determine the optimal combinations and doses, together with specific lifestyle modifications and drug therapies, as well as the best time to intervene in MetS. Importantly, studies must include not only relevant clinical outcomes but also measures of oxidative stress and related pathways such as inflammation. These measures not only will serve to provide a biological basis for the mechanisms of action but will also help to identify individual differences between patients and the nature of responders and nonresponders for each intervention.

REFERENCES

1. Reaven, G. M. 1988. Banting lecture 1988: Role of insulin resistance in human disease. *Diabetes* 37:1595.
2. World Health Organization. 1999. Definition, diagnosis, and classification of diabetes mellitus and its complications. Report of a WHO Consultation, Department of Noncommunicable Disease Surveillance, Geneva, Switzerland.
3. Expert Panel on the Detection, Evaluation, and Treatment of High Blood Cholesterol in Adults. 2001. Executive Summary of the Third Report of the National Cholesterol Education Program (NCEP) Expert Panel on Detection, Evaluation, and Treatment of High Blood Cholesterol in Adults (Adult Treatment Panel III). *JAMA* 285:486.
4. Grundy, S. M. et al. 2004. National Heart, Lung, and Blood Institute; American Heart Association, Definition of metabolic syndrome: Report of the National Heart, Lung, and Blood Institute/American Heart Association conference on scientific issues related to definition. *Circulation* 109:433.
5. Ford, E. S. 2004. The metabolic syndrome and mortality from cardiovascular disease and all-causes: Findings from the National Health and Nutrition Examination Survey II Mortality Study. *Atherosclerosis* 173:309.
6. Ford, E. S., Giles, W. H., and Dietz, W. H. 2002. Prevalence of the metabolic syndrome among U.S. adults: Findings from the third National Health and Nutrition Examination Survey. *JAMA* 287:356.
7. Grundy, S. M. 2005. Metabolic syndrome scientific statement by the American Heart Association and the National Heart, Lung, and Blood Institute. *Arterioscler Thromb Vasc Biol* 25:2243.
8. Brownlee, M. 2001. Biochemistry and molecular cell biology of diabetic complications. *Nature* 414:813.
9. Turko, I. V., Marcondes, S., and Murad, F. 2001. Diabetes-associated nitration of tyrosine and inactivation of succinyl-CoA:3-oxoacid CoA-transferase. *Am J Physiol Heart Circ Physiol* 281:H2289.
10. Maritim, A. C., Sanders, R. A., and Watkins III, J. B. 2003. Diabetes, oxidative stress, and antioxidants: A review. *J Biochem Mol Toxicol* 17:24.
11. Griffiths, H. R. et al. 2002. Biomarkers. *Mol Aspects Med* 23:101.
12. Requena, J. R., Levine, R. L., and Stadtman, E. R. 2003. Recent advances in the analysis of oxidized proteins. *Amino Acids* 25:221.

13. Tarpey, M. M., Wink, D. A., and Grisham, M. B. 2004. Methods for detection of reactive metabolites of oxygen and nitrogen: *In vitro* and *in vivo* considerations. *Am J Physiol Regul Integr Comp Physiol* 286:R431.

14. Cadet, J. et al. 2003. Oxidative damage to DNA: Formation, measurement and biochemical features. *Mutat Res* 531:5.

15. Collins, A. R. 2004. The comet assay for DNA damage and repair: Principles, applications, and limitations. *Mol Biotechnol* 26:249.

16. Abuja, P. M. and Albertini, R. 2001. Methods for monitoring oxidative stress, lipid peroxidation and oxidation resistance of lipoproteins. *Clin Chim Acta* 306:1.

17. Montague, C. T. and O'Rahilly, S. 2000. The perils of portliness: Causes and consequences of visceral adiposity. *Diabetes* 49:883.

18. Matsuzawa, Y., Funahashi, T., and Nakamura, T. 1999. Molecular mechanism of metabolic syndrome X: Contribution of adipocyte-derived bioactive substances. *Ann NY Acad Sci* 892:146.

19. Kahn, B. B. and Flier, J. S. 2000. Obesity and insulin resistance. *J Clin Invest* 106:473.

20. Fenster, C. P. et al. 2002. Obesity, aerobic exercise, and vascular disease: The role of oxidant stress. *Obes Res* 10:964.

21. Furukawa, S. et al. 2004. Increased oxidative stress in obesity and its impact on metabolic syndrome. *J Clin Invest* 114:1752.

22. Keaney Jr., J. F. et al. 2003. Obesity and systemic oxidative stress: Clinical correlates of oxidative stress in the Framingham Study. *Arterioscler Thromb Vasc Biol* 23:434.

23. Urakawa, H. et al. 2003. Oxidative stress is associated with adiposity and insulin resistance in men. *J Clin Endocrinol Metab* 88:4673.

24. Couillard, C. et al. 2005. Circulating levels of oxidative stress markers and endothelial adhesion molecules in men with abdominal obesity. *J Clin Endocrinol Metab* 90:6454.

25. Oliver, S. R., Rosa, J. S., Milne, G. L., Pontello, A. M., Borntrager, H. L., Heydari, S., and Galassetti, P. R. 2010. Increased oxidative stress and altered substrate metabolism in obese children. *Int J Pediatr Obes* 5:436–444.

26. Chiavaroli, V., Giannini, C., D'Adamo, E., de Giorgis, T., Chiarelli, F., and Mohn, A. 2009. Insulin resistance and oxidative stress in children born small and large for gestational age. *Pediatrics* 124:695–702.

27. Visentin, V. et al. Alteration of amine oxidase activity in the adipose tissue of obese subjects. *Obes Res* 12:547.

28. Davi, G. et al. 2002. Platelet activation in obese women: Role of inflammation and oxidant stress. *JAMA* 288:2008 2014.

29. Johansen, J. S. et al. 2005. Oxidative stress and the use of antioxidants in diabetes: Linking basic science to clinical practice. *Cardiovasc Diabetol* 4:5.

30. Koska, J. et al. 2000. Insulin, catecholamines, glucose and antioxidant enzymes in oxidative damage during different loads in healthy humans. *Physiol Res* 49(Suppl. 1):S95.

31. Facchini, F. S. et al. 2000. Relation between insulin resistance and plasma concentrations of lipid hydroperoxides, carotenoids, and tocopherols. *Am J Clin Nutr* 72:776.

32. Koska, J. et al. 1999. Malondialdehyde, lipofuscin and activity of antioxidant enzymes during physical exercise in patients with essential hypertension. *J Hypertens* 17:529.

33. Guxens, M., Fitó, M., Martínez-González, M. A., Salas-Salvadó, J., Estruch, R., Vinyoles, E., Fiol, M., Corella, D., Arós, F., Gómez-Gracia, E., Ruiz-Gutiérrez, V., Lapetra, J., Ros, E., Vila, J., and Covas, M. I. 2009. Hypertensive status and lipoprotein oxidation in an elderly population at high cardiovascular risk. *Am J Hypertens* 22:68–73.

34. Konukoglu, D. et al. 2003. Plasma homocysteine levels in obese and non-obese subjects with or without hypertension; its relationship with oxidative stress and copper. *Clin Biochem* 36:405.

35. Stojiljkovic, M. P. et al. 2002. Increasing plasma fatty acids elevates F2-isoprostanes in humans: Implications for the cardiovascular risk factor cluster. *J Hypertens* 20:1215.

36. Hansel, B. et al. 2004. Metabolic syndrome is associated with elevated oxidative stress and dysfunctional dense high-density lipoprotein particles displaying impaired antioxidative activity. *J Clin Endocrinol Metab* 89:4963.

37. Sjogren, P. et al. 2005. Measures of oxidized low-density lipoprotein and oxidative stress are not related and not elevated in otherwise healthy men with the metabolic syndrome. *Arterioscler Thromb Vasc Biol* 25:2580.

38. Witztum, J. L. 1994. The oxidation hypothesis of atherosclerosis. *Lancet* 344:793.

39. Myara, I. et al. 2003. Lipoprotein oxidation and plasma vitamin E in nondiabetic normotensive obese patients. *Obes Res* 11:112.

40. Kassi, E., Dalamaga, M., Faviou, E., Hroussalas, G., Kazanis, K., Nounopoulos, C. H., and Dionyssiou-Asteriou, A. 2009. Circulating oxidized LDL levels, current smoking and obesity in postmenopausal women. *Atherosclerosis* 205:279–283.

41. Kopprasch, S. et al. 2002. *In vivo* evidence for increased oxidation of circulating LDL in impaired glucose tolerance. *Diabetes* 51:3102.

42. Mizuno, T. et al. 2004. Insulin resistance increases circulating malondialdehyde-modified LDL and impairs endothelial function in healthy young men. *Int J Cardiol* 97:455.

43. Park, K., Gross, M., Lee, D. H., Holvoet, P., Himes, J. H., Shikany, J. M., and Jacobs Jr., D. R. 2009. Oxidative stress and insulin resistance: The coronary artery risk development in young adults study. *Diabetes Care* 32:1302–1307.

44. Schwenke, D. C. et al. 2003. Insulin resistance atherosclerosis study: Differences in LDL oxidizability by glycemic status: The insulin resistance atherosclerosis study. *Diabetes Care* 26:1449.

45. Holvoet, P. et al. 2004. The metabolic syndrome, circulating oxidized LDL, and risk of myocardial infarction in well-functioning elderly people in the health, aging, and body composition cohort. *Diabetes* 53:1068.

46. Kotani, K., Satoh, N., Kato, Y., Araki, R., Koyama, K., Okajima, T., Tanabe, M., Oishi, M., Yamakage, H., Yamada, K., Hattori, M., and Shimatsu, A. 2009. Japan Obesity and Metabolic Syndrome Study Group. A novel oxidized low-density lipoprotein marker, serum amyloid A-LDL, is associated with obesity and the metabolic syndrome. *Atherosclerosis* 204:526–531.

47. Fagerberg, B., Bokemark, L., and Hulthe, J. 2001. The metabolic syndrome, smoking, and antibodies to oxidized LDL in 58-year-old clinically healthy men. *Nutr Metab Cardiovasc Dis* 11:227.

48. Sigurdardottir, V., Fagerberg, B., and Hulthe, J. 2002. Circulating oxidized low-density lipoprotein (LDL) is associated with risk factors of the metabolic syndrome and LDL size in clinically healthy 58-year old men (AIR study). *J Intern Med* 252:440.

49. Beckman, J. S. and Koppenol, W. H. 1996. Nitric oxide, superoxide, and peroxynitrite: The good, the bad, and ugly. *Am J Physiol* 271:C1424.

50. Ceriello, A. et al. 2001. Detection of nitrotyrosine in the diabetic plasma: Evidence of oxidative stress. *Diabetologia* 44:834.

51. Ceriello, A. et al. 2002. Role of hyperglycemia in nitrotyrosine postprandial generation. *Diabetes Care* 25:1439.

52. Marfella, R. et al. 2001. Acute hyperglycemia induces an oxidative stress in healthy subjects. *J Clin Invest* 108:635.

53. Bo, S. et al. 2005. Relationships between human serum resistin, inflammatory markers and insulin resistance. *Int J Obes (Lond.)* 29:1315.

54. Ford, E. S., Mokdad, A. H., Giles, W. H., and Brown, D. W. 2003. The metabolic syndrome and antioxidant concentrations: Findings from the Third National Health and Nutrition Examination Survey. *Diabetes* 52:2346–2352.

55. Sugiura, M., Nakamura, M., Ogawa, K., Ikoma, Y., Matsumoto, H., Ando, F., Shimokata, H., and Yano, M. 2008. Associations of serum carotenoid concentrations with the metabolic syndrome: Interactions with smoking. *Br J Nutr* 100:1297–1306.

56. Coyne, T., Ibiebele, T. I., Baade, P. D., McClintock, C. S., and Shaw, J. E. 2009. Metabolic syndrome and serum carotenoids: Findings of a cross-sectional study in Queensland, Australia. *Br J Nutr* 102:1668–1677.

57. Sluijs, I., Beulens, J. W., Grobbee, D. E., and van der Schouw, Y. T. 2009. Dietary carotenoid intake is associated with lower prevalence of metabolic syndrome in middle-aged and elderly men. *J Nutr* 139:987–992.

58. Beydoun, M. A., Shroff, M. R., Chen, X., Beydoun, H. A., Wang, Y., and Zonderman, A. B. 2011. Serum antioxidant status is associated with metabolic syndrome among US adults: Findings from recent national surveys. *J Nutr* 141:903–913.

59. Botella-Carretero, J. I., Balsa, J. A., Vázquez, C., Peromingo, R., Díaz-Enriquez, M., and Escobar-Morreale, H. F. 2010. Retinol and alpha-tocopherol in morbid obesity and nonalcoholic fatty liver disease. *Obes Surg* 20:69–76.

60. Menke, T. et al. 2004. Comparison of coenzyme Q10 plasma levels in obese and normal weight children. *Clin Chim Acta* 349:121.

61. Konukoglu, D. et al. 1997. The erythrocyte glutathione levels during oral glucose tolerance test. *J Endocrinol Invest* 20:471.

62. Ma, S. W., Tomlinson, B., and Benzie, I. F. 2005. A study of the effect of oral glucose loading on plasma oxidant:antioxidant balance in normal subjects. *Eur J Nutr* 44:250.

63. Csabi, G. et al. 2000. Presence of metabolic cardiovascular syndrome in obese children. *Eur J Pediatr* 159:91.
64. Molnar, D., Decsi, T., and Koletzko, B. 2004. Reduced antioxidant status in obese children with multi-metabolic syndrome. *Int J Obes Relat Metab Disord* 28:1197.
65. Miles, M. V. et al. 2004. Coenzyme Q10 changes are associated with metabolic syndrome. *Clin Chim Acta* 344:173.
66. Ozata, M. et al. 2002. Increased oxidative stress and hypozincemia in male obesity. *Clin Biochem* 35:627.
67. Ji, L. L. 2002. Exercise-induced modulation of antioxidant defense. *Ann NY Acad Sci* 959:82.
68. Shin, M. J. and Park, E. 2006. Contribution of insulin resistance to reduced antioxidant enzymes and vitamins in nonobese Korean children. *Clin Chim Acta* 365(1–2):200.
69. Pedro-Botet, J. et al. 2000. Decreased endogenous antioxidant enzymatic status in essential hypertension. *J Hum Hypertens* 14:343.
70. Durrington, P. N., Mackness, B., and Mackness, M. I. 2001. Paraoxonase and atherosclerosis. *Arterioscler Thromb Vasc Biol* 21:473.
71. Watson, A. D. et al. 1995. Protective effect of high density lipoprotein associated paraoxonase. Inhibition of the biological activity of minimally oxidized low density lipoprotein. *J Clin Invest* 96:2882.
72. Ferretti, G. et al. 2005. Paraoxonase activity in high-density lipoproteins: A comparison between healthy and obese females. *J Clin Endocrinol Metab* 90:1728.
73. Chen, X., Wu, Y., Liu, L., Su, Y., Peng, Y., Jiang, L., Liu, X., and Huang, D. 2010. Relationship between high density lipoprotein antioxidant activity and carotid arterial intima-media thickness in patients with essential hypertension. *Clin Exp Hypertens* 32:13–20.
74. Garin, M. C. et al. 2005. Small, dense lipoprotein particles and reduced paraoxonase-1 in patients with the metabolic syndrome. *J Clin Endocrinol Metab* 90:2264.
75. Boemi, M. et al. 2001. Serum paraoxonase is reduced in type 1 diabetic patients compared to non-diabetic, first degree relatives: Influence on the ability of HDL to protect LDL from oxidation. *Atherosclerosis* 155:229.
76. Hashemi, M., Kordi-Tamandani, D. M., Sharifi, N., Moazeni-Roodi, A., Kaykhaei, M. A., Narouie, B., and Torkmanzehi, A. 2011. Serum paraoxonase and arylesterase activities in metabolic syndrome in Zahedan, southeast Iran. *Eur J Endocrinol* 164:219–222.
77. Senti, M. et al. 2003. Antioxidant paraoxonase 1 activity in the metabolic syndrome. *J Clin Endocrinol Metab* 88:5422.
78. Tabur, S., Torun, A. N., Sabuncu, T., Turan, M. N., Celik, H., Ocak, A. R., and Aksoy, N. 2010. Non-diabetic metabolic syndrome and obesity do not affect serum paraoxonase and arylesterase activities but do affect oxidative stress and inflammation. *Eur J Endocrinol* 162(3):535–541.
79. Grundy, S. M. et al. 2005. American Heart Association; National Heart, Lung, and Blood Institute, Diagnosis and management of the metabolic syndrome: An American Heart Association/National Heart, Lung, and Blood Institute Scientific Statement. *Circulation* 112:2735.
80. Franklin, B. A. et al. 2004. A cardioprotective 'polypill'? Independent and additive benefits of lifestyle modification. *Am J Cardiol* 94:162.
81. Dumortier, M. et al. 2003. Low intensity endurance exercise targeted for lipid oxidation improves body composition and insulin sensitivity in patients with the metabolic syndrome. *Diabetes Metab* 29:509.
82. Petrella, R. J. 2005. Can adoption of regular exercise later in life prevent metabolic risk for cardiovascular disease? *Diabetes Care* 28:694.
83. Ekelund, U. et al. 2005. Physical activity energy expenditure predicts progression toward the metabolic syndrome independently of aerobic fitness in middle-aged healthy Caucasians: The Medical Research Council Ely Study. *Diabetes Care* 28:1195.
84. Stewart, K. J. et al. 2005. Exercise and risk factors associated with metabolic syndrome in older adults. *Am J Prev Med* 28:9.
85. American College of Sports Medicine. 1993. Position stand: Physical activity, physical fitness, and hypertension. *Med Sci Sports Exerc* 25:i–x.
86. Pialoux, V., Brown, A. D., Leigh, R., Friedenreich, C. M., and Poulin, M. J. 2009. Effect of cardiorespiratory fitness on vascular regulation and oxidative stress in postmenopausal women. *Hypertension* 54:1014–1020.
87. Vasankari, T. J. et al. 1998. Reduced oxidized LDL levels after a 10-month exercise program. *Med Sci Sports Exerc* 30:1496.
88. Roberts, C. K., Vaziri, N. D., and Barnard, R. J. 2002. Effect of diet and exercise intervention on blood pressure, insulin, oxidative stress, and nitric oxide availability. *Circulation* 106:2530.

89. Roberts, C. K. et al. 2006. Effect of a diet and exercise intervention on oxidative stress, inflammation, MMP-9 and monocyte chemotactic activity in men with metabolic syndrome factors. *J Appl Physiol* 100:1657.

90. Dandona, P. et al. 2001. The suppressive effect of dietary restriction and weight loss in the obese on the generation of reactive oxygen species by leukocytes, lipid peroxidation, and protein carbonylation. *J Clin Endocrinol Metab* 86:355.

91. Hsieh, C. J. 2005. Orlistat for obesity: Benefits beyond weight loss. *Diabetes Res Clin Pract* 67:78.

92. Yesilbursa, D. et al. 2005. Lipid peroxides in obese patients and effects of weight loss with orlistat on lipid peroxides levels. *Int J Obes (Lond)* 29:142.

93. Samuelsson, L., Gottsater, A., and Lindgarde, F. 2003. Decreasing levels of tumour necrosis factor alpha and interleukin 6 during lowering of body mass index with orlistat or placebo in obese subjects with cardiovascular risk factors. *Diabetes Obes Metab* 5:195.

94. Ozcelik, O. et al. 2005. Exercise training as an adjunct to orlistat therapy reduces oxidative stress in obese subjects. *Tohoku J Exp Med* 206:313.

95. Xiang, A. H. et al. 2005. Effect of thiazolidinedione treatment on progression of subclinical atherosclerosis in premenopausal women at high risk for type 2 diabetes. *J Clin Endocrinol Metab* 90:1986.

96. Tankova, T. et al. 2003. The effect of repaglinide on insulin secretion and oxidative stress in type 2 diabetic patients. *Diabetes Res Clin Pract* 59:43.

97. Tack, C. J. et al. 1998. Troglitazone decreases the proportion of small, dense LDL and increases the resistance of LDL to oxidation in obese subjects. *Diabetes Care* 21:796.

98. Staffileno, B. A. 2005. Treating hypertension with cardioprotective therapies: The role of ACE inhibitors, ARBs, and beta-blockers. *J Cardiovasc Nurs* 20:354.

99. Saez, G. T. et al. 2004. Factors related to the impact of antihypertensive treatment in antioxidant activities and oxidative stress by-products in human hypertension. *Am J Hypertens* 17:809.

100. Muda, P. et al. 2005. Effect of antihypertensive treatment with candesartan or amlodipine on glutathione and its redox status, homocysteine and vitamin concentrations in patients with essential hypertension. *J Hypertens* 23:105.

101. Nashar, K. et al. 2004. Angiotensin receptor blockade improves arterial distensibility and reduces exercise-induced pressor responses in obese hypertensive patients with the metabolic syndrome. *Am J Hypertens* 17:477.

102. Sola, S. et al. 2005. Irbesartan and lipoic acid improve endothelial function and reduce markers of inflammation in the metabolic syndrome: Results of the Irbesartan and Lipoic Acid in Endothelial Dysfunction (ISLAND) study. *Circulation* 111:343.

103. Wollin, S. D. and Jones, P. J. 2003. Alpha-lipoic acid and cardiovascular disease. *J Nutr* 133:3327.

104. Ballantyne, C. M. et al. 2001. Influence of low high-density lipoprotein cholesterol and elevated triglyceride on coronary heart disease events and response to simvastatin therapy in 4S. *Circulation* 104:3046.

105. Deedwania, P. C. et al. 2005. STELLAR Study Group, Effects of rosuvastatin, atorvastatin, simvastatin, and pravastatin on atherogenic dyslipidemia in patients with characteristics of the metabolic syndrome. *Am J Cardiol* 95:360.

106. Oranje, W. A. et al. 2001. Effect of atorvastatin on LDL oxidation and antioxidants in normocholesterolemic type 2 diabetic patients. *Clin Chim Acta* 311:91.

107. ter Avest, E. et al. 2005. Effect of rosuvastatin on insulin sensitivity in patients with familial combined hyperlipidaemia. *Eur J Clin Invest* 35:558.

108. Kural, B. V. et al. 2004. The effects of lipid-lowering therapy on paraoxonase activities and their relationships with the oxidant-antioxidant system in patients with dyslipidemia. *Coronary Artery Dis* 15:277.

109. Palomaki, A., Malminiemi, K., and MetSa-Ketela, T. 1997. Enhanced oxidizability of ubiquinol and alphatocopherol during lovastatin treatment. *FEBS Lett* 410:254.

110. Mabuchi, H. et al. 2005. Reduction of serum ubiquinol-10 and ubiquinone-10 levels by atorvastatin in hypercholesterolemic patients. *J Atheroscler Thromb* 12:111.

111. Manuel-Keenoy, B. et al. 2004. Impact of vitamin E supplementation on lipoprotein peroxidation and composition in type 1 diabetic patients treated with atorvastatin. *Atherosclerosis* 175:369.

112. Zhang, B. et al. 2005. A comparative crossover study of the effects of fluvastatin and pravastatin (FP-COS) on circulating autoantibodies to oxidized LDL in patients with hypercholesterolemia. *J Atheroscler Thromb* 12:41.

113. Thallinger, C. et al. 2005. The ability of statins to protect low density lipoprotein from oxidation in hypercholesterolemic patients. *Int J Clin Pharmacol Ther* 43:551.

114. Shishehbor, M. H. et al. 2003. Statins promote potent systemic antioxidant effects through specific inflammatory pathways. *Circulation* 108:426.

115. Hajjar, I. M. et al. 2002. A randomized, double-blind, controlled trial of vitamin C in the management of hypertension and lipids. *Am J Ther* 9:289.
116. Ward, N. C. et al. 2005. The combination of vitamin C and grape-seed polyphenols increases blood pressure: A randomized, double-blind, placebo-controlled trial. *J Hypertens* 23:427.
117. Brockes, C. et al. 2003. Vitamin E prevents extensive lipid peroxidation in patients with hypertension. *Br J Biomed Sci* 60:5.
118. Azzi, A. et al. 2002. Non-antioxidant molecular functions of alpha-tocopherol (vitamin E). *FEBS Lett* 519:8.
119. Barbagallo, M. et al. 1999. Effects of vitamin E and glutathione on glucose metabolism: Role of magnesium. *Hypertension* 34:1002.
120. Manning, P. J. et al. 2004. Effect of high-dose vitamin E on insulin resistance and associated parameters in overweight subjects. *Diabetes Care* 27:2166.
121. McSorley, P. T. et al. 2005. Endothelial function, insulin action and cardiovascular risk factors in young healthy adult offspring of parents with type 2 diabetes: Effect of vitamin E in a randomized double-blind, controlled clinical trial. *Diabet Med* 22:703.
122. Skrha, J. et al. 1999. Insulin action and fibrinolysis influenced by vitamin E in obese type 2 diabetes mellitus. *Diabetes Res Clin Pract* 44:27.
123. Hildebrandt, W. et al. 2004. Effect of thiol antioxidant on body fat and insulin reactivity. *J Mol Med* 82:336.
124. Egert, S., Bosy-Westphal, A., Seiberl, J., Kürbitz, C., Settler, U., Plachta-Danielzik, S., Wagner, A. E., Frank, J., Schrezenmeir, J., Rimbach, G., Wolffram, S., and Müller, M. J. 2009. Quercetin reduces systolic blood pressure and plasma oxidised low-density lipoprotein concentrations in overweight subjects with a high-cardiovascular disease risk phenotype: A double-blinded, placebo-controlled cross-over study. *Br J Nutr* 102:1065–1074.
125. Basu, A., Sanchez, K., Leyva, M. J., Wu, M., Betts, N. M., Aston, C. E., and Lyons, T. J. 2010. Green tea supplementation affects body weight, lipids, and lipid peroxidation in obese subjects with metabolic syndrome. *J Am Coll Nutr* 29:31–40.
126. Czernichow, S., Vergnaud, A. C., Galan, P., Arnaud, J., Favier, A., Faure, H., Huxley, R., Hercberg, S., and Ahluwalia, N. 2009. Effects of long-term antioxidant supplementation and association of serum antioxidant concentrations with risk of metabolic syndrome in adults. *Am J Clin Nutr* 90:329–335.

15 Obesity and Type 2 Diabetes

Subhashini Yaturu, MD, FACE and Sushil K. Jain, PhD

CONTENTS

ABBREVIATIONS

ADA	American Diabetes Association
BMI	body mass index
BRFSS	Behavioral Risk Factor Surveillance System
CAD	coronary artery disease
CDC	Centers for Disease Control
CRP	C-reactive protein
CVD	cardiovascular disease
DPP	Diabetes Prevention Program
ED	endothelial dysfunction
EGO	endogenous glucose output
FFA	free fatty acid
FPG	fasting plasma glucose
HDL	high-density lipoprotein
HDL-C	high-density lipoprotein cholesterol
IGT	impaired glucose tolerance
IRS	insulin resistance syndrome
LDL	low-density lipoprotein
LDL-C	low-density lipoprotein cholesterol
NHANES	National Health and Nutrition Examination Survey
XENDOS	Xenical in the Prevention of Diabetes in Obese Subjects

DEFINITIONS

Body mass index (BMI) calculated by weight (kg)/height (m^2) and adjusted for height is used as a measure of weight standards.

Overweight is defined as a BMI of 25.0–29.9 and obesity as a BMI of ≥ 30.0.[1]

Morbid obesity is the term used for BMI > 40 kg/m^2.

Insulin resistance[2] is defined as a failure of target organs to respond normally to the action of insulin.

Insulin resistance syndrome[3] *(IRS)* refers to the cluster of abnormalities that occur more commonly in insulin-resistant individuals. These include glucose intolerance, dyslipidemia, endothelial dysfunction and elevated procoagulant factors, hemodynamic changes, elevated inflammatory markers, abnormal uric acid metabolism, increased ovarian testosterone secretion in women, and sleep-disordered breathing.

Metabolic syndrome (MS), as defined by the National Cholesterol Education Program Adult Treatment Panel III (NCEP ATP III),[4] is a cluster of metabolic abnormalities with insulin resistance as a major characteristic. The presence of any three of the five components is sufficient for diagnosis. The components of MS include (a) abdominal obesity (waist circumference >102 cm [40 in.] in men, >88 cm [35 in.] in women); (b) hypertriglyceridemia (≥ 150 mg/dL); (c) low HDL-C (<40 mg/dL in men, <50 mg/dL in women); (d) high blood pressure ($\geq 130/85$ mm Hg); and (e) high fasting glucose.

INTRODUCTION

Obesity and diabetes are emerging pandemics in the twenty-first century. The prevalence of overweight (body mass index [BMI] between 25 and 30 kg/m^2) and obesity (BMI of 30 kg/m^2 or higher) is increasing rapidly worldwide, especially in developing countries. Both are major public health problems throughout the world and are associated with significant, potentially life-threatening comorbidities. There is a strong association between obesity and type 2 diabetes. The increase in the prevalence of diabetes parallels that of obesity. Some experts call this dual epidemic diabesity. Not all subjects with type 2 diabetes are obese, and many obese subjects do not have diabetes, but most of the subjects with type 2 diabetes are overweight or obese. Overweight and obesity, as well as type 2 diabetes mellitus (T2DM), are largely preventable through changing away from lifestyles that promote sedentary habits and overconsumption of energy. The health consequences and economic costs of the overweight, obesity, and type 2 diabetes epidemics are enormous. Significant numbers of obese individuals have diabetes. Both obesity and type 2 diabetes feature insulin resistance and similar atherogenic lipid profiles such as increased triglycerides and decreased HDL-C. The genetic basis of human obesity predisposing individuals to insulin resistance and the development of type 2 diabetes is multigenic rather than monogenic. Current clinical guidelines acknowledge the therapeutic strength of exercise intervention for prevention and treatment of diabetes.

PREVALENCE

Obesity and diabetes are public health problems that have raised concern worldwide. The prevalence of diabetes parallels the increasing prevalence of obesity. The World Health Organization (WHO) projects that there are currently 2.3 billion overweight people aged 15 years and above and that there will be over 700 million obese people worldwide in 2015 (http://www.who.int/mediacentre/factsheets/fs311/en/). One consequence of obesity is an increased risk of developing type 2 diabetes. Elevated BMI and waist circumference (WC) were significantly associated with type 2 diabetes. Meta-analysis of studies that looked at this association produced pooled relative risk (RR) [95% CI] across categories of BMI of 2.40 [2.12–2.72] and 6.74 [5.55–8.19] in men, while the corresponding RR in women were 3.92 [3.10–4.97] and 12.41 [9.03–17.06].[5] The pooled RR [95% CI] across categories of WC were 2.36 [1.76–3.15] and 5.67 [4.46–7.20] in men, and the pooled RRs [95% CI] based on the same two studies were 2.27 [1.67–3.10] and 5.13 [3.81–6.90] in women, respectively.[5] The prevalence of diabetes is increasing in the United States, and the diagnosed diabetes increased from 0.9% in 1958 to 6.3% in 2008. In 2008, 18.8 million people had diagnosed diabetes, compared to only 1.6 million in 1958 (http://www.cdc.gov/diabetes/statistics/slides/long_term_trends.pdf). According to the International Diabetes Federation (IDF), it is estimated that approximately 285 million people worldwide, or 6.6%, in the age group 20–79, will have diabetes in 2010 (http://www.diabetesatlas.org/map), some 70% of whom live in low- and middle-income countries. This number is expected to increase by more than 50% in the next 20 years if preventive programs are not put in place. By 2030, some 438 million people, or 7.8% of the adult population, are projected to have diabetes (Figure 15.1). Type 2 diabetes, which is the predominant form of diabetes worldwide, constitutes 85%–95% of all diabetes. Obesity and overweight currently affect 15% and 20% of Spanish children,[6] respectively.

DIAGNOSTIC CRITERIA FOR OBESITY AND OVERWEIGHT

BMI, calculated by weight (kg)/height (m^2) and adjusted for height, is used as a measure of weight standards. The WHO defines "overweight" as a BMI equal to or more than 25 and "obesity" as a BMI equal to or more than 30. These cutoff points provide a benchmark for individual assessment, but there is evidence that risk of chronic disease in population increases progressively from a BMI of 21.

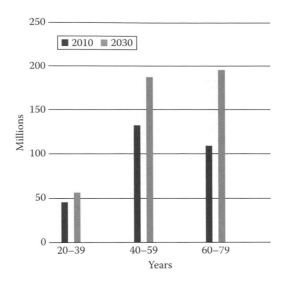

FIGURE 15.1 Number of people with diabetes by age group, 2010 and 2030. (From *IDF Diabetes Atlas*, 4th edn., International Diabetes Federation, Brussels, Belgium 2009.)

DIAGNOSTIC CRITERIA FOR DIABETES

The criteria for diagnosis of diabetes mellitus as recommended by the American Diabetes Association[7] include $A_{1C} \geq 6.5\%$ or fasting plasma glucose (FPG) value after an 8 h fast ≥ 126 mg/dL, or 2 h postload glucose (PG) ≥ 200 mg/dL (11.1 mmol/L) during an oral glucose tolerance test (OGTT), or symptoms of diabetes mellitus and a random plasma glucose concentration ≥ 200 mg/dL (11.1 mmol/L).

IMPACT OF OBESITY ON TYPE 2 DIABETES

BMI, Visceral Adiposity, and Type 2 Diabetes

The increasing prevalence of obesity is said to play a significant role in the increase in cases of type 2 diabetes. The relative risk of type 2 diabetes increases as BMI increases above 23,[8] and the association was found to be stronger in younger age groups from the Asia-Pacific region.[9] Weight gain in early adulthood is related to a higher risk and earlier onset of type 2 diabetes than is weight gain between 40 and 55 years of age.[10] Data from the Third National Health and Nutrition Examination Survey (NHANES III) indicate that two-thirds of adults, (Figure 15.2) both men and women, had BMI values >27 kg/m[2].[11] The risk of diabetes increases linearly with BMI; the prevalence of diabetes increased from 2% in those with a BMI of 25–29.9 kg/m[2], to 8% in those with a BMI of 30–34.9 kg/m[2], and finally to 13% in those with a BMI greater than 35 kg/m[2].[12] Although the prevalence of diagnosed diabetes has increased significantly over the last decade, the prevalences of undiagnosed diabetes and impaired fasting glucose (IFG) have remained relatively stable.[12,13] The risk of type 2 diabetes increases with an increase in BMI >22 kg/m[2].[7,14] More than generalized obesity, the risk of obesity increases with increase in WC, waist-to-hip ratio (WHR) visceral adiposity (VAT), or abdominal obesity.[15–18] In a review of 17 prospective and 35 cross-sectional studies in adults aged 18–74 years, either BMI or WC and WHR was predicted or was associated with type 2 diabetes independently.[19]

Although an increase in weight and/or BMI is a risk factor for diabetes, an increase in BMI is a better predictor of diabetes. Prospective studies in nondiabetic overweight adults noted a 49% increase in the incidence of diabetes in 10 years for every 1 kg/year increase in body weight, and similarly, each kg of weight lost annually over 10 years was associated with a 33% lower risk of

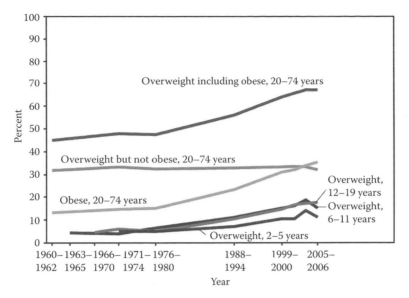

FIGURE 15.2 Overweight and obesity. (CDC/NCHS, *Health United States*, 2009. Data from the National Health Survey and the National Health and Nutrition Examination Survey.)

diabetes in the subsequent 10 years. Similar studies in Pima Indians reported that weight gain was significantly related to diabetes incidence only in those who were not initially overweight (BMI <27.3 kg/m²).[20,21] Similarly, in the Behavioral Risk Factor Surveillance System (BRFSS) for 1991–1998, Mokdad et al.[22] reported that every 1 kg increase in average self-reported weight was associated with a 9% increase in the prevalence of diabetes.[23]

Waist Circumference and Risk of Diabetes

Studies find that visceral fat mass is more strongly associated with an abnormal metabolic profile than upper body subcutaneous fat. The National Institutes of Health (NIH) cutoff uses WC to identify those at increased risk as the health risk is greater in individuals with high WC values in the normal weight, overweight, and class I obese BMI categories compared with those with normal WC values, as shown in Table 15.1.[24] In a recent Jackson heart study, abdominal VAT and subcutaneous adipose tissue are both associated with adverse cardiometabolic risk factors, but VAT remains more strongly associated with these risk factors.[25] Potential mechanisms of this increased risk may include increased free fatty acid (FFA) release and alterations in adipokines. Evidence from studies that manipulate FFA concentrations suggests that a number of these metabolic abnormalities are caused by elevated FFAs, because the most consistent abnormality in FFA metabolism is failure to suppress FFA in response to insulin/meal ingestion.[26] In people with visceral obesity, omental and mesenteric fat may play a special role in delivering both excess FFA and interleukin-6 (IL-6) to the liver.[26]

IMPACT OF CHILDHOOD OBESITY ON TYPE 2 DIABETES

Obesity now affects 15% of children and adolescents in the United States. Similar to the situation observed in adults, diseases that are commonly associated with obesity such as type 2 diabetes, hypertension (HTN), hyperlipidemia, gallbladder disease, nonalcoholic steatohepatitis,[27,28] sleep apnea, and orthopedic complications are now increasingly observed in children.[29,30] There is evidence that the prenatal, early childhood, and adolescent periods are critical in the development of obesity. There are significant negative health outcomes associated with childhood obesity, including the presence of cardiovascular risk factors, and greater prevalence of various medical problems including insulin resistance, T2DM, metabolic syndrome (MS), orthopedic problems, and

TABLE 15.1
ORs for Metabolic Diseases Comparing High vs. Normal WC within Different BMI Categories[a]

| | BMI Categories | | | | | |
| | Normal Weight | | Overweight | | Class I Obese | |
	Unadjusted OR (95% CI)	Adjusted OR (95% CI)[b]	Unadjusted OR (95% CI)	Adjusted OR (95% CI)[b]	Unadjusted OR (95% CI)	Adjusted OR (95% CI)[b]
Men						
HTN	8.56 (2.60–28.20)[c]	2.26 (0.58–8.70)	2.71 (2.16–3.41)[c]	1.47 (1.08–1.96)[c]	2.60 (1.21–5.61)[c]	1.09 (0.40–2.97)
Type 2 diabetes	5.97 (3.17–11.22)[c]	2.16 (1.11–4.21)[c]	4.26 (2.52–7.17)[c]	1.99 (0.75–5.07)	2.53 (0.81–7.89)	0.97 (0.30–3.19)
Hypercholesterolemia	2.07 (0.79–5.39)	1.31 (0.46–3.72)	2.06 (1.49–2.86)[c]	1.48 (1.00–2.16)[c]	1.23 (0.65–2.33)	0.91 (0.42–1.97)
High LDL cholesterol level	2.54 (0.52–12.59)	1.71 (0.33–8.81)	1.56 (1.02–2.38)[c]	1.31 (0.83–2.08)	0.85 (0.25–2.92)	0.71 (0.16–3.23)
Low HDL cholesterol level	0.63 (0.18–2.15)	0.54 (0.16–1.75)	1.77 (1.19–2.59)[c]	1.55 (1.07–2.31)[c]	1.35 (0.80–2.27)	1.80 (0.90–3.58)
Hypertriglyceridemia	1.33 (0.39–4.53)	0.93 (0.26–3.34)	2.06 (1.49–2.89)[c]	1.90 (1.34–2.75)[c]	1.86 (0.96–3.60)	1.55 (0.69–3.47)
MS	1.76 (0.33–9.62)	0.67 (0.12–3.69)	3.21 (2.33–4.42)[c]	2.13 (1.49–3.16)[c]	3.37 (1.79–6.32)[c]	2.90 (1.25–6.75)[c]
Women						
HTN	5.69 (4.46–7.27)[c]	1.87 (1.27–2.77)[c]	4.27 (3.10–5.86)[c]	2.04 (1.41–2.98)[c]	33.52 (8.44–133.23)[c]	15.85 (4.17–60.26)[c]
Type 2 diabetes	4.51 (2.43–8.37)[c]	1.52 (0.68–3.43)	6.79 (3.45–13.37)[c]	4.07 (1.91–8.70)[c]	34.20 (4.14–282.30)[c]	14.82 (1.69–130.10)[c]
Hypercholesterolemia	3.69 (2.56–5.31)[c]	1.71 (1.08–2.71)[c]	2.25 (1.67–3.04)[c]	1.43 (1.07–1.91)[c]	3.83 (0.54–26.83)	2.27 (0.29–17.67)
High LDL cholesterol level	3.26 (1.83–5.82)[c]	1.67 (0.96–2.91)	2.29 (1.27–4.71)[c]	1.50 (0.85–2.65)	37.76 (4.65–306–63)[c]	29.17 (3.44–247.00)[c]
Low HDL cholesterol level	2.09 (1.31–3.37)[c]	1.93 (1.13–3.30)[c]	1.58 (1.06–2.35)[c]	1.46 (0.95–2.26)	2.42 (0.56–10.45)	2.27 (0.48–10.74)
Hypertriglyceridemia	5.56 (3.76–8.21)[c]	3.11 (1.78–5.43)[c]	2.34 (1.55–3.55)[c]	1.90 (1.22–2.96)[c]	3.23 (0.42–25.14)	2.04 (0.28–14.98)
MS	4.90 (3.41–7.03)[c]	1.76 (1.09–2.86)[c]	5.18 (3.03–8.85)[c]	2.20 (1.24–3.92)[c]	74.27 (8.99–613.52)[c]	28.60 (3.71–220.23)[c]

Source: Janssen, I. et al. *Arch. Intern. Med.*, 162, 2074, 2002.

[a] Subjects with a normal waist WC value were used for the reference category (OR, 1.00). The WC and BMI categories are described in the "Definition of Groups and Terms" subsection of the "Subjects and Methods" section; CI indicates confidence interval. Other abbreviations are explained in the first footnote to Table 15.1.

[b] Adjusted for age, race, physical activity, smoking, alcohol intake, and the poverty–income ratio.

[c] *P* < .05, compared with the normal WC group.

pseudotumor cerebri. Of further concern is the increased risk for obesity in adulthood with its attendant comorbidities. BMI in childhood changes substantially with age and is not applicable when defining childhood obesity.[31–33] In the United States, the 85th and 95th percentiles of BMI for age and sex based on nationally representative survey data have been recommended as cutoff points to identify overweight and obesity.[34] Pathophysiologic studies in youth are limited and in some cases conflicting. T2DM in children and adolescents is an important public health problem directly related to the epidemic of childhood obesity. The increasing rates of youth T2DM parallel the escalating rates of obesity, which is the major risk factor affecting insulin sensitivity.[35] Altered glucose metabolism, manifested as impaired glucose tolerance (IGT), appears early in obese children and adolescents. The prevalence of the MS is considerable among obese adolescents.[36,37] Obese young people with IGT are characterized by marked peripheral insulin resistance and a relative beta-cell failure.[38] Lipid deposition in muscle and the visceral compartment, and not only adiposity per se, is related to increased peripheral insulin resistance, the "driving force" of the MS. Other elements of the MS, such as dyslipidemia and HTN, are already present in obese youngsters and worsen with the degree of obesity.[39] Altered glucose metabolism in obese youth represents an element of the "insulin resistance syndrome," comprising obesity, dyslipidemia, and HTN. The dynamics of glucose tolerance status in these youngsters seems to be more rapid than in adults, thus representing a narrow window of opportunity for successful intervention to prevent diabetes.[40] White adolescent subjects with obesity without DM were noted to have approximately 50% lower levels of adiponectin.[40,41] In addition, the study noted that hypoadiponectinemia was a strong and independent correlate of insulin resistance, β-cell dysfunction, and increased abdominal adiposity.[41] It is hypothesized that abdominal obesity leads to insulin resistance partly through decreased adiponectin.[42]

NEONATAL SIZE AND IMPACT OF CATCH-UP GROWTH

Neonatal size and body composition are influenced by parental size, maternal food intake, physical activity, and circulating concentrations of nutrients and metabolites (folate, glucose, triglycerides, cholesterol, etc.). Maternal insulin resistance promotes transfer of nutrients to the fetus. Childhood growth seems to be more influenced by paternal genetic factors, whereas intrauterine growth is more influenced by maternal factors (intrauterine environment).[43] Accelerated childhood growth is another risk factor for adiposity and insulin resistance, especially in children with low birth weight.[42] Low birth weight predicts central obesity. High BMI at birth and low socioeconomic status of the population in the Child Health Centres (CHC) were shown to be independent determinants for overweight.[44] Low maternal weight[45] as well as overweight and obese women have increased risks of preterm birth and induced preterm birth.[46] Premature infants are at increased risk for persistent growth failure, neurodevelopmental impairment, HTN, and diabetes.[47] The risk of type 2 diabetes is high among adults with low birth weight (small for gestational age) who were also overweight during childhood. The increased risk for type 2 diabetes associated with small size at birth is further increased by high growth rates after 7 years of age.[48] There is an association between thinness in infancy and the presence of IGT or diabetes in young adulthood.[49] Low birth weight and accelerated postnatal catch-up growth during early life are independent risk factors for adult disease, including diabetes, obesity, and cardiovascular disease (CVD).[50] Prevention of early catch-up growth reversed the development of glucose intolerance and obesity in the mouse model of LBW-associated diabetes.[51] Crossing into higher categories of BMI after the age of 2 years is also associated with these disorders.[51]

OBESITY AND DYSLIPIDEMIA

The prevalence of HTN, diabetes, dyslipidemia, and MS substantially increases with increasing BMI. Obesity and insulin resistance often coexist along with other abnormalities such as HTN and dyslipidemia. The original description of MS by Reaven consisted of obesity, insulin resistance, HTN, IGT or diabetes, hyperinsulinemia, and dyslipidemia characterized by elevated triglyceride and low HDL concentrations.[3,52] The NHANES study noted that with increasing overweight and obesity class, there is an increase in the prevalence of dyslipidemia, from about 8.9% for normal weight to 19.0% for obesity class 3. With normal weight individuals as a reference, individuals with obesity class 3 had an adjusted odds ratio (OR) of 2.2 (95% CI 1.7–2.4) for dyslipidemia.[53] Insulin resistance is a key feature of the MS and often progresses to type 2 diabetes. Recent evidence suggests that a fundamental defect is an overproduction of large very-low-density-lipoprotein (VLDL) particles, which initiates a sequence of lipoprotein changes, resulting in higher levels of remnant particles, smaller LDL, and lower levels of high-density-lipoprotein (HDL) cholesterol. These atherogenic lipid abnormalities precede the diagnosis of type 2 diabetes by several years, and it is thus important to elucidate the mechanisms involved in the overproduction of large VLDL particles.[54] The dyslipidemia associated with obesity no doubt plays a major role in the development of atherosclerosis and CVD. All of the components of dyslipidemia, including higher triglycerides, decreased HDL levels, and increased small, dense LDL particles, have been shown to be atherogenic. Combined weight loss and exercise, even if they do not result in normalization of body weight, can improve dyslipidemia and thus reduce CVD risk. In obesity and type 2 diabetes, the altered communication between adipose tissue and the liver results in the altered regulation of VLDL production. A number of studies indicate that adipocytokines, in particular adiponectin, may be seminal players in the regulation of fat metabolism in the liver.[55]

PATHOPHYSIOLOGY OF OBESITY, TYPE 2 DIABETES, AND INSULIN RESISTANCE

Normal glucose homeostasis is maintained by a delicate balance between insulin secretion by the pancreatic β-cells and insulin sensitivity of the peripheral tissues (muscle, liver, and adipose tissue). The NHANES study noted that with increasing overweight and obesity class, there is an increase in the prevalence of diabetes, from 2.4% for normal weight to 14.2% for obesity class 3. With normal weight individuals as a reference, individuals in obesity class 3 had an adjusted OR of 5.1 (95% CI 3.7–7.0) for diabetes.[53]

FREE FATTY ACIDS

Most obese individuals have elevated plasma levels of FFAs, which are known to cause peripheral (muscle) insulin resistance. They do this by inhibiting insulin-stimulated glucose uptake and glycogen synthesis. The mechanism involves intramyocellular accumulation of diacylglycerol and activation of protein kinase C. FFAs also cause hepatic insulin resistance. They do this by inhibiting insulin-mediated suppression of glycogenolysis.[56–59] In most obese subjects, plasma FFA levels are increased. FFAs have been shown to have an important contributing role in the pathogenesis of insulin resistance in human obesity.[59] Physiologic increases in plasma FFA levels cause insulin resistance in both diabetic and nondiabetic subjects by producing several metabolic defects: (1) FFAs inhibit insulin-stimulated glucose uptake at the level of glucose transport or phosphorylation (or both); (2) FFAs inhibit insulin-stimulated glycogen synthesis; and (3) FFAs inhibit insulin-stimulated glucose oxidation. (This last-mentioned defect probably does not contribute to insulin resistance.) The stimulatory effect of FFAs on hepatic glucose production (HGP) would then become unchecked, resulting in hyperglycemia. Hence, continuously elevated levels of plasma FFAs may play a key role in the pathogenesis of non insulin dependent diabetes (NIDDM) in predisposed individuals by impairing peripheral glucose utilization and by promoting hepatic glucose overproduction.[60] Studies have shown that both obesity and type 2 diabetes impair insulin-induced suppression of glycogenolysis and gluconeogenesis and that the degree of impairment correlates with plasma FFA concentrations.[60,61] Plasma FFA concentrations correlate with rates of gluconeogenesis and glycogenolysis, suggesting that they influence the regulation of both processes. The hepatic insulin resistance associated with obesity and type 2 diabetes results in impaired insulin-induced suppression of glycogenolysis and gluconeogenesis. There is a growing body of evidence indicating that obesity and diabetes both cause hepatic insulin resistance.[61–64]

VISCERAL ADIPOSITY, OBESITY, INSULIN RESISTANCE, AND TYPE 2 DIABETES

Many studies have pointed to an association between insulin resistance and intra-abdominal fat accumulation (visceral obesity).[65] The Look AHEAD (Action for Health in Diabetes) trial of patients with type 2 diabetes demonstrated adipose tissue distribution that was significantly altered, with more visceral adipose tissue and intermuscular adipose tissue, depots known to exacerbate insulin resistance, and less subcutaneous adipose tissue in people with diabetes than in healthy control subjects.[66] In obesity, the initial deposition of triglycerides occurs in subcutaneous adipose tissue, and as this increases in size, insulin resistance will rise and limit further subcutaneous lipid accumulation. Triglycerides will then be diverted to the visceral fat depot as well as to ectopic sites. This leads to a substantial rise in insulin resistance and the prevalence of its associated disorders. Evidence supporting this hypothesis includes studies showing that in lean subjects, the prime determinant of insulin resistance is BMI, that is, subcutaneous fat, while in overweight and obese subjects, it is WC and VAT. It has also been shown that the MS suddenly increases in prevalence at high levels of insulin resistance, and it is suggested that this is due to the diversion of lipids from the subcutaneous to the visceral depot.[67] Accumulation of fat in abdomen regions has major implications for metabolism and particularly for insulin sensitivity.[68–70] This high prevalence of comorbidities relates more to WC than to BMI. Visceral or abdominal obesity is associated with an increased risk of CVD and type 2 diabetes. A high prevalence of obesity and abdominal obesity in Mexicans is associated with a markedly increased incidence of diabetes and HTN.[71] VAT is considered a risk factor for insulin resistance MS[72] and type 2 diabetes in adults,[73] as well as in first-degree relatives of patients with type 2 diabetes with normal glucose levels.[74] Adipocytokines, hormones secreted by the visceral adipocytes, generate the insulin-resistant state and the chronic inflammatory profile that frequently goes along with visceral obesity.[75]

VISCERAL ADIPOSITY AND CHILDREN

The prevalence of obesity is also on the rise in children and adolescents. As defined by a BMI greater than the 95th percentile for age and gender from the revised National Center for Health Statistics growth charts, 10%–15% of 6–17-year-old children and adolescents are overweight in the United States and worldwide.[76] VAT is considered a risk factor for insulin resistance in children.[38,77–82] Visceral fat has been shown to have many properties different from those of subcutaneous fat, and children with central adiposity can develop the MS with insulin resistance, HTN, and dyslipidemia.[83]

VISCERAL FAT TISSUE AS A PROINFLAMMATORY TISSUE AND ITS ROLE IN INSULIN RESISTANCE

When analyzed using stepwise multivariate analysis, age, sex, FPG, and BMI seem to be the most important factors contributing to the variation of vascular reactivity.[84] Visceral fat exhibits accelerated lipolytic activity with increased release of FFAs, which can adversely affect insulin action and glucose disposal in several tissues.[85–89] A strong correlation between intramyocellular triacylglycerol concentrations and the severity of insulin resistance has been found, which led to the assumption that lipid oversupply to skeletal muscle contributes to reduced insulin action.[85,90] These increases in circulating FFA levels may also result in the development of triglyceride reservoirs in both muscle and liver, depressing the actions of insulin and increasing hepatic VLDL output.[91–93] VLDL assembly in the liver is catalyzed by microsomal triglyceride transfer protein (MTP). A study by Wolfrum and Stoffel[94] showed that the forkhead protein Foxa2 stimulates hepatic VLDL production in concert with the coactivator PGC-1beta and that insulin inhibits this process by inactivating Foxa2. MTP is a target of the transcription factor FoxO1, and it appears that excessive VLDL production associated with insulin resistance is caused by the inability of insulin to regulate FoxO1 transcriptional activation of MTP.[95,96] Plasma phospholipid transfer protein (PLTP) that facilitated lipid transfer activity is related to HDL and LDL metabolism, as well as lipoprotein lipase activity, adiposity, and insulin resistance.[96,97] Conversely, declines in VAT and reduced FFA levels following weight-loss diets have been associated with enhanced insulin sensitivity.[98,99] Conversion of LDL subclass pattern B (individuals with a predominance of small, dense LDL) to pattern A (individuals with a predominance of large LDL) and reversal of alkaline phosphatase can be achieved in a high proportion of overweight men by normalization of adiposity.[100] Pattern B men who converted to pattern A with weight loss may have an underlying impairment in fat oxidation that predisposes to both dyslipidemia and an impaired ability to achieve weight loss by energy restriction.[101] Adipose tissue is known to express and secrete a variety of products known as "adipokines," including leptin, adiponectin, resistin, and visfatin, as well as cytokines and chemokines such as TNF-α, IL-6, and monocyte chemoattractant protein-1. The release of adipokines by either adipocytes or adipose tissue–infiltrated macrophages leads to a chronic subinflammatory state that could play a central role in the development of insulin resistance and type 2 diabetes, and the increased risk of CVD associated with obesity.[102] TNF-α and IL-6 are expressed in adipose tissues, with visceral fat responsible for more TNF-α production than subcutaneous fat. These cytokines inhibit insulin signaling, and TNF-α may play a crucial role in the systemic insulin resistance of type 2 diabetes.[103,104] TNF-α inhibits tyrosine kinase phosphorylation of the insulin receptor, resulting in defects in insulin signaling and ultimately leading to insulin resistance and impaired glucose transport.[105,106] An imbalance in favor of proinflammatory cytokines from adipose tissue (hypoadiponectinemia and increased levels of IL-6) and other sources may trigger CRP secretion. CRP levels are related strongly to insulin resistance and adiposity, and elevated levels of TNF-α correlate with impaired endothelial dysfunction (ED) and CAD. This in turn can exacerbate mild insulin resistance and accentuate other metabolic abnormalities that together constitute MS. Thus, insulin resistance, itself, appears to be an ED risk equivalent. The pathways are clearly intertwined with and sparked by obesity, in large part by excess adipokine production. Abnormalities in vascular reactivity and biochemical markers of endothelial cell activation are present early in individuals at risk of developing type 2 diabetes. The association of ED with insulin resistance in the absence of overt diabetes or MS provides evidence that the atherosclerosis may actually begin earlier in the spectrum of insulin resistance, ultimately resulting in a progression of MS to prediabetes and then to type 2 diabetes.[107,108] Lipocalin-2 (LCN2) is a novel adipokine with potential roles in obesity, insulin resistance, and inflammation.

INSULIN RESISTANCE IN TYPE 2 DIABETES AND OBESITY

Insulin is a critical regulator of virtually all aspects of adipocyte biology, and adipocytes are one of the most highly insulin-responsive cell types. Insulin resistance is a fundamental aspect of the etiology of type 2 diabetes and is also linked to a wide array of other pathophysiologic sequelae including HTN, hyperlipidemia, atherosclerosis (i.e., MS, or syndrome X), and polycystic ovarian disease. The association between obesity and type 2 diabetes has been well recognized for decades, and the major link is insulin resistance. In the natural history of diabetes, obesity and insulin resistance precede abnormal glucose (Figure 15.3). Insulin resistance in both obesity and type 2 diabetes is manifested by decreased insulin-stimulated glucose transport and metabolism in adipocytes and skeletal muscle and by impaired suppression of hepatic glucose output.[109] Type 2 diabetes is characterized by four major metabolic abnormalities: obesity, impaired insulin action, insulin secretory dysfunction, and increased endogenous glucose output (EGO).[69,110] Insulin resistance is the earliest observable abnormality in individuals who are predisposed to, and who later develop, type 2 diabetes. Decreased insulin sensitivity and impaired β-cell function are the two key components in type 2 diabetes pathogenesis based on long-term experience in adults.[111–114] Emerging evidence supports the potentially unifying hypothesis that the insulin responsiveness of skeletal muscle and liver, as well as the glucose-stimulated insulin secretion by pancreatic beta cells in type 2 diabetes, is caused by mitochondrial dysfunction.[115]

ADIPOCYTE HORMONES, OBESITY, INSULIN RESISTANCE, AND PROGRESSION TO DIABETES

Adipose tissue is a highly active metabolic and endocrine organ. Adipocytes secrete protein with biological activity, called adipokines. The adipokines regulating insulin sensitivity are TNF-α, adiponectin, IL-6, resistin, and leptin,[102] all of which also play important roles in the pathogenesis

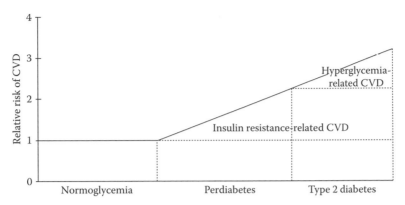

FIGURE 15.3 Relative risk of CVD in normoglycemia, prediabetes, and type 2 diabetes. (From Laakso, M., *Diabetes Care*, 33, 442, 2010.)

of diabetes, dyslipidemia, inflammation, and atherosclerosis.[102,116,117] During the progression from normal weight to obesity and then to overt diabetes, adipocyte-derived factors contribute to the occurrence and development of β-cell dysfunction and type 2 diabetes.[118] In addition to inducing insulin resistance in insulin-responsive tissues, adipocyte-derived factors play an important role in the pathogenesis of β-cell dysfunction. Leptin, FFAs, adiponectin, TNF-α, and IL-6 are all produced and secreted by adipocytes, and may directly influence aspects of β-cell function, including insulin synthesis and secretion, insulin cell survival, and apoptosis.[118] Leptin is almost exclusively expressed and produced by white adipose tissue—specifically, by differentiated adipocytes. Subcutaneous fat is responsible for 80% of total leptin production. This was shown in cultures *ex vivo* where the production of leptin was higher in subcutaneous adipocytes than in those of deeper origin.[119]

Leptin improves insulin sensitivity through activation of AMP protein kinase (AMPK), which controls cellular concentrations of malonyl-CoA, thereby inhibiting acetyl-CoA carboxylase (the enzyme involved in malonyl-CoA transformation).[120] While a deficiency of leptin is very likely to contribute to insulin resistance when adipose tissue is lacking, leptin resistance is a main feature of human obesity. TNF-α is a proinflammatory cytokine produced by numerous cells, but adipocytes also produce TNF-α. TNF-α is overexpressed in adipose tissue from obese animals and humans, and obese mice lacking either TNF-α or its receptor show protection against developing insulin resistance. TNF-α induces a state of insulin resistance in terms of glucose uptake in myocytes and adipocytes that impair insulin signaling at the level of the insulin receptor substrate proteins. The mechanism involves Ser phosphorylation of IRS-2 mediated by TNF-α activation of MAPKs.[121] Protein-Tyr phosphatase (PTP) 1B acts as a physiological, negative regulator of insulin signaling by dephosphorylating the phosphotyrosine residues of the insulin receptor and IRS-1, and PTP1B expression is increased in muscle and white adipose tissue of obese and diabetic humans and rodents. Downregulation of PTP1B activity is possible by the use of pharmacological agonists of the nuclear receptors that restore insulin sensitivity in the presence of TNF-α. The lack of PTP1B in muscle and brown adipocytes increases insulin sensitivity and glucose uptake and could confer protection against insulin resistance induced by adipokines.[105]

IL-6, one of the adipokines, has emerged as one of the potential mediators linking obesity-derived chronic inflammation with insulin resistance. Adipose tissue contributes to up to 35% of circulating IL-6, the systemic effects of which have been best demonstrated in the liver, where a STAT3-SOCS3 pathway mediates IL-6 impairment of insulin actions. In contrast to its role in liver, IL-6 is believed to be beneficial for insulin-regulated glucose metabolism in muscle.[122]

Adiponectin is a protein highly expressed in adipose tissue. Its plasma levels are between 5 and 30 mg/L in lean subjects and represent 0.01% of plasma proteins. Like leptin, adiponectin enhances insulin sensitivity through activation of AMPK.[123] Functional analyses including generation of adiponectin transgenic or knockout mice have revealed that adiponectin serves as an insulin-sensitizing adipokine. Obesity-linked downregulation of adiponectin is a mechanism that explains how obesity could cause insulin resistance and diabetes.[124] Adiponectin also affects HGP by decreasing the mRNA expression of two essential gluconeogenesis enzymes: phosphoenolpyruvate carboxykinase and glucose-6-phosphatase. It appears that high-molecular-weight adiponectin may be the most insulin sensitizing.[124] Adiponectin correlates with blood concentrations of FFAs and reduced BMI or body weight, and may be the molecular link between obesity and insulin resistance, and may serve as a biomarker for the MS.[125] Interventions to reduce insulin resistance by increasing adiponectin concentrations may be effective particularly in obese, insulin-resistant individuals.[125] Plum treatment (plum juice) significantly increased plasma adiponectin concentrations and PPAR-γ mRNA expression in adipose tissue from Wistar fatty rats.[126]

Visfatin (also known as pre-B-cell colony-enhancing factor or PBEF) is a newly discovered adipocyte hormone, highly expressed in visceral fat, with a direct relationship existing between plasma visfatin levels and T2DM. There are inconsistencies in the reported literature. Visfatin binds to the insulin receptor at a site distinct from that of insulin and causes hypoglycemia by reducing glucose release from liver cells and stimulating glucose utilization in adipocytes and myocytes.[127] Serum visfatin levels were reported to be elevated in type 2 diabetes independent of insulin resistance.[128] Increased visfatin levels have been shown to be associated with BMI and insulin resistance in obese children.[129] Visfatin is not related to insulin resistance either as assessed by a homeostasis model assessment or during lipid infusion.[130] LCN2 belongs to the lipocalin subfamily of low-molecular mass-secreted proteins that bind small hydrophobic molecules. LCN2 has been characterized recently as an adipose-derived cytokine, and its expression is upregulated in adipose tissue. LCN2 has been shown to play a critical role in the regulation of body fat mass, lipid metabolism, and insulin resistance, especially as it attenuates diet-induced insulin resistance.[131] It is a novel adipokine with potential roles in obesity, insulin resistance, and inflammation.

Increases in adiposity trigger metabolic and inflammatory changes that interfere with insulin action in peripheral tissues, culminating in beta-cell failure and overt diabetes. The cAMP response element–binding protein (CREB) is activated in adipose cells under obese conditions, where it promotes insulin resistance by triggering expression of the transcriptional repressor ATF3 and thereby downregulating expression of the adipokine hormone adiponectin as well as the insulin-sensitive glucose transporter 4 (GLUT4).[132] LCN2 is a novel adipokine with potential roles in obesity, insulin resistance, and inflammation. LCN2 is associated with MMP-2 and MMP-9 activities as well as with proinflammatory markers, suggesting its potential involvement in the low-grade chronic inflammation accompanying obesity.[133]

Nonalcoholic Fatty Liver Disease

The prevalence of nonalcoholic fatty liver disease (NAFLD) is increasing worldwide with approximately 30% of the population affected in industrialized, Western countries. With the continuing epidemics of obesity and diabetes, NAFLD has received increased attention. NAFLD is characterized by hepatic steatosis in the absence of a history of significant alcohol use or other known liver diseases. Compared with healthy controls, risk for steatosis is increased 4.6-fold in obese subjects. Primary NAFLD emerges due to the MS. Subjects with NAFLD have a twofold greater risk of diabetes.[134] Histopathologically, NAFLD can appear as simple steatosis (nonalcoholic fatty liver), or with an inflammatory reaction defined as NASH, with or without portal fibrosis, that may lead to fatty liver–associated cirrhosis (NASH-induced cirrhosis). Approximately 10% of patients with NAFLD develop NASH, and about 8%–26% of individuals with NASH progress to cirrhosis.[135] FFAs play a pivotal role in the development of simple hepatic steatosis. The development of NAFLD is closely linked to an excess flow of FFAs arising from visceral adipose tissue. Multiple mechanisms including proinflammatory cytokines and pathways have been implicated in the pathogenesis of NAFLD. Understanding the role of obesity and lipotoxicity in patients with liver disease as part of a broader metabolic disorder is likely to improve the management of these challenging diseases. In an 11-year follow-up study, NAFLD with elevated aminotransaminase (ALT) levels was a risk factor for incident diabetes or the MS.[136] Insulin resistance is the basis of both NAFLD and MS.[137,138] Obesity results in marked enlargement of the intra-abdominal visceral fat depots. The development of insulin resistance leads to continuous lipolysis within these depots, releasing fatty acids into the portal circulation, where they are rapidly translocated to the liver and reassembled into triglycerides. Reactive oxygen species, generated in the liver from oxidation of fatty acids, are precipitating factors in the cascade of events leading from simple steatosis to NASH.[27] Circulating FFAs may be cytotoxic by inducing lipid peroxidation and hepatocyte apoptosis. Insulin resistance is often associated with chronic low-grade inflammation, and numerous mediators released from immune cells and adipocytes may contribute to liver damage and liver disease progression.[138]

BENEFITS OF WEIGHT LOSS IN TYPE 2 DIABETES AND OBESITY

Recommendations from an NIH consensus conference indicate that a weight loss of 5%–10% can significantly improve risk factors for obesity-related diseases.[139] Weight reduction has been shown to improve glycemic control and cardiovascular risk factors associated with insulin resistance in obese individuals with type 2 diabetes. Clinical studies demonstrate that the therapeutic benefit rises with increasing weight loss, but that losses as low as 0.45–4 kg (1–9 lb) have positive effects on metabolic control, cardiovascular risk factors, and mortality rates. The current data support a continued focus on weight loss, including moderate weight loss, as a key component of good care for overweight patients with type 2 diabetes.[140] The list of benefits is shown in Table 15.2. The most effective interventions include comprehensive behavioral management, dietary modification, exercise, pharmacotherapy, and bariatric surgery. The most widely investigated drugs, sibutramine and orlistat, result in modest, clinically worthwhile weight loss, with demonstrable improvements in comorbidities, among which is type 2 diabetes.

Nutrition in the management of obesity and type 2 diabetes: Observational and interventional studies have clearly shown that type 2 diabetes can be prevented by lifestyle measures, including reduced energy intake to induce a modest but sustained weight reduction, together with changes in diet composition.[141] Even in elderly individuals, diet-induced weight loss results in improved insulin sensitivity and improved β-cell function.[142] In short-term[143] as well as long-term studies,[144] the use of a low carbohydrate diet in obese subjects with type 2 diabetes has improved glucose profiles, insulin sensitivity, and decreased plasma triglyceride and cholesterol levels.

TABLE 15.2
Benefits of Weight Loss in Type 2 Diabetes

1. Improved glucose levels
2. Improved glycemic control
3. Reduced fasting insulin
4. Increased insulin sensitivity
5. Reduced upper body adiposity
6. Less atherogenic lipid profile
   a. Decreased triglycerides
   b. Increased HDL cholesterol
   c. Larger, less small, dense LDL cholesterol particles
7. Reduced blood pressure
8. Improved mortality

Prevention of Type 2 Diabetes by Weight Reduction

Several interventional studies have demonstrated that significant weight reduction could lead to a decreased incidence of progression to type 2 diabetes.

Finnish Study[145]

This study from Finland included middle-aged obese subjects with impaired glucose tolerance who were randomized to receive either brief diet and exercise counseling (control group) or intensive individualized instruction on weight reduction, food intake, and guidance on increasing physical activity (intervention group). After an average follow-up of 3.2 years, there was a 58% relative reduction in the incidence of diabetes in members of the intervention group compared with the control subjects.

Diabetes Prevention Program[146]

This was a multicenter study that enrolled subjects with impaired glucose tolerance who were slightly younger and more obese. Approximately 45% of study subjects were recruited from minority groups (e.g., African American, Hispanic), and 20% of subjects were aged ≥ 60 years. Subjects were randomized to one of three intervention groups: the intensive nutrition and exercise counseling ("lifestyle") group, or either of two masked medication treatment groups, the metformin group or the placebo group. Participants in both the placebo group and the metformin group received standard diet and exercise recommendations. After an average follow-up of 2.8 years, compared with the control group, a 58% relative reduction in the progression to diabetes was observed in the lifestyle group and a 31% relative reduction in the metformin group. On an average, 50% of the subjects in the lifestyle group achieved the goal of $\geq 7\%$ weight reduction, and about 74% maintained at least 150 min/week of moderately intense activity. During follow-up after DPP at 10 years, incidences in placebo and metformin groups fell to equal those in the former lifestyle group, but the cumulative incidence of diabetes remained lowest in the lifestyle group, indicating that prevention or delay of diabetes with lifestyle intervention or metformin can persist for at least 10 years.[146,147] Progression to diabetes is more common in women with a history of gestational diabetes (GDM) compared with those without a history of GDM, despite equivalent degrees of IGT at baseline. Both intensive lifestyle changes and metformin use are highly effective in delaying or preventing diabetes in women with IGT and a history of GDM.[148]

Da Qing Study[149]

This study from China included subjects with IGT determined by oral glucose tolerance tests, who were randomized by clinic to a control group or to one of three active treatment groups: diet only, exercise only, or diet plus exercise. Subjects were followed biannually. After an average of 6 years' follow-up, the diet, exercise, and diet plus exercise interventions were associated with 31%, 46%, and 42% reductions in risk of developing type 2 diabetes, respectively.

Xenical in the Prevention of Diabetes in Obese Subjects (XENDOS) Study[150]

This study addressed the benefit of weight reduction achieved by the addition of orlistat to lifestyle change, to delay the progression of type 2 diabetes in a group with BMI $\geq 30 \, kg/m^2$ with or without IGT. After 4 years of treatment, the effect of orlistat addition corresponded to a 45% reduction in risk factors in the IGT group, with no effect observed in those without IGT.[150]

Look AHEAD[151]

This was a multicenter randomized study of 5145 participants randomized between 2001 and 2004, whose ethnicities paralleled the ethnic distribution of DM in the NHANES 1999–2000 survey, with a mean age of 59 ± 6.8 years (mean ± SD), and of whom 60% were women. Furthermore, 65.0%

of participants had a first-degree relative with diabetes. Overall, BMI averaged 36 ± 5.9 kg/m² at baseline, with 83.6% of the men and 86.1% of women having a BMI >30 kg/m² and 17.9% of men and 25.4% of women having a BMI >40 kg/m². Intensive lifestyle intervention (ILI) participants had a greater percentage of sustained weight loss (−6.15% vs. −0.88%; P < 0.001) and improvements in fitness, glycemic control, and CVD risk factors in individuals with type 2 diabetes.[152]

In a recent Japanese randomized control trial to test the feasibility and effectiveness of a lifestyle intervention program in the primary care setting, in 30–60 year old subjects, a significant improvement in insulin sensitivity and BMI >22.5 kg/m² was observed representing a significant reduction in the cumulative incidence of progression to diabetes.[153]

PHARMACOTHERAPY FOR OBESITY AND IMPROVEMENT IN METABOLIC RISK FACTORS AND DIABETES

Orlistat, a gastrointestinal (GI) lipase inhibitor drug, has been used effectively and safely in the treatment of obesity.[154] Orlistat significantly reduces body weight and improves glycemic control and several cardiovascular risk factors in overweight and obese subjects with type 2 diabetes.[155,156] In type 2 diabetic patients, orlistat also attenuates postprandial increases in triglycerides, remnant-like particles, cholesterol, and FFAs.[157] Orlistat is an effective treatment modality in obese patients with type 2 diabetes with respect to clinically meaningful weight loss and maintenance of weight loss, improved glycemic control, and improved lipid profile.[158] The antihyperglycemic effect of orlistat has been attributed to a weight loss–associated decrease in insulin resistance[155] and augmentation of the postprandial increases in plasma levels of glucagon-like peptide-1 (GLP-1).[159]

Rimonabant in Obesity–Lipids Study[162]

Rimonabant is a selective cannabinoid-1 receptor (CB1) blocker with both central and peripheral actions.[160] A 20 mg/day dose of rimonabant, along with a low calorie diet, resulted in significant weight reduction and improvement in cardiovascular risk factors such as WC, HDL cholesterol, triglycerides, insulin resistance, and the incidences of MS. In addition, it was shown to increase in plasma adiponectin levels that were partly independent of weight loss alone.

Sibutramine[163]

Sibutramine is an antiobesity drug that induces satiety and thermogenesis.[163] Sibutramine use has been shown to reduce weight, lower the levels of nonesterified fatty acids, decrease hyperinsulinemia, and reduce insulin resistance. It has been used as an effective adjunct to oral hypoglycemic therapy in obese subjects with type 2 diabetes.[164] However, the magnitude of weight loss was modest, and the long-term health benefits and safety remain unclear.[165]

Pharmacotherapy for Diabetes and Weight Reduction

Weight loss is an important therapeutic objective for individuals with type 2 diabetes.[166] Both short[167]- and long-term[168] weight loss in overweight or obese type 2 diabetic subjects on very low calorie diets was shown to decrease insulin resistance, improve measures of glycemic control, improve lipid abnormalities, and reduce blood pressure.[167,169] Metformin, an oral hypoglycemic agent, decreases calorie intake in a dose-dependent manner and leads to a reduction in body weight in subjects with type 2 diabetes and obesity.[170–172] Exenatide is a member of a new class of agents known as incretin mimetics currently in development for the treatment of type 2 diabetes. In short-term studies, exenatide improved glycemic control and helped to reduce body weight over 28 days in patients with type 2 diabetes treated with diet/exercise or metformin.[173]

Bariatric surgery for obesity and effect on type 2 diabetes: Bariatric surgery for severe obesity results in long-term weight loss, which leads to an improved lifestyle and recovery from diabetes,[174,175] hypertriglyceridemia, low levels of HDL cholesterol, HTN, and hyperuricemia.[175–177]

POTENTIAL ROLE OF ADIPONECTIN IN THE TREATMENT OF OBESITY, DIABETES, AND INSULIN RESISTANCE

Studies have shown that adiponectin administration in rodents has insulin-sensitizing, antiatherogenic, and anti-inflammatory effects and under certain settings also decreases body weight. Therefore, adiponectin replacement in humans may represent a promising approach to prevent and/or treat obesity, insulin resistance, and type 2 diabetes; however, clinical studies with adiponectin administration need to be conducted to confirm this hypothesis.

PHARMACOGENETICS: POTENTIAL ROLE IN THE TREATMENT OF DIABETES AND OBESITY

The prevalence of obesity and diabetes, which are heritable traits that arise from the interactions of multiple genes and lifestyle factors, continues to rise worldwide. Until recently, candidate gene and genome-wide linkage studies have been the main genetic epidemiological approaches to identify genetic loci for obesity and diabetes, yet progress has been slow, with limited success. Recent advances have transformed the situation, and there has been progress in understanding how genetic variation predisposes individuals to diabetes and obesity, and how candidate genes may alter drug response. The discovery of causal genes includes family-based linkage analyses and focused candidate-gene studies; among them, large-scale surveys of association between common DNA sequence variants and disease were most successful. The current total of approximately 40 confirmed type 2 diabetes loci includes variants in or near WFS1 (wolframin) and the hepatocyte nuclear factors HNF1A and HNF1B (genes that also harbor rare mutations responsible for monogenic forms of diabetes);[178–181] the melatonin-receptor gene MTNR1B (which highlights the link between circadian and metabolic regulation);[182–184] and IRS1 (encoding insulin-receptor substrate 1), one of the limited number of type 2 diabetes loci with a primary effect on insulin action rather than on secretion.[185] Genetic discoveries have provided a molecular basis for the clinically useful classification of monogenic forms of diabetes and obesity.[186,187] Genome-wide association (GWA) studies of population-based samples undertaken to examine the full range of BMI values have identified approximately 30 loci influencing BMI and the risk of obesity. The strongest signal remains the association with variants within FTO (the fat-mass and obesity–related gene).[184,188–190] Other signals near BDNF, SH2B1, and NEGR1 (all implicated in aspects of neuronal function) reinforce the view of obesity as a disorder of hypothalamic function.[191–194] There are insufficient genetic data to support management decisions for common forms of type 2 diabetes and obesity.[195] Although the TCF7L2 genotype variants influence therapeutic response to sulfonylureas but not metformin,[196] the effect is too modest to guide the care of individual patients. Three large GWA studies on obesity, together involving more than 150,000 individuals, were published in *Nature Genetics* last year. The results suggested the involvement of a large number of genetic variants in disease susceptibility and have identified 19 loci for common obesity and 18 for common type 2 diabetes. The combined contribution of these loci to the variation in obesity and diabetes risk is small, and their predictive value is typically low. One of these loci, variants in the FTO-associated gene, influences susceptibility to type 2 diabetes via an effect on adiposity/obesity.[197] The EPIC-Norfolk study is a population-based, ethnically homogeneous, white European cohort study of 25,631 residents living in the city of Norwich, United Kingdom, and its surrounding area. Of these, 12,201 had complete genotype data for all 12 single nucleotide polymorphisms (SNPs). The FTO locus represented the largest.[198] Variants that predispose to common obesity also result in altered susceptibility to PCOS, probably mediated through adiposity.[199] One SNP associated with weight is located close to monoacylglycerol acyltransferase 1 (MGAT1), the MGAT enzyme family known to be involved in dietary fat absorption.[200] Genetic studies offer two main avenues for clinical translation. First, the identification of new pathways involved in disease predisposition—for example, those influencing zinc transport and pancreatic islet regeneration in the case of type 2 diabetes—offers opportunities for the development of novel therapeutic and preventive approaches. Second, with

TABLE 15.3
Major GWA Studies of Type 2 Diabetes

Reference	Sample Size		Major Ethnic Groups	Study Type	Main Findings
	GWA	Replication			
Sladek et al. [12]	1,363	5,511	French	Single GWA study	*HHEX* and *SLC30A8* associations with type 2 diabetes
Scott et al. [14]	2,335	2,473	Finnish	Single GWA study	*CDKAL1, CDKN2A,* and *IGF2BP2* associations with type 2 diabetes
Diabetes Genetics Initiative et al. [15]	2,931	10,850	Swedish, Finnish	Single GWA study	*CDKAL1, CDKN2A,* and *IGF2BP2* associations with type 2 diabetes
Zeggini et al. [16,18]	4,862	9,103	British	Single GWA study	*CDKAL1, CDKN2A,* and *IGF2BP2* associations with type 2 diabetes
Steinthorsdottir et al. [17]	6,674	14,138	Icelandic	Single GWA study	*CDKAL1* association with type 2 diabetes and insulin secretion
Zeggini et al. [19]	10,128	79,792	European	GWA meta-analysis	Six new loci for type 2 diabetes (*NOTCH2, JAZF1, ADAMTS9, TSPAN8, THADA,* and *CDC123*)
Yasuda et al. [23]	1,691	18,239	Japanese, Korean, Chinese	Single GWA study	*KCNQ1* association with type 2 diabetes in East Asians
Unoki et al. [24]	1,752	19,489	Japanese, Singaporean	Single GWA study	*KCNQ1* association with type 2 diabetes in East Asians
Rung et al. [25]	1,376	27,033	French, Danish	Single GWA study	*IRS1* association with type 2 diabetes
Prokopenko et al. [26]	36,610	82,689 For type 2 diabetes	European	Follow-up of signals for type 2 diabetes from GWA scan for fasting glucose	*MTNR1B* association with type 2 diabetes and fasting glucose
Lyssenko et al. [27]	2,931	18,831 For type 2 diabetes	Swedish, Finnish	Follow-up of signals for type 2 diabetes from GWA scan for fasting glucose	*MTNR1B* association with type 2 diabetes and fasting glucose
Bouatia-Naji et al. [28]	2,151	15,464 For type 2 diabetes	French, Danish, Finnish	Follow-up of signals for type 2 diabetes from GWA scan for fasting glucose	*MTNR1B* association with type 2 diabetes and fasting glucose
Dupuis et al. [20]	46,186	127,677 For type 2 diabetes	European	Follow-up of signals for type 2 diabetes from GWA scan for fasting glucose	*ADCY5, PROX1, GCK, GCKR,* and *DGKB* associations with type 2 diabetes and fasting glucose
Tsai et al. [29]	1,889	3,276	Taiwanese	Single GWA study	*SRR* and *PTPRD* associations with type 2 diabetes in Taiwanese
Qi et al. [21]	5,643	84,605	European	GWA meta-analysis	*RBMS1* association with type 2 diabetes
Voight et al. [22]	47,117	94,337	European	GWA meta-analysis	12 new loci for type 2 diabetes including *DUSP9, KLF14, CENTD2, HMGA2,* and *HNF1A*

Source: McCarthy, M.I., *N. Engl. J. Med.,* 363, 2339, 2010.

Note: Only studies in which there were significant GWAs with type 2 diabetes are listed.

continuing efforts to identify additional genetic variants, it may become possible to use patterns of predisposition to tailor individual management of these conditions (Table 15.3).

BARIATRIC SURGERY FOR OBESITY AND IMPROVEMENT IN DIABETES CONTROL

Bariatric surgery as a modality to treat obesity in the United States is reserved for patients with BMI $\geq 35\,kg/m^2$ and the presence of serious comorbidities (T2DM, moderate or severe obstructive sleep apnea [OSA], pseudotumor cerebri, and severe steatohepatitis), or BMI $>40\,kg/m^2$ and minor comorbidities (mild OSA, HTN, insulin resistance, glucose intolerance, dyslipidemia, impaired quality of life, or activities of daily living). Gastric bypass surgery appears to have significant increased therapeutic potential for treating obesity and type 2 diabetes. In view of the growing enthusiasm for surgical interventions to treat T2DM, the first diabetes surgery summit (DSS) was held in Rome in March 2007. Trends in mortality in bariatric surgery were reported by Buchwald et al. in 2007[201] in a systemic review that included meta-analysis of 361 studies and a total of 85,048 patients with a mean BMI of $47.4\,kg/m^2$. The early and late mortality rates after bariatric surgery were reported as low.

A review by Cunneen reported that all studies reporting on comorbidities showed significant resolution or improvement of T2DM (> or = 60%), HTN (> or = 43%), and dyslipidemia (> or = 70%). One meta-analysis study reported that surgery was found to be superior to medical therapy in resolving T2DM, HTN, and dyslipidemia. Sleep apnea was significantly resolved/improved in $\geq 85\%$ across procedures in the one meta-analysis that addressed this comorbidity.[202] Studies have shown that those who undergo bariatric surgery for obese diabetic patients experience complete remission of diabetes, maintaining euglycemia without medications for more than 10 years.[203] Additionally, following some GI procedures, T2DM resolves within days to weeks, long before the occurrence of major weight loss. T2DM resolution or remission has usually been defined as HbA_{1C} values ranging from <6% to <7% in the absence of antidiabetic medications. Meta-analysis of bariatric surgery by Buchwald et al.[204] included 136 studies for a total of 22,094 patients; mean baseline BMI was $46.9\,kg/m^2$ (32.3–68.8). The studies that reported resolution of T2DM included a total of 1846 patients. Diabetes resolution rates were 98.9% after biliopancreatic diversion (BPD), 83.7% after Roux-en-Y gastric bypass (RYGB), and 47.9% after AGB. Another systematic review by Levy et al.[205] confirmed that bariatric surgery was highly effective in obtaining weight reduction in morbidly obese patients with losses of up to 60% of the excess weight, along with resolution of preoperative diabetes in more than 75% of the cases.

PHARMACOTHERAPY FOR DIABETES THAT HELPS WEIGHT REDUCTION

Pramlintide is an analogue of amylin, a naturally occurring hormone produced by pancreatic β-cells. The major mechanism of action appears to be inhibition of gastric emptying and suppression of glucagon release. Clinically, it also suppresses appetite in patients who receive it.

GLP-1 is recognized as an important regulator of glucose homeostasis. Exenatide and liraglutide are analogues of GLP-1, a naturally occurring incretin produced by the L-cells of the distal ileum. GLP-1 stimulates insulin release from the pancreatic β-cells, suppresses glucagon release from the pancreatic α-cells, slows gastric emptying, and acts on the brain to increase satiety. Increases in GLP-1 may be responsible for some of the weight loss following Roux-en-Y gastric bypass surgery in patients with type 2 diabetes.[206] The improvement in overall glucose control has been modest in clinical trials, at around 0.3%. However, those using the medication have also experienced weight reduction of ~1–1.5 kg in patients with type 1 diabetes and ~2.0–2.5 kg in patients with type 2 diabetes. Administration of exenatide in patients with type 2 diabetes has similar effects. Clinically, the result is an A_{1C} reduction of ~1%. Preliminary studies suggest that a significant proportion of insulin-treated patients with type 2 diabetes may be successfully transitioned from insulin to exenatide in addition to their oral agents. Most patients experience significant weight loss of ~2.5 kg when exenatide is used in addition to metformin and ~1 kg when it is added to a sulfonylurea.[207,208]

Exenatide was associated with a significant reduction in mean (SD) body weight from baseline (−2.1 [0.2] kg), with progressive reductions after 2 years (−4.7 [0.3] kg; P < 0.001 vs. baseline).[209]

Liraglutide works in a manner similar to that of exenatide but has a longer half-life, which allows for once daily (rather than twice daily) dosing. Some studies, including one meta-analysis, suggest that it may have a slightly greater A_{1C}-lowering effect than exenatide, although more investigation is warranted to substantiate such findings. In a meta-analysis, it is noted that exenatide and liraglutide resulted in greater weight loss (from 2.3 to 5.5 kg) with improvements in HbA_{1C} similar to that obtained with sulfonylureas.[210] Neither exenatide nor liraglutide is indicated for simple weight loss.

MULTIPLE RISK FACTORS FOR CARDIOVASCULAR DISEASE AND DIABETES MELLITUS

The MS is a constellation of central adiposity, impaired fasting glucose, elevated blood pressure, and dyslipidemia (high triglyceride and low HDL cholesterol). When three of these four criteria are present, the risk of CVD and diabetes is increased 1.5- to 2-fold.[211,212]

OBESITY AND COMORBIDITIES

Obesity is becoming a major public health problem throughout the world and is associated with significant, potentially life-threatening comorbidities. Either obesity itself or the comorbidities that accompany obesity are responsible for increased cardiovascular risk. Obesity is associated with most of the components of MS, the leading cause of type 2 diabetes. The comorbidities of obesity and type 2 diabetes associated with insulin resistance syndrome include obstructive sleep apnea, HTN, polycystic ovary syndrome, NAFLD, and certain forms of cancer.

IMPACT OF DIABETES AND OBESITY ON CARDIOVASCULAR DISEASE

CVD is a major cause of morbidity and mortality among subjects with type 2 diabetes and is responsible for up to 75% of deaths among them. The risk of CVD mortality in type 2 diabetic patients is more than double compared with that in age-matched subjects[213] (Figure 15.3). The risk of coronary artery disease (CAD) in subjects with type 2 diabetes is considered equivalent to that of nondiabetic subjects who have CAD,[214,215] especially women.[216] The association of obesity with clinically significant CAD is blatant in two classical prospective studies highly consulted: the Framingham Heart Study[217] and the Nurses Health Study.[218] Elevated proinflammatory cytokine levels found in obese patients relate mainly to obesity rather than to T2DM. Moreover, surgery-induced weight loss reduces circulating concentrations of key proinflammatory factors, which contribute to the improvement in the cardiovascular comorbidity following excess weight loss.[219] Obesity and overweight are often defined by WHO in terms of excess weight for a given height.[1,220] Overweight was defined as a BMI of 25.0–29.9 and obesity as a BMI of ≥30.0. BMI, calculated by weight (kg)/height (m²) and adjusted for height is used as a measure of weight standards.

MOUSE MODELS FOR OBESITY-INDUCED DIABETES

Obesity-driven type 2 diabetes (diabesity) involves complex genetic and environmental interactions that trigger the disease. Most obese humans do not develop diabetes, indicating that diabetogenesis entails a complex interaction between obesity genes and other predisposing susceptibility traits. The possible nature of some of these background modifiers is being elucidated by analysis of genetically obese mice. Among the various animal models available, mice are the most commonly used for several reasons. There are several spontaneously occurring obese mouse strains, and high-fat feeding requires only months to induce MS. It is relatively easy to study the effects of single genes by developing transgenic or gene knockouts to determine the influence of a gene. The three most commonly used spontaneously mutant obese mouse models are Lep$^{ob/ob}$, LepR$^{db/db}$, and A^y/a. They display insulin resistance and can even develop diabetes depending on the background strain. In addition, A^y/a mice have intact leptin signaling and display a delayed onset obesity that can be amplified by high-fat feeding, making them a good model for human obesity. The MC4R-deficient mouse model is similar to that of the A^y/a mice and is important because obesity in humans can be a result of mutations in the MC4R gene.[221]

The New Zealand Obese mouse (NZO/HlLt) represents one such model. These mice are hyperphagic and develop juvenile-onset obesity, even when fed a low-fat (4%–6%) diet. Approximately 50% of NZO/HlLt males transition from IGT to diabetes by 24 weeks of age.[222] The new mouse models of obesity-induced diabetes (diabesity models) have been created by combining independent diabetes risk-conferring quantitative trait loci (QTL) from two unrelated parental strains: New Zealand Obese (NZO/HlLt) and Nonobese Nondiabetic (NON/Lt).[223–225] Recombinant congenic strains (RCSs) are particularly useful for the analysis of polygenic syndromes. The NZO strain, selected for polygenic obesity, is known to contribute obesity/diabetes QTL on chromosomes (Chr) 1, 2, 4, 5, 6, 7, 11, 12, 13, 15, 17, and 18. RCS-10 recreates the 100% incidence seen in (NZOxNON) F1 males, but with less weight gain. Similarly, RCS-6, RCS-7, RCS-8, and RCS-9 represent diabetes-prone strains with different combinations of diabetogenic QTL.[222] M16 mice represent an outbred animal model used to facilitate gene discovery and elucidate the pathways controlling early-onset polygenic obesity and type 2 diabetic phenotypes. Phenotypes prevalent in the M16 model, with obesity and diabesity exhibited at a young age, closely mirror current trends in human populations.[226]

CONCLUSION

Obesity has become an epidemic worldwide. Diabetes is the fastest growing disease in the world. Obesity-driven type 2 diabetes (diabesity) involves complex genetic and environmental interactions. Behavioral changes leading to increased body weight are a major contributing factor to the rising incidence of diabetes. Measures to decrease weight will improve co-morbid conditions such as diabetes, cardiovascular disease, NAFLD and sleep apnea.

ACKNOWLEDGMENTS

The author Subhashini Yaturu was supported by VA merit review grant at the time of preparation of the chapter. The author Subhashini Yaturu receives salary support from VHA. Sushil K. Jain is supported by grants from NIDDK and the Office of Dietary Supplements of the NIH RO1 DK072433 and Malcolm Feist Endowed Chair in Diabetes. The authors thank Barbara Youngberg, MS, for excellent proofread of this chapter.

REFERENCES

1. Obesity: Preventing and managing the global epidemic. Report of a WHO consultation. World Health Organ Tech Rep Ser 2000;894:i–xii, 1–253.
2. Cefalu WT. Insulin resistance: Cellular and clinical concepts. *Exp Biol Med (Maywood)* 2001;226:13–26.
3. Reaven G. The metabolic syndrome or the insulin resistance syndrome? Different names, different concepts, and different goals. *Endocrinol Metab Clin North Am* 2004;33:283–303.
4. Erkelens DW. Insulin resistance syndrome and type 2 diabetes mellitus. *Am J Cardiol* 2001;88:38J–42J.
5. Guh DP, Zhang W, Bansback N, Amarsi Z, Birmingham CL, Anis AH. The incidence of co-morbidities related to obesity and overweight: A systematic review and meta-analysis. *BMC Public Health* 2009;9:88.
6. Franco M, Sanz B, Otero L, Dominguez-Vila A, Caballero B. Prevention of childhood obesity in Spain: A focus on policies outside the health sector. SESPAS report 2010. *Gac Sanit* 2010;24 Suppl 1:49–55.
7. American Diabetes Association. Diagnosis and classification of diabetes mellitus. *Diabetes Care* 2011; 34 Suppl 1:S62–S69.
8. Colditz GA, Willett WC, Stampfer MJ et al. Weight as a risk factor for clinical diabetes in women. *Am J Epidemiol* 1990;132:501–513.

9. Ni Mhurchu C, Parag V, Nakamura M, Patel A, Rodgers A, Lam TH. Body mass index and risk of diabetes mellitus in the Asia-Pacific region. *Asia Pac J Clin Nutr* 2006;15:127–133.

10. Schienkiewitz A, Schulze MB, Hoffmann K, Kroke A, Boeing H. Body mass index history and risk of type 2 diabetes: Results from the European Prospective Investigation into Cancer and Nutrition (EPIC)-Potsdam Study. *Am J Clin Nutr* 2006;84:427–433.

11. Flegal KM, Troiano RP. Changes in the distribution of body mass index of adults and children in the US population. *Int J Obes Relat Metab Disord* 2000;24:807–818.

12. Harris MI, Flegal KM, Cowie CC et al. Prevalence of diabetes, impaired fasting glucose, and impaired glucose tolerance in U.S. adults. The Third National Health and Nutrition Examination Survey, 1988–1994. *Diabetes Care* 1998;21:518–524.

13. Cowie CC, Rust KF, Byrd-Holt DD et al. Prevalence of diabetes and impaired fasting glucose in adults in the U.S. population: National Health and Nutrition Examination Survey 1999–2002. *Diabetes Care* 2006;29:1263–1268.

14. Colditz GA, Willett WC, Rotnitzky A, Manson JE. Weight gain as a risk factor for clinical diabetes mellitus in women. *Ann Intern Med* 1995;122:481–486.

15. Snijder MB, Dekker JM, Visser M et al. Associations of hip and thigh circumferences independent of waist circumference with the incidence of type 2 diabetes: The Hoorn Study. *Am J Clin Nutr* 2003;77:1192–1197.

16. Cassano PA, Rosner B, Vokonas PS, Weiss ST. Obesity and body fat distribution in relation to the incidence of non-insulin-dependent diabetes mellitus. A prospective cohort study of men in the normative aging study. *Am J Epidemiol* 1992;136:1474–1486.

17. Lundgren H, Bengtsson C, Blohme G, Lapidus L, Sjostrom L. Adiposity and adipose tissue distribution in relation to incidence of diabetes in women: Results from a prospective population study in Gothenburg, Sweden. *Int J Obes* 1989;13:413–423.

18. Ohlson LO, Larsson B, Svardsudd K et al. The influence of body fat distribution on the incidence of diabetes mellitus. 13.5 years of follow-up of the participants in the study of men born in 1913. *Diabetes* 1985;34:1055–1058.

19. Qiao Q, Nyamdorj R. Is the association of type II diabetes with waist circumference or waist-to-hip ratio stronger than that with body mass index? *Eur J Clin Nutr* 2010;64:30–34.

20. Aucott LS. Influences of weight loss on long-term diabetes outcomes. *Proc Nutr Soc* 2008;67:54–59.

21. Resnick HE, Valsania P, Halter JB, Lin X. Relation of weight gain and weight loss on subsequent diabetes risk in overweight adults. *J Epidemiol Community Health* 2000;54:596–602.

22. Mokdad AH, Ford ES, Bowman BA et al. Diabetes trends in the U.S.: 1990–1998. *Diabetes Care* 2000;23:1278–1283.

23. Mokdad AH, Ford ES, Bowman BA et al. Prevalence of obesity, diabetes, and obesity related health risk factors, 2001. *JAMA* 2003;289:76–79.

24. Janssen I, Katzmarzyk PT, Ross R. Body mass index, waist circumference, and health risk: Evidence in support of current National Institutes of Health guidelines. *Arch Intern Med* 2002;162:2074–2079.

25. Liu J, Fox CS, Hickson DA et al. Impact of abdominal visceral and subcutaneous adipose tissue on cardiometabolic risk factors: The Jackson Heart Study. *J Clin Endocrinol Metab* 2010;95:5419–5426.

26. Jensen MD. Role of body fat distribution and the metabolic complications of obesity. *J Clin Endocrinol Metab* 2008;93:S57–S63.

27. Verna EC, Berk PD. Role of fatty acids in the pathogenesis of obesity and fatty liver: Impact of bariatric surgery. *Semin Liver Dis* 2008;28:407–426.

28. Hoppin AG. Obesity and the liver: Developmental perspectives. *Semin Liver Dis* 2004;24:381–387.

29. Whitlock EP, Williams SB, Gold R, Smith PR, Shipman SA. Screening and interventions for childhood overweight: A summary of evidence for the US Preventive Services Task Force. *Pediatrics* 2005;116:e125–e144.

30. Barlow SE, Dietz WH. Obesity evaluation and treatment: Expert Committee recommendations. The Maternal and Child Health Bureau, Health Resources and Services Administration and the Department of Health and Human Services. *Pediatrics* 1998;102:E29.

31. Roelants M, Hauspie R, Hoppenbrouwers K. References for growth and pubertal development from birth to 21 years in Flanders, Belgium. *Ann Hum Biol* 2009;36:680–694.

32. de Onis M, Garza C, Onyango AW, Rolland-Cachera MF. [WHO growth standards for infants and young children.] *Arch Pediatr* 2009;16:47–53.

33. Rolland-Cachera MF, Sempe M, Guilloud-Bataille M, Patois E, Pequignot-Guggenbuhl F, Fautrad V. Adiposity indices in children. *Am J Clin Nutr* 1982;36:178–184.

34. Cole TJ, Flegal KM, Nicholls D, Jackson AA. Body mass index cut offs to define thinness in children and adolescents: International survey. *BMJ* 2007;335:194.

35. Tfayli H, Arslanian S. Pathophysiology of type 2 diabetes mellitus in youth: The evolving chameleon. *Arq Bras Endocrinol Metabol* 2009;53:165–174.

36. Aboul Ella NA, Shehab DI, Ismail MA, Maksoud AA. Prevalence of metabolic syndrome and insulin resistance among Egyptian adolescents 10 to 18 years of age. *J Clin Lipidol* 2010;4:185–195.

37. Holst-Schumacher I, Nunez-Rivas H, Monge-Rojas R, Barrantes-Santamaria M. Components of the metabolic syndrome among a sample of overweight and obese Costa Rican schoolchildren. *Food Nutr Bull* 2009;30:161–170.

38. Weiss R, Caprio S. The metabolic consequences of childhood obesity. *Best Pract Res Clin Endocrinol Metab* 2005;19:405–419.

39. Weiss R, Caprio S. Altered glucose metabolism in obese youth. *Pediatr Endocrinol Rev* 2006;3:233–238.

40. Lee S, Bacha F, Gungor N, Arslanian SA. Racial differences in adiponectin in youth: Relationship to visceral fat and insulin sensitivity. *Diabetes Care* 2006;29:51–56.

41. Bacha F, Saad R, Gungor N, Arslanian SA. Adiponectin in youth: Relationship to visceral adiposity, insulin sensitivity, and beta-cell function. *Diabetes Care* 2004;27:547–552.

42. Rasmussen-Torvik LJ, Pankow JS, Jacobs DR Jr., Steinberger J, Moran AM, Sinaiko AR. Influence of waist on adiponectin and insulin sensitivity in adolescence. *Obesity (Silver Spring)* 2009;17:156–161.

43. Yajnik CS. Early life origins of insulin resistance and type 2 diabetes in India and other Asian countries. *J Nutr* 2004;134:205–210.

44. Thorn J, Waller M, Johansson M, Marild S. Overweight among four-year-old children in relation to early growth characteristics and socioeconomic factors. *J Obes* 2010;2010:580642.

45. Han Z, Mulla S, Beyene J, Liao G, McDonald SD. Maternal underweight and the risk of preterm birth and low birth weight: A systematic review and meta-analyses. *Int J Epidemiol* 2011;40:65–101.

46. McDonald SD, Han Z, Mulla S, Beyene J. Overweight and obesity in mothers and risk of preterm birth and low birth weight infants: Systematic review and meta-analyses. *BMJ* 2010;341:c3428.

47. Hermann GM, Miller RL, Erkonen GE et al. Neonatal catch up growth increases diabetes susceptibility but improves behavioral and cardiovascular outcomes of low birth weight male mice. *Pediatr Res* 2009;66:53–58.

48. Forsen T, Eriksson J, Tuomilehto J, Reunanen A, Osmond C, Barker D. The fetal and childhood growth of persons who develop type 2 diabetes. *Ann Intern Med* 2000;133:176–182.

49. Bhargava SK, Sachdev HS, Fall CH et al. Relation of serial changes in childhood body-mass index to impaired glucose tolerance in young adulthood. *N Engl J Med* 2004;350:865–875.

50. Jimenez-Chillaron JC, Patti ME. To catch up or not to catch up: Is this the question? Lessons from animal models. *Curr Opin Endocrinol Diabetes Obes* 2007;14:23–29.

51. Jimenez-Chillaron JC, Hernandez-Valencia M, Lightner A et al. Reductions in caloric intake and early postnatal growth prevent glucose intolerance and obesity associated with low birthweight. *Diabetologia* 2006;49:1974–1984.

52. Grundy SM. United States Cholesterol Guidelines 2001: Expanded scope of intensive low-density lipoprotein-lowering therapy. *Am J Cardiol* 2001;88:23J–27J.

53. Nguyen NT, Magno CP, Lane KT, Hinojosa MW, Lane JS. Association of hypertension, diabetes, dyslipidemia, and metabolic syndrome with obesity: Findings from the National Health and Nutrition Examination Survey, 1999 to 2004. *J Am Coll Surg* 2008;207:928–934.

54. Adiels M, Olofsson SO, Taskinen MR, Boren J. Overproduction of very low-density lipoproteins is the hallmark of the dyslipidemia in the metabolic syndrome. *Arterioscler Thromb Vasc Biol* 2008;28:1225–1236.

55. Taskinen MR. Type 2 diabetes as a lipid disorder. *Curr Mol Med* 2005;5:297–308.

56. Boden G. Effects of free fatty acids (FFA) on glucose metabolism: Significance for insulin resistance and type 2 diabetes. *Exp Clin Endocrinol Diabetes* 2003;111:121–124.

57. Lam TK, Yoshii H, Haber CA et al. Free fatty acid-induced hepatic insulin resistance: A potential role for protein kinase C-delta. *Am J Physiol Endocrinol Metab* 2002;283:E682–E691.

58. Boden G, Cheung P, Stein TP, Kresge K, Mozzoli M. FFA cause hepatic insulin resistance by inhibiting insulin suppression of glycogenolysis. *Am J Physiol Endocrinol Metab* 2002;283:E12–E19.

59. Boden G. Free fatty acids—The link between obesity and insulin resistance. *Endocr Pract* 2001;7:44–51.

60. Boden G. Role of fatty acids in the pathogenesis of insulin resistance and NIDDM. *Diabetes* 1997;46:3–10.

61. Basu R, Chandramouli V, Dicke B, Landau B, Rizza R. Obesity and type 2 diabetes impair insulin-induced suppression of glycogenolysis as well as gluconeogenesis. *Diabetes* 2005;54:1942–1948.

62. Basu R, Singh RJ, Basu A et al. Obesity and type 2 diabetes do not alter splanchnic cortisol production in humans. *J Clin Endocrinol Metab* 2005;90:3919–3926.

63. Bonadonna RC, Groop L, Kraemer N, Ferrannini E, Del Prato S, DeFronzo RA. Obesity and insulin resistance in humans: A dose-response study. *Metabolism* 1990;39:452–459.

64. Kolterman OG, Insel J, Saekow M, Olefsky JM. Mechanisms of insulin resistance in human obesity: Evidence for receptor and postreceptor defects. *J Clin Invest* 1980;65:1272–1284.

65. Frayn KN. Visceral fat and insulin resistance—Causative or correlative? *Br J Nutr* 2000;83 Suppl 1:S71–S77.

66. Gallagher D, Kelley DE, Yim JE et al. Adipose tissue distribution is different in type 2 diabetes. *Am J Clin Nutr* 2009;89:807–814.

67. Ali AT, Ferris WF, Naran NH, Crowther NJ. Insulin resistance in the control of body fat distribution: A new hypothesis. *Horm Metab Res* 2011;43:77–80.

68. Wiklund P, Toss F, Weinehall L et al. Abdominal and gynoid fat mass are associated with cardiovascular risk factors in men and women. *J Clin Endocrinol Metab* 2008;93:4360–4366.

69. Yamashita S, Nakamura T, Shimomura I et al. Insulin resistance and body fat distribution. *Diabetes Care* 1996;19:287–291.

70. Kaplan NM. The deadly quartet. Upper-body obesity, glucose intolerance, hypertriglyceridemia, and hypertension. *Arch Intern Med* 1989;149:1514–1520.

71. Sanchez-Castillo CP, Velasquez-Monroy O, Lara-Esqueda A et al. Diabetes and hypertension increases in a society with abdominal obesity: Results of the Mexican National Health Survey 2000. *Public Health Nutr* 2005;8:53–60.

72. Merino-Ibarra E, Artieda M, Cenarro A et al. Ultrasonography for the evaluation of visceral fat and the metabolic syndrome. *Metabolism* 2005;54:1230–1235.

73. Hayashi T, Boyko EJ, McNeely MJ, Leonetti DL, Kahn SE, Fujimoto WY. Visceral adiposity, not abdominal subcutaneous fat area, is associated with an increase in future insulin resistance in Japanese Americans. *Diabetes* 2008;57:1269–1275.

74. Nyholm B, Nielsen MF, Kristensen K et al. Evidence of increased visceral obesity and reduced physical fitness in healthy insulin-resistant first-degree relatives of type 2 diabetic patients. *Eur J Endocrinol* 2004;150:207–214.

75. Vettor R, Milan G, Rossato M, Federspil G. Review article: Adipocytokines and insulin resistance. *Aliment Pharmacol Ther* 2005;22 Suppl 2:3–10.

76. Aylin P, Williams S, Bottle A. Obesity and type 2 diabetes in children, 1996–7 to 2003–4. *BMJ* 2005;331:1167.

77. Lee S, Guerra N, Arslanian S. Skeletal muscle lipid content and insulin sensitivity in black versus white obese adolescents: Is there a race differential? *J Clin Endocrinol Metab* 2010;95:2426–2432.

78. Chiarelli F, Marcovecchio ML. Insulin resistance and obesity in childhood. *Eur J Endocrinol* 2008;159 Suppl 1:S67–S74.

79. Bacha F, Saad R, Gungor N, Janosky J, Arslanian SA. Obesity, regional fat distribution, and syndrome X in obese black versus white adolescents: Race differential in diabetogenic and atherogenic risk factors. *J Clin Endocrinol Metab* 2003;88:2534–2540.

80. Goran MI, Bergman RN, Gower BA. Influence of total vs. visceral fat on insulin action and secretion in African American and white children. *Obes Res* 2001;9:423–431.

81. Caprio S, Tamborlane WV. Metabolic impact of obesity in childhood. *Endocrinol Metab Clin North Am* 1999;28:731–747.

82. Gower BA, Nagy TR, Goran MI. Visceral fat, insulin sensitivity, and lipids in prepubertal children. *Diabetes* 1999;48:1515–1521.

83. Abrams P, Levitt Katz LE. Metabolic effects of obesity causing disease in childhood. *Curr Opin Endocrinol Diabetes Obes* 2011;18:23–27.

84. Caballero AE, Arora S, Saouaf R et al. Microvascular and macrovascular reactivity is reduced in subjects at risk for type 2 diabetes. *Diabetes* 1999;48:1856–1862.

85. Timmers S, Schrauwen P, de Vogel J. Muscular diacylglycerol metabolism and insulin resistance. *Physiol Behav* 2008;94:242–251.

86. Boden G, Shulman GI. Free fatty acids in obesity and type 2 diabetes: Defining their role in the development of insulin resistance and beta-cell dysfunction. *Eur J Clin Invest* 2002;32 Suppl 3:14–23.

87. Yu C, Chen Y, Cline GW et al. Mechanism by which fatty acids inhibit insulin activation of insulin receptor substrate-1 (IRS-1)-associated phosphatidylinositol 3-kinase activity in muscle. *J Biol Chem* 2002;277:50230–50236.

88. Mittelman SD, Van Citters GW, Kirkman EL, Bergman RN. Extreme insulin resistance of the central adipose depot in vivo. *Diabetes* 2002;51:755–761.

89. Griffin ME, Marcucci MJ, Cline GW et al. Free fatty acid-induced insulin resistance is associated with activation of protein kinase C theta and alterations in the insulin signaling cascade. *Diabetes* 1999;48:1270–1274.

90. Homko CJ, Cheung P, Boden G. Effects of free fatty acids on glucose uptake and utilization in healthy women. *Diabetes* 2003;52:487–491.

91. Koo SH, Montminy M. Fatty acids and insulin resistance: A perfect storm. *Mol Cell* 2006;21:449–450.

92. Ginsberg HN, Stalenhoef AF. The metabolic syndrome: Targeting dyslipidaemia to reduce coronary risk. *J Cardiovasc Risk* 2003;10:121–128.

93. Ginsberg HN. Insulin resistance and cardiovascular disease. *J Clin Invest* 2000;106:453–458.

94. Wolfrum C, Stoffel M. Coactivation of Foxa2 through Pgc-1beta promotes liver fatty acid oxidation and triglyceride/VLDL secretion. *Cell Metab* 2006;3:99–110.

95. Kamagate A, Dong HH. FoxO1 integrates insulin signaling to VLDL production. *Cell Cycle* 2008;7:3162–3170.

96. Sparks JD, Sparks CE. Overindulgence and metabolic syndrome: Is FoxO1 a missing link? *J Clin Invest* 2008;118:2012–2015.

97. Murdoch SJ, Carr MC, Hokanson JE, Brunzell JD, Albers JJ. PLTP activity in premenopausal women. Relationship with lipoprotein lipase, HDL, LDL, body fat, and insulin resistance. *J Lipid Res* 2000;41:237–244.

98. Brunzell JD, Ayyobi AF. Dyslipidemia in the metabolic syndrome and type 2 diabetes mellitus. *Am J Med* 2003;115 Suppl 8A:24S–28S.

99. Purnell JQ, Kahn SE, Albers JJ, Nevin DN, Brunzell JD, Schwartz RS. Effect of weight loss with reduction of intra-abdominal fat on lipid metabolism in older men. *J Clin Endocrinol Metab* 2000;85:977–982.

100. Siri-Tarino PW, Williams PT, Fernstrom HS, Rawlings RS, Krauss RM. Reversal of small, dense LDL subclass phenotype by normalization of adiposity. *Obesity (Silver Spring)* 2009;17:1768–1775.

101. Siri-Tarino PW, Woods AC, Bray GA, Krauss RM. Reversal of small, dense LDL subclass phenotype by weight loss is associated with impaired fat oxidation. *Obesity (Silver Spring)* 2011;19:61–68.

102. Antuna-Puente B, Feve B, Fellahi S, Bastard JP. Adipokines: The missing link between insulin resistance and obesity. *Diabetes Metab* 2008;34:2–11.

103. Greenfield JR, Campbell LV. Relationship between inflammation, insulin resistance and type 2 diabetes: 'Cause or effect'? *Curr Diabetes Rev* 2006;2:195–211.

104. Hotamisligil GS, Spiegelman BM. Tumor necrosis factor alpha: A key component of the obesity-diabetes link. *Diabetes* 1994;43:1271–1278.

105. Lorenzo M, Fernandez-Veledo S, Vila-Bedmar R, Garcia-Guerra L, De Alvaro C, Nieto-Vazquez I. Insulin resistance induced by tumor necrosis factor-alpha in myocytes and brown adipocytes. *J Anim Sci* 2008;86:E94–E104.

106. Feinstein R, Kanety H, Papa MZ, Lunenfeld B, Karasik A. Tumor necrosis factor-alpha suppresses insulin-induced tyrosine phosphorylation of insulin receptor and its substrates. *J Biol Chem* 1993;268:26055–26058.

107. Hartge MM, Unger T, Kintscher U. The endothelium and vascular inflammation in diabetes. *Diab Vasc Dis Res* 2007;4:84–88.

108. Hsueh WA, Quinones MJ. Role of endothelial dysfunction in insulin resistance. *Am J Cardiol* 2003;92:10J–17J.

109. Reaven GM. Pathophysiology of insulin resistance in human disease. *Physiol Rev* 1995;75:473–486.

110. Weyer C, Bogardus C, Mott DM, Pratley RE. The natural history of insulin secretory dysfunction and insulin resistance in the pathogenesis of type 2 diabetes mellitus. *J Clin Invest* 1999;104:787–794.

111. Kaiser N, Leibowitz G. Failure of beta-cell adaptation in type 2 diabetes: Lessons from animal models. *Front Biosci* 2009;14:1099–1115.

112. Lowell BB, Shulman GI. Mitochondrial dysfunction and type 2 diabetes. *Science* 2005;307:384–387.

113. Kahn SE. Clinical review 135: The importance of beta-cell failure in the development and progression of type 2 diabetes. *J Clin Endocrinol Metab* 2001;86:4047–4058.

114. DeFronzo RA. Lilly lecture 1987. The triumvirate: Beta-cell, muscle, liver. A collusion responsible for NIDDM. *Diabetes* 1988;37:667–687.

115. Kahn BB, Flier JS. Obesity and insulin resistance. *J Clin Invest* 2000;106(4):473–481.

116. Kralisch S, Sommer G, Deckert CM et al. Adipokines in diabetes and cardiovascular diseases. *Minerva Endocrinol* 2007;32:161–171.

117. Arner P. Insulin resistance in type 2 diabetes—Role of the adipokines. *Curr Mol Med* 2005;5:333–339.

118. Zhao YF, Feng DD, Chen C. Contribution of adipocyte-derived factors to beta-cell dysfunction in diabetes. *Int J Biochem Cell Biol* 2006;38:804–819.

119. Considine RV, Sinha MK, Heiman ML et al. Serum immunoreactive-leptin concentrations in normal-weight and obese humans. *N Engl J Med* 1996;334:292–295.

120. Minokoshi Y, Kim YB, Peroni OD et al. Leptin stimulates fatty-acid oxidation by activating AMP-activated protein kinase. *Nature* 2002;415:339–343.

121. Nieto-Vazquez I, Fernandez-Veledo S, Kramer DK, Vila-Bedmar R, Garcia-Guerra L, Lorenzo M. Insulin resistance associated to obesity: The link TNF-alpha. *Arch Physiol Biochem* 2008;114:183–194.

122. Kim JH, Bachmann RA, Chen J. Interleukin-6 and insulin resistance. *Vitam Horm* 2009;80:613–633.

123. Yamauchi T, Kamon J, Minokoshi Y et al. Adiponectin stimulates glucose utilization and fatty-acid oxidation by activating AMP-activated protein kinase. *Nat Med* 2002;8:1288–1295.

124. Kadowaki T, Yamauchi T. Adiponectin and adiponectin receptors. *Endocr Rev* 2005;26:439–451.

125. Schondorf T, Maiworm A, Emmison N, Forst T, Pfutzner A. Biological background and role of adiponectin as marker for insulin resistance and cardiovascular risk. *Clin Lab* 2005;51:489–494.

126. Utsunomiya H, Yamakawa T, Kamei J, Kadonosono K, Tanaka S. Anti-hyperglycemic effects of plum in a rat model of obesity and type 2 diabetes, Wistar fatty rat. *Biomed Res* 2005;26:193–200.

127. Adeghate E. Visfatin: Structure, function and relation to diabetes mellitus and other dysfunctions. *Curr Med Chem* 2008;15:1851–1862.

128. Esteghamati A, Alamdari A, Zandieh A et al. Serum visfatin is associated with type 2 diabetes mellitus independent of insulin resistance and obesity. *Diabetes Res Clin Pract* 2011;91:154–158.

129. Davutoglu M, Ozkaya M, Guler E et al. Plasma visfatin concentrations in childhood obesity: Relationships with insulin resistance and anthropometric indices. *Swiss Med Wkly* 2009;139:22–27.

130. Pagano C, Pilon C, Olivieri M et al. Reduced plasma visfatin/pre-B cell colony-enhancing factor in obesity is not related to insulin resistance in humans. *J Clin Endocrinol Metab* 2006;91:3165–3170.

131. Guo H, Jin D, Zhang Y et al. Lipocalin-2 deficiency impairs thermogenesis and potentiates diet-induced insulin resistance in mice. *Diabetes* 2010;59:1376–1385.

132. Qi L, Saberi M, Zmuda E et al. Adipocyte CREB promotes insulin resistance in obesity. *Cell Metab* 2009;9:277–286.

133. Catalan V, Gomez-Ambrosi J, Rodriguez A et al. Increased adipose tissue expression of lipocalin-2 in obesity is related to inflammation and matrix metalloproteinase-2 and metalloproteinase-9 activities in humans. *J Mol Med* 2009;87:803–813.

134. Musso G, Gambino R, Cassader M, Pagano G. Meta-analysis: Natural history of non-alcoholic fatty liver disease (NAFLD) and diagnostic accuracy of non-invasive tests for liver disease severity. *Ann Med* 2011;43:617–649.

135. Matteoni CA, Younossi ZM, Gramlich T, Boparai N, Liu YC, McCullough AJ. Nonalcoholic fatty liver disease: A spectrum of clinical and pathological severity. *Gastroenterology* 1999;116:1413–1419.

136. Adams LA, Waters OR, Knuiman MW, Elliott RR, Olynyk JK. NAFLD as a risk factor for the development of diabetes and the metabolic syndrome: An eleven-year follow-up study. *Am J Gastroenterol* 2009;104:861–867.

137. Bugianesi E, Moscatiello S, Ciaravella MF, Marchesini G. Insulin resistance in nonalcoholic fatty liver disease. *Curr Pharm Des* 2010;16:1941–1951.

138. Fan JG. Impact of non-alcoholic fatty liver disease on accelerated metabolic complications. *J Dig Dis* 2008;9:63–67.

139. Clinical Guidelines on the Identification, Evaluation, and Treatment of Overweight and Obesity in Adults—The Evidence Report. National Institutes of Health. *Obes Res* 1998;6 Suppl 2:51S–209S.

140. Fujioka K. Benefits of moderate weight loss in patients with type 2 diabetes. *Diabetes Obes Metab* 2010;12:186–194.

141. Riccardi G, Capaldo B, Vaccaro O. Functional foods in the management of obesity and type 2 diabetes. *Curr Opin Clin Nutr Metab Care* 2005;8:630–635.

142. Utzschneider KM, Carr DB, Barsness SM, Kahn SE, Schwartz RS. Diet-induced weight loss is associated with an improvement in beta-cell function in older men. *J Clin Endocrinol Metab* 2004;89:2704–2710.

143. Boden G, Sargrad K, Homko C, Mozzoli M, Stein TP. Effect of a low-carbohydrate diet on appetite, blood glucose levels, and insulin resistance in obese patients with type 2 diabetes. *Ann Intern Med* 2005;142:403–411.

144. Stern L, Iqbal N, Seshadri P et al. The effects of low-carbohydrate versus conventional weight loss diets in severely obese adults: One-year follow-up of a randomized trial. *Ann Intern Med* 2004;140:778–785.

145. Tuomilehto J, Lindstrom J, Eriksson JG et al. Prevention of type 2 diabetes mellitus by changes in lifestyle among subjects with impaired glucose tolerance. *N Engl J Med* 2001;344:1343–1350.

146. Knowler WC, Barrett-Connor E, Fowler SE et al. Reduction in the incidence of type 2 diabetes with lifestyle intervention or metformin. *N Engl J Med* 2002;346:393–403.

147. Knowler WC, Fowler SE, Hamman RF et al. 10-year follow-up of diabetes incidence and weight loss in the Diabetes Prevention Program Outcomes Study. *Lancet* 2009;374:1677–1686.

148. Ratner RE, Christophi CA, Metzger BE et al. Prevention of diabetes in women with a history of gestational diabetes: Effects of metformin and lifestyle interventions. *J Clin Endocrinol Metab* 2008;93:4774–4779.

149. Pan XR, Li GW, Hu YH et al. Effects of diet and exercise in preventing NIDDM in people with impaired glucose tolerance. The Da Qing IGT and Diabetes Study. *Diabetes Care* 1997;20:537–544.

150. Torgerson JS, Hauptman J, Boldrin MN, Sjostrom L. XENical in the prevention of diabetes in obese subjects (XENDOS) study: A randomized study of orlistat as an adjunct to lifestyle changes for the prevention of type 2 diabetes in obese patients. *Diabetes Care* 2004;27:155–161.

151. Ryan DH, Espeland MA, Foster GD et al. Look AHEAD (Action for Health in Diabetes): Design and methods for a clinical trial of weight loss for the prevention of cardiovascular disease in type 2 diabetes. *Control Clin Trials* 2003;24:610–628.

152. Wing RR. Long-term effects of a lifestyle intervention on weight and cardiovascular risk factors in individuals with type 2 diabetes mellitus: Four-year results of the Look AHEAD trial. *Arch Intern Med* 2010;170:1566–1575.

153. Sakane N, Sato J, Tsushita K et al. Prevention of type 2 diabetes in a primary healthcare setting: Three-year results of lifestyle intervention in Japanese subjects with impaired glucose tolerance. *BMC Public Health* 2011;11:40.

154. Sjostrom L, Rissanen A, Andersen T et al. Randomised placebo-controlled trial of orlistat for weight loss and prevention of weight regain in obese patients. European Multicentre Orlistat Study Group. *Lancet* 1998;352:167–172.

155. Shi YF, Pan CY, Hill J, Gao Y. Orlistat in the treatment of overweight or obese Chinese patients with newly diagnosed Type 2 diabetes. *Diabet Med* 2005;22:1737–43.

156. Rowe R, Cowx M, Poole C, McEwan P, Morgan C, Walker M. The effects of orlistat in patients with diabetes: Improvement in glycaemic control and weight loss. *Curr Med Res Opin* 2005;21:1885–1890.

157. Tan KC, Tso AW, Tam SC, Pang RW, Lam KS. Acute effect of orlistat on post-prandial lipaemia and free fatty acids in overweight patients with Type 2 diabetes mellitus. *Diabet Med* 2002;19:944–948.

158. Hollander PA, Elbein SC, Hirsch IB et al. Role of orlistat in the treatment of obese patients with type 2 diabetes. A 1-year randomized double-blind study. *Diabetes Care* 1998;21:1288–1294.

159. Damci T, Yalin S, Balci H et al. Orlistat augments postprandial increases in glucagon-like peptide 1 in obese type 2 diabetic patients. *Diabetes Care* 2004;27:1077–1080.

160. Yanovski SZ. Pharmacotherapy for obesity—Promise and uncertainty. *N Engl J Med* 2005;353:2187–2189.

161. Van Gaal LF, Rissanen AM, Scheen AJ, Ziegler O, Rossner S. Effects of the cannabinoid-1 receptor blocker rimonabant on weight reduction and cardiovascular risk factors in overweight patients: 1-year experience from the RIO-Europe study. *Lancet* 2005;365:1389–1397.

162. Despres JP, Golay A, Sjostrom L. Effects of rimonabant on metabolic risk factors in overweight patients with dyslipidemia. *N Engl J Med* 2005;353:2121–2134.

163. McNeely W, Goa KL. Sibutramine. A review of its contribution to the management of obesity. *Drugs* 1998;56:1093–1124.

164. Gokcel A, Karakose H, Ertorer EM, Tanaci N, Tutuncu NB, Guvener N. Effects of sibutramine in obese female subjects with type 2 diabetes and poor blood glucose control. *Diabetes Care* 2001;24:1957–1960.

165. Norris SL, Zhang X, Avenell A et al. Efficacy of pharmacotherapy for weight loss in adults with type 2 diabetes mellitus: A meta-analysis. *Arch Intern Med* 2004;164:1395–1404.

166. Consensus development conference on diet and exercise in non-insulin-dependent diabetes mellitus. National Institutes of Health. *Diabetes Care* 1987;10:639–644.

167. Hughes TA, Gwynne JT, Switzer BR, Herbst C, White G. Effects of caloric restriction and weight loss on glycemic control, insulin release and resistance, and atherosclerotic risk in obese patients with type II diabetes mellitus. *Am J Med* 1984;77:7–17.

168. Redmon JB, Reck KP, Raatz SK et al. Two-year outcome of a combination of weight loss therapies for type 2 diabetes. *Diabetes Care* 2005;28:1311–1315.

169. Henry RR, Wiest-Kent TA, Scheaffer L, Kolterman OG, Olefsky JM. Metabolic consequences of very-low-calorie diet therapy in obese non-insulin-dependent diabetic and nondiabetic subjects. *Diabetes* 1986;35:155–164.

170. Lee A, Morley JE. Metformin decreases food consumption and induces weight loss in subjects with obesity with type II non-insulin-dependent diabetes. *Obes Res* 1998;6:47–53.

171. Genuth S. Implications of the United Kingdom prospective diabetes study for patients with obesity and type 2 diabetes. *Obes Res* 2000;8:198–201.

172. Greenway F. Obesity medications and the treatment of type 2 diabetes. *Diabetes Technol Ther* 1999;1:277–287.

173. Poon T, Nelson P, Shen L et al. Exenatide improves glycemic control and reduces body weight in subjects with type 2 diabetes: A dose-ranging study. *Diabetes Technol Ther* 2005;7:467–477.

174. Pories WJ, MacDonald KG Jr., Flickinger EG et al. Is type II diabetes mellitus (NIDDM) a surgical disease? *Ann Surg* 1992;215:633–642; discussion 43.

175. O'Leary JP. Overview: Jejunoileal bypass in the treatment of morbid obesity. *Am J Clin Nutr* 1980;33:389–394.

176. Sjostrom L, Lindroos AK, Peltonen M et al. Lifestyle, diabetes, and cardiovascular risk factors 10 years after bariatric surgery. *N Engl J Med* 2004;351:2683–2693.

177. Aucott L, Poobalan A, Smith WC et al. Weight loss in obese diabetic and non-diabetic individuals and long-term diabetes outcomes—A systematic review. *Diabetes Obes Metab* 2004;6:85–94.

178. Franks PW, Rolandsson O, Debenham SL et al. Replication of the association between variants in WFS1 and risk of type 2 diabetes in European populations. *Diabetologia* 2008;51:458–463.

179. Gudmundsson J, Sulem P, Steinthorsdottir V et al. Two variants on chromosome 17 confer prostate cancer risk, and the one in TCF2 protects against type 2 diabetes. *Nat Genet* 2007;39:977–983.

180. Sandhu MS, Weedon MN, Fawcett KA et al. Common variants in WFS1 confer risk of type 2 diabetes. *Nat Genet* 2007;39:951–953.

181. Winckler W, Weedon MN, Graham RR et al. Evaluation of common variants in the six known maturity-onset diabetes of the young (MODY) genes for association with type 2 diabetes. *Diabetes* 2007;56:685–693.

182. Bouatia-Naji N, Bonnefond A, Cavalcanti-Proenca C et al. A variant near MTNR1B is associated with increased fasting plasma glucose levels and type 2 diabetes risk. *Nat Genet* 2009;41:89–94.

183. Lyssenko V, Nagorny CL, Erdos MR et al. Common variant in MTNR1B associated with increased risk of type 2 diabetes and impaired early insulin secretion. *Nat Genet* 2009;41:82–88.

184. Prokopenko I, Langenberg C, Florez JC et al. Variants in MTNR1B influence fasting glucose levels. *Nat Genet* 2009;41:77–81.

185. Rung J, Cauchi S, Albrechtsen A et al. Genetic variant near IRS1 is associated with type 2 diabetes, insulin resistance and hyperinsulinemia. *Nat Genet* 2009;41:1110–1115.

186. O'Rahilly S. Human genetics illuminates the paths to metabolic disease. *Nature* 2009;462:307–314.

187. Jafar-Mohammadi B, McCarthy MI. Genetics of type 2 diabetes mellitus and obesity—a review. *Ann Med* 2008;40:2–10.

188. Scuteri A, Sanna S, Chen WM et al. Genome-wide association scan shows genetic variants in the FTO gene are associated with obesity-related traits. *PLoS Genet* 2007;3:e115.

189. Dina C, Meyre D, Gallina S et al. Variation in FTO contributes to childhood obesity and severe adult obesity. *Nat Genet* 2007;39:724–726.

190. Frayling TM, Timpson NJ, Weedon MN et al. A common variant in the FTO gene is associated with body mass index and predisposes to childhood and adult obesity. *Science* 2007;316:889–894.

191. Speliotes EK, Willer CJ, Berndt SI et al. Association analyses of 249,796 individuals reveal 18 new loci associated with body mass index. *Nat Genet* 2010;42:937–948.

192. Willer CJ, Speliotes EK, Loos RJ et al. Six new loci associated with body mass index highlight a neuronal influence on body weight regulation. *Nat Genet* 2009;41:25–34.

193. Thorleifsson G, Walters GB, Gudbjartsson DF et al. Genome-wide association yields new sequence variants at seven loci that associate with measures of obesity. *Nat Genet* 2009;41:18–24.

194. Loos RJ, Lindgren CM, Li S et al. Common variants near MC4R are associated with fat mass, weight and risk of obesity. *Nat Genet* 2008;40:768–775.

195. Tong Y, Lin Y, Zhang Y, Yang J, Liu H, Zhang B. Association between TCF7L2 gene polymorphisms and susceptibility to type 2 diabetes mellitus: A large Human Genome Epidemiology (HuGE) review and meta-analysis. *BMC Med Genet* 2009;10:15.

196. Pearson ER, Donnelly LA, Kimber C et al. Variation in TCF7L2 influences therapeutic response to sulfonylureas: A GoDARTs study. *Diabetes* 2007;56:2178–2182.

197. Lindgren CM, McCarthy MI. Mechanisms of disease: Genetic insights into the etiology of type 2 diabetes and obesity. *Nat Clin Pract Endocrinol Metab* 2008;4:156–163.

198. Li S, Zhao JH, Luan J et al. Cumulative effects and predictive value of common obesity-susceptibility variants identified by genome-wide association studies. *Am J Clin Nutr* 2009;91:184–190.

199. Barber TM, Bennett AJ, Groves CJ et al. Association of variants in the fat mass and obesity associated (FTO) gene with polycystic ovary syndrome. *Diabetologia* 2008;51:1153–1158.

200. Johansson A, Marroni F, Hayward C et al. Linkage and genome-wide association analysis of obesity-related phenotypes: Association of weight with the MGAT1 gene. *Obesity (Silver Spring)* 2010;18:803–808.

201. Buchwald H, Estok R, Fahrbach K, Banel D, Sledge I. Trends in mortality in bariatric surgery: A systematic review and meta-analysis. *Surgery* 2007;142:621–632; discussion 32–35.

202. Cunneen SA. Review of meta-analytic comparisons of bariatric surgery with a focus on laparoscopic adjustable gastric banding. *Surg Obes Relat Dis* 2008;4:S47–S55.

203. Buchwald H, Avidor Y, Braunwald E et al. Bariatric surgery: A systematic review and meta-analysis. *JAMA* 2004;292:1724–1737.

204. Buchwald H, Estok R, Fahrbach K et al. Weight and type 2 diabetes after bariatric surgery: Systematic review and meta-analysis. *Am J Med* 2009;122:248–256 e5.

205. Levy P, Fried M, Santini F, Finer N. The comparative effects of bariatric surgery on weight and type 2 diabetes. *Obes Surg* 2007;17:1248–1256.

206. Laferrere B, Heshka S, Wang K et al. Incretin levels and effect are markedly enhanced 1 month after Roux-en-Y gastric bypass surgery in obese patients with type 2 diabetes. *Diabetes Care* 2007;30:1709–1716.

207. Kendall DM, Riddle MC, Rosenstock J et al. Effects of exenatide (exendin-4) on glycemic control over 30 weeks in patients with type 2 diabetes treated with metformin and a sulfonylurea. *Diabetes Care* 2005;28:1083–1091.

208. Buse JB, Henry RR, Han J, Kim DD, Fineman MS, Baron AD. Effects of exenatide (exendin-4) on glycemic control over 30 weeks in sulfonylurea-treated patients with type 2 diabetes. *Diabetes Care* 2004;27:2628–2635.

209. Buse JB, Klonoff DC, Nielsen LL et al. Metabolic effects of two years of exenatide treatment on diabetes, obesity, and hepatic biomarkers in patients with type 2 diabetes: An interim analysis of data from the open-label, uncontrolled extension of three double-blind, placebo-controlled trials. *Clin Ther* 2007;29:139–153.

210. Shyangdan DS, Royle PL, Clar C, Sharma P, Waugh NR. Glucagon-like peptide analogues for type 2 diabetes mellitus: Systematic review and meta-analysis. *BMC Endocr Disord* 2010;10:20.

211. Smith SC Jr. Multiple risk factors for cardiovascular disease and diabetes mellitus. *Am J Med* 2007;120:S3–S11.

212. Bray GA, Bellanger T. Epidemiology, trends, and morbidities of obesity and the metabolic syndrome. *Endocrine* 2006;29:109–117.

213. Laakso M. Cardiovascular disease in type 2 diabetes from population to man to mechanisms: The Kelly West Award Lecture 2008. *Diabetes Care* 2010;33:442–449.

214. Haffner SM, Lehto S, Ronnemaa T, Pyorala K, Laakso M. Mortality from coronary heart disease in subjects with type 2 diabetes and in nondiabetic subjects with and without prior myocardial infarction. *N Engl J Med* 1998;339:229–234.

215. Executive Summary of the Third Report of the National Cholesterol Education Program (NCEP) Expert Panel on Detection, Evaluation, and Treatment of High Blood Cholesterol in Adults (Adult Treatment Panel III). *JAMA* 2001;285:2486–2497.

216. Juutilainen A, Lehto S, Ronnemaa T, Pyorala K, Laakso M. Type 2 diabetes as a "coronary heart disease equivalent": An 18-year prospective population-based study in Finnish subjects. *Diabetes Care* 2005;28:2901–2907.

217. Manson JE, Colditz GA, Stampfer MJ et al. A prospective study of obesity and risk of coronary heart disease in women. *N Engl J Med* 1990;322:882–889.

218. Manson JE, Willett WC, Stampfer MJ et al. Body weight and mortality among women. *N Engl J Med* 1995;333:677–685.

219. Catalan V, Gomez-Ambrosi J, Ramirez B et al. Proinflammatory cytokines in obesity: Impact of type 2 diabetes mellitus and gastric bypass. *Obes Surg* 2007;17:1464–1474.

220. Physical status: The use and interpretation of anthropometry. Report of a WHO Expert Committee. *World Health Organ Tech Rep Ser* 1995;854:1–452.

221. Kennedy AJ, Ellacott KL, King VL, Hasty AH. Mouse models of the metabolic syndrome. *Dis Model Mech* 2010;3:156–166.

222. Reifsnyder PC, Leiter EH. Deconstructing and reconstructing obesity-induced diabetes (diabesity) in mice. *Diabetes* 2002;51:825–832.

223. Leiter EH, Reifsnyder PC, Zhang W, Pan HJ, Xiao Q, Mistry J. Differential endocrine responses to rosiglitazone therapy in new mouse models of type 2 diabetes. *Endocrinology* 2006;147:919–926.

224. Mathews CE, Bagley R, Leiter EH. ALS/Lt: A new type 2 diabetes mouse model associated with low free radical scavenging potential. *Diabetes* 2004;53 Suppl 1:S125–129.

225. Leiter EH, Reifsnyder PC. Differential levels of diabetogenic stress in two new mouse models of obesity and type 2 diabetes. *Diabetes* 2004;53 Suppl 1:S4–11.

226. Allan MF, Eisen EJ, Pomp D. The M16 mouse: An outbred animal model of early onset polygenic obesity and diabesity. *Obes Res* 2004;12:1397–1407.

227. International Diabetes Federation. *IDF Diabetes Altas*, 4th edn., Brussels, Belgium.

16 Inflammation
A Hallmark of Obesity in Conflict with Wound Healing

Sashwati Roy, PhD and Chandan K. Sen, PhD

CONTENTS

INTRODUCTION

Physical trauma represents one of the most primitive challenges that threatened survival. In other words, injury eliminated the unfit. A Sumerian clay tablet (c. 2150 BC) described early wound care that included washing the wound in beer and hot water, using poultices from substances such as wine dregs and lizard dung, and bandaging the wound. Ancient scriptures depicting the science of life or *Ayurveda* report refined clinical surgical procedures such as rhinoplasty and cheek flaps as early as sixth to seventh century BC. This was the beginning of planned physical injury with the intent to cure (Wangensteen, 1975; Mehra, 2002).

Hippocrates (c. 400 BC) detailed the importance of draining pus from the wound, and Galen (c. AD 130–200) described the principle of first- and second-intention healing (Broughton et al., 2006). Wound healing advanced slowly over the centuries, with major advances in the nineteenth century in the importance of controlling infection, hemostasis, and necrotic tissue (Eming et al., 2007a). Today, surgical trauma taken together with injury caused during accidents and secondary to other clinical conditions, e.g., diabetes, represents a substantial cost to society (Sen et al., 2009). Any solution to wound healing problems will require a multifaceted comprehensive approach. First and foremost, the wound environment will have to be made receptive to therapies. Second, the appropriate therapeutic regimen needs to be identified and provided while managing systemic limitations that could secondarily limit the healing response.

In the United States, chronic wounds affect around 6.5 million patients. The annual wound care products market is projected to reach US$15.3 billion by 2010. Chronic wounds are rarely seen in individuals who are otherwise healthy. It is claimed that an excess of US$25 billion is spent annually on treatment of chronic wounds; and the burden is growing rapidly due to increasing health-care costs, an aging population, and a sharp rise in the incidence of diabetes and obesity worldwide (Sen et al., 2009). According to the Centers for Disease Control and Prevention (CDC), about one-third of U.S. adults (33.8%) are obese. During the past 20 years, there has been a dramatic increase in obesity in the United States and rates remain high. In 2010, no state had a prevalence of obesity less than 20%. Obesity, commonly associated with increased subcutaneous depot of fat, profoundly affects skin health (Shipman and Millington, 2011). Several clinical conditions are common to the majority of obese patients, e.g., striae distensae, plantar hyperkeratosis, and an increased risk of skin infections. However, it is associated with malignant melanoma and an increased risk of inflammatory dermatoses, such as psoriasis, as well as some rarer disorders. Dysregulated inflammation represents a key mechanism by which obesity complicates wound healing. This chapter will present an overview of the mechanisms underlying obesity-dependent complication of wound healing with emphasis on inflammation.

WOUND INFLAMMATION

Timely mounting and resolution of inflammation are required for successful wound healing. Tissue injury triggers an acute-phase inflammation (Latin, *inflammare*, to set on fire) response that is meant to prepare the wound site for subsequent wound closure. Inflammation encompasses a series of response of vascularized tissues of the body to injury. Local chemical mediators biosynthesized during acute inflammation give rise to the macroscopic events characterized by Celsus in the first century, namely, rubor (redness), tumor (swelling), calor (heat), and dolor (pain). At the cellular and molecular level, inflammation results from the coordination of manifold systems of receptors and sensors that affect transcriptional and posttranslational programs necessary for host defense and resolution of infection. During normal healing, the inflammatory response is characterized by spatially and temporally changing patterns of specific leukocyte subsets.

PLATELETS

Formation of the clot or thrombus is dependent on platelet activation. The platelet-rich blood clot also entraps polymorphonuclear leukocytes (PMN, neutrophils). This helps amplify blood coagulation and lays the foundation for the subsequent acute-phase inflammatory response. In a matter of hours after injury, large numbers of neutrophils extravasate by transmigrating across the endothelial cell wall of blood capillaries to the wound site. To enable this, local blood vessels are activated by pro-inflammatory cytokines such as interleukin (IL)-1β, tumor necrosis factor alpha (TNF-α), and IFN-γ. These cytokines induce the expression of adhesion molecules necessary for adhesion of leukocytes and diapedesis. Adhesion molecules such as integrins as well as P-selectin and E-selectin play a central role in enabling diapedesis of neutrophils. These adhesion molecules bind with integrins expressed on the cell surface of neutrophils such as CD11a/CD18 (LFA), CD 11b/CD18 (MAC-1), CD11c/CD18 (gp150, 95), and CD11d/CD18. Alongside cytokines, chemokines play a major role in mounting acute-phase inflammation after injury. Chemokines include IL-8, macrophage chemoattractant protein-1 (MCP-1), and growth-related oncogene-α. In the case of an infected wound, bacterial products such as lipopolysaccharide and formyl-methionyl peptides can enhance neutrophils recruitment to the wound site.

NEUTROPHILS

Neutrophils traverse postcapillary venules at sites of inflammation, degrade pathogens within phagolysosomes, and undergo apoptosis. Neutrophils serve a wide range of functions ranging from phagocytosis of infectious agents to cleansing of devitalized tissue. When coated with opsonins (generally complement and/or antibody), microorganisms bind to specific receptors on the surface of the phagocyte, and invagination of the cell membrane occurs with the incorporation of the microorganism into an intracellular phagosome. There follows a burst of oxygen consumption, and much, if not all, of the extra oxygen consumed is converted to highly reactive oxygen species. This is called respiratory burst. In addition, the cytoplasmic granules discharge their contents into the phagosome, and death of the ingested microorganism soon follows. Among the antimicrobial systems formed in the phagosome is the one consisting of myeloperoxidase (MPO), released into the phagosome during the degranulation process; hydrogen peroxide (H_2O_2), formed by the respiratory burst; and a halide, particularly chloride. The initial product of the MPO-H_2O_2-chloride system is hypochlorous acid, and subsequent formation of chlorine, chloramines, hydroxyl radicals, singlet oxygen, and ozone has been proposed. These same toxic agents can be released to the outside of the cell, where they may attack normal tissue and thus contribute to the pathogenesis of disease (Klebanoff, 2005). Other products delivered by neutrophils to the wound site include antimicrobials such as cationic peptides and eicosanoids as well as proteases such as elastase, cathepsin G, proteinase 3, and urokinase-type plasminogen activator. As it relates to the overall inflammatory process elicited in response to injury, neutrophils are major players because they can modify macrophage function and therefore regulate innate immune response during wound healing (Daley et al., 2005). In the absence of neutrophils, wound-site macrophages seem to lack guidance in conducting the healing process (Peters et al., 2005).

In a healing wound, neutrophil infiltration ceases after few days of injury. Expended neutrophils are programmed to die, and the dying neutrophils are recognized by wound-site macrophages and phagocytosed. The wound site contains a small portion of macrophages that are resident. Majority of the macrophages at the wound site are recruited from peripheral circulation. Extravasation of peripheral blood monocytes is enabled by the interaction between endothelial vascular cell adhesion molecule-1 and monocyte very late antigen-4 ($\alpha 4\beta 1$ integrin). Factors that guide the extravasated monocyte to the wound site include growth factors, chemotactic proteins, pro-inflammatory cytokines, and chemokines such as macrophage inflammatory protein 1α, MCP-1, and RANTES. The source of these chemoattractants includes clot-associated platelets, wound-edge hyperproliferative keratinocytes, wound-tissue fibroblasts, and subsets of leukocytes already at the wound site. Once the monocyte leaves the blood vessel to transmigrate into the wound site through the extracellular matrix microenvironment, the process of monocyte differentiation to macrophages has started.

Mediators present in the microenvironment that the monocyte traverses to reach the wound site interact with receptors on the monocyte cell surface, bringing forth major changes in the transcriptomic as well as proteomic make of the cell. Major examples of such receptors present on the monocyte surface include toll-like receptors (TLRs), complement receptors, and Fc receptors. At the wound site, macrophages function as antigen-presenting cells and phagocytes scavenging dead cells and debris. In addition, they deliver a wide range of growth factors that are known for their abilities to execute the wound healing process. Such growth factors include TGFβ, TGFα, basic fibroblast growth factor, vascular endothelial growth factor, and platelet-derived growth factor. These growth factors enable wound healing by causing cell proliferation, synthesis of extracellular matrix, and inducing angiogenesis. Macrophages play a crucial role in enabling wound healing. Macrophage depletion is known to markedly impair wound closure (DiPietro, 1995; Eming et al., 2007a).

Mast Cells

Mast cells are best known for their central role in mediating allergic responses. Beyond that function, it is now known that mast cells are physiologically significant in recognizing pathogens and in regulating immune response (de Vries and Noelle, 2010). Mast cells may instantly release several pro-inflammatory mediators from intracellular stores. In addition, they are localized in the host–environment interface. These properties make mast cells key players in fine-tuning immune responses during infection. Recent studies using mast cell activators as effective vaccine adjuvants show the potential of harnessing these cells to confer protective immunity against microbial pathogens (Abraham and St John, 2010). Mast cell activation helps initiate the inflammatory phase of wound healing. In response to injury, mast cells at the wound site degranulate within a matter of hours and therefore become histologically silent at the wound tissue. After about 48 h of injury, mast cells are again seen in the wound tissue and their number increases as healing progresses (Trautmann et al., 2000). On the one hand, impaired wound healing has been reported in mast cell–deficient mice (Shiota et al., 2010). On the other hand, mast cells have been implicated in skin wound fibrosis (Gallant-Behm et al., 2008). With the aid of a wide array of newly formed or preformed mediators released by degranulation, the activated mast cell controls the key events of the healing phases: triggering and modulation of the inflammatory stage, proliferation of connective cellular elements, and final remodeling of the newly formed connective tissue matrix. The importance of the mast cell in regulating healing processes is also demonstrated by the fact that a surplus or deficit of degranulated biological mediators causes impaired repair, with the formation of exuberant granulation tissue (e.g., keloids and hypertrophic scars), delayed closure (dehiscence), and chronicity of the inflammatory stage (Noli and Miolo, 2001).

Macrophages

Macrophages represent the predominant cell type in a healing wound 3–5 days following injury. The primary acute function of wound macrophages, which arrive at an injury site hours later than neutrophils, is to operate as voracious phagocytes cleansing the wound of all matrix and cell debris, including fibrin and apoptotic neutrophils. Macrophages also produce a range of cytokines and growth and angiogenic factors that drive fibroblast proliferation and angiogenesis (Rappolee et al., 1988; Martin, 1997; Martin and Leibovich, 2005; Eming et al., 2007a,b). In a classic study, Leibovich and Ross (Leibovich and Ross, 1975) demonstrated that antimacrophage serum combined with hydrocortisone diminished the accumulation of macrophages in healing skin wounds of adult guinea pigs. Such depletion resulted in impaired disposal of damaged tissue and provisional matrix, compromised fibroblast count, and delayed healing. Today, macrophages have emerged to be a pivotal driver of efficient skin repair (Goren et al., 2009; Mirza et al., 2009). Macrophages are plastic and heterogeneous cells broadly categorized into two groups: classically activated or type I macrophages, which are pro-inflammatory effectors, and alternatively activated or type II macrophages (Martinez et al., 2009). In the inflamed tissue, it is unclear whether the type II macrophages that appear during the healing phase originate from newly attracted monocytes or from a switch in the activation state of previously pro-inflammatory macrophages. Macrophage population first taking part in inflammation may change its phenotype and assume the role to resolve inflammation (Porcheray et al., 2005; Grinberg et al., 2009). Macrophages from diabetic wounds display dysfunctional inflammatory responses (Khanna et al., 2010). Persistent inflammatory state of diabetic wound macrophages is caused by impairment in the ability of these cells to phagocytose apoptotic cells at the wound site which in turn prevents the switch from M1 to M2 phenotype (Khanna et al., 2010).

Resolution of Inflammation

Inflammatory responses elicited by injury are only helpful to the healing process if it is timely and transient. Dysregulated inflammation complicates wound healing (Khanna et al., 2010). Complete resolution of an acute inflammatory response is the ideal outcome following an insult. For resolution to ensue, further leukocyte recruitment must be halted and accompanied by removal of leukocytes from inflammatory sites. Resolution of inflammation is executed by a number of key factors. At the wound site, successful phagocytosis of dead neutrophils by macrophages is a key factor. Impairments in macrophage function at the wound site derail the resolution of inflammation (Khanna et al., 2010). Lipid mediators, such as the lipoxins, resolvins, protectins, and newly identified maresins, have emerged as a novel genus of potent and stereoselective players that counterregulate excessive acute inflammation and stimulate molecular and cellular events that define resolution (Spite and Serhan, 2010). Successful resolution paves the path for the healing process to progress toward successful wound closure. Prolonged inflammation may not only compromise wound closure but may also worsen scar outcomes (Gordon et al., 2008; Li et al., 2011).

OBESITY: A PRO-INFLAMMATORY CONDITION

Epidemiological observations and metabolic investigations have consistently demonstrated that the accumulation of excess visceral fat is related to several metabolic and inflammatory perturbations. The expanded visceral fat is infiltrated by macrophages that conduct "cross talk" with adipose tissue. The differentiation of preadipocytes into mature adipocytes represents the foundation of adipose tissue generation. During positive energy balance, e.g., energy-dense diet, hypertrophic adipocytes are formed. These adipocytes feature large triglyceride stores and high lipolytic rate and produce more leptin and less adiponectin. Leptin and adiponectin are recognized as two important adipokines that influence inflammation and overall carbohydrate and lipid metabolism. Furthermore, fat cell hypertrophy causes infiltration of the adipose tissue by macrophages. Cross talk between adipocytes and macrophages contributes to the production of pro-inflammatory cytokines triggering a vicious cycle that augments inflammatory processes and resists resolution of inflammation (Figure 16.1).

IMBALANCE BETWEEN PRO- AND ANTI-INFLAMMATORY CYTOKINES

Bulky visceral adipose tissue is commonly associated with elevated circulating levels of IL-6, TNF-α, and C-reactive protein (CRP) (Despres, 2003; Blackburn et al., 2006; Cartier et al., 2008). On the other hand, adipose tissue of the obese is compromised in its ability to produce the anti-inflammatory cytokine adiponectin (Matsuzawa, 2006; Gustafson et al., 2009). The net outcome of such imbalance is the abundant presence of macrophages in the adipose tissue of the obese. The number of macrophages within the adipose tissue tightly correlates with insulin resistance. Such macrophages,

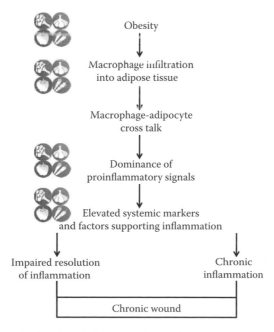

FIGURE 16.1 Obesity is associated with inflammation which complicates wound healing. Appropriate nutritional countermeasures may help directly target weight loss, suppress recruitment of inflammatory cells, attenuate pro-inflammatory signals, and lower systemic levels of pro-inflammatory agents and biomarkers.

resident within the adipose tissue, generate copious amounts of pro-inflammatory cytokines such as IL-6 and TNF-α (Matsuzawa, 2006). An area of outstanding interest in this regard is the cross talk between adipocytes and macrophages resident in the adipose tissue of the obese. Hypertrophic bulky adipocytes, as noted in the obese, produce more free fatty acids (FFAs), which activate toll-like receptor-4 (TLR4) (Mathieu et al., 2006). TLR4 reads such FFA as "danger signals" and thus leads to activation of the NF-κB pathway followed by the production of pro-inflammatory TNF-α (Nguyen et al., 2007). This signaling loop between the adipocyte and resident macrophages amplifies a detrimental pro-inflammatory cascade throughout the body. TNF-α activates lipolysis as well as the synthesis of IL-6 and MCP-1, a potent chemokine that allows the recruitment of more macrophages (Lyngso et al., 2002). IL-6 also stimulates production of CRP by the liver (Abeywardena et al., 2009). Of interest, visceral fat is infiltrated by macrophages to a greater extent than is subcutaneous fat. Abdominal fat drains into the portal system. Thus, cytokines produced by this fat depot have direct access to the liver, where they may promote the production of acute-phase proteins, including CRP. It is thus not surprising that elevated CRP levels, indicative of a pro-inflammatory state, are commonly noted in obese subjects (Arsenault et al., 2009).

Adipokines are specific adipose tissue–derived peptides representing a heterogeneous family of molecules that regulate metabolism and inflammation. Some of these adipose tissue–derived peptides have a broad range of actions (Harle and Straub, 2006). One group of such peptides are the adipokines leptin, adiponectin, and resistin. Leptin and resistin are considered to mainly confer pro-inflammatory properties, in contrast to adiponectin. Adiponectin acts in an antagonistic way to leptin, being negatively correlated with the BMI. It is also negatively correlated with the degree of hyperinsulinemia and insulin resistance. Lower adiponectin and higher leptin and resistin in the adipose tissue of the obese favors prolonged inflammation and is in conflict with resolution of inflammation—an environment that opposes wound healing.

IMPAIRED WOUND HEALING IN THE OBESE

Obese persons, subjected to surgery or trauma, often develop chronic wounds (Wilson and Clark, 2004). Length of hospital stay after burn injury is longer for the obese (Patel et al., 2010). Bariatric surgery is the most effective treatment for morbid obesity. High rate of wound complication is common in previously obese population (D'Ettorre et al., 2010). Incisional hernias represent a common delayed clinical complication in the obese (Nguyen et al., 2000; Puzziferri et al., 2006). Laparotomy wound healing is also impaired in obese rats (Xing et al., 2011). Excess body weight gained as a consequence of ovariectomy also compromises wound healing (Holcomb et al., 2009). A number of clinical factors have been implicated, including an increased incidence of surgical wound infection, technical failure, and hemorrhage (Puzziferri et al., 2006). Leptin resistance, associated with obesity, may contribute to the pathophysiology of impaired wound repair (Goren et al., 2006; Seitz et al., 2010). The Zucker diabetic fatty rats, suffering a mutation in leptin receptor, exhibit dysregulated inflammatory response and impaired healing (Slavkovsky et al., 2011). Diet-induced overweight rats exhibit delayed cutaneous healing (Paulino do Nascimento and Monte-Alto-Costa, 2011). The genetically obese (ob/ob) and diabetes (db/db) mouse strains have been commonly used to study skin repair (Seitz et al., 2010). Upon wounding, ob/ob and db/db mice develop severely disordered wound conditions. Seminal studies using these animals identified substantial mechanisms that contributed to the observed failure of tissue regeneration. The most severe defects in terms of impaired re-epithelialization and granulation tissue formation were strongly associated with a loss of function of diverse growth factors that drive keratinocyte, fibroblast, and endothelial cell functions in the presence of a greatly augmented wound inflammatory response (Wetzler et al., 2000; Goren et al., 2003, 2007). As discussed earlier, adipose tissue–driven activation of macrophages has emerged as a central cause of insulin-resistance under conditions of severe obesity. The same mechanism is implicated in diabetes-impaired healing in obese mice, as specific depletion of macrophages from sites of injury markedly improved tissue repair upon wounding and transplantation

(Goren et al., 2007; Schurmann et al., 2010). Impaired wound-healing conditions in ob/ob mice have been proven to be driven by TNF-expressing macrophages, which occurred as a consequence of metabolic disorders in the animals (Goren et al., 2007). Thus, TNF neutralization strategy may prove to be beneficial in correcting wound healing in the obese. In another study investigating inflammatory response patterns in caudally pedicled skin flaps, it was noted that distal regions of necrotic skin flap tissue were infiltrated by excess numbers of neutrophils and macrophages, and the latter were polarized toward a pro-inflammatory state as they expressed COX-2 and iNOS. Experimental depletion of inflammatory macrophages inhibited necrotic destruction of the distal skin flap tissue in diabetic mice despite the persistence of neutrophil infiltration and inflammation. It was thus concluded that wound macrophages play a pivotal role in determining the survival or loss of skin flap tissue under disturbed wound healing conditions in obese diabetic mice (Schurmann et al., 2010). The state of chronic inflammation and associated metabolic dysregulation observed in visceral obese patients negatively influences postoperative outcomes and represents a potential target for nutritional countermeasures (Doyle et al., 2010).

NUTRITIONAL COUNTERMEASURES

Poor dietary habits represent one major factor underlying the rapid spread of obesity. Nutritional intervention and supplementation may help curb some of these potential adverse affects. In order to achieve improved wound healing outcomes in the obese, emphasis should be directed on weight loss, bolstering immune defenses, and curbing inflammation. For specific surgical wounds, antioxidant supplementation may be useful to manage the increased burden of oxidative stress posed by the extensive use of anesthetics as well as analgesics. Furthermore, herbal preparations may be topically beneficial in achieving improved wound outcomes (Gupta et al., 2008; Aslam et al., 2010; Eshghi et al., 2010).

Obese nonbariatric and postbariatric patients are at nutritional risk for many primary ingredients of wound healing and immune system competency. Appropriate nutritional supplementation is an effective means for correcting these nutritional parameters and can significantly reduce surgical complications associated with obesity and bariatric surgery (Agha-Mohammadi and Hurwitz, 2010). In a study examining the preoperative nutritional parameters of 90 body-contouring patients, 38% of postbariatric patients ($n = 48$) had low pre-albumin (<20 mg/dL), 33% had vitamin A deficiency, 32.6% had low hemoglobin (<12 g/dL), 16.3% had iron deficiency, 9.5% had vitamin B12 deficiency, and 12% had hyperhomocystinemia. In comparison, in the nonbariatric patient group ($n = 42$), only 10% had low pre-albumin and 11.5% had vitamin A deficiency (Agha-Mohammadi and Hurwitz, 2010).

Carica papaya Linn is widely known as a medicinal fruit. The effects of a standardized fermented papaya preparation (FPP) have been examined for its effects on wound healing in adult obese diabetic (db/db) mice. FPP blunted the gain in blood glucose and improved the lipid profile after 8 weeks of oral supplementation. However, FPP did not influence weight gain during the supplementation period. FPP (0.2 g/kg body weight) supplementation for 8 weeks before wounding was effective in correcting wound closure. Studies on viable macrophages isolated from the wound site demonstrated that FPP supplementation improved respiratory-burst function as well as inducible NO production. Reactive oxygen species support numerous aspects of wound healing. NO availability in diabetic wounds is known to be compromised, and FPP corrects this loss. Diabetic mice supplemented with FPP showed a higher abundance of CD68 as well as CD31 at the wound site, suggesting effective recruitment of monocytes and an improved pro-angiogenic response. Thus, obese diabetic-wound outcomes may benefit from FPP supplementation by specifically influencing the response of wound-site macrophages and the subsequent angiogenic response. Given that FPP has a long track record of safe human consumption, testing of the beneficial effects of FPP on diabetic wound-related outcomes in a clinical setting is warranted (Collard and Roy, 2010).

The list of nutritional supplements that claim to be effective in causing weight loss, strengthening the immune system, and curbing inflammation is long and steadily growing. Promise, as posed by experimental observations, is substantial, but validations of such promises in human studies are few. Dietetics professionals should also consult authoritative sources for new data on efficacy as it becomes available (ods.od.nih.gov). Dietary supplements are used for two purposes in weight reduction: (a) providing nutrients that may be inadequate in calorie-restricted diets and (b) for their potential benefits in stimulating weight loss. The goal in planning weight-reduction diets is that total intake from food and supplements should meet recommended dietary allowance or adequate intake levels without greatly exceeding them for all nutrients, except energy. If nutrient amounts from food sources in the reducing diet fall short, dietary supplements containing a single nutrient or element or a multivitamin-mineral combination may be helpful. On hypocaloric diets, the addition of dietary supplements providing nutrients at a level equal to or below recommended dietary allowance or adequate intake levels or 100% daily value, as stated in a supplement's facts box on the label, may help dieters to achieve nutrient adequacy and maintain electrolyte balance while avoiding the risk of excessive nutrient intakes. Many botanical and other types of dietary supplements are purported to be useful for stimulating or enhancing weight loss. Evidence of their efficacy needs additional human studies. To date, there is little or no evidence supporting that carnitine or hydroxycitrate supplementation is of any value for weight loss in humans. Supplements such as pyruvate have been shown to be effective at high dosages, but there is little mechanistic information to explain its purported effect or data to indicate its effectiveness at lower dosages. Conjugated linoleic acid has been shown to stimulate fat utilization and decrease body fat content in mice but has not been tested in humans. The effects of ephedrine, in conjunction with methylxanthines and aspirin, in humans appear unequivocal but include various cardiovascular side effects. These supplements need to be tested for their effectiveness or safety over prolonged periods of time. Although there are few examples of safety concerns related to products that are legal and on the market for this purpose, there is also a paucity of evidence on safety for this intended use. Ephedra and ephedrine-containing supplements, with or without caffeine, have been singled out in recent alerts from the Food and Drug Administration because of safety concerns, and use of products containing these substances cannot be recommended. Dietitians should periodically check the Food and Drug Administration website (www.cfsan.fda.gov) for updates and warnings and alert patients or clients to safety concerns (Dwyer et al., 2005).

Nutritional interventions may prove to be effective in resolving or attenuating chronic inflammation. There is a considerable body of research addressing the immunomodulatory effects of several nutrients, such as fatty acids, antioxidants, carbohydrates, specific amino acids, micronutrients, and alcohol, which play a crucial role in the maintenance of an "optimal" immune response. In addition, specific dietary patterns, such as the Mediterranean diet, are evolving as protective against cardiovascular disease because of their anti-inflammatory properties.

Fish consumption is independently inversely associated with the circulating levels of several inflammatory markers (Zampelas et al., 2005). Fatty fish contain ω-3 fatty acids (eicosapentaenoic [EPA] and docosahexaenoic [DHA] acids). Apart from the lipid-lowering effects of ω-3 fatty acids, EPA and DHA may improve endothelial function by altering the metabolism of adhesion molecules, such as VCAM-1, E-selectin, and ICAM-1, and by decreasing pro-inflammatory cytokine production, including IL-6 and TNF-α (Kris-Etherton et al., 2003; Din et al., 2004). The anti-inflammatory effects of ω-3 fatty acids seem to be mediated by eicosanoids. Increasing the intake of EPA and DHA results in an increase of these fatty acids in tissue, cellular, and circulating lipids, along with a parallel reduction in ω-6 fatty acids (Dewailly et al., 2001). EPA competes with arachidonic acid (AA) in acting as substrate for both cyclooxygenase (COX) and 5-lipoxygenase (5-LOX). In this way, EPA minimizes the production of AA-derived pro-inflammatory metabolites. Replacement of the AA by ω-3 fatty acids also results in reduced formation of thromboxane-2 (TxA2) and prostacyclin I2 (PGI2) (both deriving from AA), thus inhibiting platelet aggregation and reducing thrombotic tendency (Caughey et al., 1997; Holub, 2002).

There is major interest in the effects of the different types of dietary fatty acid on several parameters of the immune system. This is partly because AA is the precursor of 2-series prostaglandins and 4-series leukotrienes, which have potent roles in regulating inflammatory and immune responses. ω-3 Polyunsaturated fatty acids (PUFAs), e.g., α-linolenic acid (ALA), EPA, and DHA, inhibit mitogen-stimulated proliferation of human lymphocytes (Santoli et al., 1990; Calder and Newsholme, 1992; Soyland et al., 1993; Purasiri et al., 1997). ALA intervention may lower TNF-α, IL-1β, TxB2, and prostaglandin E2 production by human monocytes (Caughey et al., 1996). Marked increase in ALA intake, resulting in a linolenic acid (LA):ALA ratio of approximately 1:1, may induce anti-inflammatory effects in humans. Supplementing the diet of dyslipidemic patients with 8.1 g of ALA per day for 12 weeks and subsequently changing the ratio of LA:ALA from approximately 13.0:1.0 to 1.3:1.0 resulted in a decrease in serum concentrations of CRP, serum amyloid A protein (SAA), and IL-6 (Rallidis et al., 2003, 2004; Paschos et al., 2004). Both a high-ALA diet and a high-LA diet can lower circulating VCAM-1 and E-selectin levels, an effect that was more pronounced after the high-ALA diet. ALA supplementation lowered circulating CRP levels (Zhao et al., 2004).

Dietary carbohydrates may influence inflammatory markers. Diets which promote relatively low diurnal insulin levels by inducing a relatively low postprandial insulin response, while promoting muscle insulin sensitivity is associated with lower serum levels of IL-6 and CRP, independent of the long-term impact of such diets on adipose mass. Thus, it may be possible to moderate CRP by avoiding high-insulin-response starchy foods (most notably, wheat flour products other than pasta) and preferring whole foods rich in amylose and soluble fiber (McCarty, 2005). Dietary fiber intake alone is another significant factor that may lower serum CRP concentrations (Ajani et al., 2004; King, 2005). Human studies testing the significance of antioxidants against inflammation are promising. Serum vitamin C has been inversely associated with CRP levels in healthy subjects and stroke patients (Sanchez-Moreno et al., 2004; van Herpen-Broekmans et al., 2004). Also, vitamin E supplementation decreased CRP levels in smokers with acute coronary syndrome as well as in patients with stable acute coronary artery disease (Murphy et al., 2004; Singh and Jialal, 2004). The beneficial effects of vitamin A in immunocompromised states, such as burns and surgery, are known for many years (Cohen et al., 1979; Fusi et al., 1984). Early studies demonstrating the ability of dietary carotenoids (abundant in dark green or deep orange vegetables) to prevent infections have left open the possibility that the action of these carotenoids may also be through their prior conversion to vitamin A. Subsequent studies, however, using carotenoids without provitamin A activity, such as lutein, canthaxanthin, lycopene, and astaxanthin, showed that they were actually as active as, and at times more active than, beta-carotene in enhancing cell-mediated and humoral immune response in animals and humans. In a study of healthy subjects, serum lutein and lycopene were inversely associated with ICAM-1 levels, suggesting anti-inflammatory functions (van Herpen-Broekmans et al., 2004). Plant polyphenols represent another group of phytonutrient with proven anti-inflammatory properties. Plant polyphenols are a group of chemicals that may play a beneficial role in human nutrition but are not considered essential for human health. The most significant dietary sources are fruits, nuts, vegetables, soya, curcumin, red wine, and green tea. Certain polyphenols may decrease expression of pro-inflammatory cytokines and adhesion molecules by endothelial cells and reduce monocyte adhesion (Labinskyy et al., 2006; Aquilano et al., 2008; Biswas and Rahman, 2008). Studies in chronic and degenerative disease conditions (such as thalassemia, cirrhosis, diabetes, and aging) and performance sports show that FPP favorably modulates immunological, hematological, inflammatory, vascular, and oxidative stress damage parameters (Aruoma et al., 2010). The aging process is paralleled by two- to fourfold increase in plasma/serum levels of inflammatory mediators, such as cytokines and acute-phase proteins. FPP has demonstrated beneficial functions in managing pro-inflammatory outcomes associated with aging (Marotta et al., 2007).

SUMMARY

The pro-inflammatory responses associated with obesity are in direct conflict with successful wound healing. It is therefore necessary that wound care in the obese include a productive strategy to subdue or resolve inflammation. Nutritional countermeasures represent a safe and reasonable strategy to manage excessive inflammation associated with obesity. Therapeutic options in that direction are many and must be dealt with critically and with caution. Dietary pattern rich in nutrients with favorable anti-inflammatory properties and poor in pro-inflammatory nutrients represents a prudent choice.

ACKNOWLEDGMENT

Work on wound healing in the authors' laboratory is supported by NIH RO1 grants GM069589, GM077185, and DK076566.

LITERATURE CITED

Abeywardena, M.Y., Leifert, W.R., Warnes, K.E., Varghese, J.N., and Head, R.J. (2009). Cardiovascular biology of interleukin-6. *Curr Pharm Des 15*, 1809–1821.

Abraham, S.N. and St John, A.L. (2010). Mast cell-orchestrated immunity to pathogens. *Nat Rev Immunol 10*, 440–452.

Agha-Mohammadi, S. and Hurwitz, D.J. (2010). Enhanced recovery after body-contouring surgery: Reducing surgical complication rates by optimizing nutrition. *Aesthetic Plast Surg 34*, 617–625.

Ajani, U.A., Ford, E.S., and Mokdad, A.H. (2004). Dietary fiber and C-reactive protein: Findings from national health and nutrition examination survey data. *J Nutr 134*, 1181–1185.

Aquilano, K., Baldelli, S., Rotilio, G., and Ciriolo, M.R. (2008). Role of nitric oxide synthases in Parkinson's disease: A review on the antioxidant and anti-inflammatory activity of polyphenols. *Neurochem Res 33*, 2416–2426.

Arsenault, B.J., Pibarot, P., and Despres, J.P. (2009). The quest for the optimal assessment of global cardiovascular risk: Are traditional risk factors and metabolic syndrome partners in crime? *Cardiology 113*, 35–49.

Aruoma, O.I., Hayashi, Y., Marotta, F., Mantello, P., Rachmilewitz, E., and Montagnier, L. (2010). Applications and bioefficacy of the functional food supplement fermented papaya preparation. *Toxicology 278*, 6–16.

Aslam, M.N., Warner, R.L., Bhagavathula, N., Ginsburg, I., and Varani, J. (2010). A multi-component herbal preparation (PADMA 28) improves structure/function of corticosteroid-treated skin, leading to improved wound healing of subsequently induced abrasion wounds in rats. *Arch Dermatol Res 302*, 669–677.

Biswas, S. and Rahman, I. (2008). Modulation of steroid activity in chronic inflammation: A novel anti-inflammatory role for curcumin. *Mol Nutr Food Res 52*, 987–994.

Blackburn, P., Despres, J.P., Lamarche, B., Tremblay, A., Bergeron, J., Lemieux, I., and Couillard, C. (2006). Postprandial variations of plasma inflammatory markers in abdominally obese men. *Obesity (Silver Spring) 14*, 1747–1754.

Broughton, G. 2nd, Janis, J.E., and Attinger, C.E. (2006). A brief history of wound care. *Plast Reconstr Surg 117*, 6S–11S.

Calder, P.C. and Newsholme, E.A. (1992). Polyunsaturated fatty acids suppress human peripheral blood lymphocyte proliferation and interleukin-2 production. *Clin Sci (Lond) 82*, 695–700.

Cartier, A., Lemieux, I., Almeras, N., Tremblay, A., Bergeron, J., and Despres, J.P. (2008). Visceral obesity and plasma glucose-insulin homeostasis: Contributions of interleukin-6 and tumor necrosis factor-alpha in men. *J Clin Endocrinol Metab 93*, 1931–1938.

Caughey, G.E., Mantzioris, E., Gibson, R.A., Cleland, L.G., and James, M.J. (1996). The effect on human tumor necrosis factor alpha and interleukin 1 beta production of diets enriched in n-3 fatty acids from vegetable oil or fish oil. *Am J Clin Nutr 63*, 116–122.

Caughey, G.E., Pouliot, M., Cleland, L.G., and James, M.J. (1997). Regulation of tumor necrosis factor-alpha and IL-1 beta synthesis by thromboxane A2 in nonadherent human monocytes. *J Immunol 158*, 351–358.

Cohen, B.E., Gill, G., Cullen, P.R., and Morris, P.J. (1979). Reversal of postoperative immunosuppression in man by vitamin A. *Surg Gynecol Obstet 149*, 658–662.

Collard, E. and Roy, S. (2010). Improved function of diabetic wound-site macrophages and accelerated wound closure in response to oral supplementation of a fermented papaya preparation. *Antioxid Redox Signal 13*, 599–606.

D'Ettorre, M., Gniuli, D., Iaconelli, A., Massi, G., Mingrone, G., and Bracaglia, R. (2010). Wound healing process in post-bariatric patients: An experimental evaluation. *Obes Surg 20*, 1552–1558.

Daley, J.M., Reichner, J.S., Mahoney, E.J., Manfield, L., Henry, W.L. Jr., Mastrofrancesco, B., and Albina, J.E. (2005). Modulation of macrophage phenotype by soluble product(s) released from neutrophils. *J Immunol 174*, 2265–2272.

de Vries, V.C. and Noelle, R.J. (2010). Mast cell mediators in tolerance. *Curr Opin Immunol 22*, 643–648.

Despres, J.P. (2003). Inflammation and cardiovascular disease: Is abdominal obesity the missing link? *Int J Obes Relat Metab Disord 27* (Suppl 3), S22–S24.

Dewailly, E., Blanchet, C., Lemieux, S., Sauve, L., Gingras, S., Ayotte, P., and Holub, B.J. (2001). n-3 Fatty acids and cardiovascular disease risk factors among the Inuit of Nunavik. *Am J Clin Nutr 74*, 464–473.

Din, J.N., Newby, D.E., and Flapan, A.D. (2004). Omega 3 fatty acids and cardiovascular disease—Fishing for a natural treatment. *BMJ 328*, 30–35.

DiPietro, L.A. (1995). Wound healing: The role of the macrophage and other immune cells. *Shock 4*, 233–240.

Doyle, S.L., Lysaght, J., and Reynolds, J.V. (2010). Obesity and post-operative complications in patients undergoing non-bariatric surgery. *Obes Rev 11*, 875–886.

Dwyer, J.T., Allison, D.B., and Coates, P.M. (2005). Dietary supplements in weight reduction. *J Am Diet Assoc 105*, S80–S86.

Eming, S.A., Krieg, T., and Davidson, J.M. (2007a). Inflammation in wound repair: Molecular and cellular mechanisms. *J Invest Dermatol 127*, 514–525.

Eming, S.A., Werner, S., Bugnon, P., Wickenhauser, C., Siewe, L., Utermohlen, O., Davidson, J.M., Krieg, T., and Roers, A. (2007b). Accelerated wound closure in mice deficient for interleukin-10. *Am J Pathol 170*, 188–202.

Eshghi, F., Hosseinimehr, S.J., Rahmani, N., Khademloo, M., Norozi, M.S., and Hojati, O. (2010). Effects of Aloe vera cream on posthemorrhoidectomy pain and wound healing: Results of a randomized, blind, placebo-control study. *J Altern Complement Med 16*, 647–650.

Fusi, S., Kupper, T.S., Green, D.R., and Ariyan, S. (1984). Reversal of postburn immunosuppression by the administration of vitamin A. *Surgery 96*, 330–335.

Gallant-Behm, C.L., Hildebrand, K.A., and Hart, D.A. (2008). The mast cell stabilizer ketotifen prevents development of excessive skin wound contraction and fibrosis in red Duroc pigs. *Wound Repair Regen 16*, 226–233.

Gordon, A., Kozin, E.D., Keswani, S.G., Vaikunth, S.S., Katz, A.B., Zoltick, P.W., Favata, M., Radu, A.P., Soslowsky, L.J., Herlyn, M., and Crombleholme, T.M. (2008). Permissive environment in postnatal wounds induced by adenoviral-mediated overexpression of the anti-inflammatory cytokine interleukin-10 prevents scar formation. *Wound Repair Regen 16*, 70–79.

Goren, I., Allmann, N., Yogev, N., Schurmann, C., Linke, A., Holdener, M., Waisman, A., Pfeilschifter, J., and Frank, S. (2009). A transgenic mouse model of inducible macrophage depletion: Effects of diphtheria toxin-driven lysozyme M specific cell lineage ablation on wound inflammatory, angiogenic, and contractive processes. *Am J Pathol 175*, 132–147.

Goren, I., Kampfer, H., Podda, M., Pfeilschifter, J., and Frank, S. (2003). Leptin and wound inflammation in diabetic ob/ob mice: Differential regulation of neutrophil and macrophage influx and a potential role for the scab as a sink for inflammatory cells and mediators. *Diabetes 52*, 2821–2832.

Goren, I., Muller, E., Pfeilschifter, J., and Frank, S. (2006). Severely impaired insulin signaling in chronic wounds of diabetic ob/ob mice: A potential role of tumor necrosis factor-alpha. *Am J Pathol 168*, 765–777.

Goren, I., Muller, E., Schiefelbein, D., Christen, U., Pfeilschifter, J., Muhl, H., and Frank, S. (2007). Systemic anti-TNFalpha treatment restores diabetes-impaired skin repair in ob/ob mice by inactivation of macrophages. *J Invest Dermatol 127*, 2259–2267.

Grinberg, S., Hasko, G., Wu, D., and Leibovich, S.J. (2009). Suppression of PLCbeta2 by endotoxin plays a role in the adenosine A(2A) receptor-mediated switch of macrophages from an inflammatory to an angiogenic phenotype. *Am J Pathol 175*, 2439–2453.

Gupta, A., Upadhyay, N.K., Sawhney, R.C., and Kumar, R. (2008). A poly-herbal formulation accelerates normal and impaired diabetic wound healing. *Wound Repair Regen 16*, 784–790.

Gustafson, B., Gogg, S., Hedjazifar, S., Jenndahl, L., Hammarstedt, A., and Smith, U. (2009). Inflammation and impaired adipogenesis in hypertrophic obesity in man. *Am J Physiol Endocrinol Metab 297*, E999–E1003.

Harle, P. and Straub, R.H. (2006). Leptin is a link between adipose tissue and inflammation. *Ann N Y Acad Sci 1069*, 454–462.

Holcomb, V.B., Keck, V.A., Barrett, J.C., Hong, J., Libutti, S.K., and Nunez, N.P. (2009). Obesity impairs wound healing in ovariectomized female mice. *In Vivo 23*, 515–518.

Holub, B.J. (2002). Clinical nutrition: 4. Omega-3 fatty acids in cardiovascular care. *CMAJ 166*, 608–615.

Khanna, S., Biswas, S., Shang, Y., Collard, E., Azad, A., Kauh, C., Bhasker, V., Gordillo, G.M., Sen, C.K., and Roy, S. (2010). Macrophage dysfunction impairs resolution of inflammation in the wounds of diabetic mice. *PLoS One 5*, e9539.

King, D.E. (2005). Dietary fiber, inflammation, and cardiovascular disease. *Mol Nutr Food Res 49*, 594–600.

Klebanoff, S.J. (2005). Myeloperoxidase: Friend and foe. *J Leukoc Biol 77*, 598–625.

Kris-Etherton, P.M., Harris, W.S., and Appel, L.J. (2003). Fish consumption, fish oil, omega-3 fatty acids, and cardiovascular disease. *Arterioscler Thromb Vasc Biol 23*, e20–e30.

Labinskyy, N., Csiszar, A., Veress, G., Stef, G., Pacher, P., Oroszi, G., Wu, J., and Ungvari, Z. (2006). Vascular dysfunction in aging: Potential effects of resveratrol, an anti-inflammatory phytoestrogen. *Curr Med Chem 13*, 989–996.

Leibovich, S.J. and Ross, R. (1975). The role of the macrophage in wound repair. A study with hydrocortisone and antimacrophage serum. *Am J Pathol 78*, 71–100.

Li, P., Liu, P., Xiong, R.P., Chen, X.Y., Zhao, Y., Lu, W.P., Liu, X., Ning, Y.L., Yang, N., and Zhou, Y.G. (2011). Ski, a modulator of wound healing and scar formation in the rat skin and rabbit ear. *J Pathol 223*, 659–671.

Lyngso, D., Simonsen, L., and Bulow, J. (2002). Metabolic effects of interleukin-6 in human splanchnic and adipose tissue. *J Physiol 543*, 379–386.

Marotta, F., Koike, K., Lorenzetti, A., Naito, Y., Fayet, F., Shimizu, H., and Marandola, P. (2007). Nutraceutical strategy in aging: Targeting heat shock protein and inflammatory profile through understanding interleukin-6 polymorphism. *Ann N Y Acad Sci 1119*, 196–202.

Martin, P. (1997). Wound healing—Aiming for perfect skin regeneration. *Science 276*, 75–81.

Martin, P. and Leibovich, S.J. (2005). Inflammatory cells during wound repair: The good, the bad and the ugly. *Trends Cell Biol 15*, 599–607.

Martinez, F.O., Helming, L., and Gordon, S. (2009). Alternative activation of macrophages: An immunologic functional perspective. *Annu Rev Immunol 27*, 451–483.

Mathieu, P., Pibarot, P., and Despres, J.P. (2006). Metabolic syndrome: The danger signal in atherosclerosis. *Vasc Health Risk Manag 2*, 285–302.

Matsuzawa, Y. (2006). The metabolic syndrome and adipocytokines. *FEBS Lett 580*, 2917–2921.

McCarty, M.F. (2005). Low-insulin-response diets may decrease plasma C-reactive protein by influencing adipocyte function. *Med Hypotheses 64*, 385–387.

Mehra, R. (2002). Historical survey of wound healing. *Bull Indian Inst Hist Med Hyderabad 32*, 159–175.

Mirza, R., DiPietro, L.A., and Koh, T.J. (2009). Selective and specific macrophage ablation is detrimental to wound healing in mice. *Am J Pathol 175*, 2454–2462.

Murphy, R.T., Foley, J.B., Tome, M.T., Mulvihill, N.T., Murphy, A., McCarroll, N., Crean, P., and Walsh, M.J. (2004). Vitamin E modulation of C-reactive protein in smokers with acute coronary syndromes. *Free Radic Biol Med 36*, 959–965.

Nguyen, M.T., Favelyukis, S., Nguyen, A.K., Reichart, D., Scott, P.A., Jenn, A., Liu-Bryan, R., Glass, C.K., Neels, J.G., and Olefsky, J.M. (2007). A subpopulation of macrophages infiltrates hypertrophic adipose tissue and is activated by free fatty acids via Toll-like receptors 2 and 4 and JNK-dependent pathways. *J Biol Chem 282*, 35279–35292.

Nguyen, N.T., Ho, H.S., Palmer, L.S., and Wolfe, B.M. (2000). A comparison study of laparoscopic versus open gastric bypass for morbid obesity. *J Am Coll Surg 191*, 149–155; discussion 155–147.

Noli, C. and Miolo, A. (2001). The mast cell in wound healing. *Vet Dermatol 12*, 303–313.

Paschos, G.K., Rallidis, L.S., Liakos, G.K., Panagiotakos, D., Anastasiadis, G., Votteas, V., and Zampelas, A. (2004). Background diet influences the anti-inflammatory effect of alpha-linolenic acid in dyslipidaemic subjects. *Br J Nutr 92*, 649–655.

Patel, L., Cowden, J.D., Dowd, D., Hampl, S., and Felich, N. (2010). Obesity: Influence on length of hospital stay for the pediatric burn patient. *J Burn Care Res 31*, 251–256.

Paulino do Nascimento, A. and Monte-Alto-Costa, A. (2011). Both obesity-prone and obesity-resistant rats present delayed cutaneous wound healing. *Br J Nutr 106*, 603–611.

Peters, T., Sindrilaru, A., Hinz, B., Hinrichs, R., Menke, A., Al-Azzeh, E.A., Holzwarth, K., Oreshkova, T., Wang, H., Kess, D., Walzog, B., Sulyok, S., Sunderkotter, C., Friedrich, W., Wlaschek, M., Krieg, T., and Scharffetter-Kochanek, K. (2005). Wound-healing defect of CD18(-/-) mice due to a decrease in TGF-beta1 and myofibroblast differentiation. *EMBO J 24*, 3400–3410.

Porcheray, F., Viaud, S., Rimaniol, A.C., Leone, C., Samah, B., Dereuddre-Bosquet, N., Dormont, D., and Gras, G. (2005). Macrophage activation switching: An asset for the resolution of inflammation. *Clin Exp Immunol 142*, 481–489.

Purasiri, P., McKechnie, A., Heys, S.D., and Eremin, O. (1997). Modulation in vitro of human natural cytotoxicity, lymphocyte proliferative response to mitogens and cytokine production by essential fatty acids. *Immunology 92*, 166–172.

Puzziferri, N., Austrheim-Smith, I.T., Wolfe, B.M., Wilson, S.E., and Nguyen, N.T. (2006). Three-year follow-up of a prospective randomized trial comparing laparoscopic versus open gastric bypass. *Ann Surg 243*, 181–188.

Rallidis, L.S., Paschos, G., Liakos, G.K., Velissaridou, A.H., Anastasiadis, G., and Zampelas, A. (2003). Dietary alpha-linolenic acid decreases C-reactive protein, serum amyloid A and interleukin-6 in dyslipidaemic patients. *Atherosclerosis 167*, 237–242.

Rallidis, L.S., Paschos, G., Papaioannou, M.L., Liakos, G.K., Panagiotakos, D.B., Anastasiadis, G., and Zampelas, A. (2004). The effect of diet enriched with alpha-linolenic acid on soluble cellular adhesion molecules in dyslipidaemic patients. *Atherosclerosis 174*, 127–132.

Rappolee, D.A., Mark, D., Banda, M.J., and Werb, Z. (1988). Wound macrophages express TGF-alpha and other growth factors in vivo: Analysis by mRNA phenotyping. *Science 241*, 708–712.

Sanchez-Moreno, C., Dashe, J.F., Scott, T., Thaler, D., Folstein, M.F., and Martin, A. (2004). Decreased levels of plasma vitamin C and increased concentrations of inflammatory and oxidative stress markers after stroke. *Stroke 35*, 163–168.

Santoli, D., Phillips, P.D., Colt, T.L., and Zurier, R.B. (1990). Suppression of interleukin 2-dependent human T cell growth in vitro by prostaglandin E (PGE) and their precursor fatty acids. Evidence for a PGE-independent mechanism of inhibition by the fatty acids. *J Clin Invest 85*, 424–432.

Schurmann, C., Seitz, O., Sader, R., Pfeilschifter, J., Goren, I., and Frank, S. (2010). Role of wound macrophages in skin flap loss or survival in an experimental diabetes model. *Br J Surg 97*, 1437–1451.

Seitz, O., Schurmann, C., Hermes, N., Muller, E., Pfeilschifter, J., Frank, S., and Goren, I. (2010). Wound healing in mice with high-fat diet- or ob gene-induced diabetes-obesity syndromes: A comparative study. *Exp Diabetes Res 2010*, 476969.

Sen, C.K., Gordillo, G.M., Roy, S., Kirsner, R., Lambert, L., Hunt, T.K., Gottrup, F., Gurtner, G.C., and Longaker, M.T. (2009). Human skin wounds: A major and snowballing threat to public health and the economy. *Wound Repair Regen 17*, 763–771.

Shiota, N., Nishikori, Y., Kakizoe, E., Shimoura, K., Niibayashi, T., Shimbori, C., Tanaka, T., and Okunishi, H. (2010). Pathophysiological role of skin mast cells in wound healing after scald injury: Study with mast cell-deficient W/W(V) mice. *Int Arch Allergy Immunol 151*, 80–88.

Shipman, A.R. and Millington, G.W. (2011). Obesity and the skin. *Br J Dermatol 165* (4), 743–750.

Singh, U. and Jialal, I. (2004). Anti-inflammatory effects of alpha-tocopherol. *Ann N Y Acad Sci 1031*, 195–203.

Slavkovsky, R., Kohlerova, R., Tkacova, V., Jiroutova, A., Tahmazoglu, B., Velebny, V., Rezacova, M., Sobotka, L., and Kanta, J. (2011). Zucker diabetic fatty rat: A new model of impaired cutaneous wound repair with type II diabetes mellitus and obesity. *Wound Repair Regen 19*, 515–525.

Soyland, E., Nenseter, M.S., Braathen, L., and Drevon, C.A. (1993). Very long chain n-3 and n-6 polyunsaturated fatty acids inhibit proliferation of human T-lymphocytes in vitro. *Eur J Clin Invest 23*, 112–121.

Spite, M. and Serhan, C.N. (2010). Novel lipid mediators promote resolution of acute inflammation: Impact of aspirin and statins. *Circ Res 107*, 1170–1184.

Trautmann, A., Toksoy, A., Engelhardt, E., Brocker, E.B., and Gillitzer, R. (2000). Mast cell involvement in normal human skin wound healing: Expression of monocyte chemoattractant protein-1 is correlated with recruitment of mast cells which synthesize interleukin-4 in vivo. *J Pathol 190*, 100–106.

van Herpen Broekmann, W.M., Klopping-Ketelaars, I.A., Bots, M.L., Kluft, C., Princen, H., Hendriks, H.F., Tijburg, L.B., van Poppel, G., and Kardinaal, A.F. (2004). Serum carotenoids and vitamins in relation to markers of endothelial function and inflammation. *Eur J Epidemiol 19*, 915–921.

Wangensteen, O.H. (1975). Surgeons and wound management: Historical aspects. *Conn Med 39*, 568–574.

Wetzler, C., Kampfer, H., Stallmeyer, B., Pfeilschifter, J., and Frank, S. (2000). Large and sustained induction of chemokines during impaired wound healing in the genetically diabetic mouse: Prolonged persistence of neutrophils and macrophages during the late phase of repair. *J Invest Dermatol 115*, 245–253.

Wilson, J.A. and Clark, J.J. (2004). Obesity: Impediment to postsurgical wound healing. *Adv Skin Wound Care 17*, 426–435.

Xing, L., Culbertson, E.J., Wen, Y., Robson, M.C., and Franz, M.G. (2011). Impaired laparotomy wound healing in obese rats. *Obes Surg 21* (12), 1937–1946.

Zampelas, A., Panagiotakos, D.B., Pitsavos, C., Das, U.N., Chrysohoou, C., Skoumas, Y., and Stefanadis, C. (2005). Fish consumption among healthy adults is associated with decreased levels of inflammatory markers related to cardiovascular disease: The ATTICA study. *J Am Coll Cardiol 46*, 120–124.

Zhao, G., Etherton, T.D., Martin, K.R., West, S.G., Gillies, P.J., and Kris-Etherton, P.M. (2004). Dietary alpha-linolenic acid reduces inflammatory and lipid cardiovascular risk factors in hypercholesterolemic men and women. *J Nutr 134*, 2991–2997.

17 Angiogenesis-Targeted Redox-Based Therapeutics

Shampa Chatterjee, PhD,
Debasis Bagchi, PhD, MACN, CNS, MAIChE,
Manashi Bagchi, PhD, and Chandan K. Sen, PhD

CONTENTS

INTRODUCTION

Obesity is now a worldwide epidemic.[1–3] The prevalence of overweight and obesity in the United States and other industrialized and developing countries is increasing exponentially.[1–6] Approximately half a billion of the world's population is now considered overweight (BMI 25–29 kg/m^2) or obese (BMI >30 kg/m^2) (Table 17.1).[1–3,7,8] Genetic predisposition, inadequate energy expenditure, increased caloric intake, environmental and social factors, and sedentary lifestyle represent major contributors to obesity.[1–10]

Recent studies have shown that approximately a third of the variance in adult body weights is secondary to genetic influences.[11] Leptin, an adipocyte- and placenta-derived circulating protein, regulates, to some extent, the magnitude of fat stores in the body causing obesity.[12] Gastrointestinal peptides, neurotransmitters, and adipose tissue may also have an etiologic role in obesity.[13] Low-caloric diets with or without exercise can help with temporary weight loss. Nevertheless, diet and exercise alone have not proven universally successful for long-term solutions in weight management. In addition, supplementation with drugs that suppress appetite, reduce food intake, increase energy expenditure, and/or influence nutrient partitioning or metabolism has potential efficacy but is unfortunately accompanied by adverse side effects—including some life threatening one.[14,15]

The genesis and development of metabolic syndromes such as obesity is directly fed by angiogenesis. Angiogenesis, the growth or formation of new blood vessels by capillary sprouting from preexisting vessels, is critical to the expansion of adipose tissue. New blood vessels, by providing nutrients and oxygen deep into the adipose tissue, spur the development and maturation of adipocytes.[16–19] These vessels also supply plasma which is enriched in growth factors and which helps

TABLE 17.1
Percentage of Obese Population Worldwide

Country	Adults (%)	Children (%)
United Kingdom	22	22
Spain	13	30
Finland	11	13
Denmark	10	18
Sweden	9	18
France	9	18
Italy	9	36
United States	31	15

maintain adipocyte homeostasis.[19a] In addition, newly formed vessels supply circulating stem cells, derived from bone marrow and other tissues, that are capable of differentiating into preadipocytes, adipocytes, and vascular cells.[19b] Adipocytes further induce angiogenic factors such as vascular endothelial growth factor (VEGF), monobutyrin, and leptin to accelerate angiogenesis.[16] In addition, adipocytes also induce endothelial cell (EC)-specific mitogens that cause proliferation of ECs lining the vasculature of these vessels. Such EC proliferation and differentiation within the fat tissue is presumed to be involved in the development and maintenance of adipose tissue.[16–19] ECs also interact with adipocytes and promote their maturation and proliferation. These cells secrete basic fibroblast growth factors, platelet-derived EC growth factor, and other soluble matrix-bound preadipocyte mitogens, which stimulate preadipocyte replication and promote differentiation.[16–19] Thus, newly formed adipose tissue depends on continued angiogenesis for further growth.[16] The interaction between microvascular ECs and preadipocytes promotes the expansion of adipose tissue.[17,19,20] Thus, the development of adipose tissue, also known as adipogenesis, is intrinsically associated with angiogenesis. In other words, the expanding adipose tissue in adults represents one of the few sites of active angiogenesis.

Since nonpharmacological management of obesity, such as lifestyle changes and exercise, and fat-eliminating surgical procedures are often insufficient to reduce weight, pharmacological tools are gaining new acceptance. As angiogenesis has been shown to have a crucial role in the modulation of adipogenesis and obesity, antiangiogenic drugs are being evaluated and used for obesity. Here we discuss the role of angiogenesis in adipose tissue development, growth and metabolism, and its potential to be therapeutically modulated as a possible future treatment approach for obesity and associated disorders.

ADIPOKINES, ADIPOKINOMES, INFLAMMATION, AND WHITE ADIPOSE TISSUE

Conventionally, white adipose tissue or fat was known to provide thermal and mechanical insulation to the body.[18,21] In addition, it serves as an energy storage depot for mammals.[17] The white adipose tissue has now emerged as a dynamic, multifunctional endocrine organ involved in a wide range of physiological and metabolic processes.[16–18] The tissue acts as a central reservoir of lipids subject to deposition and release of fatty acids.[16–19,21]

White adipocytes secrete several major hormones, most importantly leptin and adiponectin, and a diverse range of signaling mediators, collectively known as "adipokines" or "adipocytokines."[18–21] The total number of adipokines is now well over fifty, and their main functional categories include appetite and energy balance, immunity, insulin sensitivity, angiogenesis, homeostasis, lipid metabolism, and blood pressure.[17,21] Furthermore, there is a growing list of adipokines involved in inflammation, namely, tumor necrosis factor-α (TNF-α), interleukin 1β (IL-1β), IL-6, IL-8, IL-10, transforming growth factor-β (TGF-β), plasminogen activator inhibitor-1 (PAI-1), haptoglobin, and serum amyloid A.[16–20] Under conditions of obesity, the production of these inflammatory adipokines by adipose tissue increases. This has led to the hypothesis that obesity is characterized by a state of chronic low-grade inflammation and that this provides a link to insulin resistance and metabolic syndrome.[16,18] The term "adipokinome" refers to proteins involved in lipid metabolism, insulin sensitivity, the alternative complement system, vascular homeostasis, regulation of blood pressure and energy balance, and angiogenesis.[17,18,21] However, the extent to which adipose tissue contributes quantitatively to the elevated circulating levels of these inflammatory adipokines in obesity is unclear. Moreover, it is also unknown whether this is a generalized or local state of inflammation.[18,21] Overall, an increased production of inflammatory cytokines and acute-phase proteins by the adipose tissue in obesity primarily relates to localized events within the expanding fat depots.[17]

HYPOXIA, CANCER, AND ANGIOGENESIS

Hypoxia or low levels of oxygen availability to the adipose tissue, as might happen to the peripheral white fat mass ahead of angiogenesis, could be a key trigger for the inflammation-related events in white adipose tissue in obesity.[18–21] Adipose-derived inflammatory cytokines may directly stimulate of angiogenic factors, such as VEGF and leptin, or induce them through the activation of the transcription factor hypoxia inducible factor-1 (HIF-1).[19,21] HIF-1 controls the cellular response to hypoxia by activating numerous genes as a recent study of global gene expression using DNA microarrays has shown.[22] Immunohistochemical analysis of human tumor biopsies has revealed stabilization of HIF-1α in neoplastic tissues.[23] High HIF-1α levels in tumors reflect the frequent presence of intratumoral hypoxia and the fact that many common genetic alterations in cancer cells affect HIF-1α expression.[24] Because HIF-1α binds to and activates transcription of the gene encoding VEGF,[24] there seems to be a link between HIF, oncogene gain-of-function, and tumor vascularization. In addition, the remarkable frequency with which common genetic alterations in cancer cells are associated with increased HIF-1α expression suggests that HIF-1α stabilization could contribute to the accumulation of mutations during tumor progression. This hypothesis is supported both by mechanistic studies in animal models of cancer and by clinical studies demonstrating that HIF-1α stabilization is associated with increased risk of mortality in a variety of human cancers.[25] HIF-1α also plays critical roles in angiogenesis by directly activating the transcription of the VEGF gene.[26] HIF-1α-controlled VEGF production leads to autocrine signal transduction that is critical for angiogenesis, and many of the biological processes in angiogenesis, extracellular matrix invasion, and tube formation by ECs are stimulated through HIF-1α.[22,27]

ROLE OF LEPTIN, THE PRODUCT OF OB GENE, IN ANGIOGENESIS

Leptin, an adipocyte-derived 16,000-molecular-weight cytokine-like hormone, plays a pivotal role in the regulation of body weight and obesity, as well as on the control of food consumption, sympathetic nervous system activation, thermogenesis, and proinflammatory immune responses.[28] Because angiogenesis and adipogenesis are integrally linked during embryonic development of adipose tissue mass, Bouloumie et al.[28] evaluated the regulatory role of leptin in the growth of the vasculature using human umbilical venous endothelial cells (HUVECs) and porcine aortic ECs. Leptin, via activation of the endothelial Ob-R, generates a growth signal involving a tyrosine kinase–dependent intracellular pathway and promotes angiogenic processes.[17,28] This leptin-mediated stimulation of angiogenesis is viewed as a prime event in the development of obesity.[16,17,28] Leptin also contributes to the modulation of growth under physiological and pathophysiological conditions in other tissues.[16–18,28]

ANTIANGIOGENIC THERAPEUTIC STRATEGIES TO REGULATE OBESITY

Rupnick et al.[29] explored the corelationship between adipose tissue growth, angiogenesis, and leptin levels in ob/ob mice, which rapidly accumulate adipose tissue and develop spontaneous obesity because of a lack of functional leptin. The authors also examined EC proliferation, apoptotic cell death in adipose tissue, and metabolic consequences in these mice following treatment with anti-angiogenic inhibitor TNP-470, a synthetic analog of fumagillin, which is also an inhibitor of EC proliferation *in vitro.*[29] TNP-470-treated ob/ob mice dose-dependently lost body and adipose tissue weights as compared to the control animals. Obesity-associated hyperglycemia, serum glucose levels, and appetite level were also reduced. TNP-470-treated mice also had the lowest average lean mass.[29] A number of angiogenesis inhibitors, including endostatin, Bay12-9566 (a matrix metal-loproteinase inhibitor), thalidomide, angiostatin, and TNP-470, were tested on ob/ob mice, and all treatment groups gained less or lost weight compared to the control animals.[29] Mice from other obesity models also yielded similar results. The authors also treated 3T3-L1 preadipocytes with different concentrations of TNP-470 to evaluate whether suppression of preadipocyte proliferation contributes to this effect, and the results demonstrate that both endothelial-mediated mechanism and preadipocyte suppression are involved in this pathophysiology.[29] Cell proliferation and apoptosis were assessed in epididymal fat sections from TNP-470-treated and control ob/ob mice; TNP-470 decreased EC proliferation and increased apoptosis. Furthermore, basal metabolic rate (as measured by oxygen consumption, VO_2 max) was also increased in TNP-470-treated ob/ob mice.[29]

Brakenhielm et al.[30] evaluated the effect of TNP-470 on high-fat-diet-fed C57Bl/6 wt and ob/ob mice. Systemic administration of TNP-470 prevented obesity in high-caloric-diet-fed C57Bl/6 wt mice as well as in genetically leptin-deficient ob/ob mice. This containment of obesity in mice was accompanied by a reduction of vascularity in the adipose tissue.[30] TNP-470 selectively affected the growth of adipose tissue as measured by the ratio between total fat and lean body mass, as well as decreased serum levels of low-density lipoprotein cholesterol.[30] Furthermore, TNP-470 increased insulin sensitivity as demonstrated by reduced insulin levels, suggesting the therapeutic role of a potent angiogenesis inhibitor in the prevention of type 2 diabetes.[16,30] The investigators demonstrated that adipose tissue growth is dependent on angiogenesis and that potent antiangiogenic compounds may serve as novel therapeutic agents for the prevention of obesity and symptoms of metabolic syndrome.[30]

Voros et al.[31] studied the intricate aspects on the development of vasculature and mRNA expression of 17 pro- and antiangiogenic factors during adipose tissue development in nutritionally induced or genetically predisposed murine obesity models. Male C57Bl/6 mice were maintained either on standard food diet (SFD) or on high-fat diet (HFD), and male ob/ob mice were maintained on SFD over a period of 15 weeks. Ob/ob mice and male C57BL/6 mice on HFD had significantly larger subcutaneous and gonadal fat pads, accompanied by significantly higher blood content, increased total blood vessel volume, and higher number of proliferating cells.[31] Fat pad growth was accompanied by increased vascularization. mRNA and protein levels of angiopoietin-1 were downregulated, whereas those of thrombospondin-1 were upregulated in the developing adipose tissue in both obesity models. Angiopoietin-1 mRNA levels correlated negatively with adipose tissue weight in the early phase of nutritionally induced obesity as well as in genetically predisposed obesity.[31] Placental growth factor and angiopoietin-2 expression were increased in subcutaneous adipose tissue of ob/ob mice, and thrombospondin-2 expression was increased in both subcutaneous and gonadal fat pads. No changes were observed in the mRNA levels of VEGF-A isoforms; VEGF-B; VEGF-C; VEGF receptor-1, receptor-2, and receptor-3; and neuropilin-1.[31]

Neels et al.[19] examined the angiogenic process using the 3T3-F442A model of adipose tissue development. These investigators subcutaneously implanted 3T3-F442A preadipocytes into athymic Balb/c nude mice to study the neovascularization of developing adipose tissue.[19] These cells developed into highly vascularized fat pads over the next 14–21 days, and these fat pads were morphologically similar to normal subcutaneous adipose tissue. Histological studies demonstrated that

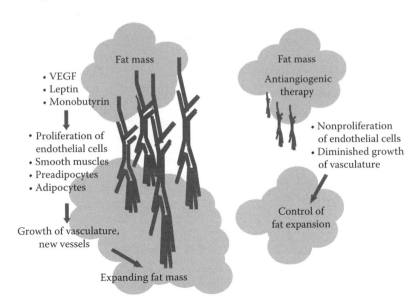

FIGURE 17.1 Pathophysiology of angiogenesis in expanding fat mass and significance of antiangiogenic therapy.

a new microvasculature comes up as early as 5 days after cell implantation, and real-time quantitative RT-PCR analyses exhibited the expression of EC markers, and adipogenesis markers increased simultaneously in parallel during fat pad development.[14] Thus, neovasculature originates by sprouting from larger host-derived blood vessels that run parallel to peripheral nerves, and the endothelial progenitor cells play minor role in this process.[19] Figure 17.1 demonstrates the key factors involved in adipose tissue development and the influence of antiangiogenic therapy.

VEGF RECEPTOR BLOCKADE AS A STRATEGY TO LIMIT ADIPOSE TISSUE EXPANSION

VEGF, a regulator of both physiological and pathological angiogenesis, binds to VEGFR1 or VEGFR2 and promotes endothelial growth and migration. VEGFR1 is expressed by various cell types including macrophages and inflammatory cells, while VEGFR2 is expressed by ECs. VEGF is reported to be upregulated during adipogenesis,[31a] and de novo adipogenesis (from transplanted preadipocytes) and neovascularization are regulated via a VEGFR2-mediated mechanism.[31b] Studies on diet-induced obesity in mice show that new vessel formation occurs by angiogenesis from preexisting fat vessels. Blocking VEGFR2 but not VEGFR1 in mice reportedly reduced their food intake and fat tissue expansion.[31c]

In addition, other pathways that promote expression of VEGF, its receptors and regulators, play a role in angiogenesis and the promotion of obesity. Blocking these inducers of VEGF may be another strategy to target angiogenesis-associated obesity.

REDOX CONTROL OF ANGIOGENESIS: OXIDANTS AS INDUCERS OF ANGIOGENIC FACTORS AND ANGIOGENESIS

ECs lining the blood vessels generate reactive oxygen species (ROS) such as $O_2^{\bullet-}$ and H_2O_2 which play a role in physiological and pathophysiological responses. High concentrations of ROS cause apoptosis and cell death.[32] Besides, ROS-induced oxidative stress is associated with the cardiovascular diseases including atherosclerosis and diabetes. However, low levels of ROS, as maybe produced in response to growth factor, hypoxia or ischemia, function as signaling molecules to mediate EC proliferation and migration which may contribute to angiogenesis *in vivo*.[33,34]

Cellular ROS can be generated from a number of sources including the mitochondrial electron transport system, xanthine oxidase, the cytochrome p450, the NADPH oxidase, and nitric oxide synthase (NOS). NADPH oxidase is one of the major sources of ROS in vasculature.[32] The neutrophil NADPH oxidase releases large amounts of $O_2^{\cdot-}$ in bursts, whereas the vascular NADPH oxidase(s) continuously produce low levels of $O_2^{\cdot-}$ intracellularly in basal state, yet it can be further stimulated acutely by various agonists and growth factors.[32] NADPH oxidase is activated by numerous stimuli such as VEGF, angiopoietin-1, cytokines, shear stress, hypoxia, and G-protein-coupled receptor agonists including angiotensin II in ECs.[32,35,36] ROS produced via activation of NADPH oxidase stimulate diverse redox signaling pathways leading to angiogenic responses in ECs as well as postnatal neovascularization *in vivo*.[34]

Besides ECs, ROS stimulates the induction of VEGF in various other cell types including vascular smooth muscle cells to promote cell proliferation and migration,[33,37] cytoskeletal reorganization, and tubular morphogenesis in ECs.[38] Hypoxia and adhesion of activated polymorphonuclear leukocytes to ECs cause ROS production, which results in capillary tube formation.[39,40] Angiogenesis growth factors such as VEGF and angiopoietin-1 increase ROS and thus induce EC migration and/or proliferation.[32,35,36]

Compounds that cause ROS formation often stimulate angiogenesis. Ethanol stimulates actin cytoskeletal reorganization, cell motility, and tube formation in an ROS-dependent manner in ECs.[41] Leptin, a circulating adipocytokine, upregulates VEGF mRNA and stimulates cell proliferation through an increase in ROS in ECs.[42]

There is strong correlation between ROS production, neovascularization, and VEGF expression in eyes of diabetics[43,44] and in balloon-injured arteries.[45] The generation of ROS during ischemia–reperfusion can also lead to angiogenesis. Reperfusion of the ischemic retina has been reported to upregulate VEGF mRNA.[46] Short periods of ischemia–reperfusion induce an increase in ROS, thereby stimulating myocardial angiogenesis in the ischemic noninfarcted heart.[47]

ANTIANGIOGENIC FUNCTION OF ANTIOXIDANTS

Since ROS is involved in angiogenesis, antioxidants that scavenge ROS should inhibit formation of new vessels. There have been reports that antioxidants such as pyrrolidine dithiocarbamate[48]; epigallocatechin-3-gallate[49]; resveratrol, a novel phytoalexin found in grapes, red wine, and diverse functional foods; and other natural polyphenols inhibit neovascularization in the mouse model.[50,51] Green tea catechins, vitamin E, etc., also inhibit angiogenic responses in ECs.[52] Antiangiogenic therapy also reduces plaque growth and intimal neovascularization,[53] and antioxidants such as vitamins C and E are reported to reduce vascular VEGF and VEGFR-2 expression in apolipoprotein-E-deficient (ApoE−/−) mice.[54] ROS are also involved in neovascularization during tumor growth. The thiol antioxidant, N-acetylcysteine (NAC), attenuates EC invasion and angiogenesis in a tumor model *in vivo*.[55]

ANTIANGIOGENIC ANTIOXIDANT NUTRIENTS

Tumor vascularization is a key step in the development of solid tumors, and the vast majority of pharmaceutical activity surrounding angiogenesis relates to the development of therapeutic strategies to destroy existing tumor vasculature and to prevent neovascularization.[17–20] Thus, antiangiogenic approaches to treat cancer represent a prime area in vascular tumor biology. Antioxidant nutrients demonstrate potent antiangiogenic functions. Catechin derivatives exhibited novel antiangiogenic properties in three different *in vitro* bioassays with concentrations ranging from 1.56 to 100 μM.[56,57] Epigallocatechin-3-gallate (EGCG) exhibited the most potent antiangiogenic activity in all the three assays among all catechins tested. EGCG inhibited the binding of VEGF to HUVECs in a concentration-dependent manner.[56,57] Resveratrol, a novel phytoalexin found in grapes, red wine, and diverse functional foods, and quercetin exhibited antiangiogenic properties in a concentration-dependent manner (6–100 μM). Pure flavonoids including rutin, kaempferol, ferrulic acid, genistein, fisetin, and luteolin also exhibited novel antiangiogenic properties.[58,59] These studies demonstrate that functional foods are effective in limiting angiogenesis *in vivo*.[56–59]

OptiBerry, a blend of six edible berry extracts including blueberry, bilberry, cranberry, elderberry, raspberry seeds, and strawberry extracts, was recently developed in our laboratories.[59,60] OptiBerry possessed high antioxidant capacity, low cytotoxicity, and potent antiangiogenic properties. In terms of antiangiogenic properties, OptiBerry was superior to individual berry anthocyanins, thus highlighting the synergistic power of the blend. OptiBerry significantly inhibited both H_2O_2 as well as TNF-α-induced VEGF expression by human keratinocytes.[59,60] Angiogenesis as monitored by Matrigel assay using human microvascular ECs was also impaired in the presence of OptiBerry.[59,60] In addition to these *in vitro* cell models, OptiBerry significantly inhibited inducible transcription factor NF-κB in an *in vivo* model.[36] In 129 P3 mice, endothelioma cells pretreated with OptiBerry showed a diminished growth of neoplastic vasculature by more than 50%.[60] These studies highlight the novel antiangiogenic and anticarcinogenic potential of select natural food constituents including catechin derivatives; curcumin (comprising about 40% of the spice turmeric); selected flavonoids including quercetin, rutin, kaempferol, ferrulic acid, genistein, fisetin, and luteolin; resveratrol; and berry anthocyanins.[56–60]

OBESITY, ANGIOGENESIS, AND CANCER

The link between obesity and angiogenesis illuminates the complex association between obesity and cancer. As mentioned earlier, adipocytes can accelerate tumor vascularization by triggering an angiogenic signaling cascade. However, the exact mechanisms behind its multifaceted functions remain unknown. Obesity itself develops via complex mechanisms involving interplay between heredity, nutrition, and physical lifestyle. In addition to the role of adipocytes in increasing vascularization and inflammation, fat deposits can also cause hormonal imbalances. High levels of estrogens contribute to the proclivity toward cancer. The increased risk of breast cancer after menopause in obese women is believed to be caused by increased levels of estrogens as fat tissues replace ovaries to become the primary source of estrogen.[61]

Obesity is often associated with the development of insulin resistance with high circulating levels of insulin and insulin-like hormones.[62] Insulin is known to stimulate cell proliferation, suggesting that an overproduction or high concentrations may be responsible, at least to some extent, for cancer development. High insulin and insulin-like hormone levels tightly associate with increased risk for breast cancer and poorer survival after breast cancer diagnosis.[63]

CONCLUSIONS

Overweight and obesity pose epidemic threats to human health, especially in the Western world. Healthy diet, proper nutrition, and exercise represent the fundamental prerequisites to fight such threat. Growth of adipose tissue depends on the blood vessels that feed the fat mass. Emergent studies reveal that the growth of adipose tissue may be regulated by inhibiting the development of vasculature. Antiangiogenic therapeutics show significant promise to manage undesired expansion of fat mass. Given that oxidants stimulate angiogenesis, it is understandable why antioxidants also possess antiangiogenic properties. Antiangiogenic nutrients provide a safe and potentially effective strategy to directly fight obesity and thus have an effect on controlling cancer. Several polyphenolic antioxidants, especially berry anthocyanins, possess potent antiangiogenic properties and should be considered as countermeasures for managing obesity in humans.

REFERENCES

1. Wyatt, S.B., Winters, K.P., Dubbert, P.M., Overweight and obesity: Prevalence, consequences, causes of a growing public health problem. *Am. J. Med. Sci.*, 331, 166, 2006.
2. Sjostrom, L.V., Mortality of severely obese subjects. *Am. J. Clin. Nutr.*, 55, S165, 1992.
3. Bray, G.A., Obesity. In: Ziegler, E.E., Filer, L.J., Jr. (eds.), *Present Knowledge in Nutrition*. ILSI Press, Washington, DC, pp. 19–32, 1996.
4. Guterman, L., Obesity problem swells worldwide. The Chronicle of Higher Education, A18, March 8, 2002.
5. U.S. Department of Health and Human Services, *The Surgeon General's Call to Action to Prevent and Decrease over Weight and Obesity 2001*. U.S. General Printing Office, Washington, DC, 2001.
6. World Health Organization, Report: Controlling the global obesity epidemic. Available at www.who.int/nut/obs.htm. Updated August 15, 2003.
7. Jequier, E., Pathways to obesity. *Int. J. Obes. Relat. Metab. Disord.*, 260, S12, 2002.
8. Frier, H.I., Greene, H.L., Obesity and chronic disease: Impact of weight reduction. In: Bendich, A., Deckelbaum, R.J. (eds.), *Preventive Nutrition: The Comprehensive Guide for Health Professionals*. Humana Press, Totowa, NJ, pp. 383–401, 2005.
9. Campbell, I., The obesity epidemic: Can we turn the tide? *Heart*, 89, 35, 2003.
10. Critser, G., Fat land: How Americans became the fattest people in the world. Houghton Mifflin, Boston, pp. 232, 2003. *New Engl. J. Med.*, 348, 2161, 2003.
11. Brownell, K.D., Obesity: Understanding and treating a serious, prevalent, and refractory disorder. *J. Consult. Clin. Psychol.*, 50, 820, 1992.
12. Frederich, R.C. et al., Leptin levels reflect body lipid content in mice: Evidence for diet-induced resistance to leptin action. *Nat. Med.*, 1, 1311, 1995.
13. Bandini, L.G. et al., Validity of reported energy intake in obese and nonobese adolescents. *Am. J. Clin. Nutr.*, 52, 421, 1990.
14. Volmar, K.E., Hutchins, G.M., Aortic and mitral fenfluramine-phenteramine valvulopathy in 64 patients treated with anorectic agents. *Arch. Pathol. Lab. Med.*, 125, 1555, 2001.
15. Cheng, T.O., Fen/Phen and valvular heart disease: The final link has now been established. *Circulation*, 102, E180, 2000.
16. Wasserman, F., The development of adipose tissue. In: Renold, A.E., Cahill, G.F. (eds.), *Handbook of Physiology*. American Society of Physiology, Washington, DC, Section 5, p. 87, 1965.
17. Hausman, G.J., Richardson, R.L., Adipose tissue angiogenesis. *J. Anim. Sci.*, 82, 925, 2004.
18. Dallabrida, S.M., Zurakowski, D., Shih, S.C., Smith, L.E., Folkman, J., Moulton, K.S., Rupnick, M.A., Adipose tissue growth and regression are regulated by angiopoietin-1. *Biochem. Biophys. Res. Commun.*, 311, 563, 2003.
19. Neels, J.G., Thinnes, T., Loskutoff, D.J., Angiogenesis in an in vivo model of adipose tissue development. *FASEB J.*, 18, 983, 2004. (a). Cao, Y., Angiogenesis modulates adipogenesis and obesity. *J. Clin. Invest.*, 117, 2362–2368, 2007. (b). Tang, W. et al., White fat progenitor cells reside in the adipose vasculature. *Science*, 322, 583–586, 2008.
20. Mandrup, S., Lane, M.D., Regulating adipogenesis. *J. Biol. Chem.*, 272, 5367, 1997.
21. Trayhurn, P., Wood, I.S., Adipokines: Inflammation and pleiotropic role of white adipose tissue. *Br. J. Nutr.*, 92, 347, 2004.
22. Manalo, D.J., Rowan A., Lavoie, T., Natarajan, L., Kelly, B.D., Ye, S.Q., Garcia, J.G.N., Semenza G.L., Transcriptional regulation of vascular endothelial cell responses to hypoxia by HIF-1. *Blood*, 105, 659, 2005.
23. Zhong, H., De Marzo, A.M., Laughner, E., Lim, M., Hilton, D.A., Zagzag, D., Buechler, P., Isaacs, W.B., Semenza, G.L., Simons, J.W., Overexpression of hypoxia-inducible factor 1α in common human cancers and their metastases. *Cancer Res.*, 59, 5830, 1999.
24. Talks, K.L., Turley, H., Gatter, K.C., Maxwell, P.H., Pugh, C.W., Ratcliffe, P.J., Harris, A.L., The expression and distribution of the hypoxia-inducible factors HIF-1α and HIF-2α in normal human tissues, cancers, and tumor-associated macrophages. *Am. J. Pathol.*, 157, 411, 2000.
25. Semenza, G.L., Targeting HIF-1 for cancer therapy. *Nat. Rev. Cancer*, 3, 721–732, 2003.
26. Forsythe, J.A., Jiang, B.H., Iyer, N.V., Agani, F., Leung, S.W., Koos, R.D., Semenza, G.L., Activation of vascular endothelial growth factor gene transcription by hypoxia-inducible factor 1. *Mol. Cell. Biol.*, 16, 4604, 1996.
27. Tang, N., Wang, L., Esko, J., Giordano, F.J., Huang, Y., Gerber, H.P., Ferrara, N., Johnson, R.S., Loss of HIF-1α in endothelial cells disrupts a hypoxia-driven VEGF autocrine loop necessary for tumorigenesis. *Cancer Cell*, 6, 485, 2004.

28. Bouloumie, A., Drexler, H.C.A., Lafontan, M., Busse, R., Leptin, the product of Ob gene, promotes angiogenesis. *Circ. Res.*, 83, 1059, 1998.

29. Rupnick, M.A., Panigrahy, D., Zhang, C.-Y., Dallabrida, S.M., Lowell, B.B., Langer, R., Folkman, M.J., Adipose tissue mass can be regulated through the vasculature. *Proc. Natl. Acad. Sci. USA*, 99, 10730, 2002.

30. Brakenhielm, E., Cao, R., Gao, B., Angelin, B., Cannon, B., Parini, P., Cao, Y., Angiogenesis inhibitor, TNP-470, prevents diet-induced and genetic obesity in mice. *Circ. Res.*, 94, 1579, 2004.

31. Voros, G., Maquoi, E., Demeulemeester, D., Clerx, N., Collen, D., Lijnen, H.R., Modulation of angiogenesis during adipose tissue development in murine models of obesity. *Endocrinology*, 146, 4545, 2005. (a). Claffey, K.P., Wilkison, W.O., Spiegelman, B.M., Vascular endothelial growth factor. Regulation by cell differentiation and activated second messenger pathways. *J. Biol. Chem.*, 267, 16317–16322, 1992. (b). Fukumura, D., Ushiyama, A., Duda, D.G., Xu, L., Tam, J., Krishna, V., Chatterjee, K., Garkavtsev, I., Jain, R.K., Paracrine regulation of angiogenesis and adipocyte differentiation during in vivo adipogenesis. *Circ. Res.*, 93, e88–e97, 2003. (c) Tam, J., Duda, D.G., Perentes, J.Y., Quadri, R.S., Fukumura, D., Jain, R.K., Blockade of VEGFR2 and not VEGFR1 can limit diet-induced fat tissue expansion: Role of local versus bone marrow-derived endothelial cells. *PLoS One*, 4, e4974, 2009.

32. Griendling, K.K., Sorescu, D., Ushio-Fukai, M., NAD(P)H oxidase: Role in cardiovascular biology and disease. *Circ. Res.*, 86, 494, 2000.

33. Stone, J.R., Collins, T., The role of hydrogen peroxide in endothelial proliferative responses. *Endothelium*, 9, 231, 2002.

34. Ushio-Fukai, M., Tang, Y., Fukai, T., Dikalov, S., Ma Y., Fujimoto, M., Mitsuaki, Q., Mark, T., Pagano, P.J., Johnson, C., Wayne, A.R., Novel role of gp91phox-containing NAD(P)H oxidase in vascular endothelial growth factor-induced signaling and angiogenesis. *Circ. Res.*, 91, 1160, 2002.

35. Ushio-Fukai, M., Alexander, R.W., Reactive oxygen species as mediators of angiogenesis signaling: Role of NAD(P)H oxidase. *Mol. Cell. Biochem.*, 264, 85, 2004.

36. Harfouche, R., Malak, N.A., Brandes, R.P., Karsan, A., Irani, K., Hussain, S.N., Roles of reactive oxygen species in angiopoietin-1/tie-2 receptor signaling. *FASEB J.*, 19, 1728, 2005.

37. Luczak, K., Balcerczyk, A., Soszynski M., Bartosz, G., Low concentration of oxidant and nitric oxide donors stimulate proliferation of human endothelial cells in vitro. *Cell. Biol. Int.*, 28, 483, 2004.

38. Shono, T., Ono, M., Izumi, H., Jimi, S.I., Matsushima, K., Okamoto, T., Kohno, K., Kuwano, M., Involvement of the transcription factor NF-kappaB in tubular morphogenesis of human microvascular endothelial cells by oxidative stress. *Mol. Cell. Biol.*, 16, 4231, 1996.

39. Lelkes, P.I., Hahn, K.L., Sukovich, D.A., Karmiol, S., Schmidt, D.H., On the possible role of reactive oxygen species in angiogenesis. *Adv. Exp. Med. Biol.*, 454, 295–310,1998.

40. Yasuda, M., Shimizu, S., Tokuyama, S., Watanabe, T., Kinchi, Y., Yamamoto, T., A novel effect of polymorphonuclear leukocytes in the facilitation of angiogenesis. *Life Sci.*, 66 2113, 2000.

41. Qian, Y. et al., Hydrogen peroxide formation and actin filament reorganization by Cdc42 are essential for ethanol-induced in vitro angiogenesis. *J. Biol. Chem.*, 278, 16189–16197, 2003.

42. Yamagishi, S., Amano, S., Inagaki, Y., Okamoto, T., Takeuchi, M., Inoue, H., Pigment epithelium-derived factor inhibits leptin-induced angiogenesis by suppressing vascular endothelial growth factor gene expression through anti-oxidative properties. *Microvasc. Res.*, 65, 186, 2003.

43. Ellis, E.A., Guberski, D.L., Somogyi-Mann, M., Grant, M.B., Increased H_2O_2, vascular endothelial growth factor and receptors in the retina of the BBZ/Wor diabetic rat. *Free Radic. Biol. Med.*, 28, 91, 2000.

44. Ellis, E.A., Grant, M.B., Murray, F.T., Wachowski, M.B., Guberski, D.L., Kubilis, P.S., Lutty, G.A., Increased NADH oxidase activity in the retina of the BBZ/Wor diabetic rat. *Free Radic. Biol. Med.*, 24, 111, 1998.

45. Ruef, J., Hu, Z.Y., Yin, L.Y., Wu, Y., Hanson, S.R., Kelly, A.B., Harker, L.A., Rao, G.N., Runge, M.S., Patterson, C., Induction of vascular endothelial growth factor in balloon-injured baboon arteries. *Circ. Res.*, 81, 24, 1997.

46. Kuroki, M., Voest, E.E., Amano, S., Beerepoot, L.V., Takashima, S., Tolentino, M., Kim, R.Y., Rohan, R.M., Colby, K.A., Yeo, K.T., Adamis, A.P., Reactive oxygen intermediates increase vascular endothelial growth factor expression in vitro and in vivo. *J. Clin. Invest.*, 98, 1667, 1996.

47. Lakshminarayanan, V., Lewallen, M., Frangogiannis, N.G., Evans, A.J., Wedin, K.E., Michael, L.H., Entman, M.L., Reactive oxygen intermediates induce monocyte chemotactic protein-1 in vascular endothelium after brief ischemia. *Am. J. Pathol.*, 159, 1301, 2001.

48. Yoshida, A., Yoshida, S., Ishibashi, T., Kuwano, M., Inomata, H., Suppression of retinal neovascularization by the NF-kappaB inhibitor pyrrolidine dithiocarbamate in mice. *Invest. Ophthalmol. Vis. Sci.*, 40, 1624, 1999.

49. Cao, Y., Cao, R., Angiogenesis inhibited by drinking tea [letter]. *Nature*, 398, 381, 1999.

50. Brakenhielm, E., Cao, R., Cao, Y., Suppression of angiogenesis, tumor growth, and wound healing by resveratrol, a natural compound in red wine and grapes. *FASEB J.*, 15, 1798, 2001.

51. Oak, M.H., El Bedoui, J., Schini-Kerth, V.B., Antiangiogenic properties of natural polyphenols from red wine and green tea. *J. Nutr. Biochem.*, 16, 1, 2005.

52. Tang, F.Y., Meydani, M., Green tea catechins and vitamin E inhibit angiogenesis of human microvascular endothelial cells through suppression of IL-8 production. *Nutr. Cancer.*, 41, 119, 2001.

53. Moulton, K.S., Heller, E., Konerding, M.A., Flynn, E., Palinski, W., Folkman, J., Angiogenesis inhibitors endostatin or TNP-470 reduce intimal neovascularization and plaque growth in apolipoprotein E-deficient mice. *Circulation*, 99, 1726, 1999.

54. Nespereira, B., Perez-Ilzarbe, M., Fernandez, P., Fuentes, A.M., Paramo, J.A., Rodriguez, J.A., Vitamins C and E downregulate vascular VEGF and VEGFR-2 expression in apolipoprotein-E-deficient mice. *Atherosclerosis*, 171, 67, 2003.

55. Cai, T., Fassina, G., Morini, M., Aluigi, M.G., Masiello, L., Fontanini, G., D'Agostini, F., De Flora, S., Noonan, D.M., Albini, A., N-Acetylcysteine inhibits endothelial cell invasion and angiogenesis. *Lab. Invest.*, 79, 1151, 1999.

56. Annabi, B., Lee, Y.T., Martel, C., Pilorget, A., Bahary, J.P., Beliveau, R., Radiation induced-tubulogenesis in endothelial cells is antagonized by the antiangiogenic properties of green tea polyphenol (-) epigallocatechin-3-gallate. *Cancer Biol. Ther.*, 2, 642, 2003.

57. Sartippour, M.R., Shao, Z.M., Heber, D., Beatty, P., Zhang, L., Liu, C., Ellis, L., Liu, W., Go, V.L., Brooks, M.N., Green tea inhibits vascular endothelial growth factor (VEGF) induction in human breast cancer cells. *J. Nutr.*, 132, 2307, 2002.

58. Losso, J.N., Bawadi, H.A., Hypoxia inducible factor pathways as targets for functional foods. *J. Agric. Food Chem.*, 53, 3751, 2005.

59. Roy, S., Khanna, S., Alessio, H.M., Bagchi, D., Bagchi, M., Sen, C.K., Anti-angiogenic properties of berry nutrients. *Free Radic. Res.*, 36, 1023, 2002.

60. Bagchi, D., Sen, C.K., Bagchi, M., Atalay, M., Anti-angiogenic, antioxidant and anti-carcinogenic properties of a novel anthocyanin-rich berry extract formula. *Biochemistry*, 69, 75, 2004.

61. Key, T.H. et al., Body mass index, serum sex hormones, and breast cancer risk in postmenopausal women. *J. Natl. Cancer Inst.*, 95, 1218, 2003.

62. Preuss, H.G., Bagchi, D., Clouatre, D., Insulin resistance; a factor in aging. In: Ghen, M.J., Corso, N., Joiner-Bey, H., Klatz, R., Dratz, A. (eds.), *The Advanced Guide to Longevity Medicine*. Ghen, Landrum, SC, p. 239, 2001.

63. Borugian, M.J. et al., Waist-to-hip ratio and breast cancer mortality. *Am. J. Epidemiol.*, 158, 963, 2003.

18 Obese and Overweight
New Sensitive Population for Drug and Chemical Toxicities?

George B. Corcoran, PhD, ATS

CONTENTS

INTRODUCTION

Obesity is the most common disease in the United States. According to the results of the most recent National Health and Nutrition Examination Survey (NHANES) covering 2007–2008, one third of U.S. men and women are overweight, defined as body mass index (BMI) of 25 or greater, and another third of U.S. men and women are obese, defined as BMI of 30 or greater [1]. From the time of the first NHANES report for the 1976–1980 period, the prevalence of obesity has increased from 15% to 34% in adults. Obesity in children and adolescents, defined as BMI greater than 95th percentile for age or greater than 30, increased from 5% to 17% over this same time period [2]. It is becoming more broadly accepted in the medical community that obesity is a leading disease that has far-reaching negative health consequences. Despite this general agreement, the full implications of obesity, particularly its adverse impact on health and wellness, remain less than fully appreciated, and this disease frequently does not lead to aggressive approaches to limit its adverse consequences that are common today for diseases like hypertension and hypercholesterolemia.

Bray [3] noted that the current worldwide epidemic of obesity will be followed by an epidemic of diabetes, a disease closely linked to metabolic syndrome found in most obese individuals [4–7]. In investigating the surge of childhood obesity, Bray and others express concern over a direct correlation with increased consumption of beverages rich in high-fructose corn syrup [8,9], although some have argued that the latter should be considered a safe and innocuous sweetener that does not pose a unique dietary risk in healthy individuals or diabetics [10].

It is deeply concerning that the Worldwatch Institute reported in 2004, for the first time, that the number of overfed and obese people, about 1.1 billion and growing, would soon outnumber under-fed people in the world, about 1.1 billion and stable or declining. Overweight and obesity was estimated to account for 4%–9% of total annual health-care costs in 2004 [11], and 30% of the increase in health-care costs seen since 1987 [12].

Life expectancy in the United States has increased from 74 years in 1980, to 77 years in 2000, and to 78 years in 2009 [13,14]. We may live to see the first generation in this country to experience a decline in life expectancy [15]. In a study that evaluated mortality in 1.5 million white adults, BMI of 22.5–24.9 was the reference category exhibiting the lowest mortality. Increased mortality and hazard ratios of 1.13, 1.44, 1.88, and 2.51 were reported for overweight, obese, morbidly obese, and BMI > 40, respectively [16]. A similar relationship between increasing BMI and excess mortality exists for East Asians but interestingly was not observed for Indians and Bangladeshis [17]. By various estimates, obesity accounts for 5%–15% of deaths each year in the United States [18]. If past trends in obesity continue unabated, its negative effects on mortality will outweigh the positive effects of the steady decline in the incidence of smoking [19]. Obesity and morbid obesity (BMI ≥ 30 and ≥40, respectively) result in substantially increased morbidity and mortality, arising from many different sources. The death rate rises when body weight exceeds the desired value for height by a little as 20% [20]. As noted in the Framingham Heart Study [21], the risk of death in 26 years is increased by 1% for each extra pound of body weight at ages 30–41 and increased by 2% for each extra pound of body weight at ages 50–62.

It was only two and a half decades ago when obesity gained official status as a disease, distinct from the large number of well-known comorbidities including heart and liver disease, hypertension, diabetes, and cancers [22,23]. Mortality from all cancers is increased by obesity in men by a relative risk of 1.52. Specific cancers that increase with obesity include liver (4.52), pancreas (2.61), stomach (1.94), colon and rectum (1.84), and gallbladder (1.76). Total cancer mortality shows a greater increase in obese women (relative risk 1.88) than men [24]. A recent meta-analysis of prospective observational studies from around the world found that a BMI increase of 5.0 correlated strongly across populations in men with esophageal adenocarcinoma (1.5) and thyroid (1.2), colon (1.24) and renal (1.24) cancers, and in women with endometrial (1.59), gall bladder (1.59), esophageal (1.51), and renal (1.34) cancers [25]. There were many weaker positive associations of other cancers in men and women. For lung cancer, BMI was not associated with cancer risk in those who never smoked. Interestingly, BMI was inversely associated with cancer risk in smokers. Weight loss by obese postmenopausal women decreases the risk of breast cancer over those who remain obese [26].

Liver disease is a hallmark of obesity and is greatly accentuated in morbid obesity. Why many forms of liver disease are increased in the obese is not well understood, but high rates of nonalcoholic fatty liver disease may be the result of increased susceptibility to injury by drugs and chemicals. Wanless and Lentz [27] reported large differences between livers of obese versus lean humans: steatosis (70% vs. 35%), nonalcoholic steatohepatitis (18.5% vs. 3%), and cirrhosis (2%–3% vs. 0%). A factor that may contribute to increased liver disease and damage to other organs is exaggerated drug toxicity. It is well known, for example, that obese patients and rats undergoing surgical anesthesia with halothane, methoxyflurane, and enflurane suffer higher rates of liver and kidney damage due to increased toxic metabolites formed as a result of accelerated biotransformation [28–30]. Additional clinical studies show that obesity increases the clearance of many drugs that are eliminated primarily by metabolism in the liver [31,32], including acetaminophen [33] and lorazepam [31]. Increased metabolic activity is also capable of activating drugs and chemicals to toxic metabolites at increased rates in obese individuals.

This chapter will consider findings, including historical data, which support the hypothesis that obese individuals are at substantially increased risk of drug toxicity. This increased risk arises from varied sources. These sources include higher rates of toxic metabolite formation, greater accumulation of the toxic form of a drug, and increased susceptibility due to decreased defenses, including those related to glutathione, and to increased underlying pathologic conditions. The chapter will not consider or present the substantial body of evidence showing that many drugs also induce higher incidences of toxicity due to inappropriately high doses of drugs administered to obese individuals. In these cases, dosing is based on total body mass (TBM) or other values that systematically overestimate actual distribution and clearance values in obese individuals, resulting in acute or chronic exposure to higher and more prolonged drug concentrations and an increased frequency of drug-related toxicities.

ANIMAL MODELS OF HUMAN OBESITY

It can be quite difficult, and in many cases impossible, to perform studies that would be a direct test of one's working hypothesis in human volunteers or patients due to ethical and other considerations. For this and other reasons, it is often necessary to perform some or most studies with models that recapitulate the human condition. In the case of obesity, a wide variety of models exist today. Each has a different array of strengths, weaknesses, and distinguishing attributes. Models divide into those primarily of genetic origin and those primarily of environmental origin [4,34–36]. By selecting a model, the implications of study results become thus specified, as does the possible relevance of results for drug-related mortality or morbidity in obese humans. When the hypothesis that drugs are more toxic in obesity first came under examination, some key animal models that exist today were poorly characterized or were not available because they had not been developed. Although models based upon leptin defects, including the leptin null (*ob/ob*) mouse and the leptin receptor null (*db/db*) mouse, were in use, the genetic bases of these models were not understood. Some current models that exploit melatonin defects (AGR Agouti, ART Agouti-Related Protein, MC4R, POMC, carboxypeptidase, and Tubby mice) were available while others were not [36]. Other environmental models in which mice or rats "acquire" obesity included dietary models (cafeteria diet, force feeding, overfeeding), surgical models (hypothalamic lesion), and chemically induced models (gold thioglucose).

Rat models offer advantages for studying drug disposition and toxicity, including the ability to obtain multiple blood samples from the same animal for the estimation of pharmacokinetic parameters. Leading rat models of obesity include the Zucker rat, a genetic model, and the overfed rat, a model in which obesity is acquired.

ROLES OF GENETICS AND ENVIRONMENT

It is widely understood that both genetic and environmental factors contribute to the majority of human obesity. Obesity is a complex disorder in which genetic predisposition factors are believed to interact with environmental factors to produce an array of different human phenotypes of the disease [37]. Pioneering studies of Stunkard and others [38–40] who observed monozygotic and dizygotic twin pairs, and adopted twins raised apart, show that at least 50%, and possibly as high as 90%, of obesity is heritable. The heritability of obesity is polygenetic. Genome-wide searches for loci responsible for obesity across populations have identified some 30 loci that influence BMI, with the FTO locus among the earliest to show a strongest correlation [41,42]. To date, 20 genes have been shown to produce obesity upon their disruption or mutation, but they account for 5% or less of human obesity [43,44]. Thus, the development of obesity requires contributions from the environment, yet genetics is believed to account for 40%–70% of the etiology of this disease [45,46]. While some studies present data showing low rates of cultural transmission of obesity, this stands in direct opposition to a well-established body of findings showing strong socioeconomic determinants of obesity. It can be said with confidence that both genetic predisposition and environmental factors are important keys to the successful modeling of human obesity.

OVERFED RAT MODEL VERSUS ZUCKER RAT MODEL

The goal of gaining greater understanding of the bases and consequences of human obesity by using animal models should not be sidetracked by the desire to work with the best or a "near perfect" model. Rather, it is important that the model under study provide informative and relevant insights for the questions at hand. Some obesity models are better mimics of drug disposition in obese humans than others. This guided our thinking in selecting and then characterizing the overfed rat model of human obesity for pharmacokinetics and metabolism studies. This model recapitulated a key environmental factor contributing to human obesity, the increasing percentage of daily caloric

TABLE 18.1

Content of Pellet Control and Energy-Rich Diets

Diet Component[a]	Pellet Control Diet	Energy-Dense Diet
Fat	6.5	60.0
Protein	14.5	24.5
Carbohydrate	57.5	7.5
Moisture	10.0	1.0
Fiber	4.0	2.0
Ash	7.5	5.0
Energy content (kcal/g)[b]	3.47	6.68

Source: Adapted from Schemmel, R. et al., *J. Nutr.,* 100, 1041, 1970.

[a] Shown as percentage (w/w) and based upon representative lot analysis of Prolab R-M-H 1000 by manufacturer (Agway, Inc., Syracuse, NY) and a description of energy dense diet adapted from Schemmel et al. [47].

[b] Calculated from 9, 4, and 4 kcal/g for fat, protein, and carbohydrate, respectively.

intake that has been represented by dietary fat over the past five decades. Sprague-Dawley rats become obese when maintained for more than 12 weeks on an energy-dense diet developed by Schemmel et al. [47] (Table 18.1, Figure 18.1).

Overfed rats that became obese on an energy-rich diet were compared to Zucker rats, genetically obese rodents that inherit obesity through an autosomal recessive trait caused by a mutation of the leptin receptor gene [48]. The latter mechanism accounts for no more than a fraction of a percent of human obesity. Comparisons showed that overfed rats resembled obese humans in 11 of 12 characteristics selected for their importance to drug disposition and toxicity, including those

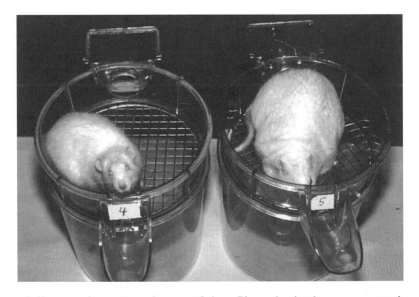

FIGURE 18.1 Pellet control rat versus obese overfed rat. Pictured animals are representative of groups of rats that were fed standard pellet diet (#4) or an obesity-inducing energy-rich diet (#5) for 57 weeks. TBM differed significantly between the group fed the pellet diet (705 ± 110 g, $n = 7$) versus the energy-dense diet (1086 ± 186 g, $n = 9$) at $p < 0.05$. Other pharmacokinetic characteristics differed substantially between pellet control and obese rats. (From Schemmel, R. et al., *J. Nutr.,* 100, 1041, 1970.)

that control drug clearance and volume of distribution. Zucker rats resembled obese humans in only 5 of 12 characteristics, and the discrepancies were highly meaningful. Zucker rats showed no increase in fat-free mass (FFM) or creatinine clearance, while thyroid function was abnormally depressed [49]. Differences of the greatest significance involved hepatic cytochrome P-450, which increased in proportion to TBM in obese overfed rats but which remained unchanged in obese Zucker rats and refractory to induction by phenobarbital. Although P450 status is not fully characterized in obese humans, many reports show increased drug oxidation in obese individuals, consistent with increased P450 levels.

TOXICITY OF DRUGS AND CHEMICALS

Being ill more often, obese individuals receive drug treatment more frequently, beginning earlier in life than those of normal weight. Ironically, information to guide the appropriate treatment of this substantial and growing population has only recently begun to accrue, and tools to adjust drug dosing for obese patients remain limited in number and application. Uncertainty in selecting the correct dose of a drug for an obese patient is a problem that has become more acute rather than becoming better understood. Because of their higher rates of morbidity, obese individuals are overrepresented among those receiving medical attention, multiple medications, and drugs with high inherent toxicity and narrow therapeutic indexes.

Studies with the obese overfed rat consistently show that representative drugs and chemicals are more toxic to obese animals, even when dosing biases are eliminated by normalizing dose according to fat-free body mass. Experiments with acetaminophen (Table 18.2) show this analgesic produces greater liver and kidney necrosis in obese overfed rats when compared to pellet-fed control rats, independent of whether animals are dosed according to TBM or to FFM [50]. The latter indicates that obese rats are intrinsically more susceptible to acetaminophen-induced necrosis in both of these organs. Rats maintained on the energy-dense diet showed increased

---

TABLE 18.2

Increased Acetaminophen-Induced Liver and Kidney Necrosis in Obese Overfed Rats

		Relative Incidence and Extent of Necrosis (%)								
		Liver				Kidney				
Group	48-h Survival	0	1+	2+	3+	0	1+	2+	3+	4+
Pellet control[a]	9/9	100				89	11			
Energy-dense lean	7/9	86		14		43	29	14	14	
Energy-dense obese[a] dosed to TBM	4/9	25	25	25	25				50	50
Energy-dense obese[b] dosed to FFM	4/9	25	25	50			33		33	33

Source: Reprinted from Wong, B.K. et al., *Drug Metab. Dispos.*, 14, 674, 1986. With permission.

Notes: Three groups of rats received 710 mg/kg acetaminophen *i.p.* and resided in metabolism cages for 24 h. The last group (dosed to FFM) received the same dose as energy-dense lean animals on an FFM basis (i.e., 955 mg/kg of FFM). Animals were sacrificed at 48 h, and portions of liver and kidney were prepared for light microscopic analysis. Hepatic and renal necrosis in surviving animals was graded from 0 (absent) to 4+ (>50%) according to the abundance of dead parenchymal or renal epithelial cells in sections stained with hematoxylin and eosin. Values represent the percentage of surviving animals within a group exhibiting each grade of injury. Differences in distribution of enumerated necrosis scores were detected by nonparametric analysis of variance and Tukey-like multiple comparison test.

[a] Values bearing the same superscript were different at $p < 0.05$. Both liver and kidney scores differed between pellet control and obese animals dosed to TBM.

[b] One kidney histology sample was lost during processing.

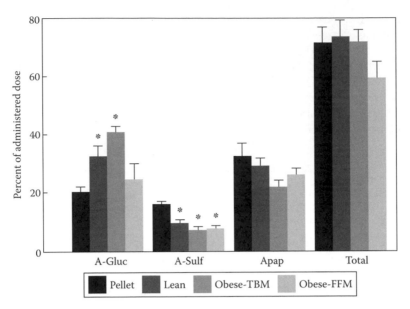

FIGURE 18.2   Effects of obesity and dosing normalization on metabolic rate of acetaminophen. Values are the sum of acetaminophen and metabolites that were excreted into urine plus those remaining in carcass at the time of sacrifice. The latter values were estimated based by multiplying the terminal plasma concentration times the volume of distribution. Differences were detected by analysis of variance and Tukey's multiple comparison test (* = $p < 0.05$). Results are expressed as mean ± SEM. (Reprinted from Raucy, J.L. et al., *Mol. Pharmacol.*, 39, 275, 1991. With permission.)

glucuronidation and decreased sulfation of acetaminophen (Figure 18.2) [51]. Prior studies demonstrated that these dosing regimens produced peak acetaminophen plasma concentrations that were not statistically different, but that the elimination profile differed between obese and control animals. Increased metabolic clearance in obese rats reproduced increased metabolic clearance seen in obese humans [33]. Acetaminophen activation to its toxic metabolite is increased in the obese overfed rat by 28% per mg hepatic microsomal protein over control rats, and immunodetectable CYP2E1, the primary catalyst of acetaminophen bioactivation, is substantially elevated in the obese overfed rat [51] and the obese Zucker rat [52]. Importantly, the obese overfed rat model directly mirrors obese humans, who have significant increases in CYP2E1 protein, enzyme activity, and drug metabolism [53,54].

Oxidation of ethanol by the MEOS system is elevated by 28% in hepatic microsomes from obese overfed rats compared to rates in microsomes from pellet control animals (Table 18.2) [55]. It is possible that this elevation in ethanol oxidation by the MEOS system contributes to the high incidence of abnormal liver pathology in obese individuals. This potential relationship bears further investigation.

The loop diuretic, furosemide (Lasix), also undergoes hepatic metabolism to a toxic metabolite that accounts for both liver and kidney necrosis and organ failure. In the obese overfed rat, furosemide is more toxic when dosed on a TBM basis as well as on a fat-free body mass basis, again indicating greater intrinsic susceptibility of the obese liver to damage by drugs undergoing P450 bioactivation [56] (Table 18.3).

Gentamicin, a powerful aminoglycoside antibiotic that is reserved for the treatment of severe or life-threatening Gram-negative infection, has a narrow therapeutic index due to nephrotoxicity and ototoxicity. For this reason, its use is typically reserved for critically ill patients. An analysis of critically ill patients treated with aminoglycoside antibiotics shows that the incidence of renal injury is higher than normal in patients who are substantially overweight [57]. This raised the possibility that drugs that do not require bioactivation by P450 also are more toxic in obese individuals. Because the diet provided to obese overfed rats produces urinary acidification, which could alter gentamicin

TABLE 18.3
Increased Furosemide-Induced Liver and Kidney Necrosis in Obese Overfed Rats Dosed according to Fat-Free Mass

| | | Relative Incidence and Extent of Necrosis (%) | | | | | | | |
| | 24-h | Liver[a] | | | | Kidney | | | |
Group	Survival	0	1+	2+	3+	0	1+	2+	3+
Pellet control[a]	6/6	83	17			67	17	17	
Energy-dense obese[a] dosed to FFM	9/9		44	44	11	33	22	22	22

Source: Reprinted from Corcoran, G.B. et al., *Toxicol. Appl. Pharmacol.*, 98, 12, 1989. With permission.

Notes: (519 ± 82 g vs. 589 ± 36 g, respectively). Animals were sacrificed at 24 h, and portions of liver and kidney were prepared for light microscopic analysis. Hepatic and renal necrosis in surviving animals was graded from 0 (absent) to 4+ (>50%) according to the abundance of dead parenchymal or renal epithelial cells in sections stained with hematoxylin and eosin. Values represent the percentage of surviving animals within a group exhibiting each grade of injury. Differences in distribution of enumerated necrosis scores were detected by nonparametric analysis of variance and Tukey-like multiple comparison test.

[a] Liver but not kidney scores differed between pellet control dosed according to FFM and energy-dense obese dosed according to FFM at $p < 0.05$.

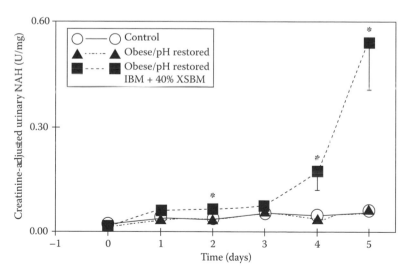

FIGURE 18.3 The effects of obesity on creatinine-adjusted urinary excretion of N-acetyl hexosaminidase (NAH) after chronic gentamicin dosing based on ideal body mass plus 40% excess body mass. Creatinine-adjusted urinary excretion of NAH was determined over time for three groups of animals. Control rats were treated with 30 mg/kg gentamicin *i.p.* twice daily for 5 days based on ideal body mass (○). Urine pH of obese rats was restored to control values (7.25 ± 0.24) by placing animals on pellet diet for 7 days. These obese, pH-restored rats were treated with gentamicin based on ideal body mass (▲) or ideal body mass plus 40% of excess body mass (■). Results are expressed as mean ± SD of six to eight animals per group (* $p < 0.05$ vs. control by analysis of variance and Tukey's test). (Reprinted from Aubert, J. et al., *Clin. Res. Hepatol. Gastroenterol.,* doi:10.1016/j.clinre.2011.04.015, 2011. With permission.)

renal accumulation and therefore toxicity, a group of obese rats was returned to the control pellet diet for 7 days to restore normal urinary pH. pH-normalized animals were dosed with gentamicin according to ideal body mass plus 40% of excess body mass, the dosing adjustment typically used in the clinic for obese patients. We tracked N-acetyl-hexosaminidase activity, a sensitive biomarker of renal epithelial necrosis. When this index of injury was normalized to creatinine excretion, obese rats demonstrated greater renal injury than pellet-fed control rats and than obese rats dosed to FFM (Figure 18.3) [58]. Increased toxicity was accompanied by increased renal accumulation of gentamicin over pellet controls. Again, obesity was found to potentiate drug-induced organ injury.

PERSPECTIVE

Obesity is a mounting public health problem in the United States and many other countries. This chapter offers consistent findings that obesity predisposes rats to liver and kidney damage by chemicals and drugs acting through different mechanisms of toxicity. These findings also offer several lines of evidence that support the hypothesis that obesity predisposes humans to drug and chemical toxicities. The latter may explain high incidences of liver, kidney, and other organ damage in obese humans. The higher rates of injury in obese overfed rats do not appear to arise because obese organs were exposed to higher drug concentrations than organs of lean controls. This latter observation points to the importance of underlying susceptibility factors, such as demonstrated increases in cytochrome P450 activities [51,53,59], diminished defenses by glutathione [60] and other protective mediators, and other relevant mechanisms such as increased rates of reactive oxygen species formation in livers with steatosis and NASH [61]. It is a reasonable notion that increased liver damage, and perhaps even the shortened life span of obese humans, may arise from greater susceptibility to chemical and drug toxicity. It would be valuable if concepts established with the obese overfed rat were pursued in the clinical setting where the uncertainty of animal model extrapolation would be obviated. Obesity will continue to grow in its negative impact on human health, and on health-care expenditures, over the next decades. Do obese and overweight individuals constitute a new sensitive population? Research resources should be marshaled to reach a definitive answer to this important question. Obesity is the most common preventable human disease in the United States. The time is now to accelerate the pace of research into the bases for this disease, and the search for new means to reverse its progression and morbidities, and prevent associated premature mortality.

ACKNOWLEDGMENTS

The author acknowledges the valuable contribution made by his many colleagues and students, as well as generous support from the NIH (NIH GM20852, NIH GM41564, NIH 2S07RR05454) and the Research Foundation of SUNY.

REFERENCES

1. Flegal, K.M., Carroll, M.D., Ogden, C.L., and Curtin, L.R. Prevalence and trends in obesity among US adults. 1999–2008. *JAMA* 303, 235, 2010.
2. Ogden, C.L., Carroll, M.D., Curtin, L.R., Lamb, M.M., and Flegal, K.M. Prevalence of high body mass index in US children and adolescents. 2007–2008. *JAMA* 303, 242, 2010.
3. Bray, G.A. The epidemic of obesity and changes in food intake: The fluoride hypothesis. *Physiol. Behav.* 82, 115, 2004.
4. Sclafani, A. Animal models of obesity: Classification and characterization. *Int. J. Obes.* 8, 419, 1984.
5. Kahn, S.E., Sinman, B., Haffner, S.M., O'neill, M.C., Kravitz, B.G., Yu, D., Freed, M.I., Herman, W.H., Holman, R.R., Jones, N.P., Lachin, J.M., and Viberti, G.C., Obesity is a major determinant of the association between C-reactive protein levels and the metabolic syndrome in type 2 diabetes. *Diabetes* 55, 2357, 2006.

6. Grundy, S.M., Brewer Jr., H.B., Cleeman, J.I., Smith Jr., S.C., and L'Enfant, C., Definition of metabolic syndrome: Report of the National Heart, Lung, and Blood Institute/American Heart Association conference on scientific issues related to definition. *Circulation* 109, 433, 2004.

7. Bray, G.A., Nielsen, S.J., and Popkin, B.M., Consumption of high-fructose corn syrup in beverages may play a role in the epidemic of obesity. *Am. J. Clin. Nutr.* 79, 537, 2004.

8. Bray, G.A., Fructose: Pure, white, and deadly? Fructose, by any other name, is a health hazard. *J. Diab. Sci. Technol.* 4, 1003, 2010.

9. McCaffree, M.A., Fryhofer, S.A., Gitlow, S., Head, C.A., Khan, M.K., Kridel, R.W., Levin, I.R., Morisy, L.R., Osbahr, A.J., Robinowitz, C.B., Sabbatini, A., Woods, G.L., and Dickinson, B.D., The effects of high fructose syrup. *J. Am. Coll. Nutr.* 28, 619, 2009.

10. White, J.S. Misconceptions about high-fructose corn syrup: Is it uniquely responsible for obesity, reactive dicarbonyl compounds, and advanced glycation endproducts? *J. Nutr.* 139, 1219S, 2009.

11. Wee, C.C., Phillips, R.S., Legedza, A.T.R., Davis, R.B., Soukup, J.R., Colditz, G.A., and Hamel, M.B., Health care expenditures associated with overweight and obesity among US adults: Importance of age and race. *Am. J. Pub. Health* 95, 159, 2005.

12. Roszak, D. Obesity accounts for nearly 30 percent of health care spending increase since '87. *Hosp. Health Netw.* 78, 58, 2004.

13. National Center for Health Statistics. *Health, United States, 2004 with Chartbook on Trends in the Health of Americans*. Hyattsville, MD: National Center for Health Statistics; 2004. Available at: http://www.cdc.gov/nchs/data/hus/hus04.pdf. Accessed March, 2005.

14. Thanne, J.H., Americans living longer, but obesity and diabetes are rising. *BMJ* 342, d1143, 2011.

15. Olshansky, S.J., Passaro, D.J., Hershow, R.C., Layden, J., Barnes, B.A., Brody, J., Hayflick, L., Butler, R.N., Allison, D.B., and Ludwig, D.S., A potential decline in life expectancy in the United States in the 21st century. *N. Engl. J. Med.* 352, 1138, 2005.

16. Berrington de Gonzalez, A., Hartage, P., Cerhan, J.R., Flint, A.J. et al., Body-mass index and mortality among 1.46 million white adults. *N. Engl. J. Med.* 363, 23, 2010.

17. Zheng, W., CeLerran, D.F., Rolland, B., Zhang, X. et al., Association between body-mass index and risk of death in more than 1 million Asians. *N. Engl. J. Med.* 364, 8, 2011.

18. Flegal, K.M., Graubard, B.I., Williamson, D.F., and Gail, M.H., Excess deaths associated with underweight, overweight and obesity. *JAMA* 293, 1861, 2005.

19. Stewart, S.T., Cutler, D.M., and Rosen, A.B., Forecasting the effects of obesity and smoking on U.S. life expectancy. *N. Engl. J. Med.* 361, 2252, 2009.

20. Society of Actuaries and Association of Life Insurance Medical Directors, Build study, 1979. Society of Actuaries and Association of Life Insurance Medical Directors, Chicago, IL, 1979.

21. Hubert, H.B. Framingham Heart Study. *Annu. Rev. Public Health* 7, 493, 1986.

22. Kolalta, G., Obesity declared a disease. *Science* 227, 1019, 1985.

23. Andersen, T., Christoffersen, R., and Gluud, C., The liver in consecutive patients with morbid obesity: A clinical, morphological and biochemical study. *Int. J. Obes.* 8, 107, 1984.

24. Calle, E.E., Rogriguez, C., Walker-Thurmond, K., and Thun, M.J., Overweight, obesity, and mortality from cancer in prospectively studied cohort of U.S. adults. *N. Engl. J. Med.* 348, 1625, 2003.

25. Renehan, A.G., Tyson, M., Egger, M., Heller, R.F., and Zwahlen, M., Body mass index and incidence of cancer: A systematic review and meta-analysis of prospective observational studies. *Lancet* 371, 569, 2008.

26. Wolin, K.Y., Carson, K., and Colditz, G.A., Obesity and cancer. *Oncologist* 15, 556, 2010.

27. Wanless, I.R. and Lentz, J.S., Fatty liver hepatitis (steatohepatitis) and obesity: An autopsy study with analysis of risk factors. *Hepatology* 12, 1106, 1990.

28. Miller, M.S., Gandolfi, A.J., Vaughan, R.W., and Bentley, J.B., Disposition of enflurane in obese patients. *J. Pharmacol. Exp. Ther.* 215, 292, 1980.

29. Rice, S.A. and Fish, K.J., Anesthetic metabolism and renal function in obese and non-obese Fisher 344 rats following enflurane and isoflurane anesthesia. *Anesthesiology* 65, 28, 1986.

30. Samuelson, P.N., Berin, R.G., Taves, D.R., Freeman, R.B., Calimlim, J.F., and Kumazawa, T., Toxicity following methoxyflurane anaesthesia. IV. The role of obesity and the effect of low does anesthesia on fluoride metabolism and renal function. *Can. Anesth. Soc.* 23, 465, 1976.

31. Abernethy, D.R. and Greenblatt, D.J., Drug disposition in obese humans: An update. *Clin. Pharmacokinet.* 11, 199, 1986.

32. McLean, A.J., Lalka, D., Corcoran, G.B., and Melander, A., Drug-nutrient interactions. *Rec. Adv. Clin. Nutr.* 2, 1, 1986.

33. Abernethy, D.R., Divoll, M., Greenblatt, D.J., and Ameer, B., Obesity, sex, and acetaminophen disposition. *Clin. Pharmacol. Ther.* 31, 783, 1982.
34. Kanasaki, K. and Koy, D., Biology of obesity: Lessons from animal models of obesity. *J. Biomed. Biotech.* doi: 10.1155/2011/197636, 2011.
35. Hariri, N. and Thibault, L., High-fat diet-induced obesity in animal models. *Nutr. Res. Rev.* 23, 270, 2010.
36. Caroll, L., Voisey, J., and Van Daal, A., Mouse models of obesity. *Clin. Dermatol.* 22, 245, 2004.
37. Comuzzie, A.G., Williams, J.T., Martin, L.J., and Blangero, J., Searching for genes underlying normal variation in human adiposity. *J. Mol. Med.* 79, 57, 2001.
38. Bouchard, C., Tremblay, A., Despres, J.P., Nadeau, A., Lupien, P.J., Theriault, G., Dussault, J., Moorjani, S., Pinault, A., and Fournier, G., The response to long-term overfeeding of identical twins. *N. Engl. J. Med.* 322, 1477, 1990.
39. Stunkard, A.J., Sorensen, T.I., Hanis, C., Teasdale, T.W., Chakraborty, R., Shull, W.J., and Schulsinger, F., An adoption study of human obesity. *N. Engl. J. Med.* 314, 193, 1986.
40. Price, R.A. and Gottesman, I.I., Body fat in identical twins reared apart: Roles for genes and environment. *Behav. Genet.* 21, 1, 1991.
41. Lindgren, C.M., Heid, I.M., Randall, J.C. et al., Genome-wide association scan meta-analysis identifies three Loci influencing adiposity and fat distribution. *PLoS Genet* 5, e1000508, 2009.
42. Frayling, T.M., Timpson, N.J., Weedon, M.N. et al., A common variant in the FTO gene is associated with body mass index and predisposes to childhood and adult obesity. *Science* 316, 889, 2007.
43. O'Rahilly, S., Human genetics illuminates the paths to metabolic disease. *Nature* 462, 307, 2009.
44. Rankinen, T., Zuberi, A., Chagnon, Y.C., Weisnagel, S.J., Argyropoulos, G., Walts, B., Perusse, L., and Bouchard, C., The human obesity gene map: The 2005 update. *Obesity* 14, 529, 2006.
45. Herrera, B.M. and Lindgren, C.M., The genetics of obesity. *Curr. Diab. Rep.* 10, 498, 2010.
46. Feero, W.G. and Gutmacher, A.E., Genomics, type 2 diabetes, and obesity. *N. Engl. J. Med.* 363, 214, 2010.
47. Schemmel, R., Mickelson, O., and Gill, J.L., Body weight and body fat accretion in seven strains of rat. *J. Nutr.* 100, 1041, 1970.
48. Chua Jr., S.C., Cheung, W.K., Wu-Peng, X.S., Zhang, Y., Liu, S.-M., Tartaglia, L., and Leibel, R.L., Phenotypes of mouse *diabetes* and rat *fatty* due to mutations in the OB [Leptin] receptor. *Science* 271, 994, 1996.
49. Corcoran, G.B., Salazar, D.E., and Sorge, C.L., Pharmacokinetic characteristics of the obese overfed rat. *Intl. J. Obes.* 13, 69, 1988; Corcoran, G.B. and Wong, B.K. Obesity as a risk factor in drug-induced organ injury: Increased liver and kidney damage from acetaminophen in the obese overfed rat. *J. Pharmacol. Exp. Ther.* 241, 921, 1987.
50. Wong, B.K., U, E.S.-W., and Corcoran, G.B., An overfed rat model that reproduces acetaminophen disposition in obese humans. *Drug Metab. Dispos.* 14, 674, 1986.
51. Raucy, J.L., Lasker, J.M., Kraner, J.C., Salazar, D.E., Lieber, C.S., and Corcoran, G.B., Induction of cytochrome P450IIE1 in the obese overfed rat. *Mol. Pharmacol.* 39, 275, 1991.
52. Khemawoot, P., Yokogawa, K., Shimada, T., and Miyamoto, K., Obesity-induced increase of CYP2E1 activity and its effect on disposition kinetics of chlorzoxazone in Zucker rats. *Biochem. Pharmacol.* 73, 155, 2007.
53. O'Shea, D., Davis, S.N., Kim, R.B., and Wilkinson, G.R., Effect of fasting and obesity in humans on the 6-hydroxylation of chlorzoxazone: A putative probe of CYP2E1 activity. *Clin. Pharmacol. Ther.* 56, 35, 1994.
54. Varela, N.M., Quinones, L.A., Orellana, M., Poniachik, J., Csendes, A., Smok, G. et al., Study of cytochrome P450 2E1 and its allele variants in liver injury of nondiabetic, nonalcoholic steatohepatitis obese women. *Biol. Res.* 41, 8, 2008.
55. Salazar, D.E., Sorge, C.L., and Corcoran, G.B., Obesity as a risk factor for drug-induced organ injury. VI. Increased hepatic P450 concentration and microsomal ethanol oxidizing activity in the obese overfed rat. *Biochem. Biophys. Res. Comm.* 157, 315, 1988.
56. Corcoran, G.B., Salazar, D.E., and Chan, H.H., Obesity as a risk factor in drug-induced organ injury. III. Increased liver and kidney injury by furosemide in the obese overfed rat. *Toxicol. Appl. Pharmacol.* 98, 12, 1989.
57. Corcoran, G.B., Salazar, D.E., and Schentag, J.J., Excessive aminoglycoside toxicity in obese patients. *Am. J. Med.* 85, 279, 1988.

58. Corcoran, G.B. and Salazar, D.E., Obesity as a risk factor for drug-induced organ injury. IV. Increased gentamicin nephrotoxicity in the obese overfed rat. *J. Pharmacol. Exp. Ther.* 248, 17, 1989.

59. Aubert, J., Begriche, K., Knockaert, L., Robin, M.A., Froment, B. et al., Increased expression of cytochrome P450 2E1 in nonalcoholic fatty liver disease: Mechanisms and pathophysiological role. *Clin. Res. Hepatol. Gastroenterol.* doi: 10.1016/, 2011.

60. Salazar, D.E., Sorge, C.L., Jordan, S.W., and Corcoran, G.B., Obesity decreases hepatic glutathione and increases allyl alcohol-induced periportal necrosis in the obese overfed rat. *Intl. J. Obes.* 18, 25, 1994.

61. Buechler, C. and Weiss, T., Does steatosis affect drug metabolizing enzymes in the liver? *Curr. Drug. Metab.* 12, 24, 2011.

19 Genomic Imprinting Disorders in Obesity

Merlin G. Butler, MD, PhD, FFACMG

CONTENTS

INTRODUCTION AND BACKGROUND

Genetic factors are known to contribute to adipogenesis and obesity. These factors may be influenced before birth by genomic imprinting or the differential expression of genetic information depending on the parent of origin. Obesity-related disorders such as Prader–Willi syndrome (PWS) and Albright hereditary osteodystrophy (AHO) (pseudohypoparathyroidism [PHP] and pseudopseudohypoparathyroidism [PPHP]) are examples of errors in genomic imprinting due to epigenetics. Epigenetics refers to heritable but reversible regulation of various genetic functions including gene expression, which may be influenced by environmental factors. The epigenetic status of a gene can be tissue specific and developmentally regulated but essential for normal cellular development and differentiation. It is mediated through DNA modification and histone interactions through mechanisms usually involving methylation but without altering the DNA sequence.

Genomic imprinting is an epigenetic phenomenon that evolved about 150 million years ago where the phenotype of an individual is modified depending on the parent contributing the allele. A very small percentage (about 1%) of mammalian genes are imprinted with the first imprinted gene (H19) reported in 1992 in humans [1]. Many imprinted genes are candidates for human diseases including cancer, obesity, and diabetes. A genome-wide search in humans identified over 150 imprinted genes for at least 100 conditions [2–4].

Methylation of cytosine bases occurs in the CpG dinucleotides of the DNA molecule involving key regulatory elements of genes. Nearly all imprinted genes have a CpG-rich differentially methylated region (DMR), which usually relates to allele repression. Imprinting genes appear to provide the paternal and maternal genomes with the ability to exert opposite effects on the developing embryo, that is, paternal genes lead to overgrowth and maternal genes cause growth suppression. Many imprinted genes are arranged in clusters (imprinted domains) on different chromosomes under control of an imprinting center affecting growth, development, and viability in mammals. Imprinted genes may contribute to behavior and language development, alcohol dependency, schizophrenia, and possibly bipolar affective disorders. In addition, the phenomena of genomic imprinting with abnormal imprinting and loss of heterozygosity contributes to a wide range of malignancies [2–5].

Epigenetic changes (such as methylation) to genes arise during gametogenesis and alters gene expression, dependent on the parent of origin, by producing monoallelic expression of either the maternal or paternal allele of a particular imprinted locus. This process is reversible in gametogenesis by marking a parent-specific genomic sequence. The expression of imprinted genes may also be specific for each tissue and developmental stage. The transcription rate of genes that influence growth can be regulated by the imprinting process through a fine balance between the expressions of the two parental alleles. However, genomic imprints are erased in both germlines and reset accordingly, which leads to differential expression in the course of development. DNA methylation patterns are established and maintained during development by three distinct DNA cytosine methyltransferases (Dnmt1, Dnmt3a, and Dnmt3b). In mammalian somatic cells, cytosine methylation occurs in 60%–80% of all CpG dinucleotides but is not randomly distributed in the genome. Heavily methylated heterochromatin and repetitive sequences appear to contribute to gene silencing, while most CpG islands located at the promoter regions of active genes are methylation free [3,5,6]. Many imprinted genes regulate growth by controlling gene expression such as the insulin-like growth factors (e.g., *IGF2* in Beckwith–Wiedemann syndrome). Paternally expressed genes are thought to enhance growth, while maternally expressed genes appear to suppress growth. Thus, imprinting disorders are due to disruption of DNA methylation within the imprinting controlling regions for a specific class of genes.

Animal studies have shown that mouse embryos containing only diploid paternal or maternal chromosomes have different outcomes. Embryos containing only a paternal genome have reduced fetal growth, and a proliferative extraembryonic (placenta) growth occurs. Embryos containing only a diploid set of maternal chromosomes show relatively normal growth patterns but exhibit poor extraembryonic growth. The process of turning on and off genes, particularly developmental genes, is ongoing throughout the life cycle in mammals influenced by tissue specificity and timing [6,7–9].

Recently, studies in the field of assisted reproductive technology (ART) have shown an influence on genomic imprinting particularly in embryo development or embryogenesis. Manipulating the cellular environment using this technology in *in vitro* processing of gametes could interfere with regulation of expression patterns of imprinted genes thereby producing abnormal outcomes. For example, Williadsen et al. in 1991 [10] reported that when newborn calves are produced by embryo cloning, abnormalities are seen in the growth pattern thereby producing malformations. These alterations are apparently due to the inability to reprogram the somatic nucleus used in the cloning process. Accelerated embryo growth, increased body weight, and birth complications were reported, which related to a large size. The number of perinatal deaths was also reportedly increased [11]. It was proposed that the large size of the offspring was due to disturbed expression of the insulin-like growth factor receptor (Igf2r) gene [12] from gamete manipulation or alterations in early embryo development through inadequate *in vitro* culturing conditions [13–15].

Imprinted genes are also targets for environmental factors that influence expression through the epigenetic process whereby the expression level is altered without changing the DNA nucleotide structure. When a gene is methylated (inactivated), it can be reactivated in either male or female gametogenesis. For example, a maternally imprinted gene (inactivated by methylation) can be unmethylated by male meiosis and transmitted as an active gene in the sperm. Imprinting disturbances reported in genetic disorders are uncommon but include Beckwith–Wiedemann syndrome, Angelman syndrome (AS), and PWS. The incidence of these disorders is thought to be increased in those individuals conceived with the use of ART [16], but more awareness and studies are needed to confirm the association between ART and imprinting disorders and to determine which disorders are at the highest risk by identifying factors involved with the methylation contributing to this process.

Genes are clustered together under the regulation of a single imprinting-controlling element suggesting possible involvement of higher-order regulatory elements showing allelic specific DNA replication. Genes contributed by the mother generally replicate or express at different rates than genes contributed by the father. However, inappropriate methylation may contribute to tumor formation by silencing tumor-suppressing genes or by activating growth-stimulating genes. Understanding the functions of DNA methylation and its regulation in mammalian development will help to elucidate how epigenetic mechanisms play a role in human diseases such as neurobehavioral problems, cancer, and obesity. Classical examples of human disorders due to errors in genomic imprinting, besides PWS and AS (involving chromosome 15) and Beckwith–Wiedemann and Silver–Russell syndromes (involving chromosome 11), are AHO and McCune–Albright syndrome involving the complex *GNAS* gene locus on chromosome 20 and uniparental chromosome 14 disomy (both paternal and maternal forms). Several of these disorders with obesity as a major feature will be discussed in the following.

EXAMPLES OF CLINICAL EPIGENETIC DISORDERS WITH OBESITY

PRADER–WILLI SYNDROME

Genetics

PWS is a complex neurodevelopmental disorder first reported in 1956 [17] that leads to life-threatening obesity if not controlled. PWS is characterized by infantile hypotonia; early onset of childhood obesity; mental deficiency (average IQ of 65); behavioral problems such as temper tantrums, outbursts, and skin picking; short stature with growth hormone deficiency; small hands and feet; hypogenitalism or hypogonadism; an atypical face (e.g., narrow bifrontal diameter, almond-shaped eyes, triangular mouth); oral findings (sticky saliva and enamel hypoplasia); and an interstitial deletion of chromosome 15q11-q13 region in about 70% of the cases [18,19]. PWS is estimated to occur in 1 in 10,000–25,000 live births and is considered to be the most common syndromal cause of marked human obesity. PWS is generally sporadic with the chance of recurrence at less than 1%. This syndrome affects 350,000–400,000 people worldwide and includes all ethnic and racial groups [20,21].

Ledbetter and others reported in 1981 [22] that an interstitial deletion of the proximal long arm of chromosome 15 or the 15q11-q13 region was present in PWS by using high-resolution chromosome analysis. The deletion was found in about 70% of PWS subjects. Later, Butler and Palmer in 1983 [23] reported that the deletion of chromosome 15 was *de novo* in origin, but the chromosome 15 was always donated by the father, which led to the deletion. In 1989, Nicholls, Butler, and others [24] were the first to report maternal disomy 15 (both 15s from the mother) in PWS subjects with normal appearing chromosomes. PWS and AS were the first examples of genomic imprinting in humans.

Maternal disomy 15 is considered the second most frequent genetic finding in PWS and seen in 25% of cases thought due to an error in meiosis with two maternal chromosome 15s in the oocyte and fertilized by a sperm containing one chromosome 15. This leads to a zygote with trisomy 15, which is not compatible with development. Trisomy 15 is a relatively common cause of early miscarriages. Through a trisomy rescue event, one of the two maternal chromosome 15s will be lost from the trisomic cell in two-thirds of the trisomic 15 pregnancies and one-third with loss of the paternal 15 resulting in a normal number of chromosomes. The fetus with loss of the paternal 15 is delivered with PWS and normal cytogenetic findings, but with maternal disomy 15. The remaining PWS subjects (less than 5%) have defects of the imprinting center, which controls the activity of the imprinted genes in the 15q11-q13 region. However, if the father carries an imprinting defect (e.g., microdeletion of the imprint center on his mother's chromosome 15), then the chance of recurrence is 50%.

Maternal disomy 15 in PWS is of two types: heterodisomy and isodisomy. Most PWS subjects with maternal disomy 15 have the heterodisomic form. Maternal heterodisomy occurs when the baby inherits each of the mother's two chromosome 15s. Maternal isodisomy results when two identical chromosome 15s are inherited from the mother as a result of nondisjunction in meiosis II. Segmental heterodisomy may also result from nondisjunction in meiosis I with a crossover event or possibly due to somatic recombination in cells in early embryo development leading to partial isodisomy for only a region of chromosome 15. This may lead to the PWS fetus with maternal isodisomy 15 having a second genetic disorder. For example, if the mother is a carrier of an autosomal recessive gene located on chromosome 15 for a genetic condition, then isodisomy or sharing two identical gene alleles would result in the fetus having PWS due to maternal disomy 15 and the second disorder by inheriting both of the mother's recessive alleles. The risk of maternal disomy 15 appears to increase with maternal age [25–27].

Butler et al. [27] reported gestational age data in PWS pregnancies grouped by genetic subtypes and found that postterm deliveries (>42 weeks gestation) were more common in the maternal disomy group compared to the chromosome 15q deletion group, suggesting that delivery date may be impacted by placental structure or function. This could be secondary to the abnormal chromosomal number in the placental cells or in mechanisms leading to the maternal disomy status. Although there are no recognized growth factor genes in the proximal long arm of chromosome 15 that are known to affect placental growth or other imprinted genes on chromosome 15, disturbances of growth factors influenced by maternal disomy 15 may contribute to abnormalities of placental growth or function in PWS leading to abnormal pregnancy outcomes.

One could speculate that differences in gestational age in PWS subjects with maternal disomy 15 compared with those PWS subjects with the 15q11-q13 deletion could be triggered by maternal disomy 15 and/or trisomy 15 rescue events in early pregnancy on placenta and fetal growth. To further investigate the trisomy rescue event and timing in abnormal cells from early pregnancy in PWS, the X chromosome inactivation ratio can be calculated using the polymorphic androgen receptor (*AR*) gene located at Xq11.2 to access X inactivation patterns in those females informative for the polymorphic CAG repeat site following DNA digestion with methyl-sensitive restriction enzymes (e.g., *HpaII*) and PCR amplification. X chromosome skewness (i.e., one X chromosome may be more or less active compared with the second X chromosome in somatic cells) is assigned at an arbitrary ratio of highly skewed (e.g., >80%:20%) and is considered to be an uncommon event [28,29]. The inactivation of the X chromosome in females is generally considered random with regard to which X is inactivated to allow for equal gene dosage for X-linked genes in normal females and males. In certain cases, the X chromosome inactivation skewness is no longer random but is skewed. X chromosome skewness occurs in X-autosomal chromosome rearrangements, mutations of the gene controlling the X inactivation process (i.e., *XIST*), or in certain X-linked disorders (e.g., Rett syndrome).

Butler et al. [29] reported on a relatively large group of PWS females having either the 15q11-q13 deletion or maternal disomy 15 and compared findings with female controls using the *AR* gene assay system in peripheral blood and found significantly larger numbers of PWS females with maternal disomy with extreme X chromosome skewness (95%:5%) compared with PWS deletion or control females. These results indicated that if a trisomy rescue event occurred in early embryo development and a small number of cells survived, then a selective advantage for cell proliferation occurs, leading to extreme X chromosome skewness in the PWS female with maternal disomy 15. Because of extreme X chromosome skewness, these PWS females could be at risk for X-linked recessive gene disorders carried by the mother if the X-linked gene mutation is present on the skewed active X chromosome.

PWS is also thought to be a contiguous gene syndrome with several imprinted (paternally expressed) genes in the 15q11-q13 region [30,31]. This region contains between 7 and 8 million DNA base pairs including a large cluster of imprinted genes but also a nonimprinted domain. Novel DNA sequences with low copy repeats are clustered at or near the two major proximal chromosome breakpoints (breakpoint 1 [BP1] and breakpoint 2 [BP2]) and the distal breakpoint (BP3) in the 15q11-q13 region. The typical PWS deletion consists of two classes, type I (TI) and type II (TII). The larger TI deletion involves BP1 nearest the centromere, while the smaller TII deletion involves BP2. BP3 is located distally in the 15q11-q13 region and is common to both typical deletion subgroups (see Figure 19.1). Using high-resolution array comparative genomic hybridization (aCGH) in PWS subjects, Butler et al. [32] reported that TI deletions ranged in size from 5.7 to 8.1 Mb (mean 6.6) and the TII deletion from 4 to 6.4 Mb (mean 5.3). Four genes are recognized between BP1 and BP2 (i.e., *GCP5*, *CYFIP1*, *NIPA1*, and *NIPA2*), and patients have been reported recently with behavioral problems and autistic features with a deletion involving only BP1 and BP2 [33]. PWS subjects with the larger typical TI deletion (involving BP1 and BP3) have more clinical problems such as obsessive-compulsive disorders, self-injury, and poorer academic performance as discussed later than those PWS subjects with the

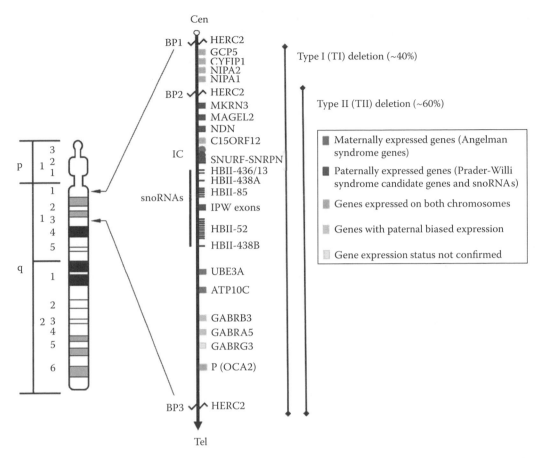

FIGURE 19.1 High-resolution chromosome 15 ideogram, location, and order of genes in the 15q11-q13 region and patterns of expression. Gene order according to the UCSC Genome Bioinformatics site: http://genome.ucsc.edu (Adapted from Bittel, D.C. and Butler, M.G., *Expert. Rev. Mol. Med.,* 7(14), 1, 2005. Reproduced with permission.)

smaller TII deletions (involving BP2 and BP3) [34]. Atypical deletions that are greater or smaller than the typical TI or TII deletion have been reported and generally occur in about 5% of PWS subjects.

There are fewer than 100 genes/transcripts in the 15q11-q13 region with about 10 imprinted genes that are paternally expressed. Methylation DNA testing that measures the methylation status of genes in the region can be used for laboratory diagnosis and is considered to be 99% accurate for the diagnosis of PWS but will not identify the specific genetic subtype (deletion, maternal disomy, or an imprinting defect). Additional testing is needed such as fluorescence *in situ* hybridization (FISH), genotyping with informative DNA markers from the 15q11-q13 region, DNA sequencing, or chromosomal microarray studies to identify the specific genetic subtypes.

The *SNRPN* (small nuclear ribonucleoprotein N), and a second protein coding sequence (*SNURF*, or *SNRPN* upstream reading frame), as well as multiple copies of C/D box small nucleolar RNAs (snoRNAs) or *SNORDs* are involved in RNA processing. Other genes in the region include *MKRN3, MAGEL2, NDN,* and *C15orf2* (located from centromere to telomere) involved in brain development and function. Exons 4–10 of the complex bicistronic *SNURF–SNRPN* gene encode a core spliceosomal protein (SmN) involved in mRNA splicing in the brain, whereas exons 1–3 encode a 71-amino-acid protein enriched in arginine residues. A disruption of this complex locus will cause loss of function of paternally expressed genes in this region, leading to PWS [30,31].

Necdin (*NDN*) is a paternally expressed gene shown to be essential for axonal outgrowth and is expressed in specific brain structures (hypothalamus, thalamus, and pons) suggesting a developmental role. Mice deficient for necdin show delayed migration of the sympathetic neurons, neonatal lethality, and respiratory problems [35]. The *MAGEL2* gene is paternally expressed in various brain regions (e.g., hypothalamus) and appears to play an important role in circadian rhythm, brain structure, behavior, and maintenance of fertility in humans [36]. The *MKRN3* gene or *ZNF127* is a member of the makorin (MKRN) RING finger protein gene family encoding proteins (makorins) and present in a wide variety of eukaryotes. The *MKRN3* is encoded in the complex imprinted area of chromosome 15q11-q13 region and is abundantly expressed in the developing brain and nervous system [37].

Two additional novel genes (*PWRN1* and *PWRN2*) are located between *NDN* and *C15orf2* in the 15q11-q13 region. *PWRN1* is a novel alternative start site for *SNURF–SNRPN* while *PWRN2* is a male germ cell–specific gene expressed from the haploid genome. Encoded within the *SNURF–SNRPN* transcript are multiple C/D box snoRNAs including single copy snoRNA genes (*SNORD64, SNORD107, SNORD108, SNORD109A,* and *SNORD109B* previously referred to as HBII-13, HBII-436, HBII-437, HBII-438A, and HBII-438B, respectively). Deletions of snoRNAs have also been implicated in causing a PWS phenotype [38,39], specifically *SNORD115* and *SNORD116*.

Two imprinted but maternally expressed genes that are paternally silenced (*UBE3A, ATP10C*) are also present in this chromosome region. The *UBE3A* gene causes AS. Other genes located in the distal area of the 15q11-q13 region include several gamma-aminobutyric acid (GABA) receptor subunits called *GABRB3, GABRA5,* and *GABRG3,* which are paternally biased. Loss of the paternal allele for these genes results in reduction in expression of greater than 50% [40]. The disturbances of receptor subunit genes for GABA, a major inhibitory neurotransmitter, have been implicated in a number of symptoms associated with PWS including hunger, obsessive-compulsive disorder, and altered visual perception and memory. The *P* gene for pigment production is also located in this chromosome region and mutations are known to cause oculocutaneous albinism II. The *P* gene is not imprinted and is expressed equally from both alleles.

The three breakpoint sites (BP1, BP2, BP3) located at the ends of the 15q11-q13 region contains copies of a large transcribed gene (*HERC2*). *HERC2* repeated sequences have been implicated in unequal crossing over in meiosis and may participate in the development of the typical 15q11-q13 and the two deletion subtypes (TI and TII) seen in both PWS and AS subjects. Although the typical deletion involving BP1 or BP2 and BP3 is seen in the majority of PWS or AS subjects, atypical larger or smaller deletions have been reported. For example, Butler et al. [41] reported a 5 year old white female with a PWS phenotype and a submicroscopic deletion of the 15q11-q13 region approximately 100–200 kb in size. High-resolution chromosome analysis was normal but molecular genetic testing showed a *de novo* paternal deletion of *SNRPN* gene. Recent unpublished data from this subject indicate that the snoRNA *SNORD116* was deleted. She did not present at 5 years of age with behavioral problems, hyperphagia, or hypopigmentation, which are characteristics of PWS, but presented with the other classical features of this disorder.

Kanber et al. [42] also reported a female subject with an atypical deletion involving the chromosome 15q11-q13 region due to an unbalanced translocation involving only a deletion of the *MKRN3, MAGEL2,* and *NDN* genes. She presented with obesity, mental retardation, and a high-pain threshold, but lacked other features of PWS. They concluded that a paternal deficiency of *MKRN3, MAGEL2,* and *NDN* in this rare patient was not sufficient to cause the complete phenotype of PWS.

Recently, Sahoo et al. [39] described a male child with several features of PWS, such as neonatal hypotonia, feeding problems, obesity, and hypogenitalism. In addition, he had atypical features including a high birth weight (macrosomia), macrocephaly, lack of mental retardation, and an atypical face. A paternal deletion was present in the snoRNAs *SNORD109A,* the *SNORD116* gene cluster, and half of the *SNORD115* cluster. Smith et al. [43] also reported a 19 year old male with hyperphagia and severe obesity, mild learning difficulties, and hypogonadism along with a 187 kb microdeletion of chromosome 15q11-q13 encompassing the noncoding small nucleolar RNAs (i.e., *SNORD116*). Therefore, paternal loss of *SNORD116* may contribute to energy homeostasis, poor growth, and reproduction, all abnormal findings seen in PWS.

Larger than anticipated deletions have also been reported involving the proximal long arm of chromosome 15 in individuals with features of PWS. The most recent report was by Butler et al. [44] in an infant girl with a *de novo* interstitial deletion of the chromosome 15q11-q14 region, larger than the typical deletion seen in PWS. She presented with hypotonia, poor suck, feeding problems, mild micrognathia, preauricular ear tags, a high-arched palate, edematous feet, and coarctation of the aorta; several of these features are not typical for PWS. G-banded chromosome analysis showed a large *de novo* deletion of the proximal long arm of chromosome 15, and methylation testing was consistent for PWS. Because of the large appearing deletion by karyotype analysis, an array comparative genomic hybridization (CGH) was performed and a 12.3 Mb deletion was found involving the 15q11-q14 region with approximately 60 protein coding genes. This rare deletion was approximately twice the size of the typical deletion seen in PWS and involved the typical proximal breakpoint BP1, but the distal breakpoint was located in the 15q14 band between previously recognized breakpoints BP5 and BP6. The deletion extended slightly more distal to the *AVEN* gene and included the neighboring *CHRM5* gene.

The recent clinical reports of very small atypical deletions appear to contribute to several PWS features and involve the paternally expressed snoRNAs (e.g., *SNORD115* and *SNORD116*). In mice, the snoRNA equivalent of *SNORD116* causes hyperphagia and growth deficiency. Furthermore, Kishore and Stamm [45] also reported that the paternally expressed snoRNA *SNORD115* regulates alternative splicing of the serotonin 5-HT$_{2C}$ receptor. If *SNORD115* is not present or functional on chromosome 15, then an alternative form of the serotonin receptor is produced with altered and reduced function. This serotonin receptor is involved with behavior influencing eating patterns. Thus, PWS is not caused by a single locus defect but by a deficiency of several genes in the region that include *SNURF–SNRPN* and the *SNORD* genes. Deficiencies of *MKRN3*, *MAGEL2*, and/or *NDN* are necessary, although not sufficient, to generate the full PWS phenotype. In addition, loss of function of paternally expressed genes in the 15q11-q13 region may affect activity of other genes. Among these genes is *SGNE1* that encodes the secretory granule neuroendocrine protein-1 or pituitary polypeptide 7B2, a specific chaperone for proprotein convertase-2 (PC2) found in neuroendocrine cells. This gene is located in the 15q13-q14 region.

Clinical Presentation

PWS is a complex genomic imprinting disorder characterized by mental, behavioral, and physical findings. Obesity is the most significant health problem and PWS is considered the most common syndromic cause of life-threatening obesity in humans [18]. Neuroendocrine peptides produced by the gastrointestinal system including ghrelin (stimulates eating) and peptide YY (inhibits eating) are involved with regulating eating that can lead to obesity in PWS. Plasma ghrelin levels are elevated in PWS, which significantly contributes to the hyperphagia, a cardinal feature in PWS.

PWS is generally divided into two major stages of clinical course development. The first stage is characterized by infantile hypotonia, temperature instability, a weak cry and poor suck, feeding difficulties, developmental delay, and hypogonadism or hypogenitalism. The second stage occurs in early childhood (2–5 years of age) and is characterized by an insatiable appetite, food seeking, rapid weight gain and subsequent obesity if diet is not controlled, short stature and growth hormone deficiency, continued developmental delay, speech articulation problems, rumination, unmotivated sleepiness, physical inactivity, decreased pain sensitivity, self-injurious behavior particularly skin picking, small hands and feet, strabismus, hypopigmentation, scoliosis, sleep apnea, enamel hypoplasia, and decreased saliva. Minor facial anomalies include almond-shaped palpebral fissures, downturned corners of the mouth, narrow bifrontal diameter, a short nose and a small chin, and lighter hair, eye, and skin color (hypopigmentation) (see Figure 19.2).

Weight control through dietary restrictions and increased physical activity are key management issues. Caloric intake is restricted to 6–8 cal/cm of height for weight loss beginning in early childhood and to 10–12 cal/cm of height to maintain weight for nongrowth-hormone-treated

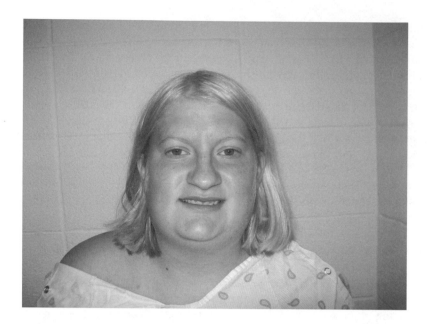

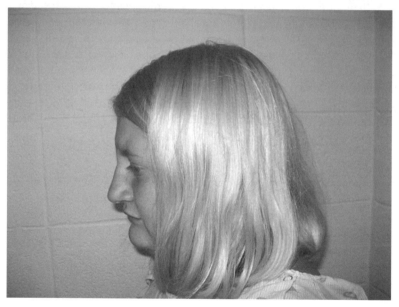

FIGURE 19.2 Frontal and profile views of the face of an 18 year old female with Prader–Willi syndrome. She has the typical 15q11-q13 TII deletion and shows common features seen in this disorder including a round face, bifrontal narrowing, almond-shaped eyes, hypopigmentation, sticky salivary secretions, small hands and feet, short stature, and obesity. Her height was 150 cm (2nd centile), weight was 98.4 kg (97th centile), head circumference was 53.2 cm (25th centile), and a shoe size of 5. She had mild learning problems, skin picking, food seeking, and hoarding. She had mild hypotonia and mild to moderate scoliosis.

PWS subjects during childhood. For PWS adolescents or adults, a general recommendation for dietary intake would be approximately 800 cal/day to lose weight or 1000–1200 cal/day to maintain weight if food seeking is closely monitored and controlled. This caloric intake is about 60% of normal. A diet plan with restricted caloric intake may include calories from protein at 25%, 50% for carbohydrates, and 25% for fat. Calcium and vitamin supplements to avoid osteoporosis are also recommended [21]. Human recombinant growth hormone therapy in PWS is currently used during infancy, which results in decreased fat levels, an increase in muscle mass, and increased physical activity and metabolism leading to a higher quality of life [21].

Clinical Findings Associated with Typical Type I versus Type II Deletions in PWS

Butler et al. [34] reported differences in psychological, cognitive, and behavioral test results in young adults with PWS with the longer TI deletion involving breakpoints BP1 and BP3 versus those with shorter TII deletions involving BP1 and BP3. PWS individuals with the longer TI deletions scored significantly worse in self-injurious and maladaptive behavior assessments compared with PWS subjects with the smaller TII deletions. Obsessive-compulsive behavior was also more common in PWS subjects with TI deletions.

Several academic achievement scores differed between those with shorter or longer typical deletions, supporting that loss of genetic material between BP1 and BP2 increases the severity of behavioral and psychological problems in PWS. Adaptive behavior scores were generally worse in individuals with PWS and the TI deletion, specifically obsessive-compulsive behaviors. PWS subjects with TI deletions also had poorer reading and math skills as well as visual-motor integration, poorer adaptive behavior, and more compulsions than subjects with TII deletions, particularly relating to grooming and bathing and compulsions more disruptive to daily living. Intellectual ability and academic achievement were poorer in subjects with TI deletions. Visual processing was also noted to be poor in subjects with TI deletions compared with TII deletions.

Other differences relate to more severely delayed speech development in TI deletions and significantly more seizures in those PWS subjects with typical deletions versus those with maternal disomy 15. More recently, reports of nine cases with microdeletions between BP1 and BP2 involving nonimprinted *GCP5, CYFIP1, NIPA2,* and *NIPA1* genes have shown behavioral problems including autism. Bittel et al. [46] also showed that the expression of these four genes can account for behavior and intellectual ability differences in those with TI or TII deletions; specifically, three of these genes are implicated in central nervous system development and/or function. For example, *NIPA1* is associated with spastic paraplegia, and the related *NIPA2*, which has recently been identified as a magnesium transporter gene, is widely expressed in the central nervous system. The *CYFIP1* gene codes for a protein that is present in synaptosomal extracts and interacts with FMRP, the protein product of the *FMR1* gene, which is responsible for fragile X syndrome. *GCP5* is a member of the cytoskeleton tubulin complex in cells. Although all four of the genes examined may contribute, *NIPA2* seemed to have the greatest impact with a large number of phenotypic parameters noted with significant correlations with *NIPA2* gene expression levels in lymphoblasts. Understanding the influence of gene expression on behavioral and cognitive characteristics in humans is in the early stage of research development and additional studies are needed.

ALBRIGHT HEREDITARY OSTEODYSTROPHY (PSEUDOHYPOPARATHYROIDISM AND PSEUDOPSEUDOHYPOPARATHYROIDISM)

AHO was first reported in 1942 [47] and is due to an end-organ resistance to parathyroid hormone (PTH) and other hormones. Obesity is a major manifestation. In addition to obesity, other clinical features of AHO consist of small stature, mild mental deficiency with an average IQ of 60, a round face with a short nose, a short neck, delayed dental eruption and enamel hypoplasia, short metacarpals and metatarsals especially of the fourth and fifth digits, and short distal phalanges of the thumb. Other features seen in this disorder include osteoporosis; areas of subcutaneous mineralization with calcium deposits including the basal ganglia, along with variable low plasma calcium levels and/or high phosphate levels; and seizures. Occasionally, hypothyroidism, hypogonadism, lens opacity or cataracts, optic atrophy, ocular degeneration, and vertebral anomalies are seen [48,49].

There are two major clinical variants referred to as PHP (PHP-Ia or PHP-Ib) and PPHP depending on the presence or absence of additional hormone resistance, the presence of the AHO phenotype, and the pattern of inheritance. Individuals with PHP-Ia have features of AHO, hypocalcemia, hyperphosphatemia, mild hypothyroidism, and hypogonadism and respond abnormally to growth hormone releasing hormone. They also have elevated serum parathyroid hormone levels. Individuals with PPHP have the characteristic features of AHO but without identified resistance to parathyroid or other hormones. PHP-Ia and PPHP have been reported in the same families but are dependent on the parent of origin indicating genomic imprinting. Both disease variants result from decreased activity of the alpha subunit of the membrane-bound trimeric G subunit-regulatory signaling protein (GNAS). GNAS is involved in several complex cellular pathways and mechanisms. Individuals with PHP who present with PTH resistance but lack AHO features including obesity are defined as having the PHP-Ib subtype. Most PHP-Ib cases are sporadic and typically lack GNAS gene mutations. Individuals with PHP-Ia and features of AHO also have mutations of the *GNAS* gene or cytogenetic deletions of chromosome 20q including *GNAS*. Those with PPHP (or those AHO patients without evidence of hormone resistance) also carry heterozygous inactivating *GNAS* gene mutations. Maternal inheritance of a mutation can lead to PHP-Ia (AHO with hormone resistance), while paternal inheritance of the same mutation leads to PPHP or AHO alone. PHP-Ia and PPHP are caused by heterozygous inactivating mutations in exons of the *GNAS* gene producing Gs-alpha, and the autosomal dominant form of PHP-Ib is caused by heterozygous mutations disrupting the long-range imprinting control element of *GNAS*. When the altered gene is inherited from the affected father with either PHP-Ia or PPHP, PPHP occurs in the offspring. If the same *GNAS* mutation is present in the mother affected with either PHP-Ia or PPHP, then the offspring will be affected with PHP-Ia [50,51].

GNAS is a complete imprinted locus on chromosome 20q13.11. Multiple transcripts are produced through the use of alternative promoters and splice sites. When altered, these transcripts can lead to several disorders. The best characterized *GNAS* transcript encodes the stimulatory guanine nucleotide-binding protein (G protein) subunit alpha (Gs-alpha). Gs-alpha is biallelically expressed in most tissues but expressed on one allele (maternal) in the gonads, pituitary and thyroid glands, and the proximal renal tubules. Other *GNAS* transcripts are expressed exclusively from either the paternal or the maternal *GNAS* allele.

The *GNAS* locus encodes four main transcripts. These are Gs-alpha, *XLAS, NESP55,* and the A/B transcript, as well as an antisense transcript (*GNASAS*). Gs-alpha is expressed ubiquitously and encodes a protein that stimulates adenyl cyclase when coupled with a membrane receptor that generates the second messenger cyclic AMP (cAMP). Many hormones and neurotransmitters exert their actions through receptors coupled to Gs-alpha. Gs-alpha is involved in AHO, *XLAS* is paternally expressed, *NESP55* is maternally expressed and encodes a chromogranin-like neuroendocrine secretory protein, while the A/B transcript is derived from the paternal *GNAS* allele, all involved in cellular processes and, when disturbed, can lead to disease [50,51].

UNIPARENTAL DISOMY 14

Human chromosome uniparental disomy 14 (UPD14) was described in 1991 and different clinical phenotypes are now recognized depending on either paternal or maternal disomy chromosome 14, that is, both chromosome 14s from the father or from the mother [52,53]. The human chromosome 14q32.2 band is in the distal region of the long arm of chromosome 14 and carries a cluster of imprinted genes including paternally expressed genes (PEGs) and maternally expressed genes (MEGs) that encompass the DMRs. The germline-derived primary *DLK1-MEG3* intergenic differentially methylated region (*IG-DMR*) and the postfertilization-derived secondary *MEG3-DMR* along with multiple imprinted genes are located in this region. The MEGs *GTL2,* gene trap locus 2; *DIO3;* and *RTL1* and a large micro-RNA cluster, as well as PEGs *DLK1, RTL1as,* and *MEG8,* are also present [54,55].

Individuals with maternal disomy 14, either through a nondisjunction event in meiosis with a normal karyotype or due to chromosome 14 translocations, have features in common with PWS, specifically obesity. Maternal disomy 14 is characterized by postnatal growth retardation, hypotonia, joint laxity, gross motor delay with mild intellectual disability, early onset of puberty, truncal obesity, small hands and feet, minor dysmorphic facial features, and occasionally hydrocephaly. The facial features include a prominent forehead and supraorbital ridges, a short philtrum, and downturned corners of the mouth. Over 30 cases have been reported [56,57].

Mitter et al. [57] reported on a cohort of 33 subjects with low birth weight, feeding difficulties, and obesity in which PWS was excluded by methylation analysis. Four (12%) of their subjects were found to have maternal disomy 14. Therefore, they recommended testing for maternal disomy 14 in those individuals with normal testing for PWS but having low birth weight, growth retardation, neonatal feeding problems, hypotonia, motor delay, precocious puberty, and truncal obesity. Additionally, Hosoki et al. [58] examined 78 subjects with a PWS-like phenotype who lacked molecular defects for PWS and performed a *MEG3* gene methylation test to detect maternal disomy 14 or other abnormalities affecting the 14q32.2-imprinted region. They identified four subjects with maternal disomy 14 and one subject with an epimutation in the 14q32.2 imprinted region. Of the four subjects with maternal disomy 14, three had complete maternal disomy 14 and one had mosaicism. They concluded that the *MEG3* gene methylation test should be performed for all undiagnosed infants with hypotonia.

Paternal disomy 14 is a more severe condition than maternal disomy 14 [59]. It is characterized by polyhydramnios, placental anomalies, thoracic deformities and rib anomalies, abdominal wall defects, growth retardation, and severe developmental delay. Irving et al. [60] reported segmental paternal disomy of 14q32-14q32.33 region and found abnormal methylation of a 3.5 Mb area in the distal 14q chromosome region involving the imprinting cluster controlling the maternally expressed *GTL2* gene promoter and the DMR between the *GTL2* and *DLK1* genes.

In summary, an imprinted locus existing at 14q32 appears to be under the control of a paternally methylated region. Imprinted genes in this region include the paternally expressed *DLK1* (delta, Drosophila homologue-like 1). This gene encodes a transmembrane signaling protein that is a growth regulator homologous to proteins in the Notch/delta pathway. The data suggest for *DLK1-GTL2* that IG-DMR functions as a regulator for the maternally inherited imprinted region and excessive *RTL1* expression, while decreased *DLK1* and *RTL1* expressions play a major role in the development of paternal disomy 14–like and maternal disomy 14–like phenotypes, respectively [61,62].

REFERENCES

1. Zhang, Y. and B. Tycko. 1992. Monoallelic expression of the human H19 gene. *Nat Genet* 1 (1):40–44.
2. Zakharova, I. S., A. I. Shevchenko, and S. M. Zakian. 2009. Monoallelic gene expression in mammals. *Chromosoma* 118 (3):279–290.
3. Murphy, S. K. and R. L. Jirtle. 2003. Imprinting evolution and the price of silence. *Bioessays* 25 (6):577–588.
4. Butler, M. G. 2009. Genomic imprinting disorders in humans: A mini-review. *J Assist Reprod Genet* 26 (9–10):477–486.
5. Delaval, K., A. Wagschal, and R. Feil. 2006. Epigenetic deregulation of imprinting in congenital diseases of aberrant growth. *Bioessays* 28 (5):453–459.
6. Cattanach, B. M., C. V. Beechey, and J. Peters. 2006. Interactions between imprinting effects: Summary and review. *Cytogenet Genome Res* 113 (1–4):17–23.
7. Cattanach, B. M. and M. Kirk. 1985. Differential activity of maternally and paternally derived chromosome regions in mice. *Nature* 315 (6019):496–498.
8. Barton, S. C., M. A. Surani, and M. L. Norris. 1984. Role of paternal and maternal genomes in mouse development. *Nature* 311 (5984):374–376.
9. McGrath, J. and D. Solter. 1984. Inability of mouse blastomere nuclei transferred to enucleated zygotes to support development in vitro. *Science* 226 (4680):1317–1319.
10. Willadsen, S. M., R. E. Janzen, and R. J. McAlistre. 1991. The viability of late morulae and blastocysts produced by nuclear transplantation in cattle. *Theriogenol* 35:161–170.
11. Walker, S. K., K. M. Hartwich, and R. F. Seamark. 1996. The production of unusually large offspring following embryo manipulation: Concepts and challenges. *Theriogenol* 45:111–120.

12. Young, L. E., K. Fernandes, T. G. McEvoy et al. 2001. Epigenetic change in IGF2R is associated with fetal overgrowth after sheep embryo culture. *Nat Genet* 27 (2):153–154.

13. Doherty, A. S., M. R. Mann, K. D. Tremblay et al. 2000. Differential effects of culture on imprinted H19 expression in the preimplantation mouse embryo. *Biol Reprod* 62 (6):1526–1535.

14. DeBaun, M. R., E. L. Niemitz, and A. P. Feinberg. 2003. Association of in vitro fertilization with Beckwith-Wiedemann syndrome and epigenetic alterations of LIT1 and H19. *Am J Hum Genet* 72 (1):156–160.

15. Maher, E. R., L. A. Brueton, S. C. Bowdin et al. 2003. Beckwith-Wiedemann syndrome and assisted reproduction technology (ART). *J Med Genet* 40 (1):62–64.

16. Niemitz, E. L. and A. P. Feinberg. 2004. Epigenetics and assisted reproductive technology: A call for investigation. *Am J Hum Genet* 74 (4):599–609.

17. Prader, A., A. Labhart, and H. Willi. 1956. Ein syndrome von adipositas, kleinwuchs, kryptorchismus and oligophrenie nach myatonieartigem zustand im neugeborenenalter. *Schweizerische Medzinische Wochenschrift* 86:1260–1261.

18. Butler, M. G. 1990. Prader-Willi syndrome: Current understanding of cause and diagnosis. *Am J Med Genet* 35 (3):319–332.

19. Cassidy, S. B. and D. J. Driscoll. 2009. Prader-Willi syndrome. *Eur J Hum Genet* 17 (1):3–13.

20. Butler, M. G. and T. Thompson. 2000. Prader-Willi syndrome: Clinical and genetic finding. *The Endocrinol* 10:3S-16S.

21. Butler, M. G., P. D. K. Lee, and B. Y. Whitman. 2006. *Management of Prader-Willi Syndrome*. 3rd edn. New York: Springer-Verlag Publishers.

22. Ledbetter, D. H., V. M. Riccardi, S. D. Airhart et al. 1981. Deletions of chromosome 15 as a cause of the Prader-Willi syndrome. *N Engl J Med* 304 (6):325–329.

23. Butler, M. G. and C. G. Palmer. 1983. Parental origin of chromosome 15 deletion in Prader-Willi syndrome. *Lancet* 1 (8336):1285–1286.

24. Nicholls, R. D., J. H. Knoll, M. G. Butler et al. 1989. Genetic imprinting suggested by maternal heterodisomy in nondeletion Prader-Willi syndrome. *Nature* 342 (6247):281–285.

25. Cassidy, S. B., L. W. Lai, R. P. Erickson et al. 1992. Trisomy 15 with loss of the paternal 15 as a cause of Prader-Willi syndrome due to maternal disomy. *Am J Hum Genet* 51 (4):701–708.

26. Christian, S. L., A. C. Smith, M. Macha et al. 1996. Prenatal diagnosis of uniparental disomy 15 following trisomy 15 mosaicism. *Prenat Diagn* 16 (4):323–332.

27. Butler, M. G., J. Sturich, S. E. Myers et al. 2009. Is gestation in Prader-Willi syndrome affected by the genetic subtype? *J Assist Reprod Genet* 26 (8):461–466.

28. Lau, A. W., C. J. Brown, M. Penaherrera et al. 1997. Skewed X-chromosome inactivation is common in fetuses or newborns associated with confined placental mosaicism. *Am J Hum Genet* 61 (6):1353–1361.

29. Butler, M. G., M. F. Theodoro, D. C. Bittel et al. 2007. X-chromosome inactivation patterns in females with Prader-Willi syndrome. *Am J Med Genet A* 143 (5):469–475.

30. Nicholls, R. D. and J. L. Knepper. 2001. Genome organization, function, and imprinting in Prader-Willi and Angelman syndromes. *Annu Rev Genomics Hum Genet* 2:153–175.

31. Bittel, D. C. and M. G. Butler. 2005. Prader-Willi syndrome: Clinical genetics, cytogenetics and molecular biology. *Expert Rev Mol Med* 7 (14):1–20.

32. Butler, M. G., W. Fischer, N. Kibiryeva, and D. C. Bittel. 2008. Array comparative genomic hybridization (aCGH) analysis in Prader-Willi syndrome. *Am J Med Genet A* 146 (7):854–860.

33. Burnside, R. D., R. Pasion, F. M. Mikhail et al. 2011. Microdeletion/microduplication of proximal 15q11.2 between BP1 and BP2: A susceptibility region for neurological dysfunction including developmental and language delay. *Hum Genet* 130 (4):517–528.

34. Butler, M. G., D. C. Bittel, N. Kibiryeva et al. 2004. Behavioral differences among subjects with Prader-Willi syndrome and type I or type II deletion and maternal disomy. *Pediatrics* 113 (3 Pt 1):565–573.

35. Miller, N. L., R. Wevrick, and P. L. Mellon. 2009. Necdin, a Prader-Willi syndrome candidate gene, regulates gonadotropin-releasing hormone neurons during development. *Hum Mol Genet* 18 (2):248–260.

36. Kozlov, S. V., J. W. Bogenpohl, M. P. Howell et al. 2007. The imprinted gene Magel2 regulates normal circadian output. *Nat Genet* 39 (10):1266–1272.

37. Gray, T. A., L. Hernandez, A. H. Carey et al. 2000. The ancient source of a distinct gene family encoding proteins featuring RING and C(3)H zinc-finger motifs with abundant expression in developing brain and nervous system. *Genomics* 66 (1):76–86.

38. Ding, F., H. H. Li, S. Zhang et al. 2008. SnoRNA Snord116 (Pwcr1/MBII-85) deletion causes growth deficiency and hyperphagia in mice. *PLoS One* 3 (3):e1709.

39. Sahoo, T., D. del Gaudio, J. R. German et al. 2008. Prader-Willi phenotype caused by paternal deficiency for the HBII-85 C/D box small nucleolar RNA cluster. *Nat Genet* 40 (6):719–721.

40. Bittel, D. C., N. Kibiryeva, Z. Talebizadeh, and M. G. Butler. 2003. Microarray analysis of gene/transcript expression in Prader-Willi syndrome: Deletion versus UPD. *J Med Genet* 40 (8):568–574.

41. Butler, M. G., S. L. Christian, T. Kubota, and D. H. Ledbetter. 1996. A 5-year-old white girl with Prader-Willi syndrome and a submicroscopic deletion of chromosome 15q11q13. *Am J Med Genet* 65 (2):137–141.

42. Kanber, D., J. Giltay, D. Wieczorek et al. 2009. A paternal deletion of MKRN3, MAGEL2 and NDN does not result in Prader-Willi syndrome. *Eur J Hum Genet* 17 (5):582–590.

43. de Smith, A. J., C. Purmann, R. G. Walters et al. 2009. A deletion of the HBII-85 class of small nucleolar RNAs (snoRNAs) is associated with hyperphagia, obesity and hypogonadism. *Hum Mol Genet* 18 (17):3257–3265.

44. Butler, M. G., D. C. Bittel, N. Kibiryeva, L. D. Cooley, and S. Yu. 2010. An interstitial 15q11-q14 deletion: Expanded Prader-Willi syndrome phenotype. *Am J Med Genet A* 152A (2):404–408.

45. Kishore, S. and S. Stamm. 2006. The snoRNA HBII-52 regulates alternative splicing of the serotonin receptor 2C. *Science* 311 (5758):230–232.

46. Bittel, D. C., N. Kibiryeva, and M. G. Butler. 2006. Expression of 4 genes between chromosome 15 breakpoints 1 and 2 and behavioral outcomes in Prader-Willi syndrome. *Pediatrics* 118 (4):e1276–e1283.

47. Albright, F., C. H. Burnett, P. H. Smith, and W. Parson. 1942. Pseudo-hypoparathyroidism—an example "Seabright-Bantam syndrome": Report of three cases. *Endocrinology* 30:922–932.

48. Levine, M. A. 2000. Clinical spectrum and pathogenesis of pseudohypoparathyroidism. *Rev Endocr Metab Disord* 1 (4):265–274.

49. Jones, K. L. 1997. *Smith's Recognizable Patterns of Human Malformation*, 5th edn. Philadelphia, PA: W.B. Saunders Company.

50. Bastepe, M. 2008. The GNAS locus and pseudohypoparathyroidism. *Adv Exp Med Biol* 626:27–40.

51. GNAS complex locus. 2010. Available from www.ncbl/nlm.nih.gov/OMIM (accessed on September 29, 2010).

52. Wang, J. C., M. B. Passage, P. H. Yen, L. J. Shapiro, and T. K. Mohandas. 1991. Uniparental heterodisomy for chromosome 14 in a phenotypically abnormal familial balanced 13/14 Robertsonian translocation carrier. *Am J Hum Genet* 48 (6):1069–1074.

53. Temple, I. K., A. Cockwell, T. Hassold, D. Pettay, and P. Jacobs. 1991. Maternal uniparental disomy for chromosome 14. *J Med Genet* 28 (8):511–514.

54. Ogata, T., M. Kagami, and A. C. Ferguson-Smith. 2008. Molecular mechanisms regulating phenotypic outcome in paternal and maternal uniparental disomy for chromosome 14. *Epigenetics* 3 (4):181–187.

55. Kagami, M., M. J. O'Sullivan, A. J. Green et al. 2010. The IG-DMR and the MEG3-DMR at human chromosome 14q32.2: Hierarchical interaction and distinct functional properties as imprinting control centers. *PLoS Genet* 6 (6):e1000992.

56. Berends, M. J., R. Hordijk, H. Scheffer, J. C. Oosterwijk, D. J. Halley, and N. Sorgedrager. 1999. Two cases of maternal uniparental disomy 14 with a phenotype overlapping with the Prader-Willi phenotype. *Am J Med Genet* 84 (1):76–79.

57. Mitter, D., K. Buiting, F. von Eggeling et al. 2006. Is there a higher incidence of maternal uniparental disomy 14 [upd(14)mat]? Detection of 10 new patients by methylation-specific PCR. *Am J Med Genet A* 140 (19):2039–2049.

58. Hosoki, K., M. Kagami, T. Tanaka et al. 2009. Maternal uniparental disomy 14 syndrome demonstrates Prader-Willi syndrome-like phenotype. *J Pediatr* 155 (6):900–903. e1.

59. Cotter, P. D., S. Kaffe, L. D. McCurdy, M. Jhaveri, J. P. Willner, and K. Hirschhorn. 1997. Paternal uniparental disomy for chromosome 14: A case report and review. *Am J Med Genet* 70 (1):74–79.

60. Irving, M. D., K. Buiting, D. Kanber et al. 2010. Segmental paternal uniparental disomy (patUPD) of 14q32 with abnormal methylation elicits the characteristic features of complete patUPD14. *Am J Med Genet A* 152A (8):1942–1950.

61. Kagami, M., Y. Sekita, G. Nishimura et al. 2008. Deletions and epimutations affecting the human 14q32.2 imprinted region in individuals with paternal and maternal upd(14)-like phenotypes. *Nat Genet* 40 (2):237–242.

62. Murphy, S. K., A. A. Wylie, K. J. Coveler et al. 2003. Epigenetic detection of human chromosome 14 uniparental disomy. *Hum Mutat* 22 (1):92–97.

Part IV

Novel Concept in Obesity Drug Development

20 Adipose Drug Targets for Obesity Treatment

Olivier Boss, PhD, Lorenz Lehr, PhD, and Jean-Paul Giacobino, PhD

CONTENTS

ABBREVIATIONS

CNS	Central nervous system
DGAT1	Acyl-CoA:diacylglycerol acyltransferase 1
SCD1	Stearoyl-CoA desaturase-1
RBP4	Retinol binding protein-4
TNFα	Tumor necrosis factor-α
IL-6	Interleukin-6
PTP-1B	Protein tyrosine phosphatase-1B
PPAR	Peroxisome proliferator-activated receptor
KO	Knockout
TZD	Thiazolidinediones

SPPARM	Selective PPAR modulators
ASO	Antisense oligonucleotides
ACC2	Acetyl-CoA carboxylase 2
β-AR	β-adrenergic receptor
TRβ	Thyroid hormone receptor β
UCP1	Uncoupling protein-1
PGC-1	PPARγ coactivator 1
ERR	Estrogen-related receptor

INTRODUCTION

PIVOTAL ROLE OF ADIPOSE TISSUE

It is well known that diet and exercise can be, in most individuals, effective means to treat obesity. However, the steadily increasing prevalence of obesity in most countries undoubtedly shows that knowing this is not sufficient to avoid or cure this disease. Indeed, obesity is still in need of effective treatments that have a long-term impact on the course of the disease and its associated cardiovascular risk factors.

In the last few years, adipose tissue has been recognized as a very important endocrine organ, communicating with the brain and peripheral tissues to balance energy intake and expenditure with the level of energy stored in adipocytes. Recent studies have shown that during the development of obesity, macrophages infiltrate the adipose tissue and generate an inflammation-like state [1]. Macrophages residing in adipose tissue, and possibly also enlarged adipocytes, then produce cytokines that are believed to play a role in the development of pathologies associated with obesity, that is, insulin resistance, type 2 diabetes, dyslipidemia, and cardiovascular disease. Adipose tissue plays a key role in the regulation of energy metabolism, as a source of both fuel (e.g., fatty acids) and hormones (e.g., leptin), and in the metabolic adaptations to body weight or fat loss observed upon food restriction in both animals and humans [2–5]. There seems to be at least two energy balance sensor systems: one that responds to acute changes in adipose mass and another that monitors long-term levels of fat stores. The former seems to involve leptin and the sympathetic nervous system (SNS) as regulators of appetite and metabolic rate. The chronic "adipostat" system, on the other hand, likely plays a key role in the regain of fat stores after weight loss, and its mechanism remains obscure. Adipose tissue must be the source of factors informing other tissues of the status of fat stores [6].

GENERAL CRITERIA FOR ANTIOBESITY DRUG DEVELOPMENT

Treatment of obesity will require induction, for a certain period of time, of a state of negative energy balance. This can be achieved through a decrease in the entry of energy (food intake), an increase in the output of energy (metabolic rate), or a combination of both. In most instances, a modification of the activity of a single target with a drug will need to trigger additional effects in another part of the system controlling energy balance in order to result in a state of negative energy balance. For example, drug inhibition of an enzyme involved in triglyceride (fat) synthesis will have to cause a decrease in food intake and/or an increase in energy expenditure to have a therapeutic effect on obesity. This requirement might seem hard to fulfill unless several drugs are used simultaneously. The endocrinological nature of the control of energy balance implies that metabolic adaptations develop when one part of the system is altered. Some adaptations prevent long-term weight loss (as the drop in metabolic rate appearing upon body weight loss with food restriction), whereas other adaptations help weight loss. In fact, in the last few years, a number of genetic animal models have shown that inhibition of lipid synthesis by targeted disruption of a key enzyme in the lipogenic pathway (e.g., stearoyl-CoA desaturase-1 [SCD1] or acyl-CoA:diacylglycerol acyltransferase 1 [DGAT1]) can lead to an increase in metabolic rate. These models thus provide biological validation of novel potential drug targets that are expressed in adipose tissue. However, we must keep in mind that disruption of the gene encoding a target will not necessarily predict the effects of inhibition of that target by a drug in adult animals, let alone in humans.

Novel drugs to treat obesity should possess some key features [7]. They must be devoid of significant side effects over the long term, as treatments will be of long duration. To improve appreciably on presently available medications, future treatments should aim to induce, and sustain, a weight loss of at least 10% of body weight. Finally, as lifelong therapy will probably be necessary, the cost associated with therapy must be affordable. In this chapter, we discuss the potential of various adipose targets for the development of drugs to treat obesity and insulin resistance.

ADIPOSE TARGETS

Two categories of adipose drug targets can be distinguished: targets that reside in adipocytes (e.g., cell-surface receptors, enzymes, and nuclear receptors) and targets that are secreted by adipocytes, that is, adipokines, that act on other tissues (e.g., brain, skeletal muscle, and liver). Adipokines stand for any factors released by adipose tissue, including adipocytes and stromavascular cells [8,9]. In the past 10 years, numerous adipokines have been discovered [8,10–15] that influence the regulation of body weight, insulin sensitivity, and glucose metabolism, as well as the cardiovascular system, and it is likely that additional adipokines that have an impact on energy metabolism remain to be uncovered [12,16,17]. Additional adipokines of importance in the development of insulin resistance, type 2 diabetes, dyslipidemia, and cardiovascular disease (e.g., retinol binding protein-4 [RBP4], tumor necrosis factor-α [TNFα], resistin, visfatin, interleukin-1β [IL-1β], and interleukin-6 [IL-6]) will not be discussed here as they do not seem to represent direct drug target candidates for obesity treatment [18].

Leptin

Most people add about a pound of fat per year in adulthood, which represents a lower than 1% inaccuracy in energy balance. This indicates that there is an amazingly tight coupling between food intake and energy expenditure. An afferent signal secreted from the adipose tissue to the central nervous system (CNS) was discovered in leptin a decade ago [19]. The amount of leptin secreted into the circulation is usually proportional to the fat mass [20,21], and it is now well established that leptin plays a major role in coordinating the regulation of food intake and metabolic rate [22]. The effects seen in rodents led to great hopes for leptin as a means to treat obesity. Unfortunately, leptin's effects on food intake and body weight have not been as strong in humans as in mice. A very strong response to leptin was seen in a few people with a mutation causing a lack of leptin [23]. However, in the majority of cases, it seems that obese patients exhibit resistance to the action of leptin rather than a deficiency of leptin.

Nonetheless, several clinical studies showed a significant effect of leptin in obese patients [24,25]. The short half-life of leptin in humans (25 min) [26] and the route of administration (injection) present pharmacodynamic hurdles for the use of leptin as a therapeutic agent. To address this issue, some studies used a long-acting, polyethylene glycol-modified recombinant human leptin [25]. Results from human studies highlight a very similar role for leptin in humans and rodents. However, the prevalent leptin resistance seen in obese patients blunts the response to leptin, as observed in certain obese rodent models. The most disappointing clinical results together with the high cost of production of the recombinant protein and the inconvenient route of administration have broadly reduced the interest in leptin as a therapeutic agent (reviewed in [27]). Nevertheless, a few clinical trials are ongoing that investigate the use of recombinant leptin as treatment for severe insulin resistance and lipodystrophy [28]. The clinical validation of the action of leptin does make the leptin system a very interesting target, and a long-acting, orally available small-molecule leptin receptor agonist would be of tremendous value. However, developing a small molecule that mimics the activating effects of leptin (a protein) will be a daunting task. Part of the challenge is due to the fact that the leptin receptor is a cytokine receptor, a class of drug targets that has traditionally been very difficult to activate with small molecules.

On the other hand, reversing the resistance to the action of leptin on food intake and energy metabolism, which seems to develop with age [29], looks like a very promising strategy for treating obesity. Unfortunately, like insulin resistance, leptin resistance is not yet well understood. Interestingly, protein tyrosine phosphatase-1B (PTP-1B) (reviewed in this chapter) has been shown to be implicated in leptin resistance [30–32], even further increasing the biological validation of PTP-1B, a pharmacologically very challenging target. Very recent results suggest that C-reactive protein (CRP), a blood plasma marker of inflammation present in higher levels in obese and insulin resistant patients, could play a role in the leptin resistance seen in obese patients [33]. If this mechanism operates in most patients, inhibitors of CRP binding to leptin might represent novel agents with clear potential to treat obesity and insulin resistance.

ADIPONECTIN

Adiponectin (also known as adipocyte complement-related protein of 30 kDa [Acrp30], adipoQ, or adipose most abundant gene transcript [apM1]) was discovered a few years ago as a 30 kDa protein abundantly produced by adipocytes [34–36]. It is present in the circulation as two major oligomeric forms with molecular weights of about 180 kDa (hexamer) and 400 kDa (higher-order structure), and the respective levels of these two forms has been suggested to be key in the action of this adipokine [37]. Several studies found that circulating adiponectin levels in humans were positively correlated with the degree of insulin sensitivity [38]. In addition, increases in the expression of adiponectin in white adipose tissue, as well as in the plasma levels of adiponectin, have been shown after treatment with PPARγ agonists, which could contribute to the insulin-sensitizing effects of PPARγ agonists [11,12,38–42].

Adiponectin knockout (KO) mice were shown by one group [43], but not another [44], to display severe diet-induced insulin resistance. This apparent discrepancy suggests that the genetic background influences compensatory mechanisms regarding the effect of adiponectin on insulin action [38]. Administration of adiponectin to mice was reported to increase fatty acid oxidation in muscle, decrease hepatic glucose production, and induce weight loss [45–48], suggesting that this hormone could represent a therapeutic agent to treat insulin resistance, type 2 diabetes, and obesity. In fact, a recombinant adiponectin fragment (Famoxin from Genset, now part of Serono) has been tested in early clinical trials in recent years, but the results of these investigations have not been published.

Due to the apparent complexity of adiponectin biology (with multiple complexes having potentially different effects) and the cost and inconvenience associated with recombinant protein treatments, the development of small-molecule adiponectin mimetics seems preferable. For this purpose, knowledge of the receptors mediating the effects of adiponectin is essential. Recently, adiponectin cell-surface receptors (AdipoR1, AdipoR2, and T-cadherin) expressed in skeletal muscle and liver have been described [42,49,50], and signaling pathways downstream of adiponectin receptors have the potential to uncover novel molecular targets amenable to small-molecule drug development.

Given the phenotype of the mouse genetic model and the effects of adiponectin treatment in mice, it seems that adiponectin and its signaling pathway represent potential therapeutic agent and drug targets for the treatment of insulin resistance or type 2 diabetes, dyslipidemia, and cardiovascular disease, rather than obesity *per se* [11].

PEROXISOME PROLIFERATOR–ACTIVATED RECEPTORS

Peroxisome proliferator–activated receptors (PPARs) are a family of three (α, β or δ, and γ) nuclear receptors that affect the transcription and expression level of target genes. PPARs act in conjunction with the retinoid X receptor; their activity is controlled by the recruitment of coactivators and corepressors, and they can be modulated by ligands [12,51] (Figure 20.1).

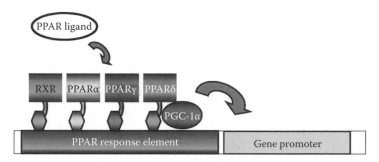

FIGURE 20.1 PPAR nuclear hormone family. PPARs and PGC-1α play a key role in energy dissipation.

PPARγ

PPARγ is mostly expressed in adipose tissue (white and brown), and it plays an essential role in adipogenesis (i.e., adipocyte differentiation) [52]. Ligands that activate PPARγ improve insulin resistance in obese, insulin-resistant animals and humans. Thiazolidinediones (TZD) are a class of PPARγ agonists currently on the market for the treatment of type 2 diabetes, which include rosiglitazone (Avandia from GlaxoSmithKline) and pioglitazone (Actos from Takeda and Eli Lilly). Unfortunately, as full activation of PPARγ enhances adipocyte differentiation (and mildly increases metabolic efficiency), animals and humans treated with TZD tend to gain weight. It is now clear, however, that the beneficial effects of PPARγ ligands on insulin sensitivity are not dependent on their effects on adipogenesis [53,54]. Thus, it should be possible to develop agents that modulate the activity of PPARγ in such a way that the compounds improve insulin sensitivity but have no effects on adipogenesis (and metabolic efficiency). Several companies are currently trying to achieve this with new compounds that do not fully activate PPARγ but modulate its activity (selective PPAR modulators, or SPPARM) [53]. Such agents should induce PPARγ to recruit a different set of coactivators and corepressors in the adipocytes than those induced by full PPARγ agonists, ultimately leading to improvement of insulin resistance without increasing adipogenesis and body weight [12,55,56]. In addition, mouse models where the PPARγ gene was disrupted (gene KO mice), and studies with PPARγ antagonists, show that inhibition of PPARγ can also improve insulin resistance and, contrary to what is observed with full activation of PPARγ, cause a decrease in fat mass [12,53,54,57–62] (Figure 20.2).

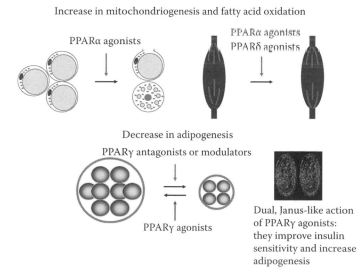

FIGURE 20.2 PPAR ligands might improve insulin sensitivity and treat obesity.

PPARδ

PPARδ (also called PPARβ) is the lesser known member of the PPAR family. This protein is abundantly expressed in most tissues, and it was recently shown to play a key role in mitochondriogenesis and fatty acid oxidation in adipose tissue and skeletal muscle in mice [14,52,55,63,64]. Overexpression of PPARδ in skeletal muscle was found to increase muscle mitochondrial content and oxidative capacity and to decrease diet-induced obesity and insulin resistance [65,66]. Also, overexpression of a constitutively active PPARδ in adipose tissue of mice was reported to enhance uncoupling protein-1 (UCP1) gene expression and fatty acid oxidation and, as a result, prevents the development of obesity induced by a high-fat diet [67]. PPARδ-deficient mice, on the other hand, were found to be more prone to obesity [52,67]. In addition, treatment of obese mice with the PPARδ agonist GW501516 induced a reduction in body fat, apparently by promoting fatty acid oxidation in skeletal muscle and adipose tissue and by increasing adaptive thermogenesis [12,63,66,68]. These results suggest that activation of PPARδ might represent a promising strategy for the treatment of obesity and insulin resistance [69–71] (Figure 20.2).

An alternative to activating a single PPAR is to develop "dual PPAR agonists" or "pan PPAR agonists" that activate both PPARα and PPARγ or all three PPARs, respectively, hoping that the PPARα or PPARδ part (which might both activate fatty acid oxidation) will balance out the adipogenic effects of PPARγ activation [14,55]. This strategy has the potential to produce agents that treat the metabolic syndrome as a whole (obesity, type 2 diabetes, dyslipidemia, atherosclerosis, and hypertension) and not only obesity.

Potential Unwanted Side Effects of PPAR Ligand Treatments

There is currently high hopes that PPARδ agonists, SPPARMs, dual PPARα/PPARγ agonists, or pan PPAR agonists will develop into successful drugs to treat obesity and type 2 diabetes. However, prolonged treatment with reasonable doses (10 mg/kg) of the PPARδ agonist GW501516 was found to cause hepatomegaly in diet-induced obese C57BL/6J mice [68]. In fact, it is well known that pure PPARα agonists (e.g., fibrates) induce peroxisome proliferation and hepatomegaly in rodents but appear well tolerated in humans, where peroxisome proliferation is not observed [52,72]. There is precedence of hepatotoxic effects of PPAR agonists, as the first PPARγ agonist of the TZD family that went to market, troglitazone, was withdrawn following cases of acute liver failure. However, more recent TZDs currently on the market for the treatment of type 2 diabetes, rosiglitazone and pioglitazone, have shown extremely rare (and reversible) signs of hepatotoxicity [73]. PPARγ agonists have been reported to promote the growth of colon cancer tumors in mice, although the effects on human colon cancer cell lines showed conflicting results [52]. Similarly, the PPARδ agonist GW501516 was shown to accelerate the growth of small intestine polyp in cancer-prone mice [52]. Recent phase 3 clinical studies with the dual PPARα/PPARγ agonist muraglitazar showed encouraging therapeutic efficacy but also revealed a dose-related higher incidence of weight gain, edema, and congestive heart failure.

In summary, the potential toxicity on liver, heart, and skeletal muscle, and the carcinogenicity of PPAR agonists will have to be carefully investigated in the evaluation of drug candidates for chronic treatments. The United States Food and Drug Administration (FDA) now requires the completion of 2 year carcinogenicity studies before clinical studies of more than 6-month duration with PPAR agonists can be initiated [56,72].

STEAROYL-COA DESATURASE-1

SCD1 is an essential enzyme for the desaturation of long-chain fatty acids to generate monounsaturated fatty acids, mainly oleic acid (C18:1). This fatty acid desaturation seems to be key for triglyceride synthesis and body fat accumulation [74,75]. Indeed, lines of mice with either a targeted disruption of the SCD1 gene (SCD1 KO) or a natural inactivating mutation in the SCD1 gene (asebia) show a decrease in high-fat-diet-induced obesity and insulin resistance, apparently as a consequence of an elevated metabolic rate as compared to wild-type mice. In addition, treatment of mice with antisense oligonucleotides

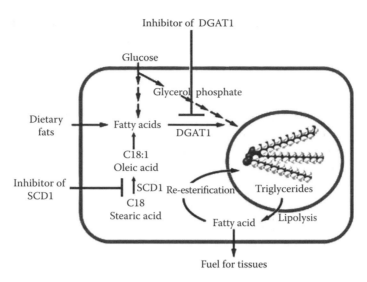

FIGURE 20.3 Inhibitors of triglyceride synthesis that might help treat obesity. DGAT1, acyl-CoA:diacylglycerol acyltransferase 1; SCD1, stearoyl-CoA desaturase-1.

(ASO) repressing the expression of SCD1 in liver and adipose tissue resulted in prevention of high-fat-diet-induced obesity, hepatic steatosis, and insulin resistance without affecting food intake [76]. In this latter study, SCD1 ASO also reduced *de novo* fatty acid synthesis, decreased the expression of lipogenic enzymes, and increased the expression of genes potentially promoting energy dissipation in liver and adipose tissue. Interestingly, SCD1 has been shown to be a major effector of leptin action on fatty acid metabolism in liver [77–79], and it could play a similar role in adipose tissue and skeletal muscle. These results strongly support, from a biological point of view, SCD1 as a high-potential target to treat obesity. In addition, the fact that SCD1 is an enzyme that would have to be inhibited by therapeutic drugs represents a very attractive avenue from a drug development point of view.

Mice that completely lack SCD1 (homozygous KO) have abnormal skin, eyelid, and hair due to deficiency in triglycerides and cholesterol ester synthesis. However, mice lacking only one allele of the SCD1 gene (heterozygous KO) [75] or treated with an SCD1 ASO [76] showed no such abnormalities despite a 50% to 75% reduction in SCD1 expression and SCD activity. These results suggest that partial inhibition of SCD1 might have beneficial metabolic effects without significant repercussions on skin, eyelid, and hair development [79]. This last point is very encouraging for the development of SCD1 inhibitors for the treatment of obesity and insulin resistance. Importantly, inhibition of other enzymes also involved in triglyceride synthesis, that is, ACC2 (acetyl-CoA carboxylase 2) and DGAT1 (see the following section), is also associated with enhanced energy expenditure and resistance to the development of obesity in mice, suggesting that triglyceride synthesis is a promising target pathway for the development of antiobesity drugs [79] (Figure 20.3).

ACYL COA:DIACYLGLYCEROL ACYLTRANSFERASE 1

DGAT1 is a microsomal enzyme that catalyzes the final and committed step in the glycerol phosphate pathway. Targeted disruption of the DGAT1 gene produced mice that are resistant to high-fat-diet-induced obesity and hepatic steatosis [80], apparently as a consequence of an increase in energy expenditure and physical activity [81]. DGAT1-deficient mice also highlighted enhanced insulin and leptin sensitivity [82]. Intriguingly, the protection against obesity and insulin resistance was not seen in ob/ob (leptin-deficient) mice (crossed with DGAT1 KO mice), possibly due to an increase in DGAT2 expression in the white adipose tissue of this animal model [83]. These data support the value of DGAT1 as a molecular target for the development of antiobesity drugs.

A total lack of DGAT1 was reported to cause alopecia and to impair the development of the mammary gland, abnormalities that were not seen in animals with only partial DGAT1 deficiency [80]. Importantly, obesity resistance and enhanced insulin sensitivity were also observed in wild-type mice transplanted with white fat pads from DGAT1 KO mice, suggesting that adipose tissue lacking DGAT1 secretes a factor that can decrease fat stores and enhance glucose disposal [16,83]. Thus, partial inhibition of the enzyme seems sufficient to produce desired effects on adiposity, suggesting that pharmacological inhibition of the enzyme should be a productive therapeutic strategy for human obesity and type 2 diabetes (Figure 20.3). Furthermore, identification of the putative factor secreted by adipose tissue lacking DGAT1 that improves blood glucose homeostasis could provide additional target candidates for drug development.

PROTEIN TYROSINE PHOSPHATASE-1B

PTP-1B is a protein tyrosine phosphatase expressed in most tissues that can interrupt insulin signaling by dephosphorylating Tyr residues on the insulin receptor and possibly also on the insulin receptor substrate-1 [84]. PTP-1B has also been shown to dephosphorylate JAK2 and interrupt leptin signaling in hypothalamus [30–32]. Thus, inhibition of PTP-1B has the potential to reverse the resistance to the action of both insulin (type 2 diabetes) and leptin (obesity) [85].

With the exception of the β3-adrenergic receptor (β3-AR), no other adipose target has been as strongly validated (in animals) as PTP-1B in the field of obesity and insulin resistance. Mice that lack the PTP-1B gene were found to be resistant to high-fat-diet-induced obesity and insulin resistance through an increase in skeletal muscle, and possibly liver, insulin sensitivity and an increase in resting and total daily metabolic rate (expressed per gram of body weight) [86,87]. The phenotype of these mice suggested that PTP-1B plays a critical role in the action of insulin on glucose metabolism in muscle and liver. Recent studies using RNA inhibition technology to repress the normal expression of PTP-1B in mice suggest that PTP-1B plays a significant role in adipose tissue, too [88,89]. In fact, the PTP-1B ASO, which, in mice, reached the adipose tissue and liver, where they strongly decreased the expression of PTP-1B but did not reach the skeletal muscle or the brain [89–91], induced improvements in glucose metabolism and insulin sensitivity and a decrease in body weight in obese, insulin-resistant ob/ob and db/db mice [88–91]. These studies suggested that inhibition of PTP-1B expression in adipose tissue and liver can lead to improvements in glucose metabolism and insulin sensitivity and a decrease in body weight in obese, insulin-resistant ob/ob and db/db mice [88–91]. At this point, it is not yet clear what the main target tissues for PTP-1B inhibition are. Results from the gene KO mice suggest that skeletal muscle and liver, but not adipose tissue, are responsible for the enhanced action of insulin (anti-insulin resistance), whereas the mechanism underlying the lower body fat or weight (antiobesity) is uncertain [87]. The results from the PTP-1B ASO studies, on the other hand, suggest that adipose tissue and liver play a key role in increased insulin sensitivity, as inhibition of PTP-1B expression in these two tissues only was sufficient to improve insulin resistance [89–91]. The lack of PTP-1B in parts of the brain involved in the control of body weight and glucose metabolism might play an important role in the phenotype of PTP-1B KO mice [30,32]. Investigation of the impact of brain-specific disruption of the PTP-1B gene might clarify the role of central PTP-1B on energy metabolism.

The development of PTP-1B inhibitors that are active *in vivo* (animals) turned out to be a major challenge, in part because the protein tyrosine phosphatase family represents a new, largely unexplored, class of drug targets and because it seems that compounds that bind to the enzymatic active site are highly charged and do not readily permeate the cell membrane or show poor oral bioavailability [85]. Nonetheless, some reports have recently described remarkable effects of small-molecule PTP-1B inhibitors (e.g., IDD-3, PTP-3848, and KR61639) in obese, insulin-resistant ob/ob, db/db, KKAy, and C57BL mice [92–98]. In fact, these effects were quite similar to those observed with ASOs repressing the expression of PTP-1B. Interestingly, the inhibitor IDD-3 was shown to improve insulin sensitivity and glucose homeostasis only after 3 days of treatment in ob/ob mice and after a single dose in high-fat-fed, insulin-resistant Wistar rats [99]. This pharmacodynamic profile suggests that, if the mechanism of action is similar in humans, proof-of-concept early clinical studies could be performed quite rapidly and give valuable indications regarding the validity of PTP-1B as a drug target in human obesity and type 2 diabetes.

In summary, inhibition of PTP-1B is one of the most promising approaches for treating obesity and insulin resistance, and we will soon know whether the challenges met by many companies in their efforts to develop small-molecule inhibitors for this enzyme can be overcome.

β_3-ADRENERGIC RECEPTOR

The pharmacological effects of β_3-AR agonists developed so far represent a classical example of the risks of extrapolating the effects observed in rodent models to clinical effects in humans.

Rodent adipose tissues (brown and white) express high levels of β_3-AR, and β_3-AR agonists are well known to be effective in these animals in terms of reducing body weight or fat stores and improving insulin resistance and blood glucose homeostasis. However, human adipose tissue has been shown to express very low levels of β_3-AR [100–102], possibly because humans live at thermoneutrality and, unlike rodents kept at room temperature, do not need to rely on nonshivering thermogenesis to maintain their body temperature. Because of this low expression level, it is hardly surprising that β_3-AR agonists have very weak effects on energy metabolism in humans [103,104].

There remains the possibility that the expression of β_3-AR in human adipose tissue could be upregulated by future treatment strategies. However, there is currently no clear target candidate to achieve this effect [104,105]. A different but related approach would be to induce the conversion of white to brown-like adipocytes with significant levels of expression of β_3-AR in human adipose tissue (see the following section).

OTHER TARGET CANDIDATES

Thyroid hormones have been used to treat obesity in the past, but their use showed unacceptable adverse effects on the heart function and skeletal muscle mass. However, recent data suggest that selective activation of thyroid hormone receptor β (TRβ) can induce an increase in metabolic rate and a decrease in body weight in rodents and nonhuman primates without adverse effects on the heart function [106,107]. Thus, new TRβ-selective agonists, or possibly TRβ modulators, represent a new class of therapeutic candidates against obesity [108]. The realization that the activity of nuclear receptors (e.g., PPARs) can be modified in different ways (and not only by full activation or inhibition) opens up new avenues in drug discovery for thyroid hormone receptors.

ADIPOSE TISSUE REMODELING: CONVERSION OF WHITE TO BROWN-LIKE ADIPOCYTES

The main effector of cold- and diet-induced thermogenesis in rodents is the brown adipose tissue (BAT). Thermogenesis in this tissue is mainly regulated by the SNS. Sympathetic activation leads to the local release of catecholamines by the sympathetic nerve terminals. Catecholamines then mediate their effects through α- and β-adrenergic receptors (α- and β-AR). The β-AR family consists of β_1-, β_2-, and β_3-AR subtypes, and the three β subtypes coexist in the BAT. In contrast to rodents maintained at room temperature (i.e., below their thermoneutrality temperature), adult humans do not possess significant amounts of BAT. Induction of brown adipocyte differentiation with drugs might be possible, although no druggable molecular target has yet been identified to achieve this in humans [7,104,109].

Various studies have shown that the white and brown preadipocytes differentiate *in vitro* in characteristic white and brown adipocytes, respectively [110–112]. Multilocular fat cells, expressing UCP1 and rich in mitochondria, have been observed for the first time in a white adipose tissue

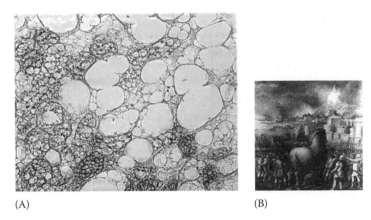

(A)   (B)

FIGURE 20.4   Cold-exposure recruitment, in the mouse WAT, of brown adipocyte-like multilocular cells expressing UCP1 (A). Thermogenic cells act as a "Trojan horse" to transform the lipid-storing WAT into an energy dissipating tissue (B). (From Jimenez, M. et al., *Eur. J. Biochem.*, 270, 699, 2003. With permission.)

(WAT) depot by Young et al. [113]. The emergence of these so-called ectopic brown adipocytes in the WAT was found to be induced by cold acclimation in rats [114,115] and mice [116–118] (Figure 20.4). This phenomenon is generally called recruitment. The new cells were found to be sympathetically innervated [119] and to remain present as long as a sympathetic stimulation persisted [117].

Several reports showed that in mice the administration of selective β_3-AR agonists like CL 316243 induced the emergence of brown adipocytes in WAT depots [118,120–122] and that this phenomenon was strongly dependent on the mouse genetic background [118,121,123]. It was, however, recently shown that transgenic overexpression of the human β_1-AR in the WAT of mice also induced the appearance of abundant brown adipocytes in this tissue [124]. These results suggested that the β_3-AR might not be the only β-subtype controlling the emergence of brown adipocytes in the WAT. However, administration of β_1-AR agonists would not be appropriate for the treatment of obesity due to the well-known effects of these agents on the heart.

UCP1-expressing cells should, by dissipating energy, provide heat and therefore contribute with the BAT to maintain body temperature and energy balance. The administration of the β_3-AR agonist CL 316243 was found to induce the recruitment of brown adipocytes in WAT depots and, at the same time, to reduce adiposity in the Zucker *fa/fa* rat [122]. Important information on the physiological importance of brown adipocyte recruitment in the WAT was obtained by comparing obesity-prone and obesity-resistant strains of mice. Chronic treatment with CL 316243 prevented obesity induced by a high-fat diet in the obesity-resistant A/J but not in the obesity-prone C57BL/6J mice. As CL 316243 also induced a marked UCP1 expression in the WAT depots of the A/J but not of the C57BL/6J mice, it could be postulated that the ability of the β_3-AR agonist to prevent diet-induced obesity depended on the recruitment phenomenon [121]. A strong correlation was found, in response to cold exposure or CL 316243 treatment in various mouse strains, between body weight loss and UCP1 levels in the retroperitoneal WAT [118].

Transgenic mice ectopically expressing UCP1 in their WAT displayed an increase in the oxygen consumption of this tissue and were protected from genetic and dietary obesity [125]. Surprisingly, their BAT was atrophied and the animals were cold-sensitive [126]. On the other hand, mice with a genetic ablation of their BAT were cold sensitive and obese [127]. This raises the possibility of distinct functions for brown adipocytes depending on their presence in BAT or in WAT depots. BAT brown adipocytes would convey both cold and obesity resistance, whereas WAT brown adipocytes would be associated only with obesity resistance. However, the phenotype of the UCP1 KO mice, which are cold sensitive but not obese [128,129] does not support a role for UCP1 in obesity resistance.

The origin and the real nature of the multilocular cells rich in mitochondria and expressing UCP1 that appeared in WAT upon cold acclimation or β_3-AR stimulation has yet to be determined. The presence of brown adipocyte progenitors in the WAT has been suggested by studies showing that 10%–15% of the precursor cells isolated from mouse WAT differentiate into brown adipocytes in culture [130] and that brown adipocyte progenitors are present in human WAT depots [131]. Another hypothesis suggests that a few unilocular white adipocytes are indeed "masked" brown adipocytes that can recover a brown phenotype in response to an SNS stimulation such as that induced by cold exposure. Himms-Hagen et al. [132], studying the effect of CL 316243 in rats, suggested that the multilocular cells expressing UCP1 that appeared in the WAT were different from the classical brown adipocytes and postulated that they might derive, at least in part, from preexisting unilocular adipocytes. Orci et al. [133] showed that hyperleptinemia in rats induces the transformation of white adipocytes into so-called postadipocytes (or fat-oxidizing machines), which have the phenotype of brown adipocytes.

Gene expression studies have shown different responses to various stimuli of WAT vs. BAT brown adipocytes. It has been observed that in the BAT of β_3-AR KO mice, UCP1 expression levels were normal at 24°C as well as after 10 days of cold exposure, whereas in the WAT of β_3-AR KO mice UCP1 expression levels and the density of multilocular cells were strongly depressed at 24°C and after a 10 day cold exposure as compared to wild-type mice [134]. These results confirm that β_3-ARs play a major role in the appearance of brown adipocytes in WAT and suggest that the multilocular cells recruited in the WAT differ from genuine brown adipocytes. Recently, Coulter et al. [135] have evaluated whether the quantitative trait loci controlling UCP1 expression also modulate PGC-1α expression levels, by analysis of backcross progeny from the A/J and C57BL/6J mouse strains. They found, comparing mice on a low- or high-fat diet, allelic variations modulating the expression of UCP1 and PGC-1α in brown adipocytes in the WAT but not in the BAT. These results suggested fundamentally different regulatory mechanisms for the control of UCP1 expression in WAT vs. BAT.

Several studies using transgenic animals have shown the strong implication of various genes in the occurrence of ectopic brown adipocytes in the WAT. Among them we have selected a few possible early target candidates for antiobesity drugs.

4E-BP1 was found to play an important inhibitory role on the recruitment of brown adipocytes in the WAT. Indeed, in 4E-BP1 KO mice, there was a robust recruitment of ectopic brown adipocytes in the inguinal and retroperitoneal WAT. Consistently, in 4E-BP1 KO mice, WAT PGC-1α and UCP1 expression levels were increased, and body fat mass was decreased [136]. Thus, a specific inhibitor of 4E-BP1 in the WAT could stimulate the resurgence of brown adipocytes in this tissue.

Forkhead C2 (FoxC2), a member of the Fox family of transcription factors, has been shown to have an effect on the switch between WAT and BAT in rodents. Its expression in mice is restricted to adipose tissues, and mice with adipose tissue–targeted overexpression of FoxC2 displayed an atrophy of the WAT and a hypertrophy of the BAT [137]. Those mice also exhibited an increase in insulin sensitivity and a more efficient signaling through β-adrenergic receptors. Further analysis showed that the overexpression of FoxC2 prevented diet-induced insulin resistance and intracellular lipid accumulation in the skeletal muscle [138]. It was therefore postulated that FoxC2 could be a novel therapeutic target for the treatment of obesity and insulin resistance.

Yet another approach would be to induce the conversion of white adipocytes to brown-like adipocytes, that is, cells rich in mitochondria with multilocular lipid droplets, not necessarily expressing UCP1 [109,132,139]. Induction of mitochondriogenesis in WAT, assuming that it would trigger an elevation of adipocyte metabolic rate through partial uncoupling of oxidative phosphorylation and an increase in thermogenesis, should favor fatty acid oxidation (possibly also glucose utilization) and decrease fat deposition or promote weight loss [140]. The nuclear receptor coactivators PGC-1α and PGC-1β have been shown to increase mitochondriogenesis when overexpressed in cells or in mice [141–147]. This increase in cellular or tissue oxidative capacity was accompanied, in most cases, by an increase in metabolic rate. Direct activation of PGC-1α (a coactivator) is hardly a possibility with a small-molecule drug, and it might not be a fruitful strategy to treat obesity and insulin resistance as this would probably enhance PGC-1α-mediated hepatic glucose production [148]. However, a possible avenue to activate PGC-1α in adipose tissue would be to interfere with a tissue-specific factor that inhibits PGC-1α. An inhibitor of PGC-1α activity, p160MBP, was recently described [149,150], and this factor could represent an interesting drug target to activate PGC-1α as long as it does not affect the activity of PGC-1α on hepatic gluconeogenesis. In addition, the nuclear receptor estrogen-related receptor, ERRα, and possibly ERRγ, has been shown to play a key role in the effects of PGC-1α on mitochondriogenesis [151–154]. Thus, ERRα and ERRγ could represent novel drug targets for the treatment of obesity and insulin resistance. These nuclear receptors, as yet orphan, would be *a priori* more amenable to drug development [155,156] than a coactivator like PGC-1α, even though the active conformation of ERRα (but not ERRγ) was shown to possess a very small ligand-binding pocket [155].

Activation of lipolysis, if it enhances metabolic rate, for example, by increasing fatty acid cycling, could represent a strategy to induce weight loss [157]. Alternatively, activation of lipolysis could, through a locally increased efflux of fatty acids possibly providing ligands to nuclear receptors involved in mitochondriogenesis, trigger a remodeling of white adipocytes into brown-like adipocytes. This effect has recently been reported after a few days of treatment with the selective β_3-AR agonist CL 316243 in mice [102] and shown to be mediated by PPARα [102,158]. This suggests that PPARα agonists (e.g., fibrates) could have direct antiobesity properties in addition to their well-known effects on dyslipidemia. Alternatively, PPARα modulators (rather than full agonists) might recapitulate some of the effects seen with β_3-AR agonists in rodent WAT. Interestingly, a PPARα agonist (K-111, formerly BM 17.0744) was shown to produce, in addition to improvements of dyslipidemia and insulin resistance, body weight loss in nonhuman primates [159,160].

CONCLUSIONS

Obesity and insulin resistance or type 2 diabetes are pathologies with rapidly growing prevalence in most of the world and with dire, unmet medical needs. Novel, effective long-term treatments of these medical conditions are urgently needed to help decrease patient suffering as well as contain the rapidly increasing cost of health care. Fortunately, remarkable progress in the understanding of the mechanisms controlling energy balance has been achieved in the last decade. Much remains to be learned until we have a complete understanding of these complex systems, but we are very optimistic that the near future will bring efficacious treatments of obesity for most patients.

However, it is unlikely that a single drug against obesity will be effective in most patients. Rather, an assortment of drugs will probably be necessary to treat a large proportion of patients, who almost certainly present heterogeneous mechanistic etiologies of obesity. In this regard, a better characterization of obese patient subcategories could help stratify patient populations for clinical trials and therapeutic strategies.

MOLECULAR TARGETS WITH SMALL-MOLECULE LEADS OR DRUGS SUCCESSFULLY DEVELOPED (PPARS)

A few molecular targets bear the most hopes for antiobesity therapeutics. These targets have been quite well validated biologically (in animals) and are known to be reachable with small molecules since there already exist drugs acting on targets from the same family. PPARs and possibly other nuclear hormone receptors are part of this category. For PPARs, the key for success will be to find the optimal combination of PPAR subtype activation or inhibition to obtain the desired effect on body fat stores and glucose metabolism.

PPARα is the target for the fibrate family compounds used for years to treat dyslipidemia linked to cardiovascular disease. Fibrates activate PPARα in the liver and adipose tissue, but they do not usually have a strong impact on body weight, fat mass, or blood glucose levels. PPARδ agonists have shown interesting effects on body fat stores in mice, and these agents could represent a new generation of antiobesity drugs. Modulation (partial activation or inhibition) of PPARγ, rather than full activation, has a promising future, as does the dual activation of PPARγ and PPARα (or PPARδ). Modulation of the activity of nuclear receptors (e.g., PPARs, thyroid hormone receptors, and orphan nuclear receptors) by affecting the recruitment of their coactivators or corepressors represent a new avenue for future drug development to treat obesity and type 2 diabetes. Potential safety issues of PPAR ligands as regards organ toxicity and carcinogenicity will have to be carefully monitored.

KEY TARGETS FROM THE LIPID SYNTHESIS PATHWAY (SCD1 AND DGAT1)

SCD1 as well as other enzymes playing a critical role in triglyceride synthesis are promising targets for antiobesity drugs. Even though it might appear odd that inhibiting an enzyme needed to store excess energy as fat would help in the treatment of obesity without causing metabolic problems, rodent models show that lacking these key enzymes can induce an adaptive increase in metabolic rate that dissipates the excess energy instead of storing it as fat.

NEW, HIGH-POTENTIAL MOLECULAR TARGET (PTP-1B)

PTP-1B is a molecular target with very high potential for the development of drugs that could be very effective in the treatment of obesity and diabetes. PTP-1B inhibitors would represent an important innovation in drug discovery, as there exist no drugs acting on protein tyrosine phosphatases yet. Hence, PTP-1B inhibitors would establish a precedent for this new class of drug targets. In summary, PTP-1B is a high-risk but very high-potential drug target that could generate unmatched gratification to the successful creators of an orally active inhibitor.

Adipocytes have provided several novel potential targets for the development of therapeutic drugs against obesity and diabetes in recent years. Research and development efforts are still needed for these recent target candidates to be validated and drugs to be developed. In addition, novel adipose factors having an impact on energy metabolism will almost certainly be identified in the near future and will provide additional opportunities for the development of antiobesity drugs.

ACKNOWLEDGMENT

We thank Nils Bergenhem for his contribution to a recent review article containing information that was used when writing this chapter.

REFERENCES

1. Wellen KE, Hotamisligil GS. Obesity-induced inflammatory changes in adipose tissue. *J Clin Invest* 2003;112:1785–1788.
2. Hansen BC, Bodkin NL, Ortmeyer HK. Calorie restriction in nonhuman primates: Mechanisms of reduced morbidity and mortality. *Toxicol Sci* 1999;52:56–60.
3. Blanc S, Schoeller D, Kemnitz J, Weindruch R, Colman R, Newton W, Wink K, Baum S, Ramsey J. Energy expenditure of rhesus monkeys subjected to 11 years of dietary restriction. *J Clin Endocrinol Metab* 2003;88:16–23.
4. Poehlman ET. Reduced metabolic rate after caloric restriction-can we agree on how to normalize the data? *J Clin Endocrinol Metab* 2003;88:14–15.
5. Dulloo AG. A role for suppressed skeletal muscle thermogenesis in pathways from weight fluctuations to the insulin resistance syndrome. *Acta Physiol Scand* 2005;184:295–307.
6. Dulloo AG, Jacquet J. An adipose-specific control of thermogenesis in body weight regulation. *Int J Obes Relat Metab Disord* 2001;25:S22–S29.
7. Ravussin E, Kozak L. Energy Homeostasis. In: Hofbauer KG, Keller U, Boss O, eds. *Pharmacotherapy of Obesity: Options and Alternatives*. Boca Raton, FL: CRC Press, 2004, Chapter 1, pp. 3–23.

8. Fain JN, Madan AK, Hiler ML, Cheema P, Bahouth SW. Comparison of the release of adipokines by adipose tissue, adipose tissue matrix, and adipocytes from visceral and subcutaneous abdominal adipose tissues of obese humans. *Endocrinology* 2004;145:2273–2282. Epub January 15, 2004.

9. Hauner H. Secretory factors from human adipose tissue and their functional role. *Proc Nutr Soc* 2005;64:163–169.

10. Saltiel AR. You are what you secrete. *Nat Med* 2001;7:887–888.

11. Rajala MW, Scherer PE. Minireview: The adipocyte–At the crossroads of energy homeostasis, inflammation, and atherosclerosis. *Endocrinology* 2003;144:3765–3773.

12. Farmer SR, Auwerx J. Adipose tissue: New therapeutic targets from molecular and genetic studies–IASO Stock Conference 2003 report. *Obes Rev* 2004;5:189–196.

13. Lau DC, Dhillon B, Yan H, Szmitko PE, Verma S. Adipokines: Molecular links between obesity and atherosclerosis. *Am J Physiol Heart Circ Physiol* 2005;288:H2031–H2041. Epub January 14, 2005.

14. Moller DE, Kaufman KD. Metabolic syndrome: A clinical and molecular perspective. *Annu Rev Med* 2005;56:45–62.

15. Yang Q, Graham TE, Mody N, Preitner F, Peroni OD, Zabolotny JM, Kotani K, Quadro L, Kahn BB. Serum retinol binding protein 4 contributes to insulin resistance in obesity and type 2 diabetes. *Nature* 2005;436:356–362.

16. Chen HC, Rao M, Sajan MP, Standaert M, Kanoh Y, Miura A, Farese RV, Jr., Farese RV. Role of adipocyte-derived factors in enhancing insulin signaling in skeletal muscle and white adipose tissue of mice lacking Acyl CoA:diacylglycerol acyltransferase 1. *Diabetes* 2004;53:1445–1451.

17. Lafontan M. Fat cells: Afferent and efferent messages define new approaches to treat obesity. *Annu Rev Pharmacol Toxicol* 2005;45:119–146.

18. Gimeno RE, Klaman LD. Adipose tissue as an active endocrine organ: Recent advances. *Curr Opin Pharmacol* 2005;5:122–128.

19. Zhang Y, Proenca R, Maffei M, Barone M, Leopold L, Friedman JM. Positional cloning of the mouse obese gene and its human homologue. *Nature* 1994;372:425–432.

20. Halaas JL, Gajiwala KS, Maffei M, Cohen SL, Chait BT, Rabinowitz D, Lallone RL, Burley SK, Friedman JM. Weight-reducing effects of the plasma protein encoded by the obese gene. *Science* 1995;269:543–546.

21. Pelleymounter MA, Cullen MJ, Baker MB, Hecht R, Winters D, Boone T, Collins F. Effects of the obese gene product on body weight regulation in ob/ob mice. *Science* 1995;269:540–543.

22. Friedman JM, Halaas JL. Leptin and the regulation of body weight in mammals. *Nature* 1998;395:763–770.

23. Farooqi IS, Matarese G, Lord GM, Keogh JM, Lawrence E, Agwu C, Sanna V, Jebb SA, Perna F, Fontana S, Lechler RI, DePaoli AM, O'Rahilly S. Beneficial effects of leptin on obesity, T cell hyporesponsiveness, and neuroendocrine/metabolic dysfunction of human congenital leptin deficiency. *J Clin Invest* 2002;110:1093–1103.

24. Heymsfield SB, Greenberg AS, Fujioka K, Dixon RM, Kushner R, Hunt T, Lubina JA, Patane J, Self B, Hunt P, McCamish M. Recombinant leptin for weight loss in obese and lean adults: A randomized, controlled, dose-escalation trial. *JAMA* 1999;282:1568–1575.

25. Hukshorn CJ, Saris WH, Westerterp-Plantenga MS, Farid AR, Smith FJ, Campfield LA. Weekly subcutaneous pegylated recombinant native human leptin (PEG-OB) administration in obese men. *J Clin Endocrinol Metab* 2000;85:4003–4009.

26. Klein S, Coppack SW, Mohamed-Ali V, Landt M. Adipose tissue leptin production and plasma leptin kinetics in humans. *Diabetes* 1996;45:984–987.

27. Campfield LA, Smith FJ. Leptin and other appetite suppressants. In: Hofbauer KG, Keller U, Boss O, eds. *Pharmacotherapy of Obesity: Options and Alternatives*. Boca Raton, FL: CRC Press, 2004, Chapter 16, pp. 321–344.

28. National Institutes of Health website, http://clinicalstudies.info.nih.gov/cgi/processqry3.pl?sort=1&search=leptin&searchtype=0&patient_type=All&protocoltype=All&institute=%25&conditions=All (accessed October 15, 2005).

29. Wang ZW, Pan WT, Lee Y, Kakuma T, Zhou YT, Unger RH. The role of leptin resistance in the lipid abnormalities of aging. *Faseb J* 2001;15:108–114.

30. Cheng A, Uetani N, Simoncic PD, Chaubey VP, Lee-Loy A, McGlade CJ, Kennedy BP, Tremblay ML. Attenuation of leptin action and regulation of obesity by protein tyrosine phosphatase 1B. *Dev Cell* 2002;2:497–503.

31. Kaszubska W, Falls HD, Schaefer VG, Haasch D, Frost L, Hessler P, Kroeger PE, White DW, Jirousek MR, Trevillyan JM. Protein tyrosine phosphatase 1B negatively regulates leptin signaling in a hypothalamic cell line. *Mol Cell Endocrinol* 2002;195:109–118.

32. Zabolotny JM, Bence-Hanulec KK, Stricker-Krongrad A, Haj F, Wang Y, Minokoshi Y, Kim YB, Elmquist JK, Tartaglia LA, Kahn BB, Neel BG. PTP1B regulates leptin signal transduction in vivo. *Dev Cell* 2002;2:489–495.

33. Chen K, Li F, Li J, Cai H, Strom S, Bisello A, Kelley DE, Friedman-Einat M, Skibinski GA, McCrory MA, Szalai AJ, Zhao AZ. Induction of leptin resistance through direct interaction of C-reactive protein with leptin. *Nat Med* 2006;12(4):425–432.

34. Scherer PE, Williams S, Fogliano M, Baldini G, Lodish HF. A novel serum protein similar to C1q, produced exclusively in adipocytes. *J Biol Chem* 1995;270:26746–26749.

35. Hu E, Liang P, Spiegelman BM. AdipoQ is a novel adipose-specific gene dysregulated in obesity. *J Biol Chem* 1996;271:10697–10703.

36. Maeda K, Okubo K, Shimomura I, Funahashi T, Matsuzawa Y, Matsubara K. cDNA cloning and expression of a novel adipose specific collagen-like factor, apM1 (AdiPose Most abundant Gene transcript 1). *Biochem Biophys Res Commun* 1996;221:286–289.

37. Pajvani UB, Du X, Combs TP, Berg AH, Rajala MW, Schulthess T, Engel J, Brownlee M, Scherer PE. Structure-function studies of the adipocyte-secreted hormone Acrp30/adiponectin. Implications fpr metabolic regulation and bioactivity. *J Biol Chem* 2003;278:9073–9085. Epub December 20, 2002.

38. Havel PJ. Update on adipocyte hormones: Regulation of energy balance and carbohydrate/lipid metabolism. *Diabetes* 2004;53:S143–S151.

39. Bajaj M, Suraamornkul S, Piper P, Hardies LJ, Glass L, Cersosimo E, Pratipanawatr T, Miyazaki Y, DeFronzo RA. Decreased plasma adiponectin concentrations are closely related to hepatic fat content and hepatic insulin resistance in pioglitazone-treated type 2 diabetic patients. *J Clin Endocrinol Metab* 2004;89:200–206.

40. Miyazaki Y, Mahankali A, Wajcberg E, Bajaj M, Mandarino LJ, DeFronzo RA. Effect of pioglitazone on circulating adipocytokine levels and insulin sensitivity in type 2 diabetic patients. *J Clin Endocrinol Metab* 2004;89:4312–4319.

41. Bouskila M, Pajvani UB, Scherer PE. Adiponectin: A relevant player in PPARgamma-agonist-mediated improvements in hepatic insulin sensitivity? *Int J Obes (Lond)* 2005;29:S17–S23.

42. Kadowaki T, Yamauchi T. Adiponectin and adiponectin receptors. *Endocr Rev* 2005;26:439–451.

43. Maeda N, Shimomura I, Kishida K, Nishizawa H, Matsuda M, Nagaretani H, Furuyama N, Kondo H, Takahashi M, Arita Y, Komuro R, Ouchi N, Kihara S, Tochino Y, Okutomi K, Horie M, Takeda S, Aoyama T, Funahashi T, Matsuzawa Y. Diet-induced insulin resistance in mice lacking adiponectin/ACRP30. *Nat Med* 2002;8:731–737. Epub June 17, 2002.

44. Ma K, Cabrero A, Saha PK, Kojima H, Li L, Chang BH, Paul A, Chan L. Increased beta -oxidation but no insulin resistance or glucose intolerance in mice lacking adiponectin. *J Biol Chem* 2002;277:34658–34661. Epub July 31, 2002.

45. Berg AH, Combs TP, Du X, Brownlee M, Scherer PE. The adipocyte-secreted protein Acrp30 enhances hepatic insulin action. *Nat Med* 2001;7:947–953.

46. Combs TP, Berg AH, Obici S, Scherer PE, Rossetti L. Endogenous glucose production is inhibited by the adipose-derived protein Acrp30. *J Clin Invest* 2001;108:1875–1881.

47. Fruebis J, Tsao TS, Javorschi S, Ebbets Reed D, Erickson MR, Yen FT, Bihain BE, Lodish HF. Proteolytic cleavage product of 30-kDa adipocyte complement-related protein increases fatty acid oxidation in muscle and causes weight loss in mice. *Proc Natl Acad Sci USA* 2001;98:2005–2010. Epub 2001 Feb 6.

48. Heilbronn LK, Smith SR, Ravussin E. The insulin-sensitizing role of the fat derived hormone adiponectin. *Curr Pharm Des* 2003;9:1411–1418.

49. Yamauchi T, Kamon J, Ito Y, Tsuchida A, Yokomizo T, Kita S, Sugiyama T, Miyagishi M, Hara K, Tsunoda M, Murakami K, Ohteki T, Uchida S, Takekawa S, Waki H, Tsuno NH, Shibata Y, Terauchi Y, Froguel P, Tobe K, Koyasu S, Taira K, Kitamura T, Shimizu T, Nagai R, Kadowaki T. Cloning of adiponectin receptors that mediate antidiabetic metabolic effects. *Nature* 2003;423:762–729.

50. Hug C, Wang J, Ahmad NS, Bogan JS, Tsao TS, Lodish HF. T-cadherin is a receptor for hexameric and high-molecular-weight forms of Acrp30/adiponectin. *Proc Natl Acad Sci USA* 2004;101:10308–10313. Epub June 21, 2004.

51. Lazar MA. PPAR gamma, 10 years later. *Biochimie* 2005;87:9–13.

52. Evans RM, Barish GD, Wang YX. PPARs and the complex journey to obesity. *Nat Med* 2004;10:355–361.

53. Berger JP, Petro AE, Macnaul KL, Kelly LJ, Zhang BB, Richards K, Elbrecht A, Johnson BA, Zhou G, Doebber TW, Biswas C, Parikh M, Sharma N, Tanen MR, Thompson GM, Ventre J, Adams AD, Mosley R, Surwit RS, Moller DE. Distinct properties and advantages of a novel peroxisome proliferator-activated protein [gamma] selective modulator. *Mol Endocrinol* 2003;17:662–676. Epub January 16, 2003.

94. Liu G, Szczepankiewicz BG, Pei Z, Janowick DA, Xin Z, Hajduk PJ, Abad-Zapatero C, Liang H, Hutchins CW, Fesik SW, Ballaron SJ, Stashko MA, Lubben T, Mika AK, Zinker BA, Trevillyan JM, Jirousek MR. Discovery and structure-activity relationship of oxalylarylaminobenzoic acids as inhibitors of protein tyrosine phosphatase 1B. *J Med Chem* 2003;46:2093–2103.

95. Umezawa K, Kawakami M, Watanabe T. Molecular design and biological activities of protein-tyrosine phosphatase inhibitors. *Pharmacol Ther* 2003;99:15–24.

96. Cheon HG, Kim SM, Yang SD, Ha JD, Choi JK. Discovery of a novel protein tyrosine phosphatase-1B inhibitor, KR61639: Potential development as an antihyperglycemic agent. *Eur J Pharmacol* 2004;485:333–339.

97. Dean D, Orlowski L, Coverdale S, Whitehouse D, Fan C, Balkan B. Chronic treatment with IDD-3, a Novel PTP1b inhibitor, results in sustained improvements in glucose homeostasis in ob/ob and db/db mice. *Diabetes* 2004;53:516P.

98. Fan C, Dean D, Whitehouse DL, Coverdale S, Balkan B. The protein tyrosine phosphase-1B (PTP1B) inhibitor, IDD-3, acutely improves glucose homeostasis in ob/ob mice and insulin action in the euglycemic-hyperinsulinemic clamp in high fat fed rats. *Diabetes* 2004;53:650P.

99. Balkan B, Beeler S, Fan C, Orlowski L, Whitehouse D, Dean DJ. Pharmacological inhibition of PTP1B prevents development of diet-induced obesity and insulin resistance. *Diabetes* 2004;53:618P.

100. Granneman JG. Why do adipocytes make the beta 3 adrenergic receptor? *Cell Signal* 1995;7:9–15.

101. Deng C, Paoloni-Giacobino A, Kuehne F, Boss O, Revelli JP, Moinat M, Cawthorne MA, Muzzin P, Giacobino JP. Respective degree of expression of beta 1-, beta 2- and beta 3-adrenoceptors in human brown and white adipose tissues. *Br J Pharmacol* 1996;118:929–934.

102. Granneman JG, Li P, Zhu Z, Lu Y. Metabolic and cellular plasticity in white adipose tissue I: Effects of beta3-adrenergic receptor activation. *Am J Physiol Endocrinol Metab* 2005;289:E608–E616. Epub June 7, 2005.

103. Larsen TM, Toubro S, van Baak MA, Gottesdiener KM, Larson P, Saris WH, Astrup A. Effect of a 28-d treatment with L-796568, a novel beta(3)-adrenergic receptor agonist, on energy expenditure and body composition in obese men. *Am J Clin Nutr* 2002;76:780–788.

104. Harper M-E, Dent R, Tesson F, McPherson R. Targeting thermogenesis in the development of antiobesity drugs. In: Hofbauer KG, Keller U, Boss O, eds. *Pharmacotherapy of Obesity: Options and Alternatives.* Boca Raton, FL: CRC Press, 2004, Chapter 18, pp. 363–383.

105. Collins S, Cao W, Robidoux J. Learning new tricks from old dogs: Beta-adrenergic receptors teach new lessons on firing up adipose tissue metabolism. *Mol Endocrinol* 2004;18:2123–2131. Epub July 8, 2004.

106. Grover GJ, Mellstrom K, Ye L, Malm J, Li YL, Bladh LG, Sleph PG, Smith MA, George R, Vennstrom B, Mookhtiar K, Horvath R, Speelman J, Egan D, Baxter JD. Selective thyroid hormone receptor-beta activation: A strategy for reduction of weight, cholesterol, and lipoprotein (a) with reduced cardiovascular liability. *Proc Natl Acad Sci USA* 2003;100:10067–10072. Epub July 29, 2003.

107. Grover GJ, Mellstrom K, Malm J. Development of the thyroid hormone receptor beta-subtype agonist KB-141: A strategy for body weight reduction and lipid lowering with minimal cardiac side effects. *Cardiovasc Drug Rev* 2005;23:133–148.

108. Lazar MA. A sweetheart deal for thyroid hormone. *Endocrinology* 2000;141:3055–3056.

109. Himms-Hagen J. Exercise in a pill: Feasibility of energy expenditure targets. *Curr Drug Targets CNS Neurol Disord* 2004;3:389–409.

110. Kopecky J, Baudysova M, Zanotti F, Janikova D, Pavelka S, Houstek J. Synthesis of mitochondrial uncoupling protein in brown adipocytes differentiated in cell culture. *J Biol Chem* 1990;265:22204–22209.

111. Rehnmark S, Nechad M, Herron D, Cannon B, Nedergaard J. Alpha- and beta-adrenergic induction of the expression of the uncoupling protein thermogenin in brown adipocytes differentiated in culture. *J Biol Chem* 1990;265:16464–16471.

112. Ailhaud G, Grimaldi P, Negrel R. Cellular and molecular aspects of adipose tissue development. *Annu Rev Nutr* 1992;12:207–233.

113. Young P, Arch JR, Ashwell M. Brown adipose tissue in the parametrial fat pad of the mouse. *FEBS Lett* 1984;167:10–14.

114. Cousin B, Cinti S, Morroni M, Raimbault S, Ricquier D, Penicaud L, Casteilla L. Occurrence of brown adipocytes in rat white adipose tissue: Molecular and morphological characterization. *J Cell Sci* 1992;103(Pt 4):931–942.

115. Cousin B, Bascands-Viguerie N, Kassis N, Nibbelink M, Ambid L, Casteilla L, Penicaud L. Cellular changes during cold acclimatation in adipose tissues. *J Cell Physiol* 1996;167:285–289.

116. Loncar D. Convertible adipose tissue in mice. *Cell Tissue Res* 1991;266:149–161.

117. Loncar D. Development of thermogenic adipose tissue. *Int J Dev Biol* 1991;35:321–333.

118. Guerra C, Koza RA, Yamashita H, Walsh K, Kozak LP. Emergence of brown adipocytes in white fat in mice is under genetic control. Effects on body weight and adiposity. *J Clin Invest* 1998;102:412–420.

119. Giordano A, Morroni M, Santone G, Marchesi GF, Cinti S. Tyrosine hydroxylase, neuropeptide Y, substance P, calcitonin gene-related peptide and vasoactive intestinal peptide in nerves of rat periovarian adipose tissue: An immunohistochemical and ultrastructural investigation. *J Neurocytol* 1996;25:125–136.

120. Nagase I, Yoshida T, Kumamoto K, Umekawa T, Sakane N, Nikami H, Kawada T, Saito M. Expression of uncoupling protein in skeletal muscle and white fat of obese mice treated with thermogenic beta 3-adrenergic agonist. *J Clin Invest* 1996;97:2898–2904.

121. Collins S, Daniel KW, Petro AE, Surwit RS. Strain-specific response to beta 3-adrenergic receptor agonist treatment of diet-induced obesity in mice. *Endocrinology* 1997;138:405–413.

122. Ghorbani M, Himms-Hagen J. Appearance of brown adipocytes in white adipose tissue during CL 316,243-induced reversal of obesity and diabetes in Zucker fa/fa rats. *Int J Obes Relat Metab Disord* 1997;21:465–475.

123. Kozak LP, Koza RA. Mitochondria uncoupling proteins and obesity: Molecular and genetic aspects of UCP1. *Int J Obes Relat Metab Disord* 1999;23(Suppl 6):S33–S37.

124. Soloveva V, Graves RA, Rasenick MM, Spiegelman BM, Ross SR. Transgenic mice overexpressing the beta 1-adrenergic receptor in adipose tissue are resistant to obesity. *Mol Endocrinol* 1997;11:27–38.

125. Kopecky J, Clarke G, Enerback S, Spiegelman B, Kozak LP. Expression of the mitochondrial uncoupling protein gene from the aP2 gene promoter prevents genetic obesity. *J Clin Invest* 1995;96:2914–2923.

126. Stefl B, Janovska A, Hodny Z, Rossmeisl M, Horakova M, Syrovy I, Bemova J, Bendlova B, Kopecky J. Brown fat is essential for cold-induced thermogenesis but not for obesity resistance in aP2-Ucp mice. *Am J Physiol* 1998;274:E527–E533.

127. Lowell BB, V SS, Hamann A, Lawitts JA, Himms-Hagen J, Boyer BB, Kozak LP, Flier JS. Development of obesity in transgenic mice after genetic ablation of brown adipose tissue. *Nature* 1993;366:740–742.

128. Enerback S, Jacobsson A, Simpson EM, Guerra C, Yamashita H, Harper ME, Kozak LP. Mice lacking mitochondrial uncoupling protein are cold-sensitive but not obese. *Nature* 1997;387:90–94.

129. Liu X, Rossmeisl M, McClaine J, Riachi M, Harper ME, Kozak LP. Paradoxical resistance to diet-induced obesity in UCP1-deficient mice. *J Clin Invest* 2003;111:399–407.

130. Klaus S, Ely M, Encke D, Heldmaier G. Functional assessment of white and brown adipocyte development and energy metabolism in cell culture. Dissociation of terminal differentiation and thermogenesis in brown adipocytes. *J Cell Sci* 1995;108(Pt 10):3171–3180.

131. Digby JE, Montague CT, Sewter CP, Sanders L, Wilkison WO, O'Rahilly S, Prins JB. Thiazolidinedione exposure increases the expression of uncoupling protein 1 in cultured human preadipocytes. *Diabetes* 1998;47:138–141.

132. Himms-Hagen J, Melnyk A, Zingaretti MC, Ceresi E, Barbatelli G, Cinti S. Multilocular fat cells in WAT of CL-316243-treated rats derive directly from white adipocytes. *Am J Physiol Cell Physiol* 2000;279:C670–C681.

133. Orci L, Cook WS, Ravazzola M, Wang MY, Park BH, Montesano R, Unger RH. Rapid transformation of white adipocytes into fat-oxidizing machines. *Proc Natl Acad Sci USA* 2004;101:2058–2063.

134. Jimenez M, Barbatelli G, Allevi R, Cinti S, Seydoux J, Giacobino JP, Muzzin P, Preitner F. Beta 3-adrenoceptor knockout in C57BL/6J mice depresses the occurrence of brown adipocytes in white fat. *Eur J Biochem* 2003;270:699–705.

135. Coulter AA, Bearden CM, Liu X, Koza RA, Kozak LP. Dietary fat interacts with QTLs controlling induction of Pgc-1 alpha and Ucp1 during conversion of white to brown fat. *Physiol Genomics* 2003;14:139–147.

136. Tsukiyama-Kohara K, Poulin F, Kohara M, DeMaria CT, Cheng A, Wu Z, Gingras AC, Katsume A, Elchebly M, Spiegelman BM, Harper ME, Tremblay ML, Sonenberg N. Adipose tissue reduction in mice lacking the translational inhibitor 4E-BP1. *Nat Med* 2001;7:1128–1132.

137. Cederberg A, Gronning LM, Ahren B, Tasken K, Carlsson P, Enerback S. FOXC2 is a winged helix gene that counteracts obesity, hypertriglyceridemia, and diet-induced insulin resistance. *Cell* 2001;106:563–573.

138. Kim JK, Kim HJ, Park SY, Cederberg A, Westergren R, Nilsson D, Higashimori T, Cho YR, Liu ZX, Dong J, Cline GW, Enerback S, Shulman GI. Adipocyte-specific overexpression of FOXC2 prevents diet-induced increases in intramuscular fatty acyl CoA and insulin resistance. *Diabetes* 2005;54:1657–1663.

139. Granneman JG, Burnazi M, Zhu Z, Schwamb LA. White adipose tissue contributes to UCP1-independent thermogenesis. *Am J Physiol Endocrinol Metab* 2003;285:E1230–E1236. Epub September 3, 2003.

140. Rossmeisl M, Flachs P, Brauner P, Sponarova J, Matejkova O, Prazak T, Ruzickova J, Bardova K, Kuda O, Kopecky J. Role of energy charge and AMP-activated protein kinase in adipocytes in the control of body fat stores. *Int J Obes Relat Metab Disord* 2004;28:S38–S44.

141. Wu Z, Puigserver P, Andersson U, Zhang C, Adelmant G, Mootha V, Troy A, Cinti S, Lowell B, Scarpulla RC, Spiegelman BM. Mechanisms controlling mitochondrial biogenesis and respiration through the thermogenic coactivator PGC-1. *Cell* 1999;98:115–124.

142. Spiegelman BM, Puigserver P, Wu Z. Regulation of adipogenesis and energy balance by PPARgamma and PGC-1. *Int J Obes Relat Metab Disord* 2000;24:S8–S10.

143. Lin J, Wu H, Tarr PT, Zhang CY, Wu Z, Boss O, Michael LF, Puigserver P, Isotani E, Olson EN, Lowell BB, Bassel-Duby R, Spiegelman BM. Transcriptional co-activator PGC-1 alpha drives the formation of slow-twitch muscle fibres. *Nature* 2002;418:797–801.

144. Kamei Y, Ohizumi H, Fujitani Y, Nemoto T, Tanaka T, Takahashi N, Kawada T, Miyoshi M, Ezaki O, Kakizuka A. PPARgamma coactivator 1beta/ERR ligand 1 is an ERR protein ligand, whose expression induces a high-energy expenditure and antagonizes obesity. *Proc Natl Acad Sci USA* 2003;100:12378–12383. Epub October 6, 2003.

145. Meirhaeghe A, Crowley V, Lenaghan C, Lelliott C, Green K, Stewart A, Hart K, Schinner S, Sethi JK, Yeo G, Brand MD, Cortright RN, O'Rahilly S, Montague C, Vidal-Puig AJ. Characterization of the human, mouse and rat PGC1 beta (peroxisome-proliferator-activated receptor-gamma co-activator 1 beta) gene in vitro and in vivo. *Biochem J* 2003;373:155–165.

146. St-Pierre J, Lin J, Krauss S, Tarr PT, Yang R, Newgard CB, Spiegelman BM. Bioenergetic analysis of peroxisome proliferator-activated receptor gamma coactivators 1alpha and 1beta (PGC-1alpha and PGC-1beta) in muscle cells. *J Biol Chem* 2003;278:26597–26603. Epub May 6, 2003.

147. Lin J, Handschin C, Spiegelman BM. Metabolic control through the PGC-1 family of transcription coactivators. *Cell Metab* 2005;1:361–370.

148. Yoon JC, Puigserver P, Chen G, Donovan J, Wu Z, Rhee J, Adelmant G, Stafford J, Kahn CR, Granner DK, Newgard CB, Spiegelman BM. Control of hepatic gluconeogenesis through the transcriptional coactivator PGC-1. *Nature* 2001;413:131–138.

149. Knutti D, Kressler D, Kralli A. Regulation of the transcriptional coactivator PGC-1 via MAPK-sensitive interaction with a repressor. *Proc Natl Acad Sci USA* 2001;98:9713–9718. Epub July 31, 2001.

150. Fan M, Rhee J, St-Pierre J, Handschin C, Puigserver P, Lin J, Jaeger S, Erdjument-Bromage H, Tempst P, Spiegelman BM. Suppression of mitochondrial respiration through recruitment of p160 myb binding protein to PGC-1alpha: Modulation by p38 MAPK. *Genes Dev* 2004;18:278–289. Epub January 26, 2004.

151. Schreiber SN, Knutti D, Brogli K, Uhlmann T, Kralli A. The transcriptional coactivator PGC-1 regulates the expression and activity of the orphan nuclear receptor estrogen-related receptor alpha (ERRalpha). *J Biol Chem* 2003;278:9013–9018. Epub January 8, 2003.

152. Mootha VK, Handschin C, Arlow D, Xie X, St Pierre J, Sihag S, Yang W, Altshuler D, Puigserver P, Patterson N, Willy PJ, Schulman IG, Heyman RA, Lander ES, Spiegelman BM. Erralpha and Gabpa/b specify PGC-1alpha-dependent oxidative phosphorylation gene expression that is altered in diabetic muscle. *Proc Natl Acad Sci USA* 2004;101:6570–6575. Epub April 20, 2004.

153. Schreiber SN, Emter R, Hock MB, Knutti D, Cardenas J, Podvinec M, Oakeley EJ, Kralli A. The estrogen-related receptor alpha (ERRalpha) functions in PPARgamma coactivator 1alpha (PGC-1alpha)-induced mitochondrial biogenesis. *Proc Natl Acad Sci USA* 2004;101:6472–6477. Epub April 15, 2004.

154. Willy PJ, Murray IR, Qian J, Busch BB, Stevens Jr. WC, Martin R, Mohan R, Zhou S, Ordentlich P, Wei P, Sapp DW, Horlick RA, Heyman RA, Schulman IG. Regulation of PPARgamma coactivator 1alpha (PGC-1alpha) signaling by an estrogen-related receptor alpha (ERRalpha) ligand. *Proc Natl Acad Sci USA* 2004;101:8912–8917. Epub June 7, 2004.

155. Kallen J, Schlaeppi JM, Bitsch F, Filipuzzi I, Schilb A, Riou V, Graham A, Strauss A, Geiser M, Fournier B. Evidence for ligand-independent transcriptional activation of the human estrogen-related receptor alpha (ERRalpha): Crystal structure of ERRalpha ligand binding domain in complex with peroxisome proliferator-activated receptor coactivator-1alpha. *J Biol Chem* 2004;279:49330–49337. Epub August 26, 2004.

156. Schulman IG, Heyman RA. The flip side: Identifying small molecule regulators of nuclear receptors. *Chem Biol* 2004;11:639–646.

157. Langin D, Lucas S, Lafontan M. Millennium fat-cell lipolysis reveals unsuspected novel tracks. *Horm Metab Res* 2000;32:443–452.
158. Li P, Zhu Z, Lu Y, Granneman JG. Metabolic and cellular plasticity in white adipose tissue II: Role of peroxisome proliferator-activated receptor-alpha. *Am J Physiol Endocrinol Metab* 2005;289:E617–E626. Epub June 7, 2005.
159. Bodkin NL, Pill J, Meyer K, Hansen BC. The effects of K-111, a new insulin-sensitizer, on metabolic syndrome in obese prediabetic rhesus monkeys. *Horm Metab Res* 2003;35:617–624.
160. Schafer SA, Hansen BC, Volkl A, Fahimi HD, Pill J. Biochemical and morphological effects of K-111, a peroxisome proliferator-activated receptor (PPAR)alpha activator, in non-human primates. *Biochem Pharmacol* 2004;68:239–251.

21 History and Regulation of Prescription and Over-the-Counter Weight Loss Drugs

Susan M. Schwartz, PhD and David M. Savastano, PhD

CONTENTS

INTRODUCTION

Drug therapy for obesity has experienced a very checkered past. Starting in the 1930s, over 10 drugs with various mechanisms of action have been approved in the United States for weight loss including three for long-term therapy, yet in 2011 only one drug remains on the market [1]. Nonprescription weight loss medications such as phenylpropanolamine hydrochloride (PPA) have had a similar fate.

Both prescription and over-the-counter (OTC) medications are intended to be used in conjunction with a program of diet control, physical activity, and behavioral modification. However, the setting under which these drugs are used is quite different. The former must be administered and used under the guidance of a physician, whereas OTC products are available without a gatekeeper to a much broader audience and involve self-medication.

The chapter examines the history of prescription and nonprescription drugs indicated for weight loss, the regulatory pathways and challenges with each, and the future role for medications in the treatment of overweight and obesity. Although the greatest proportion of the OTC category for weight loss is dietary supplements, these are not covered in the discussion as dietary supplement products are not formally evaluated and/or recognized as safe and effective by the Food and Drug Administration (FDA). There are several papers, however, which have reviewed dietary supplements for weight loss [2–4].

HISTORY OF PRESCRIPTION MEDICATIONS

In the past, there have been a number of drug therapies for weight loss, most of which have been removed from the market due to safety concerns (Table 21.1). In 1938, the first clinical study showing the efficacy of amphetamine (Benzedrine) on weight loss was published in the *New England Journal of Medicine* [5]. Unfortunately, although effective, the weight loss was accompanied with addiction. As we learned more about the role of the hypothalamus on appetite and energy metabolism, new groups of drugs to treat obesity were developed. These included drugs that acted on the

phenylpropanolamine. PPA was removed from the market in 2005 and reclassified as nonmonograph, not generally recognized as safe and effective [21]. In addition, FDA has encouraged manufacturers to remove benzocaine products from the market due to lack of efficacy data in weight reduction; it remains to be reevaluated as part of FDA's OTC drug review [22]. Most recently, there have been safety concerns raised with benzocaine topical products [23].

In 2005, the first new drug application (NDA) submitted to FDA for an OTC weight loss indication was for orlistat 60 mg. This dose had been shown to inhibit absorption of ~25% of ingested fat compared with the prescription dose of orlistat 120 mg which inhibits ~30% of dietary fat [24]. Although half the therapeutic dose, orlistat 60 mg exhibits about 85% the efficacy of the prescription drug [25,26].

The efficacy of orlistat at the 60 mg dose was evaluated in three randomized, double-blind, multicenter, placebo-controlled clinical trials [25–27]. In all three studies, subjects were instructed to take orlistat 60 mg or placebo three times a day (TID) with main meals in conjunction with a reduced calorie diet in which 30% of the calories were from fat. Two studies were conducted in subjects who were primarily obese [25,26], whereas a 4 month study was conducted in overweight subjects (BMI 25–28 kg/m^2) [27].

In all three studies, orlistat 60 mg–treated subjects lost significantly more weight than placebo-treated subjects after 4 months [27], 6 months, or 1 year of treatment [25,26]. In both the longer-term studies, the percentage of subjects who achieved a weight loss of ≥5% was significantly greater than placebo at the end of year 1 [25,26]. In addition, when examined following 6 months of treatment, similar results were observed, demonstrating a greater percent of orlistat subjects achieving a ≥5% weight loss compared with placebo [28].

Orlistat 60 mg was approved by the FDA for OTC use in February 2007. To date, it is the only FDA-approved OTC weight loss product indicated for weight loss in overweight adults who are ≥18 years of age. It is marketed by GlaxoSmithKline with educational booklets and an online behavior support program. The 60 mg dose also is available as a nonprescription drug in Europe and an increasing number of other markets globally.

REGULATORY GUIDELINES FOR PRESCRIPTION DRUGS

The regulation of prescription weight loss drugs can be considered as three separate chapters. From 1947 to 1973, drugs approved for weight loss were amphetamines and amphetamine derivatives. These drugs were indicated for treatment of obesity in any patient including adolescent, geriatric, and pregnant.

In the 1960s, the FDA commissioned a psychiatric drug panel and conducted a meta-analysis on all trials of amphetamines and derivatives. Based on the outcomes of these events, in 1973, the FDA issued an official position on these anorectic weight loss drugs concluding that although effective, these drugs had limited usefulness in treating obesity. There also was an overriding concern about the growing abuse of these drugs. Beginning around 1974, FDA established weight loss drugs as a short-term adjunct for the management of obesity in conjunction with caloric restriction.

The indication and role of long-term treatment for obesity was first considered at an NIH consensus conference [29] followed by a workshop on pharmacologic treatment of obesity [30]. Moreover, in 1992, the results of the phentermine and fenfluramine trials were published, demonstrating the efficacy of long-term treatment [6]. The FDA issued a draft Guidance for the Clinical Evaluation of Weight-Loss Drugs in 1996 [31]. The guidance provided recommendations on clinical drug development programs to examine the safety and efficacy of drugs intended to improve "health and self-esteem by reducing body fat" ([31, p. 1]). The document included guidance on duration and size, patient population, and efficacy criteria. Specifically, criteria were defined: a mean weight loss ≥5% in the drug versus placebo-treated patients or the proportion of subjects losing ≥5% is significantly greater in subjects on drug than in those on placebo. The guidance encouraged measuring the drug's effect on quality of life and obesity-associated cardiovascular risk factors during treatment, which could help in assessing the benefit-risk balance.

The 1996 guidance was never finalized, and in 2004, FDA issued a request for public comment on the 1996 draft guidance in order to understand recent scientific and clinical advances in weight management drug development. Some of the major considerations raised involved the size and duration of studies, efficacy criteria, and patient populations. As a result of the public comment and a subsequent advisory committee meeting, a revised draft guidance was issued in February 2007, which included several areas of interest that were not incorporated into in the 1996 guidance [32]. These included guidelines on the development of products for weight management in pediatric patients, patients with medication-induced weight gain, and recommendations on the development of combinations of weight-management products. No further revisions to the guidance have been published since the 2007 version.

REGULATORY GUIDELINES FOR OTC DRUGS

The regulatory path for OTC weight loss drugs involved two different pathways: the monograph system and NDA. Up until recently, the only drugs for weight loss were defined in the OTC monograph [14]. The 1982 monograph for weight control drug products provided information on the definition of a weight loss product, indication statements, target population, and duration of use. In particular, the monograph defined the target population as "adult obese persons free of known underlying organic diseases" and defined obesity as an increase in body weight as a result of an "excessive accumulation of fat in the body." One was considered obese if he or she were over 10% of the ideal body weight based on Metropolitan Life Insurance tables. There were no BMI criteria included. Duration of use, similar to the prescription products at the time, was only for 3 months and in conjunction with a reduced-calorie diet. Based on the monograph, a product could be marketed if accepted ingredients were included and the labeling of the product complied with the monograph.

Quite distinct from the OTC monograph process, a drug may be approved as OTC by switching a prescription drug to an OTC indication (Rx-to-OTC "switch"). This requires submission of an NDA which includes efficacy and safety results from controlled clinical trials, postmarketing data on the prescription drug, and consumer behavior studies. In recent years, only the switch route is available for approval of an OTC weight loss drug since the monograph system is no longer applicable; PPA is no longer on the market and benzocaine is not generally considered effective for weight loss [22].

Although all new OTC drugs had to be proven safe and properly labeled before they could be marketed [33], during earlier switches, there were no criteria to distinguish between prescription and OTC drugs. Consequently, products with the same ingredients were often marketed as both OTC and prescription [33]. As a result, in 1951 the Durham–Humphrey amendment provided specific criteria for distinguishing between prescription and OTC drugs. The amendment specified that addictive drugs and medicines that needed to be used under the supervision of a licensed health-care professional based on safety criteria could only be sold as prescription. Also, drugs which were approved for use under professional supervision would require a prescription for purchase.

In 1962, regulatory requirements were expanded by the Kefauver–Harris amendment. This regulation required FDA review of both nonprescription and prescription drugs applications. Thus, OTC drugs needed to demonstrate efficacy when used without supervision of a health-care provider. It is important to note that if a prescription drug is approved for OTC marketing, the prescription medicine can only remain on the market if it has a different indication or dose from the OTC version.

Although a drug application for an OTC indication requires demonstration of efficacy and safety based on randomized controlled clinical trials, additional criteria must be addressed if the drug is to be made available under an OTC setting (Table 21.2). The consumer must be able to recognize and diagnose the condition specified in the proposed indication; the consumer must be able to read the label and pull out the key information in order to use the drug properly, and the drug must be effective and safe when used as instructed [34].

Three types of consumer research studies are conducted as part of the switch process in order to predict the consumer's behavior to an OTC drug. These include label comprehension, self-selection, and actual use studies [33].

TABLE 21.2
Criteria for Rx-to-OTC Switch

Criteria	Requirements	Endpoint/Objective
Clinical data to support efficacy and safety	Clinical data of prescription drug evaluated; additional studies may be required with proposed OTC dose	Support benefit/risk in OTC environment
Proposed labeling	Label is directed to the consumer with words that are easily understood. Follows standard format of OTC drug facts: active ingredients, purpose, use (indication), specific warnings, directions, and inactive ingredients	Provides information that allows consumers to determine whether the drug is appropriate for their condition and how it should be used and clearly communicates safety considerations
Clinical safety U.S. and worldwide adverse event data	The likely total patient exposure to the prescription drug should be more than sufficient in both time and extent to satisfy any potential FDA safety concerns	Support benefit/risk in OTC environment
Label comprehension	A series of consumer research studies in which individuals are asked to read the label and answer questions to test their ability to read and comprehend the label's key messages	Demonstration that consumers can read and comprehend the information that details the safe and effective use of the OTC product
Self-selection	Consumer research studies in which individuals are provided with label and asked questions to determine whether the drug is appropriate for them to use; often incorporated into label comprehension and/or actual use studies	A label which clearly communicates who should or should not use the product
AUT	An open label study conducted under simulated OTC conditions in which subjects are provided with the drug to determine their ability to follow the label's directions for use, warnings, etc.	Demonstration that consumers can correctly self-select the product and use it appropriately

Label comprehension studies (LCSs) measure the ability of a consumer to read and extract the key information on a label (i.e., drug facts label): Is the drug appropriate for the treatment of their condition? Do they understand how to use the drug? Are they at risk for adverse events associated with the drug? and Do they know what to do if adverse events occur when taking the drug? [34]. In order for the drug to be used safely and effectively, the consumer must not only understand the information but know where the information is located. Data derived from an LCS can identify areas on the label that would benefit from clearer or simpler presentation of important consumer information.

Often, LCSs are designed to test the consumer's ability to apply label information to a hypothetical scenario in which the drug should or should not be used [34]. Since the label will be available to a very wide audience, subjects enrolled in these types of studies include both the general population and an enriched group of individuals with low literacy (<8th grade literacy).

Developing the final label is an iterative process in which each successive label study builds upon the previous one until a final label is considered "satisfactory" [42]. However, unlike randomized, controlled efficacy studies in which results are either positive or negative based on the hypothesis being tested, in an LCS, it can be difficult to determine when the label is good enough. There are multiple key messages on the label, some of which may be clinically more important than others. For example, the failure of an adult consumer to notice the age restriction on the label may not be clinically critical, whereas not paying attention to a certain warning could have major health risk. Thus, analysis and interpretation of results can be difficult [35].

The self-selection study is similar to LCSs in that the consumer must be able to recognize and comprehend the information [34]. However, this type of study tests the consumer's behavior to the label information. Specifically, it assesses whether the consumer can correctly decide whether the drug is appropriate for him or her to use based on the individual's health condition and label warnings and indication. Recruited subjects usually are individuals who might purchase the drug for their own use. With little cueing or assistance, subjects are provided with the package and proposed label and are asked whether the drug is appropriate for them. Whether they answer correct or incorrect is determined by the subject's self-reported medical history and the information on the label. In some cases, certain warnings on the label could have a greater medical consequence than other information and may be weighted differently in determining adequate self-selection [33].

Once a final label has been developed based on sufficient label comprehension and self-selection, an actual use trial (AUT) is usually conducted to directly assess consumer behavior by simulating OTC use [35]. Importantly, the AUT provides evidence of how the drug will be used once it is available OTC. In this type of trial, the consumer can purchase the drug, take it home, and use it without physician supervision. Unlike prescription drugs in which it is assumed that patients will be compliant and use the drug appropriately under medical guidance, an AUT observes consumer behavior in the OTC setting with regard to self-selection and purchase, adherence, safety, and in some cases, efficacy [33].

Although certain design aspects of AUTs may differ, almost all tend to be single arm, multicenter, uncontrolled, and open label. One of the most recent AUTs was conducted for the orlistat 120 mg to 60 mg switch process. This study was designed to monitor any safety concerns and answer several questions: Do subjects dose correctly? Do they complian? and can they lose weight? [36]. Conducted in 18 pharmacies, it was a 3 month, open-label, naturalistic trial and was designed to be as unobtrusive as possible to minimize affecting the behaviors being measured. Consumers were allowed to purchase orlistat packages containing a bottle of orlistat 60 mg plus educational materials, which provided lifestyle information and tools to encourage successful weight loss.

For those subjects who used and purchased the product (n = 237), most individuals followed the dosing directions (3 capsules/d with meals containing fat) throughout the study, and the majority of subjects took a daily multivitamin, as instructed on the label. In addition, 80% reported following a diet 14 days after enrollment (reduced calorie and/or low fat), and over the study duration, 51% of subjects reported more frequent or longer exercise relative to enrollment [36]. Although not designed as an efficacy trial, measured and self-reported relative median weight loss was approximately 5% after ≥60 days of using orlistat (Figure 21.1). The safety profile for orlistat in this trial was consistent with the results from randomized, placebo-controlled trials, and no unexpected adverse events were observed.

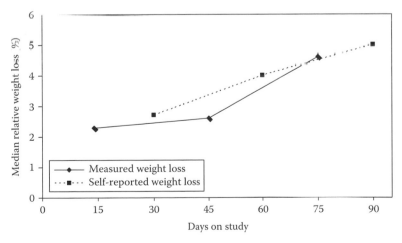

FIGURE 21.1 Measured and self-reported relative weight change in AUT of 60 mg orlistat. ♦: Sample size for measured weight loss is the number of subjects who were weighed at each time point. ■: Sample size for self-reported weight loss is the number of subjects at each time point who responded yes or no to the question, "Since you started using the study medication have you lost any weight?" (Reprinted from Schwartz, S.M. et al., *Obesity*, 16, 623, 2008.)

As part of the regulatory review process, findings from the AUT helped to provide assurance that orlistat 60 mg could be used appropriately and safely without physician supervision or dietary counseling.

These types of consumer studies can be challenging, often requiring novel trial design and measurement of multiple behavioral endpoints. Several papers have addressed some of these issues [34,35]. In response to these concerns, in August 2010, FDA issued a guidance on LCSs for nonprescription drug products based on advice obtained from a 2006 meeting of the FDA Nonprescription Drug Advisory Committee and comments received regarding the draft guidance published in May, 2009 [37]. The guidance covers circumstances in which LCSs may be required, for example, approval of a new drug product, new indication or target population, and significant labeling changes. In addition, it provides recommendations on study design and conduct, study population as well as statistical analysis and interpretation of study results.

FUTURE OF PRESCRIPTION AND OTC DRUGS

The past 30 years have been a difficult time for prescription weight loss drugs. There is a great need for new treatments, but since the approval of orlistat in 1998, no drugs have been approved in the United States. A major hurdle for antiobesity drugs has been the benefit-to-risk ratio. Every drug carries risks, and when a drug is used by so many people, potentially one-third of a population, that risk is magnified.

Drawing upon the history of effective combination drug therapies in treating conditions such as diabetes and hypertension, one approach for obesity treatment is to combine drugs in order to improve the weight loss effect. The first combination of drugs used for obesity were caffeine and ephedrine [38] followed by the Fen/Phen combination [6]. Both combinations together had an additive or synergistic effect on weight loss, but due to safety concerns, two of the drugs are no longer available. Other combinations have been examined including PPA and benzocaine, orlistat and sibutramine, and orlistat and metformin; none of the combinations were shown to enhance weight loss as compared to the drug(s) alone [39]. Recently, a study combining sibutramine or phentermine with pramlintide demonstrated greater weight loss with both combinations as compared to pramlintide or placebo alone [40]. However, the study design did not include single arms for sibutramine or phentermine, which are both antiobesity drugs. Pramlintide is not an approved weight loss drug, and in this study, weight loss was not significantly different from placebo in the evaluable population.

In 2010 and 2011, FDA denied the approval of two weight loss drug combinations—phentermine and topiramate (Qnexa) and bupropion and naltrexone (Contrave)—despite the FDA's Endocrine and Metabolic Drugs Advisory Committee's endorsement of Contrave. A third new drug, lorcaserin hydrochloride (Lorgess), also was not approved by FDA. All the combination candidates are approved drugs: bupropion is widely used for depression and smoking cessation, naltrexone is used to treat addiction, phentermine is for short-term weight loss, and topiramate is indicated as an anticonvulsant [1].

In all cases, the FDA did not feel the drugs had enough of a benefit to justify the risks. FDA had concerns about cardiovascular risks and birth defects for Qnexa, and for Contrave, the FDA required a long-term study to examine cardiovascular risk. There also were concerns about an increased cancer rate in rats with lorcaserin.

Despite setbacks, combination therapy continues to be an avenue of future drug development. Phase II and III clinical trials have been conducted using combination drug therapy for weight loss including Empatic, a combination of zonisamide, which is used in the treatment of partial seizures, and bupropion and pramlintide/metreleptin, a combination of an approved drug for treatment of diabetes and an analog of human leptin [1].

Pharmaceutical and biotech companies continue to investigate new therapeutic candidates based on pathophysiological mechanisms which modulate food intake including peptides of the gut, pancreas, and fat, and the involvement of multiple pathways within the nervous system. For example, ZGN-433 is a methionine aminopeptidase inhibitor which targets adipose tissue, and ezlopitant is a neurokinin receptor-1 (NK1R) antagonist [41]. The NK1R system has been implicated in both learned appetitive behaviors and addiction to alcohol and opioids. Several approved antidiabetes drugs are also being examined as possible antiobesity drugs: pramlintide, a synthetic analog of the pancreatic hormone amylin, and liraglutide and exenatide, glucagon-like peptide-1 (GLP-1) receptor agonists [1,41].

Within the OTC market, it is unlikely there will be any new FDA-approved drugs in the near future. The benefit to risk is even more critical since an OTC medicine can be used without professional supervision and is accessible to anyone. Moreover, an Rx-to-OTC switch first requires the prescription drug to have a number of years of postmarketing data and is usually considered in the late life cycle of the drug.

In a recent editorial in *Obesity Reviews*, Anti-obesity drugs: to be or not to be?, [42] the authors conclude, "Decisions that will only serve to stifle further drug development for one of the most important unmet needs of our times should concern us all." Given the recent trends, there is increased skepticism about the feasibility of obtaining market approval for antiobesity drugs in the United States and globally. Coupled with the enormous investment of time and resources in bringing an antiobesity drug to market, new drug candidates may wane.

Obesity continues to be a major health issue globally, and prevention strategies are critical to curb this epidemic. However, for those overweight and obese individuals who are not able to respond effectively to diet and physical activity, other options in conjunction with lifestyle changes are essential. There needs to be greater medical acceptance that obesity is a disease that needs available treatments, rather than a lifestyle change that people can make. Rather than hurdles, we hope the future will bring more medical, regulatory, and economic support so that novel weight loss drugs with greater efficacy and safety can be developed and approved for weight management.

REFERENCES

1. Ioannides-Demos LL, Piccenna L, McNeil JJ. Pharmacotherapies for obesity: Past, current, and future therapies. *Journal of Obesity* 2011;2011:1–18.
2. Alraei RG. Herbal and dietary supplements for weight loss. *Topics in Clinical Nutrition* 2010;25:136–150.
3. Pittler MH, Ernst E. Complementary therapies for reducing body weight: A systematic review. *International Journal of Obesity* 2005;29:1030–1038.
4. Gibson-Moore H. Do slimming supplements work? *Nutrition Bulletin* 2010;35:300–303.
5. Lesses MF, Myerson A. Human autonomic pharmacology. XVI. Benzedrine sulfate as an aid in the treatment of obesity. *New England Journal of Medicine* 1938;218:119–124.
6. Weintraub M. Long-term weight control: The National Heart, Lung, and Blood Institute funded multimodal intervention study: Introduction. *Clinical Pharmacology & Therapeutics* 1992;51:581–585.
7. Connolly HM, Crary JL, McGoon MD, Hensrud DD, Edwards BS, Edwards WD, Schaff HV. Valvular heart disease associated with fenfluramine phentermine. *New England Journal of Medicine* 1997;337:581–588.
8. Garfield AS, Heisler LK. Pharmacological targeting of the serotonergic system for the treatment of obesity. *Journal of Physiology* 2009;587:49–60.
9. Buckett WR, Thomas PC, Luscombe GP. The pharmacology of sibutramine hydrochloride (BTS 54 524), a new antidepressant which induces rapid noradrenergic down-regulation. *Progress in Neuro-Psychopharmacology and Biological Psychiatry* 1988;12:575–584.
10. Ryan DH, Kaiser P, Bray GA. Sibutramine: A novel new agent for obesity treatment. *Obesity Research* 1995;3(Suppl 4):553S–559S.
11. Padwal R, Rucker D, Li SK, Curionni C, Lau DC. Long-term pharmacotherapy for obesity and overweight. *Cochrane Database of Systematic Reviews* 2003 (4):CD004094.
12. Christensen R, Kristensen PK, Bartels EM, Bliddal H, Astrup A. Efficacy and safety of the weight-loss drug rimonabant: A meta-analysis of randomised trials. *Lancet* 2007;370:1706–1713.
13. James WPT, Caterson ID, Coutinho W, Finer N, Van Gaal LF, Maggioni AP, Torp-Pedersen C, Sharma AM, Shepherd GM, et al. Effect of sibutramine on cardiovascular outcomes in overweight and obese subjects. *New England Journal of Medicine* 2010;363:905–917.

Part V

Safety of Obesity Drugs

22 Safety of Obesity Drugs

Alok K. Gupta, MD, FAAFP, FASH and Frank L. Greenway, MD

CONTENTS

BACKGROUND

During the early development of mankind, acquisition of food for sustenance was a major physical endeavor. It was also a difficult task due to the paucity of food. Humans have thus evolved by adapting to famine more than plenty [1]. An increased availability of food without the need for physical activity to acquire it is thought to have favored weight gain: a mismatch between energy intake (easy availability of energy dense foods) and energy expenditure (increased sedentary life style). This trend toward overweight and the obese state began increasing dramatically in the United States around the 1980s [2] and is currently being observed worldwide [3,4] affecting not only the adults [5] but also children and adolescents [6]. Which environmental change(s) explain this recent increased prevalence of obesity is not clear, but genetic mutations (being slow to manifest) are unlikely to be responsible. Obesity predisposes to cardiovascular disease, diabetes mellitus, and other medical conditions [7], all of which have both medical and economic consequences. Obesity alone is clearly a major public health problem in the United States [8,9] with an estimated cost of $100 billion per year.

It has only been since the NIH consensus conference of 1985 classified obesity as a chronic disease [2] that drugs have been approved for the long-term obesity treatment. It was, however, the discovery of leptin in 1994 that spurred scientific inquiry into the mechanisms of obesity. Despite the new scientific interest in obesity, we are at the same place with obesity drugs today as we were with hypertension drugs in the 1950s. In the 1950s, we had thiazide diuretics that caused a loss of sodium in urine and centrally acting drugs like reserpine that had side effects related to their upstream mechanisms. With the recent withdrawal of sibutramine from the market, orlistat is the only obesity drug that remains approved for long-term use. Orlistat causes loss of fat in the stool and can be likened to thiazides that cause urinary sodium loss in hypertension. Sibutramine with its suppression of central noradrenergic neuronal reuptake prevented the improvement in blood pressure and heart rate that was usually associated with weight loss. The Food and Drug Administration (FDA) requested a voluntary withdrawal of this drug due to an increase in cardiovascular events associated with its use in participants with established cardiovascular disease.

Since 1994, there has been active investigation into the mechanisms of obesity, and many potential drug targets have progressed through the developmental pipeline. Just as hypertension drugs now act upon peripheral blood vessel targets with minimal side effects [10], it is likely that by targeting peripheral, instead of central mechanisms, a similar evolution will be seen in the development of safe drugs for the treatment of obesity. Since the scientific tools available for drug development are far more advanced today than those that were available in the 1950s, it is reasonable to believe that the road to safer and more effective obesity drugs will be not only quicker but also more efficient than was for drugs treating hypertension.

Not only does obesity represent a public health concern, but it is also a stigmatized condition, especially for women in Western societies [11]. Since the stigma may compel some to take unwarranted risks to lose weight, the safety of obesity drugs takes on a particular concern. We will review the safety of obesity drugs, pointing out that the history of obesity drugs is littered with safety disasters [12]. We will review the safety of currently available drugs for the treatment of obesity and of those obesity drugs that were and are in the approval process with the U.S. FDA. We will then discuss the safety of drugs that are available for other indications but result in weight loss and touch on the potential for herbs in the development of safe and effective obesity drugs.

OBESITY DRUGS: A HISTORICAL PRESCRIPTIVE

THYROID HORMONE

As early as 1893, thyroid hormone was used to induce weight loss [13]. Thyroxine at 150mcg/day increases weight loss, but 75% of this additional weight loss occurs from the loss of lean tissue, rather than from the loss of fat. A loss of lean tissue increases mortality, while a loss of fat decreases mortality [14].

Thyroid hormone stimulates cardiac muscular inotropy and chronotropy and causes cardiac muscular hypertrophy. Since obesity itself increases the cardiac work load, this aspect of thyroid hormone action adds to that burden. Thyroid hormone, appropriately, is no longer used as a treatment for obesity.

DINITROPHENOL

During World War I, French munitions workers, using a mixture of dinitrophenol and trinitrophenol, were noted to have toxic symptoms and even death from hyperthermia [15]. Animal studies demonstrated a stimulation of respiration along with a rise in body temperature with dinitrophenol [16,17]. Dinitrophenol is a weak acid that binds to protons. It can cross membranes protonated and return as an anion to repeat the cycle. Thus, it increases the basal proton conductance in the mitochondria, uncouples oxidative phosphorylation from ATP generation, and increases the loss of calories as heat. In the 1930s, a series of controlled studies with dinitrophenol were undertaken at Stanford University. A dinitrophenol dose–response relationship was demonstrated, where every dose increase of 100 mg resulted in an 11% increase in the resting metabolic rate. Patients taking dinitrophenol experienced warmth and sweating, but tolerated dosages from 500 mg up to 1 g a day, when attention was given to the individualization of drug dose based on the increase in metabolic rate. Dosages of dinitrophenol between 300 and 500 mg/day induced a 40% increase in resting metabolic rate, an increase which was sustained over 10 weeks. Unlike the thyroid hormone, which was in use for weight loss at the same time, dinitrophenol did not increase nitrogen excretion [18], suggesting that weight loss resulted from the loss of fat and not of lean tissue. Dinitrophenol caused edema in some people, offsetting some of the weight loss. This edema resolved and the weight loss became manifest after the drug was discontinued. Dinitrophenol did not increase blood pressure but indeed lowered blood pressure and improved glucose metabolism with continued treatment. It was released to an enthusiastic populace (100,000 people took dinitrophenol in 1934) as a weight loss drug without the need for diet modification [19]. Dinitrophenol was sold directly to the public in patent medicines. This resulted in accidental and intentional overdoses causing deaths from hyperthermia. Rashes, loss of the ability to taste sweet or salt, and cataracts were also reported. In addition, a small number of cases of agranulocytosis were reported. In 1938, the FDA acquired new powers to regulate drug manufacture. The sales of dinitrophenol were halted due to threats of prosecution by the FDA.

AMPHETAMINES

Amphetamine was first synthesized in 1887. The psychopharmacological properties of amphetamine, however, were not described until 1927. Amphetamine was found to induce euphoria, increase energy, wakefulness, and alertness in addition to decreasing fatigue. During clinical testing in 1937, weight loss was reported [9,20]. Amphetamines and related compounds cause weight loss by inhibiting food intake through the release of norepinephrine in nerve terminals centrally. Alpha-methyl-para-tyrosine, an inhibitor of noradrenaline synthesis, increased feeding when injected into the perifornical area of the hypothalamus [21]. Weight loss was reported in response to amphetamine in both obese adults and children in 1938 [22].

Amphetamine has stimulatory effects on blood pressure and heart rate and causes the release of free fatty acids through its adrenergic mechanism. It also has a potential for addiction and abuse. Amphetamine is a Drug Enforcement Administration (DEA) schedule II drug, as are dextroamphetamine and methamphetamine. They are, therefore, rarely used any longer for the treatment of obesity.

RAINBOW PILLS

Diet pills containing thyroid hormone, digitalis, diuretics, laxatives, and amphetamine became popular in the 1960s. Since different colors were to be taken at different times of the day, they were called rainbow pills. The potential for drug interactions and toxicity should be obvious from

Rimonabant was studied in phase III clinical trials with over 6000 patients, including those with dyslipidemia, and received an approvable letter for treatment of obesity from the FDA in February 2006 [51]. Published trials have shown a reduction in triglycerides, small dense low-density lipoprotein particles, and an increase in high-density lipoprotein–cholesterol in patients meeting the criteria for the metabolic syndrome, with numbers which were in excess of those expected from the weight loss induced by the drug [52]. Rimonabant at 20 mg/day has a weight loss efficacy similar to sibutramine. Nausea and diarrhea are prominent side effects and consistent with CB-1 receptors being present in the gastrointestinal tract. Anxiety, insomnia, dizziness, and depression are also seen, and might be expected, since they are the opposite emotions associated with marijuana smoking.

The European Medicines Agency approved the use of rimonabant for the treatment of obesity in 2006, but not for smoking cessation. The approval letter by the FDA triggered a review process which was followed by an advisory panel meeting in 2007. The advisory panel voted against the approval of rimonabant which prompted the sponsor to suspend the new drug application (NDA). The European Medicines Agency, citing the risks outweighing the benefits for use of rimonabant in the European Union, directed that its sales be stopped in October 2008. The drug development program was completely abandoned in November 2008. The results from the trials, STRADIVARIUS—detailing progression of atherosclerosis in patients with abdominal obesity and coronary artery disease, and CRESCENDO—elucidating the prevention of cardiovascular events, have since been published [53,54]. Although rimonabant did not slow the progression of atherosclerosis or lead to a reduction in cardiovascular events, it did provide significant improvement of cardiometabolic risk factors. The neuropsychiatric, serious psychiatric side effects, including suicide, appeared to be common to all members of this drug class and with the withdrawal of rimonabant. All other CB-1 receptor antagonist drugs under development were abandoned.

SIBUTRAMINE

Sibutramine is a noradrenaline and serotonin (5-HT) reuptake inhibitor that was approved for the long-term treatment of obesity in 1997. Since sibutramine causes an increase in the concentration of noradrenaline and serotonin in the intraneuronal cleft in response to food intake, it increases satiety. Sibutramine increases thermogenesis to a lesser degree [55]. Like most other obesity drugs, sibutramine-associated weight loss occurs over 6 months of treatment and plateaus after this 6 month period in the registration studies lasting up to 2 years [56,57]. Sibutramine reduces serum triglycerides, increases high-density lipoprotein cholesterol [58], and improves glucose control in patients with diabetes [59,60]. Sibutramine does not provide the decrease in blood pressure and heart rate expected with weight loss, and it is contraindicated in patients with uncontrolled hypertension, coronary heart disease, cardiac dysrhythmias, congestive heart failure, or stroke [61]. It is distributed as capsules of 5, 10, and 15 mg taken once a day and is typically started at 10 mg/day. The dose can be adjusted up to 15 mg/day or down to 5 mg/day depending on response while monitoring the blood pressure and pulse. The rise in blood pressure is modest and is usually offset by the decrease in weight. Sibutramine is associated with dry mouth, insomnia, constipation, headache, and dizziness. These symptoms are similar to some of those seen with the amphetamine derivatives since both medications increase noradrenergic activity. Although there is no evidence of abuse, sibutramine carries a DEA schedule IV due to its structural similarities with amphetamine [62].

Sibutramine is contraindicated in patients receiving monoamine oxidase inhibitors (MAOIs), patients who have a hypersensitivity to sibutramine or any of the inactive ingredients, in the presence of a major eating disorder (anorexia nervosa or bulimia nervosa), and in patients taking other centrally acting weight loss drugs. Sibutramine should be used with caution in patients with a history of hypertension, coronary artery disease, congestive heart failure, arrhythmias, stroke, narrow-angle glaucoma, or pulmonary hypertension. The use of sibutramine comes with a warning relative to blood pressure and pulse since sibutramine substantially increases blood pressure and/or pulse rate in some patients. Blood pressure and pulse rate should be measured prior to starting therapy and should be monitored at regular intervals thereafter. For patients who experience a sustained increase in blood pressure or pulse rate, either a dose reduction or discontinuation of therapy should be considered. Sibutramine should not be given to patients with uncontrolled or poorly controlled hypertension.

A post-marketing study—the Sibutramine Cardiovascular Morbidity/Mortality Outcomes Study in Overweight or Obese Subjects at Risk of a Cardiovascular Event (SCOUT trial)—evaluated the long-term effects of sibutramine compared with placebo on the incidence of cardiovascular disease and death among high-risk subjects concurrently participating in a diet and exercise program [63]. Subjects participating in the SCOUT trial either had diabetes (a condition for which the drug was approved) or established cardiovascular disease (a condition for which the drug was not approved). A 16% increase in the risk of serious cardiovascular events such as nonfatal heart attack, nonfatal stroke, the need for resuscitation after cardiac arrest, and death were noted in the sibutramine group with established cardiovascular disease compared to the placebo group. The drug was removed from the European market in 2009 after the results of this 10,000-person post-marketing safety study requested by the European regulatory authorities were announced. The initial response of the U.S. FDA was to put a black box warning: not to use sibutramine in the face of established cardiovascular disease. On October 8, 2010, following the recommendation of their advisory panel, the U.S. FDA requested that sibutramine be voluntarily removed from the market. Abbott Laboratories complied with this request. The enrollment of people with contraindications to sibutramine in the SCOUT trial, the low incidence of cardiovascular events which drove the decision to do so, and letting subjects remain on the drug for years without a clinically significant weight loss have alerted the obesity field to the need for reevaluation of the design of any future cardiovascular safety studies for obesity drugs.

OBESITY DRUGS PRESENTLY AVAILABLE

AMPHETAMINE DERIVATIVES

The amphetamine derivatives benzphetamine and phendimetrazine are in DEA schedule III, while phentermine and diethylpropion are in DEA schedule IV. All four are currently available in the United States for treatment of obesity. They have less abuse and addiction potential than amphetamine itself. The abuse of these drugs during treatment of obesity has rarely been a problem, but these drugs have been sold and abused on the street for recreational purposes. Although benzphetamine and phendimetrazine are rarely used today, phentermine is the most commonly prescribed obesity medication [64]. These drugs were approved for continuous use up to 12 weeks when obesity was still considered to be the result of bad habits. The mechanism by which amphetamine-related drugs reduce weight is through the central release of noradrenaline which has the potential for CNS stimulation [65]. The potential for addiction is related to the ability of these drugs to also release dopamine in the CNS. As might be expected from their mechanism of action, these drugs can increase blood pressure and heart rate and stimulate lipolysis.

All amphetamine derivatives are contraindicated in the presence of hyperthyroidism, advanced arteriosclerotic vascular disease, moderate to severe hypertension, symptomatic cardiovascular disease, agitated states, a history of drug abuse, glaucoma, pregnancy (due to an association with fetal toxicity), lactation, within 14 days of MAOI drug use, and in the presence of a known sensitivity to sympathetic amines.

All the amphetamine derivatives should be used with caution when using hazardous machinery, since they could impair mental alertness and coordination. They should also be used with caution in the presence of mild to moderate hypertension or in people younger than 12 years of age, and its potential for addiction must be kept in mind.

BENZPHETAMINE

Benzphetamine was first used in 1960, is available as 25 mg tablets, and has similar but less frequent side effects than amphetamine. The contraindications and caution for the use of benzphetamine have been listed previously.

DIETHYLPROPION

Diethylpropion is available as 25 mg immediate-release and 75 mg sustained-release tablets. The potential for CNS stimulation and a rise in blood pressure is minimal due to the keto substitution on the β-carbon of phenethylamine side chain. Diethylpropion should be used with caution in people younger than 12 years of age and in people with epilepsy since it has initiated seizures in epileptic patients. The contraindications and caution for the use of diethylpropion have been listed previously.

PHENDIMETRAZINE

Phendimetrazine is available as 35 mg tablets with side effects similar to benzphetamine. Abnormal heart valves and PPH have been reported with phendimetrazine, and it should not be used with other anorectics. The contraindications and caution for the use of phendimetrazine have been listed previously.

PHENTERMINE

Phentermine is available as a resin in 15 and 30 mg tablets, and it is also available in 37.5 mg tablets. Phentermine has an α-methyl substitution on the phenethylamine side chain, resulting in a lower CNS stimulation potential. It can, however, increase blood pressure and heart rate, in addition to causing insomnia and dry mouth. Phentermine is the most prescribed obesity drug in the United States, and treatment on alternate months has been shown to be as efficacious as continuous treatment. Alternate month treatment allows the drug to be used for prolonged periods of time, while remaining within the constraints of the package insert limits the drug to no more than 12 weeks of continuous use [66].

Phentermine should not be used with selective serotonin reuptake inhibitors (SSRIs), and the drug should be stopped for symptoms of PPH or valvulopathy. These symptoms include dyspnea, angina, syncope, ankle edema, and deterioration in exercise tolerance. The contraindications and caution for the use of phentermine have been listed previously.

ORLISTAT

Orlistat is a reversible gastrointestinal lipase inhibitor (both gastric and pancreatic) that impairs the absorption of dietary fat from the intestinal lumen. It is approved for long-term use (since 1999) and acts entirely within the gastrointestinal tract. Orlistat treatment results in significant and sustained weight reduction in clinical trials lasting 2 years [67]. Orlistat improves low-density lipoprotein cholesterol more than expected from the weight loss it induces, possibly due to enforcing a low-fat diet [68,69]. Other lipid parameters improve in the manner expected with weight loss. Orlistat improves glucose metabolism in obese patients with and without diabetes [70,71] and reduces blood pressure in proportion to the weight loss it induces [72,73]. It is supplied by prescription as 120 mg capsules to be taken three times a day with meals. It is recommended that the drug be used with a 30% fat diet. Orlistat use can result in adverse gastrointestinal events including flatus with discharge, fatty stools, oily stools, oily spotting, oily evacuation, fecal urgency, fecal incontinence, increased defecation, and abdominal pain. These symptoms usually occur early in the course of treatment, are exaggerated in patients who eat a high-fat diet, and are rarely severe enough to cause discontinuation in clinical trials. A nightly multivitamin supplementation is recommended to compensate for impaired absorption of fat-soluble vitamins (A, D, E, and K). Despite the demonstrated benefits of orlistat, its use in clinical practice has been disappointing. This lack of use may be due to fear of side effects resulting from the FDA mandated warnings in direct to consumer advertising and the potential for fecal incontinence becoming fodder for late-night television comedians. An over-the-counter preparation of orlistat with a reduced dosage of 60 mg three times a day became available in 2007. Orlistat is contraindicated in patients with chronic malabsorption syndrome or cholestasis and in patients with known hypersensitivity to orlistat.

In August 2009, FDA announced an ongoing review of the potential for severe liver injury associated with the use of orlistat. With one case in the United States and 12 cases noted elsewhere, during a 10 year period of use by an estimated 40 million users worldwide, the FDA directed a revised label to include new safety information about cases of severe liver injury in May 2010. The users of orlistat are advised to stop its use if itching, yellow eyes or skin, fever, weakness, vomiting, fatigue, dark urine, light-colored stools, or loss of appetite occur. They are further advised to see their physician in follow-up at the earliest possible opportunity should these symptoms occur.

DRUGS APPROVED FOR OTHER REASONS THAT ARE ASSOCIATED WITH WEIGHT LOSS

BUPROPION

Bupropion is a norepinephrine and dopamine reuptake inhibitor that is approved for the treatment of depression and smoking cessation. It has been used in weight loss studies ranging from 8 to 48 weeks in doses of 300–400 mg/day. The largest trials included subjects with depressive symptoms [74] and subjects with uncomplicated obesity [75] enrolled across multiple centers. Weight loss in subjects with depressed symptoms treated with 300–400 mg of bupropion per day over a 6 month period was 6.0% in the bupropion group compared to 2.8% in the placebo group in those that completed the trial [74]. Weight loss in subjects with uncomplicated obesity was 5%, 7.2%, and 10.1% of initial body weight in subjects on placebo, 300 mg bupropion, and 400 mg bupropion groups, respectively [75]. Dropouts from the two trials were 45% and 30% at 6 months in the subjects with depressive symptoms and the uncomplicated obesity, respectively.

Bupropion can induce epilepsy (0.1% with doses up to 300 mg/day and 0.4% at a dose of 400 mg/day) and is contraindicated in patients with a seizure disorder. Patients with bulimia have a higher risk of seizures, and the use of bupropion in this patient group is contraindicated. Due to its association with epilepsy, bupropion should be administered with extreme caution in patients with a lowered seizure threshold (alcohol or drug withdrawal, history of head trauma, or the use of drugs such as theophylline). Due to its adrenergic mechanism, bupropion can be associated with hypertension and is contraindicated for use with MAOIs. Allergic reactions, agitation, tinnitus, pharyngitis, insomnia, psychosis, confusion, mania, neuropsychiatric phenomenon, and an increased risk for suicide in depressed patients have also been associated with bupropion use. Caution is advised if bupropion is used in subjects with hepatic or renal insufficiency.

EXENATIDE

Glucagon-like peptide-1 (GLP-1), or enteroglucagon, is a protein derived from proglucagon and secreted by L-cells in the terminal ileum and colon in response to a meal. GLP-1 decreases food intake and has been postulated to be responsible for the superior weight loss and substantial improvement in diabetes seen with obesity bypass surgery [76,77]. Increased GLP-1 inhibits glucagon secretion and stimulates insulin secretion and glycogenogenesis along with delaying the gastric emptying [78]. GLP-1 is rapidly degraded by dipeptidyl peptidase-4 (DPP-4), an enzyme that is elevated in the obese. Gastric bypass operations for obesity increase GLP-1 but do not change the levels of DPP-4 [79].

Exendin-4 is a 39-amino-acid peptide that is produced in the salivary gland of the Gila monster lizard. It has 53% homology with GLP-1 and has a much longer half-life. Exendin-4 induces satiety and weight loss in Zucker rats with peripheral administration and crosses the blood-brain barrier to act in the CNS [80,81]. It decreases food intake and body weight gain while lowering glycosylated hemoglobin [82]. It also increases beta-cell mass to a greater extent than would be expected for the degree of insulin resistance [83].

In humans, exendin-4 reduces fasting and postprandial glucose levels, slows gastric emptying, and decreases food intake by 19% [84]. It was tested in a placebo-controlled trial where 377 subjects with type 2 diabetes who were failing maximal sulfonylurea therapy were given 10 mcg subcutaneously per day for 30 weeks. The fasting glucose decreased, glycosylated hemoglobin fell 0.74% more than placebo, and there was a progressive weight loss of 1.6 kg [85]. The side effects are headache and nausea and vomiting, which can be lessened by gradual dose escalation [86]. Thus, exendin-4 shows promise of being an effective treatment for diabetes with a favorable weight loss profile.

Exenatide is contraindicated in patients with known hypersensitivity to this product or any of its components. Exenatide should be used with caution in subjects with severe gastrointestinal disease since exenatide can cause nausea, vomiting, and diarrhea. As with all drugs for the treatment of diabetes, one must be vigilant for hypoglycemia. Providing new information with regard to the following, the FDA has required post-marketing studies as follows:

1. Renal injury: http://www.fda.gov/safety/MedWatch/SafetyInformation/SafetyAlertsfor HumanMedicalProducts/ucm188703.htm
2. Pancreatitis: http://www.prescriber.org.uk/2008/08/exenatide-safety-warning/
3. Thyroid cancer and pancreatic cancer: http://www.fda.gov/Drugs/DrugSafety/ PostmarketDrugSafetyInformationforPatientsandProviders/Drug SafetyInformationfor HeathcareProfessionals/ucm190406.htm
4. Here is the safety concerns link from the FDA and New England Journal, respectively: http:// www.fda.gov/Drugs/DrugSafety/PostmarketDrugSafetyInformationforPatientsandProviders/ ucm198543.htm, http://www.nejm.org/doi/full/10.1056/NEJMp1001578

BYDURION

Bydurion is the once-weekly form of exenatide under development for treatment of diabetes mellitus. In a 26 week clinical study comparing sitagliptin, pioglitazone, or metformin, the three commonly prescribed oral type 2 diabetes medications, bydurion monotherapy, besides reducing glycosylated hemoglobin by 1.5%, resulted in a 4.5 lb weight loss (similar to 1.5% reduction and a 4.4 lb weight loss with metformin). The most frequently reported adverse events were nausea (withdrawal rate less than 1%) and diarrhea. The FDA has requested an electrocardiographic QT interval study prior to its approval [87]. This drug was approved by the US FDA January 27, 2012.

LIRAGLUTIDE

Liraglutide is another GLP-1 agonist approved as Victoza for treatment of diabetes. A study was published in Lancet by Astrup et al. which highlights its development for treatment of obesity [88]. In a 20 week double-blind, placebo-controlled clinical trial, liraglutide produced 2.1 kg (95% CI 0.6–3.6) to 4.4 kg (2.9–6.0) greater than that with placebo, with 76% of participants losing more than 5% of their body weight. Adverse events of nausea and vomiting occurred more often in individuals on liraglutide than in those on placebo, but these were mainly transient and rarely led to discontinuation of study drug.

FLUOXETINE AND SERTRALINE

Fluoxetine and sertraline are both SSRIs approved for the treatment of depression. Fluoxetine at a dose of 60 mg/day has been used in the treatment of obesity. Goldstein et al. reviewed these trials: a 36 week trial in type 2 diabetic subjects, a 52 week trial in subjects with uncomplicated obesity, and two 60 week trials in subjects with dyslipidemia, diabetes, or both [89]. There were a total of 1441 subjects in these trials, and approximately 70% completed 6 months of treatment (comment: this dropout rate is not unusual for weight loss trials). Weight loss in the fluoxetine and placebo groups at 6 months and 1 year was a modest 2.2, 4.8 and 1.8, 2.4 kg, respectively. The regain of 50% of the lost weight during the second 6 months of treatment on fluoxetine made it an inappropriate drug for the treatment of obesity, a condition which requires chronic treatment. Sertraline provided an average weight loss of 0.45–0.91 kg in clinical trials lasting 8–16 weeks for depression. Fluoxetine and sertraline may be preferred over tricyclic antidepressants in the obese for the treatment of depression, as the latter are associated with significant weight gain. Fluoxetine and sertraline by themselves are not good drugs for the treatment of obesity.

Fluoxetine is contraindicated in patients with known hypersensitivity. Thioridazine and MAOIs are contraindicated with its use. The neuroleptic malignant syndrome, a serious and sometimes fatal reaction, can occur with its use. It has been also reported with sertraline. Sertraline is contraindicated with the concomitant use of MAOIs. Sertraline has been associated with inappropriate antidiuretic hormone secretion and altered platelet function. When used for depression, an increased suicide risk can occur with both medications.

Fluoxetine should be used with caution in subjects with chest pain or who have attempted suicide. Sertraline use has been associated with delayed ejaculation, palpitations, chest pain, and sexual dysfunction.

METFORMIN

Metformin is a biguanide which is approved for the treatment of diabetes mellitus. This drug reduces hepatic glucose production, decreases intestinal absorption from the gastrointestinal tract, and enhances insulin sensitivity. In clinical trials where metformin was compared with a sulfonylurea, it produced weight loss [90]. The best trial of metformin in terms of evaluating weight loss effects is the Diabetes Prevention Program (DPP), a study of individuals with impaired glucose tolerance. This three-treatment-arm study included randomly assigned participants over 25 years of age with a body mass index (BMI) above 24 kg/m^2 (except Asian Americans who only needed a BMI $\geq$ 22 kg/m^2) and impaired glucose tolerance. The three primary arms included lifestyle (N = 1079 participants), metformin (N = 1073), and placebo (N = 1082). At the end of 2.8 years (on average), the Data Safety Monitoring Board terminated the trial because the advantages of lifestyle and metformin were clearly superior to placebo. During this time, the metformin-treated group lost 2.5% of their body weight (P < 0.001 compared to placebo), and the conversion from impaired glucose tolerance to diabetes was reduced by 31% compared to placebo. In the DPP trial, metformin was more effective in reducing the development of diabetes in the subgroup who were most overweight and in the younger members of the cohort [91]. Although metformin does not produce enough weight loss (5%) to qualify as a "weight loss drug" using the FDA criteria, it would appear to be a very useful choice for overweight individuals with newly diagnosed diabetes mellitus. Metformin has also found use in the treatment of women with the polycystic ovarian syndrome, where the modest weight loss may contribute to increased fertility and a reduction in insulin resistance [92].

Metformin is known to be substantially excreted by the kidney, and the risk of metformin accumulation and lactic acidosis increases with the degree of impairment of renal function. Thus, patients with serum creatinine levels above the upper limit of normal for their age should not use metformin. Renal function should be monitored during metformin treatment, and metformin should be stopped prior to surgical procedures or procedures using x-ray contrast material. Since alcohol potentiates the effect of metformin on lactic acid metabolism, excessive alcohol intake should be avoided. Metformin should be used with caution in patients with congestive heart failure, hepatic insufficiency, hypoxic conditions, or acidosis. Metformin is also associated with a decline in vitamin B_{12} levels.

PRAMLINTIDE

Beta cells in the pancreas secrete amylin in a fixed ratio to insulin. In type 1 diabetes mellitus, immunologically damaged beta cells are deficient in amylin. Pramlintide, a synthetic amylin analog, was approved by the FDA for the treatment of insulin-requiring diabetes. Unlike insulin and many other diabetes medications, pramlintide is associated with weight loss. Maggs et al. analyzed the data from two 1 year studies in insulin-treated type 2 diabetic subjects randomized to pramlintide 120 mcg twice a day (bid) or 150 mcg three times a day [93]. Weight decreased by 2.6 kg and hemoglobin A1C decreased by 0.5%. When weight loss was then analyzed by ethnic group, African Americans lost 4 kg, Caucasians lost 2.4 kg, and Hispanics lost 2.3 kg. The improvement in diabetes correlated with the weight loss obtained, suggesting that pramlintide is most effective in the ethnic group with the greatest obesity burden. The most common adverse event was nausea which was usually mild and confined to the first 4 weeks of therapy. Pramlintide treatment in insulin-treated type 2 diabetes mellitus may offer an added benefit of weight loss in subjects with preexisting obesity.

Pramlintide is contraindicated in patients with a known hypersensitivity to pramlintide or any of its components, including metacresol. Since pramlintide delays gastric emptying, it should not be used in subjects with a confirmed diagnosis of gastroparesis. Pramlintide and insulin should always be administered as separate injections. Pramlintide should be used with caution in subjects with moderate or severe renal impairment, local allergy, and hepatic impairment.

SOMATOSTATIN

Insulin hypersecretion accompanies hypothalamic obesity [94]. Treatment with octreotide, an analog of somatostatin, results in weight loss in children with hypothalamic damage, and their weight loss correlated with reduced insulin secretion on a glucose tolerance test [95]. This open-label trial was followed by a randomized controlled trial of octreotide treatment in children with hypothalamic obesity. The subjects received octreotide 5–15 mcg/kg/day or placebo for 6 months. The children on octreotide gained 1.6 kg compared to a 9.1 kg gain for those in the placebo group [96]. A trial of 44 subjects, a subset of obese subjects with insulin hypersecretion by an oral glucose tolerance test, was undertaken. Octreotide-LAR 40 mg/month for 6 months was given. These subjects lost weight, reduced food intake, and reduced carbohydrate intake. Weight loss was greatest in those with insulin hypersecretion, and the amount of weight loss was correlated with the reduction in insulin hypersecretion [97]. Since a larger prospective study of 172 insulin-hypersensitive subjects randomized to 40 or 60 mg of long-acting octreotide versus placebo lost a maximum of 3.8% of initial body weight in the high-dose group, it does not appear that octreotide will meet the criteria for approval as a weight loss drug by the FDA [98]. Octreotide has been shown to decrease gastric emptying [99]. Octreotide treatment of patients with the Prader–Willi Syndrome who have elevated ghrelin levels does not cause weight loss but ghrelin levels are normalized. The reason for the lack of weight loss has been postulated to be the reduction of PYY, a satiating gastrointestinal hormone that also decreased [100].

Octreotide is contraindicated in the face of sensitivity to it or any of its components. It causes gall bladder stasis and is associated with gallstones, gallbladder sludge, and biliary duct dilatation. Octreotide alters the glucose counterregulatory hormones and can be associated with hypoglycemia, hyperglycemia, and hypothyroidism. Cardiac conduction abnormalities have developed on octreotide, and cases of pancreatitis have been reported. Octreotide can alter absorption of dietary fat and depress vitamin B_{12} levels.

TOPIRAMATE

Topiramate is an antiepileptic drug that was observed to result in weight loss in clinical trials for epilepsy. Weight losses of 3.9% of initial weight were seen at 3 months and losses of 7.3% of initial weight were seen at 1 year [101]. Bray et al. reported a 6 month, placebo-controlled, dose-ranging study. A total of 385 obese subjects were randomized to placebo or topiramate at 64, 96, 192, or 384 mg/day. These doses were gradually reached by a tapering increase and were reduced in a similar manner at the end of the trial. Weight loss from baseline to 24 weeks was 2.6%, 5%, 4.8%, 6.3%, and 6.3% in the placebo, 64, 96, 192, and 384 mg groups, respectively. The most frequent adverse events were paresthesia, somnolence, and difficulty with concentration, memory, and attention [102].

This trial was followed by two large multicenter trials extending for 1 year [103,104]. Despite impressive weight losses of 7%–16.5% of initial body weight, a significant improvement in blood pressure, and improvement in glucose tolerance, the sponsor terminated further study to pursue a time-released formulation of the drug. Although topiramate is still available as an antiepileptic drug, the development program to pursue an indication for obesity was terminated by the sponsor in December 2004 due to the associated adverse events.

Topiramate has been evaluated in the treatment of binge-eating disorder [105]. Sixty-one subjects were randomized to 25–600 mg/day of topiramate or placebo in a 1:1 ratio. The topiramate group had improvement in binge-eating symptoms and lost 5.9 kg at an average topiramate dose of 212 mg/day [106,107]. It has also been used to treat patients with the Prader–Willi Syndrome [108–110], subjects with nocturnal eating syndrome and sleep-related eating disorder [111].

Topiramate is a carbonic anhydrase inhibitor associated with kidney stones (1.5%) and metabolic acidosis. Topiramate has been associated with the syndrome of acute myopia and secondary angle closure glaucoma. Topiramate can decrease sweating and increase the risk of hyperthermia. CNS adverse events associated with topiramate include psychomotor slowing, difficulty in concentration, speech difficulties, language problems, word-finding difficulties, somnolence, fatigue, irritability, and depression. Peripheral nervous system adverse events consist of paresthesias. Dosage adjustment of topiramate is needed in renal and hepatic failure.

ZONISAMIDE

Zonisamide is an antiseizure drug that has been evaluated for the treatment of obesity. It has serotonergic and dopaminergic activity in addition to blocking neuronal sodium and calcium channels. In a 16 week trial of 60 subjects (92% women) administered a hypocaloric diet, zonisamide 400–600 mg/day was shown to result in greater weight loss compared with placebo, with few adverse effects [112].

Since zonisamide is a sulfonamide anticonvulsant, it can cause hypersensitivity reactions in those allergic to sulfa. Zonisamide can reduce sweating and increase the risk of hyperthermia, and there are rare but serious reported cases of aplastic anemia. The possible CNS effects of zonisamide include depression, psychosis, psychomotor slowing, difficulty with concentration, word finding difficulties, somnolence, and fatigue. Zonisamide is also associated with asthenia, vomiting, tremor, convulsions, abnormal gait, hyperesthesia, and incoordination. Since zonisamide inhibits carbonic anhydrase, it is associated with the formation of renal calculi. There is also a decrease in glomerular filtration rate associated with zonisamide which can cause an increase in the blood urea nitrogen. Rare reports of creatine phosphokinase elevation and pancreatitis have been reported with zonisamide. Zonisamide can also cause birth defects and should not be used in women with the potential for pregnancy unless the benefits are felt to outweigh this risk.

RECENT DRUG DEVELOPMENT

LORCASERIN

There are 14 known serotonin receptors; the 5HT2B is responsible for the cardiac valvular effects, while the 5HT2C is responsible for weight loss [113]. Lorcaserin, the novel selective serotonin 5HT2c-receptor agonist, provided a 5.8% weight loss compared to a 2.5% weight loss with placebo (5 kg weight loss at 52 weeks) in overweight and obese individuals [114]. The debacle of valvulopathy and PPH caused by fenfluramine and fen-phen (fenfluramine with phentermine) ensured a very thorough surveillance for cardiac valvulopathy during the clinical trials. The adverse effects included headache, nausea, dizziness, fatigue, and dry mouth. Overall, syncope, depression, and anxiety were noted in some participants with no statistically significant increase in the risk of depression or suicide ideation. Citing the marginal efficacy and the propensity for development of cancer, the FDA's Endocrinologic and Metabolic Drugs Advisory Committee voted against recommendation for approval of this drug for treatment of overweight (BMI of 27–30 kg/m^2) with one or more comorbidity and obese (BMI > 30 kg/m^2) subjects. The FDA subsequently also rejected a marketing application to obtain more data.

TESOFENSINE

Tesofensine is a new drug which inhibits the presynaptic reuptake of the neurotransmitters noradrenaline, dopamine, and serotonin and is thought to enhance the neurotransmission of all three monoamines. It resulted in twice the weight loss in obese individuals as has been seen with the currently marketed drugs. The mechanisms by which it produces weight loss in humans are unresolved. It is thought to be related to the upregulation of the neurotransmitters dopamine, serotonin, and norepinephrine in the interneuronal cleft which are known to be involved in the central regulation of appetite.

Tesofensine initially developed as a treatment for Alzheimer's and Parkinson's disease was noted to produce weight loss [115]. With tesofensine producing placebo-subtracted weight loss of approximately 4% in obese participants without any diet and lifestyle therapy, and without any adverse effects on blood pressure over 14 weeks, it was tested for the treatment of obesity [116]. In a phase II, randomized, double-blind, placebo-controlled trial after a 2 week run-in phase, obese participants were prescribed an energy-restricted diet and randomly assigned to treatment with tesofensine 0.25, 0.5, or 1.0 mg or placebo once daily for 24 weeks. After 24 weeks with 71% completing the study, the mean weight loss produced by diet and placebo was 2.0%. Tesofensine 0.25, 0.5, and 1.0 mg and diet induced a mean weight loss of 4.5%, 9.2%, and 10.6%, respectively, greater than diet and placebo. The most common adverse events caused by tesofensine were dry mouth, nausea, constipation, hard stools, diarrhea, and insomnia. After 24 weeks, tesofensine 0.25 and 0.5 mg showed no significant increases in systolic or diastolic blood pressure compared with placebo, whereas in the tesofensine 0.5 mg group heart rate was increased by 7.4 beats per min. While these findings of efficacy and safety need confirmation in phase III trials, these results suggest that tesofensine at 0.5 mg might have the potential to produce twice the weight loss of the currently approved drugs.

In a randomized, controlled trial, healthy, overweight, or moderately obese men were treated with tesofensine 2.0 mg daily for 1 week, followed by 1 mg for 1 more week or corresponding placebo. Despite efforts to keep body weight and composition constant, a 1.8 kg weight loss above placebo was noted. Higher satiety ratings of fullness resulted in a lower prospective food intake in the tesofensine group. Tesofensine increased energy expenditure during the night and increased 24 h fat oxidation.

With tesofensine having a pronounced effect on appetite sensations and a slight effect on energy expenditure at night, it can contribute to a strong weight-reducing effect [117].

COMBINATION DRUGS

The use of more than one drug in combination to achieve an additive or synergistic effect is an established strategy in the treatment of chronic diseases like diabetes and hypertension. The use of this rationale for the development of the combination drugs in treatment of obesity is described next.

BUPROPION + NALTRAXONE

The combination of bupropion and naltrexone was first shown to cause a synergistic increase in the firing rate of proopiomelanocortin (POMC) neurons present in the hypothalamus of mice. Bupropion stimulates the POMC neurons to release POMC which is subsequently cleaved into alpha melanocyte-stimulating hormone (α-MSH) and an endogenous mu-opioid. α-MSH binds to the melanocortin-4 receptor to decrease food intake and increase the metabolic rate in rodents. Naltrexone binds to an opioid inhibitory receptor on the POMC neuron and blocks the down regulation of POMC secretion. Studies in rodents have shown the same synergy of bupropion and naltrexone on food intake at the level of the hypothalamus and the reward pathway. A proof-of-concept study in humans confirmed this synergy of the bupropion and naltrexone by demonstrating body weight loss [118]. A study with PET scanning showed that 32 mg of naltrexone was sufficient to saturate the POMC receptors in the brain, and a dose-ranging study confirmed that 32 mg of naltrexone was the most efficacious dose for weight loss [119].

Bupropion has been used for the treatment of depression for over 20 years and has become the antidepressant of choice in obese patients due to the modest weight loss it provides, in contrast to the weight gain associated with tricyclic antidepressant treatment. Bupropion is also approved for smoking cessation and treatment of seasonal affective disorder. Naltrexone has been in use for over 20 years for treatment of alcohol addiction and has also, subsequently, received approval for use in the treatment of opioid addiction. The most common side effect noted with the use of this combination in the proof-of-concept study was nausea that was related to the maximal serum concentrations of naltrexone. Thus, a proprietary time-release formulation by decreasing maximal serum concentrations of naltrexone reduced this side effect. Bupropion shares a norepinephrine reuptake mechanism with sibutramine, and, as such, the reduction in blood pressure expected with weight loss does not occur unless greater than 10% body weight is lost. This occurred in a minority of the population studied in the phase III trials [120].

The naltrexone-bupropion combination met one of the two efficacy criteria set up for approval of drugs treating obesity by the FDA. Overweight and obese adults lost 4.2% more body weight in the clinical trials by last observation carried forward but having more than 35% of subjects lose 5% of their body weight which was more than twice the percentage in the placebo group. The FDA's Endocrinologic and Metabolic Drugs Advisory Committee voted 13 to 7 to recommend approval of Orexigen's NDA in December 2010. The committee, however, did express concern about the elevation of blood pressure and heart rate, and recommended that a post marketing study of cardiovascular endpoints proceed without delay with the commencement of marketing.

There were no increases in depression or suicidal ideation compared to placebo. The major side effect of nausea occurred early in the course of therapy and subsided as therapy is continued. Other side effects were those known to occur with the two component drugs including headache, constipation, dizziness, vomiting, epilepsy, and dry mouth, but the use of the two drugs in combination did not create new or unexpected side effects. The sponsor is seeking FDA approval for the treatment of overweight subjects with a BMI of 27–30 kg/m^2 with one or more comorbidity and for subjects with obesity (BMI > 30 kg/m^2).

PRAMLINTIDE + METRELEPTIN

Since obesity seems to engender a resistance to the effects of leptin, the developmental testing of leptin for the treatment of obesity was dropped, [121,122]. Amylin and leptin are secreted by the pancreas and the adipose tissue, respectively, and act on the CNS. Studies indicate that amylin and insulin work together to control blood sugar levels, especially after meals. Pramlintide and metreleptin are injectable synthetic analogs of naturally occurring hormones amylin and leptin. Pramlintide has been shown to reverse insulin resistance by increasing stat-3 signaling in the hypothalamus and the area postrema. Thus, the combination of pramlintide and metreleptin may realize the potential of leptin as a treatment for obesity that has been disappointing up to this point [122].

Pramlintide given alone has been demonstrated to reduce food intake [123] and reduce body weight [124]. Studies in both animals and humans have demonstrated that pramlintide together with metreleptin reduces body weight in an additive or synergistic fashion.

In a proof-of-concept study, overweight and obese subjects were given pramlintide 180 mg bid for 2 weeks before the dose was increased to 360 mg bid for an additional 2 weeks. Subjects losing 2%–8% weight loss were randomized to pramlintide 360 mg bid, metreleptin 5 mg bid, or a combination of the two for the ensuing 20 weeks. At the end of the study, the combination group lost 12.7% of initial body weight compared to 8.4% and 8.2% in the pramlintide and metreleptin groups, respectively [125]. The weight loss continued through to the end of the study with no evidence of plateau. The most robust efficacy was seen in patients with a BMI less than 35 kg/m². The combination therapy appeared to be generally well tolerated, with nausea and injection site reactions as the adverse events most commonly observed to be associated with pramlintide and metreleptin, respectively. Following initiation of therapy, these adverse events occurred at a reduced rate over time in patients continuing the combination therapy. The initiation of phase III trials is anticipated.

PHENTERMINE AND CONTROLLED-RELEASE TOPIRAMATE

Phentermine is the most prescribed obesity drug in the United States, and treatment on alternate months has been shown to be as efficacious as continuous treatment. Alternate-month treatment allows the drug to be used for prolonged periods of time, while remaining within the constraints of the package insert limits the drug to no more than 12 weeks of continuous use [66]. Phentermine has an α-methyl substitution on the phenethylamine side chain, resulting in a lower CNS stimulation potential than its parent amphetamine molecule. It can, however, increase blood pressure and heart rate, in addition to causing insomnia and dry mouth.

Topiramate is an antiepileptic drug that was observed to give weight loss in the clinical trials for epilepsy. Weight losses of 3.9% of initial weight were seen at 3 months and losses of 7.3% of initial weight were seen at 1 year [101]. The most frequent adverse events were paresthesia, somnolence, and difficulty with concentration, memory, and attention [102].

Vivus formulated a proprietary combination of immediate-release phentermine 15 mg and modified-release topiramate 92 mg, along with the combination in lower doses maintaining the same ratio. The clinical trials testing the combination lead to a NDA. The high dose phentermine–topiramate combination resulted in a 10.6% weight loss compared to a 1.7% weight loss in the placebo group meeting both of the FDA criteria for obesity drug efficacy. Despite the fact that no new adverse events were seen by combining these two drugs, the side effects from their long-term use are well known that phentermine is already approved for the treatment of obesity at twice the dose and that topiramate is approved for the prophylaxis of migraine headaches at higher doses than used in the high-dose obesity combination drug, the FDA's Endocrinologic and Metabolic Drugs Advisory Committee voted against approval of the NDA. The FDA rejected the NDA and has asked for additional data. The adverse effects that concerned the FDA advisory panel included teratogenicity, psychiatric and cognitive-related adverse events, metabolic acidosis, and cardiovascular adverse events related to an elevation of blood pressure and heart rate compared to placebo.

POTENTIAL FOR USING HERBS TO DEVELOP NEW OBESITY DRUGS

The traditional method of discovering new drugs for obesity, or for other purposes, is to screen novel compounds for activity in assays measuring a mechanism for the disease in question.

Appropriate activity in a screening assay leads to further *in vitro* testing and eventually to testing in humans. Most candidate compounds with activity in screening assays fall out of the development process due to safety considerations. As we have already reviewed, safety is of particular concern in the treatment of obesity. Another approach is to find plants used in food with folklore to suggest that they might have efficacy in treating obesity and to test these presumably safe foods for their efficacy in treating human obesity. We will give one example of such an approach.

Cissus quadrangularis (CQ) is a herb used in India to promote healing of fractures and in Cameroon as a component of rehydration fluid to treat many illnesses. Irvingia gabonensis (IG) is also known as bush mango. Its seeds are used for food flavoring and have been thought to have beneficial effects on diabetes and obesity. A supplement called Cylaris™ that contains CQ with several dietary supplements (green tea, soy, selenium, chromium, and B vitamins) was evaluated in an 8 week clinical trial involving 123 overweight and obese subjects. Ninety-two obese subjects were randomized to one of three groups—placebo bid, Cylaris™ without diet bid, and Cylaris™ with 2000–2200 kcal/day diet bid. The remaining 31 subjects were overweight and took Cylaris™ bid without a diet. The percent loss of body weight over 8 weeks was 2.4%, 6.9%, 8.5%, and 4.8% in the placebo, Cylaris™ without diet, Cylaris™ with diet, and Cylaris™ in overweight without diet groups, respectively. Placebo-subtracted reductions were seen in low-density lipoprotein cholesterol (8%–22%), triglycerides (10%–32%), fasting glucose (6.8%–11%), and C-reactive protein (17%–21%), along with a placebo-subtracted increase in high-density lipoprotein cholesterol (2%–33%) [126].

A second study compared a standardized extract of CQ (2.5% ketosteroids and 15% soluble fiber) bid to Cylaris™ with twice the amount of CQ standardized extract bid. The group on the standardized CQ extract lost 4% of their placebo-subtracted body weight which was statistically significantly different from placebo which gained 1.2% of body weight. This was not statistically different than the Cylaris™ with twice the dose of CQ which lost 8.5% of body weight. The metabolic syndrome–associated parameters were again improved [127].

The most recently reported 10 week study randomized 72 overweight and obese subjects to one of three groups: CQ 150 mg/day (standardized to 2.5% ketosteroids), IG 250 mg/day (standardized to 7% albumins), and a combination of both. The placebo, CQ, and combination groups lost 1.4 and 2%, 7.6 and 8.9%, and 8.9 and 11.9% of their initial body weight at 8 and 10 weeks, respectively. In addition, the combination group at 8 weeks had a reduction in body fat (17%), waist circumference (8%), low-density lipoprotein cholesterol (33%), and fasting blood sugar (25%). The side effects were greater in the placebo group than the groups taking the dietary herbal supplement which suggests good tolerance [128].

DISCUSSION AND CONCLUSIONS

Obesity drugs have a very poor track record for safety. Obese individuals, especially women, experience discrimination in our society [11]. This discrimination encourages some women to take unreasonable risks to lose weight. This makes drug safety all the more important for the treatment of obesity.

The situation with obesity drugs today can be compared to the situation with hypertension drugs in the 1950s. At that time, we had thiazide diuretics that caused a loss of salt in urine and drugs working at the level of the brain like reserpine that had side effects on mood. The present drugs available for the treatment of obesity have limited efficacy and, with the exception of orlistat, work on upstream targets. Orlistat, which by preventing fat absorption in the gut results in a loss of calories in the stool, has parallels with diuretics for the treatment of hypertension. Older obesity medications which were derived from the basic amphetamine chemical structure stimulate the CNS and have parallels with the antihypertensive drugs of the 1950s like reserpine which cause side effects such as depression.

The pipeline of new obesity drug candidates is rich, and the technology available to the pharmaceutical industry is much more advanced when compared with the 1950s. The future is therefore bright for much more rapid development of safe and efficacious obesity drugs which act on downstream targets. Drug acting on downstream targets have less potential for side effects than drugs acting upstream on the CNS. We now have drugs for treatment of hypertension like the angiotensin receptor blockers that have peripheral action and very few side effects. As we develop new drugs for obesity that act on downstream targets, we should see a similar advance in the safety of pharmacological treatment of obesity. Using herbs as a platform for the development of obesity drugs offers an additional strategy that may increase the safety of future obesity drugs. This serves to emphasize why a chapter on the safety of obesity drug is germane to a book on phytopharmaceuticals and the therapy of obesity.

REFERENCES

1. Prentice AM. Early influences on human energy regulation: Thrifty genotypes and thrifty phenotypes. *Physiol Behav* 2005;86:640–645.
2. Burton BT, Foster WR, Hirsch J, Van Itallie TB. Health implications of obesity: An NIH Consensus Development Conference. *Int J Obes* 1985;9:155–170.
3. Flegal KM, Carroll MD, Ogden CL, Johnson CL. Prevalence and trends in obesity among US adults, 1999–2000. *JAMA* 2002;288:1723–1727.
4. World Health Organization (WHO), Obesity and overweight facts, http://www.who.int/hpr/NPH/docs/gs_obesity.pdf (accessed on July, 2004).
5. Hedley AA, Ogden CL, Johnson CL, Carroll MD, Curtin LR, Flegal KM. Prevalence of overweight and obesity among US children, adolescents, and adults, 1999–2002. *JAMA* 2004;291:2847–2850.
6. Kushner RF, Roth JL. Assessment of the obese patient. *Endocrinol Metab Clin North Am* 2003;32:915–933.
7. International Obesity Taskforce, http://www.iotf.org (accessed on July, 2004).
8. World Health Organization (WHO), Controlling the global obesity epidemic: Nutrition, http://www.who.int/nut/obs.htm (accessed on July, 2004).
9. Yanovski SZ, Yanovski JA. Obesity. *N Engl J Med* February 21, 2002;346(8):591–602. Review.
10. Bays H, Dujovne C. Anti-obesity drug development. *Expert Opin Investig Drug* 2002;11:1189–1204.
11. Puhl RM, Brownell KD. Psychosocial origins of obesity stigma: Toward changing a powerful and pervasive bias. *Obes Rev* 2003;4:213–227.
12. Greenway FL, Caruso MK. Safety of obesity drugs. *Expert Opin Drug Saf* 2005;4:1083–1095.
13. Rozen R, Abraham G, Falcou R, Apfelbaum M. Effects of a 'physiological' dose of triiodothyronine on obese subjects during a protein-sparing diet. *Int J Obes* 1986;10:303–312.
14. Allison DB, Zannolli R, Faith MS et al. Weight loss increases and fat loss decreases all-cause mortality rate: Results from two independent cohort studies. *Int J Obes Relat Metab Disord* 1999;23:603–611.
15. Parascandola J. Dinitrophenol and bioenergetics: An historical perspective. *Mol Cell Biochem* 1974;5:69–77.
16. Magne H, Mayer A, Plantefol L. Studies on the action of dinitrophenol 1–2–4 (Thermol). *Ann Physiol Physicochem* 1932;8:1–167.
17. Cutting W, Tainter M. Actions of dinitrophenol. *Proc Soc Exp Med* 1932;29:1268.
18. Cutting W, Tainter M. Metabolic actions of dinitrophenol. *J Am Med Assoc* 1933;101:2099–2102.
19. Tainter M. Use of dinitrophenol in nutritional disorders: A critical survey of clinical results. *Am J Public Health* 1934;24:1045–1053.
20. Nathanson M. The central action of beta-aminopropylbenzene (benzedrine) clinical observations. *JAMA* 1937;108:528–531.
21. Ulrich H. Narcolepsy and its treatment with benzedrine sulfate. *N Engl J Med* 1937;217:696–701.
22. Leibowitz SF, Brown LL. Histochemical and pharmacological analysis of noradrenergic projections to the paraventricular hypothalamus in relation to feeding stimulation. *Brain Res* 1980;201:289–314.
23. Lesses M, Meyerson A. Human autonomic pharmacology XVI: Benzedrine sulfate as an aid in the treatment of obesity. *N Engl J Med* 1938;281:119–124.
24. Henry RC. Weight reduction pills. *JAMA* 1967;201:895–896.
25. Jelliffe RW, Hill D, Tatter D, Lewis E, Jr. Death from weight-control pills. A case report with objective postmortem confirmation. *JAMA* 1969;208:1843–1847.
26. Asher WL, Dietz RE. Effectiveness of weight reduction involving "diet pills". *Curr Ther Res Clin Exp* 1972;14:510–524.
27. Asher WL. Mortality rate in patients receiving "diet pills". *Curr Ther Res Clin Exp* 1972;14:525–539.

28. Byrne-Quinn E, Grover RF. Aminorex (Menocil) and amphetamine: Acute and chronic effects on pulmonary and systemic haemodynamics in the calf. *Thorax* 1972;27:127–131.

29. Michelakis ED, Weir EK. Anorectic drugs and pulmonary hypertension from the bedside to the bench. *Am J Med Sci* 2001;321:292–299.

30. Gurtner HP. Pulmonary hypertension, "plexogenic pulmonary arteriopathy" and the appetite depressant drug aminorex: Post or propter? *Bull Eur Physiopathol Respir* 1979;15:897–923.

31. Heath D, Smith P. Pulmonary vascular disease. *Med Clin North Am* 1977;61:1279–1307.

32. Weintraub M, Hasday JD, Mushlin AI, Lockwood DH. A double-blind clinical trial in weight control. Use of fenfluramine and phentermine alone and in combination. *Arch Intern Med* 1984;144:1143–1148.

33. Weintraub M. Long-term weight control: The National Heart, Lung, and Blood Institute funded multimodal intervention study. *Clin Pharmacol Ther* 1992;51:581–585.

34. Curzon G, Gibson EL, Oluyomi AO. Appetite suppression by commonly used drugs depends on 5-HT receptors but not on 5-HT availability. *Trends Pharmacol Sci* 1997;18:21–25.

35. Abenhaim L, Moride Y, Brenot F et al. Appetite-suppressant drugs and the risk of primary pulmonary hypertension. International Primary Pulmonary Hypertension Study Group. *N Engl J Med* 1996;335:609–616.

36. Connolly HM, Crary JL, McGoon MD et al. Valvular heart disease associated with fenfluramine-phentermine. *N Engl J Med* 1997;337:581–588.

37. Robiolio PA, Rigolin VH, Wilson JS et al. Carcinoid heart disease. Correlation of high serotonin levels with valvular abnormalities detected by cardiac catheterization and echocardiography. *Circulation* 1995;92:790–795.

38. Ryan DH, Bray GA, Helmcke F et al. Serial echocardiographic and clinical evaluation of valvular regurgitation before, during, and after treatment with fenfluramine or dexfenfluramine and mazindol or phentermine. *Obes Res* 1999;7:313–322.

39. Greenway F, Herber D, Raum W, Morales S. Double-blind, randomized, placebo-controlled clinical trials with non-prescription medications for the treatment of obesity. *Obes Res* 1999;7:370–378.

40. Weintraub M, Ginsberg G, Stein EC et al. Phenylpropanolamine OROS (Acutrim) vs. placebo in combination with caloric restriction and physician-managed behavior modification. *Clin Pharmacol Ther* 1986;39:501–509.

41. Kernan WN, Viscoli CM, Brass LM et al. Phenylpropanolamine and the risk of hemorrhagic stroke. *N Engl J Med* 2000;343:1826–1832.

42. Chen K. Ephedrine and related substances. *Medicine* 1930;9:1–119.

43. Greenway FL. The safety and efficacy of pharmaceutical and herbal caffeine and ephedrine use as a weight loss agent. *Obes Rev* 2001;2:199–211.

44. Shekelle PG, Hardy ML, Morton SC et al. Efficacy and safety of ephedra and ephedrine for weight loss and athletic performance: A meta-analysis. *JAMA* 2003;289:1537–1545.

45. Haller CA, Benowitz NL. Adverse cardiovascular and central nervous system events associated with dietary supplements containing ephedra alkaloids. *N Engl J Med* 2000;343:1833–1838.

46. Howlett AC, Breivogel CS, Childers SR, Deadwyler SA, Hampson RE, Porrino LJ. Cannabinoid physiology and pharmacology: 30 years of progress. *Neuropharmacology* 2004;47(Suppl 1):345–358.

47. Casu MA, Porcella A, Ruiu S et al. Differential distribution of functional cannabinoid CB1 receptors in the mouse gastroenteric tract. *Eur J Pharmacol* 2003;459:97–105.

48. Bensaid M, Gary-Bobo M, Esclangon A et al. The cannabinoid CB1 receptor antagonist SR141716 increases Acrp30 mRNA expression in adipose tissue of obese fa/fa rats and in cultured adipocyte cells. *Mol Pharmacol* 2003;63:908–914.

49. Denson TF, Earleywine M. Decreased depression in marijuana users. *Addict Behav* 2006;31:738–742.

50. Simiand J, Keane M, Keane PE, Soubrie P. SR 141716, a CB1 cannabinoid receptor antagonist, selectively reduces sweet food intake in marmoset. *Behav Pharmacol* 1998;9:179–181.

51. Van Gaal LF, Rissanen AM, Scheen AJ, Ziegler O, Rossner S, Group RI-ES. Effects of the cannabinoid-1 receptor blocker rimonabant on weight reduction and cardiovascular risk factors in overweight patients: 1-year experience from the RIO-Europe study. *Lancet* 2005;365:1389–1397.

52. Despres JP, Golay A, Sjostrom L, Rimonabant in Obesity-Lipids Study Group. Effects of rimonabant on metabolic risk factors in overweight patients with dyslipidemia. *N Engl J Med* 2005;353:2121–2134.

53. Nissen SE, Nicholls SJ, Wolski K et al. Effect of rimonabant on progression of atherosclerosis in patients with abdominal obesity and coronary artery disease: The STRADIVARIUS randomized controlled trial. *JAMA* 2008;299:1547–1560.

54. Topol EJ, Bousser MG, Fox KA et al. Rimonabant for prevention of cardiovascular events (CRESCENDO): A randomised, multicentre, placebo-controlled trial. *Lancet* 2010;376:517–523.

55. Connoley IP, Liu YL, Frost I, Reckless IP, Heal DJ, Stock MJ. Thermogenic effects of sibutramine and its metabolites. *Br J Pharmacol* 1999;126:1487–1495.
56. Wirth A, Krause J. Long-term weight loss with sibutramine: A randomized controlled trial. *JAMA* 2001;286:1331–1339.
57. James WP, Astrup A, Finer N et al. Effect of sibutramine on weight maintenance after weight loss: A randomised trial. STORM Study Group. Sibutramine Trial of Obesity Reduction and Maintenance. *Lancet* 2000;356:2119–2125.
58. Dujovne CA, Zavoral JH, Rowe E, Mendel CM, Silbutramine Study Group. Effects of sibutramine on body weight and serum lipids: A double-blind, randomized, placebo-controlled study in 322 overweight and obese patients with dyslipidemia. *Am Heart J* 2001;142:489–497.
59. Fujioka K, Seaton TB, Rowe E et al. Weight loss with sibutramine improves glycaemic control and other metabolic parameters in obese patients with type 2 diabetes mellitus. *Diabetes Obes Metab* 2000;2:175–187.
60. Finer N, Bloom SR, Frost GS, Banks LM, Griffiths J. Sibutramine is effective for weight loss and diabetic control in obesity with type 2 diabetes: A randomised, double-blind, placebo-controlled study. *Diabetes Obes Metab* 2000;2:105–112.
61. Kim SH, Lee YM, Jee SH, Nam CM. Effect of sibutramine on weight loss and blood pressure: A meta-analysis of controlled trials. *Obes Res* 2003;11:1116–1123.
62. The amphetamine appetite suppressant saga. *Prescrire Int* 2004;13:26–29.
63. James WP, Caterson ID, Coutinho W et al. Effect of sibutramine on cardiovascular outcomes in overweight and obese subjects. *N Engl J Med* 2010;363:905–917.
64. Rothman RB, Partilla JS, Dersch CM, Carroll FI, Rice KC, Baumann MH. Methamphetamine dependence: Medication development efforts based on the dual deficit model of stimulant addiction. *Ann N Y Acad Sci* 2000;914:71–81.
65. Rothman RB, Baumann MH, Dersch CM et al. Amphetamine-type central nervous system stimulants release norepinephrine more potently than they release dopamine and serotonin. *Synapse* 2001;39:32–41.
66. Munro JF, MacCuish AC, Wilson EM, Duncan LJ. Comparison of continuous and intermittent anorectic therapy in obesity. *Br Med J* 1968;1:352–354.
67. Davidson MH, Hauptman J, DiGirolamo M et al. Weight control and risk factor reduction in obese subjects treated for 2 years with orlistat: A randomized controlled trial. *JAMA* 1999;281:235–242.
68. Sjostrom L, Rissanen A, Andersen T et al. Randomised placebo-controlled trial of orlistat for weight loss and prevention of weight regain in obese patients. European Multicentre Orlistat Study Group. *Lancet* 1998;352:167–172.
69. Mittendorfer B, Ostlund RE, Jr., Patterson BW, Klein S. Orlistat inhibits dietary cholesterol absorption. *Obes Res* 2001;9:599–604.
70. Heymsfield SB, Segal KR, Hauptman J et al. Effects of weight loss with orlistat on glucose tolerance and progression to type 2 diabetes in obese adults. *Arch Intern Med* 2000;160:1321–1326.
71. Kelley DE, Bray GA, Pi-Sunyer FX et al. Clinical efficacy of orlistat therapy in overweight and obese patients with insulin-treated type 2 diabetes: A 1-year randomized controlled trial. *Diabetes Care* 2002;25:1033–1041.
72. Lindgarde F. The effect of orlistat on body weight and coronary heart disease risk profile in obese patients: The Swedish Multimorbidity Study. *J Intern Med* 2000;248:245–254.
73. Rossner S, Sjostrom L, Noack R, Meinders AE, Noseda G. Weight loss, weight maintenance, and improved cardiovascular risk factors after 2 years treatment with orlistat for obesity. European Orlistat Obesity Study Group. *Obes Res* 2000;8:49–61.
74. Jain AK, Kaplan RA, Gadde KM et al. Bupropion SR vs. placebo for weight loss in obese patients with depressive symptoms. *Obes Res* 2002;10:1049–1056.
75. Anderson JW, Greenway FL, Fujioka K, Gadde KM, McKenney J, O'Neil PM. Bupropion SR enhances weight loss: A 48-week double-blind, placebo- controlled trial. *Obes Res* 2002;10:633–641.
76. Small CJ, Bloom SR. Gut hormones as peripheral anti obesity targets. *Curr Drug Targets CNS Neurol Disord* 2004;3:379–388.
77. Greenway SE, Greenway FL, 3rd, Klein S. Effects of obesity surgery on non-insulin-dependent diabetes mellitus. *Arch Surg* 2002;137:1109–1117.
78. Patriti A, Facchiano E, Sanna A, Gulla N, Donini A. The enteroinsular axis and the recovery from type 2 diabetes after bariatric surgery. *Obes Surg* 2004;14:840–848.
79. Lugari R, Dei Cas A, Ugolotti D et al. Glucagon-like peptide 1 (GLP-1) secretion and plasma dipeptidyl peptidase IV (DPP-IV) activity in morbidly obese patients undergoing biliopancreatic diversion. *Horm Metab Res* 2004;36:111–115.

80. Rodriquez de Fonseca F, Navarro M, Alvarez E et al. Peripheral versus central effects of glucagon-like peptide-1 receptor agonists on satiety and body weight loss in Zucker obese rats. *Metabolism* 2000;49:709–717.

81. Kastin AJ, Akerstrom V. Entry of exendin-4 into brain is rapid but may be limited at high doses. *Int J Obes Relat Metab Disord* 2003;27:313–318.

82. Szayna M, Doyle ME, Betkey JA et al. Exendin-4 decelerates food intake, weight gain, and fat deposition in Zucker rats. *Endocrinology* 2000;141:1936–1941.

83. Gedulin BR, Nikoulina SE, Smith PA et al. Exenatide (exendin-4) improves insulin sensitivity and {beta}-cell mass in insulin-resistant obese fa/fa Zucker rats independent of glycemia and body weight. *Endocrinology* 2005;146:2069–2076.

84. Edwards CM, Stanley SA, Davis R et al. Exendin-4 reduces fasting and postprandial glucose and decreases energy intake in healthy volunteers. *Am J Physiol Endocrinol Metab* 2001;281:E155–E161.

85. Buse JB, Henry RR, Han J et al. Effects of exenatide (exendin-4) on glycemic control over 30 weeks in sulfonylurea-treated patients with type 2 diabetes. *Diabetes Care* 2004;27:2628–2635.

86. Fineman MS, Shen LZ, Taylor K, Kim DD, Baron AD. Effectiveness of progressive dose-escalation of exenatide (exendin-4) in reducing dose-limiting side effects in subjects with type 2 diabetes. *Diabetes Metab Res Rev* 2004;20:411–417.

87. DURATION-4 study results: BYDUREON efficacy and tolerability profile extended to monotherapy treatment, http://www.bioportfolio.com/news/pdf/22525/Duration-4-Study-Results-Bydureon-Efficacy-And-Tolerability-Profile-Extended-To-Monotherapy.pdf (accessed on June 15, 2010).

88. Astrup A, Rossner S, Van Gaal L et al. Effects of liraglutide in the treatment of obesity: A randomised, double-blind, placebo-controlled study. *Lancet* 2009;374:1606–1616.

89. Goldstein DJ, Rampey AH, Jr., Roback PJ et al. Efficacy and safety of long-term fluoxetine treatment of obesity–Maximizing success. *Obes Res* 1995;3(Suppl 4):481S–490S.

90. Bray GA, Greenway FL. Current and potential drugs for treatment of obesity. *Endocr Rev* 1999;20:805–875.

91. Knowler WC, Barrett-Connor E, Fowler SE et al. Reduction in the incidence of type 2 diabetes with lifestyle intervention or metformin. *N Engl J Med* 2002;346:393–403.

92. Ortega-Gonzalez C, Luna S, Hernandez L et al. Responses of serum androgen and insulin resistance to metformin and pioglitazone in obese, insulin-resistant women with polycystic ovary syndrome. *J Clin Endocrinol Metab* 2005;90:1360–1365.

93. Maggs D, Shen L, Strobel S, Brown D, Kolterman O, Weyer C. Effect of pramlintide on A1C and body weight in insulin treated African Americans and Hispanics with type 2 diabetes: A pooled post hoc analysis. *Metabolism* 2003;52:1638–1642.

94. Bray GA, Gallagher TF, Jr. Manifestations of hypothalamic obesity in man: A comprehensive investigation of eight patients and a review of the literature. *Medicine (Baltimore)* 1975;54:301–330.

95. Lustig RH, Rose SR, Burghen GA et al. Hypothalamic obesity caused by cranial insult in children: Altered glucose and insulin dynamics and reversal by a somatostatin agonist. *J Pediatr* 1999;135:162–168.

96. Lustig RH, Hinds PS, Ringwald-Smith K et al. Octreotide therapy of pediatric hypothalamic obesity: A double-blind, placebo-controlled trial. *J Clin Endocrinol Metab* 2003;88:2586–2592.

97. Velasquez-Mieyer PA, Cowan PA, Arheart KL et al. Suppression of insulin secretion is associated with weight loss and altered macronutrient intake and preference in a subset of obese adults. *Int J Obes Relat Metab Disord* 2003;27:219–226.

98. Lustig RH, Greenway F, Velasquez D. Weight loss in obese adults with insulin hypersecretion treated with Sandostatin LAR Depot. *Obes Res* 2003;11(Suppl):A25.

99. Foxx-Orenstein A, Camilleri M, Stephens D, Burton D. Effect of a somatostatin analogue on gastric motor and sensory functions in healthy humans. *Gut* 2003;52:1555–1561.

100. Tan TM, Vanderpump M, Khoo B, Patterson M, Ghatei MA, Goldstone AP. Somatostatin infusion lowers plasma ghrelin without reducing appetite in adults with Prader-Willi syndrome. *J Clin Endocrinol Metab* 2004;89:4162–4165.

101. Ben-Menachem E, Axelsen M, Johanson EH, Stagge A, Smith U. Predictors of weight loss in adults with topiramate-treated epilepsy. *Obes Res* 2003;11:556–562.

102. Bray GA, Hollander P, Klein S et al. A 6-month randomized, placebo-controlled, dose-ranging trial of topiramate for weight loss in obesity. *Obes Res* 2003;11:722–733.

103. Wilding J, Van Gaal L, Rissanen A, Vercruysse F, Fitchet M, Group O-S. A randomized double-blind placebo-controlled study of the long-term efficacy and safety of topiramate in the treatment of obese subjects. *Int J Obes Relat Metab Disord* 2004;28:1399–1410.

104. Astrup A, Caterson I, Zelissen P et al. Topiramate: Long-term maintenance of weight loss induced by a low-calorie diet in obese subjects. *Obes Res* 2004;12:1658–1669.

105. Shapira NA, Goldsmith TD, McElroy SL. Treatment of binge-eating disorder with topiramate: A clinical case series. *J Clin Psychiatry* 2000;61:368–372.

106. McElroy SL, Arnold LM, Shapira NA et al. Topiramate in the treatment of binge eating disorder associated with obesity: A randomized, placebo-controlled trial. *Am J Psychiatry* 2003;160:255–261.

107. McElroy SL, Shapira NA, Arnold LM et al. Topiramate in the long-term treatment of binge-eating disorder associated with obesity. *J Clin Psychiatry* 2004;65:1463–1469.

108. Shapira NA, Lessig MC, Murphy TK, Driscoll DJ, Goodman WK. Topiramate attenuates self-injurious behaviour in Prader-Willi Syndrome. *Int J Neuropsychopharmacol* 2002;5:141–145.

109. Smathers SA, Wilson JG, Nigro MA. Topiramate effectiveness in Prader-Willi syndrome. *Pediatr Neurol* 2003;28:130–133.

110. Shapira NA, Lessig MC, Lewis MH, Goodman WK, Driscoll DJ. Effects of topiramate in adults with Prader-Willi syndrome. *Am J Ment Retard* 2004;109:301–309.

111. Winkelman JW. Treatment of nocturnal eating syndrome and sleep-related eating disorder with topiramate. *Sleep Med* 2003;4:243–246.

112. Gadde KM, Franciscy DM, Wagner HR, 2nd, Krishnan KR. Zonisamide for weight loss in obese adults: A randomized controlled trial. *JAMA* 2003;289:1820–1825.

113. Smith BM, Smith JM, Tsai JH et al. Discovery and structure-activity relationship of (1R)-8-chloro-2,3,4,5-tetrahydro-1-methyl-1H-3-benzazepine (Lorcaserin), a selective serotonin 5-HT2C receptor agonist for the treatment of obesity. *J Med Chem* 2008;51:305–313.

114. Smith SR, Prosser WA, Donahue DJ et al. Lorcaserin (APD356), a selective 5-HT(2C) agonist, reduces body weight in obese men and women. *Obesity (Silver Spring)* 2009;17:494–503.

115. Astrup A, Meier DH, Mikkelsen BO, Villumsen JS, Larsen TM. Weight loss produced by tesofensine in patients with Parkinson's or Alzheimer's disease. *Obesity (Silver Spring)* 2008;16:1363–1369.

116. Astrup A, Madsbad S, Breum L, Jensen TJ, Kroustrup JP, Larsen TM. Effect of tesofensine on bodyweight loss, body composition, and quality of life in obese patients: A randomised, double-blind, placebo-controlled trial. *Lancet* 2008;372:1906–1913.

117. Sjodin A, Gasteyger C, Nielsen AL et al. The effect of the triple monoamine reuptake inhibitor tesofensine on energy metabolism and appetite in overweight and moderately obese men. *Int J Obes (Lond)* 2010;34:1634–1643.

118. Greenway FL, Whitehouse MJ, Guttadauria M et al. Rational design of a combination medication for the treatment of obesity. *Obesity (Silver Spring)* 2009;17:30–39.

119. Greenway FL, Dunayevich E, Tollefson G et al. Comparison of combined bupropion and naltrexone therapy for obesity with monotherapy and placebo. *J Clin Endocrinol Metab* 2009;94:4898–4906.

120. Greenway FL, Fujioka K, Plodkowski RA et al. Effect of naltrexone plus bupropion on weight loss in overweight and obese adults (COR-I): A multicentre, randomised, double-blind, placebo-controlled, phase 3 trial. *Lancet* 2010;376:595–605.

121. Heymsfield SB, Greenberg AS, Fujioka K et al. Recombinant leptin for weight loss in obese and lean adults: A randomized, controlled, dose-escalation trial. *JAMA* 1999;282:1568–1575.

122. Roth JD, Roland BL, Cole RL et al. Leptin responsiveness restored by amylin agonism in diet-induced obesity: Evidence from nonclinical and clinical studies. *Proc Natl Acad Sci U S A* 2008;105:7257–7262.

123. Smith SR, Blundell JE, Burns C et al. Pramlintide treatment reduces 24-h caloric intake and meal sizes and improves control of eating in obese subjects: A 6-wk translational research study. *Am J Physiol Endocrinol Metab* 2007;293:E620–E627.

124. Smith SR, Aronne LJ, Burns CM, Kesty NC, Halseth AE, Weyer C. Sustained weight loss following 12-month pramlintide treatment as an adjunct to lifestyle intervention in obesity. *Diabetes Care* 2008;31:1816–1823.

125. Ravussin E, Smith SR, Mitchell JA et al. Enhanced weight loss with pramlintide/metreleptin: An integrated neurohormonal approach to obesity pharmacotherapy. *Obesity (Silver Spring)* 2009;17:1736–1743.

126. Oben J, Kuate D, Agbor G, Momo C, Talla X. The use of a Cissus quadrangularis formulation in the management of weight loss and metabolic syndrome. *Lipids Health Dis* 2006;5:24.

127. Oben JE, Enyegue DM, Fomekong GI, Soukontoua YB, Agbor GA. The effect of Cissus quadrangularis (CQR-300) and a Cissus formulation (CORE) on obesity and obesity-induced oxidative stress. *Lipids Health Dis* 2007;6:4.

128. Oben JE, Ngondi JL, Momo CN, Agbor GA, Sobgui CS. The use of a Cissus quadrangularis/Irvingia gabonensis combination in the management of weight loss: A double-blind placebo-controlled study. *Lipids Health Dis* 2008;7:12.

23 Historical Perspective, Efficacy of Current Drugs, and Future Directions in the Management of Obesity

Birgit Khandalavala, MD and Archana Chatterjee, MD, PhD

CONTENTS

INTRODUCTION

Obesity has been described as an "epidemic in need of therapeutics" (Van der Ploeg 2000). In a recent landmark study, the global mean body mass index (BMI; reported as kg/m²) has been reported to be on the upswing since 1980 with a mean increase of 0.4 kg/m² per decade. The highest incidence is in the Oceania countries and in the United States. In this systematic analysis of 960 country-years and 9.1 million participants, it was rare to find countries without an increase (Finucane et al. 2011). The International Obesity Task Force estimates that approximately 1 billion adults are currently overweight with a BMI of 25–29.9 kg/m² and a further 475 million are obese with a BMI of over 30 kg/m² (International Obesity Task Force Press Statement, 2011). Adding the Asian-specific cutoff points for the definition of obesity (BMI > 28 kg/m²), the number of obese adults would total over 600 million. Two hundred million school-age children are either overweight or obese, and of those, nearly one in five would qualify as obese. The widespread prevalence of obesity and paucity of proven long-term effective therapeutic options has led to biomedical research in energy homeostasis and metabolic balances with the hope of eventually safe and effective pharmacological interventions that would be available to all socioeconomic strata (Bloom et al. 2008). The number of current options has been further plagued by safety concerns and the removal of agents from the market that had been already in use for a few years (Ioannides-Demos et al. 2011). The predominant concerns in the drug therapy for obesity have been safety and efficacy, and current options do not provide either adequately.

OVERVIEW

Guidelines for the clinical management of obesity in adults from the National Heart, Lung, and Blood Institute, are readily available for use in practice since 1998 and available online. A revision is expected within the year. Obesity guidelines are in addition provided by the American Gastroenterological Association (American Gastroenterological Association 2002) and the American College of Physicians (Snow et al. 2005). The latter two resources do not have as widespread a use as that from the National Heart, Lung, and Blood Institute (National Heart, Lung, and Blood Institute 1998). Separate guidelines exist for children and adolescents and can be accessed from the American Academy of Pediatrics. The foundation of any treatment recommendation is lifestyle modification incorporating aspects of physical activity and nutritional advice in conjunction with behavior modification. Medication use and surgical options have to be carefully considered on an individual basis after an evaluation of risks and benefits. Drug therapy is indicated only in concurrent use with lifestyle modification. For morbid obesity, surgical options are usually the most effective therapy.

GOALS AND APPROACH TO THERAPY

- Calculation of the BMI is an essential initial step of any guideline. Evaluation could include other measures of adiposity such as the waist circumference, the waist-to-hip ratio, waist-to-height ratio, or the abdominal height.
- Detection of comorbid conditions, such as elevated blood pressure, hyperglycemia, overt diabetes mellitus, and dyslipidemia, is considered fundamental. More recently, the high prevalence of fatty liver and sleep apnea are increasingly reported and require early recognition and appropriate intervention. Medications are indicated if the BMI is greater than $27-30\,\mathrm{kg/m^2}$. A trial of drug therapy could be indicated at a lower BMI if comorbidities or a higher waist circumference are present. Asian-specific guidelines may require lower cutoffs both for the calculation of the BMI as obesity and for the waist circumference (Yusuf et al. 2005).
- Careful assessment of the risks and benefits of therapeutic intervention must be calculated for each individual case. Concurrent cardiac and mental health conditions, particularly depression, require the foremost evaluation and subsequent supervision.
- Use of medications is an adjunct to lifestyle modification. Physical activity and diet changes are imperative and need to occur in conjunction.
- Realistic endpoints and goals need to be established since few achieve their ideal weight (Foster et al. 1997). Weight regain following cessation adds to the patients' frustrations.
- A weight loss of 4 lb within the first month of treatment is considered indicative of efficacy and the assumption that the patient is responding to therapy. In the absence of documented weight loss, the impact on risk factors and improvement in concomitant medical conditions can constitute an indication for continuation.
- 5%–10% weight loss may impact comorbid conditions to a much larger effect. (Douketis et al. 2005; Knowler et al. 2002). This is not a linear relationship. A weight loss of 10%–15% is sought as the therapeutic efficacy when the impact is being assessed in a pharmacological intervention.
- Long-term therapy may be required. Current long-term data are for 2 years on sibutramine, which was withdrawn in 2010 (James et al. 2010), and 4 years for orlistat (Torgerson et al. 2004). Informed consent is advised for long-term use, if indicated.
- Weight regain needs to be anticipated when the medication is withdrawn. Similar to hypertension and diabetes, the use of medication has an effect when in use, but this is not sustained once withdrawn. No medication currently exists that can actually maintain the adipose tissue in a permanently reduced or metabolic inactive state which would be the ultimate goal and cure of obesity. Drug therapy, however, remains a vital component of successful weight maintenance.
- Bariatric surgery is indicated in cases where drug therapy has failed. Bariatric surgery is the most validated and effective treatment for individuals with a BMI over 40 or, over 35 with two comorbid conditions.

MECHANISM OF ACTION AND HISTORICAL TIME LINE OF WEIGHT LOSS MEDICATIONS

There have been many attempts to introduce medications to induce weight loss over the last 80 years (Ioannides-Demos et al. 2011). Mechanisms of action of medications usually involve

- Appetite reduction—sibutramine and amphetamines
- Increasing satiety—sympathomimetic drugs such as phentermine and diethylpropion
- Reduction of absorption of nutrients—orlistat
- Increasing energy expenditure—thyroid hormone and dinitrophenol

Safety issues related to drug therapy have been a concern from the outset, and many of these medications have been removed from the market (Table 23.1). Currently only phentermine is indicated for short-term use and orlistat for long-term use, and even this medication has had a recently added warning regarding the potential for severe liver damage (US Food and Drug Administration [FDA] Drug Safety Communication 2010).

TABLE 23.1
Time Line of Introduction of Weight Loss Medications and Current Status

Drug	Introduced	Mechanism of Action	Status
Dinitrophenol	1930s	Increases metabolic rate	Withdrawn—risk of neuropathy and cataracts
Amphetamines dexamphetamine, methamphetamine	1936	Appetite suppression	Banned, restricted, or discouraged—dependency and abuse potential, cardiovascular adverse effects
Amphetamine-like analogues phentermine, diethylpropion, phenylpropanolamine	1959—U.S.	Appetite suppression	Diethylpropion—available for short-term use (≤12 weeks) Phentermine—available for short-term use (≤12 weeks) in some countries, withdrawn 2000 (UK) Phenylpropanolamine—withdrawn 2000, increased risk of hemorrhagic stroke
Aminorex	1965	Appetite suppression	Withdrawn 1968—pulmonary hypertension
Mazindol	1970s	Appetite suppression	Discontinued 1993—Australia
Fenfluramine	1963—Europe 1973—U.S.	Appetite suppression	Withdrawn 1997—valvular heart disease, pulmonary hypertension
Dexfenfluramine	1985—Europe 1996—U.S.	Appetite suppression	Withdrawn 1997—valvular heart disease, pulmonary hypertension
Orlistat	1998—Europe and U.S.	Decreased fat absorption	Also available *over-the-counter* in several countries
Sibutramine	1997—U.S. 2001—Europe	Appetite suppression	Temporarily withdrawn 2002 Italy—concerns of raised risk of heart attacks and strokes Increase in contraindications—U.S. and Australia Suspension of market authorization 2010
Rimonabant	2006—Europe		Withdrawn 2009—potential of serious psychiatric disorders

Source: Ioannides-Demos, L.L. et al., *J. Obes.*, 2011, 179674, 2011.

MEDICATIONS: EFFICACY AND SAFETY CONCERNS

EFFICACY AND SIDE EFFECTS OF MEDICATIONS APPROVED BY THE FDA FOR WEIGHT LOSS

Current medications that are indicated for weight loss are sparse, and only orlistat remains available for long-term therapy (Table 23.2). Concerns regarding their safety have eliminated many other medications. The common or serious effects have been highlighted along with the efficacy. Weight loss with medication is usually modest with at best 2–7.9 kg more than placebo, and no current medication provides the efficacy needed to produce and sustain adequate weight loss required for morbidly obese patients (Ioannides-Demos et al. 2011).

TABLE 23.2
Medications Approved by the FDA for Weight Loss

Drug	Dose	Weight Loss (Mean)	Common or Serious Adverse Effects
Diethylpropion • (Tenuate, Tenuate Dospan) • Rx—schedule IV • Generic available	Immediate release 25 mg tid or qid 1 h before meals and midevening Extended release 75 mg once daily, taken midmorning	3 kg (6.6 lb) more than placebo (pooled analysis, study duration 6–12 months, dose 75 mg)	Pulmonary hypertension, valvular heart disease, dependence, withdrawal, psychosis, tachyarrhythmias Increased blood pressure, seizures, CNS stimulation, tremor, euphoria, dysphoria, headache, gastrointestinal (GI) complaints, bone marrow suppression
Phentermine (Adipex-P, Phentercot, Atti-plexP, Fastin, Phentride, Pro-fast) • Rx—schedule IV • Generic available	37.5 mg tablets daily before breakfast or 1–2 h after breakfast OR 18.75 mg tablets daily OR 15–30 mg capsules 2 h after breakfast	3.6 kg (7.92 lb) more than placebo (pooled analysis; study duration 2–24 weeks; dose 15–30 mg daily)	Pulmonary hypertension, valvular heart disease, dependence, withdrawal, psychosis, tachycardia, increased blood pressure, CNS stimulation, tremor, euphoria, dysphoria, headache, GI complaints
Orlistat (Xenical, Alli) • Over the counter • Rx—Xenical • No generic available	Xenical 10 mg tid with each meal containing fat Alli 60 mg up to tid with each fat-containing meal	3.45 kg (7.6 lb) more than placebo at 1 year (pooled study data, intent-to-treat population)	Cholelithiasis, flatulence, oily spotting, fecal incontinence, urgency or frequency, oily or fatty stool, abdominal or rectal pain, nausea, hepatitis, pancreatitis
Sibutramine (Meridia) • Rx—schedule IV • No generic available	10 mg once daily, titrated after 4 weeks to 15 mg once daily if needed	4 kg (8.8 lb) more than placebo at 1 year (study completers only with 10 mg dose)	Increased blood pressure and pulse, pulmonary hypertension, seizures, bleeding, gallstones, cognitive or motor impairment, headache, tachycardia, constipation, nausea, dry mouth, dizziness, CNS stimulation UPDATE—10/8/2010 Withdrawn from U.S. and Canadian markets due to risk of serious cardiovascular events

Sources: Ioannides-Demos, L.L. et al., *J. Obes.*, 2011, 179674, 2011; James, W.P. et al., *N. Engl. J. Med.*, 363, 905, 2010; McKay, R.H., *Curr. Med. Res. Opin.*, 1, 489, 1973; Munro, J.F. et al., *Br. Med. J.*, 1, 352, 1968; Li, Z. et al., *Ann. Intern. Med.*, 142, 532, 2005; FDA Drug Safety Communication. FDA Drug Safety Communication: Completed Safety Review of Xenical/Alli (Orlistat) and Severe Liver Injury. U.S. Food and Drug Administration. http://www.fda.gov. cuhs1.creighton.edu/Drugs/DrugSafety/PostmarketDrugSafetyInformationforPatientsandProviders/ucm213038.htm Additional Information for Health Care Professionals (accessed January 24, 2011).

FDA Nonapproved Medications

These consist of medications that may have had other primary indications and were found to be useful for weight loss. Efficacy and safety are the limiting factors. A move toward combinations of previously approved medications has resulted in some unique compounds. The medications are discussed in Table 23.3. The comparative efficacy of the medications indicated for long-term use is reviewed in Table 23.4.

TABLE 23.3
Medications Used or Studied Off-Label for Weight Loss

Drug	Dose	Weight Loss	Common or Serious Adverse Effects
Buproprion (Wellbutrin SR) • Rx • Generic available	300–400 mg per day, divided twice daily	2.8 kg (6.1 lb) more than placebo (pooled analysis of three studies in obese patients, obese patients with depressive symptoms, and patients with depression [some obese]; study duration 6–12 months; dose 200 mg twice daily)	Dry mouth, nausea, CNS stimulation, tremor, palpitations, seizures, psychosis, mania, increased blood pressure
Fluoxetine (Prozac) • Rx • Generic available	60 mg per day	2.6 kg (5.7 lb) at 6 months and 0.6 kg (1.3 lb) at 12 months more than placebo	Regain of 50% of the weight during the second 6 months of treatment, sexual dysfunction
Human chorionic gonadotropin (HCG, Novarel, Pregnyl) • Rx • Generic available	125 IU IM once daily, plus fat-free 500 kcal per day diet	No reliable evidence of weight loss, fat redistribution, decreased appetite, or improved mood	Ovarian hyperstimulation, edema, ovarian cyst rupture with hemoperitoneum, multiple births, headache, irritability, restlessness, depression, fatigue, precocious puberty, gynecomastia, injection site pain, arterial thromboembolism, allergic reactions
Thyroid hormone • Rx • Generic available	Liothyronine (T3) 18–117 mcg/70 kg or levothyroxine (T4) 80 mcg/70 kg, plus caloric restriction to <800 kcal/day	Unable to assess due to study limitations	Subclinical hyperthyroidism leading to muscle wasting, weakness, cardiac effects, and decreased bone mineral density
Zonisamide (Zonegran) • Rx • Generic available	100–600 mg daily (Labeling recommends 2 weeks between dosage increases in increments of 100 mg. Take as single daily dose or divide twice daily.)	Additional 5% of baseline weight lost compared to placebo in 16 weeks	Serious skin and hematologic reactions, mood disorders, psychosis, cognitive impairment, somnolence, dizziness, headache, nausea, agitation, irritability, fatigue, kidney stones, renal impairment, muscle damage, pancreatitis

Sources: Li, Z. et al., *Ann. Intern. Med.*, 142, 532, 2005; Goldstein, D.J. et al., *Int. J. Obes. Relat. Metab. Disord.*, 18, 129, 1994; Lijesen, G.K. et al., *Br. J. Clin. Pharmacol.*, 40, 237, 1995; Kaptein, E.M. et al., *J. Clin. Endocrinol. Metab.*, 94, 3663, 2009.

TABLE 23.4

**Comparative Efficacy of Drugs and Meta-Analyses
of Long-Term Studies in Adults (12 Months or Longer)**

Drug	Number of Studies	Total Number of Subjects	Mean Difference in Weight (kg) 95% Confidence Interval
Rimonabant	4	Placebo 1600 Rimonabant 2500	4.7 (4.1, 5.3)
Orlistat	14	Placebo 4509 Orlistat 4948	2.9 (2.4, 3.2)
Sibutramine	7	Placebo 699 Sibutramine 873	4.2 (3.6, 4.8)
Sibutramine Orlistat	5	Sibutramine 229 Orlistat 249	3.4 (2.3, 4.6)
Bupropion	5	Placebo 344 Bupropion 618	2.8 (1.1, 4.5)

Sources: Li, Z. et al., *Ann. Intern. Med.,* 142, 532, 2005; Van Gaal, L. et al., *Diabetes Care,* 31, S229, 2008; Christensen, R. et al., *Ugeskr. Laeger.,* 169, 4360, 2007; Padwal, R. et al., *Cochrane Database of Systematic Reviews (Online),* 3, CD004094, 2004; Rucker, D. et al., *BMJ (Clinical Research Edition),* 335, 1194, 2007.

DIABETES DRUGS ASSOCIATED WITH WEIGHT LOSS

Certain medications used in the treatment of diabetes have been known to reduce weight (Table 23.5). Metformin was used in the Diabetes Prevention Program for glucose intolerance (Knowler et al. 2002). Metformin does not induce a sustained weight loss of at least 5% to have a weight loss indication, but it has been found to be useful in children and adolescents and been used to prevent weight gain due to antipsychotic drugs (Ellinger et al. 2010). As compared to most diabetic medications, metformin is weight neutral.

Pramlintide is only available in the parenteral form and is a peptide hormone that not only lowers blood glucose but delays gastric emptying resulting in weight loss (Maggs et al. 2003). Combinations with recombinant methyl human leptin, sibutramine, phentermine, and exenatide are under evaluation.

Exenatide is an incretin peptide that is a glucagon-like polypeptide-1 agonist and is only available for parenteral administration. Dose-dependent weight loss has been reported with its use (Ratner et al. 2006). Its effect on weight loss was determined to be independent of the nausea associated with its use.

Liraglutide has recently been introduced in the United States and indicated for diabetes. In patients without known diabetes reports of sustained weight loss has been shown in a 20 week study with this drug (Astrup et al. 2009). This is a more easily tolerated medication due to the convenience of the once-a-day dosing without regard to meals and the lower incidence of nausea as a side effect. However, this drug carries a warning about thyroid cell carcinoma that was detected in rats during studies but has yet to be reported in humans. This cancer is difficult to detect, with minimal monitoring options available and concerns regarding long-term safety remain.

TABLE 23.5

Diabetes Drugs Associated with Weight Loss

Drug	Dose	Weight Loss	Side Effects
Metformin biguanide • Rx • Generic available Oral route	500–2500 mg	2.5% of body weight after an average of 2.8 years of follow-up	GI most commonly and includes a metallic taste in the mouth, mild anorexia, nausea, abdominal discomfort and lactic acidosis (rare)
Pramlintide (Symlin) • Rx • No generic available • Injectable only	60–120 mcg just before major meals (250 kcal or 30 g carbohydrate) (diabetes dose)	1.7 kg (3.74 lb) more than placebo after 6 months (in type 2 diabetes patients in diabetes trials) with a 120 mcg dose	Severe hypoglycemia, local or systemic allergic reactions, nausea, vomiting
Exenatide (Byetta) • Rx • No generic available	5–10 mcg SQ twice daily, 1 h prior to two main meals, at least 6 h apart (diabetes dose)	2.7–2.9 kg (5.94–6.38 lb) over 24 weeks in diabetes patients in clinical trials	Nausea, hypoglycemia, vomiting, diarrhea, feeling jittery, dizziness, headache, dyspepsia, renal impairment, pancreatitis
Liraglutide • Rx • No generic • Injectable only	0.6–1.8 mg once a day SQ	4.8–7.2 kg (10.6–15.6 lb) in a 20 week study	Nausea, vomiting and diarrhea, rare pancreatitis. In rats, associated with benign and malignant thyroid C cell tumors

Sources: Knowler, W.C. et al., *N. Engl. J. Med.,* 346, 393, 2002; Maggs, D. et al., *Metabolism,* 52, 1638, 2003; Ratner, R.E. et al., *Diabetes. Obes. Metab.,* 8, 419, 2006; Astrup, A. et al., *Lancet,* 374, 1606, 2009; Li, Z. et al., *Ann. Intern. Med.,* 142, 532, 2005.

NOVEL OR INVESTIGATIONAL MEDICATIONS AND FUTURE DIRECTIONS

Obesity is increasingly thought to have a fetal origin. This may be related to the very early and critical stages of fetal and neonatal development with a focus on the connectivity of important hypothalamic circuits. Maternal overnutrition and hyperinsulinemia, along with increased energy intake in the first months of life may set up in the genetically susceptible an epigenetic programming resulting in a predisposition to obesity that persists into adulthood (Bloom et al. 2008). Control of obesity currently needs multiple expensive drugs targeting redundant energy homeostasis pathways. Though the present list of medications is sparse, a number of clinical trials of novel therapeutic agents are underway (Tables 23.6 through 23.9).

The U.S. FDA has published specific guidelines for the development of drug therapies to address obesity, which would be safe for long-term use and have a minimum efficacy profile (Food and Drug Administration 2007). These criteria have not been strictly achieved by many of the potential candidates. In spite of this, a combination of bupropion and naltrexone is close to receiving FDA approval in 2011 (Orexigen 2011b). The FDA advisory panel voted to recommend its approval for obesity management on December 7, 2010, but the FDA in January of 2011 indicated that more data needed to be studied and presented and hence did not meet approval (Orexigen 2011a). The glucagon-like peptide-1 is also being evaluated for use in obesity. However, whether in the long term an injectable drug will be found to be acceptable as a treatment option is yet to be established. An adequate safety profile in addition requires to be established. Nevertheless, optimism that these will fulfill their promise for the treatment of obesity has been expressed (Bray 2009).

TABLE 23.6

Investigational Products for Weight Loss

Drug	Mechanism	Weight Loss	Side Effects of Action
Leptin	Peptide produced from adipocytes	Weakly dose dependent from 1.4 kg in the 0.03 mg/kg dose to 7.1 kg in the 0.30 mg/kg dose group	Leptin resistance
Peptide YY	Gut hormone peptide that decreases food intake	200 mcg dose three times a day was not different from placebo 600 mcg dose not assessed due to 60% drop out rate	Nausea and vomiting
Oxyntomodulin	Peptide from the L-cells of the GI tract.	2.3 ± 0.4 kg compared to 0.5 ± treated with placebo	
Melanocortin-4 receptor agonists	Stimulates the hypothalamic-melanocortin system	In normal-weight subjects, reduced weight by 1.7 kg but not in overweight subjects	
Tensofensine	Initially developed for Parkinson's disease and inhibits the uptake of norepinephrine, dopamine, and serotonin	Dose-dependent weight loss 32.1% achieved a weight loss	Heart rate increase though blood pressure remained stable
Locarserin	Selective serotonin 2C agonist	10 mg twice a day 3.0	Headache, dizziness, nausea
Taranabant	Cannabinoid CB-1 receptor inverse agonist	6 mg dose had the highest weight loss	Due to serious psychiatric events that included depression, anxiety, anger, and aggression with dose-dependent increased risk of suicide, clinical studies were ceased; 80% experienced some adverse effect

Sources: Heymsfield, S.B. et al., *JAMA*, 282, 1568, 1999; Gantz, I. et al., *J. Clin. Endocrinol. Metab.*, 92, 1754, 2007; Wynne, K. et al., *Diabetes*, 54, 2390, 2005; Hallschmid, M. et al., *J. Clin. Endocrinol. Metab.*, 91, 522, 2006; Astrup, A. et al., *Lancet*, 372, 1906, 2008; Smith, S.R. et al., *N. Engl. J. Med.*, 363, 245, 2010; Addy, C. et al., *Cell Metab.*, 7, 68, 2008; Aronne, L.J. et al., *Int. J. Obes.*, 34, 919, 2010; Ioannides-Demos, L.L. et al., *J. Obes.*, 2011, 179674, 2011.

TABLE 23.7
Combination Therapies

Drug	Mechanism of Action	Dose Efficacy	Side Effects
Bupropion and naltrexone (Contrave)	Naltrexone blocks beta endorphin–mediated propiomelanocortin (POMC) autoinhibition + bupropion activates POMC neurons	Naltrexone 16, 32, or 48 mg with bupropion 360/400 mg	Generally well-tolerated. Nausea most common adverse effect Significant improvement in depressive symptoms Several phase III trials completed Did not receive FDA approval—more cardiovascular safety data requested
Bupropion and zonisamide	Zonisamide has biphasic dopaminergic and 5 HT activity	Bupropion (120/360 mg) with zonisamide 360 mg	Somnolence, headache, nausea, and insomnia Appears to have greater weight loss than the bupropion/naltrexone combination Three phase II trials
Topiramate and phentermine	Topiramate is a GABA agonist while phentermine is a sympathomimetic agent	Topiramate 92/46 mg with phentermine 15/7.5 mg. Weight loss of 9.2% for the combination, 6.4% for topiramate alone and 6.1% for phentermine alone	Increased heart rate, possible birth defects, and psychiatric problems. Final FDA approval was not given and new safety data have been requested by the FDA
Pramlintide and metreleptin combination therapies	Peptide hormone with leptin, an adipocyte-derived hormone. Also used in combination with sibutramine and phentermine, which are sympathomimetic agents	Greater weight loss than with a single agent Pramlintide/metreleptin 12.7% Pramlintide/sibutramine 11.1% Pramlintide/phentermine 3.7%	Nausea, increased heart rate and blood pressure

Sources: Ioannides-Demos, L.L. et al., *J. Obes.*, 2011; 179674, 2011; Orexigen Therapeutics, Inc., FDA issues complete response to new drug application for Contrave® for the management of obesity, 2011; http//ir.orexigen.com/phoenix.zhtml?c=207034&p=irol-newsArticle&ID=1505602&highlight (accessed March 30, 2011).

TABLE 23.8
Recent Randomized Controlled Trials of Weight Loss Therapies with 6 Month Follow-Up

Drug	Number of Subjects (n)	Absolute Weight Loss (kg)	≥5% Weight Loss	≥10% Weight Loss
Bupropion (400mg) plus naltrexone	Placebo (n = 85)	0.9 ± 0.5	15%	2%
	N 48 mg (n = 56) B (n = 60)	1.1 ± 0.7	10%	2%
	BN 16 mg (n = 64)	2.6 ± 0.6	26%	7%
		5.1 ± 0.6[a]	52%[a]	17%[a]
	BN 32 mg (n = 63)	5.1 ± 0.6[a]	51%[a]	19%[a]
	BN 48 mg (n = 61)	4.0 ± 0.6[a]	39%[a]	15%[a]
Bupropion (120/360 mg) plus zonisamide (360/360 mg)	Total n = 729			
	Placebo	1.4	15%	4%
	Z120	3.2	27%	9%
	Z360	5.3	44%	18%
	B360	2.3	21%	11%
	ZB120	6.1%[b]	47%[a]	25%[a]
	ZB360	7.5[b]	60%[a]	32%[a]
Rimonabant	Placebo (n = 417)	0.5	NR	NR
	R (n = 422)	4.3[b]		
Rimonabant	Total n = 3165			
	Placebo	1.6	19.7%	7.8%
	R	6.5	50.8%[b]	27%[b]
Tesofensine	Placebo (n = 52)	2.2	13 (29%)	3 (7%)
	T 0.25 mg (n = 52)	6.7[c]	29 (59%)	17 (35%)
	T 0.5 mg (n = 50)	11.3[c]	41 (87%)	25 (53%)
	T 1.0 mg (n = 49)	12.8[c]	42 (91%)	34 (74%)

Source: Modified from Ioannides-Demos, L.L. et al., *J. Obes.*, 2011, 179674, 2011.
NR, not recorded; NA, not available; B, bupropion; N, naltrexone; Z, zonisamide; R, rimonabant; T, tesofensine.

[a] P < .05.
[b] P < .001.
[c] P < .0001.

TABLE 23.9

Recent Randomized Controlled Trials of Weight Loss Therapies with 12 Month Follow-Up

Drug	Number of Subjects (n)	Absolute Weight Loss (kg)	≥5% Weight Loss	≥10% Weight Loss
Lorcaserin	Placebo (n = 716)	2.16 ± 0.14	20.3%	7.7%
	Lorcaserin (n = 883)	5.81 ± 0.16[a]	47.5%[a]	22.6%[a]
Taranabant	Placebo (n = 417)	2.6	27.2%	8.4%
	TB 2 mg (n = 415)	6.6[a]	56.5%[a]	27.9%[a]
	TB 4 mg (n = 414)	8.1[a]	64.2%[a]	35.8%[a]
Taranabant	Placebo (n = 196)	+1.7	62.2%	NR
	TB 0.5 mg (n = 196)	0.1[b]	71.8%	NR
	TB 1 mg (n = 196)	0.6[b]	78% (P < .05)	NR
	TB 2 mg (n = 196)	1.2[b]	83.3%[a]	NR
Taranabant	Placebo (n = 137)	1.4	24.3%	7.3%
	TB 0.5 mg (n = 141)	5.0[a]	44.2[a]	21.3[a]
	TB 1 mg (n = 138)	5.2[a]	45.3[a]	18.2[a]
	TB 2 mg (n = 277)	6.4[a]	53[a]	28[a]
Bupropion/naltrexone (with intensive behavior modification)	Placebo (n = 202)	7.3% ± 0.9%	60.4%	30.2%
	B/N 360/32 mg (n = 591)	11.5% ± 0.6%[a]	80.4%[a]	55.2%[a]
Bupropion/naltrexone	B (n = 60)	2.7 ± 0.9	33%	12%
	BN 16 mg (n = 64)	5.0 ± 0.9	50%	22%
	BN 32 mg (n = 63)	6.1 ± 0.8 (P < .05)	51%	25%
	BN 48 mg (n = 61)	4.6 ± 0.9	39%	20%
Pramlintide	Placebo (n = 63)	2.1 ± 0.9	3%	11%
	Pramlintide (n = 61)	3.6 ± 0.7	28%	36%
Topiramate	Placebo (n = 55)	2.5 ± 3.1	19%	2%
	T (n = 54)	6.0 ± 5.2[a]	50%[a]	20%[a]
Topiramate/phentermine	P (n = 498)	1.6	17%	NA
	TP 3.75/23 mg (n = 234)	5.1[c]	45%[c]	
	TP 15/92 mg (n = 498)	11[c]	67%[c]	
Topiramate/phentermine	P (n = 979)	1.8	21%	NA
	TP 7.5/46 mg (n = 488)	8.4[c]	62%[c]	
	TP 15/92 (n = 981)	10.4[c]	70%[c]	

Source: Modified from Ioannides-Demos L. L. et al., *J. Obes.,* 2011, 179674, 2011.

NB, naltrexone/bupropion; TB, taranabantr; T, topiramate controlled release; TP, topiramate/phentermine; NS, not significant; NA, not available.

[a] P < .001.

[b] P < .007.

[c] P < .0001.

Obesity is a long-term, chronic disease, and the modalities for treatment need to be similarly long term since pharmacological effects are difficult to sustain once the therapy is terminated and weight regain is often inevitable. Surgical options are also associated with subsequent weight regain, though usually this is slower and less dramatic. Effective public health measures are required to reduce the effects of a combination of inactivity with excess cheap calories that are readily available. This will take time and enormous effort. In the meanwhile, the development of more effective antiobesity drugs is justified for patients with physiological defects who need targeted pharmacological interventions. This subset will probably consist of those with refractory and severe obesity. Also, medications or therapeutics with a better safety profile are needed to overcome the toxic effects of the current obesogenic environment. These individuals may have already had alterations in their genetic material causing them to remain obese their entire life even if the environment around them is no longer obesogenic. Often obesity requires a combination of treatments, using all three components of lifestyle modification, pharmacological agents, and surgical options to maximize the weight loss. The modalities are not exclusive of one another. It is anticipated that the costs of obesity management will continue to rise and will require multidrug regimens to control elevated body weight and associated cardiovascular and other associated risk factors (Bloom et al. 2008).

REFERENCES

Addy, C., H. Wright, K. Van Laere, I. Gantz, N. Erondu, B. J. Musser, K. Lu et al. The acyclic CB1R inverse agonist taranabant mediates weight loss by increasing energy expenditure and decreasing caloric intake. *Cell Metabolism* 7(1) (January, 2008): 68–78.

American Gastroenterological Association. American Gastroenterological Association Medical Position Statement on Obesity. *Gastroenterology* 123(3) (September, 2002): 879–881.

Aronne, L. J., S. Tonstad, M. Moreno, I. Gantz, N. Erondu, S. Suryawanshi, C. Molony et al. A clinical trial assessing the safety and efficacy of taranabant, a CB1R inverse agonist, in obese and overweight patients: A high-dose study. *International Journal of Obesity* 34(5) (May, 2010): 919–935.

Astrup, A., S. Madsbad, L. Breum, T. J. Jensen, J. P. Kroustrup, and T. M. Larsen. Effect of tesofensine on bodyweight loss, body composition, and quality of life in obese patients: A randomised, double-blind, placebo-controlled trial. *Lancet* 372(9653) (November 29, 2008): 1906–1913.

Astrup, A., S. Rossner, L. Van Gaal, A. Rissanen, L. Niskanen, M. Al Hakim, J. Madsen, M. F. Rasmussen, M. E. Lean, and NN8022-1807 Study Group. Effects of liraglutide in the treatment of obesity: A randomised, double-blind, placebo-controlled study. *Lancet* 374(9701) (November 7, 2009): 1606–1616.

Bloom, S. R., F. P. Kuhajda, I. Laher, X. Pi-Sunyer, G. V. Ronnett, T. M. Tan, and D. S. Weigle. The obesity epidemic: Pharmacological challenges. *Molecular Interventions* 8(2) (April, 2008): 82–98.

Bray, G. A. Gastrointestinal hormones and weight management. *Lancet* 374(9701) (November 7, 2009): 1570–1571.

Christensen, R., P. K. Kristensen, E. M. Bartels, H. Bliddal, and A. V. Astrup. A meta-analysis of the efficacy and safety of the anti-obesity agent rimonabant. *Ugeskrift for Laeger* 169(50) (December 10, 2007): 4360–4363.

Douketis, J. D., C. Macie, L. Thabane, and D. F. Williamson. Systematic review of long-term weight loss studies in obese adults: Clinical significance and applicability to clinical practice. *International Journal of Obesity (2005)* 29(10) (October, 2005): 1153–1167.

Ellinger, L. K., H. J. Ipema, and J. M. Stachnik. Efficacy of metformin and topiramate in prevention and treatment of second-generation antipsychotic-induced weight gain. *The Annals of Pharmacotherapy* 44(4) (April, 2010): 668–679.

FDA Drug Safety Communication. FDA Drug Safety Communication: Completed Safety Review of Xenical/Alli (Orlistat) and Severe Liver Injury. U.S. Food and Drug Administration. http://www.fda.gov.cuhsl.creighton.edu/Drugs/DrugSafety/PostmarketDrugSafetyInformationforPatientsandProviders/ucm213038.htm#AdditionalInformationforHealthcareProfessionals (accessed January 24, 2011).

Finucane, M. M., G. A. Stevens, M. J. Cowan, G. Danaei, J. K. Lin, C. J. Paciorek et al. National, regional, and global trends in body-mass index since 1980: Systematic analysis of health examination surveys and epidemiological studies with 960 country-years and 9.1 million participants. Accessed at *www.thelancet.com*, 377(February 2011): 557–567.

Food and Drug Administration. Guidance for Industry Developing Products for Weight Management. U.S. Food and Drug Administration. 2007, http://www.fda.gov.cuhsl.creighton.edu/downloads/Drugs/GuidanceComplianceRegulatoryInformation/Guidances/ucm071612.pdf (accessed January 24, 2011).

Foster, G. D., T. A. Wadden, R. A. Vogt, and G. Brewer. What is a reasonable weight loss? Patients' Expectations and evaluations of obesity treatment outcomes. *Journal of Consulting and Clinical Psychology* 65(1) (February, 1997): 79–85.

Gantz, I., N. Erondu, M. Mallick, B. Musser, R. Krishna, W. K. Tanaka, K. Snyder et al. Efficacy and safety of intranasal peptide YY3-36 for weight reduction in obese adults. *The Journal of Clinical Endocrinology and Metabolism* 92(5) (May, 2007): 1754–1757.

Goldstein, D. J., A. H. Rampey Jr., G. G. Enas, J. H. Potvin, L. A. Fludzinski, and L. R. Levine. Fluoxetine: A randomized clinical trial in the treatment of obesity. *International Journal of Obesity and Related Metabolic Disorders: Journal of the International Association for the Study of Obesity* 18(3) (March, 1994): 129–135.

Hallschmid, M., R. Smolnik, G. McGregor, J. Born, and H. L. Fehm. Overweight humans are resistant to the weight-reducing effects of melanocortin4–10. *The Journal of Clinical Endocrinology and Metabolism* 91(2) (February, 2006): 522–525.

Heymsfield, S. B., A. S. Greenberg, K. Fujioka, R. M. Dixon, R. Kushner, T. Hunt, J. A. Lubina et al. Recombinant leptin for weight loss in obese and lean adults: A randomized, controlled, dose-escalation trial. *JAMA: The Journal of the American Medical Association* 282(16) (October 27, 1999): 1568–1575.

International Obesity Task Force. International obesity task force press statement. http://www.iotf.org/media/iotfaug25.htm (accessed January 18, 2011).

Ioannides-Demos, L. L., L. Piccenna, and J. J. McNeil. Pharmacotherapies for obesity: Past, current, and future therapies. *Journal of Obesity (Online)* 2011, (2011): 179674.

James, W. P., I. D. Caterson, W. Coutinho, N. Finer, L. F. Van Gaal, A. P. Maggioni, C. Torp-Pedersen et al. Effect of sibutramine on cardiovascular outcomes in overweight and obese subjects. *The New England Journal of Medicine* 363(10) (September 2, 2010): 905–917.

Kaptein, E. M., E. Beale, and L. S. Chan. Thyroid hormone therapy for obesity and nonthyroidal illnesses: A systematic review. *The Journal of Clinical Endocrinology and Metabolism* 94(10) (October, 2009): 3663–3675.

Knowler, W. C., E. Barrett-Connor, S. E. Fowler, R. F. Hamman, J. M. Lachin, E. A. Walker, D. M. Nathan, and Diabetes Prevention Program Research Group. Reduction in the incidence of type 2 diabetes with lifestyle intervention or metformin. *The New England Journal of Medicine* 346(6) (February 7, 2002): 393–403.

Li, Z., M. Maglione, W. Tu, W. Mojica, D. Arterburn, L. R. Shugarman, L. Hilton et al. Meta-analysis: Pharmacologic treatment of obesity. *Annals of Internal Medicine* 142(7) (April 5, 2005): 532–546.

Lijesen, G. K., I. Theeuwen, W. J. Assendelft, and G. Van Der Wal. The effect of human chorionic gonadotropin (HCG) in the treatment of obesity by means of the simeons therapy: A criteria-based meta-analysis. *British Journal of Clinical Pharmacology* 40(3) (September, 1995): 237–243.

Maggs, D., L. Shen, S. Strobel, D. Brown, O. Kolterman, and C. Weyer. Effect of pramlintide on A1C and body weight in insulin-treated African Americans and Hispanics with type 2 diabetes: A pooled post hoc analysis. *Metabolism: Clinical and Experimental* 52(12) (December, 2003): 1638–1642.

McKay, R. H. Long-Term use of diethylpropion in obesity. *Current Medical Research and Opinion* 1(8) (1973): 489–493.

Munro, J. F., A. C. MacCuish, E. M. Wilson, and L. J. Duncan. Comparison of continuous and intermittent anorectic therapy in obesity. *British Medical Journal* 1(5588) (February 10, 1968): 352–354.

National Heart, Lung, and Blood Institute. Clinical guidelines on the identification, evaluation, and treatment of overweight and obesity in adults. National Institutes of Health. http://www.nhlbi.nih.gov.cuhsl.creighton.edu/guidelines/obesity/ob_gdlns.pdf (accessed January 24, 2011).

Orexigen Therapeutics, Inc. Contrave® weight loss drug information. Orexigen, 2011a. http://www.tesofensine-information.com/contrave.html (accessed January 24, 2011).

Orexigen Therapeutics, Inc. FDA issues complete response to new drug application for Contrave® for the management of obesity, 2011b. http://ir.orexigen.com/phoenix.zhtml?c=207034&p=irol-newsArticle&ID=1505602&highlight (accessed March 30, 2011).

Padwal, R., S. K. Li, and D. C. Lau. Long-term pharmacotherapy for obesity and overweight. *Cochrane Database of Systematic Reviews (Online)* 3(3) (2004): CD004094.

Ratner, R. E., D. Maggs, L. L. Nielsen, A. H. Stonehouse, T. Poon, B. Zhang, T. A. Bicsak, R. G. Brodows, and D. D. Kim. Long-term effects of exenatide therapy over 82 weeks on glycaemic control and weight in over-weight metformin-treated patients with type 2 diabetes mellitus. *Diabetes, Obesity & Metabolism* 8(4) (July, 2006): 419–428.

Rucker, D., R. Padwal, S. K. Li, C. Curioni, and D. C. Lau. Long term pharmacotherapy for obesity and overweight: Updated meta-analysis. *BMJ (Clinical Research Edition)* 335(7631) (December 8, 2007): 1194–1199.

Smith, S. R., N. J. Weissman, C. M. Anderson, M. Sanchez, E. Chuang, S. Stubbe, H. Bays, W. R. Shanahan, and Behavioral Modification and Lorcaserin for Overweight and Obesity Management (BLOOM) Study Group. Multicenter, placebo-controlled trial of lorcaserin for weight management. *The New England Journal of Medicine* 363(3) (July 15, 2010): 245–256.

Snow, V., P. Barry, N. Fitterman, A. Qaseem, K. Weiss, and Clinical Efficacy Assessment Subcommittee of the American College of Physicians. Pharmacologic and surgical management of obesity in primary care: A clinical practice guideline from the American College of Physicians. *Annals of Internal Medicine* 142(7) (April 5, 2005): 525–531.

Torgerson, J. S., J. Hauptman, M. N. Boldrin, and L. Sjostrom. XENical in the Prevention of Diabetes in Obese Subjects (XENDOS) Study: A randomized study of orlistat as an adjunct to lifestyle changes for the prevention of type 2 diabetes in obese patients. *Diabetes Care* 27(1) (January, 2004): 155–161.

Van der Ploeg, L. H. Obesity: An epidemic in need of therapeutics. *Current Opinion in Chemical Biology* 4(4) (August, 2000): 452–460.

Van Gaal, L., X. Pi-Sunyer, J. P. Despres, C. McCarthy, and A. Scheen. Efficacy and safety of rimonabant for improvement of multiple cardiometabolic risk factors in overweight/obese patients: Pooled 1-year data from the Rimonabant In Obesity (RIO) Program. *Diabetes Care* 31(Suppl 2) (February, 2008): S229–S240.

Wynne, K., A. J. Park, C. J. Small, M. Patterson, S. M. Ellis, K. G. Murphy, A. M. Wren et al. Subcutaneous oxyntomodulin reduces body weight in overweight and obese subjects: A double-blind, randomized, controlled trial. *Diabetes* 54(8) (August, 2005): 2390–2395.

Yusuf, S., S. Hawken, S. Ôunpuu et al., on behalf of the INTERHEART Study Investigators. Obesity and the risk of myocardial infarction in 27000 participants from 52 countries: A case-control study. *Lancet* 366(9497) (November, 2005):1640–1649.

Part VI

Natural, Nutritional, and Physical Approaches of Weight Management

24 Essential Role of Exercise and Physical Activity in Weight Management

Dawn Blatt, PT, DPT, MS and Cheri L. Gostic, PT, DPT, MS

CONTENTS

GROWING OBESITY EPIDEMIC

Obesity has grown into one of the most concerning public health epidemics in the United States over the past several decades. The prevalence of obesity has doubled in adults, while the incidence of overweight children and adolescents has tripled since 1980.[1] Data from the National Health and Nutrition Examination Survey (NHANES) obtained in 2007–2008 revealed that 33.8% of adults in the United States were obese and that 68.0% were overweight or obese.[2] Data from NHANES obtained in 2005–2006 revealed 15.5% of children and adolescents were obese and 30.1% were overweight or obese.[3] In the United States, obesity is ranked second only to the use of tobacco as the leading preventable cause of death.[4]

Body mass index (BMI), defined as body weight (in kg) divided by height squared (in meters^2), has become the most commonly used indicator of obesity in recent years. Whereas a BMI equal to or greater than $30 \, kg/m^2$ signifies obesity, the National Center for Health Statistics reports that health risks actually begin to increase at a BMI greater than $27 \, kg/m^2$. Children are at risk of being overweight if their BMI falls between the 85th and 95th percentile for their sex and age and deemed obese at or above the 95th percentile.

Children and adolescents who are overweight are at risk of developing type 2 diabetes, sleep apnea, and poor self-esteem and have to deal with the social consequences of being overweight.[5] They are six times more likely to have at least one cardiovascular risk factor as compared to children of healthy weight and are at increased risk for various chronic diseases as adults.[6] In adults, the health risks associated with obesity are well established. Obesity increases the risks of cardiovascular disease, stroke, diabetes, arthritis, gall bladder disease, certain cancers, and lung pathologies.[7] Abdominal or central obesity and insulin resistance are also considered the primary risk factors associated with metabolic syndrome, a cluster of conditions that appear to directly promote the development of atherosclerotic cardiovascular disease.[8] Research by Shen et al. suggests that a measurement of waist circumference has a stronger correlation to health risks associated with metabolic syndrome than BMI or percent body fat measured by DEXA and is an important adjunct in the clinical assessment of obesity.[9] Based on recent research, Bray has proposed that men with a waist circumference between 100 and 120 cm are at high risk and, above 120 cm, at very high risk for cardiovascular disease. His new proposed risk classification designates women with a waist circumference between 90 and 109 cm at high risk, and those above 110 cm at very high risk.[10]

The problem of overweight and obesity results from an imbalance involving elevated caloric intake relative to energy expenditure and is influenced by genetic, behavioral, metabolic, and socioeconomic factors. The World Health Organization Consultation on Obesity (2002) determined that physical inactivity and overindulgence in food are primarily responsible for the obesity epidemic in the United States. Americans' devotion to television and computers, labor-saving devices, and contracted household services has contributed greatly to a more sedentary culture. Research has determined that there is a strong relationship between the amount of television an individual watches and the prevalence of obesity and diabetes.[11] The U.S. Department of Health and Human Services reports that 40% of adults in the United States engage in no leisure time physical activity, while 80% of overweight adults are completely sedentary.

A review of the literature by Blair and Brodney in 1999 demonstrated that regular physical activity attenuates many of the health risks associated with obesity. It found that overweight or obese individuals who are physically fit and active remarkably have lower morbidity and mortality than individuals of normal weight who are sedentary.[12] Research by Hu et al. concluded that a sedentary lifestyle and increased adiposity were strong and independent predictors of death, which, together, accounted for 31% of all premature deaths among the nonsmoking women involved in their study.[13] It is clear that regular exercise and physical activity result in improved fitness and health and need to be foundational elements in combating obesity in this country.

Despite national initiatives to reverse the growing problem of obesity in the United States, data collected between 1994 and 2000 by Jackson et al. revealed that the proportion of obese persons receiving advice to lose weight from primary care providers fell from 44.0% to 40.0% despite an increased prevalence of obesity during this same period. In addition, individuals who were less educated and from lower income brackets were noted to be less likely to receive advice to lose weight by health care providers than those with greater education and assets. Among obese persons not graduating from high school, advice declined from 41.4% to 31.8% from 1994 to 2000, and for those with annual household incomes below $25,000, advice dropped from 44.3% to 38.1%. In contrast, the prevalence of advice among obese persons with a college degree or in the highest income group remained relatively stable and high (>45%) over the study period.[14] It is obvious that physicians and other health-care professionals need to more consistently educate patients regarding the benefits of physical activity and weight loss if we are to effectively deal with this growing crisis.

INITIATIVE TO COMBAT OBESITY

Based on a systematic review of the literature from 1980 to 1997, the National Heart, Lung, and Blood Institute (NHLBI) released clinical guidelines in 1998 on the identification, evaluation, and treatment of overweight and obese adults. Recommendations included a call for all health professionals to address risk-factor reduction and weight management strategies with patients who are obese. The NHLBI also advocated the establishment of a modest target weight loss of 10% of body weight, at a rate of 1–2 lb/week. Studies have demonstrated that even modest weight loss results in improvement or prevention of hypertension, diabetes, and hyperlipidemia.[15] Goals related to weight management should focus on achieving and maintaining clinically meaningful weight loss and reducing the risk of obesity-related pathologies. The promotion of long-term lifestyle change in diet and physical activity in conjunction with the establishment of modest weight-loss goals provides a realistic chance of success in combating the obesity epidemic.

An approach to weight loss that combines an increase in physical activity, restriction of calories, and behavior modification has been shown to be the most effective regimen for weight loss, weight maintenance, and improved quality of life.[15] Realistic goal setting, stimulus control, problem-solving strategies, and contingency planning are all components of an effective behavioral therapy program. Self-monitoring of exercise and diet using a journal and enlisting the support of family and friends can be useful in reinforcing positive behavioral change.

ESSENTIAL ROLE OF EXERCISE IN WEIGHT MANAGEMENT

Exercise is a critical adjunct to diet and behavioral modification in a comprehensive weight-loss program. It not only increases energy expenditure but has been shown to diminish the loss of lean body mass and associated decline in resting metabolic rate that is characteristic of dieting alone.[16] Exercise improves the body's ability to burn fat, thus enhancing the loss of adipose tissue.[17] In addition, it has been shown to improve dietary adherence while reducing anxiety, stress, and depression that can trigger overeating.[18] Research confirms that the combination of diet and exercise results in greater weight loss than diet or exercise alone.[19] Extreme caloric restriction alone can produce a significant decrease in metabolic rate that can persist after the dieting period ends, often leading to rapid weight regain. Research has repeatedly demonstrated that daily physical activity and exercise adherence are the greatest determinants of weight maintenance following weight loss.[20–22]

EXERCISE PRESCRIPTION

Prior to the initiation of an exercise program, risk factors, medical history, and medications should be assessed and, when indicated, medical clearance obtained from a physician. The Physical Activity Readiness Questionnaire (PAR-Q) has been recommended by the American College of Sports Medicine (ACSM) as a minimal standard for participation in a moderate-intensity exercise program.[23] ACSM has developed risk stratification guidelines based on age, health status, coronary artery disease risk factors, and symptoms that can be utilized to determine the need for a medical exam and exercise testing prior to the initiation of an exercise program.[24] Heart rate (HR) parameters derived from an exercise stress test should be incorporated into the exercise prescription. Individuals at low risk can be counseled and provided with patient education literature to guide them in developing an exercise program that can be incorporated into their lives. It is recommended that health-care professionals follow these individuals' progress on a regular basis to improve compliance.

Information regarding an individual's previous level of activity, exercise preferences, physical impairments, and time constraints should be ascertained. Exercise should be pain-free, convenient, and enjoyable to the participant to facilitate long-term compliance. Whereas exercise classes or group settings may provide valuable support and social benefits for some, home-based exercise programs may improve compliance for others.

An exercise prescription should incorporate a warm-up, training, and cool-down program and include guidelines for progression of intensity, duration, and frequency of exercise. The warm-up and cool-down portion should be designed to address impairments in body function and structures that may contribute to activity limitations while also serving to prevent injuries and sudden changes in HR and blood pressure. Warm-up and cool-down exercises can include flexibility, resistive, or

TABLE 24.1

Indicators of Moderate Intensity Exercise

55%–69% maximum HR

Borg rating of perceived exertion scale 12–14 ("somewhat hard")

3.0–6.0 Metabolic Equivalents (METS)

Sources: Parameters from Pollock, M.L. et al., *Med. Sci. Sports Exerc.*, 30, 975, 1998; Borg,
G.A., *Med. Sci. Sports Exerc.*, 14, 377, 1982; Pate, R.R. et al., *JAMA*, 273, 402, 1995.

TABLE 24.2

Example of an Aerobic Exercise Prescription for Weight Loss

	Weeks	Duration (min)	Frequency (Times/Week)	Intensity	Time (Optional)
Initial phase	1–4	15–30	3–4	40%–55% HR max	5–10 min bouts
Improvement phase	5–24	30–45	4–5	50%–69% HR max	15–20 min bouts
Maintenance phase	25+	45–60	5–7	60%–69% HR max	Continuous

balance exercises tailored to address any impairments an individual may have. Flexibility exercises can improve posture, enhance function, and provide greater freedom of movement. Resistance exercises can be useful in improving function. An increase in strength that results in an improved level of mobility can facilitate an increase in daily physical activity. Resistance exercises should target weak muscle groups involved in functional tasks. Balance exercises can be a valuable component of a warm-up or cool-down program and reduce the risk of falls, enhance function and safety during gait, and promote a more active lifestyle. Physical therapists can play an integral role in prescribing an appropriate exercise program for patients who are overweight or obese.

Individuals should be encouraged to gradually increase the intensity of their exercise from low to moderate over time. Parameters that can be utilized to define moderate-intensity exercise are listed in Table 24.1. A gradual increase in duration and frequency of exercise should be implemented as well, based upon the individual's tolerance and prior activity level. The cumulative effect of exercise over time is substantial, and research has demonstrated a clear dose–response relationship between the amount of weekly exercise performed and the amount of weight lost in individuals who are overweight.[25] The most successful exercise programs for individuals who are obese are of moderate intensity, long duration, and are performed frequently.[26–28] Individuals should be counseled to strive for a long-term goal of 60 min of moderate-intensity physical activity over the course of a day. An example of an exercise prescription is provided in Table 24.2.

EXERCISE OPTIONS

Aerobic exercise is the preferred type of exercise for individuals initiating a weight-loss program due to its well-established cardiovascular benefits and volume of calories burned. Aerobic exercise options include walking or the use of treadmills, upper-body exercise cycles, stationary or recumbent cycles, swimming, exercise videos, and exercise classes. The selection of an appropriate mode of aerobic exercise should be made by the individual based on preferences, access to equipment, time constraints, and physical impairments. In a randomized controlled trial involving women who were overweight, having access to exercise equipment at home was associated with better exercise adherence and weight loss at 18 months when compared with women without home exercise equipment.[21] Walking can be accomplished indoors at a local mall or on a treadmill or outdoors around a neighborhood or at a local track. Pedometers can be useful to monitor activity levels and to improve compliance. Based on available evidence in the literature, it has been proposed that healthy individuals need to accrue 10,000 or more steps a day to be classified as "active."[29] America on the Move (AOM) Foundation is a nonprofit organization that has established a free pedometer-based program on the internet as a national initiative to improve health and quality of life. Members establish a baseline step count and aim to increase their daily steps by 2000/day toward a long-term goal of 10,000 or more. The website allows members to map their progress weekly and offers information, support, and dietary tips to enhance success.

Home cycle units are a relatively inexpensive and convenient aerobic option that imparts minimal stress to the joints. Recumbent cycles are more expensive but provide a comfortable alternative to upright cycles. Swimming or aquatic therapy is an excellent alternative for individuals with arthritis. Indoor pools can be found by contacting local YMCAs, school districts, health clubs, or motels for information about pool membership and class availability. Exercise classes (yoga, aquatic, aerobic, and t'ai chi) provide a social and structured environment that may improve compliance for some. Exercise videos (low-impact aerobics, dance, t'ai chi, and yoga) are a convenient and inexpensive choice for those who prefer to exercise at home. Health clubs are an option but individuals who are obese must be aware that exercise equipment such as treadmills, cycles, and elliptical trainers manufactured for the general public tend to have weight limits of 300–350 lb. Individuals who are severely obese may require specialized equipment to facilitate an increase in physical activity. Bariatric gait training systems, lift and transfer devices, walkers, and wheelchairs are available to meet the needs of these individuals.

Resistance exercises are not typically included in an exercise program for weight loss but can have an impact when addressing obesity, general physical inactivity, and predisposing risk factors in cardiovascular disease.[15] Performing resistance exercises can promote an active lifestyle by increasing lean muscle mass and muscle strength. Studies have found that resistance training results in a decrease in body fat mass and an increase in resting metabolic rate in men and women.[30,31] Resistance training may also be better tolerated by overweight and obese individuals since it involves slow, controlled movements, and exercises can be customized for comfort. The American Heart Association (AHA) recommends the following strengthening exercise regimen for persons without cardiovascular disease:[32]

- Training to begin 2 days/week, progressing to 3 days/week
- Training of 8–10 major muscle groups, including back, abdomen, lower extremities, chest, and upper extremities
- Selecting a weight that can be lifted for 8–10 repetitions initially, progressing to 12–15 repetitions

Strengthening programs should be incorporated into an exercise program that includes aerobic training and can be progressed at a pace that is not too overwhelming in regard to the time required for completion. Additional research is needed to determine the optimal mix of aerobic and resistance training for optimal weight loss and weight management.

ROLE OF DAILY PHYSICAL ACTIVITY IN WEIGHT MANAGEMENT

Daily physical activity plays a fundamental role in energy balance, weight control, and overall health. Although public health recommendations issued by the ACSM and AHA in 2007 advised adults to partake in a minimum of 30 min of moderate-intensity aerobic physical activity on 5 days each week, guidelines to prevent weight gain and prevent weight regain are higher.[33] The International Association for the Study of Obesity (IASO) concluded that 45–60 min of physical activity/day is required to prevent the transition to overweight and obesity in adults.[34] In addition, for individuals who have lost a significant amount of weight, studies generally support the need for 60–90 min of moderate-intensity physical activity/day to prevent weight regain.[34–36] Individuals should establish realistic goals that allow adequate time to steadily progress to this recommended level of daily physical activity.

The incorporation of "lifestyle activity" to a weight-loss regime can be an effective adjunct or alternative to more structured, continuous forms of exercise. Research demonstrates that intermittent, moderate-intensity physical activity is an appropriate means to achieve the recommended quantity of daily physical activity. A weight-loss program of diet with moderate-intensity lifestyle activity seems to offer similar health and weight-loss benefits as that of diet in conjunction with a structured aerobic exercise program.[12,20,27] Participation in a program of intermittent exercise or activity may appeal to individuals with time constraints or to those that dislike continuous exercise. A comparison of the effects of performing multiple 10 min bouts of exercise throughout the day with a single, longer bout in overweight subjects revealed greater adherence by those exercising in short bouts, with no negative impact on long-term weight loss or fitness.[21,37]

Participation in moderate-intensity physical activities, such as those listed in Table 24.3, satisfy the recommended guidelines as an alternative to structured, continuous exercise. Individuals should be instructed to park in distant parking spaces, climb stairs when possible, get off the bus or subway a stop early and walk the remaining distance, walk during lunch breaks, perform more of their own household chores, and participate in more active leisure time activities on a daily basis. Yard or housework, play with children, or dance can fulfill the recommended physical activity guidelines if performed at an adequate intensity. The accumulation of physical activity in intermittent, short bouts has been shown to be an effective means to achieving an adequate activity level. The literature suggests that the accumulated amount of activity is far more important than the manner in which the activity is performed.[27]

TABLE 24.3
Examples of Moderate Intensity Physical Activity (3–6 METS)

Swimming (leisurely)	6.0 METS
General health club exercise	5.5 METS
Walking 4 mph	5.0 METS
Golf (walking or carrying clubs)	4.5 METS
Mowing lawn (power mower)	4.5 METS
Home repair (painting)	4.5 METS
Gardening (weeding and cultivating)	4.5 METS
Raking the lawn	4.0 METS
Cycling (<10 mph)	4.0 METS
Yoga, t'ai chi, and stretching	4.0 METS
Water aerobics	4.0 METS
Fishing (standing in the river)	3.5 METS
Canoeing (rowing for pleasure)	3.5 METS
Childcare (bathing, feeding, and dressing)	3.5 METS
Mopping floors	3.5 METS
Walking 3 mph	3.3 METS
Housecleaning	3.0 METS
Walking the dog	3.0 METS

Source: Ainsworth, B.E. et al., *Med. Sci. Sports Exerc.*, 32(Suppl 9), S498, 2000.

CONSIDERATIONS FOR SPECIAL POPULATIONS

PEDIATRICS

Obesity in children is growing at an alarming rate. Because overweight adolescents have a 70% chance of becoming overweight or obese adults and an 80% chance if one or more parent is overweight or obese, it is of utmost importance to treat and prevent obesity in childhood.[38] The goal of intervention in this population is to promote good nutritional habits and increase daily physical activity and exercise to improve physical fitness and increase energy expenditure. For children, the school system affords an additional means to provide education and institute programs to address the problem of obesity.

Daily Activity Level and Exercise

The U.S. Department of Health and Human Services recommends that children accumulate at least 60 min of moderate physical activity on most days of the week, with more needed to prevent weight gain, lose weight, or maintain weight loss.[39] This is a goal that sedentary children can build up to gradually by incorporating small bouts of activity throughout the course of the day. Children who are overweight or obese need to strive toward a long-term goal of more than 60 min of physical activity most days of the week to facilitate or maintain weight loss. Children should progress to a level of intensity where they are "working up a sweat." If questions arise regarding the structure of a program for a particular child, referral to an intervention program or physical therapist may be warranted. Children can participate in structured activities such as team sports, dance, martial arts, or swimming. If preferred, health club memberships are options for older children (many will allow membership for ages 12 and older), and some health clubs are developing programs targeted at children under 12 as a need and interest has been identified. Research indicates that children and adolescents may safely participate in strength training activities. Recommendations for strength training include 8–15 repetitions at a moderate intensity for 1–3 sets, no more than 2 days/week with special attention to proper form to reduce risk of injury.[40] The key to foster compliance is to choose an activity that the child enjoys and one that fosters good self-esteem. Children should be cultivating interests that will allow them to maintain an improved level of fitness into adulthood.

It has been suggested that obese children are less active over the course of a day in moderate and vigorous activities when compared with nonobese children.[41] Television has been identified as a common sedentary activity that consumes hours of time each day for the average child. According to data collected during the NHANES survey in 2003–2004, the average time spent watching television for adolescents ages 12–17 is 4 h/day and in children ages 6–11 is 2 h and 13 min/day.[42] A report by the Kaiser Foundation in 2004 indicated that what was watched and how it was watched also contributes to the negative aspect of this activity. Not only are children seated in front of the screen, but they tend to snack while watching TV. It was also found that the type of advertising related to food choices, such as candy, fast food, soda, etc., have an additional negative influence beyond the sedentary act of watching television.[43] The American Academy of Pediatrics recommends limiting "total screen time," which includes television, videos, video games, and computer use, to less than 2 h/day.[44] Parents play a critical role in setting limits for children, as well as encouraging children to participate in activities that are nonsedentary. Parents should provide active choices to their children such as "going to a park *or* riding a bike," instead of choices that include sedentary activities. Parents can influence an overweight or obese child to increase overall energy expenditure by decreasing sedentary activities and enhancing accessibility to physically active alternatives. Parents must consider alternatives for their children as they look to change a child's preferences. During a 2 year study of a family-based behavioral weight program, it was found that promoting a reduction in sedentary behaviors was as effective as targeting physical activity.[45]

There are endless ways that physical activity can be made appealing to children. It is common for some children to participate in organized sports, but this must be an enjoyable option for them.

If not, they can choose activities such as jumping rope, dancing, or general outdoor play. For the child that enjoys video games, physical activity can be incorporated into this pastime as well. Most popular video game companies offer interactive systems that promote full body play. Interactive dance mats are a great option, plugging into common game systems and allowing children to set the level of difficulty, time, and mode of play. In addition, a line of stationary cycles are available that also plug into video game systems, permitting interactive play that requires physical activity to participate in the game. A child can play alone or compete against another player with either of these options.

The American Physical Therapy Association has a list of tips for families to combat obesity called "Smart Moves for Families" available online.[46] It suggests that parents set an example for their children by participating in physical activities with the child and becoming the child's "exercise buddy." Parents should plan active family activities, not just try to fit exercise in when there is time.

School-Based Intervention

The school setting provides an additional opportunity to influence children's daily activity. The percentage of public schools that provide daily physical education (PE) programs range from 17%–22% at the elementary level. Twenty-two percent of public schools offer PE only 1 day/week. Forty-three percent of first grade PE classes and 34% of fifth and sixth grade classes were found to be 30 min or less in duration.[47] The Youth Risk Behavior Summary Report 2006 by the Center for Disease Control and Prevention (CDC) found that as children reach high school, only 54.2% were enrolled in PE, and of those participating in PE, only 20% were active for 20 min or longer.[48] The school system has the ability to engage students in more vigorous activities and provide additional exposure to activities that may be of long-term interest to students. Healthy People 2020, an initiative by the CDC and President's Council on Physical Fitness, includes a goal to increase the proportion of the nation's public and private schools requiring daily PE for all students.[49] The CDC publishes a booklet titled, "Make a Difference at Your School," that offers 10 strategies for schools to utilize to aid in the battle against obesity in children and adolescents.[50] Recess is another prime time for schools to offer activities that get children moving. Curriculum in health education in the schools can promote aspects of healthy lifestyles, with changes in attitude and values instilled in children at younger ages.

GERIATRICS

The lack of physical activity is more common in the geriatric population than in any other age group and contributes to a loss of independence in later years of life.[51] The reduction in endurance and strength often attributed to aging is partly the result of reduced physical activity. Research has demonstrated that diet and exercise training improves physical function and ameliorates frailty in older adults who are obese.[52]

It is recommended that exercise programs be instituted under the supervision of a qualified health-care professional for elderly patients who are obese and have concomitant medical problems, with the long-term goal of a self-monitored, independent exercise regimen. Physical therapists are experts in developing appropriate exercise programs to address impairments in body function and structures and activity limitations in patients with cardiovascular, neurological, or musculoskeletal disorders. An assessment of strength, range of motion, function, balance, and endurance should be performed and an exercise program designed to address the deficits found. Appropriately designed exercise programs can reduce the risk of falls and facilitate a more active lifestyle through improved mobility and function. Strength training is beneficial for seniors as it prevents loss of bone mass and sarcopenia frequently observed in the elderly. Extension exercises are particularly important to consider for older adults to improve flexibility due to their tendency to develop flexed postures and tightness in hip flexors, hamstrings, and abdominal and cervical muscles. To promote compliance and minimize the risk of medical complications, exercise intensity should start low and progress gradually to a moderate level based on tolerance and HR parameters. It is recommended that a maximum HR be derived from a stress test in prescribing exercise intensity in this population due to the variability in peak HR seen in the elderly and their increased risk of underlying coronary artery disease.[53] It is also important to take into consideration the medications older adults are taking in prescribing and monitoring an exercise program.

PATIENT'S STATUS POST BARIATRIC SURGERY

Bariatric surgery rates have increased since surgery was recognized as a weight-loss intervention by the NIH for individuals with a BMI of 40 or above, or for those with a BMI of 35 and above with at least one related health problem, who have failed medical management. Between the years 1996 and 2001, bariatric procedures for obesity increased almost sevenfold, primarily due to growth of the Roux-en-Y procedures performed.[54] In December 2010, an FDA Advisory Panel voted to expand the use of lap band devices to those individuals with a BMI of 35, or a BMI of 30 with at least one associated health condition.[55] If the FDA accepts this recommendation, it will dramatically increase the number of people eligible for this procedure. There is little in the way of exercise guidelines in the literature for pre- or postoperative intervention. Individuals who are morbidly obese generally have multiple comorbidities that may affect their ability to exercise. A study by Elkins et al. examining noncompliance following bariatric surgery found that 40% and 41% of the 100 subjects at 6 and 12 months, respectively, were not exercising.[56]

The New York State Report, "Focus on Overcoming Obesity," recommends participation in a preoperative exercise program for a few months prior to bariatric surgery.[57] The preoperative program at Northwest Kaiser Permanente includes establishment of a 60–90 min daily home exercise program to improve physical fitness and prepare patients for the postoperative weight-loss program. It recommends walking for those who are able and water aerobics or "water walking" as a viable alternative. A "bigger picture" goal of the preoperative program strives for patients to find activities they can sustain following surgery.[58] Immediately postoperatively, patients are at risk for blood clots and pneumonia and should be encouraged to perform ankle pumps, deep breathing exercises, and ambulation as tolerated. In reviewing discharge instructions from various surgical programs, lifting objects greater than 15–20 lb is generally prohibited for 6 weeks following invasive surgery and 3 weeks following laparoscopic surgery. Upon discharge from the hospital, general recommendations include walking with a gradual increase in the time and distance walked. There is great variability in the specific recommendations among surgical programs with little attention to the intensity of the exercise. Generally, it is recommended that patients find an activity that is well tolerated that they enjoy and to engage in it on a regular basis at a moderate intensity. No specific contraindications for exercise were noted in the literature, except that individuals who undergo adjustable gastric banding should avoid "abdominal crunch" type machines due to a report that a port connection had become dislodged in one patient following this type of exercise.[59]

CONSIDERATIONS FOR SPECIFIC MEDICAL CONDITIONS (DIABETES, HYPERTENSION, AND OSTEOARTHRITIS)

Due to the common comorbidities associated with obesity, there are precautions that need to be considered when prescribing exercise. Initiating an exercise program will also attenuate some of the health risks associated with these disease states. For the person with diabetes who is obese, exercise is contraindicated when blood glucose is over 300 mg/dL or greater than 240 mg/dL with urinary ketone bodies. At the initiation of an exercise program, blood glucose should be monitored before, during, and after activity if insulin or oral medications have been prescribed. Exercise has an insulin-like effect and may lead to exercise-induced hypoglycemia. A carbohydrate snack may be needed either before or during exercise. It is important to review the signs of hypoglycemia (dizziness, light-headedness, confusion, and anxiety) with the individual. Exercise-induced hypoglycemia can occur up to 4–6 h after the cessation of exercise. Exercise should be planned for early to midday, avoiding the evening due to an increased risk of nocturnal hypoglycemia. As the exercise program is progressed, insulin needs may change, so close monitoring and follow-up with a physician is important. People with diabetes are at risk for autonomic neuropathies associated with silent heart ischemia and/or blunted HR response to exercise. It is important that HR monitoring be performed in conjunction with a rating of perceived exertion scale to determine a safe exercise program intensity level.[60]

Hypertension is another common comorbidity. Exercise is contraindicated if resting systolic blood pressure is greater than 200 mmHg or diastolic blood pressure is greater than 115 mmHg. For persons on alpha-1, alpha-2, or calcium channel blockers or vasodilators, the risk of postexertion hypotension exists, and the cool-down phase of the exercise program needs to be strictly adhered to.[60]

A third common comorbidity is lower extremity osteoarthritis. Between 1971 and 2002, public health records reveal an increase from 3% to 18% in arthritis due to obesity in the baby boomer population.[61] Exercises that minimize weight bearing may be best tolerated by this group. Stationary exercise cycles and water walking or water aerobics are options that place less stress on hips, knees, and ankles than walking. If exercise produces pain, compliance will be diminished. A recent study found that children who were overweight had a higher incidence of bone fractures, joint or muscle pain, and abnormal knee joint alignment.[62] This may contribute to an increase in sedentary behaviors, requiring a recommendation for non-weight-bearing exercise and physical activity to counteract this potential.

INFORMATION AVAILABLE ONLINE

There is a multitude of information available to the consumer with online access. Included in this section is a list and summary of internet sites that individuals can be referred to for education and to provide tips, strategies, and structure to improve activity levels, overall fitness, and nutrition:

- www.shapeup.org: This not-for-profit organization's mission is to increase awareness of obesity as a health issue, providing evidence-based information. They offer a 10-step program for weight loss and strategies to increase daily activity. They advocate 10,000 steps/day.
- www.americaonthemove.org: A national initiative dedicated to improve health and quality of life through healthy eating and increased activity. Participation can be on an individual basis or as part of a larger group affiliation.
- http://www.heart.org/HEARTORG/GettingHealthy/GettingHealthy_UCM_001078_SubHomePage.jsp: The AHA provides information on weight management, physical activity, and health for adults and children.
- www.mypyramid.gov: The U.S. Department of Agriculture promotes the newest food pyramid as a guide for healthy eating and includes sections for children and health professionals.
- www.nichd.nih.gov/msy: Media Smart Youth—A health promotion program instituted by the NIH to assist 11–13 year old children in learning how media influences nutrition and activity choices.
- www.wecan.nhlbi.nih.gov: NIH We Can! provides practical tools for parents of 8–13 year olds to assist in healthy weight management.
- www.cdc.gov/nccdphp/dnpa/physical/recommendations/older_adults.htm: Recommendations for physical activity for older adults from the CDC.
- www.nia.nih.gov/HealthInformation/Publications/ExerciseGuide/: Provides access to the free comprehensive book, *Exercise: A Guide from the National Institute on Aging*
- http://www.letsmove.gov/: Part of a government initiative to reduce childhood obesity, provides information to empower parents and caregivers in the areas of nutrition and physical activity.

THOUGHTS ON PREVENTION

Healthy People 2010, a statement of national health objectives developed at the turn of the century by the NIH include the following three goals:

- Reduce the proportion of children and adolescents who are overweight or obese
- Increase the proportion of adults who are at a healthy weight
- Reduce the proportion of adults who are obese

Despite our government's current efforts in combating obesity in the United States, the report of our nation's progress toward these goals, released in 2008, reveals a continued trend in the opposite direction. Data comparing statistics from 1988 to 1994 to those gathered between 2003 and 2006 reveal that the proportion of adults at a healthy weight has dropped from 42% to 32%, the proportion of adults who are obese has climbed from 24% to 33%, and the proportion of children and adolescents who are overweight or obese has increased from 11% to 17% in children and 18% in adolescents over this period of time.[63] Clearly, our efforts as a nation in this regard have so far been unsuccessful.

It is no wonder that obesity rates continue to rise when we consider our current cultural norms. Television, video games, and the widespread use of computers have contributed greatly to our sedentary lifestyles. Americans thrive on new technology and services that are developed to provide conveniences that concomitantly reduce physical activity. Take out and fast foods are an inherent part of many families' daily routine. Education about the importance of good nutrition and benefits of physical activity is a necessity if future generations are to strive toward a healthy lifestyle and reverse the growing trend toward an obese population within our culture. Physical activity and exercise need to become a routine component of our lives.

In order to make progress toward the objective of increasing the proportion of adults who are at a healthy weight, public health initiatives need to focus on prevention through education and the promotion of healthy lifestyles and behaviors beginning in childhood. It is easier to maintain a healthy, active lifestyle into adulthood if the benefits of good nutrition and physical activity are valued and practiced at a young age than it is to improve dietary choices and incorporate physical activity into daily routines of sedentary adults.

It is crucial to address prevention in the pediatric population as research demonstrates that pediatric obesity is a predictor of adult obesity. It is important that children learn about physical fitness and proper nutrition both at home and in school. Cultivating an interest in physical activities at a young age will encourage an active lifestyle as children enter adulthood. Parents should act as good role models and consistently strive to provide active choices to their children during leisure time. Physical education, health class, recess, and extracurricular activities all provide wonderful opportunities to promote physical activity in the school environment. Food and drinks available to students in the schools should reflect healthy nutritional choices and reinforce information provided in classes about proper nutrition. The "Child Nutrition and WIC Reauthorization Act of 2004" is a federal law established to address the issue of childhood obesity through the public schools. Educational systems were tasked to develop a wellness policy by 2006 to provide nutrition education, increase physical activity, and improve nutritional content of lunches and snacks sold in school.[64]

Because research indicates that a small percentage of people who lose weight are successful in maintaining their weight loss, prevention is key in combating the obesity epidemic in the United States. It is clear that changes in diet and physical activity that individuals make in order to lose weight must be maintained after the weight loss is achieved in order to sustain the weight loss. The concept that people can "go on a diet" temporarily to lose weight and expect that the weight loss is maintained when they revert to old eating habits is implausible. True weight management strategies in overweight patients need to promote long-term adherence to more healthy lifestyles.

It is critical that health-care professionals consistently intervene when dealing with overweight individuals to prevent weight progression to the level of obesity and to prevent further weight gain in individuals who have demonstrated an increase in BMI from a healthy weight to one consistent with being overweight. In order to accomplish this, health-care professionals should routinely include the determination of BMI and the measurement of waist circumference in initial examinations, introduce the topic of weight loss when warranted, provide patient information regarding the health risks associated with being overweight or obese, address risk-factor reduction, make referrals to nutritionists, and develop individualized weight-loss programs with these patients that includes an exercise prescription following medical clearance.

Weight gain seems to incorporate a detrimental cyclical component. When an individual gains weight, the weight gain often makes physical activity more of an exertion, which can cause the individual to become less active, which, in turn, leads to more weight gain. Physical activity can become more difficult due to pain, restrictive lung disease, the onset of diabetes, or the increased work of activity. It is critical that an effort is made to break this cycle for individuals before long-term health issues develop or before the excessive weight makes exercise or physical activity too challenging to achieve.

There is a window of opportunity for patients to address the problem of excessive weight before the problem itself makes weight loss extremely difficult. When patients are overweight for many years, there is a greater risk of developing cardiovascular disease, restrictive pulmonary disease, and arthritis that make the initiation of an exercise program extraordinarily difficult. This is particularly true of patients with morbid obesity. Many of these individuals require assistive devices to ambulate and have difficulty accomplishing activities of daily living, let alone initiating an exercise program. Interventions in this population need to focus on proper eating habits, reducing impairments in body structures and function, and enhancing daily activity and participation. Patients will benefit from adequate pain management, recommendations for appropriate assistive devices and equipment to enhance mobility and function, and an exercise program that addresses flexibility, balance, and strength deficits and permits pain-free physical activity. Successful long-term weight control requires that overweight or obese individuals develop an appreciation for physical activity and good nutrition as essential components of a healthy lifestyle.

In order to effectively address the obesity epidemic in the United States, public policy needs to be instituted to promote education, prevention, and wellness for both adults and children. The lack of third-party payment for intervention or prevention of obesity continues to be a major obstacle in curtailing the continued trend toward obesity in our country. Cuts in state aid for our school systems make expansion of physical education programs and extracurricular activities financially unfeasible. Strategies to address these problems include government funding of school programs and health insurance coverage or incentives for overweight individuals seeking a healthier lifestyle by joining a gym. Americans must begin to embrace physical activity as an essential component of their lives and improve their eating habits in order to reverse the growing trend toward obesity in our country.

SUMMARY

Exercise and physical activity are fundamental components of a comprehensive weight-loss program. The most successful exercise programs are those of low to moderate intensity, long duration, and performed frequently. The cumulative effect of exercise over time is substantial, and research has demonstrated a clear, dose–response relationship between the amount of weekly exercise performed and the amount of weight lost in overweight individuals.[25] Emphasizing long-term lifestyle changes in diet and physical activity and establishing modest weight-loss goals are key factors in successful weight-loss programs. Adherence to daily physical activity and exercise are the greatest determinants in weight maintenance following weight loss. Health-care professionals need to be aware of unique challenges posed by pediatric, geriatric, post bariatric surgery, and medically complex individuals when counseling for weight management. If we are to reverse the growing trend toward an obese population within our culture, physical activity and exercise need to become a routine component of daily life, and education about the importance of good nutrition and the benefits of physical activity is a necessity. Public policies and funding are needed to promote education, prevention, and wellness for both adults and children.

REFERENCES

1. National Health and Nutrition Examination Survey (NHANES), 1999–2000, US Department of Health and Human Services, Centers for Disease Control and Prevention, National Center for Health Statistics, Hyattsville, MD, 2002.
2. Flegal, K.M. et al., Prevalence and trends in obesity among US adults, 1999–2008, *JAMA*, 303, 235, 2010.
3. Ogden, C.L., Carol, M.D., and Flegal, K.M., High body mass index for age among US children and adolescents, 2003–2006, *JAMA*, 299, 2401, 2008.
4. Mokdad, A.H. et al., Actual causes of death in the United States, 2000, *JAMA*, 291, 1238, 2004.
5. Must, A. and Anderson, S.E., Effects of obesity on morbidity in children and adolescents, *Nutr Clin Care*, 6, 4, 2003.
6. Freedman, D.S. et al., The relation of overweight to cardiovascular risk factors among children and adolescents: The Bogalusa Heart Study, *Pediatrics,* 103, 1175, 1999.
7. National Heart, Lung, and Blood Institute, Obesity Education Initiative Expert Panel, The practical guide: Identification, evaluation and treatment of overweight and obesity in adults, National Institutes of Health publication No. 00-4084, Rockville, MD, October 2000.
8. Grundy, S.M. et al., Executive summary–Diagnosis and management of the metabolic syndrome: An American Heart Association/National Heart, Lung, and Blood Institute scientific statement, *Curr Opin Cardiol*, 21, 1, 2006.
9. Shen, W. et al., Waist circumference correlates with metabolic syndrome indicators better than percentage fat, *Obesity*, 14, 727, 2006.
10. Bray, G.A., Don't throw the baby out with the bath water, *Am J Clin Nutr*, 79, 347, 2004.
11. Hu, F.B. et al., Television watching and other sedentary behaviors in relation to risk of obesity and type 2 diabetes mellitus in women, *JAMA*, 289, 1785, 2003.
12. Blair, S.N. and Brodney, S., Effects of physical inactivity and obesity on morbidity and mortality: Current evidence and research issues, *Med Sci Sports Exerc*, 31, S646, 1999.
13. Hu, F.B., Willett, W.C., Li, T. et al., Adiposity as compared with physical activity in predicting mortality among women, *N Engl J Med*, 351, 2694, 2004.
14. Jackson, J.E. et al., Trends in professional advice to lose weight among obese adults, 1994 to 2000, *J Gen Intern Med*, 20, 814, 2005.
15. National Heart, Lung and Blood Institute, Clinical guidelines on the identification, evaluation, and treatment of overweight and obesity in adults-the evidence report, National Institutes of Health (published erratum appears in *Obes Res*, 6, 464, 1998) *Obes Res*, 6(Suppl 2), 51S, 1998.
16. Svendsen, O.L., Hassager, C., and Christiansen, C., Effect of an energy-restrictive diet, with or without exercise, on lean tissue mass, resting metabolic rate, cardiovascular risk factors, and bone in overweight postmenopausal women, *Am J Med*, 95, 131, 1993.
17. Racette, S.B. et al., Effects of aerobic exercise and dietary carbohydrate on energy expenditure and body composition during weight reduction in obese women, *Am J Clin Nutr*, 61, 486, 1995.
18. Racette, S.B. et al., Exercise enhances dietary compliance during moderate energy restriction in obese women, *Am J Clin Nutr,* 62, 345, 1995.
19. Orzano, J. and Scott, J.G., Diagnosis and treatment of obesity in adults: An applied evidence-based review, *J Am Board Fam Pract*, 17, 359, 2004.
20. Anderson, R.E. et al., Effects of lifestyle activity versus structured aerobic exercise in obsess women: A randomized trial, *JAMA,* 281, 335, 1999.
21. Jakicic, J.M. et al., Effects of intermittent exercise and use of home exercise equipment on adherence, weight loss, and fitness in overweight women: A randomized trial, *JAMA*, 282, 1554, 1999.
22. Anderson, J.W. et al., Long-term weight-loss maintenance: A meta-analysis of US studies, *Am J Clin Nutr*, 74, 579, 2001.
23. Canadian Society for Exercise Physiology, PAR-Q and you, Revised 2002. www.csep.ca/cmfiles/publications/parq/par-q.pdf (accessed on February 8, 2012).
24. Guthrie, J., Cardiorespiratory and health-related physical fitness assessments, in Ehrman, J.K. et al. (eds.), *ACSM's Resource Manual for Guidelines for Exercise Testing and Prescription*, 6th edn., Lippincott Williams & Wilkins, Philadelphia, PA, 2010, chapter 19.

25. Slentz, C.A. et al., Effects of the amount of exercise on body weight, body composition, and measures of central obesity, *Arch Intern Med*, 164, 31, 2004.

26. Jakicic, J.M. et al., Appropriate intervention strategies for weight loss and prevention of weight regain for adults, *Med Sci Sports Exerc*, 33, 2145, 2001.

27. Pate, R.R. et al., Physical activity and public health: A recommendation from the CDC and the ACSM, *JAMA*, 273, 402, 1995.

28. Jakicic, J.M. et al., Effect of exercise duration and intensity on weight loss in overweight, sedentary women, *JAMA*, 290, 1323, 2003.

29. Tudor-Locke, C. and Bassett Jr., D.R., How many steps/day are enough? Preliminary pedometer indices for public health, *Sports Med,* 34, 1, 2004.

30. Hunter, G.R., Bryan, D.R., Wetzstein, C.J. et al., Resistance training and intra-abdominal adipose tissue in older men and women, *Med Sci Sports Exerc*, 34, 1023, 2002.

31. Tresierras, M.A. and Balady, G.J., Resistance training and the treatment of diabetes and obesity: Mechanisms and outcomes. *J Cardiopulm Rehabil Prev*, 29, 67, 2009.

32. Braith, R.W. and Stewart, K.J., Resistance exercise training: Its role in the prevention of cardiovascular disease, *Circulation,* 113, 2642, 2006.

33. Haskell, W.L. et al., Physical activity and public health: Updated recommendation for adults from the American College of Sports Medicine and the American Heart Association, *Circulation*, 116, 1081, 2007.

34. American College of Sports Medicine, *ACSM's Guidelines for Exercise Testing and Prescription*, 7th edn., Lippincott Williams & Wilkins, Philadelphia, PA, 2006, Chapter 1.

35. Schoeller, D.A., Shay, K., and Kushner, R.F., How much physical activity is needed to minimize weight gain in previously obese women? *Am J Clin Nutr*, 66, 551, 1997.

36. Weinsier, R.L. et al., Free-living activity energy expenditure in women successful and unsuccessful at maintaining a normal body weight, *Am J Clin Nutr*, 75, 499, 2002.

37. Jakicic, J.M. et al., Prescribing exercise in multiple short bouts versus one continuous bout: Effects on adherence, cardiorespiratory fitness, and weight loss in overweight women, *Int J Obes Relat Metab Disord*, 19, 893, 1995.

38. United States Department of Health and Human Services (USDHHS), The surgeon general's call to action to prevent and decrease overweight and obesity: Overweight in children and adolescents, United States Department of Health and Human Services, Washington, DC, 2007, http://www.surgeongeneral. gov/topics/obesity/calltoaction/fact_adolescents.htm (accessed on February 8, 2012).

39. United States Department of Health and Human Services (USDHHS), Overweight and obesity: At a glance (fact sheet), United States Department of Health and Human Services, Washington, DC, 2007, www.surgeongeneral.gov/topics/obesity/calltoaction/fact_glance.htm (accessed on February 8, 2012).

40. Coe, D.P. and Fiataroni-Singh, M.A., Exercise prescription in special populations: Women, pregnancy, children, and the elderly, in Ehrman, J.K. et al. (eds.), *ACSM's Resource Manual for Guidelines for Exercise Testing and Prescription,* 6th edn., Lippincott Williams & Wilkins, Philadelphia, PA, 2010, chapter 41.

41. Page, A. et al., Physical activity patterns in nonobese and obese children assesses using minute-by-minute accelerometry, *Int J Obes*, 29, 1070, 2005.

42. Ogden, C.L. et al., Prevalence of overweight and obesity in the United States, 1999–2004, *JAMA*, 295, 1549, 2006.

43. The Henry J. Kaiser Family Foundation, *The Role of Media in Childhood Obesity*, Publication No: 7030, Washington, DC, 2004.

44. The American Academy of Pediatrics Council on Communications and Media, Policy statement, *Pediatrics*, 126, 1012, 2010.

45. Epstein, L.H. et al., Decreasing sedentary behaviors in treating pediatric obesity, *Arch Pediatr Adolesc Med*, 154, 220, 2000.

46. American Physical Therapy Association, Smart moves for families, www.moveforwardpt.com/tips/smart-moves-for-families/, accessed on December 15, 2010.

47. U.S. Department of Education, *Calories in, Calories Out: Food and Exercise in Public Elementary Schools 2005*, National Center for Educational Statistics, Washington, DC, 2006.

48. Centers for Disease Control and Prevention, Youth risk behavior surveillance—United States June 2005, *MMWR Surveill Summ*, 55(SS-5), 1–108, June 9, 2006.

49. U.S. Department of Health and Human Services, Healthy people 2020, www.healthypeople.gov/2020/topicsobjectives2020/pdfs/HP2020objectives.pdf, accessed on December 15, 2010.

50. U.S. Department of Health and Human Services, Make a difference at your school: Key strategies to prevent obesity, National Center for Chronic Disease Prevention and Health Promotion, Centers for Disease Control and Prevention, U.S. Department of Health and Human Services, Atlanta, GA, 2008, http://www.cdc.gov/HealthyYouth/keystrategies/pdf/make-a-difference.pdf (accessed on February 8, 2012).

51. Phillips, E.M., Schneider, J.C., and Mercer, G.R., Motivating elders to initiate and maintain exercise, *Arch Phys Med Rehabil*, 85(Suppl 3), S52, 2004.

52. Villareal, M.D. et al., Effect of weight loss and exercise on frailty in obese older adults, *Arch Intern Med*, 166, 860, 2006.

53. American College of Sports Medicine, *ACSM's Guidelines for Exercise Testing and Prescription*, 7th edn., Lippincott Williams & Wilkins, Philadelphia, PA, 2006, chapter 10.

54. Livingston, E.H., Procedure incidence and in-hospital complication rates of bariatric surgery in the United States, *Am J Surg*, 188, 105, 2004.

55. U.S. DHHS, Gastroenterology and urology devices panel meeting minutes, December 3, 2010, U.S. Food and Drug Administration, Silver Spring, MD, 2010, http://www.fda.gov/downloads/AdvisoryCommittees/CommitteesMeetingMaterials/MedicalDevices/MedicalDevicesAdvisoryCommittee/Gastroenterology-UrologyDevicesPanel/UCM236137.pdf, accessed on December 22, 2010.

56. Elkins, G. et al., Noncompliance with behavioral recommendations following bariatric surgery, *Obes Surg*, 15, 546, 2005.

57. New York State Department of Law, Health Care Bureau, *Focus on Overcoming Obesity*, Office of the Attorney General, Buffalo, NY, November 2004.

58. Bachman, K.H. et al., Bariatric surgery in the KP northwest region: Optimizing outcomes by using a multidisciplinary program, *Perm J*, 9, 52, 2005.

59. Felberbauer, F.X., Prager, G., and Wenzl, E., The inflatable band and exercise machines, *Obes Surg*, 11, 532, 2001.

60. American College of Sports Medicine, *ACSM's Guidelines for Exercise Testing and Prescription*, 7th edn., Lippincott Williams & Wilkins, Philadelphia, PA, 2006, Chapter 9.

61. Leveille, S.G., Wee, C.C., and Iezzoni, L.I., Trends in obesity and arthritis among baby boomers and their predecessors, 1971–2002, *Am J Pub Health,* 95, 1607, 2005.

62. Taylor, E.D. et al., Orthopedic complications of overweight in children and adolescents, *Pediatrics*, 117, 2167, 2006.

63. U.S. Department of Health and Human Services, Progress Review: Nutrition and Overweight http://www.healthypeople.gov/2010/Data/2010prog/focus19/default.htm, accessed on January 7, 2011.

64. National Conference of State Legislators, PL 108-265, http://www.ncsl.org/Portals/1/documents/immig/StIssuesCN.pdf, accessed on January 7, 2011.

25 Role of Exercise in Diet and Weight Loss

William J. Kraemer, PhD, FACSM, FNSCA, FISSN, FACN,
Courtenay Dunn-Lewis, MA, and Hui-Ying Luk, MS

CONTENTS

INTRODUCTION

As the science of exercise physiology developed over the last century, it became obvious that exercise, or planned physical activity, could have a host of therapeutic, health, and performance benefits. While exercise has become a topic of scientific inquiry, the commercial value of weight loss has popularized packaged programs in the viewing public via infomercials, health clubs, and personal trainers. These exercise programs range from those too light for meaningful benefits to extreme weight-loss programs. They are targeted indiscriminately at populations ranging from sedentary to highly motivated individuals wanting to make dramatic physical changes. What qualifies as knowledge of exercise today—even among those who instruct others on fitness—is unfortunately influenced more strongly by commercial forces than by science.

Fundamental principles (which include specificity, variation in the exercise stress, frequency, and duration) are vital to understanding exercise. Each contributes to the ultimate goals and outcomes of the program. Each program should be directed toward an individual's goals and objectives and should be realistic. The expectations that bombard the public are many times extreme; as noted in every infomercial, the mantra, "results are not typical" is put forth all of the time, making one wonder how many diet and exercise failures exist owing to misplaced expectations. Such marketed exercise programs are not individually prescribed or progressed over time—a fundamental flaw for optimal and safe implementation of any exercise program. Thus, not only are unrealistic, generic programs typically prescribed, but frequently, such commercial programs have little in the way of scientific merit.

The key question revolves around what exercise truly contributes to weight loss. Are all exercise types the same? What is the real benefit of adding an exercise program to a diet program targeted at weight loss, and finally, how can it benefit the individual trying to lose weight? These are a few of the questions we will explore in this chapter in order to give the reader a better picture of the expectations of exercise when undergoing a program focused on weight loss. We will review the fundamentals of aerobic and anaerobic exercise, how each modality is programmed, and how each impact weight loss and management. Finally, we will describe the role of diet in weight loss, aerobic exercise in weight maintenance, and resistance exercise in the maintenance of lean body tissue.

EXERCISE MODALITIES

Exercise is the formal use of body movements configured in a program that tells one what to do, how to move, and what type of activity to perform. Fundamental to this concept is the mode or *modality* of the activity. Most modes of physical activity can be categorized into aerobic/endurance exercise or anaerobic exercise (including resistance exercise). Variation in the training stimulus (both among and within modalities) is important with any exercise program as it allows the body to recover and repair and helps avoid overtraining syndromes. Ultimately, variation in exercise programs can help fight boredom and enhance adherence to a lifestyle that includes exercise.

Key to any modality is the intensity at which the exercise is performed—which is where the role of caloric expenditure comes into play. First, in order to produce muscular movement, the body must produce energy in the form of adenosine triphosphate (ATP); thus, metabolic cycles must be increased, and energy transformations take place from the breakdown of protein, carbohydrates, and fat to energy. A host of chemical reactions occur in the body to breakdown food into their constitutive components that can then enter into metabolic pathways to produce energy. There are two general metabolic pathways that have been popularly termed "aerobic" and "anaerobic." With long-term exercise, aerobic metabolism dominates the energy profile used. Conversely, with short-term higher-intensity exercise, anaerobic metabolism then dominates the energy profile of utilization. In the case of typical aerobic exercise, the total caloric expenditure is observed primarily during exercise with little increases after the workout is completed. This is different with types of anaerobic exercise as we will see later. While a great deal of detail exists on this aerobic/anaerobic continuum of metabolism, such terms provide a broad characterization related to the demands and the ability of the body to continue activity.

AEROBIC EXERCISE

Natural human locomotion involves moving from one place to another using lower body musculature. Walking, jogging, and running are therefore modalities of exercise that caught on rapidly (while cycling, swimming, and similar activities are also popular). Aerobic or endurance exercise is attractive owing to its ease of implementation (i.e., just going for a walk or run) and its submaximal nature that allows for continuous activity with lower perceptual and physiological strain in most activities, only increasing as intensity is increased (e.g., exercising at a higher percentage of one's maximal heart rate). These modalities were popularized in Dr. Ken Cooper's small paperback entitled "Aerobics," which started a revolution in exercise training genre by the late 1960s that exploded in the 1970s (Cooper 1968). From this popular excitement, research in exercise physiology demonstrated the health benefits from so-called aerobic or endurance type exercise and included preventive aspects of cardiovascular diseases (e.g., improved lipid profiles, improved cardiovascular performance, and enhanced quality of life) whether within cardiac rehabilitations programs or plain preventive fitness programs. The world of fitness was launched beyond what had ever been previously known. Research from the 1950s until the late 1980s was dominated by the scientific study of this one form of exercise. Thus, we know a great deal about this form of exercise and its role in weight loss as well as in health and well-being but comparatively little in terms of anaerobic activity.

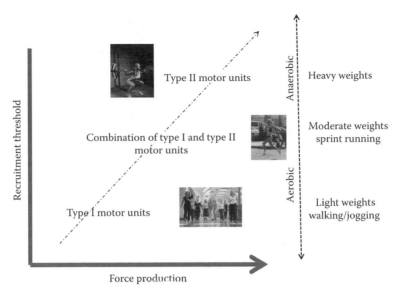

FIGURE 25.1 Size principle is one of the key theories in exercise science. It dictates what muscle fibers are recruited as part of neural activation of motor units. Motor units are recruited from the low threshold motor units, which produce less force, to higher and higher threshold motor units that produce higher levels of force in an individual muscle. Recruitment goes from low to high, and each muscle has a different array of motor units based on anatomical position in the body and its movement function. Not all individuals have the same number of motor units nor do all muscles have the same number of motor units. More external demands require higher numbers of motor units to be recruited to meet the demands for force production.

Aerobic exercise is defined as large muscle group exercises (walking, jogging, etc.) that could be repetitively performed for extended periods of time (e.g., 30 min or longer). The term *aerobic* comes for the concept that this type of exercise derives a high percentage of its energy from aerobic metabolism (the Krebs cycle and associated electron transport system). Oxygen acts as the final electron acceptor in the respiratory chain and therefore is necessary for successful energy production in this system. When muscles are recruited, oxygen is needed to fuel metabolic machinery especially as the activity continues beyond a few minutes (see Figure 25.1). The function of the heart and lungs and their ability to extract oxygen from the air and circulate it to activated muscle fibers is paramount to continuous movement. As such, repeated workouts with proper progression force the body to make adaptations to better meet the demands for such continuous exercise. This includes improving lung function to allow more oxygen to be extracted from the air one breathes, improving heart muscle function (from increased left chamber volume to increased myocardial wall size to increased extraction by the activated muscle to take and utilize more oxygen in its aerobic metabolic cycle). Collateral to this phenomenon, a host of other adaptations occur that have been shown to be beneficial to the health, well-being, and improved cardiovascular function—from improved lipid profiles due to better use of energy metabolism to improved muscle function and caloric expenditures.

Aerobic Exercise Programming

The American College of Sports Medicine (ACSM) has championed the inclusion of aerobic exercise for many years and has presented the following information in their position stand as to exercise prescription guidelines (see Table 25.1). While current updates in such guidelines are currently being formulated, the need for individualization, monitoring, and clinical observation is echoed by their published statement in their 1998 position stand (Donnelly et al. 1998). As noted in the following quote, a minimum intensity is needed to stimulate training effects—even in cardiac patients. When someone is very deconditioned or untrained for a variety of reasons (e.g., sedentary lifestyle or cardiac pathologies), one can do almost anything and see improvement in exercise

---

TABLE 25.1

Exercise Prescription Guidelines for Aerobic Exercise

Frequency: 3–5 days per week

Duration: 20–60 min of continuous aerobic activity

Intensity: 40%–50% of heart rate reserve (HRR) for individuals with very low
  level of fitness level one can start and see significant training effects

Typically: 50%–85% of maximal aerobic capacity (VO$_2$ max), or

50%–85% of HRR or

60%–90% of maximal heart rate (HR max)

The heart rate reserve is derived from the Karvonen formula as follows:

✓ Determine your resting heart rate (RHR)

✓ Determine your predicted HR max

✓ HR max = 220 – age

✓ Calculate your HRR

✓ HRR = HR max – RHR

  • Low intensity: 35%–60% of HR max or 50%–60% of HRR

  • Moderate intensity: 60%–80% of HR max or 60%–70% of HRR

  • High intensity: 80%–90% of HR max or 70%–85% of HRR

Source: Donnelly, J.E. et al., *Med. Sci. Sports Exerc.*, 30, 975, 1998.

---

performance and other physiological gains (as the window of opportunity can be very large with only the genetic ceiling above limiting improvement). We have seen cardiac patients go on to be marathon runners—but proper progression and appropriate intensity need to be carefully monitored and sequenced over time.

> …The combination of frequency, intensity, and duration of chronic exercise has been found to be effective for producing a training effect. The interaction of these factors provide the overload stimulus. In general, the lower the stimulus the lower the training effect, and the greater the stimulus the greater the effect… aerobic endurance training of fewer than 2 d.wk-1, at less than 40%–50% of VO2R, and for less than 10 min-1 is generally not a sufficient stimulus for developing and maintaining fitness in healthy adults. Even so, many health benefits from physical activity can be achieved at lower intensities of exercise if frequency and duration of training are increased appropriately. In this regard, physical activity can be accumulated through the day in shorter bouts of 10-min durations. In the interpretation of this position stand, it must be recognized that the recommendations should be used in the context of participant's needs, goals, and initial abilities.

Extensive guidelines have also been developed for the implementation of aerobic exercise and to assess who needs to be clinically screened by a physician and/or undergo a clinical graded exercise test to rule out elevated risk. As very nicely overviewed by the Georgia State University's Department of Kinesiology and Health website (http://www2.gsu.edu/~wwwfit/getstart.html) and based upon the Guidelines for Exercise Testing and Prescription, ACSM, 5th Edition, 1995, they summarize these concerns as follows and we quote:

1. Are you a man over 45 years old?
2. Are you a woman over the age of 55? Or, are you less than 55 years old and past menopause, but not taking estrogen?
3. Has any male family member died of a heart attack before age 55? Or, has any female family member died of a heart attack before age 65?
4. Do you smoke cigarettes?

5. Has a doctor ever told you have high blood pressure? Or, has your blood pressure been measured more than once at greater than 140 over 90? Or, do you take high blood pressure medicine?
6. Has your doctor ever told you that you have high cholesterol? Or, do you know if your total cholesterol is greater than 200? Or, is your HDL cholesterol less than 35?
7. Do you consider yourself physically inactive at work and during your leisure time?

If you answered "yes" to more than one of these questions, it is recommended that you see a doctor before pursuing a vigorous exercise program.

ANAEROBIC EXERCISE

Anaerobic exercise comes in many programmatic forms including sprint interval training (running, cycling, or swimming), downhill skiing, and, notably, most programs in resistance or weight training. With these forms of exercise, caloric expenditures can be seen to be somewhat small during most programs yet, during what is called the excess postexercise oxygen consumption (EPOC), can be increased in some cases over the next 24 h. Caloric expenditure is thus often increased far beyond what is observed with the activity itself. Yet as we will see, weight training is typically more important to help preserve lean tissue mass than as a method for producing weight loss.

The term *anaerobic* is used to signify that anaerobic exercise gains its ATP energy from two metabolic cycles that do not require oxygen to produce energy (namely, the phosphagen or ATP/PC system and the anaerobic glycolysis or lactic acid system). Anaerobic exercise broadly overviews a wide range of high-intensity exercise beyond the body's maximum oxygen consumption or its ability to perform continuously. The name is somewhat exaggerated, as any time muscle is recruited, it constitutes an oxidative event. Aerobic and anaerobic metabolic cycles exist on a percentage continuum, each contributing a certain amount when muscles are recruited to perform an activity. Anaerobic exercise will have both aerobic (albeit little) and anaerobic percentage contributions. Anaerobic exercise modalities typically require more force production and therefore recruit more motor units (meaning more muscle fibers) than aerobic activities (based upon the size principle). These activities therefore cannot be typically maintained for a very long duration. The intensity and the duration of the activity dictates the amount of muscle needed to produce force and the number of calories expended to meet the metabolic demands.

Resistance Training

Even in the anaerobic exercise type, not every exercise can recruit the same number of motor units (and thus muscle), which impacts muscle metabolism and caloric expenditure. A key fact in understanding exercise is that if a motor unit is not recruited, it will not adapt despite the fact that other motor units in the same region are being used in an exercise. Resistance training ranges from high-repetition training (which start to mimic aerobic training) to heavy loads, which stimulate a large number of motor units and therefore produce adaptations in a host of systems apart from what can be accomplished by aerobic exercise. Resistance training really starts to be effective as the intensity is increased, and it starts to recruit significant amounts of muscle. It is the key to muscle tissue recruitment; even sprint intervals are not able to affect all of the muscle that heavy load resistance training can (and only glycogen depletion after 2 h of high-intensity aerobic exercise can begin to cause recruitment of higher-threshold motor units).

A reduction in body weight is usually the primary focus of weight-loss programs, but the implicit goal is to lose body fat while preserving or gaining muscle mass. With the potential infinite number of combinations of resistance training programs and anaerobic programs in the public domain, it is important that fundamental principles are observed; the impact of each resistance exercise protocol may be very different in terms of its potential for increasing lean muscle tissue gain (which increases the basal metabolic rate or the EPOC of protocol). From a metabolic perspective, the ability to make healthy changes in body composition or the percentage of fat and lean tissue mass (which includes muscle) ultimately relates to whether the actions in the body are "anabolic" (meaning to build) or "catabolic" (meaning to break down). While all exercise results in various degrees of tissue breakdown (and in the case of muscle repair, rebuilds the muscle back to its former integrity or better), catabolism can impact muscle and other tissues in a more chronic negative manner by not allowing optimal remodeling and repair. While fat tissue catabolism is primarily related to the use of stored fuels (thereby reducing fat mass in adipocytes), permanent damage does not occur—as can be the case with skeletal muscle and bone. The role of resistance exercise in lean body mass (LBM) is probably its most important role in the process of weight loss.

Resistance Exercise Programming

No matter what the exercise protocol or workout presented, it can be characterized by the "acute program variables" (Fleck and Kraemer 2004). These variable domains include choice of the exercise, the order of the exercise, the intensity of the exercise, the number of sets for an exercise, and the amount of rest utilized between sets and repetitions. The choice of exercise variable domain is quite large and therefore will dictate a lot of what is observed in training adaptations (e.g., if one does not exercise the lower body and only performs exercise on the upper body musculature, the lower body will not benefit). Typically, appropriate exercise order stipulates large muscle group exercises to be placed first in a workout to optimize maximal muscle activation and stimulate metabolism. The intensity of the exercise is one of the major features of any resistance training program as this dictates the number of motor units that are activated, which determines the amount of muscle tissue mass that is utilized in exercise. The more motor units that are activated, the greater the number of fibers that will metabolically adapt to the exercise protocol. Many lightweight exercise protocols do not activate or affect type II muscle fibers and therefore are not metabolically active nor do they contribute to the caloric expenditure related to repair and remodeling.

Fundamental to resistance exercise are the terms "sets and reps." Reps dictate how many repetitions can be performed or are performed with a given intensity. Each group of reps is described as a "set," and frequently, there is a rest period between each set. The most effective repetition is the concentric/eccentric repetition where one both lifts the weight up and then resists it as one lowers it back to the starting position. Popular programs (especially for women) that use just the concentric muscle action limit the effects on bone and other connective tissue and limit effectiveness on strength gains. In the area of weight loss and exercise, the typical concentric/eccentric repetition, with multiple sets and large muscle groups complemented with the smaller ones, are most effective in maintaining the most lean tissue mass under conditions of weight loss. The intensity of the exercise interacts with the number of sets to provide a volume of work that is vital for many programs directed at maintaining lean tissue mass during a weight-loss program.

Finally, the amount of rest used between sets and reps will have a great deal of influence on the metabolic profile. Shorter rest protocols produce much higher glycolytic demands at the cost of decreased resistance and more free-radical scavenging. They have a much higher catabolic potential for activated muscle tissue. These types of short rest programs have today attained much popularity at the expense of proper recovery needed. Too often commercial resistance programs focus on extreme exercise demands to help with marketing (this was the same motivation in the aerobic world that made marathons and triathlons popular from the 1970s on). Periodization, which allows for different types of workouts (but with adequate rest planned into the workout regime), is vital (Kraemer et al. 2012). Unlike such popular models, a variety of exercise types and intensities should be programmed into a week, month, and year. Long aerobic runs should not be programmed the same day as heavy resistance exercise.

A recent position stand by the ACSM in 2009 gives detailed evidence and suggestions for the proper progression of a resistance training program in healthy adults (ACSM position stand. Progression models in resistance training for healthy adults 2009). Table 25.2 overviews some of the exercise prescription guidelines for a resistance training program. Not all resistance training workouts or programs are the same: in linear programming, participants tend to follow a set plan that proceeds in a steady, predictable progression; in a flexible nonlinear programming approach, participants may adjust workouts based on fatigue and other environmental factors. Typical schedules for linear and nonlinear programs are presented in Table 25.3.

TABLE 25.2
Basic Guidelines for Resistance Training Program Design

Choice of exercise: Choose large muscle group exercises, use both unilateral and bilateral exercises, use exercises that activate muscle on both sides of the joint, use free weight and machine exercises, include both body part and structural exercises

Order of exercise: Perform large muscle group or complex movement exercises in the beginning of a workout, in circuit training alternate from upper to lower body exercises

Intensity of exercise: Use a periodized training program that uses both heavy 85%–95% of 1 RM or a 3–6 RM zone (not going to failure), moderate intensity 65%–80% of 1 RM or 8–10 RM (not going to failure), light intensity 40%–50% of 1 RM 12–15 RM (not going to failure), and power days with proper exercises that have no deceleration and ranging in modes from plyometrics to high-velocity Olympic style exercises, which do require more teaching and instruction

Number of sets: One can start with one set of exercise and then progress to 3 or 4 sets in most exercises. Not all exercises need to be performed with the same number of sets. If power exercises are performed, more sets with a few repetitions will assure a better quality of workout (e.g., hang pulls, 6 sets of 3 repetitions with 40% of 1 RM load)

Rest period length between sets and reps: It is important that shorter rest periods are carefully monitored for symptoms of adverse responses ranging from light headedness, dizziness, nausea, to vomiting, which does NOT indicate it was a good workout; it was too much too soon

- Short rest: 1–2 min
- Moderate rest: 3–4 min
- Long rest: 5–7 min

As the resistance load gets heavier, longer rest is needed and short rest should be used with light resistance loads. The weights one can use with short rest periods are reduced, and technique can fail due to fatigue creating increased chances of injury

TABLE 25.3
Example Programs for Linear and Nonlinear Periodization Programs

Linear periodized program intensities

Microcycle 1	**Microcycle 2**
3–5 sets of 12–15 RM	4–5 sets of 8–10 RM
Microcycle 3	**Microcycle 4**
3–4 sets of 4–6 RM	3–5 sets of 1–3 RM

Nonlinear periodized program: This protocol uses a 5-day rotation

Monday	**Wednesday**
2 sets 12–15 RM	6 sets of 1–3 RM
Friday	**Monday**
3 sets of 4–6 RM	Power day—plyometrics
Wednesday	
4 sets of 8–10 RM	One cycle of workouts last for 12 weeks with 1 week rest to follow

Microcycle lengths: 2–4 weeks.

RM = RM zones, but one should not lift to failure as to avoid over-training. These sets are for the major muscle group exercises as smaller muscle groups can use and 6–12 RM range (Kraemer and Fleck 2007).

Prior to any periodization of training program, a "general preparation" phase (4–12 weeks) should be used. During this time, features of the exercise program can be taught such as exercise technique and spotting requirements. It is important that instruction be conducted by an individual with an accredited certification; a recent study (Malek et al. 2002; Malek and Coburn) found that only those certified by the National Strength and Conditioning Association (NSCA) or ACSM received a passing score on a standardized test of fitness instructor knowledge (years of experience did not contribute to knowledge, although a degree in the field did). Supervision by a certified strength and conditioning specialist (the gold standard in resistance exercise certifications) is advised to ensure a safe and effective program when the workouts are elevated to more serious levels of physical demand (Kraemer and Fleck 2005).

EXERCISE AND WEIGHT LOSS

An overview of selected studies utilizing exercise and diet to produce weight loss is shown in Table 25.4. This demonstrates some of the complexity in today's interpretation of effective weight-loss programs and cautions readers as to the futility of many infomercial claims for dramatic changes and maintenance of weight loss over time. It is evident that the exercise program types, dietary regimes, and modalities are quite complex, and the subjects utilized also add further complexity to the interpretation based on differences in sex, age, and fitness levels.

One fundamental aspect in the understanding of health and body composition is the difference between a temporary state of weight loss to reduce body fat (or acute weight loss) and weight maintenance over time. Acute weight loss is determined largely through diet but can be indiscriminant; without proper protein intake and exercise, weight loss may occur through loss of lean tissue instead of body fat. Chronic weight maintenance is the process involved in preventing the weight gain with age (or preventing weight regain in some). Chronic weight maintenance involves diet but incorporates exercise to a greater degree.

ACUTE WEIGHT LOSS AND PRESERVATION OF LBM

Diet and Catabolic Effects

The most fundamental determinant of acute weight loss is diet. As noted by the ACSM position stand (Donnelly et al. 1998, 2009), "Most weight loss programs either limit energy intake to a specific amount (e.g., 500–1500 kcal · day^{-1}) regardless of the size or gender of the individuals participating in the program or select a specific energy deficit through diet (e.g., energy restriction of 300 kcal · day^{-1}) and/or exercise (e.g., 300 kcal · day^{-1}) to bring about a total energy reduction (e.g., 600 kcal · day^{-1})." Programs that achieve greater than 10% of initial body weight typically expend 1500 kcal · week^{-1} above baseline activity values. Dietary changes, including diet-induced caloric deficit, are the primary determinants of body weight loss.

Unfortunately, body weight loss is not necessarily an indication of body fat loss. The loss of lean body tissue (such as muscle and bone) is undesirable and may even be counterproductive to weight maintenance (due to lower metabolic rate) in the long term. Aerobic exercise is unlikely to prevent such a loss; aerobic exercise typically involves slow twitch (type I) muscle fibers that are made for endurance activity. High-threshold motor units are typically not affected as they are not recruited to produce force (refer back to Figure 25.1). Kraemer et al. (1995) was the first to demonstrate that high-intensity *endurance* training (made up of both continuous running and interval training) resulted in a reduction in the size of the type I muscle fibers as well as reducing muscular power. Thus, pure aerobic training done at high intensity is catabolic not only to the fat component of body composition but also to the muscle or lean mass component. Exercise itself may increase hunger and decrease resting metabolic rate. Caloric deficit and aerobic training therefore are both acting to reduce lean body tissue during weight loss and require a countermeasure to prevent excessive muscle atrophy.

TABLE 25.4

Although Cardiovascular Exercise and Diet Result in Weight Loss, Both Decrease Lean Body Tissue. Optimal Results Are Seen When Cardiovascular Activity and Diet Are Paired with Resistance Exercise

Study	Intervention	Exercise Protocol	Results				Nutrition	
			Mean BW Change	Mean % Fat Change	Mean FFM Change	Metabolic Rate	Macro/Supplement	Calorie Intake
Bond Brill et al. (2002). 56 premenopausal overweight women	12 week intervention 1. 30 min—5 days/week 2. 60 min—5 times/week 3. Diet control	Walking	1. −5.75 kg 2. −5.85 kg 3. −4.13 kg	1. −1.2% 2. −2.3% 3. −1.02%				1. −1028.1 kcal 2. −733.1 kcal 3. −915.7 kcal
van Aggel-Leijssen et al. (2001). 40 obese men	1. Diet 2. Diet + exercise (4 times/week for 60 min)	Low-intensity cycling on an ergometer, walking and aqua-jogging (40% of VO₂ max) for 12 weeks	1. −14.7 kg 2. −15.2 kg	1. −8.7% 2. −8.5%			First 6 weeks: 2.1 MJ: 50 g CHO, 52 g protein, 7 g fat Weeks 7–8: 1.4 MJ/ day + 3.5 MJ from other food Weeks 9 and 10: 0.7 MJ/day + 4.9 MJ from other food Week 11: return to energy balance Entire week 12: visit the lab	
Saris et al. (2000). 398 moderately obese adults	G1. Control group G2. Control diet group (dietary intervention = average national intake)		G2: +0.8 G3: − 0.9 G4: − 1.8	G2: +0.6 G3: −1.3 G4: −1.8	G2: +0.1 kg G3: +0.3 kg G4: 0.0 kg		G2: P-61 ± 22 g; F-77 ± 22 g; CHO-65 ± 21 g; S. CHO-72 ± 29 g; c.CHO-60 ± 22 g	

(continued)

TABLE 25.4 (continued)

Although Cardiovascular Exercise and Diet Result in Weight Loss, Both Decrease Lean Body Tissue. Optimal Results Are Seen When Cardiovascular Activity and Diet Are Paired with Resistance Exercise

Study	Intervention	Exercise Protocol	Results				Nutrition	
			Mean BW Change	Mean % Fat Change	Mean FFM Change	Metabolic Rate	Macro/Supplement	Calorie Intake
	G3. Low-fat simple CHO (carbohydrate) G4. Low-fat high-complex CHO						G3: P-61 ± 22g; F-65 ± 22g; CHO-66 ± 19g; S. CHO-78 ± 26g; c. CHO-56 ± 24g G4: P-69 ± 21g; F-69 ± 17g; CHO- 67 ± 22g; S. CHO-5719g; c. CHO-74 ± 27g	
Fragala et al. (2009). 22 healthy overweight matched women	8 week placebo-controlled, double-blind study G1. Supplement G2. Placebo	8 week supervised exe. 4–5/week 30–60 min. Intensity of 60%–90% of age-predicted max HR	G1: −9.2 kg G2: −4.2 kg	G1: −7.3 G2: −3.7			Supplement: 400 mg of Trisynex per capsule Placebo: 400 mg of magnesium stearate per capsule	
Volek et al. (2009). 40 overweight subjects	~1500 kcal CRD—CHO restricted C:F:P—12:59:28 LFD—low-fat diet C:F:P—56:24:20		CRD: −10.1 kg LFD: −5.2 kg	CRD: −2.4% LFD: −2.2%	CRD: −3.4 kg LFD: −1 kg		Pro (g): CRD: +10 g LFD: −10 g CHO (g): CRD: −225 g LFD: −59 g Fat (g): CRD: +3 g LFD: −39 g	CRD: −847 kcal LFD: −604 kcal

Study	Intervention	Exercise					
Kraemer et al. (2007). 22M + 20F overweight	8 week intervention No exercise (No-Ex): 3000mg glucomannan Exercise (Ex): 3000mg glucomannan + resistance training (RT) and endurance	3 weekly sessions RT:1h nonlinear total body resistance exercise program (3 sets of 3–12 rep with progressive overload) + 30min endurance walking and running on a running track	BMI: Male: No-Ex: −0.8 Ex: −0.9 Female: No-Ex: −0.9 Ex: −1.3	Male: No-Ex: −1.4% Ex: −2.9% Female: No-Ex: −1.9% Ex: −2.8%	Men: No-Ex: −0.1 kg Ex: +0.6 kg Female: No-Ex: +0.4 kg Ex: +0.4 kg	Pro (g) No-Ex: +2 Ex: +3 CHO (g) No-Ex:−34 Ex: −73 Fat (g) No-Ex: −17 Ex: −20	No-Ex: −376 kcal/day Ex: −463 kcal/day
Layman et al. (2003). 24 women (BMI > 26)	10 weeks C. CHO group CHO/protein ratio of 3.5 (68 g protein/day) P. Protein group CHO/protein ratio of 1.4 (125 g protein/day)		CHO: −6.98 kg Pro: −7.53 kg	CHO: −4.8 Pro: −5.67	CHO: −1.21 kg Pro: −0.83 kg	CHO (g) CHO:−7 Pro: −7.5 Pro (g) CHO: −7 Pro: +50 Fat (g) CHO: −27 Pro: −21	CHO: −1255 kcal/day Pro: −1209 kcal/day
Kraemer et al. (1997). 31 overweight women	12 week intervention 1. Control (Con; n = 6) 2. Diet (D: n = 8): maintained normal activities + reducing calories 3. Diet + endurance (DE; n = 9):diet + performed endurance exercise 3 days/week 4. Diet + endurance + strength (DES; n = 8): diet + endurance + strength 3 days/week	Endurance: 1st week; 70%–80% targeted HR; ~30min and gradually increased to 50min; exercises such as treadmill walking or jogging, stationary cycling, seated rowing, and stationary stair climbing Strength: heavy day (5–7 RM; 2–3min rest); moderate day (8–10 RM; 1min rest) squat, additional Nautilus machine, exercise for major muscle groups	Con: − D: −6.2 kg DE: −6.8 kg DES: −7.0 kg	Con: − D: −5.8 DE: −8.0 DES: −4.3	Con: −0.04 D: +0.02 DE: −0.01 DES: −0.05	Pro: D: 15.7 ± 2.8% DE: 15.3 ± 1.3% DES: 15.2 ± 2.2% CHO: D: 71.6 ± 4.5% DE: 71.8 ± 2.5% DES: 70.0 ± 3.5% Fat: D: 12.7 ± 3.1% DE: 13 ± 1.6% DES: 14.8 ± 4.4%	D: 1246 ± 148 DE: 1139 ± 111 DES: 1179 ± 191

(continued)

TABLE 25.4 (continued)

Although Cardiovascular Exercise and Diet Result in Weight Loss, Both Decrease Lean Body Tissue. Optimal Results Are Seen When Cardiovascular Activity and Diet Are Paired with Resistance Exercise

Study	Intervention	Exercise Protocol	Results				Nutrition	
			Mean BW Change	Mean % Fat Change	Mean FFM Change	Metabolic Rate	Macro/Supplement	Calorie Intake
Geliebter et al. (1997). 65 subjects moderately obese	8 week intervention 1. Diet + ST (DS) 2. Diet + AT (DA) 3. Diet only (DO)	3 times/week energy expenditure of 150 kcal ST (~60 min): Eight stations for both upper and lower body; first 2 sets—6 rep each; 30 s rest; 3rd set—as much as possible, if >8 rep, increase resistance next time AT (~30 min): Stationary leg cycle ergometer (60 rpm, 8 min, 0 resistance); upper body ergometer (8 min, 0 resistance); leg cycling (8 min, 0 resistance). First set to be 55% of VO_2 peak; keep HR just above 70% of max HR	DS: −7.7 kg DA: −9.6 kg DO: −9.5 kg	DS: −6.7 kg^2 DA: −7.2 kg^2 DO: −6.8 kg^2	DS: −1.1 kg^2 DA: −2.3 kg^2 DO: −2.7 kg^2	DS: −532 kJ/day DA: −623 kJ/day DO: −359 kJ/day	Formula diet: Protein: 70 g CHO: 32.5 g Fat: 10 g Fiber: 2 g	70% of RMR or 5150 kJ/day for 8 weeks + 1% fat milk to provide 70% of RMR

Stella L. Volpe, PhD, Hati Kobusingye, MS, Smita Bailur, MS, Edward Stanek, PhD. N = 90 (M = 44; F = 46) BMI = 27–35 kg/m²

9 month intervention Exercise (E; N = 34) Diet and exercise (DE; N = 28) Diet (D; N = 28)

For E and DE (–3 months (phase I, supervised); 3 times/week for 1st 6 weeks; gradually increase to 4 times/week for 30 min for 2nd 6 weeks + nutrition class (aim to lose 0 5–1.0 kg of BW/ week)

4–5 months (phase II, supervised); 4 times/week; 30 min for 1st 6 weeks; 5 times/week; 30 min for 2nd 6 weeks + nutrition class

7–9 months (phase III; home based) skiing apparatus exercise

Women:
D: +0.1
E: —
DE: –1.7

Men:
D: +0.3
E: –0.8
DE: –2.6

Pro (g)
Women:
D: –8.5
E: –9.2
DE: –14.9

Men:
D: –0.8
E:+10.8
DE: +2.4

Fat (g)
Women:
D: –30.8
E: –14.1
DE: –26.6

Men:
D: –13.7
E: –1.3
DE: –8.8

CHO (g)
Women:
D: –28
E: –13.5
DE: –46.6

Men:
D: –65.4
E: +70.1
DE: +4.9

Women:
D: –1895
E: –981
DE: –1887

Men:
D: –1682
E: +1324
DE: –1

(continued)

TABLE 25.4 (continued)

Although Cardiovascular Exercise and Diet Result in Weight Loss, Both Decrease Lean Body Tissue. Optimal Results Are Seen When Cardiovascular Activity and Diet Are Paired with Resistance Exercise

Study	Intervention	Exercise Protocol	Results				Nutrition	
			Mean BW Change	Mean % Fat Change	Mean FFM Change	Metabolic Rate	Macro/Supplement	Calorie Intake
Janssen et al. (2002). N = 38 obese women; BMI > 27	16 week intervention Diet only (DO: N = 13) Diet and aerobic (DA; N = 11) Diet and resistance exe (DR; N = 14) Energy requirements were estimated by multiplying the Harris–Benedict equation by a factor of 1.5, which is within ~8% of actual energy requirement (follow it for 2 weeks before pretreatment testing) For 16 weeks treatment Goal: lose weight maintenance energy intake by 100 kcal/day Keep daily diet records Limit dietary fat intake <30%	DA: 5 times/week ~15 min at beginning → 60 min based on ability; exercise: walking on a motorized treadmill, stair stepping; intensity 50%–85% of max HR DR: 3 times/week ~30 min; 7 exercises: leg extension and flexion, super pullover, bench press, shoulder press, triceps extension and biceps curl, sit ups; 1 set of 8–12 rep to volitional fatigue; 2 s con; 4 s ecc *Finish 12 rep in good form; increase weight that permitted ~8 rep	DO: −10.0 kg DA: −11.1 kg DR: −10.0 kg	DO: −7.8 kg DA: −9.9 kg DR: −8.6 kg			Fat intakes DO: 21 ± 5% DA: 25 ± 5% DR: 22 ± 5%	Average dietary-induced energy deficit for 16 week treatment period: DO: 1222 ± 293 kcal/day DA: 1299 ± 215 kcal/day DR: 1209 ± 211 kcal/day

| Kirk et al. (2009). RT, N = 22 (16 males, 6 females) C, N = 17 (11 males, 6 females) BMI = 27.7 ± 0.5 kg/m² | 6 months of supervised minimal resistance training. Resistance training (RT; N = 22) Control (C; N = 17) | RT: 3 nonconsecutive days/week for 6 months; 1 set of 9 exercises: chest press, back extension, lateral pull-down, triceps extension, shoulder press, leg press, calf raise, leg curl, and abdominal crunch; 85%–90% of 1 RM *>6 rep for 2 consecutive training → increase weight by ~2.25 kg | C: +2.4 kg RT: +2.5 kg | C: +2.1 RT: +0.3 | C: −0.3 RT: +1.5 | C: +235 RT: +679 | |
| Volek et al. (2004). N = 28 20–55 y >25% body fat | 2 restricted diets (male with 50 days and female with 30 days for each diet). Low-fat diet (LF; Male [n = 15]; female [n = 13]) CHO: Fat: Protein 58:22:20. Very-low-carbohydrate Ketogenic (VLCK; Male [n = 15]; female [n = 13]) 9:63:28. *Subjects kept detailed food diaries during three 1 week periods (21 days total) of each diet | Men: VLCK Weight loss: 11/15 person Total fat loss: 11/15 person Trunk fat loss: 12/15 person Women: Weight loss: 8/13 person Total fat loss: 10/13 person Trunk fat loss: 12/13 person | Men: VLCK: −0.8% LF: +1.2 Women: VLCK: −0.7% LF: +0.3% | | | Men: VLCK: −140 LF: −233 Women: VLCK: −16 LF: −95 | Low-fat diet (<10% of saturated fat) CHO: Fat: Protein 58:22:20 Very low carbohydrate Ketogenic 9:63:28 | Restricted diet (−500 kcal/day) VLCK: average 1855 kcal/day LF: average 1562 kcal/day |

(continued)

TABLE 25.4 (continued)

Although Cardiovascular Exercise and Diet Result in Weight Loss, Both Decrease Lean Body Tissue. Optimal Results Are Seen When Cardiovascular Activity and Diet Are Paired with Resistance Exercise

| Study | Intervention | Exercise Protocol | Results | | | | Nutrition | |
			Mean BW Change	Mean % Fat Change	Mean FFM Change	Metabolic Rate	Macro/Supplement	Calorie Intake
LeCheminant (2007). N = 55 Overweight/obese middle-aged adults BMI > 27 kg/m²	9 month intervention Low-fat diet (LF; n = 29) Low-CHO diet (LC; n = 26) 1st 3 months (identical liquid diet): 2177 kJ/day; 5 times/day; 1 liquid diet contains 435 kJ (13–17 g CHO; 1 g fat; 10–14 g protein) *have to lose 10% of BW to proceed Month 4: reduce identical liquid diet; refeeding with solid foods; LC (green leafy vegetables, broccoli florets, lean meant and nuts); LF (fruits, vegetables, potatoes, and whole grains) Month 5 onward: (meal plan) LC: upper limit for CHO (g) to be consumed each day ~20% LF: upper limit for fat (g) to be consumed each day ~30%	Physical activity (PA) level = 1.4*REE Moderate intensity activity, for example, brisk walking (major muscle groups) lasted for ≥10 min 15 min/day; 3 times/week → 50–60 min/day; 5–6 times/ week by month 6 (overall goal PA level of 300 min/ week by month 6 and remain throughout the study)	LC: −20.3 kg LF: −19.5 kg				CHO (g): LC: −93 LF: +5 PRO (g): LC: +7 LF: −7 FAT (g): LC: −1 LF: −54	LC: −1402 LF: −2272

Donnelly (2003). N = 74 male and female 17–35 y BMI 25.0–34.9	16 month intervention Control (C; n = 33) Exercise (Exe; n = 41)	Exercise: Walking on treadmills (stationary biking and walking on elliptical should not consist of 20% of the total exe sessions; 1 of 5 days) 20 min at beginning → 45 min by month 6 60% HR reserve at baseline → 75% by month 6 (55%–70% VO² max; remain throughout the whole study) =Targeted minimum energy equivalent of exe ~400 cal/day (~2000 cal/week) (gradually achieved in the 1st 6 months and remains throughout the study)	Men: C: −0.5 Exe: −5.2 Women: C: +2.9 Exe: +0.6	Men: C: −0.8 Exe: −2.7 Women: C: +1.1 Exe: −0.7			Energy expenditure Women: C: +142 Exe: +209 Men: C: −34 Exe: +372 Energy intake Women: C: +97 Exe: +43 Men: C: −192 Exe: +12
Donnelly et al. (1991). N = 69 obese female	90 day intervention Diet (C; n = 26) Diet + endurance exercise (EE; n = 16) Diet + weight training (WT; n = 18) Diet + EE + WT (EEWT; n = 9) 90 day liquid diet (ingested 5 scheduled times/day	EE: 4 days/week 20 min at the beginning → 60 min by 90 days intensity: 13 RPE from day 1 to 14; 70% of HR reserve from day 15–90 WT: 4 days/week beginning: 2 sets/ 6–8 rep at 70% 1 RM from day 1–14→ 3 sets/ 6–8 rep at 80% 1 RM from day 15–90	C: −20.4 ± 5.7 EE: −21.4 ± 3.8 WT: −20.9 ± 6.2 EEWT: −22.9 ± 5.1	C: −7.8 EE: −9.0 WT: −9.3 EEWT: −10.1	C: −16.1 kg EE: −16.6 kg WT: −4.7 kg EEWT: −4.1 kg	C: −579 EE: −664 WT: −782 EEWT: −908	Liquid diet: Protein 50 g CHO 79 g Fat 1 g Vitamins + mineral tablet before and after bed Liquid diet 2184 kJ/day

(continued)

TABLE 25.4 (continued)

Although Cardiovascular Exercise and Diet Result in Weight Loss, Both Decrease Lean Body Tissue. Optimal Results Are Seen When Cardiovascular Activity and Diet Are Paired with Resistance Exercise

Study	Intervention	Exercise Protocol	Results				Nutrition	
			Mean BW Change	Mean % Fat Change	Mean FFM Change	Metabolic Rate	Macro/Supplement	Calorie Intake
Ryan et al. (1995). N = 15 postmenopausal female; 50–69 y Nonobese (n = 8; BMI <27) Obese (n = 7; BMI > 27)	16 week intervention of resistance training Resistance training (RT; nonobese; n = 8) Resistance training with weight loss (RTWL; obese; n = 7) 4 weeks before study (standardized diet by RD) 50%–55% CHO 15%–20% protein <30% Fat <300 mg cholesterol RT (follow the standardized diet for the remaining 16 weeks) RTWL (underwent a hypocaloric diet (0.25–0.5 kg/week weight loss)	RT: 3 times/week on nonconsecutive days for ~16 weeks; using 14 exercises on pneumatic variable-resistance machines (1st set of extension, overhead press, leg adductor, leg abductor, upper back, triceps, lower back, upper abdominals, biceps curl (dumbbells), and lower abdominals (floor). 2nd set of press, leg curl, and leg extension machine Begin with 5 RM or 90% of 3 RM for 1st 3–4 reps; from 4th to 5th rep onward, reduced weight and finish up by 15 reps *Energy expenditure for each session ~150 kcal	RT: +0.1 kg RTWL: −5.0 kg	RT: −1.2 RTWL: −4.1	RT: +1.1 kg RTWL: +0.5 kg	RT: +53 RTWL: +52	CHO (%) RT: +0.2 RTWL: +1 Protein (%) RT: −1 RTWL: +1 Fat (g) RT: −1 RTWL: −2	RT: +53 kcal/day RTWL: +52 kcal/day

Study	Intervention	Exercise					
Donnelly et al. (2000). N = 22 female; BMI > 25	18 month intervention Intermittent (INT; n = 11) Continuous (CON; n = 11) Energy intake: 3-day food records (2 week days and 1 week end for months 0/9/18 24h recalls by months 3/6/12/15	Continuous exercise: 3 days/week for 30 min; 60%–75% max aerobic capacity Intermittent exer 5 days/week; 2 * 15 min sessions with 2h elapsed; 50%–65% max aerobic capacity by using brisk walking	CON: −1.7kg INT: −0.80kg	CON: −1.75% INT: −0.54%	CON: +0.4kg INT: −0.07kg		Pro(%) CON: — INT: +1.5 CHO (%) CON: −0.3 INT: +3.6 Fat (%) CON: +0.4 INT: −5.1	CON: −132 INT: −361
Kraemer et al. (1999). N = 35 male	12 week intervention Control (C; n = 6) Diet (D; n = 8) Aerobic endurance + diet (DE; n = 11) DE+ resistance training (DES; n = 10) Diet: Attend 1h group format nutrition education (implement a healthy well balanced eating plan designed to lose body mass; objective was to create a 6–9kg weight loss in each subject by moderate caloric restriction over the 12 weeks) Subjects were given a 1-week supply of Matol (included prepackaged high-fiber meal replacement bars, shakes, and cereal which contained ~50% of the USRDA for vitamins and minerals) products at each meeting	Endurance exercise: 70%–80% target HR 1st week ~30min → 50min at the end of the study Exercise type: cross training mix of treadmill walking/jogging; stationary cycling, seated rowing, and stationary stair climbing Resistance training (nonlinear progression): (after aerobic training) Intensity: Heavy (5–7 RM; 2–3 min rest) Moderate (8–10 RM; 1 min rest); 1st 2–3 week (1–3 sets) → throughout 12 weeks to increase the amount of weight lifted within each designated rep range Exercise: military press, bench press, lat pull down, seated row, sit-ups, lower back, legpress, hamstring curls, calf raises, and arm curls	C: +0.35 D: −9.64 DE: −8.99 DES: −9.90	C: −0.76% D: −3.62% DE: −4.70% DES: −8.42%	C: +0.45 kg D: −2.96 kg DE: −2.00 kg DES: −0.33 kg	C: +0.01 D: +0.01 DE: — DES: —	Based on 3 days of food records: Pro (%): D: 18.7 ± 5.4 DE: 15.4 ± 2.3 DES: 15.7 ± 2.8 CHO (%) D: 55.2 ± 12.3 DE: 54.5 ± 8.7 DES: 61.2 ± 4.2 Fat (%) D: 20.8 ± 9.2 DE: 24.9 ± 10.4 DES: 17.8 ± 4.7	Based on 3 days of food records: D: 1551 ± 428kcal DE: 1430 ± 426kcal DES: 1449 ± 578kcal

(continued)

TABLE 25.4 (continued)

Although Cardiovascular Exercise and Diet Result in Weight Loss, Both Decrease Lean Body Tissue. Optimal Results Are Seen When Cardiovascular Activity and Diet Are Paired with Resistance Exercise

| Study | Intervention | Exercise Protocol | Results | | | | Nutrition | |
			Mean BW Change	Mean % Fat Change	Mean FFM Change	Metabolic Rate	Macro/Supplement	Calorie Intake
							Matola: consumed in place of certain meals in a 4 day rotational sequence; 1 product on day 1, 2 products on day 2, 3 products on day 3, and no products on day 4 (total 12 products/week)	
Racette et al. (1995). 23 obese women	12 week intervention: 1. Aerobic exercise (Ex) + Low fat (LF; LF/Ex) 2. Ex + Low CHO (LC; LC/Ex) 3. No exercise (Nx) + LF (LF/Nx) 4. Nx + LC (LC/Nx)	Ex: 3 times/week for 12 weeks Aerobic exercise: 45 min; 60%–65% of VO$_2$ max Treadmill; bicycle ergometer; airdyne bicycle; rowing ergometer; stairstepper 3 different exercises for 15 min	LC: −10.6 LF: −8.1 Ex: −10.5 Nx: −8.3	−7.3	−2.0 kg		Reported diet LF/Nx: CHO: 59 ± 1% PRO: 24 ± 1% Fat: 18 ± 1% LC/Nx: CHO: 27 ± 2% Pro: 24 ± 1% Fat: 49 ± 2% LF/Ex: CHO: 57 ± 4% Pro: 24 ± 1% Fat: 19 ± 3% LC/Ex: CHO: 26 ± 1% Pro: 25 ± 1% Fat: 49 ± 0%	75% of RMR LF/Nx: 5.15 ± 0.80 MJ/day LC/Nx: 4.80 ± 0.41 MJ/day LF/Ex: 4.86 ± 0.70 MJ/day LC/Ex: 4.88 ± 0.64 MJ/day

(continued)

Wadden et al. (1997). 128 obese women	48 week intervention: 1. Diet (D) 2. Diet + Endurance (DE) 3. Deit + ST (DS) 4. Diet + endurance + ST (DES)	First 28 weeks: 3 supervised exercises/week Weeks 29–48; 2 supervised exercises/week + 1 home exercise/week Endurance: Step aerobics (10 cm, 15 cm, or 20 cm step; moderate intensity or 11–15 RPE; 12 min at week 1 and add 2 min each week by week 14 (40 min) Weeks 29–48 assisted in developing a home exercise to replace the 3rd session ST: Universa Gym (Syracuse cohort); Cybex (PA cohort) Week 2: 1 set each >= 10 < 14 ~20 min Weeks 3–14 2 sets each ~40 min Weeks 14–23; 2 sets; increase resistance if >14 rep for 2 consecutive sets ST + Aerobic: 60% RT + 40% Aerobic Syracuse cohort: step aerobics PA cohort: Treadmill walking and stationary bicycling	D: −14.03 kg DE: −13.58 kg DS: −14.6 kg DES: −13.78 kg	D: −83.23% DE: −84.13% DS: −85.7% DES: 90.87%	D: −2.47 kg DE: −2.33 kg DS: −2.33 kg DES: −1.73 kg	D: −130.33 DE: −76 DS: −138 DES: −83.67	Weeks 2–17; liquid meal (150 kcal; 15 g protein; 11.2 g CHO; 5 g fat) + shelf-stable dinner (~280–300 kcal; 20 g protein; 35–40 g CHO; 7 g fat) + 2 cups of salad Week 18; decrease liquid meal; increase conventional foods → by week 20; ~1250 kcal/day Weeks 22–48; self-selected diet ~1599 kcal/day; 12%–15% protein; 55%–60% CHO; 15%–30% fat

TABLE 25.4 (continued)

Although Cardiovascular Exercise and Diet Result in Weight Loss, Both Decrease Lean Body Tissue. Optimal Results Are Seen When Cardiovascular Activity and Diet Are Paired with Resistance Exercise

Study	Intervention	Exercise Protocol	Results				Nutrition	
			Mean BW Change	Mean % Fat Change	Mean FFM Change	Metabolic Rate	Macro/Supplement	Calorie Intake
Volek (2002). N = 20 men	6 week diet intervention Carbohydrate-restricted diet (CR; n = 12) Habitual diet (Con; n = 8) CR: Reduced CHO intake to 5%–10% of energy; fat comprised ~60% of energy			CR: −3.6% Con: −0.1%	CR: +1.1 kg Con: +0.4 kg		Pro (%) CR: +13% Con: 0% CHO (%) CR: −40% Con: 0% Fat (%) CR: +29% Con: 0%	CR: −0.86% (MJ) Con: −1.0% (MJ)
Farnsworth et al. (2003). 57 subjects completed the study 14 men and 43 women (overweight with BMI: 27–43) Had fasting serum insulin concentration >12mU/L	12 weeks of energy restriction (ER) (6–6.3 MJ/day) 4 weeks of energy balance (EB) (~8.2 MJ/day) 1. Standard protein diet (SP); protein: 16%; CHO: 57%; fat: 27% 2. High-protein diet (HP); protein: 27%; CHO: 44%; fat: 29%		Men: SP: −9.6 kg HP: −11.5 kg Women: SP: −7.4 kg HP: −6.6 kg	Men: SP: −7.6 kg HP: −4.5 kg Women: SP: −7.1 kg HP: −2.9 kg			ER: SP: protein: 15.7%; CHO: 57.3%; fat: 26.8% HP: protein: 27.4%; CHO: 44.4%; fat: 27% EB: SP: protein: 15.4%; CHO: 56.9%; fat: 27.5% HP: protein: 27.3%; CHO: 44.6%; fat: 26.9%	SP: ER: 6.5 MJ/day EB: 8.2 MJ/day HP: ER: 6.3 MJ/day EB: 8.0 MJ/day

Resistance Exercise and Maintenance of LBM

While protein intake may help to prevent the loss of lean tissue, resistance exercise may also be of benefit. When a resistance training program was added to the Kraemer et al. (1995) protocol, muscle wasting (or what might be called exercise-induced atrophy) was eliminated. This supports the use of a total conditioning program where the tissue mass is to be protected, as in this study, no caloric deficit was part of the training program. Another investigation by Kraemer et al. (1997) examined women in control, diet-only, diet and endurance training, and diet and endurance and strength training groups. After 12 weeks, all of the noncontrol groups lost weight, but no differences were observed in the magnitude of body mass loss, body fat change, fat mass loss, or in resting metabolic rate. The data indicated that weight loss during moderate caloric restriction is not altered by inclusion of aerobic or aerobic + resistance exercise. At the same time, those who dieted and included training produced adaptations in muscular strength and aerobic capacity despite significant reductions in body mass. Loss in fat-free mass was not only attenuated but maintained or increased when exercise was added to dietary restriction. A follow-up study in men by Kraemer et al. (1999) using the same experimental design again showed similar results. Thus, resistance training allows for the preservation of the muscle or lean tissue biocompartment in both men and women when using a moderate calorie deficit in a weight-loss program.

Resistance Exercise and Weight Loss

Many different types of resistance training programs are hyped as part of weight-loss advertisements. This has led to confusion in the lay public. The use of exercise as part of a weight-loss program is both complex and multifaceted due to the wide variation in program designs for both aerobic and anaerobic exercise programs. A recent position stand has stated that resistance training alone does not result in weight loss. This might have some efficacy, yet again, only general weight training programs have been evaluated over short-term periods. The majority of research into this interaction has typically only looked at the more general exercise prescriptions that might be thought of as "fitness" programs, leaving the role of exercise in diet and weight loss somewhat speculative if one uses more advanced exercise prescriptions. At the same time, progressing safely to more advanced exercise prescriptions requires proper training. Many of the commercial programs that are called "extreme" provide little rest and depend upon massive catabolic responses that result not only in fat breakdown but also lean tissue breakdown (most notably, muscle). Again, careful monitoring and proper progression in periodized training is necessary for long term adherence and success.

The two mechanisms by which weight training alone might impact weight loss are the increase in muscle tissue mass (leading to a higher resting metabolic rate) or its contribution to the EPOC (which would increase the caloric consumption). Both are dependent upon the programs used and the gain potential of each individual. As such, if one does not have a high number of muscle fibers, the gain potential for lean muscle mass is limited, and even when higher numbers of fibers exist in an individual's muscle, the amount of weight gain from muscle possible only results in metabolic increases from 25 to 100 extra calories a day, making its overall contribution to weight loss less dramatic. The potential for increased caloric expenditures due to EPOC requires both large muscle mass exercises (e.g., squat) using relatively heavy loads (75%–90% of 1RM) with high enough volume of exercise (i.e., multiple sets, 4–6) and with the lighter loads shorter rest period to ramp up the metabolic machinery. This has also been observed for run training in that high speed 400 m repeats may be needed to increase this EPOC for long periods of time. Thus, it might be speculated that unless you are capable of such higher intensity workouts, weight loss from just resistance training alone would be quite challenging.

In essence, resistance training alone (without diet modification) will not mediate weight loss but rather an alteration of the body composition profiles (Kraemer et al. 1995). Thus, some type of dietary program using various methods (e.g., high fiber, caloric restriction, or macronutrient changes) is needed to see the loss of body fat or weight (Donnelly et al. 1998). It is worth mentioning that not all studies indicate no effect. In an investigation of a fiber supplement (glucomannan) on weight loss, a non-exercise group was compared to an exercise group (resistance and cardiovascular). For both the no exercise and exercise group, respectively, there were significant reductions in body mass (men, -2.7 ± 1.4 and -3.0 ± 4.0 kg; women, -2.2 ± 1.5 and -3.3 ± 1.5 kg), and for fat mass (men, -2.3 ± 1.6 and -3.9 ± 2.5 kg; women, -2.6 ± 1.4 and -3.6 ± 1.1 kg) (Kraemer et al. 2007). The combined exercise program appeared to augment the reduction in fat mass (by 63% and 50% in men and women, respectively) and waist circumference but did not affect total weight loss. Addition of a resistance and endurance exercise training program to a glucomannan diet regimen significantly improved measures of body composition, HDL-C, and TC/HDL-C ratio. It is difficult to ascertain, however, whether the added weight loss was due to resistance exercise, aerobic exercise, or the combination.

Dietary Approaches and Weight Loss

The control of macronutrient intakes may well be another important factor in diet interventions. While the so-called Atkins Diet has produced a strong message to the lay public, it still is misinterpreted as a high-protein diet, which is not true. Low-carbohydrate intakes have a new and emerging presence in the science of weight loss, obesity, and metabolic syndrome but struggles against long-held concepts entrenched within nutrition dogma. Scientific facts go beyond the emotional hype, showing "low-carbohydrate" diets to be very effective in both men and women for weight loss as well as improvements in combating metabolic syndrome symptoms or diabetes (Volek et al. 2002, 2009a,b; Westman et al. 2003; Feinman and Volek 2008; Forsythe et al. 2010).

CHRONIC WEIGHT MAINTENANCE

Maintaining weight loss over the long term takes an extreme amount of vigilance. A long-term weight loss study by the Look AHEAD research group observed the long-term effects of "an intensive lifestyle intervention program on cardiovascular morbidity and mortality in overweight or obese persons with type 2 Diabetes" as well as body image aspects. The components of the intensive lifestyle intervention included a low-calorie, low-fat diet; a goal of a minimum of 175 min per week of physical activity; and maintenance contact meetings with either groups or individual sessions (Wing 2010; Stewart et al. 2011). The results of these studies showed that the intensive lifestyle intervention was successful at producing weight loss and improving cardiovascular risk factors, but vigilance was the key. Subjects who were able to maintain their weight loss over an extended period of time all consistently maintained a low-calorie, low-fat diet; engaged in high levels of physical activity; limited their television watching; and weighed themselves daily or at least several times per week. The weight loss maintainers also exhibited a lower calorie intake, lower fat calorie intake, higher amounts of physical activity per week, lower amounts of television watched per week, and a higher weighing-in frequency than their equivalent weight controls that had not previously been overweight or obese. It is clear that increased aerobic activity can limit weight gain over time—the primary goal related to achieving a healthy lifestyle and the basis for related preventive medicine in cardiovascular disease and diabetes.

GENETIC FACTORS

Genetics is a significantly influential factor in the weight-loss process. The body's response to changes in lipid levels is partially determined by genetic components. A diet and exercise intervention study performed on pairs of identical twins showed that "genetic differences partially account for the variation in the response of lipids and lipoproteins to the negative energy protocol" (Lakka et al. 2004). The similarity within each pair of twins in response to the endurance exercise and negative energy protocol, in relation to improvement in plasma lipid profile, suggests that the response was genetically predetermined. Ruaño et al. (2006) also opened the door on a new aspect of physiogenomics in nutrition using variances in weight loss and nutritional intake profiles to gain insights into genetic basis for alterations from interventions. A strong association between weight loss induced by dietary CHO restriction and variability in genes regulating fat digestion, hepatic glucose metabolism, intravascular lipoprotein remodeling, and appetite were detected. It forwarded the concept that such discoveries could provide important clues to our understanding of the physiological adaptations underlying the body mass response to CHO restriction. Furthermore, it presents a possible future for such study and clinical approach to weight loss in medicine.

CONCLUSIONS

In summary, while diet is the primary factor involved in acute weight loss, the catabolic effects of reduced caloric intake and aerobic exercise require dietary (increased protein intake) and anaerobic (resistance exercise) approaches to preserve lean muscle tissue. Aerobic activity, while unlikely to appreciably aid acute weight loss, plays an important role in cardiovascular health and long-term weight maintenance. Sensible approaches for weight loss require proper programming and attention to the key programming concepts such as variety, intensity, and rest. Both aerobic and anaerobic exercises are essential for health, with resistance exercise playing a stronger short-term role in LBM maintenance and aerobic playing a strong role in long-term body fat maintenance. Finally, dietary approaches such as low-carbohydrate diets appear to be an important component of weight loss. Both low-carbohydrate diet approaches and genetic factors stand to provide interesting research into the future.

REFERENCES

American College of Sports Medicine position stand 2009. Progression models in resistance training for healthy adults. *Medicine and Science in Sports and Exercise* 41 (3):687–708.

Bond Brill, J., A.C. Perry, L. Parker, A. Robinson, and K. Burnett. 2002. Dose-response effect of walking exercise on weight loss. How much is enough? *International Journal of Obesity and Related Metabolic Disorders: Journal of the International Association for the Study of Obesity* 26 (11):1484–1493. http://www.ncbi.nlm.nih.gov/pubmed/12439651

Cooper, K.H. 1968. *Aerobics*. New York: M. Evans; distributed in association with Lippincott.

Donnelly, J.E., S.N. Blair, J.M. Jakicic, M.M. Manore, J.W. Rankin, and B.K. Smith. 1998. American College of Sports Medicine position stand: The recommended quantity and quality of exercise for developing and maintaining cardiorespiratory and muscular fitness and flexibility in healthy adults (Med Sci Sports Exerc Jun American College of Sports in Resistance Training for Healthy Adults). *Medicine and Science in Sports and Exercise* 30 (6 SRC GoogleScholar):975–991.

Donnelly, J.E., S.N. Blair, J.M. Jakicic, M.M. Manore, J.W. Rankin, and B.K. Smith. 2009. American College of Sports Medicine position stand: Appropriate physical activity intervention strategies for weight loss and prevention of weight regain for adults. *Medicine and Science in Sports and Exercise* 41 (2):459–471.

Donnelly, J.E., J.O. Hill, D.J. Jacobsen, J. Potteiger, D.K. Sullivan, S.L. Johnson, K. Heelan, M. Hise, P.V. Fennessey, B. Sonko, T. Sharp, J.M. Jakicic, S.N. Blair, Z.V. Tran, M. Mayo, C. Gibson, and R.A. Washburn. 2003. Effects of a 16-month randomized controlled exercise trial on body weight and composition in young, overweight men and women: The midwest exercise trial. *Archives of Internal Medicine* 163 (11):1343–1350.

Donnelly, J.E., D.J. Jacobsen, K.S. Heelan, R. Seip, and S. Smith. 2000. The effects of 18 months of intermittent vs. continuous exercise on aerobic capacity, body weight and composition, and metabolic fitness in previously sedentary, moderately obese females. *International Journal of Obesity and Related Metabolic Disorders* 24 (5):566–572.

Donnelly, J.E., N.P. Pronk, D.J. Jacobsen, S.J. Pronk, and J.M. Jakicic. 1991. Effects of a very-low-calorie diet and physical-training regimens on body composition and resting metabolic rate in obese females. *The American Journal of Clinical Nutrition* 54 (1):56–61.

Farnsworth, E., N.D. Luscombe, M. Noakes, G. Wittert, E. Argyiou, and P.M. Clifton. 2003. Effect of a high-protein, energy-restricted diet on body composition, glycemic control, and lipid concentrations in overweight and obese hyperinsulinemic men and women. *The American Journal of Clinical Nutrition* 78 (1):31–39. http://www.ncbi.nlm.nih.gov/pubmed/12816768

Feinman, R.D. and J.S. Volek. 2008. Carbohydrate restriction as the default treatment for type 2 diabetes and metabolic syndrome. *Scandinavian Cardiovascular Journal* 42 (4):256–263.

Fleck, S.J. and W.J. Kraemer. 2004. *Designing Resistance Training Programs*, 3rd edn. Champaign, IL: Human Kinetics.

Forsythe, C.E., S.D. Phinney, R.D. Feinman, B.M. Volk, D. Freidenreich, E. Quann, K. Ballard, M.J. Puglisi, C.M. Maresh, W.J. Kraemer, D.M. Bibus, M.L. Fernandez, and J.S. Volek. 2010. Limited effect of dietary saturated fat on plasma saturated fat in the context of a low carbohydrate diet. *Lipids* 45 (10):947–962.

Fragala, M.S., W.J. Kraemer, J.S. Volek, C.M. Maresh, M.J. Puglisi, J.L. Vingren et al. 2009. Influences of a dietary supplement in combination with an exercise and diet regimen on adipocytokines and adiposity in women who are overweight. *European Journal of Applied Physiology* 105 (5):665–672. http://www.ncbi.nlm.nih.gov/pubmed/19048277

Geliebter, A., M.M. Maher, L. Gerace, B. Gutin, S.B. Heymsfield, and S.A. Hashim. 1997. Effects of strength or aerobic training on body composition, resting metabolic rate, and peak oxygen consumption in obese dieting subjects. *The American Journal of Clinical Nutrition* 66 (3):557–563. http://www.ajcn.org/content/566/553/557.abstract

Janssen, I., A. Fortier, R. Hudson, and R. Ross. 2002. Effects of an energy-restrictive diet with or without exercise on abdominal fat, intermuscular fat, and metabolic risk factors in obese women. *Diabetes Care* 25 (3):431–438.

Kirk, E.P., J.E. Donnelly, B.K. Smith, J. Honas, J.D. Lecheminant, B.W. Bailey, D.J. Jacobsen, and R.A. Washburn. 2009. Minimal resistance training improves daily energy expenditure and fat oxidation. *Medicine and Science in Sports and Exercise* 41 (5):1122–1129.

Kraemer, W.J. and S.J. Fleck. 2005. *Strength Training for Young Athletes*. Champaign, IL: Human Kinetics.

Kraemer, W.J. and S.J. Fleck. 2007. *Optimizing Strength Training: Designing Nonlinear Periodization Workouts*. Champaign, IL: Human Kinetics.

Kraemer, W.J., S.J. Fleck, and M.R. Deschenes. 2012. *Exercise Physiology: Integrating Theory and Application*. Philadelphia, PA: Wolters Kluwer/Lippincott Williams & Wilkins.

Kraemer, W.J., J.F. Patton, S.E. Gordon, E.A. Harman, M.R. Deschenes, K. Reynolds, R.U. Newton, N.T. Triplett, and J.E. Dziados. 1995. Compatibility of high-intensity strength and endurance training on hormonal and skeletal muscle adaptations. *Journal of Applied Physiology* 78 (3):976–989.

Kraemer, W.J., J.L. Vingren, R. Silvestre, B.A. Spiering, D.L. Hatfield, J.Y. Ho, M.S. Fragala, C.M. Maresh, and J.S. Volek. 2007. Effect of adding exercise to a diet containing glucomannan. *Metabolism: Clinical and Experimental* 56 (8):1149–1158.

Kraemer, W.J., J.S. Volek, K.L. Clark, S.E. Gordon, S.M. Puhl, L.P. Koziris, J.M. McBride, N.T. Triplett-McBride, M. Putukian, R.U. Newton, K. Hakkinen, J.A. Bush, and W.J. Sebastianelli. 1999. Influence of exercise training on physiological and performance changes with weight loss in men. *Medicine and Science in Sports and Exercise* 31 (9):1320–1329.

Kraemer, W.J., J.S. Volek, K.L. Clark, S.E. Gordon, T. Incledon, S.M. Puhl, N.T. Triplett-McBride, J.M. McBride, M. Putukian, and W.J. Sebastianelli. 1997. Physiological adaptations to a weight-loss dietary regimen and exercise programs in women. *Journal of Applied Physiology* 83 (1):270–279.

Lakka, H.M., A. Tremblay, J.P. Després, and C. Bouchard. 2004. Effects of long-term negative energy balance with exercise on plasma lipid and lipoprotein levels in identical twins. *Atherosclerosis* 172 (1):127–133.

Layman, D.K., R.A. Boileau, D.J. Erickson, J.E. Painter, H. Shiue, C. Sather, and D.D. Christou. 2003. A reduced ratio of dietary carbohydrate to protein improves body composition and blood lipid profiles during weight loss in adult women. *Journal of Nutrition* 133 (2):411–417.

Lecheminant, J.D., C.A. Gibson, D.K. Sullivan, S. Hall, R. Washburn, M.C. Vernon, C. Curry, E. Stewart, E.C. Westman, and J.E. Donnelly. 2007. Comparison of a low carbohydrate and low fat diet for weight maintenance in overweight or obese adults enrolled in a clinical weight management program. *Nutrition Journal* 6:36.

Malek, M.H., D.P. Nalbone, D.E. Berger, and J.W. Coburn. 2002. Importance of health science education for personal fitness trainers. *Journal of Strength and Conditioning Research/National Strength & Conditioning Association* 16 (1):19–24.

Malek, M.H. and K.T. Coburn. 2008. *The Level of Exercise Science Knowledge Among Personal Fitness Trainers A Guideline*. National Strength and Conditioning Association Hot Topic. www.nsca-lift.org.

Racette, S.B., D.A. Schoeller, R.F. Kushner, K.M. Neil, and K. Herling-Iaffaldano. 1995. Effects of aerobic exercise and dietary carbohydrate on energy expenditure and body composition during weight reduction in obese women. *The American Journal of Clinical Nutrition* 61 (3):486–494.

Ruaño, G., A. Windemuth, M. Kocherla, T. Holford, M.L. Fernandez, C.E. Forsythe, R.J. Wood, W.J. Kraemer, and J.S. Volek. 2006. Physiogenomic analysis of weight loss induced by dietary carbohydrate restriction. *Nutrition & Metabolism* 3:20.

Ryan, A.S., R.E. Pratley, D. Elahi, and A.P. Goldberg. 1995. Resistive training increases fat-free mass and maintains RMR despite weight loss in postmenopausal women. *Journal of Applied Physiology* 79 (3):818–823.

Saris, W.H., A. Astrup, A.M. Prentice, H.J. Zunft, X. Formiguera, W.P. Verboeket-van de Venne et al. 2002. Randomized controlled trial of changes in dietary carbohydrate/fat ratio and simple vs complex carbohydrates on body weight and blood lipids: The CARMEN study. The Carbohydrate Ratio Management in European National Diets. *International Journal of Obesity and Related Metabolic Disorders: Journal of the International Association for the Study of Obesity*. 24 (10):1310–1318. http://www.ncbi.nlm.nih.gov/pubmed/11093293

Stewart, T.M., A.R. Bachand, H. Han, D.H. Ryan, G.A. Bray, and D.A. Williamson. 2011. Body image changes associated with participation in an intensive lifestyle weight loss intervention. *Obesity* 19 (6):1290–1295.

van Aggel-Leijssen, D.P., W.H. Saris, G.B. Hul, and M.A. van Baak. 2001. Short-term effects of weight loss with or without low-intensity exercise training on fat metabolism in obese men. *The American Journal of Clinical Nutrition* 73 (3):523–531.

Volek, J.S., K.D. Ballard, R. Silvestre, D.A. Judelson, E.E. Quann, C.E. Forsythe, M.L. Fernandez, and W.J. Kraemer. 2009a. Effects of dietary carbohydrate restriction versus low-fat diet on flow-mediated dilation. *Metabolism: Clinical and Experimental* 58 (12):1769–1777.

Volek, J.S., A.L. Gómez, D.M. Love, A.M. Weyers, R. Hesslink, J.A. Wise, and W.J. Kraemer. 2002. Effects of an 8-week weight-loss program on cardiovascular disease risk factors and regional body composition. *European Journal of Clinical Nutrition* 56 (7):585–592.

Volek, J.S., S.D. Phinney, C.E. Forsythe, E.E. Quann, R.J. Wood, M.J. Puglisi, W.J. Kraemer, D.M. Bibus, M.L. Fernandez, and R.D. Feinman. 2009b. Carbohydrate restriction has a more favorable impact on the metabolic syndrome than a low fat diet. *Lipids* 44 (4):297–309.

Volek, J., M. Sharman, A. Gomez, D. Judelson, M. Rubin, G. Watson, B. Sokmen, R. Silvestre, D. French, and W. Kraemer. 2004. Comparison of energy-restricted very low-carbohydrate and low-fat diets on weight loss and body composition in overweight men and women. *Nutrition and Metabolism (London)* 1 (1):13.

Volek, J.S., M.J. Sharman, D.M. Love, N.G. Avery, A.L. Gomez, T.P. Scheett, and W.J. Kraemer. 2002. Body composition and hormonal responses to a carbohydrate-restricted diet. *Metabolism* 51 (7):864–870.

Wadden, T.A., R.A. Vogt, R.E. Andersen, S.J. Bartlett, G.D. Foster, R.H. Kuehnel et al. 1997. Exercise in the treatment of obesity: Effects of four interventions on body composition, resting energy expenditure, appetite, and mood. *Journal of Consulting and Clinical Psychology* 65 (2):269–277. http://www.ncbi.nlm.nih.gov/pubmed/9086690

Westman, E.C., J. Mavropoulos, W.S. Yancy, and J.S. Volek. 2003. A review of low-carbohydrate ketogenic diets. *Current Atherosclerosis Reports* 5 (6):476–483.

Wing, R.R. 2010. Long-term effects of a lifestyle intervention on weight and cardiovascular risk factors in individuals with type 2 diabetes mellitus: Four-year results of the look AHEAD trial. *Archives of Internal Medicine* 170 (17):1566–1575.

26 Role of Exercise in Weight Management and Other Health Benefits

Emphasis on Pedometer-Based Program

Harry G. Preuss, MD, MACN, CNS,
Debasis Bagchi, PhD, MACN, CNS, MAIChE,
and Gilbert R. Kaats, PhD, FACN

CONTENTS

INTRODUCTION

Obesity is strongly associated with a broad spectrum of degenerative diseases. Unfortunately, there is no single magic bullet as reported by many that can control and regulate obesity. Accordingly, numerous experts favor a proper health regimen with differing elements to accomplish success. Physical exercise is an important component in such a regimen that can play a major role to keep us healthy and fit, and walking is an important part of most individuals' exercise program. Accordingly, pedometers are a unique and convenient feature that record on a daily basis step counts to estimate a major portion of our regular physical activity level.

EXERCISE

It is generally accepted by most individuals that proper exercise programs are effective interventions that make for an enhanced healthful existence with the passing of time. In addition to maintaining optimal body composition by lessening fat accumulation, building muscle, strengthening bone, and ameliorating overall functional decline, appropriate exercise may also provide a number of psychological benefits and preserve cognitive function [1]. It is virtually impossible to listen to advertisements concerning weight control programs and products without the inclusion of a requirement to "exercise regularly." A multitude of studies have substantiated the weight control and health benefits of regular exercise [2,3], and, accordingly, exercise has become a consistent component of most commercial weight control programs.

The American College of Sports Medicine in their position stand regarding exercise and physical activity in older adults believes "the benefits associated with regular exercise and physical activity contribute to a more healthy, independent lifestyle, greatly improving the functional capacity and quality of life in this population" [4]. A majority of investigators would agree that the rate of decline in aerobic capacity is higher in sedentary rather than active adults [1,5–7]. Kasch et al. [7] reported that an exercising adult loses on an average 0.25 mL/kg/min of aerobic capacity each year in contrast to a 0.71 mL/kg/min loss per year for a nonexerciser. Spirudo and Cronin [8] reported that most results consistently show that long-term physical activity postpones disability and dependent living.

In addition to weight loss, perhaps nowhere are the benefits of planned exercise regimens more important than in prevention of and rehabilitation from cardiovascular disease. Miller et al. [9] reinforced the concept that physically inactive lifestyle is associated with twice the risk of developing cardiovascular disease and, unfortunately, that more than half of the adult population is sedentary or inactive. They concluded that there is a definite need for the development of approaches to increase physical activity over the life span.

The major resistances to (or rationalizations against) exercise are a lack of time, motivation, physical difficulties, and a deficiency of financial resources [10–12]. Although the medical community has long encouraged physicians to promote exercise to their patients, few actually do [12,13]—citing lack of time, inadequate reimbursement, unfamiliarity with appropriate techniques, and repeated observations of patient noncompliance [14,15]. It is also difficult for physicians to ascertain the veracity of patient self-reports since it is generally believed that patients typically overestimate the amount of time spent exercising.

In summing up their excellent review of physical activity on health status in older adults, Buchner and colleagues [1] made some most interesting observations. "Future research… should address issues in recruiting functionally impaired older adults into exercise studies, issues in promoting long-term adherence to exercise, and whether the currently low rate of exercise-related injuries in supervised classes can be sustained in more cost-effective interventions that require less supervision."

WALKING: A GOOD EXERCISE

Considering the statement mentioned earlier [1], walking would seem to be ideal to initiate an exercise or activity program for younger, middle-aged, and older men and women whether healthy or infirmed and to be the solid foundation for a wider program [16]. It is generally accepted that walking is the most popular and prevalent form of physical activity [17,18] with low injury and relatively high adherence rates [19]. Interestingly, walking has been found to result in better adherence than more severe forms of exercise [20].

How do we get adults, both young and old, to undertake such a program? A good answer is to start out easy. As the Mayo Clinic staff reported over the Internet [21], "Walking is a gentle, low-impact exercise that can ease you into a higher level of fitness and health. Walking is a form of exercise accessible to just about everybody. It's safe, simple, and doesn't require practice. And the health benefits are many." In January 2008, the Mayo Clinic Health Letter's lead article entitled, "Moderate exercise: A little goes a long way" pointed out that moderately strenuous exercise, as little as 30 min a day, can lead to enormous benefits in weight management, overall physical health, elevation of mood, and even the ability to live longer and healthier [22]. The benefits in overall health would include lowering low-density lipoprotein (LDL) cholesterol and raising high-density lipoprotein (HDL) cholesterol, lowering blood pressure, reducing weight and the risk for diabetes, and giving one a psychological boost from a health-providing accomplishment (Table 26.1). Figure 26.1 provides a summary in graphic form of the research benefits of increasing daily activity levels to the equivalent of 3000–6000 steps per day using the data reported from the Mayo Clinic [22].

Brief advice, pedometers, computer-based programs, mobile phones, telecommunications, and different types of marketing have been used to encourage more participation in a walking program

---

TABLE 26.1

Benefits of Walking

Walking, like other exercise, can help you achieve a number
of important health benefits. Walking can help

  Improve cholesterol readings

  Improve coronary artery disease

  Lower blood pressure

  Enhance insulin sensitivity

  Reduce incidence of stroke

  Manage body weight

  Improve mood and maintain mental well-being

  Lessen depression

  Strengthen bone

  Increase energy and stamina

The Mayo Clinic has reviewed studies on the relationship between increasing and maintaining daily step
totals and the risks of disease and unhealthy conditions, e.g., blood pressure. The chart below
summarizes their findings on the effects of increasing daily step totals by 3000 and 6000.

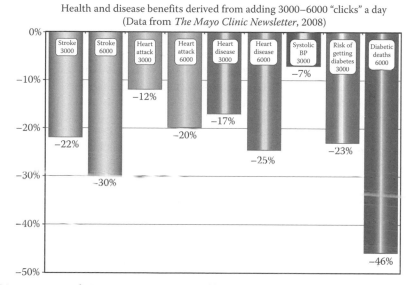

Health and disease benefits derived from adding 3000–6000 "clicks" a day
(Data from *The Mayo Clinic Newsletter*, 2008)

Using an average of 100 steps a minute means adding 30 or 60 min of activity, not "exercise", throughout
the waking hours. But even a small amount helps so another way of looking at these results is to
approximate how many clicks are needed to reduce the risk of each of these conditions by 1%. It takes
an increase of:

  200 steps a day to reduce the risk of having a stroke by 1%

  300 steps a day to reduce the risk of having a heart attack by 1%

  176 steps a day to reduce the risk of having heart disease by 1%

  857 steps a day to reduce systolic blood pressure by 1%

  130 steps a day to reduce the risk of getting diabetes by 1%

  130 steps a day for diabetics to reduce their risk of dying by 1%

The 200 steps a day needed to reduce the risk of strokes by 1% can be achieved in only
two minutes and the 1% for heart disease can be achieved in less than two minutes a day.
So get clicking! Moderate exercise: A little goes a long way.
Mayo Clinic Health Letter. 2008;12(1):1–2.

FIGURE 26.1   Mayo Clinic reports effects of increasing daily step totals and disease risks.

with some success [16,23–26]. Ogilvie et al. [23] report that the most successful interventions could increase walking among appropriate participants as much as an hour a week over the short term. This is important because a recent thorough review indicated that increasing walking levels produced a dose-dependent decrease in some risk factors for cardiovascular disease [27]. Walking duration, distance, frequency, and pace are all important considerations in developing the proper individual regimen. Many believe that if more adults began a regular walking program, heart disease costs could be lowered by millions or even billions of dollars [28–30].

Morris and Hardman [18] echoed many of the benefits mentioned earlier to walking. They describe walking as gentle start up to get people exercising that returns "a bonus of independence and social well-being." Walking can achieve favorable body composition goals listed earlier: lose fat, gain muscle, and strengthen bone. The most common advice is to recommend approximately 30 min of activity most days of the week. Taking 10,000 steps per day is approximately equivalent to 30 min of moderate exercise [31]. Unfortunately, few can attain this goal on their own and need some additional support.

The association between more extensive walking duration and intensity and reduced cardiovascular risk factors is equivalent for all ages and both genders [16].

USE OF PEDOMETERS TO PROMOTE WALKING

Pedometers are motivational tools that allow instant reporting of steps taken by those individuals who have set up goals for themselves. Wearing a pedometer and recording daily step totals capitalizes on a well-established behavior modification principle: "What gets measured, gets managed; what gets measured and tracked, gets managed better; and what gets measured, tracked and fedback, gets managed even better." Many reviews and investigations have emphasized the effectiveness of pedometers to increase walking, i.e., increase step counts. The general consensus is that pedometer-based behavioral modification programs, along with other measures like telephone support, are important means to cause behavioral changes in all ages, both genders, and in the healthy and those with certain medical maladies [32–39].

Wearing a pedometer during waking hours and tracking daily step totals goes beyond just walking. It is responsive to even small increases in walking and provides the user with a constant and objective stream of reality throughout the day. For the physician, encouraging patients to wear a pedometer throughout their waking hours and track their daily step-totals is a specific, practical, non-time-consuming recommendation. Compliance can easily be tracked by simply asking the patient to report their daily activity levels and enter the totals in the patient's medical records. The behavior change is even more likely if the physician or health-care provider uses a pedometer himself/herself and sets up a program to provide the patient feedback and encouragement [39].

Perhaps the most comprehensive review on the subject appeared in the Journal of the American Medical Association (JAMA) in 2007 [40]. In order to evaluate the association of pedometer use with activity and health in adults, the investigators reported results from 26 studies examining 2767 participants. These studies reported the use of pedometer and changes in steps per day. Results were very encouraging. The participants, 85% women, had an average age of 49 years. The most important finding was that the use of the pedometer was associated with an increase of more than 2000 steps per day over baseline. Physical activity increased, body mass index (BMI) decreased by 0.38, and systolic blood pressure was lowered by an average of 3.8 mm Hg. A final comment in this paper stated, "Our results suggest that the use of these small, relatively inexpensive devices is associated with significant increases in physical activity and improvements in some key health outcomes, at least in the short term. The extent to which these results are durable over the long term is unknown."

Shortly after the Stanford researchers published their review, researchers at the University of Michigan published their own in the Annals of Family Medicine [41]. The reviewers analyzed 9 different studies with a total of 307 participants from which they concluded that people who participate in a pedometer-based walking program could be expected to lose a modest amount of weight even without changing diet. The investigators surmised that the longer the individual stuck with the program, the more weight was lost. Participants increased their daily activity levels by the equivalent of one mile a day and lost almost 3 lb over 4 weeks to 1 year with a median duration of 16 weeks without changes in diet. The investigators concluded that pedometer-based walking programs resulted in a modest weight loss with a greater weight loss the longer the program.

Kang et al. [42] analyzed a number of "pedometer studies" to determine the effectiveness of pedometers as motivational tools to increase walking. They concluded that the overall data suggest that pedometers have a moderate, positive influence to increase physical activity. The overall mean increase of steps per day exceeded 2000. Importantly, they also concluded, "The evidence suggests that the effects of pedometer use were similar across all age groups and intervention lengths. There were greater effects in females and intervention strategy of 10,000 steps/day as a step goal."

SELECTION OF PEDOMETER

A key component of a pedometer plan is the selection of a reliable, valid, and durable pedometer [43–47]. Inaccurate or flimsy pedometers will quickly discourage users and prove to be just another gimmick that causes frustration, adverse feelings about the instrument, and poor compliance [46]. Accordingly, it is imperative that each individual find the most accurate pedometer for them.

In general, two types of pedometers exist: spring-levered and piezoelectric pedometers. Crouter et al. [48] examined the effects of BMI, waist circumference, and pedometer tilt on the accuracy of each type in 40 participants. The investigators found that the spring-loaded variety tested here was more susceptible to error from pedometer tilt, increased waist circumference, or BMI. Nevertheless, a spring-loaded pedometer, Yamax Digi-Walker SW-200 is considered the "gold-standard" against which other pedometers have been compared by many researchers [43–46,48].

CONCLUSION

A broad spectrum of evidence emphasizes the usefulness of pedometers and their proper application in promoting health benefits. It has been successfully demonstrated by a number of researchers in the field that regular walking and exercise is very important in controlling obesity and a broad spectrum of degenerative diseases. Pedometers provide us reliable estimates concerning our level of daily activities and encourage compliance in a walking program.

REFERENCES

1. Buchner DM: Effects of physical activity on health status in older adults II: Intervention studies. *Annu Rev Publ Health* 13:469–488, 1992.
2. Van Zant RS: Influence of diet and exercise on energy: A review. *Int J Sport Nutr* 2(1):1–19, 1992.
3. Stiegler P and Cunliffe A: The role of diet and exercise for the maintenance of fat-free mass and resting metabolic rate during weight loss. *Sports Med* 36:239–262, 2006.
4. American College of Sports Medicine Position Stand: Exercise and physical activity for older adults. *Med Sci Sports Exerc* 30:992–1008, 1998.
5. Buchner DM and Wagner EH: Preventing frail health. *Clin Geriatr Med* 8(1):1–17, 1992.
6. Dehn MM and Bruce RA: Longitudinal variations in maximal oxygen intake with age and activity. *J Appl Physiol* 33(6):805–807, 1972.
7. Kasch FW, Boyer JL, Van Camp SP, Verity LS, and Wallace JP: The effects of physical activity and inactivity on aerobic power in older men (a longitudinal study). *Phys Sportmed* 18:73–83, 1990.
8. Spirduso WW and Cronin DL: Exercise dose-response effects on quality of life and independent living in older adults. *Med Sci Sports Exerc* 33:S598–S608, 2001.
9. Miller TD, Balady GJ, and Fletcher GF: Exercise and its role in the prevention and rehabilitation of cardiovascular disease. *Ann Behav Med* 19(3):220–229, 1997.
10. Pender NJ and Pender AR: Attitudes, subjective norms, and intentions to engage in health behaviors. *Nurs Res* 35(1):15–18, 1986.

11. Pender NJ: Motivation for physical activity among children and adolescents. *Annu Rev Nurs Res* 16:139–172, 1998.

12. Harris AA, Caspersen CJ, DeFriese GH, and Estes EH Jr.: Physical activity counseling for healthy adults as a primary preventive intervention in the clinical setting. Report for the US preventive services task force. *JAMA* 261:3588–3598, 1989.

13. Chakravarthy MV, Joyner MJ, and Booth FW: An obligation for primary care physicians to prescribe physical activity to sedentary patients to reduce the risk of chronic health conditions. *Mayo Clin Proc* 77:165–173, 2002.

14. Abramson S, Stein J, Schaufele M, Frates E, and Rogan S: Personal exercise habits and counseling practices of primary care physicians: A national survey. *Clin J Sport Med* 10:40–48, 2000.

15. Meriwether RA, Lee JA, LaFleur AS, and Wiseman P: Physical activity counseling. *Am Fam Phys* 77:1129–1136, 2008.

16. Murtagh EM, Murphy MH, and Boone-Heinonen J: Walking: The first steps in cardiovascular disease prevention. *Curr Opinion Cardiol* 25(5):490–496, 2010.

17. Hatziendreu EI, Koplan JP, Weinstein MC, Caspersen CJ, and Werner KE: A cost-effectiveness analysis of exercise as a health promotion activity. *Am J Public Health* 78:1417–1421, 1988.

18. Morris JN and Hardman AE: Walking to health. *Sports Med* 23:306–332, 1997.

19. Pollock ML, Carroll JF, Graves JE, Leggett SH, Braith RW, Limacher M et al.: Injuries and adherence to walk/jog and resistance training programs in the elderly. *Med Sci Sports Exerc* 23(10):1194–1200, 1991.

20. Dishman RK, Ickes W, and Morgan WP: Self-motivation and adherence to habitual physical activity. *J Appl Soc Psychol* 10:115–132, 1980.

21. http://www.mayoclinic.com/health/walking/HQ01612 (accessed September 2, 2011).

22. Moderate exercise: A little goes a long way. *Mayo Clinic Health Letter* 12(1):1–2, 2008.

23. Ogilvie D, Foster CE, Rothnie H, Cavill N, Hamilton V, Fitzsimons CF, and Mutrie N: Scottish Physical Activity Research Collaboration: Interventions to promote walking: Systemic review. *BMJ* 334:1204–1207, 2007.

24. Eyler AA, Brownson RC, Bacak SJ, and Housemann RA: The epidemiology of walking for physical activity in the United States. *Med Sci Sports Exerc* 35(9):1529–1536, 2003.

25. Simpson ME, Serdula M, Galuska DA, Gillespie C, Donehoo R, Macera C, and Mack K: Walking trends among US adults: The behavioral risk factor surveillance system, 1987–2000. *Am J Prev Med* 25(2):95–100, 2003.

26. Williams DM, Matthews CE, Ruff C, Napolitano MA, and Marcus BH: Interventions to increase walking behavior. *Med Sci Sports Exerc* 40:567–573, 2008.

27. Boone-Heinonen J, Evenson KR, Taber DR, and Gordon-Larsen P: Walking for prevention of cardiovascular disease in men and women: A systematic review of observational studies. *Obes Rev* 10:204–217, 2009.

28. Jones TF and Eaton CB: Cost benefit analysis of walking to prevent coronary heart disease. *Arch Fam Med* 3(8):703–710, 1994.

29. Tsuji I, Takahashi K, Nishino Y, Ohkubo T, Kuriyama S, Watanabe Y et al.: Impact of walking upon medical care expenditure in Japan: The Ohsaki cohort study. *Int J Epidemiol* 32:809–814, 2003.

30. Zheng H, Ehrlich F, and Amin J: Economic evaluation of the direct healthcare cost savings resulting form the use of walking interventions to prevent coronary heart disease in Australia. *Int J Health Carte Finance Econ* 10(2):187–201, 2010.

31. Navratilova M, http://www.aarp.org/health/fitness/info-09-2010/martina_easiest_exercise_walking.html (visited on September 29, 2011).

32. Croteau KA: Strategies used to increase lifestyle physical activity in a pedometer-based intervention. *J Allied Health* 33:278–281, 2004.

33. Croteau KA, Richeson NE, Farmer BC, and Jones DB: Effect of a pedometer-based intervention on daily step counts of community-dwelling older adults. *Res Q Exerc Sport* 78:401–406, 2007.

34. Tudore-Locke C and Lutes L: Why do pedometers work? A reflection upon the factors related to successfully increasing physical activity. *Sport Med* 39(12):981–993, 2009.

35. Beets MW, Bornstein D, Beighle A, Cardinal BJ, and Morgan CE: Pedometer: Measured physical activity patterns of youth: A 13-country review. *Am J Prev Med* 38:208–216, 2010.

36. Snyder A, Colvin B, and Gammack JK: Pedometer use increases daily steps and functional status in older adults. *J Am Med Dir Assoc* 2010 October 7. [Epub ahead of print].

37. Sugden JA, Sniehottq FE, Donnan PT, Boyle P, Johnston DW, and McMurdo ME: The feasibility of using pedometers and brief advice to increase activity in sedentary older women: A pilot study. *BMC Heath Serv Res* 8:169, 2008, doi: 10.1186/1472-6963-8-169.

38. De Greef KP, Deforche BI, Ruige JB, Bouckaert JJ, Tudor-Locke CE, Kaufman J-M, and De Bourdeaudhuij LM: The effects of a pedometer-based behavioral modification program with telephone support on physical activity and sedentary behavior in type 2 diabetic patients. *Patient Ed and Counsel* 84:275–279, 2011.

39. Trinh L, Wilson R, MacLeod Williams H, Sum AJ, and Naylor P-J: Physicians promoting physical activity using pedometers and community partnerships: A real world trial. *Br J Sports Med*, 2011 January 31 [Epub ahead of print].

40. Bravata DM, Smith-Spangler C, Sundaram V, Gienger AL, Lin N, Lewis R, Stave CD, Olkin I, and Sirard JR: Using pedometers to increase physical activity and improve health: A systematic review. *JAMA* 298(19):2296–2304, 2007.

41. Richardson CR, Newton TL, Abraham JJ, Sen A, Jimbo M, and Swartz AM: A meta-analysis of pedometer-based walking intervention and weight loss. *Ann Fam Med* 6(1):69–77, 2008.

42. Kang M, Marshall SJ, Barreira TV, and Lee J-O: Effect of pedometer-based physical activity interventions: A meta-analysis. *Res Q Exerc Sport* 80(3):648–655, 2009.

43. Preuss HG and Gottlieb B: Step right up to weight control: Use a pedometer to walk more- and keep off weight you've lost. In: *The Natural Fat Loss Pharmacy*. Broadway Books, New York, pp. 246–260, 2007.

44. Kaats GR: The clicker: What gets measured and tracked, gets managed. In: *Restructuring Body Composition: How the Kind, Not the Amount, of Weight Loss Defines a Pathway to Optimal Health*. Taylor Publishing, Dallas, TX, pp. 223–249, 2008.

45. Kaats GR, Preuss HG, Keith SC, and Keith PL: The use of pedometers in medical and alternative care treatment plans. *The Original Internist* 14:187–190, 2008.

46. Clemes SA, O'Connell S, Rogan LM, and Griffiths PL: Evaluation of a commercially available pedometer used to promote physical activity as part of a national programme. *Br J Sports Med* 44(16):1178–1183, 2010.

47. Tudor-Locke C, Sisson SB, Lee SM, Craig CL, Plotnikoff C, and Bauman A: Evaluation of quality of commercial pedometers. *Can J Public Health* 97(Suppl 1): S10–5, S10–6, 2006.

48. Schneider PL, Crouter SE, and Bassett DR Jr.: Pedometer measures of free-living physical activity: Comparison of 13 models. *Med Sci Sports Exerc* 36:331–335, 2004.

TABLE 27.1

Common Hormone or Peptide Signals That Control Satiety and Hunger

Satiety Signals	Stimulus	Site of Production	Effects
CCK	Fat or protein	Duodenum	Decreases food intake by controlling the meal size
Glucagon-like-peptide 1 (GLP-1)	Carbohydrate or protein	Ileum	Decreases food intake, affects mobility of nutrients from stomach to intestine, and stimulates insulin secretion
Peptide YY (PYY)	Meal	Gut endocrine cells	Decreases food intake and inhibits gut mobility and gastric emptying
Ghrelin	Fasting	Gut	Increases food intake
Leptin	—	Adipocytes	Decreases food intake only during energy imbalance

HUNGER, SATIETY, AND FOOD INTAKE

Food consumption in humans is a complex process regulated by a number of factors including environmental cues, sensory stimuli, social pressures, appetite, and feelings of hunger. Physiologically, the regulation of food intake depends on direct feedback signals from the gut and adipose tissue to the hypothalamus in the brain, containing the hunger and satiety centers [11–13]. Food intake is generally in distinct bouts or episodes (i.e., meals and snacks). The meals are eaten until full (satiated) and then the next meal is not eaten for a certain time (satiety). The gastrointestinal tract, in response to meals, generates a variety of biochemical peptide signals, or satiety factors, that accumulate during eating and contribute to meal termination. These signals are transmitted to the central nervous system and are manifested as a behavioral modification of feeding [12–16]. Some peptide signals (anorexigenic signals) decrease food intake as they promote satiety, whereas other peptides signals (orexigenic signals) increase food intake as they induce appetite. Table 27.1 lists various peptide- and hormone-related signals that are generated in the gut and influence feelings of satiety and hunger.

FOOD FACTORS RELATED TO SATIETY AND CALORIE CONTROL

Physical characteristics as well as the macronutrient composition of a meal are important determinants of its satiating effects. Studies have shown that increasing the volume of a food (by adding water or air) can improve satiety and significantly reduce the calorie intake [17,18]. The energy density (ED) of a diet, or calorie value of a food per unit weight or volume, also plays a key role in satiety. Dietary ED depends mainly on the water content of the foods eaten. As a rule, high-ED foods are more palatable but less satiating, whereas low-ED foods are more satiating but less palatable [19,20]. Lowering the ED of a diet may also increase the fiber content of the diet, especially if fiber-rich fruits and vegetables or whole grains are added. Studies have demonstrated that eating low-ED foods (such as fruits, vegetables, and soups) maintains satiety while reducing energy intake and improved weight control [20–22]. Dietary Guidelines for Americans 2010 [23] also concluded that low energy dense eating patterns improve weight loss and weight maintenance and soups, particularly broth- or water-based soup, may lead to decreased calorie intake and body weight over time. Some data suggest that solid foods are more satiating than semisolid or liquid foods, and more viscous liquid foods are more satiating than less viscous liquid foods [24]. The macronutrient composition of foods also appears to be a determinant of satiety [25]. Traditionally, fats are considered to be most satiating; however, fats have the highest ED. In isocaloric preload studies, fat was found to be the least satiating macronutrient [26]. A strong body of evidence suggests that on a relative scale proteins and fiber are most satiating than carbohydrates and fat [27–33]. However, according to Dietary Guidelines 2010, there is strong evidence suggesting that only the total number of calories and not the proportion of macronutrients (protein, fat, and carbohydrate) are related to weight loss [23].

NOVEL SATIETY INGREDIENTS AND FUNCTIONAL FOODS

Several functional food ingredients are metabolically active and help improve satiety. Many of these novel ingredients have been known to function by activating the cholecystokinin (CCK) mechanism. Slendesta® (Kemin Industries, Inc.) is a protein extract from vegetables called "PI2" and is claimed to stimulate CCK [34]. Similarly, Satietrol (PacificHealth Laboratories, Inc.) is a milk-derived peptide (glycomacropeptide) and is claimed to stimulate CCK and thus improve satiety [35]. Satietrol also contains potato and guar fibers, as well as alfalfa, to help maintain the higher levels of CCK longer. Fabuless™ is a novel fat emulsion containing fractionated palm oil and fractionated oat oil in water; it has been shown to have satiating effects via a fat-induced ileal brake mechanism [36]. Gelling fibers, such as alginate and konjac fiber, are known to delay gastric emptying and increase satiety due to their gel-forming ability in the gastrointestinal tract [37,38].

FUNCTIONAL FOODS AFFECTING ENERGY METABOLISM

Many functional foods have been shown to alter energy metabolism or fat partitioning by influencing the substrate utilization or thermogenesis [39–41]. These may not influence the absorption of the nutrients, but they act postabsorptively and increase the oxidative rate:

- *Tea*—Tea is a widely consumed beverage made from the leaves and buds of the plant *Camellia sinensis*. The three types of tea are nonfermented green tea, semifermented oolong tea, and fermented black tea. Tea contains high amounts of antioxidants polyphenols (catechins, theaflavins, and thearubigins) [42]. Green tea and oolong tea are particularly rich in catechins (EGCG) and have been shown to increase fat oxidation and decrease adiposity and body weight in clinical and animal studies [43–45].
- *Medium-chain triglycerides (MCTs)*—MCTs are naturally occurring or commercially prepared dietary fats containing 6- to 12-carbon fatty acid chains. Like long-chain triglycerides (LCTs), MCTs are also digested to their fatty acids (MCFs) and absorbed in the gastrointestinal tract; however, they are not repackaged as MCTs in chylomicrons for transportation through peripheral circulation like the LCTs are. MCFs from MCTs are directly transported via the portal system to the liver for oxidation. MCTs therefore bypass the adipose tissue and do not get deposited into adipose tissue store [46].
- *Diacylglycerols (DAGs)*—DAGs are naturally occurring as minor components (1%–10%) of oils. These are glycerides in which the glycerol molecule is esterified to only two fatty-acid chains. Similar to triacylglycerol (TAG), DAGs are also absorbed in the gastrointestinal tract; however, they are transported via the portal system to the liver for oxidation, and they bypass the adipose tissue. A few human clinical studies have shown that the replacement of TAG by DAG leads to significant weight reduction [47].
- *Conjugated linoleic acid (CLA)*—CLA is a group of naturally occurring *trans*-isomers of linoleic acid. The main dietary sources are dairy products and beef. In animal studies, CLA has been found to reduce body fat, possibly through increased fat oxidation and decreased fat deposition in adipose tissue [40]; however, the human data available to support the efficacy of CLA in weight management are inconsistent [48,49].
- *Capsaicin and capsinoids*—Capsaicin is a major pungent component in capsicum and capsinoids are its nonpungent analogues. Capsaicin and capsinoids have been shown to decrease adiposity by increasing energy metabolism and fat oxidation in human and animal studies [50].

BOTANICALS AND DIETARY SUPPLEMENTS FOR WEIGHT CONTROL

Several dietary supplements and herbal products are currently being promoted for weight management [51–55]. The potential biological mechanisms include increased energy expenditure, increased fat oxidation, decreased fat absorption, and increased satiety (Table 27.2). Concerns have been

TABLE 27.2

List of Commonly Used Dietary Supplements and Herbs and Their Proposed Mechanisms for Weight Control

Dietary Supplements and Herbs	Proposed Mechanism
Ephedra, yerba mate, and caffeine	Increase energy expenditure
Psyllium, guar gum, hoodia, and pinnothin (pine extract)	Increase satiety
Chitosan	Inhibits fat absorption
Green tea and *Garcinia cambogia* (hydroxycitric acid)	Increase fat oxidation
Chromium picolinate and ginseng	Influence carbohydrate metabolism

Sources: Pittler, M.H. and Ernst, E., *Am. J. Clin. Nutr.*, 79, 529, 2004; Heber, D., *Primary Care*, 30(2), 441, 2003; Lenz, T.L. and Hamilton, W.R., *J. Am. Pharm. Assoc.*, 44(1), 59, 2004.

raised regarding the efficacy and safety of herbal products and dietary supplements promoted for weight management. The U.S. Food and Drug Administration (FDA) has taken regulatory actions against a number of dietary supplements. The scientific evidence is insufficient or conflicting, and clinical data are necessary to ensure their safety and efficacy.

CONCLUSION

Obesity has become an important health issue in the recent years. Energy imbalance is an important etiological factor, and dietary and nutritional factors, functional food ingredients, and dietary supplements may help address this issue (Figure 27.1). Readers are advised, however, to be sure of the safety and efficacy of functional food ingredients, herbs, and dietary supplements before using them.

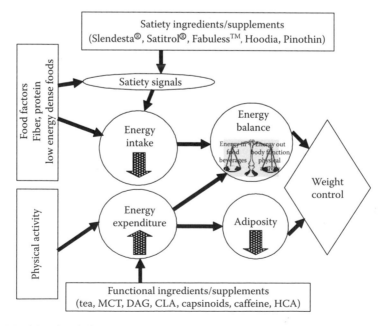

FIGURE 27.1   Nutritional and dietary mechanisms for weight control.

REFERENCES

1. Flegal KM, Carroll MD, Ogden CL, and Curtin LR. Prevalence and trends in obesity among US adults, 1999–2008. *JAMA* 303:235–241, 2010.
2. Ogden CL, Carroll MD, Curtin LR, Lamb MM, and Flegal KM. Prevalence of high body mass index in US children and adolescents, 2007–2008. *JAMA* 303:242–249, 2010.
3. Bary GA. Medical consequences of obesity. *J Clin Endocrinol Metab* 89:2583–2589, 2004.
4. Kopelman PG. Obesity as a medical problem. *Nature* 404:635–643, 2000.
5. Pi-Sunyer FX. The medical risk of obesity. *Postgrad Med* 121:21–33, 2009.
6. Mokdad AH, Marks JS, Stroup DF, and Gerberding JL. Actual causes of death in United States, 2000. *JAMA* 291:1238–1245, 2004.
7. Stein CJ and Colditz GA. The epidemic of obesity. *J Clin Endocrinol Metab* 89:2522–2525, 2004.
8. Speakman JR. Obesity: The integrated roles of environment and genetics. *J Nutr* 134:2090S–2105S, 2004.
9. Storey ML, Forshee RA, Weaver AR, and Sansalone WR. Demographic and lifestyle factors are associated with body mass index among children and adolescents. *Int J Food Sci Nutr* 54:491–503, 2003.
10. FDA. *Calorie Count: Report of the Working Group on Obesity*. US Food and Drug Administration. Washington, DC, 2004.
11. Schwartz MW, Woods SC, Porte Jr. D, Seeley RJ, and Baskin DG. Central nervous system control of food intake. *Nature* 404:661–671, 2000.
12. Woods SC, Seeley RJ, Porte Jr. D, and Schwartz MW. Signals that regulate food intake and energy homeostasis. *Science* 280:1378–1383, 1998.
13. Moran TH and Dailey MJ. Intestinal feedback signaling and satiety. *Physiol Behav* 105(1):77–81. Doi:10.1016/j.physbeh.2011.02.005, 2011.
14. Murphy KG and Bloom SR. Gut hormone in the control of appetite. *Exp Physiol* 89:507–516, 2004.
15. Chaudhri OB, Field BC, and Bloom SR. Gastrointestinal satiety signals. *Int J Obes (Lond)* 32:S28–S31, 2008.
16. Woods SC. Gastrointestinal satiety signals. 1. An overview of gastrointestinal signals that influence food intake. *Am J Gastrointest Liver Physiol* 286:G7–G13, 2004.
17. Rolls BJ, Bell EA, and Waugh BA. Increasing the volume of a food by incorporating air affects satiety in men. *Am J Clin Nutr* 72:361–368, 2000.
18. Rolls B. *The Volumetrics Eating Plan*, HarperCollins Publishers, New York, 2005.
19. Drewnowski A, Almiron-Roig E, Marmonier C, and Lluch A. Dietary energy density and body weight: Is there a relationship? *Nutr Rev* 62:403–413, 2004.
20. Rolls BJ. The relationship between dietary energy density and energy intake. *Physiol Behav* 97(5):609–615, 2009.
21. Savage JS, Marini M, and Birch LL. Dietary energy density predicts women's weight change over 6 y. *Am J Clin Nutr* 88(3):677–684, 2008.
22. Ledikwe JH, Rolls BJ, Smiciklas-Wright H, Mitchell DC, Ard JD, Champagne C, Karanja N, Lin P-H, Stevens VJ, and Appel LJ. Reductions in dietary energy density are associated with weight loss in overweight and obese participants in the PREMIER trial. *Am J Clin Nutr* 85:1212–1221, 2007.
23. USDA. *Dietary Guidelines for Americans 2010*, U.S. Department of Agriculture, Washington, DC, 2010.
24. Hulshof T, DeGraaf C, and Weststrate JA. The effects of preloads varying in physical state and fat content on satiety and energy intake. *Appetite* 21(3):273–286, 1993.
25. Kundrat S. Satiety: Why we feel full. *Inform* 17:200–202, 2006.
26. Rolls BJ. Carbohydrates, fats, and satiety. *Am J Clin Nutr* 61(Suppl 4):960S–967S, 1995.
27. Slavin J and Green H. Dietary fibre and satiety. *Nutr Bull* 32(Suppl 1):32–42, 2007.
28. Blundell JE and MacDiarmid JI. Fat as a risk factor for over consumption: Satiation, satiety and patterns of eating. *J Am Diet Assoc* 97(Suppl 7):S63–S69, 1997.
29. Howarth NC, Saltzman E, and Roberts SB. Dietary fiber and weight regulation. *Nutr Rev* 59(5):129–139, 2001.
30. Anderson GH and Moore SE. Dietary proteins in the regulation of food intake and body weight in humans. *J Nutr* 134:974S–979S, 2004.
31. Halton TL and Hu FB. The effects of high protein diets on thermogenesis, satiety and weight loss: A critical review. *J Am Coll Nutr* 23(5):373–385, 2004.
32. Paddon-Jones D, Westman E, Mattes RD, Wolfe RR, Astrup A, and Westerterp-Plantenga M. Protein, weight management, and satiety. *Am J Clin Nutr* 87:1558S–1561S, 2008.
33. Astrup A, Kristensen M, Gregersen NT, Belza A, Lorenzen JK, Due A, and Larsen TM. Can bioactive foods affect obesity? *Ann N Y Acad Sci* 1190:25–41, 2010.

34. Slendesta®: Feel nothing but satisfied. Kemin Industries, Inc., http://www.kemin.com/nutraceuticals/slendesta (accessed 2005).

35. Satrietrol®: The appetite control protein. Pacific Health Laboratories Inc., http://www.satietrol.com/pages/appetite_control.html (accessed 2005).

36. Burns AA, Livingstone MB, Welch RW, Dunne A, and Rowland IR. Dose-response effects of a novel fat emulsion (Olibra) on energy and macronutrient intakes up to 36 h post-consumption. *Eur J Clin Nutr* 56(4):368–377, 2002.

37. European Food Safety Authority, Scientific opinion on the substantiation of health claims related to konjac mannan (glucomannan) and reduction of body weight. *EFSA J* 8(10):1798, 2010.

38. Peters HP, Koppert RJ, Boers HM, Ström A, Melnikov SM, Haddeman E, Schuring EA, Mela DJ, and Wiseman SA. Dose-dependent suppression of hunger by a specific alginate in a low-viscosity drink formulation. *Obesity (Silver Spring)* 19(6):1171–1176. Doi:10.1038/oby,2011.63, 2011.

39. St.-Onge MP. Dietary fats, teas, dairy, and nuts: Potential functional foods for weight control? *Am J Clin Nutr* 81:7–15, 2005.

40. Kovacs EM and Mela DJ. Metabolically active functional food ingredients for weight control. *Obes Rev* 7(1):59–78, 2006.

41. Hursel R and Westerterp-Plantenga MS. Thermogenic ingredients and body weight regulation. *Int J Obes (Lond)* 34(4):659–669, 2010.

42. McKay DL and Blumberg JB. The role of tea in human health: An update. *J Am Coll Nutr* 21(1):1–13, 2002.

43. Rumpler W, Seale J, Clevidenc B, Judd J, Wiley E et al. Oolong tea increases metabolic rate and fat oxidation in men. *J Nutr* 131:2848–2852, 2001.

44. Westerterp-Plantenga MS. Green tea catechins, caffeine and body-weight regulation. *Physiol Behav* 100:42–46, 2010.

45. Rains TM, Agarwal S, and Maki K. Antiobesity effects of green tea catechins: A mechanistic review. *J Nutr Biochem* 22(1):1–7, 2011.

46. St.-Onge MP, Ross R, Parsons WD, and Jones PJ. Medium-chain triglycerides increase energy expenditure and decrease adiposity in overweight men. *Obes Res* 11:395–402, 2003.

47. Katsuragi Y, Yasukawa T, Matsuo N, Flickinger BD, Tokimitsu I, and Matlock MG, (Eds.). *Diacylglycerol Oil*, AOCS Press, Champaign, IL, 2004.

48. Larsen TM, Toubro S, and Astrup A. Efficacy and safety of dietary supplements containing CLA for the treatment of obesity: Evidence from animal and human studies. *J Lipid Res* 44:2234–2241, 2003.

49. Kennedy A, Martinez K, Schmidt S, Mandrup S, LaPoint K, and McIntosh M. Antiobesity mechanisms of action of conjugated linoleic acid. *J Nutr Biochem* 21(3):171–179, 2010.

50. Josse AR, Sherriffs SS, Holwerda AM, Andrews R, Staples AW, and Phillips SM. Effects of capsinoid ingestion on energy expenditure and lipid oxidation at rest and during exercise. *Nutr Metab (Lond)* 7:65, 2010.

51. Pittler MH and Ernst E. Dietary supplements for body weight reduction: A systematic review. *Am J Clin Nutr* 79:529–536, 2004.

52. Heber D. Herbal preparations for obesity: Are they useful? *Primary Care* 30(2):441–463, 2003.

53. Lenz TL and Hamilton WR. Supplemental products used for weight loss. *J Am Pharm Assoc* 44(1):59–67, 2004.

54. Saper RB, Eisenberg DM, and Phillips RS. Common dietary supplements for weight loss. *Am Fam Physician* 70:1731–1738, 2004.

55. Onakpoya IJ, Wider B, Pittler MH, and Ernst E. Food supplements for body weight reduction: A systematic review of systematic reviews. *Obesity (Silver Spring)* 19(2):239–244, 2011.

28 Gender Effects on Adiposity

Sanja Cvitkusic, BS, David J. Baer, MS, PhD,
and Gabriel Keith Harris, MS, PhD

CONTENTS

INTRODUCTION

During the late nineteenth and throughout the twentieth century, numerous experiments were conducted to determine the effects of diet on human health. Notable examples include the work of Goldberg, who studied the effects of diet on pellagra in prisoners, and of Keys, who examined the effects of starvation and refeeding on conscientious objectors during the Second World War.[1,2] Without delving into the ethical dilemmas associated with those studies, one thing is clear: the majority of these early studies were conducted on young or middle-aged men, but the results were often extrapolated to men and women, without respect to factors such as age, ethnicity, activity level, and health status. Now, at the beginning of the twenty-first century, it is becoming increasingly apparent that men and women differ considerably in their response to diet, physical activity, and other factors that may affect changes in body fat.

The increasing prevalence of obesity throughout the world is often referred to as an "obesity epidemic."[3] Studies supporting the concept of an "obesity epidemic" include the 1999–2000 National Health and Nutrition Examination Survey (NHANES), which reported that an estimated 30.5% of U.S. citizens were obese as compared to 22.9% from the 1988–1994 survey.[4] Obesity was estimated using BMI, or body mass index, a measure of weight in kilograms divided by the square of an individual's height in meters (kg/m^2). Individuals with a BMI greater than 30 are considered obese since weight for a given height is associated with body fat content. This has created controversy, however, given that very muscular individuals may have a BMI of 30 or greater but may still be very lean.

Regardless of the source of the data, it appears that an increasing proportion of the world's population is now either overweight or overfat or both. Although the problem of obesity *seems* to be an exceedingly simple one to solve (consume fewer calories and increase physical activity), controlling obesity has proven to be exceedingly difficult. One facet of this problem that has received little attention is the role that gender plays in obesity and fat gain or loss. The purpose of this chapter is to outline the known differences in fat gain, loss, and maintenance between men and women and, perhaps more importantly, highlight how little is known about the subject. To this end, we discuss the reported effects of gender differences on body fat distribution, fat use as an energy source, and exercise-related fat loss. Additionally, we relate the effects of gender differences in adiposity with age, ethnicity, and health status.

FAT DISTRIBUTION

One of the most obvious distinctions between men and women is the difference in body fat percentage and distribution. Across all races and cultures, women have greater adipose stores than men, even after correcting for BMI, and carry on average 1.8 kg more subcutaneous abdominal fat than men for any given waist circumference.[5] The mean percentage of body fat for normal-weight women (BMI 18–25 kg/m^2) is similar to that of men who are classified as obese (BMI ≥30 kg/m^2).[6] Another obvious difference between the sexes is that men tend to store fat in the abdominal region to a greater degree, while women tend to store fat in the gluteal and femoral (thigh) areas. Less obvious is that men have a greater tendency to store visceral (internal, organ-associated) abdominal fat, whereas women tend to store fat in subcutaneous tissues (between skin and muscle).[7,8] This means that for a given waist circumference, men store a higher percentage of visceral fat.[9]

Gender-based differences in fat distribution appear to be due, at least partially, to the tendency to store fat in or recruit stored fat from distinct areas. For example, men tend to recruit more free fatty acids (FFAs) from the thigh region than women during weight loss and exercise. Under the same conditions, total body fat mobilization from upper body stores appears to be similar between genders, although men tend to recruit a larger percentage of fat from subcutaneous tissue.[10] The net result is a protection of subcutaneous lower body fat in women. This effect is clearly evident in male and female bodybuilders, where body fat loss is essential to display maximum muscularity. Male competitors tend to display an equal degree of upper and lower body leanness, while female competitors tend to retain more lower body fat.[11] A study comparing lipolysis (conversion of stored triglycerides to glycerol and fatty acids) rates in the subcutaneous abdominal fat of morbidly obese men and women undergoing bariatric surgery found that lipolysis rates were only elevated in women. This finding may indicate that women have an increased resistance to the accumulation of abdominal fat relative to men, even in cases of extreme obesity.[12] In summary, gender-specific differences in body fat storage and mobilization tend to favor the preservation of lower body and subcutaneous fat in women and of abdominal (and in particular visceral abdominal) fat in men.

METABOLIC RATE

In addition to differences in fat distribution, men and women also differ with respect to basal metabolic rate and the use of macronutrients as energy sources. Gender differences in body fat distribution rise from metabolic and hormonal differences between the sexes, and contribute to differences between women and men in health risks attributable to obesity. The hormones leptin and insulin regulate appetite, reduce food intake, and may play a role in increasing energy metabolism.[13] However, circulating levels of leptin and insulin appear to reflect different fat stores in that leptin concentration affect subcutaneous fat depots, whereas insulin concentrations target visceral fat stores. With gender differences in the proportion of visceral to subcutaneous fat, leptin is generally better correlated with total fat mass in women, while insulin is more highly correlated to total fat mass in men.[13]

Basal metabolic rate is primarily influenced by fat-free mass.[14] Since men tend to possess more muscle mass both in absolute terms and as a percentage of body weight, they also tend to burn more calories at rest than women. Women appear to use stored body fat differently than men, both at rest and during exercise. At rest and in a fed state, women tend to use a smaller percentage of fat as an energy source than men. Conversely, during exercise, women have been reported to use twice as much fat as a fuel source than men.[15,16] In the fasted state, men and women use fat similarly, although women appear to switch more quickly from the use of glucose to fat as an energy source.[17] Since energy burned at rest (basal metabolic rate) represents the majority of total daily energy expenditure in Western societies, the overall effect of these gender differences on metabolic rate and macronutrient usage appears to be a tendency toward body fat conservation in women.[14] With that said, the fact that the "obesity epidemic" is not restricted to women indicates that a great number of both men and women in many countries around the world are consuming an excess amount of energy, not exercising enough, or both.

FOOD INTAKE

In addition to gender differences in the use of stored body fat as an energy source, men and women have also been reported to differ with regard to responses to food consumption in general. Not surprisingly, food intake tends to reduce the use of stored fat as an energy source in both genders. This feeding effect is more pronounced in women than in men, since men continue to use small amounts of stored fat as an energy source even in a fed state. The result of this gender difference is a greater tendency to maintain established fat stores in women.[18] In keeping with previously mentioned differences in body fat distribution, men tend to store a higher percentage of dietary fatty acids in visceral tissue after meals. For nonobese men, their efficiency of FFA storage per gram of fat has been reported to be 30% greater in abdominal subcutaneous fat than in femoral subcutaneous fat.[19] Women tend to store relatively larger percentages of dietary fat in subcutaneous tissues.[10] Healthy-weight women show no difference between the subcutaneous fat and the femoral subcutaneous fat depots, whereas obese women are 40% more efficient in directly storing FFAs in the femoral rather than in the abdominal region.[19] The efficiency of FFA storage increases as a function of leg fat mass in premenopausal women.[20] However, both normal-weight men and women tend to store more meal fatty acids (per gram adipose fat) in abdominal fat than in leg fat.[21] The differences in regional efficiency of direct FFA uptake support gender-related variations in body fat distribution: women tend to store more fat in the lower body and men in the upper body. Looking at total body fat, overconsumption of food appears to favor greater total body fat gains in women, primarily in subcutaneous tissues, and a greater degree of visceral fat gain in men than in women.

With regard to the effects of specific macronutrients on stored body fat, a recent study reported that the ratios of dietary carbohydrate and fat were related to body fat levels in women, but not in men. In women, carbohydrate intake was reported to be negatively associated with body fat percentage, while fat intake was reported to have a positive association with body fat percentage. Additionally, following the consumption of high-fat, high-calorie meals, it was reported that women store an increased proportion of dietary fat in leg fat as compared to men. This is associated with greater activity of lipoprotein lipase, an enzyme responsible for hydrolyzing triglycerides and uptake of FFAs in femoral adipose tissue in women.[22] The direct FFA storage pathway might play a role in favoring lower-body fat accumulation in women.[20]

The reasons for the association between fatty food consumption and higher percent total body fat in women are not entirely clear. One reason suggested for this is the high energy density of fatty foods, making overindulgence a stronger possibility.[23] In a separate study, carbohydrate intake was found to induce higher peak glucose levels and higher insulin responses in women.[24] The significance of this finding with regard to body fat stores is unclear, although one role of insulin is to facilitate fat storage. Although the data are limited, they appear to suggest that gender-specific differences in the body fat storage and utilization is a function not only of total calories consumed but also of macronutrient ratios.

EXERCISE EFFECTS

Traditional wisdom would say that the best way to affect changes in body fat is a combination of calorie control or restriction combined with exercise, regardless of gender. In theory, exercise should generate an energy deficit and result in weight or fat loss, but in fact, the association between physical activity and body fat is not as straightforward as one might expect. For men, increased physical activity does appear to be an effective means of weight loss or weight maintenance.[23,25] Exercise alone seems less effective as a means of fat reduction for women than for men. Multiple studies have examined the role of gender on fat loss in men and women. One study reported no effect of physical activity on body fat percentage in women.[21] A second study found that exercise produced significant fat losses in men, but not women.[26] A third study found that exercise was effective for body fat maintenance, but not fat loss, in women.[27] Interestingly enough, strength training does not seem to change subcutaneous or intermuscular fat, regardless of gender, and although men exhibit a greater muscle hypertrophic (muscle cell enlargement) response to strength training than do women, the difference is small.[28] With regard to weight loss, women may find exercise to be a less effective tool than men because men have less body fat and more muscle mass to help them metabolize fat.[29]

There are at least two proposed mechanisms for the observed lack of effect of exercise on body fat stores in women. The first is a compensatory increase in calorie intake in response to increased energy expenditure in women, but not in men.[30,31] The only study that measured actual food intake did not find any compensation effect in women, however.[23] In this study, total energy expenditure (resting energy expenditure combined with energy expended during physical activity) was positively associated with body fat in women. The same study reported that physical activity was negatively associated with body fat in men only. Taken together, these studies raise several interesting questions. First, if women do not compensate for energy used during exercise, why does it appear to have little to no effect on fat loss? Perhaps it is because voluntary exercise represents a relatively small fraction of total daily energy expenditure relative to basal metabolic rate. Second, why would energy expenditure be positively associated with body fat in women? Is this counterintuitive finding simply reflective of the increased energy expenditure associated with weight gain? Based on the current literature, there are no obvious answers to these questions. Further studies are needed to determine the role of exercise on fat loss in women.

A second proposed mechanism for gender effects on fat use and storage is the differential activation of adrenergic receptors in men versus women. Exercise causes the releases of the catecholamines epinephrine and norepinephrine, which interact with adrenergic receptors. In women, only beta-adrenergic receptors, which promote fat mobilization, are activated. In contrast, both the pro-lipolysis beta receptors and the antilipolysis alpha-adrenergic receptors are activated in men.[16,32] These gender differences appear to be due to the relative amounts of epinephrine and norepinephrine released during exercise. Exercise-induced epinephrine levels are twice as high in men as in women. Epinephrine has a greater affinity for alpha–adrenergic receptors, which inhibit the use of stored fat as an energy source. This difference may be one reason that women, more so than men, use fat as an energy source during exercise. In contrast, men tend to use a higher percentage of stored carbohydrate during exercise.[33] Even if exercise was definitively shown to have a lesser effect on body weight in women versus men, achieving a negative energy balance can still result in body weight or fat loss for both genders.

AGE AND ETHNICITY

Aside from gender, age and ethnicity lead to differences in abdominal shape and fat distribution in men and women. Although differences in adiposity are present at birth, both boys and girls have comparable waist-to-hip ratios (WHRs) before reaching puberty. After puberty, however, women deposit more fat on the hips, which leads to a significant reduction in their WHR.[34] The typical range of the WHR for healthy premenopausal women and healthy adult men lies between 0.67–0.80 and 0.85–0.95, respectively.[34] Women maintain lower WHRs than men throughout their reproductive age, but after menopause, a reduction in estrogen production causes their WHR range to approach that of men.[35] Higher levels of testosterone increase the WHR, while elevated levels of estrogen lower the WHR.[36]

In both men and women, visceral fat relative to total body fat tends to increase with age, but this effect is especially apparent in men.[37,38] A study conducted on healthy Japanese adults confirmed that subcutaneous fat decreases with age in men with BMIs greater than $23.0\,kg/m^2$, but not in women. Even with these age-related changes in abdominal fat distribution, women retained the subcutaneous dominant type of fat distribution up to the age of 70.[39] It is important to note that Asians have more body fat for any given BMI than do Caucasians or individuals of sub-Saharan African descent,[40] with a greater percentage of fat as visceral fat.[41,42] A higher proportion of fat as visceral adipose tissue may pose a significant risk for the metabolic syndrome (insulin resistance, dyslipidemia, and hypertension) in older men and women, even among those of normal weight.[43] Insulin resistance increases with age, most importantly due to the steady increase in bodyweight and the reduction in physical activity.[44] With increasing age, body fat percentage in men tends to increase initially and then level off; this effect is also observed in elderly women, but to a lesser extent than in elderly men. This age-related change is due to an accelerated decrease in lean mass and an initial increase and a later decrease in fat mass.[45] Albeit a weak correlation between total body fat percentage and disability in men and women, it was demonstrated that an increase in total body fat is indicative of greater likelihood of disability, slightly more so in women.[46]

OBESITY AND COMORBIDITIES

Although it is unclear as to why fat distribution varies with gender, gaining an understanding of this occurrence is important, because fat distribution relates to disease risk. Obesity tends to alter ratios of visceral and subcutaneous fat in both men and women. While the amount of visceral fat remains much lower than subcutaneous fat in obese women, the ratio of visceral to subcutaneous fat will be larger compared to that of normal-weight women as the amounts of visceral fat will have increased. Obese men will have simultaneously gained large amounts of visceral fat and subcutaneous fat on their legs so that the overall ratio of visceral to subcutaneous fat is slightly smaller compared to that of healthy-weight males.[6]

Body fat distribution is also an important predictor of metabolic abnormalities in obese humans. The WHR is an indicator of significant risk factors for comorbidities of obesity. In the context of obesity, a predominantly upper body fat distribution, defined as a WHR of >0.85 in women and >0.95 in men, is associated with larger postabsorptive and postprandial (postmeal) plasma FFA concentrations.[18] Circulating FFAs appear to play a significant role in the development of type 2 diabetes and cardiovascular disease.

CONCLUSIONS

It is important to emphasize that the findings presented in this chapter are based on limited data and, as such, require further study. Figure 28.1 provides an overview of the known gender-specific differences in fat utilization under various physical conditions. There are many unanswered questions with regard to the effects of gender on fat metabolism. These include the interaction of gender with long-term fat loss and with weight cycling. The majority of fat/weight-loss studies are short term in nature (less than 1 year in duration). This fact raises the possibility that the health effects observed are a result of the *process* of weight loss and are not reflective of the effects of long-term weight loss.[12] The effects of weight cycling (repeated gain and loss of body weight and or body fat) on body fat percentage are unclear and are complicated by the fact that weight cycling in young men may be related to "making weight" in athletics via heavy exercise and strict diets, while, in women, it is most often a result of repetitive calorie restriction related to self-esteem and body image.[47,48] Some studies have reported a decreased basal metabolic rate across genders as a result of weight cycling, but this result is by no means an established fact. Based on the existing body of literature, the following conclusions may be drawn with regard to differences in body fat changes between men and women:

1. Women have lower basal metabolic rates than men due to a lower fat-free mass.
2. Women preferentially store subcutaneous fat; men preferentially store visceral fat.
3. Visceral fat is more easily gained or lost by men than by women.
4. During fat loss, women preferentially retain lower body fat; men mobilize upper and lower body fat more equally but tend to retain abdominal fat.

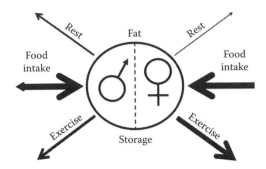

FIGURE 28.1   The gender-specific effects of activity level and food intake on fat storage and utilization. The left of the figure illustrates the predominating effects in men, while the right side shows predominating effects in women under the same conditions. The arrows indicate the movement of fat into or out of storage, while their size approximates the magnitude of the effect.

5. Women more readily use fat as an energy source during exercise; men more readily use fat as an energy source at rest.
6. Exercise appears to be more effective for weight loss and maintenance in men than in women for reasons that are not clear.
7. With increasing age, body fat percentage tends to increase initially and then level off, and this effect is more apparent in men than in women.
8. Obesity tends to alter ratios of visceral and subcutaneous fat in both men and women.

REFERENCES

1. Kalm, L.M. and Semba, R.D. They starved so that others be better fed: Remembering Ancel keys and the Minnesota experiment. *J Nutr*, 135, 1347–1352, 2005.
2. Spies, T.D. Observations on the treatment of pellagra. *J Clin Invest*, 13, 807, 1934.
3. James, P.T. et al. The worldwide obesity epidemic. *Obes Res*, 9(Suppl 4), 228S–233S, 2001.
4. Flegal, K.M. et al. Prevalence and trends in obesity among us adults, 1999–2000. *JAMA*, 288(14), 1723, 2002.
5. Kuk, J.L., Lee, S.J., Heymsfield, S.B., and Ross, R. Waist circumference and abdominal adipose tissue distribution: Influence of age and sex. *Am J Clin Nutr*, 81(6), 1330–1334, 2005.
6. Nielson, S., Guo, Z.K., Johnson, M., Hensrud, D.D., and Jensen, M.D. Splanchic lipolysis in human obesity. *J Clin Invest*, 113, 1582–1588, 2004.
7. Rodrıguez, G., Samper, M.P., Olivares, J.L., Ventura, P., Moreno, L.A., and Perez-Gonzalez, J.M. Skinfold measurements at birth: Sex and anthropometric influence. *Arch Dis Child Fetal Neonatal Ed*, 90(3), F273–F275, 2005.
8. Conway, J.M., Yanovski, S.Z., Avila, N.A., and Hubbard, V.S. Visceral adipose tissue differences in black and white women. *Am J Clin Nutr*, 61, 765–771, 1995.
9. Blaak, E. Gender differences in fat metabolism. *Curr Opin Clin Nutr Metab Care*, 4(6), 499–502, 2001.
10. Power, M.L. and Schulkin, J. Sex differences in fat storage, fat metabolism, and the health risks from obesity: Possible evolutionary origins. *Brit J Nutr*, 99(5), 931–940, 2008.
11. Sandoval, W.M., Heyward, V.H., and Lyons, T.M. Comparison of body composition, exercise and nutritional profiles of female and male body builders at competition. *J Sports Med Phys Fitness*, 29(1), 63–70, 1989.
12. Woods, S.C., Gotoh, K., and Clegg, D.J. Gender differences in the control of energy homeostasis. *Exp Biol Med*, 228(10), 1175–1180, 2003.
13. Lofgren, P., Hoffstedt, J., Ryden, M., Thörne, A., Holm, C., Wahrenberg, H., and Arner, P. Major gender differences in the lipolytic capacity of abdominal subcutaneous fat cells in obesity observed before and after long-term weight reduction. *J Clin Endocrinol Metab*, 87(2), 764–771, 2002.
14. Robertson, M.D., Livesey, G., and Mathers, J.C. Quantitative kinetics of glucose appearance and disposal following a 13C-labelled starch-rich meal: Comparison of male and female subjects. *Br J Nutr*, 87(6), 569–577, 2002.

15. Johnstone, A.M. et al. Factors influencing variation in basal metabolic rate include fat-free mass, fat mass, age, and circulating thyroxine but not sex, circulating leptin, or triiodothyronine. *Am J Clin Nutr*, 82, 941–948, 2005.

16. Mittendorfer, B., Horowitz, J.F., and Klein, S. Effect of gender on lipid kinetics during endurance exercise of moderate intensity in untrained subjects. *Am J Physiol Endocrinol Metab*, 283, E58–E64, 2002.

17. Hellstrom, L., Blaak, E., and Hagstrom-Toft, E. Gender differences in adrenergic regulation of lipid mobilization during exercise. *Int J Sports Med*, 17, 439–447, 1996.

18. Steinberg, H.O., Tarshoby, M., Monestel, R., Hook, G., Cronin, J., Johnson, A., Bayazeed, B., and Baron, A.D. Elevated circulating free fatty acid levels impair endothelium-dependent vasodilation. *J Clin Invest*, 100, 1230–1239, 1997.

19. Votruba, S.B., Mattison, R.S., Dumesic, D.A., Koutsari, C., and Jensen, M.D. Meal fatty acid uptake in visceral fat in women. *Diabetes*, 56(10), 2589–2597, 2007.

20. Mittendorfer, B., Horowitz, J.F., and Klein, S. Gender differences in lipid and glucose kinetics during short-term fasting. *Am J Physiol Endocrinol Metab*, 281, E1333–E1339, 2001.

21. Jensen, M.D. Gender differences in regional fatty acid metabolism before and after meal ingestion. *J Clin Invest*, 96, 2297–2303, 1995.

22. Koutsari, C., Dumesic, D.A., Patterson, B.W., Votruba, S.B., and Jensen, M.D. Plasma free fatty acid storage in subcutaneous and visceral adipose tissue in postabsorptive women. *Diabetes*, 57(5), 1186–1194, 2008.

23. Santosa, S. and Jensen, M.D. Why are we shaped differently, and why does it matter? *Am J Physiol Endocrinol Metab*, 295(3), E531–E535, 2008.

24. Paul, D.R., Novotny, J.A., and Rumpler, W.V. Effects of the interaction of sex and food intake on the relation between energy expenditure and body composition. *Am J Clin Nutr*, 79(3), 385–389, 2004.

25. Westerterp, K.R. and Goran, M.I. Relationship between physical activity related energy expenditure and body composition: A gender difference. *Int J Obes Relat Metab Disord*, 21(3), 184–188, 1997.

26. Westerterp, K.R. et al. Long-term effect of physical activity on energy balance and body composition. *Br J Nutr*, 68, 21–30, 1992.

27. Donnelly, J.E. et al. Effects of a 16-month randomized controlled exercise trial on body weight and composition in young, overweight men and women: The midwest exercise trial. *Arch Intern Med*, 163(11), 1343, 2003.

28. Donnelly, J.E. and Smith, B.K. Is exercise effective for weight loss with ad libitum diet? Energy balance, compensation, and gender differences. *Exerc Sport Sci Rev*, 33, 169–174, 2005.

29. Stubbs, R.J. et al. The effect of graded levels of exercise on energy intake and balance in free-living women. *Int J Obes Relat Metab Disord*, 26(6), 866–869, 2002.

30. Stubbs, R.J. et al. The effect of graded levels of exercise on energy intake and balance in free-living men, consuming their normal diet. *Eur J Clin Nutr*, 56, 129–140, 2002.

31. Lafontan, M., Berlan, M., and Villeneuve, A. Preponderance of alpha 2-over beta 1-adrenergic receptor sites in human fat cells is not predictive of the lipolytic effect of physiological catecholamines. *J Lipid Res*, 24(4), 429–440, 1983.

32. Bouchard, C., Despres, J.P., and Mauriege, P. Genetic and nongenetic determinants of regional fat distribution. *Endocr Rev*, 14(1), 72–93, 1993.

33. Marti, B., Tuomilehto, J., Soloman, V., Kartovaara, L., Korhonen, H.J., and Pietinen, P. Body fat distribution in the Finish population: Environmental determinants and predictive power for cardiovascular risk factor levels. *J Epidemiol Commun Health*, 45, 131–137, 1991.

34. Kirschner, M.A. and Samojlik, E. Sex hormone metabolism in upper and lower body obesity. *Int J Obes*, 15(Suppl 2), 101–108, 1991.

35. Singh, D. Shape and significance of feminine beauty: An evolutionary perspective. *Sex Roles*, 64, 723–731, 2011.

36. Kotani, K. et al. Sexual dimorphism of age-related changes in whole-body fat distribution in the obese. *Int J Obes Relat Metab Disord*, 18, 207–212, 1994.

37. Sugihara, M., Oka, R., Sakurai, M., Nakamura, K., Moriuchi, T., Miyamoto, S., Takeda, Y., Yagi, K., and Yamagishi, M. Age-related changes in abdominal fat distribution in Japanese adults in the general population. *Intern Med*, 50(7), 679–685, 2011.

38. Deurenberg, P., Deurenberg-Yap, M., and Guricci, S. Asians are different from Caucasians and from each other in their body mass index/body fat percent relationship. *Obes Rev*, 3, 141–146, 2002.

39. Park, Y.-W., Allison, D.B., Heymsfield, S.B., and Gallagher, D. Larger amounts of visceral adipose tissue in Asian Americans. *Obes Res*, 9(7), 381–387, 2001.

40. Yajnik, C.S. Early life origins of insulin resistance and type 2 diabetes in India and other Asian countries. *J Nutr*, 134, 205–210, 2004.
41. Goodpaster, B.H., Krishnaswami, S., Harris, T.B., Katsiaras, A., Kritchevsky, S.B., Simonsick, E.M., Nevitt, M., Holvoet, P., and Newman, A.B. Obesity, regional body fat distribution, and the metabolic syndrome in older men and women. *Arch Intern Med*, 165(7), 777–783, 2005.
42. Amati, F., Dube, J.J., Coen, P.M., Stefanovic-Racic, M., Toledo, F.G., and Goodpaster, B.H. Physical inactivity and obesity underlie the insulin resistance of aging. *Diabetes Care*, 32(8), 1547–1549, 2009.
43. Ding, J., Kritchevsky, S.B., Newman, A.B., Taaffe, D.R., Nicklas, B.J., Visser, M., Lee, J.S., Nevitt, M., Tylavsky, F.A., Rubin, S.M., Pahor, M., and Harris, T.B. Effects of birth cohort and age on body composition in a sample of community-based elderly. *Am J Clin Nutr*, 85(2), 405–410, 2007.
44. Foster, N.A., Segal, N.A., Clearfield, J.S., Lewis, C.E., Keysor, J., Nevitt, M.C., and Torner, J.C. Central versus lower body obesity distribution and the association with lower limb physical function and disability. *PM R*, 2(12), 1119–1126, 2010.
45. Saarni, S.E. et al. Weight cycling of athletes and subsequent weight gain in middleage. *Int J Obes (Lond)*, 30(11), 1639–1644 2006.
46. Devlin, M.J. et al. Metabolic abnormalities in Bulimia nervosa. *Arch Gen Psychiatry*, 47, 144–148, 1990.
47. Walts, C.T., Hanson, E.D., Delmonico, M.J., Yao, L., Wang, M.Q., and Hurley, B.F. Do sex or race differences influence strength training effects on muscle or fat? *Med Sci Sports Exerc*, 40(4), 669–676, 2008.
48. Zehnder, M., Ith, M., Kreis, R., Saris, W., Boutellier, U., and Boesch, C. Gender-specific usage of intramyocellular lipids and glycogen during exercise. *Med Sci Sports Exerc*, 37(9), 1517–1524, 2005.

29 Beyond Obesity Prevention
The Antiaging Effects of Caloric Restriction

Kurt W. Saupe, PhD and Jacob D. Mulligan, PhD

CONTENTS

This chapter contrasts with much of the book in that instead of focusing on treating obesity, we discuss the effects of lowering body mass in animals that are not overweight or obese to start with. For the purposes of this chapter, caloric restriction (CR) is defined as limiting caloric intake while providing adequate micronutrients. It should be emphasized that we are not treating obesity but making relatively lean animals very lean while avoiding any malnourishment by increasing nutrient density of the diet. CR is unique in that it significantly increases mean and maximal life span of a population. An important aspect of CR is that it does not simply prolong the survival of the organism in an aged or decrepit state—it actually confers a "young" phenotype to the organism. No other nongenetic interventions have emerged that produce similar benefits.

CR AND LIFE SPAN

While people throughout history have unsuccessfully looked for a "fountain of youth," in the early decades of the twentieth century, several groups reported that life span in rodents could be significantly lengthened by restricting the amount of food they were given [46,48,51]. Over the subsequent years, this observation that a CR diet could extend life span was built upon several fundamental observations:

1. CR extends both mean and maximal life spans of a colony of animals, causing a parallel rightward shift in the survival curve as shown in Figure 29.1 [72]. Particularly noteworthy is the increase in survival of the oldest members of the colony. The fact that CR does not just "square off" the survival curve by preventing early deaths is a strong indication that

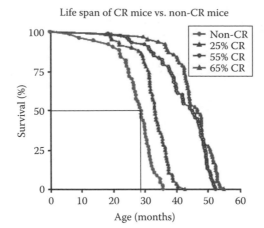

FIGURE 29.1   Effects of increasing levels of CR on survival in mice. CR causes a parallel rightward shift in the survival curve, increasing both average and maximal life span. (From Weindruch, R. et al., *J. Nutr.*, 116, 641, 1986.)

    CR actually retards aging. Subsequent studies have established that the improved survival of CR animals appears to be caused by a delayed onset of age-associated diseases including cancer and neurodegenerative diseases.

2. The amount of life span extension afforded by CR is related to two main dosing factors: the age at which CR is initiated and the severity of CR. Regarding this first factor, if CR is initiated either too early or late in life, beneficial effects of CR are lessened. For example, if CR is initiated before an animal is mature (prior to weaning in a rodent), any benefits of CR may be obscured. On the other hand, the later in life (after maturity) CR is initiated, the less life span will be extended. For example, an equivalent level of CR (approximately 40% less than *ad libitum* calories) will increase life span in a mouse by approximately 9, 6, and 3 months when it is started at 3, 14, or 19 months of age [14,41,72]. In other words, starting CR during late-middle age yields only approximately a third of the life span extension as does starting CR during early adulthood. A second critical dosing factor is the degree to which food intake is restricted [72]. It is interesting to note that there is generally a linear increase in mean and maximal life span as caloric intake is reduced, with no minimal point defined where further reduction in caloric intake causes no further benefit, or even harm (Figure 29.2). While at some point, reduction of caloric intake must decrease life span, this point, often assumed to be approximately a 65% reduction, has not been empirically defined.

3. The increase in life span is not simply due to preventing obesity. While preventing obesity clearly has many health benefits, even when very lean mice are used as the basis of comparison (such as the 25% restriction group in Figure 29.1), further restriction of food intake substantially increases life span. It bears repeating that the antiaging and life span extension afforded by CR are in addition to benefits of preventing obesity. Surprisingly, the retardation of aging and extension of life span is not due simply to maintaining a low body weight or low body fat percentage. This is most directly demonstrated by Holloszy et al. who reported that exercise-induced weight loss extended mean life span slightly but did not extend maximal life span [28,29]. The retardation of aging and life span extension with CR seems to be caused by metabolic adjustments to chronic lack of food.

4. The beneficial effects of CR on life span occur in all species studied to date, including yeast, worms, mice, rats, and large mammals. In fact, the effects of CR are so robust that even in genetically long- or short-lived mice, the effects of CR are preserved [32]. Thus, the effect of CR appears to superimpose on animals with a wide range of genetic backgrounds (Figure 29.3). An overriding unanswered question is to what extent will CR affect aging in long-lived mammals such as humans (see "Will CR work in humans?" section).

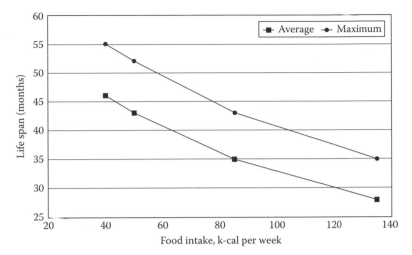

FIGURE 29.2 Effects of decreasing food intake on average and maximal survival. There is a linear increase in life span with decreasing levels of food intake. Note that even at very low levels of food intake, life span is further increased by lessening food intake. (From Weindruch, R. et al., *J. Nutr.*, 116, 641, 1986.)

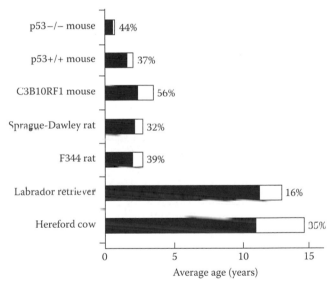

FIGURE 29.3 Effects of moderate CR on survival across mammalian species. Even in relatively long-lived mammals and mice genetically engineered to have short or long lives, CR significantly increases life span. (From Hursting, S.D. et al., *Annu. Rev. Med.*, 54, 131, 2003.)

5. The effects of CR have rapid on and off kinetics. Dhahbi et al. have recently shown that within the first 8 weeks of starting a CR diet, survival is improved in aged mice [14]. They also noted that the pattern of gene expression is altered within the first 2 weeks of CR. Thus, the key molecular "trigger" events that ultimately lead to the CR phenotype must occur within this time window, possibly as soon as the first restricted day. Conversely, when a CR diet is stopped and animals are allowed to eat *ad libitum*, the benefits of CR disappear quickly. The rapid kinetics of CR-mediated changes is a boost to the practicality of CR research. Depending on the endpoint being studied, it is possible to collect meaningful data in a timely manner rather than conducting long-term studies. In fact, a current priority in this area of research is identifying biomarkers of longevity as "surrogate endpoints"

and alternatives to life span. Furthermore, the time frame of CR-mediated changes gives important clues as to the molecular causes. It seems likely that many of the effects of CR may be in common with those effects that follow a short-term fast.

The kinetics of CR effects is also of interest to those—both researchers and subjects—considering CR diet as treatment. While the rapid onset of these effects might be encouraging, unfortunately, the benefits of CR accumulate relatively slowly, and it may take many months or years on the CR regimen to have a noticeable impact on health. The emerging field of CR mimetic drugs, however, may eventually decrease that time, or at least make the "treatment" period more feasible. CR mimetics are discussed in "CR mimetic drugs" section.

6. The increase in life span with CR can be seen using any one of a number of dietary regimens. The key common factor is a reduction in caloric intake without sacrificing micronutrients. Interestingly, some data suggest that even intermittent fasting protocols that do not produce a profound weight loss still provide many of the benefits of CR [4,7].

7. Life span extension with CR is due largely to the retardation of age-associated diseases, most importantly cancer. In rodents and other species that die largely of neoplastic disease, much of the life span extension can be attributed to anticancer effects [32,70]. This inhibitory action of CR on carcinogenesis is effective in multiple species for a variety of tumor types and for both spontaneous and chemically induced neoplasms. Fortunately, even relatively mild CR (20%–30% less calories than *ad libitum*) can significantly delay and lower the incidence rate of late-life neoplasms [58,72]. Also encouraging from the standpoint of applicability to humans is the fact that CR even initiated as late as middle age retards the development of tumors [71]. While there are numerous theories as to the molecular basis for how CR prevents and slows cancer, (see [32,70] for reviews), the actual mechanism(s) remains unclear.

CAUSES AND EFFECTS OF CR

Given the difficulty of voluntarily restricting food intake, there is a great deal of interest in understanding the molecular mechanisms underlying the effects of CR well enough to harness the powerful effects. However, finding a clear, universally satisfying explanation for how CR works has remained elusive. One major issue is that so many molecular and physiological variables are altered with CR that it is hard to tell the effects of CR from causes. For example, it has been widely observed that chronic CR causes a decrease in core body temperature (see [52]). However, the extent to which lowered body temperature and other CR-induced changes contributes to the CR phenotype of retarded aging is unknown. While many theories of aging and CR have been well discussed over the past three decades, here we will highlight two recent areas of investigation into the basis for the CR phenotype.

EFFECT OF CR ON STEM CELLS AND THE REGENERATIVE POTENTIAL OF TISSUES

One theory of aging is that loss of tissue regenerative potential with age contributes to the aging phenotype. Aged tissues heal less effectively in response to acute injury, and there is also a gradual decline in regeneration regarding basal tissue maintenance [13,34,59]. This has been shown in both proliferative and "postmitotic" tissues [9,13,39,45]. It is thought that the decline in tissue regeneration with age occurs when stem or precursor cell function decreases to the point where the production of new cells can no longer match cellular turnover in the tissue, leading to a net loss of tissue function. Aging decreases the functional capacity of circulating stem cells of the hematopoietic and mesenchymal lineages, [19,35] as well as resident tissue-specific precursors, such as the satellite cells in skeletal muscle [13].

Recent evidence has suggested that in some types of tissue, CR increases regenerative potential and/or stem cell function. CR-mediated improvements in tissue function following acute injury include rescue of cardiac function in postischemic hearts [2,43] and enhanced hepatic regeneration following toxin-induced injury [6]. In the latter study, CR was thought to enhance hepatic regeneration by inducing apoptosis of damaged cells and promitotic signaling in healthy cells.

The effect of CR on stem or primitive cells has been studied directly. In bone marrow-derived hematopoietic stem cells, CR not only slowed aging of the stem cells but also enhanced function to the extent that in a repopulation assay, stem cells from old CR mice outperformed stem cells from young mice fed *ad libitum* [12]. CR has also been shown to attenuate the age-associated reduction in T-cell precursors [50], while, in another study, CR reduced the number of senescent T-cells [64]. This suggests that CR may strengthen the regenerative potential of tissues in part by increasing the potency of the progenitor-type cell population.

Recent evidence suggests that CR may exert its effects on regeneration via the circulation. Conboy et al. demonstrated that regeneration capacity in liver and muscle from old mice can be restored by cross-circulation with a young mouse [13]. The simplest interpretation of this result is that the "CR effect" is carried in the blood stream—at least the part of the effect that is involved in enhancing cellular rejuvenation. Since CR confers a "young" phenotype on many aspects of the hormonal milieu (decreases insulin and IGF-1), it is not surprising that CR may improve tissue regeneration through the circulation [37]. Furthermore, hematopoietic stem cells, which are functionally improved by CR, move through the circulation to sites where they may be involved in tissue regeneration.

EFFECTS OF CR ON FAT AND ADIPOKINES

The recent recognition that white adipose tissue plays a central role in age-related pathologies such as type 2 diabetes and cancer, combined with the fact that white adipose tissue is dramatically remodeled by CR, has led to the suggestion that CR-induced changes in white adipose tissue may play a key role in the CR phenotype [38,56]. Recent experimental evidence indicates that fat is a dynamic endocrine organ that can become "dysfunctional" and not only secrete hormones that contribute to pathology but also shunt lipids to be stored in other organs, resulting in insulin resistance [24]. Our understanding of the biological significance of the peptides and other substances secreted by adipose tissue (sometimes referred to as adipokines) and how they are affected by CR is in its infancy.

HOW DOES CR AFFECT A REPRESENTATIVE ORGAN SYSTEM (CARDIOVASCULAR SYSTEM)?

While CR has long been established as having powerful antineoplastic effects, more recently, there has been interest in determining how CR affects other major causes of human mortality, especially cardiovascular diseases. This question has become particularly important with the dramatic increase in age-associated cardiovascular disease in recent decades. In evaluating the effects of CR on the cardiovascular system, the large majority of studies have been performed on rodents. However, several reports have studied nonhuman primates or human subjects despite the many methodological difficulties and limitations. The findings of these studies in rodents and primates can be divided into three broad categories, the effect of CR on (1) systemic hemodynamics and cardiac contractile function, (2) oxidative damage, and (3) gene expression.

HEMODYNAMICS AND CARDIAC CONTRACTILE FUNCTION

CR has been reported to decrease blood pressure (BP) and heart rate (HR) in rodents [31,69] and BP in nonhuman primates [47]. This HR and BP lowering occurs in normotensive as well as hypertensive animal models and seems to be secondary to increases and decreases in parasympathetic and sympathetic tone, respectively. Mager et al. showed that the decrease in HR and BP caused by either CR or intermittent fasting was quickly reversed by switching the animal to an *ad libitum* diet [44].

The most relevant data from humans come from the study of a cohort that voluntarily underwent a CR diet regimen for a mean of 6 years [49]. In this study, Meyer et al. compared 25 CR volunteers

(BMI = 20, %fat = 9) and 25 age-matched, nonobese controls (BMI = 27, %fat = 26). The CR group had lower systolic (102 vs. 113 mmHg) and diastolic (61 vs. 83 mmHg) BP compared to the control group. Another study using similar subjects revealed an improved blood lipid profile in the CR group [20]. CR increased HDL-cholesterol (48 mg/dL vs. 63 mg/dL) and decreased LDL-cholesterol (127 mg/dL vs. 86 mg/dL) and triglyceride (147 mg/dL vs. 48 mg/dL). It should be noted that these studies—as is true of all studies on humans—carry important limitations; for example, small sample size and lack of strict control over subject diet intake. Furthermore, these subjects volunteered for CR rather than being randomly placed on CR by the investigators. This, at the very least, suggests a difference in lifestyle between the groups. Another important limitation of this study was age of the subjects. At the relatively young age of 53, neither group would be expected to display a large age-associated decline in cardiovascular function.

The effects of CR on cardiac contractile function are most often studied in the context of testing the ability of CR to reverse age-associated changes in left ventricular function. In rodents, CR generally attenuated age-associated changes in echocardiographically measured left ventricular function. Specifically, CR decreased peak atrial filling velocity and fraction [67], and intermittent fasting improved cardiac output, pressure work, and efficiency [65], and prevented the age-associated reduction in left ventricular contractility [11]. It should be noted that in mice and rats age-associated changes in the heart are relatively small and of unknown significance since mice do not die of heart disease. Thus, the extent to which CR-induced changes in left ventricular function contribute to life span extension is probably minimal.

In humans, however, the age-associated decline in cardiovascular function is a major health issue. Cardiovascular function was tested in the same voluntary CR cohort introduced earlier [49]. CR had no effect on systolic function—which declines little if at all with age—but caused improvement in diastolic function, an age-dependent parameter. Specifically, CR decreased peak A-wave velocity (53 cm/s vs. 46 cm/s) and increased the E/A wave ratio (1.2 vs. 1.6). CR also improved left ventricular chamber viscoelasticity and stiffness compared to control subjects.

A critical aspect of the healthy heart is its ability to mitigate and recover from stress-induced damage. CR has proven beneficial in this regard. In rodents, CR was shown to lower HR following ischemia [8,43] and swimming stress [69] and to blunt the hypertension-induced increase in left ventricular weight to body weight ratio [66]. Experimentally, one way to lessen ischemic damage is to subject the heart to short periods of ischemia prior to a prolonged period of ischemia (ischemic preconditioning). Aged hearts are especially sensitive to damage from ischemia and do not respond to this ischemic preconditioning [1,26]. CR has been shown to restore the beneficial effect of pre-ischemic conditioning in the aged heart, as interpreted by improved developed pressure recovery and increased cardiac output following ischemia [2,43]. This effect of CR has been combined with exercise to achieve an additive result [3].

OXIDATIVE DAMAGE

A key hypothesis for the cause of cellular aging is the accumulation of oxidative damage to proteins, lipids, and DNA. The majority of oxidative damage is caused by the production of reactive oxygen species (ROS) in the mitochondria. It is thought that with aging, ROS production is increased and/or removal of ROS is decreased [25]. Although there is some disagreement on the details, considerable evidence exists that CR improves control over oxidative damage in the heart. For example, the production of ROS was shown to be decreased by 6 weeks of CR [62], though another study showed no change after 4 months of CR [54]. There is more agreement on the expression of enzymes that remove ROS. CR has been demonstrated to increase the levels of catalase, glutathione peroxidase, thioredoxin reductase, and superoxide dismutase [10,16,18,60]. Oxidative damage is also reduced by the presence of antioxidant or reducing molecules in the cell. CR corrects the age-associated decline in reduced glutathione and coenzyme Q [10,36,57], though one study showed a surprising decline in α-tocopherol levels with CR [36].

Importantly, CR has been shown to reduce not only ROS levels but also actual oxidative damage to protein [42,53], lipids [16,18], and DNA [63]. Some studies showed duration dependence. Gredilla et al. demonstrated a decrease in oxidative damage to DNA with 12 months of CR, but not with 8 weeks [22]. Forster et al. showed that 12 months of CR decreased protein oxidation, but 6 weeks was less effective. This group also showed that the CR effect was completely lost with a few weeks of being switched back to an *ad libitum* diet [21].

GENE EXPRESSION

Two research groups have measured the effects of CR on global cardiac gene expression in mice using microarrays. The scope of these studies makes them exceptionally useful for seeing the larger picture of how CR affects the biochemical landscape of the heart. Lee et al. found that of over 5000 genes analyzed in the heart 312 were altered by at least 50% with age and 831 were altered by at least 50% with CR [40]. This study revealed a gene expression pattern that suggests that aging results in a downregulation of fatty acid metabolism—the preferred fuel substrate in the healthy heart—and a subsequent upregulation of glucose metabolism. CR, however, reversed much of this age-dependent "fuel switching" pattern. Additionally, CR was shown to induce genes involved in DNA repair and to downregulate genes involved in programmed cell death (apoptosis).

Recently, Dhahbi et al. compared gene expression in both short- and long-term CR and the effect of going back to an *ad libitum* diet after the CR diet [15]. Eight weeks of CR produced 19% of the gene expression changes as 22 months of CR, in line with studies showing that, although many changes occur quickly, the benefit of CR increases with time. Interestingly, 97% of CR-induced changes in gene expression were completely reversed within only 8 weeks of the animals switching back to an *ad libitum* diet.

In summary, CR has a profound effect on the physiology and biochemistry of the heart. By and large, the available data suggest that this effect is a positive one. However, many important details about how CR affects the human cardiovascular system are lacking due to the sparse human data available being primarily from observations of overweight subjects in experiments that were not strictly controlled. While the benefit of CR is quite robustly illustrated in many experimental models in nonhumans, more meaningful insights should come from additional well-controlled studies in nonobese humans.

WILL CR WORK IN HUMANS?

One of the most frequently asked questions in the field of CR is "will a CR diet work in humans, and if it does, will the sacrifices be worth it?" Much of the answer to this question depends on whether one is discussing disease prevention or antiaging and extension of maximal life span. It is clear that some level of CR would provide most Americans with an important degree of disease prevention as the data in Table 29.1 indicates [20]. However, the question of whether CR retards aging and extends maximal life span in humans is more complicated. There are several theoretical reasons to believe that CR will not provide these kinds of benefits to humans that are discussed extensively elsewhere [17,55]. They include the suspicion that humans will not be willing or able to restrict calories to the needed levels at an early enough age to garner any significant benefits. Since it is unlikely that survival curves such as shown in Figure 29.1 will ever be generated to directly answer this question, we must look at available data.

Additionally, the question of "is it worth it" can only be answered when the cost and benefits of various CR regimens are known. The obvious costs include nearly constant hunger that does not seem to dissipate with time. This issue raises the interesting philosophical question of would you extend life by a few years if it meant being hungry almost constantly? Clearly, different people would answer this question very differently, and the hope is that they could make informed choice based on complete knowledge of costs/benefits. However, currently we have only a poor idea of either the benefits or costs in humans. It should be recognized that the importance of studying the basic biological causes of CR-induced retardation of aging does not depend on a "yes" answer to the question of "is it worth it," since this area of research may lead to a pharmacological way of reproducing some of the benefits of CR.

EFFECTS OF CR IN HUMANS

Recently, it has been demonstrated that humans can voluntarily submit to a CR diet in at least two settings. The first is self-selected individuals who have decided to follow a CR diet [20,49]. Despite the obvious methodological problems, this approach has provided some intriguing data, particularly when longitudinal data are available from before the CR was initiated in the individual (Table 29.1) [20]. It would be difficult to argue that these changes in BP and blood chemistry are not desirable consequences of voluntary restriction of caloric intake. Note that the pre-CR BMI is within the nonobese normal range, suggesting that these individuals reflect the general American population prior to initiating CR in an important way. These 50 year olds had on average only been on CR for 6 years, revealing the increased motivation that may be too late. Data from these individuals is intriguing but relatively uncontrolled with regard to some factors, such as composition of the diet, that may contribute to improved cardiovascular health. However, these individuals clearly demonstrate that at least some people can restrict caloric intake to low chronic levels with impressive cardiovascular benefits.

A second group of individuals that has voluntarily undergone CR are those involved in an NIH/NIA-sponsored randomized multicenter trial (Comprehensive Assessment of the Long Term Effects of Reducing Intake of Energy, CALERIE) [27]. In part of this long-term research effort, 48 healthy, sedentary adults, 27–49 year old, were randomized to one of four groups: controls (weight maintenance), 25% CR, 12.5% CR plus exercise, or 890 kcal/day until 15% decrease in body weight. Importantly, the subjects entered the study overweight (BMI of 28 and body fat percentage of 32) so some of the effects noted may be due to normalization of body weight. Over the 6 months of the study, the CR and CR plus exercise groups lost weight at a rate of approximately 3 lb/month, whereas the 890 kcal/day group lost approximately 23 lb in 10 weeks after which body weight was maintained. There are several noteworthy findings from this study. First, under these carefully controlled circumstances, the highly motivated volunteers were able to tolerate a moderate degree of CR. Second, some but not all biomarkers of CR established in rodents changed as predicted. For example, CR did not affect blood glucose or DHEA levels as one might expect from rodent data,

TABLE 29.1
Effects of Chronic CR on BP and Blood Lipids in Humans

Parameter	Pre-CR	∞1 Year CR	Present
	Value		
BMI, kg/m²	24.5 ± 2.6	20.9 ± 2.4	19.5 ± 2.1
Total cholesterol, mg/dL	194 ± 45	161 ± 31	157 ± 38
LDL-C, mg/dL	122 ± 36	89 ± 24	86 ± 17
HDL-C, mg/dL	43 ± 8	58 ± 13	65 ± 24
Total cholesterol/HDL-C ratio	4.1 ± 1	2.8 ± 0.5	2.5 ± 0.4
Triglycerides, mg/dL	149 ± 87	72 ± 35	54 ± 15
Systolic BP, mmHg	132 ± 15	112 ± 12	97 ± 8
Diastolic BP, mmHg	80 ± 11	69 ± 7	59 ± 5

Source: Fontana, L. et al., *Proc. Natl. Acad. Sci. USA*, 101, 6659, 2004.

Note: Values are means ± SD for 12 individuals.

whereas 6 months of CR significantly decreased insulin levels in all three groups. Intriguingly, DNA damage, but not the levels of protein carbonyls, was decreased in all three CR groups. Longer-term studies should yield interesting information.

CR MIMETIC DRUGS

Given the difficulties mentioned earlier and uncertainties regarding CR in humans, there is intense interest in trying to reproduce some of the beneficial effects of CR pharmacologically [33,61]. As more information about the molecular basis for CR's effects is available, the search for compounds that mimic the effects of CR becomes more rational and focused. Since the benefits of CR are not directly linked to weight loss, a weight-loss drug per se is not the goal. In general, there have been two pharmacological strategies for CR mimetics: finding drugs that reproduce the general metabolic state of food deprivation and finding agonists/antagonists of specific molecules that are thought to be "upstream" in the pathway by which CR retards aging. In the first category is the structural analog of glucose, 2-deoxy-D-glucose (2-DG) that acts as a competitive inhibitor of glycolysis. While 2-DG has shown great therapeutic potential in some settings, the extent to which it mimics the effects of CR at nontoxic doses appears limited [33].

A second member of this category is insulin sensitizers such as the commonly used antidiabetes drug metformin. The rationale for this approach centers on the observation that CR causes a broad insulin sensitization of tissues that has been implicated in the antiaging phenotype of CR animals. Consistent with a central role of endocrine effects of CR, studies in species including *C. elegans*, *Drosophila*, and rodents suggest that CR-induced life span extension may be related to alterations in insulin and/or insulin-like growth factor signaling that retard cellular aging [5,68]. Using microarray analysis of the liver, Dhabi et al. found that 8 weeks of metformin treatment in mice produced 75% of the changes in gene expression that were produced by long-term CR. To put this number in perspective, 8 weeks of CR only produced 71% of the changes in expression observed during long-term CR. This dramatic mimicking of CR by metformin was observed to a much weaker degree with other putative CR mimetics such as glipizide (16%), rosiglitazone (17%), or soy isoflavone extract (11%). Thus, metformin not only shows great potential as a CR mimetic, but it can be inferred that insulin sensitization is relatively far upstream in causing the broad changes in gene expression observed with long-term CR.

In addition to drugs that reproduce the general effects of food deprivation, exciting recent work has also focused on agonists of specific molecules. Most notably, Howitz et al. found that resveratrol (a naturally occurring polyphenol that is present in red grape skins and red wine) increases the replicative life span of yeast by stimulating the histone deacetylase Sir2 [30]. This group also reported that resveratrol extends life span in *Drosophila melanogaster* and stimulates the mammalian homologue SIRT1. The extent to which this finding is applicable to mammals has not yet been determined. Some have speculated that the effects of CR on aging and longevity in mammals may be caused by a CR-induced increase in SIRT1 activity [23]. While the extent to which CR affects SIRT1 in mammals has not been clearly defined, this is an area of great scientific interest.

REFERENCES

1. Abete P, Cioppa A, Ferrara P, Caccese P, Ferrara N, and Rengo F. Reduced aerobic metabolic efficiency in postischemic myocardium dysfunction in rats: Role of aging. *Gerontology* 41: 187–194, 1995.
2. Abete P, Testa G, Ferrara N, De Santis D, Capaccio P, Viati L, Calabrese C, Cacciatore F, Longobardi G, Condorelli M, Napoli C, and Rengo F. Cardioprotective effect of ischemic preconditioning is preserved in food-restricted senescent rats. *Am J Physiol Heart Circ Physiol* 282: H1978–H1987, 2002.
3. Abete P, Testa G, Galizia G, Mazzella F, Della Morte D, de Santis D, Calabrese C, Cacciatore F, Gargiulo G, Ferrara N, Rengo G, Sica V, Napoli C, and Rengo F. Tandem action of exercise training and food restriction completely preserves ischemic preconditioning in the aging heart. *Exp Gerontol* 40: 43–50, 2005.

4. Anson RM, Guo Z, de Cabo R, Iyun T, Rios M, Hagepanos A, Ingram DK, Lane MA, and Mattson MP. Intermittent fasting dissociates beneficial effects of dietary restriction on glucose metabolism and neuronal resistance to injury from calorie intake. *Proc Natl Acad Sci USA* 100: 6216–6220, 2003.

5. Antebi A. Inside insulin signaling, communication is key to long life. *Sci Aging Knowledge Environ* 2004: pe25, 2004.

6. Apte UM, Limaye PB, Desaiah D, Bucci TJ, Warbritton A, and Mehendale HM. Mechanisms of increased liver tissue repair and survival in diet-restricted rats treated with equitoxic doses of thioacetamide. *Toxicol Sci* 72: 272–282, 2003.

7. Berrigan D, Perkins SN, Haines DC, and Hursting SD. Adult-onset calorie restriction and fasting delay spontaneous tumorigenesis in p53-deficient mice. *Carcinogenesis* 23: 817–822, 2002.

8. Broderick TL, Belke T, and Driedzic WR. Effects of chronic caloric restriction on mitochondrial respiration in the ischemic reperfused rat heart. *Mol Cell Biochem* 233: 119–125, 2002.

9. Capogrossi MC. Cardiac stem cells fail with aging: A new mechanism for the age-dependent decline in cardiac function. *Circ Res* 94: 411–413, 2004.

10. Chandrasekar B, Nelson JF, Colston JT, and Freeman GL. Calorie restriction attenuates inflammatory responses to myocardial ischemia-reperfusion injury. *Am J Physiol Heart Circ Physiol* 280: H2094–H2102, 2001.

11. Chang KC, Peng YI, Lee FC, and Tseng YZ. Effects of food restriction on systolic mechanical behavior of the ventricular pump in middle-aged and senescent rats. *J Gerontol A Biol Sci Med Sci* 56: B108–B114, 2001.

12. Chen J, Astle CM, and Harrison DE. Hematopoietic senescence is postponed and hematopoietic stem cell function is enhanced by dietary restriction. *Exp Hematol* 31: 1097–1103, 2003.

13. Conboy IM, Conboy MJ, Wagers AJ, Girma ER, Weissman IL, and Rando TA. Rejuvenation of aged progenitor cells by exposure to a young systemic environment. *Nature* 433: 760–764, 2005.

14. Dhahbi JM, Kim HJ, Mote PL, Beaver RJ, and Spindler SR. Temporal linkage between the phenotypic and genomic responses to caloric restriction. *Proc Natl Acad Sci USA* 101: 5524–5529, 2004.

15. Dhahbi JM, Tsuchiya T, Kim HJ, Mote PL, and Spindler SR. Gene expression and physiologic responses of the heart to the initiation and withdrawal of caloric restriction. *J Gerontol A Biol Sci Med Sci* 61: 218–231, 2006.

16. Diniz YS, Cicogna AC, Padovani CR, Silva MD, Faine LA, Galhardi CM, Rodrigues HG, and Novelli EL. Dietary restriction and fibre supplementation: Oxidative stress and metabolic shifting for cardiac health. *Can J Physiol Pharmacol* 81: 1042–1048, 2003.

17. Dirks AJ and Leeuwenburgh C. Caloric restriction in humans: Potential pitfalls and health concerns. *Mech Ageing Dev* 127: 1–7, 2006.

18. Faine LA, Diniz YS, Almeida JA, Novelli EL, and Ribas BO. Toxicity of ad lib. Overfeeding: Effects on cardiac tissue. *Food Chem Toxicol* 40: 663–668, 2002.

19. Fehrer C and Lepperdinger G. Mesenchymal stem cell aging. *Exp Gerontol* 40: 926–930, 2005.

20. Fontana L, Meyer TE, Klein S, and Holloszy JO. Long-term calorie restriction is highly effective in reducing the risk for atherosclerosis in humans. *Proc Natl Acad Sci USA* 101: 6659–6663, 2004.

21. Forster MJ, Sohal BH, and Sohal RS. Reversible effects of long-term caloric restriction on protein oxidative damage. *J Gerontol A Biol Sci Med Sci* 55: B522–B529, 2000.

22. Gredilla R, Sanz A, Lopez-Torres M, and Barja G. Caloric restriction decreases mitochondrial free radical generation at complex I and lowers oxidative damage to mitochondrial DNA in the rat heart. *Faseb J* 15: 1589–1591, 2001.

23. Guarente L. Calorie restriction and SIR2 genes–towards a mechanism. *Mech Ageing Dev* 126: 923–928, 2005.

24. Guerre-Millo M. Adipose tissue and adipokines: For better or worse. *Diabetes Metab* 30: 13–19, 2004.

25. Harper ME, Bevilacqua L, Hagopian K, Weindruch R, and Ramsey JJ. Ageing, oxidative stress, and mitochondrial uncoupling. *Acta Physiol Scand* 182: 321–331, 2004.

26. Headrick JP. Aging impairs functional, metabolic and ionic recovery from ischemia-reperfusion and hypoxia-reoxygenation. *J Mol Cell Cardiol* 30: 1415–1430, 1998.

27. Heilbronn LK, de Jonge L, Frisard MI, DeLany JP, Larson-Meyer DE, Rood J, Nguyen T, Martin CK, Volaufova J, Most MM, Greenway FL, Smith SR, Deutsch WA, Williamson DA, and Ravussin E. Effect of 6-month calorie restriction on biomarkers of longevity, metabolic adaptation, and oxidative stress in overweight individuals: A randomized controlled trial. *JAMA* 295: 1539–1548, 2006.

28. Holloszy JO. Mortality rate and longevity of food-restricted exercising male rats: A reevaluation. *J Appl Physiol* 82: 399–403, 1997.

29. Holloszy JO and Schechtman KB. Interaction between exercise and food restriction: Effects on longevity of male rats. *J Appl Physiol* 70: 1529–1535, 1991.

30. Howitz KT, Bitterman KJ, Cohen HY, Lamming DW, Lavu S, Wood JG, Zipkin RE, Chung P, Kisielewski A, Zhang LL, Scherer B, and Sinclair DA. Small molecule activators of sirtuins extend *Saccharomyces cerevisiae* lifespan. *Nature* 425: 191–196, 2003.

31. Hunt LM, Hogeland EW, Henry MK, and Swoap SJ. Hypotension and bradycardia during caloric restriction in mice are independent of salt balance and do not require ANP receptor. *Am J Physiol Heart Circ Physiol* 287: H1446–H1451, 2004.

32. Hursting SD, Lavigne JA, Berrigan D, Perkins SN, and Barrett JC. Calorie restriction, aging, and cancer prevention: Mechanisms of action and applicability to humans. *Annu Rev Med* 54: 131–152, 2003.

33. Ingram DK, Zhu M, Mamczarz J, Zou S, Lane MA, Roth GS, and deCabo R. Calorie restriction mimetics: An emerging research field. *Aging Cell* 5: 97–108, 2006.

34. Juhaszova M, Rabuel C, Zorov DB, Lakatta EG, and Sollott SJ. Protection in the aged heart: Preventing the heart-break of old age? *Cardiovasc Res* 66: 233–244, 2005.

35. Kamminga LM and de Haan G. Cellular memory and hematopoietic stem cell aging. *Stem Cells* 24: 1143–1149, 2006.

36. Kamzalov S and Sohal RS. Effect of age and caloric restriction on coenzyme Q and alpha-tocopherol levels in the rat. *Exp Gerontol* 39: 1199–1205, 2004.

37. Katic M and Kahn CR. The role of insulin and IGF-1 signaling in longevity. *Cell Mol Life Sci* 62: 320–343, 2005.

38. Kloting N and Bluher M. Extended longevity and insulin signaling in adipose tissue. *Exp Gerontol* 40: 878–883, 2005.

39. Kuhn HG, Dickinson-Anson H, and Gage FH. Neurogenesis in the dentate gyrus of the adult rat: Age-related decrease of neuronal progenitor proliferation. *J Neurosci* 16: 2027–2033, 1996.

40. Lee CK, Allison DB, Brand J, Weindruch R, and Prolla TA. Transcriptional profiles associated with aging and middle age-onset caloric restriction in mouse hearts. *Proc Natl Acad Sci USA* 99: 14988–14993, 2002.

41. Lee CK, Pugh TD, Klopp RG, Edwards J, Allison DB, Weindruch R, and Prolla TA. The impact of alpha-lipoic acid, coenzyme Q10 and caloric restriction on life span and gene expression patterns in mice. *Free Radic Biol Med* 36: 1043–1057, 2004.

42. Leeuwenburgh C, Wagner P, Holloszy JO, Sohal RS, and Heinecke JW. Caloric restriction attenuates dityrosine cross-linking of cardiac and skeletal muscle proteins in aging mice. *Arch Biochem Biophys* 346: 74–80, 1997.

43. Long P, Nguyen Q, Thurow C, and Broderick TL. Caloric restriction restores the cardioprotective effect of preconditioning in the rat heart. *Mech Ageing Dev* 123: 1411–1413, 2002.

44. Mager DE, Wan R, Brown M, Cheng A, Wareski P, Abernethy DR, and Mattson MP. Caloric restriction and intermittent fasting alter spectral measures of heart rate and blood pressure variability in rats. *Faseb J* 20: 631–637, 2006.

45. Martin K, Potten CS, Roberts SA, and Kirkwood TB. Altered stem cell regeneration in irradiated intestinal crypts of senescent mice. *J Cell Sci* 111 (Pt 16): 2297–2303, 1998.

46. Masoro EJ. Subfield history: Caloric restriction, slowing aging, and extending life. *Sci Aging Knowledge Environ* 2003: RE2, 2003.

47. Mattison JA, Lane MA, Roth GS, and Ingram DK. Calorie restriction in rhesus monkeys. *Exp Gerontol* 38: 35–46, 2003.

48. McCay CM, Crowell MF, and Maynard LA. The effect of retarded growth upon the length of life span and upon the ultimate body size. *Nutrition* 5: 155–171; discussion 172, 1989.

49. Meyer TE, Kovacs SJ, Ehsani AA, Klein S, Holloszy JO, and Fontana L. Long-term caloric restriction ameliorates the decline in diastolic function in humans. *J Am Coll Cardiol* 47: 398–402, 2006.

50. Miller RA and Harrison DE. Delayed reduction in T cell precursor frequencies accompanies diet-induced lifespan extension. *J Immunol* 134: 1426–1429, 1985.

51. Osborne TB, Mendel LB, and Ferry EL. The effect of retardation of growth upon the breeding period and duration of life in rats. *Science* 45: 294–295, 1917.

52. Overton JM and Williams TD. Behavioral and physiologic responses to caloric restriction in mice. *Physiol Behav* 81: 749–754, 2004.

53. Pamplona R, Barja G, and Portero-Otin M. Membrane fatty acid unsaturation, protection against oxidative stress, and maximum life span: A homeoviscous-longevity adaptation? *Ann N Y Acad Sci* 959: 475–490, 2002.

54. Pamplona R, Portero-Otin M, Requena J, Gredilla R, and Barja G. Oxidative, glycoxidative and lipoxidative damage to rat heart mitochondrial proteins is lower after 4 months of caloric restriction than in age-matched controls. *Mech Ageing Dev* 123: 1437–1446, 2002.

55. Phelan JP and Rose MR. Why dietary restriction substantially increases longevity in animal models but won't in humans. *Ageing Res Rev* 4: 339–350, 2005.

56. Picard F and Guarente L. Molecular links between aging and adipose tissue. *Int J Obes (Lond)* 29 (Suppl 1) S36–S39, 2005.

57. Rebrin I, Kamzalov S, and Sohal RS. Effects of age and caloric restriction on glutathione redox state in mice. *Free Radic Biol Med* 35: 626–635, 2003.

58. Rehm S, Rapp KG, and Deerberg F. Influence of food restriction and body fat on life span and tumour incidence in female outbred Han: NMRI mice and two sublines. *Z Versuchstierkd* 27: 240–283, 1985.

59. Roh C and Lyle S. Cutaneous stem cells and wound healing. *Pediatr Res* 59: 100R–103R, 2006.

60. Rohrbach S, Gruenler S, Teschner M, and Holtz J. The thioredoxin system in aging muscle: Key role of mitochondrial thioredoxin reductase in the protective effects of caloric restriction? *Am J Physiol Regul Integr Comp Physiol* 291: R927–R935, 2006.

61. Roth GS, Lane MA, and Ingram DK. Caloric restriction mimetics: The next phase. *Ann NY Acad Sci* 1057: 365–371, 2005.

62. Sanz A, Gredilla R, Pamplona R, Portero-Otin M, Vara E, Tresguerres JA, and Barja G. Effect of insulin and growth hormone on rat heart and liver oxidative stress in control and caloric restricted animals. *Biogerontology* 6: 15–26, 2005.

63. Sohal RS, Agarwal S, Candas M, Forster MJ, and Lal H. Effect of age and caloric restriction on DNA oxidative damage in different tissues of C57BL/6 mice. *Mech Ageing Dev* 76: 215–224, 1994.

64. Spaulding CC, Walford RL, and Effros RB. The accumulation of non-replicative, non-functional, senescent T cells with age is avoided in calorically restricted mice by an enhancement of T cell apoptosis. *Mech Ageing Dev* 93: 25–33, 1997.

65. Starnes JW and Rumsey WL. Cardiac energetics and performance of exercised and food-restricted rats during aging. *Am J Physiol* 254: H599–H608, 1988.

66. Swoap SJ, Boddell P, and Baldwin KM. Interaction of hypertension and caloric restriction on cardiac mass and isomyosin expression. *Am J Physiol* 268: R33–R39, 1995.

67. Taffet GE, Pham TT, and Hartley CJ. The age-associated alterations in late diastolic function in mice are improved by caloric restriction. *J Gerontol A Biol Sci Med Sci* 52: B285–B290, 1997.

68. Tatar M, Bartke A, and Antebi A. The endocrine regulation of aging by insulin-like signals. *Science* 299: 1346–1351, 2003.

69. Wan R, Camandola S, and Mattson MP. Intermittent fasting and dietary supplementation with 2-deoxy-D-glucose improve functional and metabolic cardiovascular risk factors in rats. *Faseb J* 17: 1133–1134, 2003.

70. Weindruch R. Effect of caloric restriction on age-associated cancers. *Exp Gerontol* 27: 575–581, 1992.

71. Weindruch R and Walford RL. Dietary restriction in mice beginning at 1 year of age: Effect on life-span and spontaneous cancer incidence. *Science* 215: 1415–1418, 1982.

72. Weindruch R, Walford RL, Fligiel S, and Guthrie D. The retardation of aging in mice by dietary restriction: Longevity, cancer, immunity and lifetime energy intake. *J Nutr* 116: 641–654, 1986.

30 Carbohydrate Digestion Inhibitors
A Focus on Natural Products

Jay K. Udani, MD and Marilyn L. Barrett, PhD

CONTENTS

INTRODUCTION

Obesity is a major health hazard, with increased risk for cardiovascular disease (mainly heart disease and stroke), type 2 diabetes, musculoskeletal disorders (especially osteoarthritis), and certain types of cancer (endometrial, breast, and colon).[1] The World Health Organization (WHO) estimated that in 2005, approximately 1.6 billion adults worldwide were overweight and at least 400 million were obese. Further, the WHO estimated that at least 20 million children under the age of 5 years were overweight. The projected numbers for 2015 are larger, with 2.3 billion adults expected to be overweight and 700 million expected to be obese.[1]

The cause of excess body weight is an imbalance between energy intake and expenditure. The WHO has identified a global shift in diet toward increased intake of energy-dense foods that are high in fat and sugars but low in vitamins, minerals, and other micronutrients. At the same time, there is a trend toward decreased physical activity due to the increasingly sedentary nature of many forms of work, changing modes of transportation, and increasing urbanization.[1]

Control of diet and exercise are cornerstones of the management of excess weight. A number of nutritional approaches and diets with difference proportions of lipids, proteins, and carbohydrates have been prescribed for weight loss. Initial guidance on weight loss was a restriction in saturated fats. However, diets low in saturated fats did not necessarily result in weight loss as expected. More recently, there has been a shift toward a reduction in carbohydrates, particularly refined carbohydrates, as an approach to reduce weight and the incidence or related disease risk.[2]

CARBOHYDRATE DIGESTION

In most diets, carbohydrates are the greatest source of calories. Carbohydrates are polyhydroxy aldehydes, ketones, alcohols, and acids that range in size from single monomeric units (monosaccharides) to polymers (polysaccharides). Before being absorbed by the body, carbohydrates must be broken down into monosaccharides. This breakdown occurs due to two major enzymes: amylase and glucosidase.[3]

Digestion of carbohydrates begins in the mouth, with amylase secreted by salivary glands. This action accounts for only about 5% of the breakdown of carbohydrates. The process is halted in the stomach due to the high-acid environment destroying the amylase activity. When the food enters the intestine, the acidic pH is neutralized by the release of bicarbonate by the pancreas and by the mucous that lines the walls of the intestine. Amylase is secreted into the small intestines by the pancreas. Alpha-glucosidase enzymes are located in the brush border of the small intestines. Amylase breaks down the carbohydrates into oligosaccharides. The glucosidase enzymes (including lactase, maltase, and sucrose) complete the breakdown to monosaccharide units. It is only the monosaccharide units that are absorbed into the body. Glucose and other monosaccharides are transported via the hepatic portal vein to the liver. Monosaccharides not immediately utilized for energy are stored as glycogen in the liver or as fat (triglycerides) in adipose tissue, liver, and plasma. Carbohydrates that are resistant to digestion in the intestine enter the colon, where they are fermented by colonic bacteria to produce short-chain fatty acids, carbon dioxide, and methane.

GLYCEMIC INDEX

Dietary carbohydrates that are composed mostly of monosaccharide units are absorbed quickly and are said to have a "high glycemic index." Carbohydrates in polymeric form are absorbed more slowly and said to have a "low glycemic index." The glycemic index (GI) is defined as the incremental area under the blood glucose curve following ingestion of a test food, expressed as a percentage of the corresponding area following an equivalent load of a reference carbohydrate, either glucose or white (wheat) bread.[4] Factors that influence the GI besides the composition of the carbohydrate are the fat and protein content of the food, the acidity of the food, and the presence of fiber.[5] Low-GI foods (<55) include vegetables, unsweetened yogurt, and protein-enriched spaghetti. High-GI foods (>70) include white bread, baked potato, and dates.

After consumption of high-GI foods, there is a large, rapid increase in blood sugar levels and, in response, a rapid increase in insulin levels. Insulin promotes the uptake of glucose from the blood into cells in the liver and skeletal muscle tissue, storing it as glycogen. Insulin also increases fatty acid synthesis and can result in the accumulation of lipids. Accumulation of lipids in skeletal muscle and the liver is associated with a decrease in insulin sensitivity. Insulin resistance increases the chance of developing type 2 diabetes and heart disease. Postprandial hyperglycemia and insulin resistance are thought to play a central role in the development and progression of cardiovascular disease in subjects with impaired glucose tolerance. Postprandial hyperglycemia is associated with endothelial dysfunction and an increase in intima-media thickness as well as a higher prevalence of atherosclerotic plaques. High glucose levels have been shown to stimulate the expression of adhesion molecules (intercellular adhesion molecule-1, vascular adhesion molecule-1, E-selectin) and cytokines in *in vitro* models. Hyperglycemia causes an increase in oxidative stress with associated oxidation of low-density lipoprotein (LDL), platelet activation, and thrombin generation.[5,6] A body of evidence, including prospective cohort studies, randomized controlled trials, and mechanistic experiments, supports a role for low-GI diets in the prevention of obesity, diabetes, and cardiovascular disease.[7–9] Three large-scale epidemiological studies on women reported a correlation between a high-GI diet and the incidence of type 2 diabetes.[10–12] The populations studied were 59,000 U.S. black women, 65,000 Chinese women, and 91,249 U.S. nurses who were each followed for a period of 5–8 years. Another prospective cohort study in Europe, which included 25,000 men and women, concluded that high cereal fiber was inversely associated with the risk of developing diabetes.[13]

As previously indicated, the choice of the type of carbohydrate foods in the diet, with their varying glycemic properties, will determine the rate of absorption of sugars into the body. One means of reducing the GI of a meal is the inclusion of resistant starches. Resistant starches are those that resist digestion in the small intestine, thereby passing into the large intestine, where they act like dietary fiber.[14] These starches are naturally found in seeds, legumes, and unprocessed whole grains. The amount of resistant starch in food is influenced by processing, which can either increase or decrease the amounts found in the raw substance. Resistant starch can be added to foods, such as bread, biscuits, sweet goods, pasta, nutritional bars, and cereal, in order to lower their GI index without affecting taste or texture.[15,16]

DIGESTIVE ENZYME INHIBITION

An alternative to a low-GI diet are products that slow the absorption of carbohydrates through the inhibition of enzymes responsible for their digestion. These products include alpha-amylase and alpha-glucosidase inhibitors. Acarbose (Prandase®, Precose®) is a prescription drug, which inhibits alpha-glucosidase enzymes in the brush border of the small intestines and pancreatic alpha-amylase. Other drugs that belong to this class are miglitol and voglibose. Acarbose reduces postprandial hyperglycemia and is used to treat type 2 diabetes. Clinical studies with subjects with impaired glucose tolerance have demonstrated not only an improvement in postprandial hyperglycemia but also cardiovascular benefits. Acarbose has been shown to slow the progression of thickening of the intima-media in the carotid arteries, reduce the incidence of cardiovascular disease, and reverse newly diagnosed hypertension. Recently, acarbose has been reported to improve insulin resistance in subjects with impaired glucose tolerance or type 2 diabetes. Due to these findings, acarbose has been suggested as treatment to reduce cardiovascular risk in subjects with metabolic syndrome (a cluster of risk factors including high triglycerides, low high-density lipoprotein [HDL] cholesterol, and hypertension).[6]

NATURAL SOURCES OF INHIBITORS

ACARBOSE

Acarbose is a natural product produced in large-scale fermentation from strains of *Actinoplanes* sp., a bacterium. Alpha-glucosidase and alpha-amylase inhibitors with activity against mammalian forms of the enzyme have also been identified in plants. It has been suggested that this activity in select plants may be, at least in part, the basis for their use in traditional medicine for the treatment of diabetes.[17]

BOTANICAL SOURCES OF CARBOHYDRATE INHIBITORS

Screening of plant extracts for *in vitro* activity against alpha-glucosidase and alpha-amylase has produced numerous "hits," with compounds classified as polyphenolics, terpenoids, and tannins identified as being active.[17] Specifically, anthocyanins and ellagitannins have been reported to inhibit alpha-glucosidase and alpha-amylase activity, respectively.[18] Alpha-glucosidase activity has been reported in anthocyanin-rich extracts of blueberry and black currant. While extracts of raspberry and strawberry, containing ellagitannins, were active against alpha-amylase. Other researchers investigated the ability of teas (green, oolong, and black) to inhibit alpha-amylase and alpha-glucosidase. Fully fermented black teas were the most potent in an *in vitro* model of starch digestion. The authors suggested that the theaflavins (and to a lesser extent the oxidized catechins) were responsible for the activity.[19]

Spondias mombin L "hog plum" leaves have been used by traditional healers in southwest Nigeria to manage diabetes. Studies in alloxan-induced diabetic rats demonstrated the ability of a preparation of the leaves to lower experimentally induced hyperglycemia. Activity-guided fractionation of the extract indicated that alpha-sitosterol may be the active constituent.[20] Investigations into *Salacia reticulata*, a plant traditionally used in the treatment of type 2 diabetes in Ayurvedic medicine, demonstrated that the constituents salacinol, kotalanol, and de-O-sulfonated kotalanol were effective inhibitors of maltase-glucoamylase (an intestinal glucosidase) *in vitro*.[21] A recent review covered 60 extracts prepared from plants using different solvents and 66 natural compounds that have demonstrated alpha-amylase and/or alpha-glucosidase inhibitory activity.[17]

ALPHA-AMYLASE INHIBITORS FROM GRAINS

Alpha-amylase inhibitors are also present in grains, including wheat and rice.[17] The alpha-amylase inhibiting activity in wheat was identified as a protein named 0.19-albumin, referring to its identifying location using gel electrophoresis. This protein makes up nearly 25% of wheat albumin (WA) but contributed 80% of the inhibitory activity *in vitro* against amylases from salivary glands and the pancreas.[22] The effects of this inhibitor were measured clinically in healthy subjects and those with type 2 diabetes. A single dose of 0, 0.25, 0.5, and 1.0 g was administered to healthy subjects along with a test meal. As a result, there was a dose-dependent reduction, 31%, 47%, and 50%, in peak postprandial blood glucose levels with the three respective dosages. This study was followed with a double-blind randomized controlled study with 24 type 2 diabetic subjects that studied the effects of 3 months administration of placebo or 0.5 g WA before each meal. This procedure did not lower fasting blood glucose levels but did lower hemoglobin HbA_{1c} levels (a measurement of average blood sugar levels over 3 months time). This effect was greater for those with an initial HbA_{1c} level of 7–8 than it was for those with an initial level of 6–7.[22] Follow-up studies in insulin-resistant rats indicated that WA inhibited the increase in plasma insulin and triacylglycerol which followed administration of starch.[23] In the human studies, administration of WA was not associated with hypoglycemia or gastrointestinal symptoms such as diarrhea, flatulence, or abdominal pain.[22] The study authors considered that WA is proteinous and could be digested by proteinases in the digestive tract, thereby losing its amylase-inhibiting activity. They considered that WA might delay the absorption of carbohydrate but not reduce the total amount of carbohydrate absorption. This rationale might account for the lack of hypoglycemia and deleterious effects on the gastrointestinal tract. A potential limitation of this treatment is that WA is an allergen for many people, and for those with this allergy, the use of WA would not be an option.

ALPHA-AMYLASE INHIBITORS FROM BEANS

The greatest body of research has gone into glycoproteins extracted from kidney beans (*Phaseolus vulgaris*). Common beans have three isoforms of alpha-amylase inhibitor (alpha-AI, alpha-AI2, alpha-AIL). The alpha-AI isoform has antiamylase activity in humans. This enzyme is found in the embryonic axes and cotyledons in the seed and not in other organs of the plant. It is not active against plant alpha-amylases and is therefore classified as an antifeedant or seed defense protein.[24]

The alpha-amylase inhibitor prevents starch digestion by completely blocking access to the active site of the alpha-amylase enzyme. Factors that affect the activity of the alpha-AI isoform inhibitor are pH, temperature, incubation time, and the presence of particular ions. The optimum pH for the inhibitor is 4.5–5.5 and the optimal temperature is 22°C–37°C. There is no activity at 0°C, and the inhibitor is completely inactivated by boiling for 10 min. The ideal incubation period has been recorded as 10, 40, and 120 min by three different researchers.[3] The different incubation times are thought to be due to the use of different test conditions, namely, a pH of 6.9 for the longer incubation periods and a pH of 4.5 for the shortest.[3]

Background Experiments in Humans

In the early 1980s, several products containing crude preparations of bean amylase inhibitors were marketed in the United States. However, early clinical studies were disappointing, and it was discovered that the preparations had insufficient enzyme-inhibiting activity, as well as issues with potency and stability. Subsequently, a research group at the Mayo Clinic developed a partially purified white bean product and published a series of studies exploring the activity of inhibitor in human clinical studies. The test product was described as a concentrate: six- to eightfold by total protein content and 30- to 40-fold by dry weight.[25] The product was found to inactivate salivary, intraduodenal, and intraileal amylase activity *in vitro*. Its activity was not affected by exposure to gastric juice and only minimally by duodenal juice (by 15%). *In vitro* studies demonstrated that the inhibitor decreased digestion of dietary starch in a dose-dependent manner.[25] Perfusion of the white bean product into the duodenum of human subjects completely inhibited the activity of intraluminal amylase activity (5 mg/mL at 5 mL/min).[25] Subsequent experiments were conducted with volunteers intubated with an oroileal tube in order to obtain duodenal, jejunal, and terminal ileal samples.[26] After intubation, the subjects ingested 50 g rice starch, and on the subsequent day, they ingested starch with the amylase inhibitor (5 or 10 g white bean extract). The white bean extract significantly reduced duodenal, jejunal, and ileal intraluminal amylase activity by more than 95%; it acted as quickly as 15 min and for as long as 2 h. It increased the postprandial delivery of carbohydrates to the distal small bowel by 22%–24% (as measured by oroileal tube aspiration) and increased hydrogen concentrations in the breath from 30 to 90 min after the meal. Hydrogen breath testing is an accepted method of determining carbohydrate malabsorption as colonic bacteria ferment carbohydrates into organic acids, carbon dioxide, and hydrogen. A percentage of these gases are absorbed into the portal blood stream and subsequently expired through the lungs.[27–29] The white bean extract also reduced the postprandial plasma glucose rose by 85% and eliminated the subsequent fall of glucose level to below fasting levels. The extract significantly lowered the postprandial plasma levels of insulin, C-peptide, and gastric inhibitory polypeptide.[26]

A follow-up study using subjects with diabetes mellitus demonstrated a decrease in the postprandial increases in plasma glucose and insulin levels.[30] Further studies revealed that a dose of 3.8 g white bean inhibitor could cause more than twice the amount of hydrogen in the breath following a standard spaghetti meal. The percentage of malabsorbed carbohydrate increased from 4.7% to 7.0% (p < 0.05). Also, the form of the inhibitor (powder, tablet) had no effect on the activity when taken with the spaghetti.[31] Follow-up studies found that a dose of 2.9 g was sufficient to significantly inhibit the postprandial increases in blood glucose, C-peptide, and gastric inhibitory polypeptide following 650-calorie meal containing carbohydrate, fat, and protein.[32] A longer-term study was conducted over 3 weeks with six non-insulin-dependent diabetics. The subjects were given sufficient white bean inhibitor to reduce the increase in postprandial plasma glucose by more than 30%: a dose of 4–6 g with each meal. As a result, there were significant decreases in postprandial glucose, C-peptide, insulin, and gastric inhibitory polypeptide along with a significant increase in hydrogen excretion in the breath. Diarrhea and gastrointestinal symptoms occurred the first day of administration of the inhibitor and resolved over the next couple of days.[33] A further experiment with 18 healthy subjects reported that carbohydrates perfused into the ileum delayed emptying of a meal infused into the stomach. In one-half of the subjects, the amylase inhibitor was added to the ileum perfusate. The inhibitor significantly reduced the absorption of carbohydrate from the ileum and enhanced the delay in gastric emptying. Plasma concentrations of C-peptide, glucagon, motilin, gastrin, and human pancreatic polypeptide were not influenced by changes in gastric emptying or by the ileal perfusates. However, the delay in gastric emptying was significantly associated with a decrease in plasma concentrations of gastric inhibitory polypeptide and neurotensin along with an increase in concentrations of peptide YY. This effect was caused by the delay in gastric emptying, rather than the other way around. Human polypeptide levels were not changed and the authors concluded that the hormonal changes were not mediated via the vagus nerve.[34]

Phase 2 Specifications

The Phase 2® product is a water extract of the white kidney bean (*Phaseolus vulgaris*) standardized to alpha-amylase (8;12;15;39) inhibiting units (Pharmachem Laboratories, Inc., Kearny, NJ). Phase 2 is produced from non-GMO whole white kidney beans, which are ground and then extracted for 4 h. The liquid is filtered and concentrated under vacuum. The extract is filtered again and then pasteurized before being spray dried. Phase 2 is odorless and tasteless. Each lot of Phase 2 has at least 3000 alpha-amylase inhibiting units (AAIU) per g when tested at a pH 6.8 using potato starch as the substrate and pancreatin as the enzyme source. The Phase 2 extraction process was designed to make it more potent and stable than the white bean product tested by the Mayo Clinic.

Phase 2 is used as a dietary supplement in various forms, including powders, tablets, capsules, and chewables. There are approximately 200 brands of nutritional supplement or weight-loss products in the worldwide market that contain Phase 2. A typical dose is one to two capsules, each containing 500 mg, taken before each of three daily meals, for a total of 1500–3000 mg per day. A private safety panel approved a maximum daily intake of 10,000 mg (10 g).[35]

Experiments conducted incorporating Phase 2 into food products have found that it can be incorporated into chewing gum, mashed potatoes, and yeast-raised dough (bread, pizza, etc.) without losing activity or altering the appearance, texture, or taste of the food.[36–38]

Clinical Studies Conducted with Phase 2

Ten clinical studies have demonstrated weight loss over time following administration of Phase 2. Three studies demonstrated significant loss of body weight with Phase 2 compared to a placebo control in people who are overweight or obese. The doses ranged from 445 mg for 4 weeks to 3000 mg for 8–12 weeks.[39–41] A placebo-controlled study showed a comparative loss in body weight only when subjects were stratified by dietary carbohydrate intake. Those who consumed the greatest amount of carbohydrate lost significant body weight in comparison to the placebo group.[42] Six additional studies reported a loss of weight over time.[43–48] Three clinical studies reported a reduction in serum triglycerides over time (Table 30.1).[44,45,48]

Weight Loss: Compared to Placebo

A 12 week randomized, double-blind, placebo-controlled trial included 60 overweight individuals (BMI between 24 and 32 kg/m²). The subjects consumed two soft chewables before each meal containing either Phase 2 (500 each mg) or placebo for 12 weeks. The Phase 2 group consumed a total of 3000 mg Phase 2 per day. A total of 88 men and women enrolled in the study, while 60 completed the study and were included in the analyses. There was a statistically significant weight reduction in the active group compared with the placebo group at weeks 6, 8, and 12. The amount of weight lost by the active group at 12 weeks was 6.9 ± 7.9 lb (average of 0.575 lb per week), while the placebo group gained 0.8 ± 6.1 lb (p = 0.029 between groups). There were no significant differences between groups in body fat, lean body mass, or body measurements (waist–hip circumferences). No adverse events were reported.[40]

A randomized, double-blind, placebo-controlled study was conducted with 60 slightly overweight subjects (5–15 kg overweight). The subjects were required to have a stable weight for the past 6 months and underwent a 2 week single-blinded, run-in period prior to randomization. The subjects took one tablet (active or placebo) per day for 30 consecutive days before a meal rich in carbohydrates (2000- to 2200-calorie diet). The active tablet contained 445 mg Phase 2 and 0.5 mg chromium picolinate (≈55 mcg elemental chromium). After 30 days, the active group had a significant reduction in body weight, BMI, fat mass, adipose tissue thickness, and waist/hip/thigh circumferences while maintaining lean body mass. The active group lost an average of 2.93 kg

TABLE 30.1

Phase 2 Clinical Data

Author, Date [Reference]	Study Design/Duration	Subjects	Purpose	Preparation/Dose	Main Results
Thom (2000)[43]	RPCT, 12 weeks	n = 40 (BMI 28–39)	Weight loss	400 mg Phase 2 three times after meals, total 1200 mg/day (other ingredients: inulin and *Garcinia* extract)	↓ Body weight, BMI, and % body fat in active group (p < 0.05); no effect in placebo group; no between-group analysis
Erner (2003)[44]	RPCT, 12 weeks, then open 12 weeks	n = 54 (BMI 24–36)	Weight loss	Thera-Slim: 1000 mg Phase 2 before two meals, total 2000 mg/day	Trend toward ↓ body weight, three times decrease in triglycerides; no between-group analysis
Rothacker (2003)[40]	RPCT, 12 weeks	n = 88 (BMI 24–32)	Weight loss	StarchAway chews: 1000 mg Phase 2 before three meals, total 3000 mg/day	↓ Body weight comparison to placebo (p < 0.05)
Udani (2004)[48]	RPCT, 8 weeks	n = 39 (BMI 30–43)	Weight loss	Phase 2 1500 mg two times, 3000 mg/day	↓ Body weight comparison to placebo (ns) ↓ triglycerides(ns)
Koike (2005)[45]	Open, 8 weeks	n = 10 (BMI 23–30)	weight loss	Three capsules Phaseolamin® 1600 diet two times daily; 750 mg Phase 2 daily	↓ Body weight (p = 0.002), calorie intake, BMI, triglycerides, and HDL (all p < 0.05)
Osorio (2005)[46]	Open, 30 days	n = 39 (overweight and obese)	Weight loss	PreCarb capsules: 1000 mg Phase 3 with meals, total 3000 mg/day	↓ Body weight and ↓ waist-to-hip ratio over time (both p < 0.001)
Celleno (2007)[39]	RPCT, 30 days	n = 60 (BMI avg 26)	Weight loss	Phase 2 + chromium; 445 mg extract daily	↓ Body weight (p < 0.001), BMI, body fat (both p < 0.01)
Vinson (2009)[49]	PCT, X-over, single dose	Part 1: n = 11, Part 2: n = 7	Plasma glucose	Phase 2 mixed with margarine or gravy, 750 or 1500 mg	↓ AUC postprandial blood glucose; higher dose (p < 0.05)
Udani (2009)[50]	RPC, X-over, single dose	n = 13 (BMI 18–25)	Plasma glucose	Phase 2 capsules or mixed with butter. 1500, 2000, 3000 mg	↓ AUC postprandial blood glucose; 3000 mg with butter (p < 0.05)
Wu (2010)[41]	RPCT, 60 days	n = 101 (BMI 25–40)	Weight loss	Phase 2; 1000 mg three times daily	↓ Body weight, waist circumference (both p < 0.01)

Note: DB, double-blind; PCT, placebo-controlled trial; RPCT, randomized placebo-controlled trial; X-over, crossover.

(6.45 lb) in 30 days compared with an average of 0.35 kg (0.77 lb) in the placebo group (p < 0.001). BMI in the test group was reduced from an initial 25.9 ± 2.0 (SEM) to 24.9 ± 1.9 (p < 0.01). The placebo showed no significant change from the initial 26.0 ± 2.3 (SEM). Body composition was measured with bioelectrical impedance. The active group demonstrated a 10.45% reduction in body fat compared with a 0.16% reduction in the placebo group (p < 0.001). Waist and hip circumferences measured in a standard way showed the same pattern as well. The active group demonstrated 2.93 and 1.48 cm reductions, respectively, compared with 0.46 and 0.11 cm reductions in the placebo group (p < 0.001). No adverse events were reported.[39]

A randomized, double-blind, placebo-controlled study was conducted in China with 101 volunteers who had a BMI between 25 and 40. The subjects were given a single capsule containing 1000 mg Phase 2 or placebo three times per day, just before meals, for 60 days. The active group ingested a total of 3000 mg Phase 2 per day. As a result, there was significant weight loss in the active groups compared to the placebo group after 30 and 60 days. After 60 days, the average weight loss in the active group was 1.9 ± 0.15 kg compared to 0.4 ± 0.13 kg in the placebo group (p < 0.001). There was also a significant reduction in waist measurement in the active group compared to the placebo group (1.9 ± 0.32 cm compared to 0.4 ± 0.26 [p < 0.001]). There was no effect on hip measurements. Blood chemistries did not change significantly over the 2 month study and no adverse side effects were reported.[41]

A 4 week, randomized, double-blind, placebo-controlled study conducted with 25 healthy overweight (BMI 25–30) subjects.[42] The subjects took 1000 mg of Phase 2 or an identical placebo twice a day (before breakfast and lunch) as part of a weight loss program, which included diet, exercise, and behavioral intervention. The subjects were given nutritional guidelines to standardize their calorie intake at 1800 kcal/day. Breakfast and lunch were provided to increase compliance. In addition, subjects met with a personal trainer to establish an exercise program and had a counseling session with a behavioral psychologist to identify psychological barriers to weight loss. As a result of this intervention, both groups reduced weight and waist size significantly compared to baseline, but there were no significant differences between groups. After 4 weeks, the active group lost 6.0 lb and the placebo group lost 4.7 lb compared to baseline (p = 0.0002 active and p = 0.0016 placebo). The active group lost a mean of 2.2 in. from their waists and the control group lost 2.1 in. from their waists compared to baseline (p = 0.050 and 0.0001, respectively). For exploratory analysis, subjects were stratified by dietary carbohydrate intake. In this analysis, the tertile that took in the most carbohydrates demonstrated significantly greater loss of body weight compared with the placebo group (8.7 lb vs. 1.7 lb, p = 0.04). This group also had a significantly greater loss in inches around the waist (3.3 vs. 1.3 in.; p = 0.01). There were no significant changes from baseline in hip circumference, triglycerides, fasting glucose, total cholesterol, appetite control, hunger, energy level, and percent body fat, nor were there any significant differences between groups. No side effects or adverse events were reported.[42]

Weight Loss: Over Time

In a randomized, double-blind, placebo-controlled trial, forty healthy overweight (BMI 27.5–39.0) were randomized and instructed to take two tablets of the test product immediately after all three meals (breakfast, lunch, and dinner) for 12 weeks.[43] Subjects were also instructed to follow a 1200 kcal/day low-fat diet. The tablets, 650 mg each, contained a proprietary blend (Suco-Bloc®) including 200 mg of Phase 2 (Leuven Bioproducts, Belgium), 200 mg of inulin (from chicory root), and 50 mg of Garcinia cambogia extract. The remaining 200 mg in the tablets were not described. All subjects were included in an intent-to-treat analysis, including seven subjects who dropped out of the study (six in the placebo arm, one in the active arm). After 12 weeks, the active group had a significant reduction in weight, BMI, and percent body fat compared to baseline, whereas there was no significant change in the placebo group. The active group lost an average of 3.5 kg (7.7 lb; p = 0.001) and the placebo group lost 1.3 kg (2.9 lb). BMI decreased by 1.3 kg/m^2 (p = 0.01) in the active group and by 0.5 kg/m^2 in the placebo group. Percent body fat (measured by bioelectrical impedance) decreased by 2.3% (p = 0.01) in the active group and by 0.7% in the placebo. Body mass analyses showed that the weight loss in the active group consisted mainly of fat loss as >85% of the weight loss was accounted for by fat. Between-group analysis was not provided for any of the variables. No adverse events were reported in either group.[43]

A 12 week, double-blind, placebo-controlled study was conducted, and this period was followed by additional 12 weeks wherein all the participants received active treatment.[44] In the first part of the study, the subjects took two capsules twice a day of placebo or Thera-Slim™. Thera-Slim™ capsules contained 500 mg Phase 2 plus 250 mg fennel seed powder. The placebo contained cellulose and fennel seed powder. The active group received a total of 2000 mg Phase 2 per day. The subjects were asked to eat a diet in which lunch and dinner contained 100–200 g of carbohydrates. Sixty overweight and obese adult subjects (BMI 24–36) were randomized and 54 completed the study. After the first 12 weeks, the active group lost an average of 1.4 lb and the placebo gained an average of 0.6 lb. Serum triglyceride levels dropped by almost 3.3 times in the active group compared to the placebo group (−38.1 vs. −11.9). The levels of total cholesterol and HDL were similar in both groups. No between-group analyses were included in the report. There were no adverse events reported after 24 weeks of usage.

A randomized, double-blind, placebo-controlled study was conducted with 39 obese subjects (BMI 30–43) who were randomly allocated to receive either 1500 mg of Phase 2 or an identical placebo twice daily with lunch and dinner for 8 weeks.[48] The active group received a total of 3000 mg Phase 2 per day. Subjects were instructed to consume a controlled high-fiber/low-fat diet that provided 100–200 g of complex carbohydrate intake per day. Subjects were also instructed to eat the majority of their carbohydrates during lunch and dinner since those were the meals at which the Phase 2 or placebo were taken. The amount of carbohydrate intake was determined for the subjects on the basis of their estimated daily maintenance carbohydrate requirement. Twenty-seven subjects completed the study (14 active and 13 placebo). After 8 weeks, the active group lost an average of 3.79 lb. (an average of 0.47 lb per week) compared with the placebo group which lost an average of 1.65 lb. (an average of 0.21 lb per week). The difference was not statistically significant with a two-tailed p-value of 0.35. Triglyceride levels in the Phase 2 group were reduced by an average of 26.3 mg/dL. This reduction was more than three times the average reduction of 8.2 mg/dL seen in the placebo group (p = 0.07).

Several secondary outcomes were measured during the study including body fat percentage, waist and hip circumferences, energy level, hunger, appetite, HbA_{1c}, and total cholesterol. For each of these secondary measures, no clinically or statistically significant differences were identified between the active and the placebo group. No adverse events occurred that were felt to be due to the active product. One placebo subject experienced abdominal pain, bloating, and gas, while one active group subject complained of an increased incidence of tension headaches. There were no clinically significant changes in biochemical indicators of safety, including serum electrolytes, and markers of kidney and liver function.[48]

Weight Loss: Open Studies

An open study was conducted with 10 healthy subjects (five men and five women) with a BMI between 23 and 30 and a body fat ratio of over 25% for men and over 30% for women.[45] The subjects took three capsules of Phaseolamin® 1600 diet twice a day, 30 min before lunch and dinner, for 8 weeks. The six capsules (1.5 g) contained 750 mg Phase 2, 200 mg clove, 20 mg lysine, 20 mg arginine, and 20 mg alanine.

Over the course of 8 weeks, calorie intake decreased from 1742 ± 254 kcal/day to 1525 ± 249 kcal/day (p = 0.01), and the subjects lost a significant amount of weight (2.4%; 74.5 ± 7.3 to 72.7 ± 7.8; p = 0.002). There were also a significant reduction in body fat (p < 0.001) and BMI (p = 0.002). There were reductions in waist and hip circumferences without a significant change in the ratio of waist-to-hip circumference. Over the 8 weeks, there were significant reductions in systolic and diastolic blood pressure (p = 0.01 and p < 0.001). There were also significant reductions in triglycerides (p = 0.019) and HDL cholesterol (p = 0.001), but not in total cholesterol or LDL cholesterol. There was no change in blood glucose levels, and no adverse events were reported.[45]

An open study was conducted with 50 healthy adult subjects who were overweight or obese. They were given Precarb (Natrol's Carb Intercept 500 mg capsules) containing Phase 2.[46] The subject took 1 g Precarb (two capsules) three times daily with high-carbohydrate meals for 30 days. A per-protocol analysis was conducted on the 37–39 subjects who completed the study. There was a significant reduction in mean body weight of 2.34 ± 2.21 kg (n = 37; p < 0.001) and a significant reduction in mean waist-to-hip ratio 2.77 ± 2.55 (n = 39; p < 0.001).

In an open-label study, 23 adult men and women (BMI 22) took "Super Bows Diet Type B," a granular food available in Japan that contains 500 mg Phase 2, Coleus forskohlii extract, and mushroom chitosan (Plus fort Barrious®) for a period of 8 weeks.[47] Super Bows Diet Type B was taken as one packet of powder in a glass of water 20 min before lunch and dinner. After 8 weeks, the product caused a significant decrease in body weight (0.78 ± 0.20 kg, p < 0.01) and percent body fat (1.19 ± 0.37%; p < 0.01). There was no change in calorie intake during this period. In 10 subjects who had a BMI over 24 and a total cholesterol over 220 mg/dL, there was a significant decrease in cholesterol after 4 and 8 weeks (25.3 ± 7.1 and 11.3 ± 4.0 mg/dL, respectively; both p < 0.05). There were temporary gastrointestinal symptoms such as bloating and constipation, but these symptoms disappeared following a few days of continuous intake of the product.

Glycemic Index

Four crossover clinical studies addressed the potential effect of Phase 2 on postprandial increases in blood sugar. All four studies indicated that Phase 2 could reduce postprandial spikes in blood sugar with a suggestion that the effect is dose related.

In the first study, a placebo-controlled, crossover study, 11 fasting subjects (men and women aged 21–57) were given four slices of white bread and 42 g (3 tbs.) of margarine with or without 1500 mg of Phase 2 (Phase 2 was added to the margarine).[49] The food contained a total of 610 calories, 60.5 of which came from carbohydrate. The tests were administered a week apart. Absorption and metabolism of carbohydrate was measured as levels of plasma glucose over time. In comparison to control, the glucose levels following the consumption of Phase 2 returned to baseline 20 min earlier. The area under the plasma glucose vs. time curve was 66% lower with Phase 2 compared to the control (p < 0.05). The authors concluded that this indicated that one-third of the carbohydrate in the bread was absorbed. However, actual absorption and subsequent excretion was not measured.

The second study, published in the same paper, was also a placebo-controlled, crossover study. Seven subjects (men and women 23–43 years old) were given a frozen dinner containing country fried steak, mash potatoes, green beans, and cherry-apple pie (630 cal with 64 g carbohydrate) with and without 750 mg Phase 2. In this study, the Phase 2 was mixed with the gravy. The effect of Phase 2 was to reduce the average plasma glucose vs. time curve by 28%, and the authors concluded that two-thirds of the carbohydrate in the meal was absorbed. The authors noted that there appeared to be a dose-related effect with the 1500 mg dose of Phase 2 being twice as effective as the 750 mg dose.[49]

A six-arm crossover study was conducted with 13 randomized subjects (BMI 18–25) to determine whether the addition of Phase 2 would lower the GI of a commercially available high-glycemic food (white bread).[50] Standardized GI testing was performed using capillary blood glucose measurements following ingestions of white bread with butter, with and without the addition of Phase 2 in capsule or powder form. In both formulations, Phase 2 was given in dosages of 1500, 2000, and 3000 mg. The powdered form was mixed with the butter. Statistical analysis was performed by one-way ANOVA of all seven treatment groups using unadjusted multiple comparisons (t-tests) to the white bread control. For the capsule formulation, the 1500 mg dose had no effect on the GI, and the 2000 and 3000 mg capsule doses caused insignificant reductions in GI. For the powder, the 1500 and 2000 mg doses caused insignificant reductions in the GI, while the 3000 mg dose caused a significant reduction in postprandial glucose levels (a reduction of 34.11%; p = 0.023).

A single-dose, double-blind, crossover test was conducted on the effects of Super Bows Diet Type B on blood sugar levels.[47] As previously stated, this product is a granular food available in Japan that contains 500 mg Phase 2, Coleus forskohlii extract, and mushroom chitosan. The experiment included 13 men and women with a fasting blood glucose level above 126 mg/dL. In two test periods 1 week apart, the subjects took a packet of product or placebo along with a glass of water 5 min before eating 300 g polished rice. Blood samples were taken before the intake of the rice and 30, 60, 90, and 120 min afterward. Blood sugar levels 30 min after eating the rice were significantly lower with the test product (p < 0.01). Plasma insulin levels were significantly lower compared to the control at 30 and 60 min after consuming the rice (p < 0.01).

Safety of Phase 2

In the human clinical studies reviewed earlier, there were no reports of serious side effects resulting from ingestion of white bean extracts. Clinical efficacy studies using doses of Phase 2 up to 3000 mg per day in divided doses for periods of 30 days to 24 weeks also reported no significant adverse events. An acute animal toxicity study was conducted in rats with Phase 2 at doses of 500–5000 mg/kg body weight along with a subchronic study of 90 days with doses of 200–1000 mg/kg. In response, there were no adverse reactions and signs of toxicity in biochemical and histopathological analysis.[51] A 28 day toxicity study conducted with male and female rats reported a no-adverse-effect level (NOAEL) of 2500 mg/kg/day.[52] Cantox Health Sciences International conducted a safety review of published and unpublished data on Phase 2, and the panel of experts concluded that it could be safely consumed at doses up to 10 g per day.[35]

Since alpha-amylase inhibitors prevent the degradation of complex carbohydrates into oligosaccharides, those carbohydrates will pass through the intestine into the colon. In the colon, bacteria will digest the complex carbohydrates, and this may initially cause gastrointestinal side effects such as flatulence and diarrhea. In the study conducted with Super Bows Diet Type B that contained Phase 2 along with other ingredients, there were temporary gastrointestinal symptoms including bloating and constipation, but these symptoms resolved with continued intake of the product.[47]

Raw beans contain phytohemagglutinin (PHA) at high levels which have been associated with toxic effects in animals and severe gastrointestinal disturbances in humans.[3] However, PHA levels in beans are drastically reduced by cooking. In addition, white beans have negligible amounts of PHA compared to colored beans. Phase 2 is a standardized white bean extract prepared using a specialized process which substantially inactivates hemagglutinating activity (HA) and trypsin-inhibiting activity (TIA). The finished product contains less than 700 HA units per g and less than 20 TIA units per mg dry weight.[35]

SUMMARY

Spikes in blood sugar and corresponding spikes in plasma insulin levels resulting from the intake of simple carbohydrates are associated with an increased risk of insulin resistance which can lead to the development and progression of cardiovascular disease. Low-carbohydrate diets (carbohydrate intake of 30–130 g/day) can assist in weight loss, glucose and insulin response, and cardiovascular risk factors in normal healthy subjects as well as those with metabolic syndrome and other diseases. Low-carbohydrate diets are associated with better glycemic control, lower serum levels of triglycerides and HDL cholesterol.[53] Low-carbohydrate diets may however be hard to maintain. An alternative to a low-carbohydrate diet is to emphasize carbohydrates with a low GI. Resistant starches are found naturally in seeds, legumes, and unprocessed whole grains. However, for individuals who are reluctant to change their diet, ingestion of carbohydrate digestion inhibitors might be more feasible.

Acarbose (Prandase®, Precose®), a prescription drug used to treat type 2 diabetes, inhibits alpha-glucosidase enzymes and thus delays the absorption of carbohydrate from the small intestine. Acarbose has also been shown to improve insulin resistance.[6] Screening of plant extracts for *in vitro* activity against alpha-glucosidase and alpha-amylase has produced numerous "hits." There is a correlation between plants containing these enzyme inhibitors and those used in traditional medicine systems to treat or prevent diabetes.[17] Other sources of inhibitors of carbohydrate digestion are common foods such as raspberries, strawberries, blueberries, and black currant.[54] An alpha-amylase inhibitor that has been isolated from wheat has shown promise in lowering average blood sugars (measured via HbA$_{1c}$) in type 2 diabetics.[22] However, the largest body of research has been conducted on an alpha-amylase inhibitor isolated from white beans (*Phaseolus vulgaris*) and a specific proprietary product called Phase 2. Clinical experiments conducted with the Phase 2 indicate that it reduces the rate of absorption of carbohydrates, thereby reducing the GI of foods. Clinical evidence also indicates that Phase 2 promotes weight loss when taken concurrently with meals containing carbohydrates. [55] Experiments conducted incorporating Phase 2 into food and beverage products have found that it can be integrated into various products without losing activity or altering the appearance, texture, or taste of the food. There have been no serious side effects reported following consumption of Phase 2. Gastrointestinal side effects are rare and diminish upon extended use of the product.

In conclusion, research to date indicates that inhibitors of carbohydrate digestion have the potential to play an important role in improving the health of those with impaired glucose tolerance and merit further development.

REFERENCES

1. World Health Organization. Obesity and overweight. http://www.who.int/mediacentre/factsheets/fs311/en/index.html. 2006. Accessed: August 2011.
2. Preuss HG. Bean amylase inhibitor and other carbohydrate absorption blockers: Effects on diabesity and general health. *J Am Coll Nutr* 2009;28:266–276.
3. Obiro WC, Zhang T, Jiang B. The nutraceutical role of the Phaseolus vulgaris alpha-amylase inhibitor. *Br J Nutr* 2008;100:1–12.
4. Food and Agriculture Organization, World Health Organization. Carbohydrates in human nutrition: Report of a joint FAO/WHO report. *FAO Food and Nutr Pap* 1998;66:1–140.
5. Radulian G, Rusu E, Dragomir A, Posea M. Metabolic effects of low glycaemic index diets. *Nutr J* 2009;8:5.
6. Yamagishi S, Matsui T, Ueda S, Fukami K, Okuda S. Clinical utility of acarbose, an alpha-glucosidase inhibitor in cardiometabolic disorders. *Curr Drug Metab* 2009;10:159–163.
7. Brand-Miller J, McMillan-Price J, Steinbeck K, Caterson I. Dietary glycemic index: Health implications. *J Am Coll Nutr* 2009;28 Suppl 1:446S–449S.
8. Barclay AW, Petocz P, McMillan-Price J et al. Glycemic index, glycemic load, and chronic disease risk–a meta-analysis of observational studies. *Am J Clin Nutr* 2008;87:627–637.
9. Thomas DE, Elliott EJ, Baur L. Low glycaemic index or low glycaemic load diets for overweight and obesity. *Cochrane Database Syst Rev* 2007;CD005105.
10. Krishnan S, Rosenberg L, Singer M et al. Glycemic index, glycemic load, and cereal fiber intake and risk of type 2 diabetes in US black women. *Arch Intern Med* 2007;167:2304–2309.
11. Villegas R, Liu S, Gao YT et al. Prospective study of dietary carbohydrates, glycemic index, glycemic load, and incidence of type 2 diabetes mellitus in middle-aged Chinese women. *Arch Intern Med* 2007;167:2310–2316.
12. Schulze MB, Liu S, Rimm EB, Manson JE, Willett WC, Hu FB. Glycemic index, glycemic load, and dietary fiber intake and incidence of type 2 diabetes in younger and middle-aged women. *Am J Clin Nutr* 2004;80:348–356.
13. Schulze MB, Schulz M, Heidemann C, Schienkiewitz A, Hoffmann K, Boeing H. Fiber and magnesium intake and incidence of type 2 diabetes: A prospective study and meta-analysis. *Arch Intern Med* 2007;167:956–965.
14. Englyst KN, Englyst HN. Carbohydrate bioavailability. *Br J Nutr* 2005;94:1–11.
15. Grabitske HA, Slavin JL. Low-digestible carbohydrates in practice. *J Am Diet Assoc* 2008;108:1677–1681.
16. Higgins JA. Resistant starch: Metabolic effects and potential health benefits. *J AOAC Int* 2004;87:761–768.
17. Tundis R, Loizzo MR, Menichini F. Natural products as alpha-amylase and alpha-glucosidase inhibitors and their hypoglycaemic potential in the treatment of diabetes: An update. *Mini Rev Med Chem* 2010;10:315–331.
18. McDougall GJ, Stewart D. The inhibitory effects of berry polyphenols on digestive enzymes. *Biofactors* 2005;23:189–195.
19. Koh LW, Wong LL, Loo YY, Kasapis S, Huang D. Evaluation of different teas against starch digestibility by mammalian glycosidases. *J Agric Food Chem* 2010;58:148–154.

20. Fred-Jaiyesimi AA, Wilkins MR, Abo KA. Hypoglycaemic and amylase inhibitory activities of leaves of Spondias mombin Linn. *Afr J Med Med Sci* 2009;38:343–349.

21. Sim L, Jayakanthan K, Mohan S et al. New glucosidase inhibitors from an ayurvedic herbal treatment for type 2 diabetes: Structures and inhibition of human intestinal maltase-glucoamylase with compounds from Salacia reticulata. *Biochemistry* 2010;49:443–451.

22. Kodama T, Miyazaki T, Kitamura I et al. Effects of single and long-term administration of wheat albumin on blood glucose control: Randomized controlled clinical trials. *Eur J Clin Nutr* 2005;59:384–392.

23. Murayama Y, Mochizuki K, Shimada M et al. Dietary supplementation with alpha-amylase inhibitor wheat albumin to high-fat diet-induced insulin-resistant rats is associated with increased expression of genes related to fatty acid synthesis in adipose tissue. *J Agric Food Chem* 2009;57:9332–9338.

24. Moreno J, Altabella T, Chrispeels MJ. Characterization of alpha-amylase-inhibitor, a lectin-like protein in the seeds of phaseolus vulgaris. *Plant Physiol* 1990;92:703–709.

25. Layer P, Carlson GL, DiMagno EP. Partially purified white bean amylase inhibitor reduces starch digestion in vitro and inactivates intraduodenal amylase in humans. *Gastroenterology* 1985;88:1895–1902.

26. Layer P, Zinsmeister AR, DiMagno EP. Effects of decreasing intraluminal amylase activity on starch digestion and postprandial gastrointestinal function in humans. *Gastroenterology* 1986;91:41–48.

27. Strocchi A, Corazza GR, Anania C et al. Quality control study of H2 breath testing for the diagnosis of carbohydrate malabsorption in Italy. The "Tenue Club" group. *Ital J Gastroenterol Hepatol* 1997;29:122–127.

28. Strocchi A, Corazza G, Ellis CJ, Gasbarrini G, Levitt MD. Detection of malabsorption of low doses of carbohydrate: Accuracy of various breath H2 criteria. *Gastroenterology* 1993;105:1404–1410.

29. Brummer RJ, Karibe M, Stockbrugger RW. Lactose malabsorption. Optimalization of investigational methods. *Scand J Gastroenterol Suppl* 1993;200:65–69.

30. Layer P, Rizza RA, Zinsmeister AR, Carlson GL, DiMagno EP. Effect of a purified amylase inhibitor on carbohydrate tolerance in normal subjects and patients with diabetes mellitus. *Mayo Clin Proc* 1986;61:442–447.

31. Brugge WR, Rosenfeld MS. Impairment of starch absorption by a potent amylase inhibitor. *Am J Gastroenterol* 1987;82:718–722.

32. Boivin M, Zinsmeister AR, Go VL, DiMagno EP. Effect of a purified amylase inhibitor on carbohydrate metabolism after a mixed meal in healthy humans. *Mayo Clin Proc* 1987;62:249–255.

33. Boivin M, Flourie B, Rizza RA, Go VL, DiMagno EP. Gastrointestinal and metabolic effects of amylase inhibition in diabetics. *Gastroenterology* 1988;94:387–394.

34. Jain NK, Boivin M, Zinsmeister AR, Brown ML, Malagelada JR, DiMagno EP. Effect of ileal perfusion of carbohydrates and amylase inhibitor on gastrointestinal hormones and emptying. *Gastroenterology* 1989;96:377–387.

35. Nicolosi R, Hughes D, Bechtel D. Evaluation of the generally recognized as safe (GRAS) status of Phase 2® white bean (*Phaseolus vulgaris*) extract. http://www.phase2info.com/pdf/science-dossier/phase2-gras-expert-report.pdf, 3-5-2007. Bridgewater, NJ, Cantox Health Sciences International.

36. Udani K. The mighty bean. *European Baker* 2005. Available at: http://www.phase2info.com/pdf/Phase2Study11.pdf

37. Das Y. Phase 2/starch lite. http://www.phase2info.com/pdf/Phase2_Study13.pdf ISSI no. P25036, pp. 1–7, 2007. Piscataway, NJ, ISSI Laboratories, Inc. Accessed: August 2011.

38. Das Y. Phase 2/starch lite in chewing gum. http://www.phase2info.com/pdf/Phase2_Study14.pdf ISSI no. P25036-B, pp. 1–4, 2007. Piscataway, NJ, ISSI Laboratories, Inc. Accessed: August 2011.

39. Celleno L, Tolaini MV, D'Amore A, Perricone NV, Preuss HG. A dietary supplement containing standardized Phaseolus vulgaris extract influences body composition of overweight men and women. *Int J Med Sci* 2007;4:45–52.

40. Rothacker D. Reduction in body weight with a starch blocking diet aid: Starch away comparison with placebo. http://www.phase2info.com/pdf/Phase2_Study6.pdf, 2003. Leiner Health Products. Accessed: August 2011.

41. Wu X, Xu X, Shen J, Perricone N, Preuss H. Enhanced weight loss from a dietary supplement containing standardized Phaseolus vulgaris extract in overweight men and women. *J Appl Res* 2010;10:73–79.

42. Udani J, Singh BB. Blocking carbohydrate absorption and weight loss: A clinical trial using a proprietary fractionated white bean extract. *Altern Ther Health Med* 2007;13:32–37.

43. Thom E. A randomized, double-blind, placebo-controlled trial of a new weight-reducing agent of natural origin. *J Int Med Res* 2000;28:229–233.

44. Erner S, Meiss D. Thera-slim for weight loss: A randomized double-blind placebo controlled study. http://www.phase2info.com/pdf/Phase2_Study8.pdf, 2003. Accessed: August 2011.

45. Koike T, Koizumi Y, Tang L, Takahara K, Saitou Y. The antiobesity effect and the safety of taking "Phaseolamin® 1600 diet". *J New Rem Clin* 2005;54:1–16.

46. Osorio L, Gamboa J. Random multicenter evaluation to test the efficacy of Phaseolus vulgaris (Precarb) in obese and overweight individuals. http://www.phase2info.com/pdf/Phase2_Study10.pdf Internal Report, 2005. Accessed: August 2011.

47. Yamada J, Yamamoto T, Yamaguchi T. Effects of combination of functional food materials on body weight, body fat percentage, serum triglyceride and blood glucose. http://www.phase2info.com/pdf/Phase2_Study15.pdf, 2007. Accessed: August 2011.

48. Udani J, Hardy M, Madsen DC. Blocking carbohydrate absorption and weight loss: A clinical trial using Phase 2 brand proprietary fractionated white bean extract. *Altern Med Rev* 2004;9:63–69.

49. Vinson J, Al Kharrat H, Shuta D. Investigation of an amylase inhibitor on human glucose absorption after starch consumption. *Open Nutraceut J* 2009;2:88–91.

50. Udani JK, Singh BB, Barrett ML, Preuss HG. Lowering the glycemic index of white bread using a white bean extract. *Nutr J* 2009;8:52.

51. Harikumar KB, Jesil AM, Sabu MC, Kuttan R. A preliminary assessment of the acute and subchronic toxicity profile of phase2: An alpha-amylase inhibitor. *Int J Toxicol* 2005;24:95–102.

52. Chokshi D. Subchronic oral toxicity of a standardized white kidney bean (Phaseolus vulgaris) extract in rats. *Food Chem Toxicol* 2007;45:32–40.

53. Hite AH, Berkowitz VG, Berkowitz K. Low-carbohydrate diet review: Shifting the paradigm. *Nutr Clin Pract* 2011;26:300–308.

54. McDougall GJ, Shpiro F, Dobson P, Smith P, Blake A, Stewart D. Different polyphenolic components of soft fruits inhibit alpha-amylase and alpha-glucosidase. *J Agric Food Chem* 2005;53:2760–2766.

55. Barrett ML, Udani JK. A proprietary alpha-amylase inhibitor from white bean (Phaseolus vulgaris): A review of clinical studies on weight loss and glycemic control. *Nutr J* 2011;10:24.

31 Vegetarian Diets in the Prevention and Treatment of Obesity

Kathryn T. Knecht, PhD, Hayden T. Cale, BS,
Hien T. Bui, PharmD, Don K. Tran, PharmD,
and Joan Sabate, MD, PhD

CONTENTS

INTRODUCTION

Vegetarian diets of varying degrees of restriction may be adopted for cultural, religious, or health reasons. In 2009, an estimated 3.4% of adults in the United States reported no consumption of meat, poultry, or seafood and thus could be described as vegetarian, while 0.8% omitted all animal-derived products (including milk, eggs, and honey) and could be described as vegan [1]. The official position statement of the American Dietetic Association states that "Appropriately planned vegetarian diets, including total vegetarian or vegan diets, are healthful, nutritionally adequate, and may provide health benefits in the prevention and treatment of certain diseases" [2]. Specifically, vegetarian diets have been linked with a decrease in the risk of ischemic heart disease and other obesity-related disorders [3,4] in some but not all studies. The topic of vegetarian diets and obesity has been reviewed by one of the authors and others; in general, body mass index (BMI) has been found to be lower in both men and women in vegetarians vs. nonvegetarians [5–8]. The discussion that follows in this chapter emphasizes results published within the last 10 years. This chapter first describes observational studies of populations who have self-selected either vegetarian or nonvegetarian diets, then factors that might affect the outcome of these observational studies. Subsequently, intervention studies of vegetarian diets are discussed, followed by an elaboration of potential mechanisms by which vegetarian diets might affect body weight.

STUDIES OF VEGETARIAN DIETS AND OBESITY

OBSERVATIONAL STUDIES

In Europe, the Oxford cohort of the European Prospective Investigation into Cancer and Nutrition (EPIC) recruited a significant proportion of vegetarians among its 65,000 subjects [9]. Categories studied included meat-eaters (omnivores), fish eaters (fish but no meat or poultry), lacto-ovo vegetarians (milk and eggs but no flesh foods), and vegans. Several analyses of these data indicated that meat-eaters had a higher mean BMI and higher incidence of being overweight ($25 > \text{BMI} > 29.9 \, \text{kg/m}^2$) or obese ($\text{BMI} > 30 \, \text{kg/m}^2$), even when correction was made for nondietary factors [4,10–15]. Body weight parameters for nonvegan vegetarians (e.g., lacto-ovo) or for those who eat fish but not meat were between those for meat-eaters and vegans [10,14,15], and only the BMI of meat-eaters was within the overweight range [13,14]. During a 5 year follow-up period of subjects from the EPIC–Oxford study, all dietary groups tended to increase BMI, but vegans and fish-eating women showed less gain than did meat-eaters. Interestingly, individuals who converted to a more vegetarian diet during the 5 year period had the smallest weight gain, and those reverting from a more vegetarian diet had a weight gain greater than any other group, including meat-eaters [16].

The U.K. Women's Cohort Study, with 35,372 participants, also demonstrated a lower BMI for vegetarians than for meat-eaters, although two groups of fish eaters had average BMIs as low as or lower than those of vegetarians. Only the meat-eating group had a BMI as high as the cutoff for the definition of overweight ($25.0 \, \text{kg/m}^2$) [17]. In the 5292 subjects of the Oxford Vegetarian Study, meat-eaters had a higher prevalence of being overweight or obese than non-meat-eaters (including fish eaters) and a higher mean BMI [18]. Results from the 55,459 members of the Swedish Mammography cohort also demonstrated that omnivores were heavier than semivegetarians, lacto-vegetarians, or vegans, with a higher BMI and risk of being overweight or obese; however, in none of these diet groups was the mean $\text{BMI} > 25$ [19]. Alewaeters et al. [20] found that 326 male and female Flemish vegetarians had a lower BMI than corresponding reference populations, with only the male reference cohort having mean BMIs in the overweight range.

In the 1817-member British Columbia Nutrition Survey, the mean BMI was $2.6 \, \text{kg/m}^2$ lower in female vegetarians than in their nonvegetarian counterparts; BMI was only $0.8 \, \text{kg/m}^2$ lower in male vegetarians compared to male nonvegetarians. Only 76 female vegetarians had a mean BMI within the normal range, and female vegetarians were found to have a lower waist circumference and a lower prevalence of being overweight or obese. Increased exercise by female vegetarians may have accounted for the differences in body composition in this particular study. The 30 male vegetarians had a 0.8 cm greater waist circumference than male nonvegetarians and a slightly greater incidence of being normal or overweight but a decreased incidence of obesity [21].

Buddhism promotes a vegetarian diet [22], and predominantly Tzu-Chi Buddhist nuns comprised a cohort of 49 Taiwanese vegetarians. These women had lower BMI, body weight, and waist and hip circumference than 49 age-matched omnivorous controls who were predominantly local hospital employees [23]. However, when Korean vegetarian Buddhist nuns and omnivorous Catholic nuns were compared, BMI of the omnivores was significantly lower, although both groups were of normal weight. Interestingly, body fat tended to decrease with the length of vegetarianism, suggesting that vegetarianism did exert some effect on body weight [22]. Studies of 363 Taiwanese women and of 49 Taiwanese parents of preschool children showed lower BMI for vegetarians than omnivores, although these differences were not statistically significant [24,25]. In the latter study, the percentage obesity was higher among omnivores [25].

In the United States, studies of the Seventh-Day Adventist population have shown an inverse correlation between vegetarianism and obesity. The teachings of this denomination endorse a healthy lifestyle and support vegetarianism, and approximately 50% of a cohort of 34,192 Californian Seventh-Day Adventists ate meat less than once a week. Within this population, BMI was significantly associated with diet, with only male and female vegetarians and female semivegetarians (poultry or fish, <1/week) having mean BMIs below 25 [26]. In the subsequent Adventist Health Study-2, BMI also varied with diet, with vegans < lacto-ovo vegetarians < pesco-vegetarians < semivegetarians < nonvegetarians [3,27]. Seventh-Day Adventist vegetarians in Barbados also showed a decreased risk of obesity compared to nonvegetarian Seventh-Day Adventists [28].

Data from the 13,313 respondents in the Continuing Survey of Food Intake by Individuals in the United States showed a decreased BMI in self-defined vegetarians vs. self-defined nonvegetarians, with further decreases in BMI in self-defined vegetarians who did not eat meat vs. those who did [29]. When vegetarianism in this cohort was defined by the absence of meat (including poultry and fish) on the survey date, vegetarians so defined had a lower BMI than any other group except for those reporting a high-carbohydrate diet adhering to the U.S. Department of Agriculture (USDA) food pyramid [30]. A cohort of 12 American vegetarian men had a nearly significantly lower BMI but also lower fat-free weight than 11 nonvegetarian controls [31].

The aforementioned studies focused on adult populations. The BMI of 22 Polish vegetarian children was slightly lower than that of 13 omnivore controls (15.7 vs. 16.0 kg/m^2), although the vegetarian children were older [32]. A study of 51 vegetarian children in Hong Kong found an increase in the prevalence of obesity relative to previously reported data from the local population [33], but a lack of physical activity in these children may have been a factor. Vegetarian preschoolers in Taiwan were also heavier than their omnivorous counterparts [25], although the prevalence of obesity was higher among omnivores. Vegetarian Australian adolescents had lower BMI and waist circumference than nonvegetarians [34]. In teens and young adults in the Project EAT-II study, BMI was higher in current teen vegetarians (mean age 17.2 years) than in former or never vegetarians, but these differences were not significant. In a young adult cohort (mean age 20.4 years), however, BMI was significantly lower in current vegetarians than in former or never vegetarians, and the percentage of overweight or obesity was also lower [35]. Among Jordan University students, vegetarianism was significantly associated with lower BMI [36]. In the Continuing Survey of Food Intake by Individuals, BMI tended to be lower for vegetarians ages 6–11 and 12–19 though differences were not significant [29].

Table 31.1 provides a summary of the previously described BMI data. Other anthropomorphic parameters were available in some but not all studies and thus were not put into tabular form. For male adults, a weighted average of available data resulted in mean BMI of 25.3 kg/m^2 for meat-eaters and 23.9 kg/m^2 for vegetarians, with a total of 13,902 meat-eaters and 5198 vegetarians [4,18,20,21,28,31]. For females, corresponding weighted BMIs were 24.6 and 23.2 kg/m^2, with a total of 110,660 meat-eaters and 21,437 vegetarians [4,17–24,28,37]. For both males and females, the weighted average BMI was 25.6 for 166,907 meat-eaters and 24.4 for 47,145 vegetarians [4,17–25, 27–29,31,35,37]. In this analysis, data from only the most recent reports of the EPIC–Oxford cohort and the Continuing Survey of Food Intake by Individuals were used [4,29]. For males 6 ft in height, the calculated average difference of 1.5 kg/m^2 in BMI between vegetarians and meat-eaters would correspond to a difference of 11 lb.

In addition to studies addressing vegetarianism *per se*, studies have examined the impact of consumption of animal foods. Total meat and red meat consumption, respectively, were found to correlate with increased body weight gain in the EPIC–PANACEA study [38] and in a Chinese population [39]. In a cohort of school-aged children, increased consumption of animal foods (meat, dairy, and eggs) was associated with increased risk of overweight [40]. Clusters of food choices have been categorized as "meat and alcohol," "prudent" or "healthy," "Mediterranean," "junk food," etc. Similar to studies described for vegetarians, Kesse-Guyot et al. found that a meat and alcohol pattern correlated with low physical activity, smoking, overweight, and abdominal obesity [41]. Among the 459 members of the Baltimore Longitudinal Study of Aging, vegetarianism *per se* was not

TABLE 31.1

Observational Studies on the Differences in BMI between Vegetarian and Nonvegetarian Diets

Author, Date [Reference]	Study Population	Number of Vegetarians/Total Number	Gender	BMI (kg/m^2) Meat-Eater	Vegetarian	Vegan	Difference, Meat-Eater vs. Vegetarian
Adults							
Key et al. (2009) [4]	EPIC–Oxford	16,081/47,254	Male	25.2	24.3[a]		−0.9
			Female	24.2	23.5[a]		−0.7
Cade et al. (2004) [17]	UK Women's Cohort Study	6,478/35,372	Female	25	23.3[a]		−1.7
Appleby et al. (1998) [18]	Oxford Vegetarian Study	2,847/5,292	Male	23.18	22.05[a]		−1.1
			Female	22.32	21.32[a]		−1.0
Newby et al. (2005) [19]	Swedish Mammography cohort	242/55,459	Female	24.7	23.4[a]	23.3[a]	−1.3
Alewaeters et al. (2005) [20]	Flemish vegetarians	326/9,659	Male	25.7	22.6[a]		−3.1
			Female	24.6	22.1[a]		−2.5
Bedford and Barr (2005) [21]	British Columbia vegetarian adults	106/1,817	Male	26.7	25.9		−0.8
			Female	25.7	23.1[a]		−2.6
Lee and Krawinkel (2009) [22]	Korean nuns	54/85	Female	20.7	22.6		1.9
Hung et al. (2006) [23]	Taiwanese vegetarian women	49/98	Female	22	20.9[a]		−1.1
Chen et al. (2011) [24]	Taiwanese females	173/363	Female	23.28	22.87		−0.41
Yen et al. (2008) [25]	Taiwanese parents	21/49	Male and female	23.2	22.6		−0.6

Reference	Population	n	Subgroup				
Tonstad et al. (2009) [27]	Adventist Health Study-2	20,408 (2,731)/51,900	Male and female	28.8	25.7[a]	23.6[a]	-3.1
Brathwaite et al. (2003) [28]	Seventh-Day Adventists, Barbados	177/407	Male	25.1	24.3		-0.8
			Female	27.8	27		-0.8
Haddad and Tanzman (2003) [29]	Continuing Survey of Food Intake by Individuals		Age ≥ 20	26.1	22.8[a]		-3.3
Poehlman et al. (1988) [31]	Vegetarian men	12/23	Male	24.4	22.7		-1.7
Barr and Broughton (2000) [37]	British Columbia vegetarian women	90/193	Female	23.5	23.2		-0.3
Weighted average			Male	25.32	23.86		
			Female	24.63	23.23		
			All	25.56	24.37		
Children							
Haddad and Tanzman (2003) [29]	Continuing Survey of Food Intake by Individuals	13/1,893	Male and female, 6–11 years old	18.5	17.3		-1.2
		19/1,380	Male and female, 12–19 years old	22.3	20		-2.3
Bas et al. (2005) [45]	Turkish adolescent vegetarians	31/1,205	Male	22.9	22.1[a]		-0.8
			Female	20.8	19.8[a]		-1.0
Ambroszkiewicz et al. (2004) [32]	Polish vegetarian children	22/35	Male and Female	16	15.7		-0.3
Robinson-O'Brien et al. (2009) [35]	EAT-II adolescents	32/698	Male and female	24	25		1
Grant et al. (2008) [34]	Australian adolescents	53/207	Male and female	21.9	20.5		-1.4

[a] Statistics provided, $p < 0.05$ vs. meat-eaters.

addressed, but a diet high in fruit, vegetables, whole grains, and dairy and low in red and processed meat was associated with the lowest baselines and smallest increases in BMI and waist circumference over time [42]. Only this healthy diet resulted in a mean BMI that started and remained within the normal range.

FACTORS AFFECTING THE IMPACT OF A VEGETARIAN DIET

The effect of a vegetarian diet may be varied by the length of time spent on the diet, the strictness of the diet, and the other lifestyle factors that may accompany vegetarianism; for example, it seems plausible that the effects of a vegetarian intervention might be most clearly seen with a longer time period. If overweight or obese individuals were to adopt a vegetarian diet in the short term as a means of weight loss, their presence in the vegetarian cohort would be likely to increase the mean body weight. In the EPIC–Oxford cohort and in a population of Seventh-Day Adventists in Barbados, the BMI was lowest for those who had been vegan or vegetarian for more than 5 years [11,28]. Mortality in the form of ischemic heart disease was also lower in those who had been vegetarian for more than 5 years, and body fat decreased in vegetarian Taiwanese women with length of vegetarianism [22]. Appleby et al. [18], however, found that the BMIs of non-meat-eaters who had not eaten meat for more than 5 years were only slightly and not significantly lower than those for individuals who had adopted a nonmeat diet within the last 5 years. Similarly, individuals becoming vegetarian as adults (>20 years) were no heavier than lifelong vegetarians.

Interestingly, the BMI was higher for men and women becoming vegetarians as children than for life-long vegetarians [13].

A possible complication in analyzing the effects of a vegetarian diet is that self-reported vegetarians may not adhere strictly to a vegetarian diet. As a practical concession, the definition of vegetarian has been drawn to include a minimal level of meat consumption, for example, meat or fish less than once a week or below 10 g/day [17,28]. Even so, discrepancies remain; only 18% of a study population qualified as vegetarian under a definition that included some meat consumption, although 28% considered themselves vegetarian [17]. Multiple studies report vegetarian consumption of fish, chicken, and even red meat at varying frequencies [20,21,35,43]. Bedford and Barr reported the percentages of vegetarian women eating fish or other seafood, poultry, or red meat at least occasionally were as high as 74.9%, 57.6%, and 22.4%, respectively [21]. Smith et al. [43] found that of 59 self-reported college student vegetarians, 40 (68%) had included poultry and/or fish in their diet. Newby et al. [19] found that although groups of "semivegetarians," "lacto-vegetarians," and "vegans" all consumed some animal products, these discrepancies did not alter the conclusions of their study. However, Haddad and Tanzman [29] reported that 214 of 334 "vegetarians" ate some meat, fish, or poultry on at least one of two dietary survey days and that non-meat-eating "vegetarians" had a lower mean BMI than meat-eating "vegetarians." The possibility remains that an effect of vegetarianism on leanness could be weakened by the inclusion of meat-eating "vegetarians" in the study cohort.

Conversely, when "vegetarian" was defined as those who did not consume meat on a given study day, the numbers of vegetarians by definition were higher than for self-defined vegetarians in the same cohort [29]. The BMI appears to be lower in vegetarians by any definition, but the combination of self-defined vegetarianism and the lack of meat (including poultry and seafood) resulted in the most marked decrease [29].

Another confounding factor may be that vegetarian populations may possess characteristics other than diet that may influence body weight. Vegetarians in general and vegans in particular have a decreased incidence of smoking and higher exercise levels and tend to be younger and of a higher social class [7,10,12,13,15,17,18,20,21,35,37,38,44], though Vergnaud et al. found that the lowest quintile of meat consumption in their study was less physically active [38]. Vegetarians were also more likely to be female [1,21] and to have a higher nutritional supplement use [17,21,36] and lower prescription medication use [20]. Alcohol use was reported to be higher among meat-eaters relative to non-meat-eaters [7,12,14,18,26], although wine drinking was also reported to be higher in non-meat-eaters [29]. Decreased body weight is cited among the top reasons for choosing a vegetarian diet [35,36,43,45], and, therefore, vegetarians may have preexisting concerns about health in general and weight in particular. It could be, in other words, that vegetarianism serves as a marker of a health-seeking personality [21] and that vegetarianism *per se* confers no additional advantages. Barr and Broughton [37] found that a convenience sample of 193 current, former, and nonvegetarian women, health conscious and demographically similar except for ethnic background and parity, did not differ significantly with regard to BMI, weight, or self-assessed weight or health, although only formerly vegetarian women had BMIs in the mean overweight range. Men who became vegetarian after age 20 had a lower BMI before beginning a vegetarian diet than did a corresponding same-age group of meat-eaters [16]. Among individuals of normal body weight, it is certainly less likely that any dietary change would exert a noticeable effect since there is less body fat to be affected. No differences were seen in BMI between Taiwanese vegetarians and nonvegetarians, but BMI for both groups was already low [22]. However, in the EPIC–Oxford study, BMI was lower for vegetarians even though all participants were generally health conscious and had lower mortality than the general population [4].

Cultural differences may also make interpretation of different studies more difficult. Fraser suggests that "high" consumption of fruits and vegetables in the British EPIC study might correspond to low consumption in the Mediterranean EPIC cohort [3]. A vegetable-rich dietary pattern in Chinese adults was associated with greater weight gain than a traditional, meat-containing diet, but increased energy consumption from oil used in stir-frying and concurrent wheat consumption could be responsible [46]. Widely varying levels of meat intake among the different countries of the EPIC–Oxford cohort [38] could blunt the contrast between vegetarian and nonvegetarian groups. It may be that results may be clearer if the broad category of "vegetarian" is subdivided into specific types [3].

INTERVENTION STUDIES

A more direct analysis on the impact of vegetarian diets on body weight can be found with intervention studies (Table 31.2). Phillips et al. [47] examined the effect on 33 volunteers of a 6 month diet excluding meat but including fish. Although weight, BMI, and waist-to-hip ratio were not altered, significant decreases were seen in mid–upper arm circumference, skinfold measurements, percent body fat, and waist and hip circumferences. During a crossover study, 35 women reduced their weight and BMIs during a low-fat vegetarian diet phase lasting two menstrual cycles [48]

Barnard et al. [49,50] and Turner-McGrievy et al. [51] studied 59 obese women assigned to either a low-fat vegan diet or a diet following the National Cholesterol Education Program Step II guidelines, with limits on fat, saturated fat, and cholesterol, and percentages of energy from protein and carbohydrate at 15% and >55%, respectively. The vegan group had a greater decrease in body weight, BMI, and waist circumference over the 14 weeks period than did the Step II group, although the means of both groups remained in the obese range [50,51]. In a group of 14 women assigned to a lifestyle intervention including vegetarian diet, BMI decreased slightly but significantly more than in a group of 11 controls [52]. After 6 months of either a reduced-calorie, low-fat lacto-ovo diet or a reduced-calorie, low-fat omnivorous diet, there was no statistically significant difference in weight, BMI, or waist circumference between the two groups. However, when a distinction was made between subjects who were adherent and nonadherent to the vegetarian diet, adherent subjects had greater decreases in weight and BMI, while adherent women had greater decreases in waist circumference as well [53]. After 18 months, both vegetarians and nonvegetarians experienced weight loss, but there was no significant difference between groups [54].

As with cross-sectional studies, results may be attributable to the personal characteristics of individuals amenable to a vegetarian diet and not to the diet itself. For example, individuals who are already health conscious might show less improvement. Delgado et al. [55] found that a 2 month transition from a Mediterranean diet to a lacto-ovo vegetarian diet did not affect the body composition

TABLE 31.2
Direct Analysis on the Impact of Vegetarian Diets on Body Weight

Author, Date [Reference]	Study Population	Number in Intervention/ Control Group	Type of Study	Dietary Intervention	Control	Length of Study	Change in BMI	
							Intervention	Control
Barnard et al. (2000) [48]	Premenopausal women	35	Crossover	Low-fat vegetarian diet phase	Placebo "supplement phase"	2 menstrual cycles	0.9[a]	0.3
Barnard et al. (2005) [50] Turner-McGrievy et al. (2004) [51]	Obese postmenopausal women	29	Parallel	Low-fat vegan diet	National Cholesterol Education Program Step II guidelines	14 weeks	2.1[a]	1.4
Toobert et al. (2000) [52]	Postmenopausal women	14	Parallel	Lifestyle intervention including mostly vegan diet	Usual care	24 months	1[a]	0
Burke et al. (2006) [53]	Overweight and obese adults	35/48	Parallel	Calorie-restricted, low-fat, lacto-ovo vegetarian diet	Calorie-restricted, low-fat, omnivorous diet	6 months	3.87[a]	1.91
Burke et al. (2008) [54]	Overweight and obese adults with preferred diet	35/48	Parallel	Calorie-restricted, low-fat, lacto-ovo vegetarian diet	Calorie-restricted, low-fat, omnivorous diet	6 months	5.3	3.9
Burke et al. (2008) [54]	Overweight and obese adults with assigned diet	45/48	Parallel	Calorie-restricted, low-fat, lacto-ovo vegetarian diet	Calorie-restricted, low-fat, omnivorous diet	18 months	7.9	8
Phillips et al. (2004) [47]	Recent vegetarians	33	Pre-post	Diet excluding meat but including fish	Baseline	6 months	0.1[b]	—

[a] Results significantly different compared to control group.
[b] Other parameters of body fat show significant change.

of 14 individuals; however, study subjects were current or former physical education students who did not consume significant quantities of fast food, so nutritional changes and possible room for weight improvement may have been minimal. Barnard et al. [48] found that individuals with initial BMIs < 22.0 kg/m^2 lost less weight (in kg) than those with initial BMIs > 22 kg/m^2.

Preference could play an important role in the success of a dietary intervention [56]; however, Barnard et al. [48] found no demographic differences between 35 completers and 16 noncompleters of their dietary intervention. Burke et al. found that after 18 months, individuals assigned randomly to a diet actually lost more weight than those assigned to their diet of preference, though adherence was similar for random and preferred groups [54].

One aspect of a vegetarian diet that may be of practical benefit is that long-term adherence to a vegetarian diet may be greater than adherence to a "weight-loss" diet. Smith et al. [43] reported that the median times a group of college students adhered to weight-loss diets and vegetarian diets were 3 months and 24 months, respectively. Loss of interest was more commonly cited as a reason for quitting for the weight-loss group than for the vegetarian group. The BMI was lower for students who had been on a vegetarian diet at any time than for those who had been on a weight-loss diet at any time (whether or not they had ever tried a vegetarian diet) or neither; mean BMIs for all groups were within the normal range. Barnard et al. reported that a vegan diet had a high degree of acceptability compared to a National Cholesterol Education Program Step II diet and was comparable in adherence and acceptability to a American Diabetes Association diet [49,57]. Over an 18 month period, adherence to a lacto-ovo diet was only 38% [58], but this diet was also calorie restricted and low fat, and adherence to an omnivorous, calorie-restricted, and low-fat diet was similarly low.

NUTRITIONAL DIFFERENCES BETWEEN VEGETARIAN AND NONVEGETARIAN DIETS

Vegetarian and nonvegetarian diets are defined by the presence or absence of meat and other animal products. Vegetarians presumably eat more plant-based foods to compensate for the missing animal products; thus, the nutrient profile of vegetarian and nonvegetarian diets is likely to be different. Table 31.3 shows differences in dietary components reported for vegetarian and nonvegetarian diets. Vegetarian diets may facilitate weight loss for a number of different possible reasons, presumably mediated by the differences in composition. Lower concentrations of some dietary components and higher concentrations of others may each have their own effects. Vegetarian diets have been found for the most part to be lower in overall energy [14,17,19,23,30], protein [14,17,19,21,23,30,31,37], fat [14,17,19,21,23,25,30,31], saturated fat [14,17,19,23,30], and cholesterol [21,29,37]. Vegetarian diets tended to be higher in fiber [17,19,21–23,25,29,31,37] and carbohydrate [17,19,21,30,31,37]. Omega-3 polyunsaturated fatty acids (PUFAs) in diet and plasma, in particular eicosapentaenoic acid (EPA)

TABLE 31.3
Dietary Components Reported in Vegetarian Diets

Dietary Components Reported in Lower Concentrations in Vegetarian Diets [17,19,21,23,25,29,31,37]	Dietary Components Reported in Higher Concentrations in Vegetarian Diets [17,19,21–23,25,29–31,37]
Energy	Fiber
Protein	Carbohydrate
Fat	
Saturated fat	
Cholesterol	
(Omega-3) PUFAs	
Monounsaturated fatty acids	

---

and docosahexaenoic acid (DHA), were reported to be lower in vegetarians [2,14,19,23], although increased overall PUFA levels could be due to omega-6 fatty acids [2,14,17]. Consumption of fish by "vegetarians" may affect omega-3 fatty acid levels [29]. Monounsaturated fatty acids were lower in the diet of vegetarians [17,19,29,30]. Possible roles for each of these dietary components in affecting body weight will be discussed individually.

POSSIBLE MECHANISMS FOR SPECIFIC DIETARY COMPONENTS

ENERGY

The balance of energy intake and expenditure determines whether a person will gain or lose weight, and a low-fat, lower-calorie diet (plus exercise) is a standard behavioral treatment for obesity [56]. Indeed, as described earlier, many analyses of vegetarian diets show a decreased energy (caloric) content, and decreased energy was correlated with weight loss [37]. Kennedy et al. [30] suggested that any diet sufficiently reducing energy intake should lead to weight loss. Decreased energy intake should not be confused with consciously restricted food intake, as total energy decreased with vegetarian diets even when food portions were not deliberately limited [47,50,51]; rather, a vegetarian diet was associated with decreased hunger scores [49]. A fiber-rich vegetarian diet is therefore typically less energy-dense than a diet high in animal fats, and a high energy intake would be more difficult to achieve. A fiber-rich, low–glycemic index (GI) diet, rich in fruits and vegetables, could contribute to an earlier feeling of satiety and decreased voluntary intake [59–63]. It should be noted that leptin, one of the hormones associated with satiety, was decreased in 22 vegetarian children ages 2–10 years relative to 13 omnivore controls [32]. Leptin is primarily derived from adipocytes; thus, decreased leptin may be a consequence of decreased body fat [64].

Reports of decreased energy intake do not automatically correspond to decreased weight in those individuals [55]. Decreased energy expenditure and resting metabolic rate may counter decreased energy intake with vegetarian diets, negating some of the beneficial effect of energy reduction [50]. The effects of a decrease in energy intake might be masked if heavier individuals were to underreport intake [65], had remained on a diet for too short a time for effects on weight to be noticed, or were within normal weight range and had no excess body fat to lose [55].

Furthermore, decreased energy intake may act in conjunction with other factors, as oily-fish eaters consumed more calories than meat-eaters or vegetarians but had a lower BMI than any of the other groups [17]. Meat consumption *per se* was associated with increased weight gain in the EPIC–PANACEA study, even after correction for energy density; thus, factors other than the caloric density of meat are implicated [38]. Similarly, individuals lost more weight on a vegan diet than on a National Cholesterol Education Program Step II diet, although both had decreased energy intake [50]. Vegetarians in this latter study had less fat and more carbohydrate relative to the Step II group. It may be that macronutrient balance is important; therefore, the effects of the three main macronutrients (i.e., protein, fat, and carbohydrate) are considered individually.

PROTEINS

The removal of meat from the diet is a simple modification that is easy to implement and maintain and produces favorable changes in body composition [37,43,47,49]. The absence of red meat, primarily beef, was associated with a decreased BMI in Seventh-Day Adventists [26], while increased meat consumption is associated with weight gain [38,39]. Meat contributes significant amounts of protein as well as energy-dense saturated fat, and it could displace fiber- and nutrient-rich plant foods in the diet. Meat may also serve as a marker for general overnourishment. As described earlier, vegetarians typically eat less dietary protein than do meat-eaters. The exact mechanism of how this decrease in protein might affect weight loss is unclear. With regard to increased body weight of meat-eaters, it has been suggested that high protein consumption early in life could result in increased insulin-like growth factor, which might lead to adipocyte replication as well as decreased growth hormone [66,67]; however, individuals becoming vegetarian as children were heavier than adult-onset vegetarians, and lifelong vegetarians were no different in BMI from adult-onset vegetarians [13].

High-protein diets have in fact been used as an approach to weight loss, and it has been reported that the high-protein content increases satiety and thermogenesis [68–74]. Protein preloads increased satiety relative to a glucose preload and corresponded with decreases in the appetite-inducing hormone ghrelin and increases in satiety-inducing cholecystokinin (CCK) and glucagon-like peptide 1 (GLP-1) [75,76]. Ghrelin was decreased more by a high-protein breakfast than a high-carbohydrate breakfast [77]. Increased satiety and decreased hunger and actual or desired food intake were noted for 19 and 57 subjects placed on a high-protein diet, although in these subjects ghrelin was increased [71,78]. Raben et al. [79], however, found no effect of high protein on postprandial satiety, and Nickols-Richardson et al. [70] found no difference in actual energy intake between high-protein and high-carbohydrate diets, although hunger scores were lower in the high-protein group.

Diet-induced thermogenesis is defined as the expenditure of energy required for absorbing, processing, and storing of nutrients. Expressed as a percentage of the energy content of each macronutrient, reported values range from 20%–30% for protein to 5%–10% for carbohydrates and 0%–3% for lipids [80]. A protein-rich diet, then, requires more energy to digest and store and should therefore, in theory, generate fewer calories left over for storage. Johnston et al. [68] observed increased thermogenesis and a slightly higher postmeal body temperature in volunteers after high-protein meals vs. high-carbohydrate meals, Raben et al. [79] reported 17% higher thermogenesis after a protein meal than after fat or carbohydrate meals, and Tentolouris et al. found a threefold increase in thermogenesis after a protein-rich meal compared to a fat-rich meal. Correspondingly, it might be expected that lower-protein vegetarian diets would be less thermogenic and more conducive to weight increase. Indeed, Poehlman et al. [31] found a decreased postprandial thermic response in a group of 12 vegetarian men vs. a group of 11 normal controls. Weigle et al. [71], however, found that thermogenesis did not significantly increase with a high-protein diet, and Barnard et al. [50] found an increased thermic effect in vegetarians compared to nonvegetarians.

Thus, there appears to be no clear mechanism by which low protein *per se* could lead to decreased weight, and, in fact, an increased amount of protein might seem to be more effective in weight loss. However, plant-based and meat-based diets differ in amino acid makeup as well as protein quantity. Lin et al. found that in a Belgian population, animal protein was positively associated with BMI, while plant protein was negatively associated [81]. Similarly, a vegetable-based, low-carbohydrate diet but not an animal-based, low-carbohydrate diet was associated with lower cardiovascular mortality, which presumably would include a weight component [82]. In a study of 12 young men, pork protein produced higher total daily energy expenditure than soy protein [69], possibly because soy protein was less able to support energetically costly protein turnover. However, a comparison of meat, dairy, and soy meals found no difference in energy expenditure, only a decrease in protein oxidation with meat [74].

Plant proteins contain more nonessential amino acids than do animal proteins. A higher intake of nonessential amino acids can tend to downregulate insulin and upregulate glucagon, thereby decreasing fat synthesis and increasing fat oxidation [50,66,83]. Taiwanese vegetarians who consumed large amounts of soy-based proteins had greater insulin sensitivity [23]. Relative decreases in essential amino acids have also been associated with lower levels of insulin-like growth factor 1 (IGF-1) in vegan women [84], possibly resulting in adipocyte stimulation [66]. Correspondingly, increased risk of diabetes is correlated with increased consumption of meat, especially processed meats [44,85]. There was an increased risk of diabetes with an increase in total or animal-based protein, but not plant or cereal protein [86].

In regard to satiety, a preload of plant protein in the form of tofu and mushroom mycoprotein had a greater effect on satiety than did chicken protein, and study participants did not compensate for the lower food intake at lunch by eating more at dinner [87]. In human duodenal tissue, pea and wheat proteins were more effective in releasing satiety hormones than were egg or codfish proteins [88].

Carbohydrates

As discussed, vegetarian diets on average contain more carbohydrates than do meat-containing diets. Carbohydrate ingestion, which results in increased blood glucose, stimulates the secretion of insulin, which, in turn, removes glucose from the blood and increases fat storage. Increased insulin would also promote more rapid onset of hunger by clearing glucose from the bloodstream more quickly [89]. In the liver, increased insulin after a high-carbohydrate meal has a fat-sparing effect, decreasing fat oxidation [79,90]. Carbohydrates would therefore appear to promote weight gain via the effects of insulin; however, sources of carbohydrates differ in regard to glucose release. In a vegetarian diet, carbohydrates may be more likely to come from fruits, vegetables, and unrefined grains with a lower GI rather than from higher GI foods such as white bread [19,26,42,91]. Low-GI carbohydrates would by definition release glucose more slowly and therefore produce less of an insulin response. Dietary carbohydrate may be better than dietary fat at suppressing postprandial ghrelin and increasing leptin. Both of these changes would increase satiety and decrease food intake [71,92], although Raben et al. [79] found no difference in satiety among meals rich in protein, refined carbohydrate, or fat; however, satiety effects may be more relevant with low-GI foods. However, though there is evidence for benefit of GI on satiety, this evidence is not conclusive [93,94]. Similarly, there is some evidence that a lower glycemic load (GL), reflecting net quantity as well as quality of carbohydrate, seems to be related to reduced body weight [93,95,96]. Gaessner summarizes data indicating an inverse relationship between carbohydrate intake and BMI, possibly related to dietary fiber [96].

Fiber

Dietary fiber consists of nondigestible, plant-derived carbohydrates and lignin [97] and is increased in vegetarian diets. Data from 14 cohorts of 12 studies indicate a median increase in fiber intake of 5.5 g for vegetarians vs. meat-containing diets, with a weighted average of 28.9 g for total fiber intake of vegetarians [14,17–19,21–23,25,29,31,32,37]. In the National Health and Nutrition Examination Survey 1999–2004, decreased body weight correlated with increased whole grain and fiber consumption [98]. In the Oxford Vegetarian Study, fiber was a factor that was associated with lower BMI in both men and women [18]. Increased fiber was associated with lower BMI in 2165 women but not 2374 men in the Continuing Survey of Food Intakes by Individuals [97]. Fiber was inversely associated with weight gain over an 8 year period in a prospective cohort of 27,082 men [63] and in a cohort of 74, 091 middle-aged women [62]. Weight gain in men was decreased by 2.51 kg for every 20 g/day fruit fiber, by 0.81 kg for every 20 g/day cereal fiber, and by 0.36 kg for every 20 g/day added bran [62], and an intake of 14 g/day of fiber for 2 or more days appeared to correspond with a 10% decrease in energy intake [99]. Pereira and Ludwig [100] discuss three mechanisms by which fiber could lower body weight. First, fiber has a low energy density. Because of its bulk and because of associated fluid, fiber in the diet can lead to a fuller stomach and increased satiety. Increased satiety plus the lower palatability of fiber-rich foods could subsequently decrease energy intake. Second, changes in the consistency and movement of food in the gut can alter the generation of satiety-related hormones such as CCK, gastric inhibitory peptide (GIP), GLP-1, and insulin. Third, fiber fermentation generates short-chain fatty acids that can decrease hepatic glucose production and FFA, further affecting insulin secretion and sensitivity.

Dietary Fats

As described earlier, vegetarian diets on the average tend to be lower in fat than meat-containing diets, although Fraser [26] noted that the diet of Seventh-Day Adventist vegetarians was not necessarily low in fat. Low fat consumption and low fat in conjunction with fiber were associated with a lower BMI in men and women, respectively [101]. In the EPIC–Potsdam cohort, foods high in fat were correlated with increased weight gain in women [102]. High levels of dietary fat would not appear to be desirable with regard to weight loss. The high energy density of fats plays an important role in increasing energy intake and body weight [103], and fat as a palatable food suppresses satiety, possibly through insulin or leptin resistance [104]. Furthermore, a high-fat diet has little thermogenic effect [80]. Dietary fat upregulates acyl-CoA:monoacylglycerol acyltransferase (MGAT), an enzyme involved in fat absorption and storage [105].

It may be that the type of fat is as important as total fat content. Appleby et al. [18] found that lowered consumption of animal fat, which is high in saturated fat, was a significant factor contributing to low body mass in non-meat-eaters. Several studies have found that switching from saturated to monounsaturated fat decreased body fat [106–108]. Saturated fatty acids have been reported to produce less satiety and stimulate less fatty acid oxidation relative to unsaturated fats [109,110], although several later studies showed no difference in satiety or energy expenditure for several different sources of fatty acid [111–116]. Furthermore, saturated fat has been associated with higher insulin resistance relative to monounsaturated fat [107,117,118], although again this association has not been consistently found [115,119]. Saturated fat is lower in a vegetarian diet [14,17,19,23,30], but monounsaturated [17,19,29,30] and omega-3 PUFAs [2,14,19,23] were decreased as well. Although several mechanisms exist by which increased PUFA intake could lead to decreased obesity and insulin resistance [120], there is no clearly established role for polyunsaturated fats in obesity or insulin resistance *in vivo* [119,121].

DOES THE DECREASE IN BMI ASSOCIATED WITH A VEGETARIAN DIET IMPLY BETTER HEALTH?

A presumption of this discussion is that a decreased body weight represents a healthy change. A counterexample might be the decreased body weight associated with the unhealthful practice of smoking. Smokers, for example, tend to have lower body weight, and smoking cessation is associated with weight gain [16], but overall the practice of smoking would not be considered beneficial. It could also be that the lower BMIs result from reduced muscle mass; thus, the possibility must be considered that decreased body weight in vegetarians results from inadequate nutrition that could adversely affect health. However, the average BMI values for all vegetarian groups described earlier were within normal limits.

Although vegetarian diets are considered to be appropriate and healthful [2], a poorly planned vegetarian diet could contribute to malnutrition; for example, vegetarians can be more likely to have dietary deficiencies in a number of micronutrients including B12 and vitamin D [6,29,37,51,122]. A deficiency in B12 was cited as a possible cause of elevated homocysteine in Turkish female vegetarians [123]. Vegetarians and especially vegans have lower levels of the omega-3 PUFAs that are considered protective in cardiovascular and other diseases, yet they have less ischemic heart disease [6,14]. Perry et al. [91], however, found that adolescent vegetarians had a healthier diet than nonadolescent vegetarians, and vegetarian diets can be appropriately used to support athletic performance [6,122].

Mortality from ischemic heart disease was decreased in vegetarian populations [7], although the corresponding decrease in an EPIC–Oxford cohort was not significant and all-cause mortality increased slightly [12]. However, a study of Chinese vegetarians demonstrated poorer vascular health, possibly related in part to decreased B12 and increased sodium and carbohydrate intake [124].

A cohort of 30 male vegetarians was more likely to report heart disease than a comparison group of nonvegetarians; however, because they also were more likely to choose foods based on effects on heart disease and high blood pressure, it may be that cardiovascular problems were a cause and not a consequence of vegetarianism [21]. Similarly, individuals with higher cardiovascular risk factors may have chosen a prudent diet as a response to these risk factors [21,39,41]. Vegetarians had less self-reported illness than meat-eaters [17], higher health perception, and less prescription drug use [20], although Barr and Broughton [37] found no differences in health assessment among health-conscious women with differing dietary patterns, and a cohort with the lowest quintile of meat consumption was more likely to have reported previous illness [38].

In a negative light, vegetarianism was also linked with eating disorders in Turkish adolescents, although young vegetarians cited "taste preference" and "healthier diet" above "weight control" as reasons for their dietary practices [43,45]. Only 24% of a cohort of college students who had ever tried a vegetarian diet expected to lose weight, although 59% of the students who had at some point tried a weight-loss diet expected weight loss from a vegetarian diet [43]. Adolescent and young adult vegetarians were more likely to indulge in binge eating than nonvegetarians, and current and former vegetarians were more likely than nonvegetarians to have practiced extreme unhealthful weight-control measures such as diet pills or vomiting [35].

CONCLUSIONS

A large body of evidence suggests that vegetarian populations have a decreased body weight compared to corresponding populations of nonvegetarians, although the increased health consciousness of individuals drawn toward vegetarianism may be a contributing factor. Intervention studies suggest benefits from switching to a meatless diet, with the advantage that such diets may be more easily adopted and sustained than a standard weight-loss diet. Even periods as short as 14 weeks generated improvement; more benefit was seen at >5 years, but lifelong vegetarianism did not appear to be necessary nor was strict adherence to a vegetarian diet required, as many "vegetarians" admitted consuming some flesh foods, particularly fish and poultry. A number of possible mechanisms for the benefits of a vegetarian diet have been suggested, resulting mostly from increases or decreases in dietary macronutrients. Meat and concomitantly protein, fat, and energy are decreased, while carbohydrate and fiber are generally increased. An additional benefit of a plant-based diet is presumably increased intake of plant antioxidants, polyphenols, and other phytochemicals. Although these components may be secondary to macronutrients in regard to protection from obesity, they may contribute to the cardiovascular and other health benefits reported for vegetarian diets.

ACKNOWLEDGMENTS

The authors wish to thank Ms. Maria Knecht for assistance with references and Dr. Karen Jaceldo-Siegl for statistical advice.

REFERENCES

1. Stahler C. How many vegetarians are there? *Veg J*. 2009;22(3):8.
2. Craig WJ, Mangels AR. Position of the American Dietetic Association: Vegetarian diets. *J Am Diet Assoc*. Jul 2009;109(7):1266–1282.
3. Fraser GE. Vegetarian diets: What do we know of their effects on common chronic diseases? *Am J Clin Nutr*. May 2009;89(5):1607S–1612S.
4. Key TJ, Appleby PN, Spencer EA, Travis RC, Roddam AW, Allen NE. Mortality in British vegetarians: Results from the European Prospective Investigation into Cancer and Nutrition (EPIC-Oxford). *Am J Clin Nutr*. May 2009;89(5):1613S–1619S.
5. Berkow SE, Barnard N. Vegetarian diets and weight status. *Nutr Rev*. Apr 2006;64(4):175–188.
6. Key TJ, Appleby PN, Rosell MS. Health effects of vegetarian and vegan diets. *Proc Nutr Soc*. Feb 2006;65(1):35–41.
7. Key TJ, Fraser GE, Thorogood M et al. Mortality in vegetarians and nonvegetarians: Detailed findings from a collaborative analysis of 5 prospective studies. *Am J Clin Nutr*. Sep 1999;70 (3 Suppl):516S–524S.
8. Sabate J, Blix G. Vegetarian diets and obesity prevention. In Sabate J (ed.), *Vegetarian Nutrition*. Boca Raton, FL: CRC Press; 2001, pp. 91–107.
9. EPIC Study of Nutrition and Health. Available at http://www.epic-oxford.org/ (accessed December 16, 2010).

10. Davey GK, Spencer EA, Appleby PN, Allen NE, Knox KH, Key TJ. EPIC-Oxford: Lifestyle characteristics and nutrient intakes in a cohort of 33 883 meat-eaters and 31 546 non meat-eaters in the UK. *Public Health Nutr.* May 2003;6(3):259–269.

11. Key T, Davey G. Prevalence of obesity is low in people who do not eat meat. *BMJ.* Sep 28 1996;313(7060):816–817.

12. Key TJ, Appleby PN, Davey GK, Allen NE, Spencer EA, Travis RC. Mortality in British vegetarians: Review and preliminary results from EPIC-Oxford. *Am J Clin Nutr.* Sep 2003;78(3 Suppl):533S–538S.

13. Rosell M, Appleby P, Key T. Height, age at menarche, body weight and body mass index in life-long vegetarians. *Public Health Nutr.* Oct 2005;8(7):870–875.

14. Rosell MS, Lloyd-Wright Z, Appleby PN, Sanders TA, Allen NE, Key TJ. Long-chain n-3 polyunsaturated fatty acids in plasma in British meat-eating, vegetarian, and vegan men. *Am J Clin Nutr.* Aug 2005;82(2):327–334.

15. Spencer EA, Appleby PN, Davey GK, Key TJ. Diet and body mass index in 38000 EPIC-Oxford meat-eaters, fish-eaters, vegetarians and vegans. *Int J Obes Relat Metab Disord.* Jun 2003;27(6):728–734.

16. Rosell M, Appleby P, Spencer E, Key T. Weight gain over 5 years in 21,966 meat-eating, fish-eating, vegetarian, and vegan men and women in EPIC-Oxford. *Int J Obes.* Sep 2006;30(9):1389–1396.

17. Cade JE, Burley VJ, Greenwood DC. The UK Women's Cohort Study: Comparison of vegetarians, fish-eaters and meat-eaters. *Public Health Nutr.* Oct 2004;7(7):871–878.

18. Appleby PN, Thorogood M, Mann JI, Key TJ. Low body mass index in non-meat eaters: The possible roles of animal fat, dietary fibre and alcohol. *Int J Obes Relat Metab Disord.* May 1998;22(5):454–460.

19. Newby PK, Tucker KL, Wolk A. Risk of overweight and obesity among semivegetarian, lactovegetarian, and vegan women. *Am J Clin Nutr.* Jun 2005;81(6):1267–1274.

20. Alewaeters K, Clarys P, Hebbelinck M, Deriemaeker P, Clarys JP. Cross-sectional analysis of BMI and some lifestyle variables in Flemish vegetarians compared with non-vegetarians. *Ergonomics.* Sep 15– Nov 15 2005;48(11–14):1433–1444.

21. Bedford JL, Barr SI. Diets and selected lifestyle practices of self-defined adult vegetarians from a population-based sample suggest they are more 'health conscious'. *Int J Behav Nutr Phys Act.* Apr 13 2005;2(1):4.

22. Lee Y, Krawinkel M. Body composition and nutrient intake of Buddhist vegetarians. *Asia Pac J Clin Nutr.* 2009;18(2):265–271.

23. Hung CJ, Huang PC, Li YH, Lu SC, Ho LT, Chou HF. Taiwanese vegetarians have higher insulin sensitivity than omnivores. *Br J Nutr.* Jan 2006;95(1):129–135.

24. Chen CW, Lin CT, Lin YL, Lin TK, Lin CL. Taiwanese female vegetarians have lower lipoprotein-associated phospholipase A2 compared with omnivores. *Yonsei Med J.* Jan 1 2011;52(1):13–19.

25. Yen CE, Yen CH, Huang MC, Cheng CH, Huang YC. Dietary intake and nutritional status of vegetarian and omnivorous preschool children and their parents in Taiwan. *Nutr Res.* Jul 2008;28(7):430–436.

26. Fraser GE. Associations between diet and cancer, ischemic heart disease, and all-cause mortality in non-Hispanic white California Seventh-Day Adventists. *Am J Clin Nutr.* Sep 1999;70(3 Suppl):532S–538S.

27. Tonstad S, Butler T, Yan R, Fraser GE. Type of vegetarian diet, body weight, and prevalence of type 2 diabetes. *Diabetes Care.* May 2009;32(5):791–796.

28. Brathwaite N, Fraser HS, Modeste N, Broome H, King R. For the patient. Are vegetarians at less risk for obesity, diabetes, and hypertension? Obesity, diabetes, hypertension, and vegetarian status among Seventh-Day Adventists in Barbados: Preliminary results. *Ethn Dis.* Winter 2003;13(1):148.

29. Haddad EH, Tanzman JS. What do vegetarians in the United States eat? *Am J Clin Nutr.* Sep 2003;78(3 Suppl):626S–632S.

30. Kennedy ET, Bowman SA, Spence JT, Freedman M, King J. Popular diets: Correlation to health, nutrition, and obesity. *J Am Diet Assoc.* Apr 2001;101(4):411–420.

31. Poehlman ET, Arciero PJ, Melby CL, Badylak SF. Resting metabolic rate and postprandial thermogenesis in vegetarians and nonvegetarians. *Am J Clin Nutr.* Aug 1988;48(2):209–213.

32. Ambroszkiewicz J, Laskowska-Klita T, Klemarczyk W. Low serum leptin concentration in vegetarian prepubertal children. *Rocz Akad Med Bialymst.* 2004;49:103–105.

33. Leung SS, Lee RH, Sung RY et al. Growth and nutrition of Chinese vegetarian children in Hong Kong. *J Paediatr Child Health.* Jun 2001;37(3):247–253.

34. Grant R, Bilgin A, Zeuschner C et al. The relative impact of a vegetable-rich diet on key markers of health in a cohort of Australian adolescents. *Asia Pac J Clin Nutr.* 2008;17(1):107–115.

35. Robinson-O'Brien R, Perry CL, Wall MM, Story M, Neumark-Sztainer D. Adolescent and young adult vegetarianism: Better dietary intake and weight outcomes but increased risk of disordered eating behaviors. *J Am Diet Assoc.* 2009;109(4):648–655.

36. Suleiman AA, Alboqai OK, Kofahi S, Aughsteen AA, Masri KE. Vegetarianism among Jordan University students. *J Biol Sci*. 2009;9(3):237–242.

37. Barr SI, Broughton TM. Relative weight, weight loss efforts and nutrient intakes among health-conscious vegetarian, past vegetarian and nonvegetarian women ages 18 to 50. *J Am Coll Nutr*. Nov–Dec 2000;19(6):781–788.

38. Vergnaud AC, Norat T, Romaguera D et al. Meat consumption and prospective weight change in participants of the EPIC-PANACEA study. *Am J Clin Nutr*. Aug 2010;92(2):398–407.

39. Xu F, Yin XM, Tong SL. Association between excess bodyweight and intake of red meat and vegetables among urban and rural adult Chinese in Nanjing, China. *Asia Pac J Public Health*. 2007;19(3):3–9.

40. Sabate J, Wien M. Vegetarian diets and childhood obesity prevention. *Am J Clin Nutr*. May 2010;91(5):1525S–1529S.

41. Kesse-Guyot E, Bertrais S, Peneau S et al. Dietary patterns and their sociodemographic and behavioural correlates in French middle-aged adults from the SU.VI.MAX cohort. *Eur J Clin Nutr*. Apr 2009;63(4):521–528.

42. Newby PK, Muller D, Hallfrisch J, Qiao N, Andres R, Tucker KL. Dietary patterns and changes in body mass index and waist circumference in adults. *Am J Clin Nutr*. Jun 2003;77(6):1417–1425.

43. Smith CF, Burke LE, Wing RR. Vegetarian and weight-loss diets among young adults. *Obes Res*. Mar 2000;8(2):123–129.

44. Vang A, Singh PN, Lee JW, Haddad EH, Brinegar CH. Meats, processed meats, obesity, weight gain and occurrence of diabetes among adults: Findings from Adventist Health Studies. *Ann Nutr Metab*. 2008;52(2):96–104.

45. Bas M, Karabudak E, Kiziltan G. Vegetarianism and eating disorders: Association between eating attitudes and other psychological factors among Turkish adolescents. *Appetite*. Jun 2005;44(3):309–315.

46. Shi Z, Yuan B, Hu G, Dai Y, Zuo H, Holmboe-Ottesen G. Dietary pattern and weight change in a 5-year follow-up among Chinese adults: Results from the Jiangsu Nutrition Study. *Br J Nutr*. Nov 25 2010:1–8.

47. Phillips F, Hackett AF, Stratton G, Billington D. Effect of changing to a self-selected vegetarian diet on anthropometric measurements in UK adults. *J Hum Nutr Diet*. Jun 2004;17(3):249–255.

48. Barnard ND, Scialli AR, Bertron P, Hurlock D, Edmonds K, Talev L. Effectiveness of a low-fat vegetarian diet in altering serum lipids in healthy premenopausal women. *Am J Cardiol*. Apr 15 2000;85(8):969–972.

49. Barnard ND, Scialli AR, Turner-McGrievy G, Lanou AJ. Acceptability of a low-fat vegan diet compares favorably to a step II diet in a randomized, controlled trial. *J Cardiopulm Rehabil*. Jul–Aug 2004;24(4):229–235.

50. Barnard ND, Scialli AR, Turner-McGrievy G, Lanou AJ, Glass J. The effects of a low-fat, plant-based dietary intervention on body weight, metabolism, and insulin sensitivity. *Am J Med*. Sep 2005;118(9):991–997.

51. Turner-McGrievy GM, Barnard ND, Scialli AR, Lanou AJ. Effects of a low-fat vegan diet and a Step II diet on macro- and micronutrient intakes in overweight postmenopausal women. *Nutrition*. Sep 2004;20(9):738–746.

52. Toobert DJ, Glasgow RE, Radcliffe JL. Physiologic and related behavioral outcomes from the Women's Lifestyle Heart Trial. *Ann Behav Med*. Winter 2000;22(1):1–9.

53. Burke LE, Styn MA, Steenkiste AR, Music E, Warziski M, Choo J. A randomized clinical trial testing treatment preference and two dietary options in behavioral weight management: Preliminary results of the impact of diet at 6 months—PREFER study. *Obesity (Silver Spring)*. Nov 2006;14(11):2007–2017.

54. Burke LE, Warziski M, Styn MA, Music E, Hudson AG, Sereika SM. A randomized clinical trial of a standard versus vegetarian diet for weight loss: The impact of treatment preference. *Int J Obes*. Jan 2008;32(1):166–176.

55. Delgado M, Gutierrez A, Cano MD, Castillo MJ. Elimination of meat, fish, and derived products from the Spanish-Mediterranean diet: Effect on the plasma lipid profile. *Ann Nutr Metab*. 1996;40(4):202–211.

56. Burke LE, Choo J, Music E et al. PREFER study: A randomized clinical trial testing treatment preference and two dietary options in behavioral weight management—Rationale, design and baseline characteristics. *Contemp Clin Trials*. Feb 2006;27(1):34–48.

57. Barnard ND, Gloede L, Cohen J et al. A low-fat vegan diet elicits greater macronutrient changes, but is comparable in adherence and acceptability, compared with a more conventional diabetes diet among individuals with type 2 diabetes. *J Am Diet Assoc*. Feb 2009;109(2):263–272.

58. Burke LE, Hudson AG, Warziski MT et al. Effects of a vegetarian diet and treatment preference on biochemical and dietary variables in overweight and obese adults: A randomized clinical trial. *Am J Clin Nutr*. Sep 2007;86(3):588–596.

59. Rolls BJ, Drewnowski A, Ledikwe JH. Changing the energy density of the diet as a strategy for weight management. *J Am Diet Assoc.* May 2005;105(5 Suppl 1):S98–S103.
60. Rolls BJ, Roe LS, Meengs JS. Reductions in portion size and energy density of foods are additive and lead to sustained decreases in energy intake. *Am J Clin Nutr.* Jan 2006;83(1):11–17.
61. Warren JM, Henry CJ, Simonite V. Low glycemic index breakfasts and reduced food intake in preadolescent children. *Pediatrics.* Nov 2003;112(5):e414.
62. Liu S, Willett WC, Manson JE, Hu FB, Rosner B, Colditz G. Relation between changes in intakes of dietary fiber and grain products and changes in weight and development of obesity among middle-aged women. *Am J Clin Nutr.* Nov 2003;78(5):920–927.
63. Koh-Banerjee P, Franz M, Sampson L et al. Changes in whole-grain, bran, and cereal fiber consumption in relation to 8-y weight gain among men. *Am J Clin Nutr.* Nov 2004;80(5):1237–1245.
64. McDuffie JR, Riggs PA, Calis KA et al. Effects of exogenous leptin on satiety and satiation in patients with lipodystrophy and leptin insufficiency. *J Clin Endocrinol Metab.* Sep 2004;89(9):4258–4263.
65. Maurer J, Taren DL, Teixeira PJ et al. The psychosocial and behavioral characteristics related to energy misreporting. *Nutr Rev.* Feb 2006;64(2 Pt 1):53–66.
66. McCarty MF. The origins of western obesity: A role for animal protein? *Med Hypotheses.* Mar 2000;54(3):488–494.
67. Rolland-Cachera MF, Deheeger M, Bellisle F. Nutrient balance and body composition. *Reprod Nutr Dev.* Nov–Dec 1997;37(6):727–734.
68. Johnston CS, Day CS, Swan PD. Postprandial thermogenesis is increased 100% on a high-protein, low-fat diet versus a high-carbohydrate, low-fat diet in healthy, young women. *J Am Coll Nutr.* Feb 2002;21(1):55–61.
69. Mikkelsen PB, Toubro S, Astrup A. Effect of fat-reduced diets on 24-h energy expenditure: Comparisons between animal protein, vegetable protein, and carbohydrate. *Am J Clin Nutr.* Nov 2000;72(5):1135–1141.
70. Nickols-Richardson SM, Coleman MD, Volpe JJ, Hosig KW. Perceived hunger is lower and weight loss is greater in overweight premenopausal women consuming a low-carbohydrate/high-protein vs high-carbohydrate/low-fat diet. *J Am Diet Assoc.* Sep 2005;105(9):1433–1437.
71. Weigle DS, Breen PA, Matthys CC et al. A high-protein diet induces sustained reductions in appetite, *ad libitum* caloric intake, and body weight despite compensatory changes in diurnal plasma leptin and ghrelin concentrations. *Am J Clin Nutr.* Jul 2005;82(1):41–48.
72. Westerterp-Plantenga MS, Nieuwenhuizen A, Tome D, Soenen S, Westerterp KR. Dietary protein, weight loss, and weight maintenance. *Annu Rev Nutr.* 2009;29:21–41.
73. Halton TL, Hu FB. The effects of high protein diets on thermogenesis, satiety and weight loss: A critical review. *J Am Coll Nutr.* Oct 2004;23(5):373–385.
74. Tan SY, Batterham M, Tapsell L. Energy expenditure does not differ, but protein oxidation rates appear lower in meals containing predominantly meat versus soy sources of protein. *Obes Facts.* 2010;3(2):101–104.
75. Bowen J, Noakes M, Clifton PM. Appetite regulatory hormone responses to various dietary proteins differ by body mass index status despite similar reductions in *ad libitum* energy intake. *J Clin Endocrinol Metab.* Aug 2006;91(8):2913–2919.
76. Bowen J, Noakes M, Clifton PM. Appetite hormones and energy intake in obese men after consumption of fructose, glucose and whey protein beverages. *Int J Obes.* Nov 2007;31(11):1696–1703.
77. Blom WA, Lluch A, Stafleu A et al. Effect of a high-protein breakfast on the postprandial ghrelin response. *Am J Clin Nutr.* Feb 2006;83(2):211–220.
78. Moran LJ, Luscombe-Marsh ND, Noakes M, Wittert GA, Keogh JB, Clifton PM. The satiating effect of dietary protein is unrelated to postprandial ghrelin secretion. *J Clin Endocrinol Metab.* Sep 2005;90(9):5205–5211.
79. Raben A, Agerholm-Larsen L, Flint A, Holst JJ, Astrup A. Meals with similar energy densities but rich in protein, fat, carbohydrate, or alcohol have different effects on energy expenditure and substrate metabolism but not on appetite and energy intake. *Am J Clin Nutr.* Jan 2003;77(1):91–100.
80. Tappy L. Thermic effect of food and sympathetic nervous system activity in humans. *Reprod Nutr Dev.* 1996;36(4):391–397.
81. Lin Y, Bolca S, Vandevijvere S et al. Plant and animal protein intake and its association with overweight and obesity among the Belgian population. *Br J Nutr.* Dec 9 2010:1–11.
82. Fung TT, van Dam RM, Hankinson SE, Stampfer M, Willett WC, Hu FB. Low-carbohydrate diets and all-cause and cause-specific mortality: Two cohort studies. *Ann Intern Med.* Sep 7 2010;153(5):289–298.
83. Krajcovicova-Kudlackova M, Babinska K, Valachovicova M. Health benefits and risks of plant proteins. *Bratisl Lek Listy.* 2005;106(6–7):231–234.

84. Allen NE, Appleby PN, Davey GK, Kaaks R, Rinaldi S, Key TJ. The associations of diet with serum insulin-like growth factor I and its main binding proteins in 292 women meat-eaters, vegetarians, and vegans. *Cancer Epidemiol Biomarkers Prev.* Nov 2002;11(11):1441–1448.

85. van Dam RM, Willett WC, Rimm EB, Stampfer MJ, Hu FB. Dietary fat and meat intake in relation to risk of type 2 diabetes in men. *Diabetes Care.* Mar 1 2002;25(3):417–424.

86. Pounis GD, Tyrovolas S, Antonopoulou M et al. Long-term animal-protein consumption is associated with an increased prevalence of diabetes among the elderly: The Mediterranean Islands (MEDIS) study. *Diabetes Metab.* Dec 2010;36(6 Pt 1):484–490.

87. Williamson DA, Geiselman PJ, Lovejoy J et al. Effects of consuming mycoprotein, tofu or chicken upon subsequent eating behaviour, hunger and safety. *Appetite.* Jan 2006;46(1):41–48.

88. Geraedts MC, Troost FJ, Tinnemans R, Soderholm JD, Brummer RJ, Saris WH. Release of satiety hormones in response to specific dietary proteins is different between human and murine small intestinal mucosa. *Ann Nutr Metab.* 2010;56(4):308–313.

89. Bell SJ, Sears B. Low-glycemic-load diets: Impact on obesity and chronic diseases. *Crit Rev Food Sci Nutr.* 2003;43(4):357–377.

90. Koutsari C, Sidossis LS. Effect of isoenergetic low- and high-carbohydrate diets on substrate kinetics and oxidation in healthy men. *Br J Nutr.* Aug 2003;90(2):413–418.

91. Perry CL, McGuire MT, Neumark-Sztainer D, Story M. Adolescent vegetarians: How well do their dietary patterns meet the healthy people 2010 objectives? *Arch Pediatr Adolesc Med.* May 2002;156(5):431–437.

92. Monteleone P, Bencivenga R, Longobardi N, Serritella C, Maj M. Differential responses of circulating ghrelin to high-fat or high-carbohydrate meal in healthy women. *J Clin Endocrinol Metab.* Nov 2003;88(11):5510–5514.

93. Niwano Y, Adachi T, Kashimura J et al. Is glycemic index of food a feasible predictor of appetite, hunger, and satiety? *J Nutr Sci Vitaminol.* Jun 2009;55(3):201–207.

94. Flint A, Moller BK, Raben A et al. Glycemic and insulinemic responses as determinants of appetite in humans. *Am J Clin Nutr.* Dec 2006;84(6):1365–1373.

95. Livesey G, Tagami H. Interventions to lower the glycemic response to carbohydrate foods with a low-viscosity fiber (resistant maltodextrin): Meta-analysis of randomized controlled trials. *Am J Clin Nutr.* Jan 2009;89(1):114–125.

96. Gaesser GA. Carbohydrate quantity and quality in relation to body mass index. *J Am Diet Assoc.* Oct 2007;107(10):1768–1780.

97. Academies IoMotN. Dietary reference intakes: Proposed definition of dietary fiber. 2001. http://www.iom.edu/Reports/2001/Dietary-Reference-Intakes-Proposed-Definition-of-Dietary-Fiber.aspx (accessed December 20, 2010).

98. O'Neil CE, Zanovec M, Cho SS, Nicklas TA. Whole grain and fiber consumption are associated with lower body weight measures in US adults: National Health and Nutrition Examination Survey 1999–2004. *Nutr Res.* 2010;30(12):815–822.

99. Howarth NC, Saltzman E, Roberts SB. Dietary fiber and weight regulation. *Nutr Rev.* May 2001;59(5):129–139.

100. Pereira MA, Ludwig DS. Dietary fiber and body-weight regulation. Observations and mechanisms. *Pediatr Clin North Am.* Aug 2001;48(4):969–980.

101. Howarth NC, Huang TT, Roberts SB, McCrory MA. Dietary fiber and fat are associated with excess weight in young and middle-aged US adults. *J Am Diet Assoc.* Sep 2005;105(9):1365–1372.

102. Schulz M, Kroke A, Liese AD, Hoffmann K, Bergmann MM, Boeing H. Food groups as predictors for short-term weight changes in men and women of the EPIC-Potsdam cohort. *J Nutr.* Jun 2002;132(6):1335–1340.

103. Astrup A. The role of dietary fat in obesity. *Semin Vasc Med.* Feb 2005;5(1):40–47.

104. Erlanson-Albertsson C. How palatable food disrupts appetite regulation. *Basic Clin Pharmacol Toxicol.* Aug 2005;97(2):61–73.

105. Cao J, Hawkins E, Brozinick J et al. A predominant role of acyl-CoA:Monoacylglycerol acyltransferase-2 in dietary fat absorption implicated by tissue distribution, subcellular localization, and up-regulation by high fat diet. *J Biol Chem.* Apr 30 2004;279(18):18878–18886.

106. Fernandez de la Puebla RA, Fuentes F, Perez-Martinez P et al. A reduction in dietary saturated fat decreases body fat content in overweight, hypercholesterolemic males. *Nutr Metab Cardiovasc Dis.* Oct 2003;13(5):273–277.

107. Perez-Jimenez F, Lopez-Miranda J, Pinillos MD et al. A Mediterranean and a high-carbohydrate diet improve glucose metabolism in healthy young persons. *Diabetologia.* Nov 2001;44(11):2038–2043.

108. Piers LS, Walker KZ, Stoney RM, Soares MJ, O'Dea K. Substitution of saturated with monounsaturated fat in a 4-week diet affects body weight and composition of overweight and obese men. *Br J Nutr.* Sep 2003;90(3):717–727.

109. Lawton CL, Delargy HJ, Brockman J, Smith FC, Blundell JE. The degree of saturation of fatty acids influences post-ingestive satiety. *Br J Nutr.* May 2000;83(5):473–482.

110. Piers LS, Walker KZ, Stoney RM, Soares MJ, O'Dea K. The influence of the type of dietary fat on postprandial fat oxidation rates: Monounsaturated (olive oil) vs saturated fat (cream). *Int J Obes Relat Metab Disord.* Jun 2002;26(6):814–821.

111. Alfenas RC, Mattes RD. Effect of fat sources on satiety. *Obes Res.* Feb 2003;11(2):183–187.

112. Coelho SB, de Sales RL, Iyer SS et al. Effects of peanut oil load on energy expenditure, body composition, lipid profile, and appetite in lean and overweight adults. *Nutrition.* Jun 2006;22(6):585–592.

113. Cooper JA, Watras AC, Paton CM, Wegner FH, Adams AK, Schoeller DA. Impact of exercise and dietary fatty acid composition from a high-fat diet on markers of hunger and satiety. *Appetite.* Feb 2011;56(1): 171–178.

114. Flint A, Helt B, Raben A, Toubro S, Astrup A. Effects of different dietary fat types on postprandial appetite and energy expenditure. *Obes Res.* Dec 2003;11(12):1449–1455.

115. MacIntosh CG, Holt SH, Brand-Miller JC. The degree of fat saturation does not alter glycemic, insulinemic or satiety responses to a starchy staple in healthy men. *J Nutr.* Aug 2003;133(8):2577–2580.

116. Strik CM, Lithander FE, McGill AT, MacGibbon AK, McArdle BH, Poppitt SD. No evidence of differential effects of SFA, MUFA or PUFA on post-ingestive satiety and energy intake: A randomised trial of fatty acid saturation. *Nutr J.* 2010;9:24.

117. Panico S, Iannuzzi A. Dietary fat composition and the metabolic syndrome. *Eur J Lipid Sci Tech.* 2004;106(1):61–67.

118. Vessby B, Uusitupa M, Hermansen K et al. Substituting dietary saturated for monounsaturated fat impairs insulin sensitivity in healthy men and women: The KANWU Study. *Diabetologia.* Mar 2001;44(3):312–319.

119. McAuley K, Mann J. Thematic review series: Patient-oriented research. Nutritional determinants of insulin resistance. *J Lipid Res.* Aug 2006;47(8):1668–1676.

120. Haag M, Dippenaar NG. Dietary fats, fatty acids and insulin resistance: Short review of a multifaceted connection. *Med Sci Monit.* Dec 2005;11(12):RA359–RA367.

121. Lombardo YB, Chicco AG. Effects of dietary polyunsaturated n-3 fatty acids on dyslipidemia and insulin resistance in rodents and humans. A review. *J Nutr Biochem.* Jan 2006;17(1):1–13.

122. Venderley AM, Campbell WW. Vegetarian diets: Nutritional considerations for athletes. *Sports Med.* 2006;36(4):293–305.

123. Karabuduk E, Kiziltan G, Cigerim N. A comparison of some of the cardiovascular risk factors in vegetarian and omnivorous Turkish females. *J Hum Nutr Diet.* 2008;21(1):13–22.

124. Kwok T, Chook P, Tam L et al. Vascular dysfunction in Chinese vegetarians: An apparent paradox? *J Am Coll Cardiol.* Nov 15 2005;46(10):1957–1958.

32 Atkins Paradigm

Ariel Robarge, RD and Bernard W. Downs, BSc

CONTENTS

INTRODUCTION

In the beginning, it is important to state that this chapter is not an attempt to discredit Dr. Atkins theory. In fact, his observations were right on the mark in general terms. This chapter hopes to put Dr. Atkins contribution, as controversial as it may be, into its correct context as a catalyst and vehicle for a major paradigm shift in our understanding of and approach to the causes and treatments of obesity and related disorders. Dr. Atkins was instrumental in removing our obsessive focus that fat is the greatest enemy in regard to disease prevention and treatment. However, to gain an understanding of the premise of the Atkins program, one must first understand in what environment the Atkins program was created and what caused Dr. Atkins to pioneer this paradigm at that particular time.

Recall that following WWII, there was a sharp increase in refined and processed food production and consumption. The major characteristic of these foods was that they were rich in fats (they were also rich in sweeteners like high-fructose corn syrup, invert sugar, etc.). This led to a passive overconsumption of high-fat, high-calorie foods (and high sugar consumption). Concomitant with this increase in high-fat foods was a significant increase in CVD, diabetes, and obesity. These new dietary habits were recognized as problematic by the medical and nutrition establishment that ultimately, in response to the consequences of these dietary habits, mandated a "low-fat" lifestyle. The experts of the time stated what they believed to be the obvious conclusion; if we eat too much fat, we get fat and suffer fat-related diseases, i.e., fat begets fat and fat-related problems.

At this point, the Food Guide Pyramid was developed with an emphasis on increasing dietary carbohydrate intake while reducing fat consumption. In hindsight, the flaw with the new guidelines was that the carbohydrates emphasized (bread, rice, cereal, and pasta) were derived primarily from refined processed sources, not necessarily "whole" unprocessed grains. Americans were told that the majority of their food intake should be grain derived, and fats in any shape or form were to be avoided at all costs. All fats were thought to contribute to disease and obesity and should be avoided as much as possible.

SCIENCE SPAWNS COMMERCIAL OPPORTUNITIES

Responding to the commercial opportunities created by these new "official" guidelines, agribusiness and the food processing industry jumped on the bandwagon and began producing high-carbohydrate, low-fat refined and processed alternatives, which eventually became the dogma of mainstream nutrition. This paradigm of low fat (high carbohydrate) became a societal mantra to the point of being a phobia. New dietary laws regarding nutrition, health, weight management, and disease treatment and prevention branded dietary fats as the villainous culprit responsible for a host of pathological disorders. An increasingly fat-obsessed society, including health professionals, business interests, and consumers alike, responded by adopting this paradigm, thus inciting the shift to high (refined) carbohydrate consumption.

OUTSIDE THE BOX OF CONVENTIONAL DOGMA

Dr. Atkins, a cardiologist, saw that several decades of high carbohydrate consumption was accompanied by a significant increase in insulin-resistant problems (metabolic syndrome X), like CVD, diabetes, hypertension, hyperlipidemia (high cholesterol, high triglycerides), obesity, etc. His approach was to eliminate carbohydrates from the diet as a means of treating these disorders. Initially, his focus was improving health. It was not about obesity *per se*; it was about anything that had to do with insulin resistance and related disorders. He consistently observed remarkable improvements in all of these insulin-resistant problems, especially obesity, as a result of drastic changes made to patients' diets. He authored *Dr. Atkins' Health Revolution* in 1988 to publish this new paradigm. To keep things in perspective, Dr. Atkins never promoted an unhealthy dietary lifestyle. Contrary to antagonists' assertions, he never said, "stop eating sugar and start eating pork rinds and bacon fat." He simply recognized that refined carbohydrates were particularly bad for patients who suffered from insulin resistance and heart disease. In practice, he found that by simply removing these foods from the diet, the patients had remarkable improvements in all parameters of their health.

Atkins proposed that a high-fat, high-protein diet gave a metabolic advantage that allowed you to eat as much as you wanted and lose weight. Subsequently, some studies have shown that initially there is an increase in the amount of weight lost on low-carbohydrate diets as opposed to the traditional low-fat, high-carbohydrate diets. However, this difference apparently disappears after the initial period of approximately 12 months.[1] Also, a careful meta-analysis of popular diets revealed that it was more likely the adherence to the low-carbohydrate approach that gave rise to a greater weight loss. The research has shown that when carbohydrates are reduced so drastically people spontaneously decrease calorie intake by approximately 1000 calories a day.[2] More on the effects of dietary modifications on "sustainable" weight loss will be discussed later in this chapter.

Fat and protein intake elicits a much greater sense of satisfaction and increased ketosis, also promoting a decrease in appetite. This makes it much more manageable for the dieter to not be struggling with constant hunger pains. On the other hand, an extremely high-carbohydrate diet that is low in fat tends not to be as satisfying and may cause swings in blood sugar that make compliance and adherence extremely difficult. This difficulty is accentuated when the carbohydrates are primarily refined. A 1 year comparison of four popular diet programs, Weight Watchers, Atkins, Ornish, and The Zone, showed that at 1 year weight loss was practically identical and was independent of macronutrient ratio of the diet. It was almost exclusively correlated with (reduced) caloric intake.[3]

ATKINS CONCEPT

The Atkins diet is based on the theory that obesity is a result of carbohydrates and not calorie intake *per se*. Atkins proposed that carbohydrates are the only catalyst for insulin release. So if you are eating foods that do not cause an increase in insulin levels, you can eat all you want and lose weight. Fat and protein are allowed in unlimited quantities, and carbohydrates are significantly reduced depending on the phase of the diet you are in. Atkins suggested that because insulin is involved in fat storage, weight loss was simply a matter of reducing insulin. Therefore, if you stop eating carbohydrates, you will burn fat and lose weight more efficiently, according to Atkins. This is why the initial phase of Atkins diet is so strict. An individual is allotted only 20 g of carbohydrates per day during the induction phase, which lasts 2 weeks. This facilitates a complete depletion of glycogen stores and an associated water loss of 3–5 lb. The body then enters a state of ketosis where it burns fats and proteins for energy as opposed to glucose.

KETOSIS: HOW DOES IT WORK?

When carbohydrates are eaten, they are broken down to sugar and used as energy or stored as glycogen for later use. Insulin is released by the pancreas to carry the sugar to the cells where it can be burned for energy and stored as glycogen, and any excess is converted to fat. Atkins proposes that it is this chronic state of high blood sugar induced by our standard high-carbohydrate diet that leads to diabetes and obesity. Ketosis can be induced by carbohydrate restriction. In simple terms, you switch to burning fat instead of sugar for energy. Ketones are carbon–oxygen fragments that are released during the breakdown of fats. Most people experience ketosis when carbohydrate intake falls below 40 g a day. Side effects include breath odor, loss of appetite, and constipation. Liver and kidney distress can occur in extreme states of ketosis. Chronic long-term ketosis may lead to organ distress and/or failure. However, the brain, red blood cells, and some organs still rely on glucose for energy. The minimal amount recommended for proper functioning is 120 g a day. The body will go through a process of gluconeogenesis, conversion of proteins to glucose, to provide the essential blood sugar for those tissues. These proteins may be obtained through food, or the body will pull proteins from lean body mass to provide the essential blood glucose. Some studies have shown that low-carbohydrate diets may cause a greater loss of lean body mass for this reason.[4]

DOES KETOSIS PROPEL FAT LOSS BY A METABOLIC ADVANTAGE?

Atkins claimed that there is a metabolic advantage that occurs with ketosis, with ketones (by-products of fat metabolism) being excreted via the feces and urine, reducing metabolizable energy and allowing for greater fat loss. Therefore, you can eat more and lose weight as ketosis is metabolically efficient, so the principle asserts. Carbohydrate intake blunts ketosis because the body no longer needs to break down fats to provide energy. This is why the Atkins program does not put a limit on total caloric intake for the day and instead focuses on drastically reducing carbohydrate consumption.

More recent research has shown that the amount of energy lost as ketones is very minimal and does not make a significant contribution to a metabolic advantage. A study compared 6 weeks of a ketogenic low-carbohydrate diet (KLC: 5% of calories from carbohydrates) to a nonketogenic low-carbohydrate diet (NLC: 40% of calories from carbohydrates). The authors concluded that while both diets resulted in similar loss of weight and reduced insulin resistance, the KLC was associated with a number of adverse metabolic and emotional effects.[5] While the study duration was for only 6 weeks and may be inadequate to assess longer-term effects, it does suggest that any energy that may be lost via ketosis might not be sufficient to offer a significant enough metabolic advantage over other alternatives, especially in light of ketosis-induced metabolic consequences. Furthermore, it calls into question the proposed tactical advantages that altering energy ratios may offer in weight management.

ENERGY AND THE METABOLIC BANK ACCOUNT

Atkins also suggests that the energy cost of digesting and metabolizing a high-fat meal is greater than a meal high in carbohydrates. However, recent research examined the effects of high-carbohydrate/low-fat/high-protein meals (60:10:30) compared to low-carbohydrate/high-fat/low-protein meals

(30:60:10) on 24 h energy expenditure when consumed over a 36 h period. The authors found that high-carbohydrate meals induce greater energy expenditure when coupled with a relatively higher protein intake (than fat) over high-fat/low-carbohydrate meals. In other words, higher-fat meals resulted in a reduced thermic effect compared to the meals high in carbohydrate when the carbohydrates were accompanied by higher protein intake as well.[6] More recent research confirms that protein intake was crucial in determining the intensity of the thermic effects.[7]

The metabolic advantage of the low-carbohydrate paradigm has been difficult to consistently verify. When patients have been studied in a metabolic ward where energy is provided, this metabolic advantage ceases to exist. Earlier research has shown that isocaloric amounts of proteins, fats, and carbohydrates elicit almost identical losses in fat tissue regardless of whether those calories are derived from protein, carbohydrate, or fat.[8] It is more likely that when people are in a state of ketosis, they feel that they are eating more and losing weight because of the significant decrease in appetite.

ATKINS CONTRIBUTION

It is the authors' opinions that, among other things, Dr. Atkins program gave rise to the recognition of the importance of "glycemic indexing" (GI) as a means of evaluating the impact of carbohydrates on blood sugar, insulin, and metabolism. It is not our purpose to delve into the details of GI but just to note that this model of dietary management arose as a result of the awareness that carbohydrates have varying effects on metabolism relative to the efficiency in which they are converted to blood sugar. That sugar impact concept was the platform of the Atkins program and the reason for omitting carbohydrates from the diet to reverse insulin-resistant disorders. The prevailing belief was that carbohydrates were the only macronutrient that stimulated the release of insulin. However, according to subsequent research, we now know that that is not entirely correct. Proteins and fats also increase insulin production and release by the pancreas. However, proteins and fats did not induce a proportional and/or concomitant rise in blood sugar. For example, beef intake raised insulin levels more than brown rice and fish raised insulin more than pasta. However, neither protein source raised blood sugar more than the carbohydrate sources. Therefore, insulin is not just responsive to only carbohydrate consumption.[9]

It is clear that the interplay of hormones, lifestyle, genetics, and metabolism are much more complicated than once thought and that the causes and treatments for obesity cannot be evaluated in such a simplistic one-dimensional manner. For example, there is an interrelationship of hormones involved in digestion and regulation of metabolism. Focusing on one aspect and disregarding other variables (especially for a short term) is not comprehensive and will not lead to optimal health, which is required to effectively address chronic obesity. Initially, such a drastic change in diet may yield some positive results, but this is short term because it does not address the root cause of the initial problem. Given the multidimensional aspects of human metabolism, in addition to insulin, a number of other hormones and neurotransmitters, like ghrelin, leptin, cholecystokinin, serotonin, and dopamine (to name a few), along with genetic factors, need to be simultaneously addressed and included in the framework of a healthy metabolic and body recomposition program.

The greatest minds in medicine and science (including Atkins) have zeroed in on specific aspects of metabolism (as the culprits or solutions) and analyzed them from a standpoint that those aspects hold the key to unlocking the mysteries to successful obesity management. It is sort of like the six blind men describing the structure of an elephant, each holding on to a different part of the animal. Each blind man gives an accurate description on that part of the elephant he is holding but falls short of giving a complete and totally accurate description of the whole elephant. We in (nutrition) science tend to do the same thing.

It should be obvious that weight management, nutrition, and metabolism are interrelated, and there is more than one component contributing to the rise in obesity. Science fails to make the correlation between multiple aspects of metabolism and instead focuses on one or two mechanisms without addressing the whole picture. For instance, the fat phobia was supported by research that showed fat calories are more easily stored as fat in the body and carbohydrates are preferentially burned for energy. This led to an interpretation that you could eat as much as you wanted as long at it was low fat. People started eating generous amounts of processed, refined low-fat foods (offset mainly by high-fructose corn syrup) with the false idea that these foods did not contribute to weight gain and obesity. This mistaken dietary shift increased the momentum of the obesity epidemic.

Clearly, a dominant consumption of refined (nutrient deficient) carbohydrates can lead to many unhealthy consequences. Atkins rightly condemned this type of lifestyle. In hindsight, the flaw of the Atkins program, maybe due to more commercial forces and requirements, was that it obsessed almost solely on insulin and carbohydrate metabolism, missing other critical issues that contribute both to obesity and to long-term health.

Successful solutions to the obesity epidemic will need to encompass, in practical terms, management of the multifaceted aspects of human metabolism, their relationship to genetic expressions and lifestyle (nutrition, personality profiles, stress, and environmental factors among others), and the symbiotic relationship between all of these elements. As indicated, this includes not only physical laws but also the emotional issues and neuroendocrine effects on digestion, metabolism, and food intake.

Our focus should be long-term holistic health that emphasizes achieving optimal body composition on an individual basis. There is no "one size fits all" when it comes to weight management, and focusing on the "bathroom scale" as the primary assessment of one's health is missing the mark. The scale is a poor measure of success in regard to weight loss. Many diets cause a loss of an excessive amount of lean body mass along with the loss of fat. Then, during the nearly inevitable rebound effect, metabolism slows down, the body becomes more efficient at storing fat, and brain chemicals are altered, which lead to an increase in food cravings, irritability, and obsession with food.

Food consumed in its unprocessed whole form, as it was intended, provides the nutrients that fund the structure and function of the body. Oftentimes, science and research fail to take into consideration individual needs and lifestyle. The dieting cycle and severe restriction of calories commonly touted by weight loss programs fail to consider the long-term effects on gene expression, energy metabolism, the structural competence of cells and tissues, and overall health. History is showing us that drastically reducing calories or altering ratios and percentages is short sighted and will not work in the long run. When the body is deprived of nutrition and energy, it sets up a cascade of events that lead to mood disorders, bingeing, and weight cycling that leaves the person feeling powerless and out of control of their weight.

NUTRIGENOMICS

Obesity can also not really be attributed to an individual's lack of motivation or willpower. There is a significant genetic component, which while suspected and reported in the scientific literature during Dr. Atkins time, was not well understood nor adequately defined.[10–12] Nutrigenomics is the science that studies the effect nutrition has on gene expression and the influence that exerts on overall health. This field of science was embryonic during Dr. Atkins life and is still in its childhood owing in large part to the complexity of the human genome. But we have learned that genes play a significant role in determining all craving and acquisition behaviors, especially in regard to carbohydrates and fats.[12,13] While we cannot change our genes, we have learned that we can change gene expression. Nutritional deficits alter gene expression resulting in unhealthy behaviors and ill-health, whereas nutritional replenishment (repletion) alters gene expression toward optimal health. Much of the seminal research in the area of brain chemistry and reward satiety was done by Dr. Kenneth Blum, who is considered the father of psychiatric genetics and applied nutrigenomics. Dr. Blum, along with Dr. Noble, is credited with discovering the dopamine D2 receptor gene role in driving addictive behaviors in alcoholism and subsequently for all addicting substances, including food. Their revelation was published in JAMA in 1990.[13] Interestingly, this field of science is also providing exciting revelations about the causes and potential treatments of impulsive, compulsive, and addictive behaviors, including for foods such as carbohydrates.[14] Dr. Blum defined deficits in the reward center of the brain and coined the term "reward deficiency syndrome" (RDS). We can only speculate how Dr. Atkins would have modified his approach to his low-carb/high-protein dietary program if he had utilized a nutrigenomic approach to positively alter gene expression to reduce carb cravings and excessive food intake.

To achieve sustainable loss of fat, it is important to understand that all the cells, tissues, and organs of the body are genetically programmed for survival. This simple fact determines how the body will react (phase 2) to one-dimensional, single-locus weight loss tactics (phase 1), such as dietary restrictions or deprivation, stimulation, and/or aggressive elimination programs. These types of programs elicit a sequela of genetic, hormonal, immunological, and biochemical "defensive" responses, a sort of ripple effect, catalyzed by genetic survival instructions. The phase 1–induced phase 2 defensive survival responses can result in adverse reactions, rejection, and retaliation that includes lowering of the basal metabolic rate, increasing in fat storage, and an intensified increase in craving behaviors. This phenomenon could be accurately termed "behavioral biology" and is a common trait of RDS. While this is not the focus of this chapter, it punctuates the reasons why existing weight loss programs fail when evaluated through the eyeglass of time. Most health authorities report greater than a 95% failure rate at 5 years. Even people who followed Dr. Atkins program reported significant rebound weight gain consequences when they stopped following it. This, however, does not diminish the importance of understanding the consequences of a diet high in refined carbohydrates (and high–glycemic impact foods).

Focusing on one aspect of dietary manipulation fails to take into account that the body requires all nutrients for synergy and wellness of metabolism. The way to optimal and healthy body composition is tuning into the body and providing its essential needs for protein, carbohydrates, fats, vitamins, and minerals from whole foods. By focusing on eating a balanced diet that is primarily composed of fresh, whole, uncontaminated, and unrefined foods, and engaging in an active and vital lifestyle, the body gets the energy, nutrients, and exercise it needs for optimal performance and an ability to rid itself of unneeded fat stores. The body is "preprogrammed" to work efficiently, energetically, and effectively if it has all of its essential resources and a minimum of stressful, toxic, and burdensome challenges dismantling the scaffolding of health (at a greater rate than it can be rebuilt). We are made only of food, air, water, and sunshine. The quality of our health and metabolism is a direct result of the quality of those resources and the attitude with which we meet life's challenges.

CONCLUSIONS

Atkins offered a strategy of reducing the insulin resistance–induced metabolic insult caused by an excessive consumption of the sort of carbohydrates that distressed insulin and blood sugar metabolism. In contrast to the low-fat high-carbohydrate paradigm popular at that time and the juggernaut of failed tactics implementing that paradigm, as evidenced by the significant increase in insulin-resistant disorders, it can be concluded that Dr. Atkins was moving in the right direction. The old adage that "hindsight is 20/20 vision" certainly gives us a critical advantage in perspective over that of Dr. Atkins. More recent research reveals a few flaws in the sweeping conclusions supporting the foundations of the Atkins paradigm. However, this does not completely dismantle the scaffolding of his premise that chronic insulin resistance and related disorders, especially obesity, CVD, and diabetes, are exacerbated by the nemesis of excessive refined carbohydrate consumption as a component of a lifestyle including other poor dietary habits. Dr. Atkins did not have the benefit of research that has helped to improve our understanding of many factors, including genetics and gene expression, that contribute to obesity, some of which were spurred in response to the power and popularity of the Atkins paradigm. To that point, Dr. Atkins was a courageous pioneer who ventured outside the box against conventional dogma. And he spurred renewed investigations into and helped establish scientific merit for the insulin-related issues he championed. To that extent, we owe him well-deserved accolades and a debt of gratitude.

REFERENCES

1. Foster GD, Wyatt HR, Hill JO, McGuckin BG, Brill C, Mohammed BS, Szapary PO, Rader DJ, Edman JS, and Klein S. A randomized trial of a low-carbohydrate diet for obesity. *N Engl J Med*. May 22, 2003; 348(21):2082–2090.
2. Astrup A, Meinert Larsen T, and Harper A. Atkins and other low-carbohydrate diets: Hoax or an effective tool for weight loss? *Lancet*. September 4–10, 2004; 364(9437):897–899.
3. Dansinger ML, Gleason JA, Griffith JL, Selker HP, and Schaefer EJ. Comparison of the Atkins, Ornish, Weight Watchers, and Zone diets for weight loss and heart disease risk reduction: A randomized trial. *JAMA*. January 5, 2005; 293(1):43–53.
4. Noakes M, Foster PR, Keogh JB, James AP, Mamo JC, and Clifton PM. Comparison of isocaloric very low carbohydrate/high saturated fat and high carbohydrate/low saturated fat diets on body composition and cardiovascular risk. *Nutr Metab*. January 11, 2006; 3:7.
5. Johnston CS, Tjonn SL, Swan PD, White A, Hutchins H, and Sears B. Ketogenic low-carbohydrate diets have no metabolic advantage over nonketogenic low-carbohydrate diets. *Am J Clin Nutr*. May 2006; 83(5):1055–1061.
6. Westerterp KR, Wilson SA, and Rolland V. Diet induced thermogenesis measured over 24 h in a respiration chamber: Effect of diet composition. *Int J Obes Relat Metab Disord*. March 1999; 23(3):287–292.
7. Westerterp KR. Diet induced thermogenesis. *Nutr Metab*. 2004; 18:1(1):5.
8. Golay A, Allaz AF, Morel Y, de Tonnac N, Tankova S, and Reaven G. Similar weight loss with low- or high-carbohydrate diets. *Metabolism*. December 1994; 43(12):1481–1487.
9. Holt SHA, Brand Miller JC, and Petocz P. An insulin index of foods: The insulin demand generated by 1000-kJ portions of common foods. *Am J Clin Nutr*. 1997; 66:1264–1276.
10. Grimm ER and Steinle NI. Genetics of eating behavior: Established and emerging concepts. *Nutr Rev*. 2010; 69(1):52–60.
11. Johnson PM and Kenny PJ. Dopamine D2 receptors in addiction-like reward dysfunction and compulsive eating in obese rats. *Nature Neurosci*. 2010; 13(5):635–643.
12. Downs BW, Chen AL, Chen TJ, Waite RL, Braverman ER, Kerner M, Braverman D, Rhoades P, Prihoda TJ, Palomo T, Oscar-Berman M, Reinking J, Blum SH, DiNubile NA, Liu HH, and Blum K. Nutrigenomic targeting of carbohydrate craving behavior: Can we manage obesity and aberrant craving behaviors with neurochemical pathway manipulation by immunological compatible substances (nutrients) using a genetic positioning system (GPS) Map? *Med Hypoth*. 2009; 73:427–434.
13. Blum K, Noble EP, Sheridan PJ, Montgomery A, Ritchie T, Jagadeeswaran P, Nogami H, Briggs AH, and Cohn JB. Allelic association of human dopamine D2 receptor gene in alcoholism. *JAMA*. April 18, 1990; 263(15):2055–2060.
14. Blum K, Liu Y, Shriner R, and Gold MS. Reward circuitry dopaminergic activation regulates food and drug craving behavior. *Curr Pharm Des*. 2011; 17(12):1158–1167.

33 Nature vs. Nurture
Role of Plant-Based Diet in Obesity Management

Dilip Ghosh, PhD, FACN

CONTENTS

INTRODUCTION

The World Health Organization has recognized the epidemic of obesity as one of the top 10 global health problems [1]. In biological terms, obesity is the result of an imbalance between energy input (food intake) and energy expenditure. In most individuals, obesity appears as a multigenic, multi-factorial disease, and estimations indicate that genetic determinants account for at least 50% of the obese phenotype, whereas the rest is due to the environment [2]. The present view of obesity indicates that the environment in developed countries promotes overconsumption of energy in terms of food and reduction of energy expenditure. Obesity is related to several chronic and debilitating conditions including coronary artery disease, metabolic syndrome (MetS), hypertension, stroke, hyperlipidemia, diabetes, osteoarthritis, sleep apnea, gout, gallbladder disease, several cancers, and joint problems [3].

Recent studies predict that one in three Americans born in the year 2000 will develop diabetes in their lifetime [4], and a similar ominous future confronts nearly all developed nations. The prevalence of obesity is rising rapidly throughout the world in both rich and poor countries, and it affects all sections of society. There are several important reasons for addressing the prevention of obesity, rather than its treatment or management. The prevention of weight gain (or the reversal of small gains) and the maintenance of a healthy weight are likely to be easier, less expensive, and potentially more effective than the treatment of obesity after it has fully developed. A structured planning framework for the identification of potential interventions for the promotion of healthy weight and the prevention of weight gain is clearly required.

Drugs have been developed to ameliorate or prevent obesity, but there are the costs, efficacy, and side effects to consider. For centuries, people have used plants for healing. Written records about medicinal plants date back at least 5000 years to the Sumerians [5]. Investigating new targets and perspectives may lead to better methods in the prevention and treatment of obesity and related diseases.

The use of plants has potential to keep the increasing prevalence of MetS in check. Many people are using natural products and plant-based dietary supplements for weight loss. According to a recent survey, over 42% of adults in the United States reported using one or more forms of alternative medicines or dietary supplements [6]. More than 8000 polyphenolic compounds are found in foods of plant origin [7]. These compounds have been known for more than 20 years for their antioxidant properties, but it is now becoming clear that they may have other health benefits, including a role in energy control and weight management [5]. Dietary guidelines recommend an increase in fruit and vegetable consumption, and interpretation of epidemiological evidence infers that this may have an effect on weight management and obesity [8,9].

CAUSES OF OBESITY

Table 33.1 shows the causes identified among people who are overweight or obese (adapted from Douglas et al. 2008). Participants described their weight problems as due to (1) being lazy and gluttonous; (2) inherited, that is, either genetically, through their upbringing, or through their social environment; and (3) their response to life events or illness. Most pointed to combinations of these factors as being more or less significant at different times in their lives.

DIETARY FIBER SUPPLEMENTS IN OBESITY CONTROL

Dietary fiber (DF) is a term that reflects to a heterogenous group of natural food sources, processed grains, and commercial supplements. The classical definition of DF is "the edible parts of plants or analogous carbohydrates that resist digestion and absorption in the human small intestine, with complete or partial fermentation in the human large intestine. It includes polysaccharides, oligosaccharides, lignin, and associated plant substances. DF exhibits one or more of laxation, blood cholesterol attenuation, and/or blood glucose attenuation" [11].

Several forms of DF have been used as complementary or alternative agents in the management of manifestations of the MetS, including obesity such as nonstarch polysaccharides (polyglucoses, e.g., cellulose, hemicellulose, and β-glucans; polyfructoses [inulin]; natural gums and heteropolymers [pectin]; oligosaccharides; lignin [a noncarbohydrate complex of polyphenylpropane units functionally linked to polysaccharides, increasing resistance to digestion]; fatty acid derivatives [waxes, cutin, suberin, serving as cross-links between the main constituents]; other plant substances [mucilages, storage polysaccharides, phytates]; and analogous polysaccharides [by-products of food production affecting digestibility, or purposefully synthesized compounds]) [12,13]. Not surprisingly, there is a great variation in the biological efficacy of DF in MetS and body weight control. Diverse factors and mechanisms have been reported as mediators of the effects of DF on the MetS and obesity [14].

TABLE 33.1
Causes Identified among People Who Are Overweight or Obese

Causes of weight problems	Laziness and gluttony
	Inherited—genetics, family upbringing, or social environment
	Response to life events or illness
Barriers to weight loss	Psychological
	Social
	Environmental (economic and physical)
	Medical or biological
Enabling factors	Psychological or motivational
	Social support and work
	Environmental

Source: Douglas, F. et al., *Aust. Econ. Rev.*, 41(1), 72, 2008.

Epidemiological studies suggest an inverse relation of DF intake and body weight [15,16], and this is supported by cross-sectional studies [17,18,19] and large observational studies [20,21]. Although a number of interventional human trials have shown positive weight reduction with diets rich in DF or DF supplements [22–24], other studies failed to demonstrate any effect [25–27].

Body weight and fat-mass regulation result from a complex interplay of multiple factors, involving central nervous circuits, peripheral sensation stimuli, mechanical and chemical satiation signals arising in the gastrointestinal tract, afferent vagal input, and adiposity signals from fat tissue and liver [28]. The stomach signals satiation in response to volume and calories of the ingested meal [29]; a lower post-prandial volume predicted an increased satiation score and a decreased maximum tolerated volume of a challenge meal test [30]. In many studies, DF induced greater satiety compared with digestible polysac-charides and simple sugars [31,32]. Greater satiety may result from several factors: the intrinsic physical properties of DF (bulking, gel formation, and viscosity change of gastric contents) [33], modulation of gastric motor function, and blunting of postprandial glucose and insulin responses. Postulated effects on gut peptide hormones involved in signaling satiation (such as ghrelin, glucagon-like peptide-1 [GLP-1], cholecystokinin, peptide YY [PYY], or glucose-dependent insulinotropic peptide [GIP]) remain incom-pletely resolved [34–39]. DF may also prolong meal duration and result in increased mastication with possible cephalic and peripheral influences on satiety [40]. DF-containing meals have a lower energy density [32] and may affect palatability of food, possibly reducing energy intake [41].

ASSOCIATION BETWEEN FRUIT AND VEGETABLE CONSUMPTION AND OBESITY

There are numerous health benefits proposed to result from consuming a diet rich in fruits and vegetables. The association between fruit and vegetable intake and weight management is not well understood, and few studies have been specifically designed to address this issue. Short-term clinical studies have shown that substituting fruit and vegetables for foods with higher energy densities can be an effective weight management strategy [42]. Fruit and vegetables are high in water and fiber. Incorporating them into the diet can reduce the energy density of the diet, promote satiety, and decrease energy intake [43]. Two epidemiological studies have been carried out on children and adolescents to examine the relationship between fruit and vegetable intake and body weight. In a 3 year prospective cohort study, it was concluded that the recommendation for the consumption of fruit and vegetables may be well founded but should not be based on a beneficial effect on regulation of body mass index (BMI) in weight regulation [44]. In contrast, Lin and Morrison [45] concluded from their study that higher fruit consumption was linked with lower body weight. In a recent review of epidemiological studies, Tohill et al. [46] tabulate and discuss 16 adult studies as well as the two on children and adolescents. Of the 16 adult studies, eight reported a significant association between higher intake of fruit or vegetables and decreased weight status, but there were confounding effects. Of the 18 studies reviewed, only two examined the association between fruit and vegetable intake and anthropometric outcome of body weight as a primary objective. The authors make recommendations for future epidemiological studies to clarify the relationship. Another more recent study also demonstrated that increasing the intake of fruit and vegetables may reduce long-term risk of obesity and weight gain among middle-aged women [8]. Apple and pear intake has also been shown to be associated with weight loss in middle-aged overweight women in Brazil [47]. Participants who consumed either of the fruits for 12 weeks had a significant weight loss compared to controls. Overall, there is rea-sonable evidence emerging to support the claim that a diet enriched in fruit and vegetables may play a role in weight management. There has been a concern, however, that high intake of fruit juice could promote the development of obesity, but the results have not been consistent across studies [47,48].

Very recently, Kouki et al. [49] have studied the associations of intakes of selected food items and nutrients with the risk of having MetS. They demonstrated that the consumption of vegetables, nonroot vegetables, legumes and nuts, berries, and fish had an inverse effect, whereas the consump-tion of sausage had a direct association with the risk of having MetS in men after adjustment for age, smoking, and alcohol consumption. However, after further adjustment for maximal oxygen uptake (VO_2max), most of these associations were abolished. They concluded that the consumption of legumes and nuts, berries, and fish was inversely associated with MetS in men. Consumption of sausage was directly associated with MetS in women. VO_2max seems to be a strong confounding factor between food consumption and MetS. Interestingly, Te Velda at al. [50] observed beneficial effects of vegetable intake as a means of weight maintenance only in women, whereas no evidence was found for promoting fruit intake as a means of weight maintenance.

Unfortunately, dietary patterns, such as combinations of different fruits and vegetables, are extremely complex, and extensive randomized trials are needed to assess whether such dietary patterns will have a truly beneficial impact on weight management [51]. More intervention and epidemiological studies are needed to reach a conclusion regarding the relationship between fruit and vegetable.

COMPLEMENTARY AND ALTERNATIVE MEDICINE IN WEIGHT MANAGEMENT

Complementary and alternative therapies have long been used in the Eastern world, but recently, these therapies are being used increasingly worldwide [52]. When conventional medicine fails to treat chronic diseases and conditions such as obesity efficaciously and without adverse events, many people seek unconventional therapies including herbal medicine [53]. Although the number of randomized trials on complementary therapies has doubled every 5 years and the Cochrane library included 100 systematic reviews of unconventional interventions [54], none of these studies specifically mentioned herbal therapy in obesity or weight management.

Hasani-Ranjbar et al. [55] in their recent review identified 915 results; a total of 77 studies were included (19 human and 58 animal studies). Studies with *Cissus quadrangularis* (CQ), *Sambucus nigra*, *Asparagus officinalis*, *Garcinia atroviridis*, *Ephedra* and caffeine, and Slimax (extract of several plants including *Zingiber officinale* and *Bofutsushosan*) showed a significant decrease in body weight. In 41 animal studies, significant weight loss or inhibition of weight gain was found. No significant adverse effects or mortality were observed except in studies with supplements containing ephedra, caffeine, and *Bofutsushosan*. Compounds containing ephedra, CQ, ginseng, bitter melon, and zingiber were found to be effective in the management of obesity and open a new approach for novel therapeutic treatment [55].

DIETARY SUPPLEMENTS/FUNCTIONAL FOODS OR NUTRACEUTICALS

A recent postmarket analysis identifies 990 new food and beverage product launches globally in 2008 with weight management claims on their label. This compares to 267 new launches in 2005, 185 in 2006, and 890 in 2007 [56]. The retail market for weight management products was estimated by Euromonitor International to be worth $3.7 billion in the United States in 2008, compared to $3.93 billion in 2005. In Europe, the market was valued at $1.4 billion in 2008 compared to $0.93 billion in 2005. This includes satiety ingredients or appetite suppressants, fat burners (thermogenic ingredients), and other weight management ingredients. The slimming ingredients market can be divided into five groups based on the mechanisms of action: increasing energy expenditure, modulating carbohydrate metabolism, increasing satiety or suppressing appetite, increasing fat oxidation or reducing fat synthesis, and blocking dietary fat absorption [57].

Most of the marketing and branding experts agree that there is a fair degree of "hype" surrounding the excitement over weight management foods. The obesity issue is some sort of permanent news, and the industry follows that hype. Everybody thinks they need a product in that category because it is so hot. Data from all leading marketing agencies showed that the global market for weight management supplements and functional foods will have grown 8% a year between 2006 and 2009, which is in between "evidence-based" and "hype-based." These reports show there were 42 satiety-related products launched in the first quarter of 2008 alone. Satiety is fast becoming the focus for increasing numbers of suppliers of functional ingredients. Table 33.2 [58] describes the recent market trends in weight management ingredients or products. A mix of fiber and protein

TABLE 33.2

Weight Management Ingredients and Products

Ingredients	Source	Mechanism of Action	Regulatory Status	Commercial Brand
Hydroxycitric acid (HCA)	*Garcinia cambogia* (Indian tamarind)	Inhibits citrate lyase	GRAS in the United States Approved in the United States and some Asian countries as dietary supplement	Citrisan, SuperCitrimax
Alkaloid ephedrine	*Sida cordifolia*	Stimulates beta-receptors by increasing the levels of neurohormones that can reduce appetite by increasing thermogenic response	Not approved in most of the countries	Nil
Alkaloid piperine (capsaicin)	*Piper longum*, *Piper nigrum*	Same as alkaloid ephedrine	Capsaicin is considered to be safe for human consumption	LeanGard, Capsimax
Diterpene alkaloid forskolin	*Coleus forskohlii*	Regulates insulin secretion by stimulating cAMP and thyroid stimulating hormones	Approved as dietary supplement	Tisanax
Conjugated linoleic acid (CLA)	Seeds of flax, nut oils, fish oils, and in poultry eggs	Lowering plasma triacylglycerol via the decrease of VLDL or apolipoprotein B production	Approved as dietary supplement	Tonalin, Clarinol
Psyllium fiber	Seed of *Psyllium*	Decreases postprandial insulin, glycemic response, and gastric emptying	FDA approved as dietary supplement	Metamucil, Serutan, Vi-Siblin
Green tea (CT), oolong tea (OT), black tea (BT), and white tea (WT) extract	Leaves of *Camellia sinensis* L.	Stimulate thermogenesis and fat oxidation through sympathetic activation of the central nervous system	Approved as dietary supplement	Teavigo, Sunphenon
Chromium picolinate and nicotinate	Trace mineral in diet	Enhance the effectiveness of insulin	Novel food approval in EFSA	Chromax, ChromeMate
Decaffeinated green coffee	Coffee bean	Inhibits the activity of glucose-6-phosphatase	Approved as dietary supplement	Svetol
Gymnemic acid	Indian herb, *Gymnema sylvestre*	Modulating taste bud and intestinal receptors to prevent sugar absorption	Approved as dietary supplement	Sugarest, Genomyx Slin-Sane
Phaseolus vulgaris extract	White kidney beans	Carbohydrate blocker	Approved as dietary supplement	Phase 2, Dietrine

(*continued*)

TABLE 33.2 (continued)
Weight Management Ingredients and Products

Ingredients	Source	Mechanism of Action	Regulatory Status	Commercial Brand
Whey proteins and peptides	Milk	Modulation of satiety signals that affect food intake regulation	Approved as dietary supplement	Wide ranges of branded and nonbranded supplements
Functional oligosaccharides, such as fructo-, isomalto-, malto-, arabinoxylan-, glucose-, and galacto-oligosaccharides	DFs	Up- and downregulation of specific appetite-related hormones	Approved as dietary supplement	FOS, GOS, FenuLife
Seeds, palm and oat oil, potato extract	Korean pine nut tree, palm, oat, potato extract	Satiety	Approved as dietary supplement	PinnoThin, Fabuless, Slendesta
Resveratrol	Grape seed	Inhibitor of fatty acid synthase	Approved as dietary supplement	resVida, Resevenox

Source: Ghosh, D., *Nutrition Insight*, 22, 2010.

is a popular choice for manufacturers. The simplicity of the ingredients and the ease with which consumers understand them no doubt appeal, for example, fat burning ingredients or products such as conjugated linoleic acid (CLA), which has been shown in tests to reduce 9%–20% of body fat (depending on whether physical activity is involved) and maintain and increase lean muscle [59]. The third main kind of weight management benefit, calorie burning, appears to be the least popular. The declining consumer demand for Coca-Cola's Enviga (green tea [GT] extract and caffeine) is one of the examples.

Identification and modulation of specific neural pathways such as channelrhodopsin that control feeding is one of the hottest areas in weight management product development [60]. Also, functional imaging has recently been used to map the human brain regions that control eating. Such studies have revealed leptin-mediated changes in neural circuits that control reward-associated behavior, providing a link between neurobiology and psychology [57]. Emerging data in antiobesity therapy show that leptin and amylin together produce a potent signal to induce substantial weight loss. The aim now is to evaluate the safety and long-term efficacy of this combined therapy.

The future potential of the weight management market has already been hyped up by consultants with their wild estimates. Today, weight management is where probiotics were 10 years ago. Although the dietary supplements are commonly used for weight loss, only a few have been tested in a controlled randomized clinical trial environment. Of those dietary supplements used for weight loss having clinical support, at least several were as effective at promoting weight loss as the gold standard of producing 1–2 lb of weight loss per week [61]; the following ingredients or products are under this category [62]: chromium picolinate, hydroxycitric acid (HCA), decaffeinated green coffee extract, *Phaseolus vulgaris*, the *Acacia* blend, the HCA blend, and the CQ blend. Among satiety ingredients, protein (soy and mycoprotein) and fiber are still at the top of the list.

For companies looking to create a new brand from scratch, their road will be the hardest. Companies who already have a "healthy lifestyle" or "diet" brand will have a better basis to start from. To succeed in the global weight management ingredients market, manufacturers should find innovative ways to prolong ingredient lifespan, work toward securing favorable legislation, and introduce new functional and palatable ingredients into this market.

CONCLUSION

The American Heart Association statement emphasizes [63] the need for changes that help people make better food choices and be more physically active. Examples given in the report include things like "limiting the availability of high-fat, low-fiber foods and sugary drinks, reducing restaurant portion sizes, reconsidering the location of fast-food restaurants, and thinking more creatively about community design and infrastructure to enhance 'walkability' of neighborhoods and commutes between home, school, and recreation." Internet-based obesity prevention programs may be an effective channel for promoting healthy diet (fruits, vegetables, juices) and physical activity behaviors to youth at risk of obesity. Additional research is needed to more fully examine their effectiveness at promoting and maintaining diet and physical activity change [64].

Not a single weight management claim has been approved by the U.S. Food and Drug Administration (FDA) or the European Food Safety Authority (EFSA) and nor are any approved in any other major markets. In the United States at least, companies can take their chances with structure or function claims. There is nothing in the regulation specifically preventing general weight management claims being made. The sole restriction is that a claim cannot be made for the actual rate of weight loss, and thus, the weight management claims cannot link with disease reduction claims. This is a very debatable issue that the tightening of the rules on health claims in Europe and elsewhere will help improve consumer confidence in functional products, or this will ruin innovation and future investment in research and development [58].

REFERENCES

1. World Health Organization. 1998. Obesity, preventing and managing the global epidemic, Report of a WHO consultation on obesity, Geneva, Switzerland.
2. Comuzzie, A.G. and Allison, D.B. 1998. The search for human obesity genes. *Science* 280, 1374–1377.
3. Pi-Sunyer, X. 2003. A clinical view of the obesity problem. *Science* 299, 859–860.
4. Seaquist, E.R., Damberg, G.S., Tkac, I., and Gruetter, R. 2001. The effect of insulin on in vivo cerebral glucose concentrations and rates of glucose transport/metabolism in humans. *Diabetes* 50, 2203–2209.
5. Swerdlow, J. 2000. *Nature's Medicines*: *Plants That Heal*. Washington, DC: National Geographic Society.
6. Eisenberg, D.M. 1998. Trends in alternative medicine use in the United States. *JAMA* 280, 1569–1575.
7. Pietta, P.G. 2000. Flavonoids as antioxidants. *J Nat Product* 63, 1035–1342.
8. He, K., Hu, F.B., Colditz, G.A., Manson, J.E., Willett, W.C., and Liu, S. 2004. Changes in intake of fruits and vegetables in relation to risk of obesity and weight gain among middle-aged women. *Int J Obes Relat Metab Disord* 28, 1569–1574.
9. National Institute of Health (NIH). 1998. Clinical guidelines on the identification, evaluation, and treatment of overweight and obesity in adults: The evidence report. NIH Publication No. 98-4083.
10. Douglas, F., Greener J., and van Teijlingen, E. 2008. 'Ask Me Why I'm Fat!' The need to engage with potential recipients of health promotion policy to prevent obesity. *Aust Econ Rev* 41, 72–77.
11. Chemists, AOAC. 2001. The definition of dietary fiber. *Cereal Food World* 46, 112–129.
12. DeVries, J.W. 2003. On defining dietary fibre. *Proc Nutr Soc* 62, 37–43.
13. Trowell, H.C. and Burkitt, D.P. 1987. The development of the concept of dietary fibre. *Mol Aspects Med* 9, 7–15.
14. Papathanaso poulos, A. and Camilleri, M. 2010. Dietary fiber supplements: Effects in obesity and metabolic syndrome and relationship to gastrointestinal functions. *Gastroenterology* 138, 65–72.
15. Koh-Banerjee, P. and Rimm, E.B. 2003. Whole grain consumption and weight gain: A review of the epidemiological evidence, potential mechanisms and opportunities for future research. *Proc Nutr Soc* 62, 25–29.
16. Slavin, J.L. 2005. Dietary fiber and body weight. *Nutrition* 21, 411–418.

17. Alfieri, M.A., Pomerleau, J., Grace, D.M., and Anderson, L. 1995. Fiber intake of normal weight, moderately obese and severely obese subjects. *Obes Res* 3, 541–547.

18. van de Vijver L.P., van den Bosch, L.M., van den Branolt, P.A., and Gold Bohm, R.A. 2009. Whole-grain consumption, dietary fibre intake and body mass index in the Netherlands cohort study. *Eur J Clin Nutr* 63, 31–38.

19. Kromhout, D., Bloemberg, B., Seidell, J.C., Nissinen, A., and Menotti, A. 2001. Physical activity and dietary fiber determine population body fat levels: The Seven Countries Study. *Int J Obes Relat Metab Disord* 25, 301–306.

20. Liu, S., Willett, W.C., Manson, J.E., Hu, F.B., Rosner, B., and Colditz, G. 2003. Relation between changes in intakes of dietary fiber and grain products and changes in weight and development of obesity among middle aged women. *Am J Clin Nutr* 78, 920–927.

21. Koh-Banerjee, P., Franz, M., Sampson, L., Liu, S., Jacobs, D.R. Jr, Spiegelman, D., Willett, W., and Rimm, E. 2004. Changes in whole-grain, bran, and cereal fiber consumption in relation to 8-y weight gain among men. *Am J Clin Nutr* 80, 1237–1245.

22. Birketvedt, G.S., Aaseth, J., Florholmen, J.R., and Ryttig, K. 2000. Long-term effect of fibre supplement and reduced energy intake on body weight and blood lipids in overweight subjects. *Acta Medica (Hradec Kralove)* 43, 129–132.

23. Rigaud, D., Ryttig, K.R., Angel, L.A., and Apfelbaum, M. 1990. Overweight treated with energy restriction and a dietary fibre supplement: A 6-month randomized, double-blind, placebo-controlled trial. *Int J Obes* 14, 763–769.

24. Pittler, M.H. and Ernst, E. 2001. Guar gum for body weight reduction: Meta-analysis of randomized trials. *Am J Med* 110, 724–730.

25. Hays, N.P., Starling, R.D., Liu, X., Sullivan, D.H., Trappe, T.A., Fluckey, J.D., and Evans, W.J. 2004. Effects of an *ad libitum* low-fat, high-carbohydrate diet on body weight, body composition, and fat distribution in older men and women: A randomized controlled trial. *Arch Intern Med* 164, 210–217.

26. Jenkins, D.J., Kendall, C.W., Augustin, L.S., Martini, M.C., Axelsen, M., Faulkner, D., Vidgen, E., Parker, T., Lau, H., Connelly, P.W., Teitel, J., Singer, W., Vandenbroucke, A.C., Leiter, L.A., and Josse, R.G. 2002. Effect of wheat bran on glycemic control and risk factors for cardiovascular disease in type 2 diabetes. *Diabetes Care* 25, 1522–1528.

27. Ludwig, D.S., Pereira, M.A., Kroenke, C.H., Hilner, J.E., VanHorn, L., Slattery, M.L., and Jacobs, D.R. Jr. 1999. Dietary fiber, weight gain, and cardiovascular disease risk factors in young adults. *JAMA* 282, 1539–1546.

28. Woods, S.C. 2005. Signals that influence food intake and body weight. *Physiol Behav* 86, 709–716.

29. Deutsch, J.A., Young, W.G., and Kalogeris, T.J. 1978. The stomach signals satiety. *Science* 201, 165–167.

30. Vazquez Roque, M.I. 2006. Gastric sensorimotor functions and hormone profile in normal weight, overweight, and obese people. *Gastroenterology* 131, 1717–1724.

31. Howarth, N.C., Saltzman, E., and Roberts, S.B. 2001. Dietary fiber and weight regulation. *Nutr Rev* 59, 129–139.

32. Pereira, M.A. and Ludwig, D.S. 2001. Dietary fiber and body-weight regulation. Observations and mechanisms. *Pediatr Clin North Am* 48, 969–980.

33. Jenkins, D.J., Wolever, T.M., Leeds, A.R., Gassull, M.A., Haisman, P., Dilawari, J., Goff, D.V., Metz, Z.L., and Alberti, K.G. 1978. Dietary fibres, fibre analogues, and glucose tolerance: Importance of viscosity. *Br Med J* 1, 1392–1394.

34. Karhunen, L.J., Juvonen, K.R., Huotari, A., Purhonen, A.K., and Herzig, K.H. 2008. Effect of protein, fat, carbohydrate and fibre on gastrointestinal peptide release in humans. *Regul Pept* 149, 70–78.

35. Heini, A.F., Lara-Castro, C., Schneider, H., Kirk, K.A., Considine, R.V., and Weinsier, R.L. 1998. Effect of hydrolyzed guar fiber on fasting and postprandial satiety and satiety hormones: A double-blind, placebo controlled trial during controlled weight loss. *Int J Obes Relat Metab Disord* 22, 906–909.

36. Bourdon, I., Yokoyama, Y., Davis, P., Hudson, C., Baskus, R., Richter, B., Knuckles, B., and Schneeman, B.O. 1999. Postprandial lipid, glucose, insulin, and cholecystokinin responses in men fed barley pasta enriched with beta-glucan. *Am J Clin Nutr* 69, 55–63.

37. Flourie, B., Vidon, N., Chayvialle, J.A., Palma, R., Franchisseur, C., and Bernier, J.J. 1985. Effect of increased amounts of pectin on a solid-liquid meal digestion in healthy man. *Am J Clin Nutr* 42, 495–503.

38. Di Lorenzo, C., Williams, C.M., Hajnal, F., and Valenzuela, J.E. 1988. Pectin delays gastric emptying and increases satiety in obese subjects. *Gastroenterology* 95, 1211–1215.

39. Burton-Freeman, B.D.P. and Schneeman, B.O. 1998. Postprandial satiety: The effect of fat availability in meals. *FASEB J* 12, A650.

40. Sakata T. 1995. A very-low-calorie conventional Japanese diet: Its implications for prevention of obesity. *Obes Res* 3, 233s–239s.

41. Drewnowski, A. 1998. Energy density, palatability, and satiety: Implications for weight control. *Nutr Rev* 56, 347–353.

42. Rolls, B.J., Ello-Martin, J.A., and Tohill, B.C. 2004a. What can intervention studies tell us about the relationship between fruit and vegetable consumption and weight management? *Nutr Rev* 62, 1–17.

43. Rolls, B.J., Roe, L.S., and Meengs, J.S. 2004b. Salad and satiety: Energy density and portion size of a first-course salad affect energy intake at lunch. *J Am Diet Assoc* 104, 1570–1576.

44. Field, A.E., Gillman, M.W., Rosner, B., Rockett, H.R., and Colditz, C.A. 2003. Association between fruit and vegetable intake and change in body mass index among a large sample of children and adolescents in United States. *Int J Obes Relat Metab Disord* 27, 821–826.

45. Lin, B.H. and Morrison, R.M. 2002. Higher fruit consumption linked with lower body mass index. *Food Rev* 25, 28–32.

46. Tohill, B.C., Seymour, J., Serdula, M., Kettel-Khan, L., and Rolls, B.J. 2004. What epidemiologic studies tell us about the relationship between fruit and vegetable consumption and body weight. *Nutr Rev* 62, 365–374.

47. De Oliveiera, M., Sichieri, R., and Moura, A. 2003. Weight loss associated with a daily intake of three apples or three pears among overweight women. *Nutrition* 19, 253–256.

48. Dennison, B.A., Rockwell, H.L., and Baker, S.L. 1997. Excess fruit juice consumption by preschool-aged children is associated with short stature and obesity. *Pediatrics* 99, 15–22.

49. Kouki, R., Schwab, U., Hassinen, M., Komulainen, P., Heikkila, H., Lakka, T.A., and Rauramaa, R. 2011. Food consumption, nutrient intake and the risk of having metabolic syndrome: The DR's EXTRA Study. *Eur J Clin Nutr* 65, 368–377.

50. te Velde, S.J., Twisk, J.W.R., and Brug, J. 2007. Tracking of fruit and vegetable consumption from adolescence into adulthood and its longitudinal association with overweight. *Brit J Nutr* 98, 431–438.

51. Ghosh, D. and Skinner, M. 2007. Polyphenols from fruits and vegetables in weight management and obesity control. In *Obesity Epidemiology, Pathophysiology, and Prevention*, eds. D. Bagchi and H.G. Preuss, pp. 321–337, CRC Press, Boca Raton, FL.

52. Hasani-Ranjbar, S., Larijani, B., and Abdollahi, M. 2008. A systematic review of Iranian medicinal plants useful in diabetes mellitus. *Arch Med Sci* 4, 285–292.

53. Liu, J.P., Zhang, M., Wang, W.Y., and Grimsgard, S. 2004a. Chinese herbal medicines for type 2 diabetes mellitus. *Cochrane Database Syst Rev* 2004, CD003642.

54. Liu, J.P., Yang, M., and Du, X.M. 2004b. Herbal medicines for viral myocarditis. *Cochrane Database Syst Rev* 2004, CD003711.

55. Hasani-Ranjbar, S., Nayebi, N., Larijani., B., and Abdollahi, M. 2009. A systematic review of the efficacy and safety of herbal medicines used in the treatment of obesity. *World J Gastroenterol* 15, 3073–3085.

56. Euromonitor International. 2010. Obesity and its effect on consumer health. http://blog.euromonitor.com/2010/11/obesity and its effect on consumer health html.

57. Friedman, J.M. 2009. Causes and control of excess body fat. *Nature* 459, 340–342.

58. Ghosh, D. 2010. Natural weight management. *Nutrition Insight*, 22–25.

59. Larsen, T.M., Toubro, S., and Astrup, A. 2003. Efficacy and safety of dietary supplements containing CLA for the treatment of obesity: Evidence from animal and human studies. *J Lipid Res* 44, 2234–2241.

60. Perez, C.A., Stanley, S.A., Wysocki, R.W., Havranova, J., Ahrens-Nicklas, R., Onyimba, F., and Friedman, J.M. 2011. Molecular annotation of integrative feeding neural circuits. *Cell Metab* 13, 222–232.

61. NHLBI Working Group 2000. *The Practical Guide: Identification, Evaluation, and Treatment of Overweight and Obesity in Adults*. Bethesda, MD: National Institute of Health. http://www.nhlbi.nih.gov/guidelines/obesity/prctgd_c.pdf, accessed on July 21, 2011.

62. Ghosh, D. 2009. A botanical approach to managing obesity. In *Functional Foods for Chronic Diseases*, ed. D.M. Danik, Vol. 4, pp. 263–273, D&A Inc./FF Publishing, Dallas, TX.

63. Edmunds, M.W. 2009. Obesity requires thinking beyond the stethoscope. *J Nurse Pract* 5, 6.

64. Thompson, D., Baranowski, T., Cullen, K., Watson, K., Liu, Y., Canada, A., Bhatt, R., and Zakeri, J. 2008. Food, fun, and fitness internet program for girls: Pilot evaluation of an e-Health youth obesity prevention program examining predictors of obesity. *Prev Med* 47, 494–497.

34 Glycemic Index
Issues and Concepts

David J.A. Jenkins, MD, PhD, DSc, Krobua Srichaikul, MSc,
Arash Mirrahimi, MSc, Livia S.A. Augustin, PhD,
Laura Chiavaroli, MSc, John L. Sievenpiper, MD, PhD,
and Cyril W.C. Kendall, PhD

CONTENTS

INTRODUCTION

The glycemic index (GI) concept has been well reviewed [1], with a number of informative meta-analyses performed on the topic [2,3]. The benefits of lower GI diets appear best established in the dietary management of type 2 diabetes [2]. However even in this situation the therapeutic advantage of lower GI diets has not always been demonstrated, for example in type 2 diabetes participants with low mean HbA1C levels (6.2%) who were controlled by diet alone [4]. There are also studies that weight loss may be promoted by low-glycemic-load (GI × carbohydrate) diets, especially in those with raised 30 min insulin levels [5]. However, not all studies have shown this effect consistently. The relation of high GI diets to hyperinsulinemia and cancer promotion has also attracted attention. The concept is strong from the theoretical standpoint with type 2 diabetes being associated with more cancer [6,7] with the exception of prostate cancer and lymphoma [8]. Though the association of high-GI diets and increased cancer risk has been demonstrated in some cohort and case control studies [9–13], in others it has not [14]. The same applies to the association of low-GI diets and heart disease. For these and other reasons, the use of the GI concept has continued to be a matter of debate for 30 years. It is perhaps timely to review the concepts and issues that are relevant to this debate.

ESTABLISHED CONCEPTS IN RELATED AREAS: CHALLENGING TIMES

Before positioning the GI concept as uniquely controversial, it is probably worth bringing up other areas of contention in related fields. For a long time, there was doubt over the value of cholesterol as a predictor of coronary heart disease (CHD) risk. Much attention had to be put to the standardization of cholesterol measurement, and it was with the advent of standardized measurement of LDL-C and HDL-C that more sense has been made of this issue. Even so a recent meta-analysis concluded that the most commonly prescribed cholesterol-lowering drugs, the statins, were not associated with a reduction in all-cause mortality, as the ultimate goal, despite a significant reduction in CHD mortality [15]. It took a recent meta-analysis of 170,255 patients to demonstrate a statin-related reduction in both total (10%) and CHD mortality (20%) [16]. Tight glycemic control (the "tighter the better", as measured clinically by %HbA1C) has for decades been the objective of diabetes treatment. Diabetes is linked to heart disease, and so any improvement in diabetes management should not only be reflected by an improvement in microvascular disease but also in macrovascular disease. Nevertheless, a series of studies demonstrated either no significant benefit of intensive pharmacological treatment of diabetes on CHD risk in type 2 diabetes or, worse, a significant adverse CHD outcome [17–19]. This issue has sparked much debate over the use of thiazolidinediones, drug-induced weight gain, and increased hypoglycemic episodes. As a result, a more moderate stand on the level of HbA1C that is desirable has been taken, and even the value of HbA1C has been called into question. Together with concern over the means by which glucose levels are reduced, there has arisen debate over whether the longer acting insulin therapy may promote cancer [20]. Closer to home (nutrition), a recent meta-analysis concluded that, possibly due to the changing nature of the dietary carbohydrate, since 1980, saturated fat intake has not been associated with increased CHD risk [21]. This finding challenged a fundamental concept endorsed by all agencies internationally concerned with promoting health and CHD health specifically. Nor is there concern only with saturated fatty acids. The fish fats (n-3 fatty acids: EPA and DHA) for which there is solid international endorsement for a protective role in CHD have failed in several large randomized controlled trials to influence CHD or all-cause mortality [22,23]. It is not surprising that controversy surrounds the GI with implications it has for both diabetes and CHD.

GLYCEMIC INDEX CONCEPT

The GI concept came from the original dietary fiber hypothesis as envisioned by Denis Burkett and Hugh Trowell. They concluded that much of Western chronic disease related to the consumption of fiber-depleted processed foods by Western communities that differed from the traditional foods eaten in the African diet (Uganda in particular) [24]. This African diet, they concluded, was more similar to the original diet on which humans had evolved before they left Africa and therefore was "in tune" with human physiology and metabolism. Government regulating bodies (and many scientists) have always had difficulty with this concept since fiber is not a specific simple entity (such as sodium, bad; or docosahexaenoic acid [DHA], good) that can be clearly labeled on food packages, giving the exact content. Fiber is a physiologically defined entity, not a single chemical compound but a complex mixture of small intestinally indigestible carbohydrates and lignan with a wide range of physical states and physiological functions. For many years, this food component has defied consensus on definition and therefore on analysis [25]. Likewise, the factors that determine the GI of a food are also many, including all those factors that alter gastric emptying, small intestinal absorption, insulin secretion, and systemic carbohydrate metabolism [26]. Thus, just as one has to determine the digestibility of the carbohydrate to determine how much fiber is present, so the GI is classically tested in humans to assess the effect of that food's carbohydrate content in raising the blood glucose. The data from this test food are then compared to postprandial glucose data from a control carbohydrate source, originally glucose [27] but, more recently, white bread as a staple starchy food comparison. This physiological definition obviously gives rise to regulatory distrust and suspicion since there is no clear chemical or physical assay and the temptation for such bodies to do nothing and preserve the regulatory status quo is far stronger than to do something, with all the implications of physiological assay variability.

As with fiber, slowing the rate of digestion is a feature of many low-GI foods. Since digestion of starch starts in the mouth with salivary amylase, those foods that release their products of starch digestion more readily taste sweet and therefore more palatable [28]. This increased appeal may encourage increased consumption and may be a reason for manufacturers to produce foods with faster digestion properties (higher GI foods).

Over time, ready availability of palatable foods will promote weight gain [5] when combined with inactive Western lifestyles and as a result increase the risk of diabetes and CHD. The high-GI foods themselves will challenge the pancreatic insulin secretory capacity exacerbated by insulin resistance associated with obesity. Thus, both prevention [29,30] and treatment of type 2 diabetes [2,31,32] should be positively influenced by low-GI diets.

The same scenario applies to CHD. Low-GI-diet consumption has been associated with lower TG, higher HDL-C, and lower C-reactive protein (CRP) levels, all factors that would suggest reduced CHD risk. Furthermore, the glycemic excursion has been linked to free radical generation that in turn may damage LDL-C (oxidized LDL), a more atherogenic particle than native LDL due to its preferential uptake by the scavenger uptake system and the increased cholesterol accumulation it produces in the subendothelial space of the coronary (and other) arteries.

Finally, the increased insulin secretion resulting from the consumption of high-GI foods, together with the insulin-like growth factors (IGFI and 2), may act as promoters of transformed cells (and may actually transform cells secondary to free radical generation) thus increasing cancer risk. Some studies appear to support this hypothesis [9–13] while others do not.

GLYCEMIC INDEX ISSUES

A major issue in relation to the GI is the reliability of the GI data. The standard testing of foods, related to a reference food (glucose originally but white bread more recently as a representative starchy food) containing 50 g of carbohydrate, involves 10 subjects. Subjects are studied after an overnight fast on two occasions with finger prick blood samples taken for blood glucose at 0, 15, 30, 45, 60, 90, and 120 min for healthy subjects. The ratio of the incremented area above baseline for the food divided by the corresponding value for the control and expressed as a percentage gives the GI value (glucose or bread standardized) [33]. Apart from making sure the individuals have adequate carbohydrate intake and are not losing weight, there appears to be little advantage to controlling the previous day's activity. Such testing can detect 30 GI unit differences between foods as significant (bread scale). This will determine whether a food has a high or low GI. Further refinements that have been introduced are the use of two baseline fasting blood samples and three white bread tests (reference food) in any series of testing; such an approach has been found to give a good level of agreement between centers in a multicenter study [34].

However, since 12–14 GI units is the mean difference in diet GI that can be routinely achieved, for example, in type 2 diabetes, a better protocol for GI testing may be required for individual foods than the current ability to detect of a 30-unit difference. The review by Brouns is informative in this respect and indicated graphically that to detect a 20-unit difference requires 20 participants; a 10-unit difference, 30 participants; and a 5-unit difference, 40 participants [35]. Since on the bread scale a GI of over 100 units (100% bread scale) is considered high, between 100 and 70 units is intermediate, and less than 70 units is low, 10 participants is adequate to tell the difference between high- and low-GI foods. Smaller differences require greater numbers. These figures should be borne in mind for research studies requiring greater differentiation between foods.

The second issue is the change in the food supply, with manufactured foods being reformulated on an ongoing basis with new foods added and old foods removed from production. As a result, testing has to be done on a continuing basis, certainly for key foods intended for the diet. In addition, many foods (e.g., fruit) have never been tested, or only tested once. No indication is usually given as to whether the fruit is ripe, sweet, or has a firm or soft texture, all factors that may influence the glycemic response together with the total carbohydrate content. Much more testing is required in these areas.

Finally, some studies fail to show an effect of changing the GI of the diet while others detect differences with changes as low as 5–6 GI units (bread scale). The participant numbers in these studies vary greatly from low teens to over 100 in each study. Our own experience suggests that when using foods available in Western supermarkets, including the use of temperate climate versus tropical fruit, a 12–14-unit reduction from 82–84 to 68–70 GI units can reasonably be achieved compared to a high-fiber control [31,32]. A 0.1–0.3 reduction in HbAIC can be expected to be significant in studies of 3–6 month duration, which employ over 200 participants. Smaller numbers ($n = 120$) may also give significance using the CONTRAST statement approach (SAS) and taking two blood samples for baseline and three samples during the last month, to be used for the CONTRAST determination (a multiple test approach).

For cohort studies, a major issue may be the frequency of dietary data collection. Those studies relying on only one baseline diet history or food frequency questionnaire may require far larger numbers of individuals than those with multiple follow-up assessments.

The answer, therefore, to many of the concerns raised in relation to the GI is the use of larger numbers both in GI testing of individual foods and in assessing the effect of low-GI diets in dietary interventions, cohort, and case control studies.

CONCLUSION

The GI concept continues to show promise in a number of areas. Debate over its utility also continues, but this issue is common to many areas of pharmacology and nutrition in relation to diabetes and CHD. As with so many other debates of this sort, part of the answer lies in carrying out studies with sufficient power to detect the relatively small, but on a population basis meaningful, differences, since it is only small effects that can be expected from many diet and lifestyle modifications or interventions.

CONFLICTS OF INTEREST

David J.A. Jenkins holds an unrestricted grant from the Coca-Cola Company and has served on the scientific advisory board for or received research support, consultant fees, or honoraria from Barilla, Solae, Unilever, Hain Celestial, Loblaws Supermarkets, Sanitarium Company, Herbalife International, Pacific Health Laboratories Inc., Metagenics/MetaProteomics, Bayer Consumer Care, Oldways Preservation Trust, The International Tree Nut Council Nutrition Research & Education, The Peanut Institute, Procter and Gamble Technical Centre Limited, Griffin Hospital for the development of the NuVal System, Pepsi Company, Soy Advisory Board of Dean Foods, Alpro Soy Foundation, Nutritional Fundamentals for Health, Pacific Health Laboratories, Kellogg's, Quaker Oats, The Coca-Cola Sugar Advisory Board, Agrifoods and Agriculture Canada (AAFC), Canadian Agriculture Policy Institute (CAPI), Abbott Laboratories, the Almond Board of California, the California Strawberry Commission, Orafti, the Canola and Flax Councils of Canada, Pulse Canada, and the Saskatchewan Pulse Growers. He also holds additional grant support from the Canadian Institutes of Health Research, Canadian Foundation for Innovation, Ontario Research Fund, and Advanced Foods and Material Network. David J.A. Jenkins's spouse is a vice president and director of research at GI Laboratories (Toronto, Ontario, Canada).

Krobua Srichaikul, Arash Mirrahimi, and Livia S.A. Augustin have not declared conflicts of interest related to this article. Laura Chiavaroli is a clinical research coordinator at GI Laboratories (Toronto, Ontario, Canada). John L. Sievenpiper has received several unrestricted travel grants from the Coca-Cola Company to present research at meetings and is a co-investigator on an unrestricted research grant from the Coca-Cola Company. He has also received travel funding and honoraria from Abbott Laboratories, Archer Daniels Midland, and the International Life Sciences Institute North America, as well as research support, consultant fees, and travel funding from Pulse Canada. Cyril W.C. Kendall is a co-investigator on an unrestricted grant from the Coca-Cola Company. He has served on the scientific advisory board and received research support, travel funding, consultant fees, or honoraria from Pulse Canada, Barilla, Solae, Unilever, Hain Celestial, Loblaws Supermarkets, Oldways Preservation Trust, the Almond Board of California, the International Nut Council, Paramount Farms, the California Strawberry Commission, the Canola and Flax Councils of Canada, and Saskatchewan Pulse Growers. Cyril W.C. Kendall also receives partial salary funding from research grants provided by Unilever, Loblaws Supermarkets, and the Almond Board of California.

REFERENCES

1. Ludwig DS. The glycemic index: Physiological mechanisms relating to obesity, diabetes, and cardiovascular disease. *JAMA* 2002;287:2414–2423.
2. Brand-Miller J, Hayne S, Petocz P, and Colagiuri S. Low-glycemic index diets in the management of diabetes: A meta-analysis of randomized controlled trials. *Diabetes Care* 2003;26:2261–2267.
3. Livesey G, Taylor R, Hulshof T, and Howlett J. Glycemic response and health—A systematic review and meta-analysis: Relations between dietary glycemic properties and health outcomes. *Am J Clin Nutr* 2008;87:258S–268S.
4. Wolever TM, Gibbs AL, Mehling C et al. The Canadian Trial of Carbohydrates in Diabetes (CCD), a 1-y controlled trial of low-glycemic-index dietary carbohydrate in type 2 diabetes: No effect on glycated hemoglobin but reduction in C-reactive protein. *Am J Clin Nutr* 2008;87:114–125.
5. Ebbeling CB, Leidig MM, Feldman HA, Lovesky MM, and Ludwig DS. Effects of a low-glycemic load vs low-fat diet in obese young adults: A randomized trial. *JAMA* 2007;297:2092–2102.
6. McKeown-Eyssen G. Epidemiology of colorectal cancer revisited: Are serum triglycerides and/or plasma glucose associated with risk? *Cancer Epidemiol Biomarkers Prev* 1994;3:687–695.
7. Giovannucci E. Insulin and colon cancer. *Cancer Causes Control* 1995;6:164–179.
8. Giovannucci E, Harlan DM, Archer MC et al. Diabetes and cancer: A consensus report. *CA Cancer J Clin* 2010;60:207–221.
9. Augustin LS, Dal Maso L, La Vecchia C et al. Dietary glycemic index and glycemic load, and breast cancer risk: A case-control study. *Ann Oncol* 2001;12:1533–1538.
10. Augustin LS, Galeone C, Dal Maso L et al. Glycemic index, glycemic load and risk of prostate cancer. *Int J Cancer* 2004;112:446–450.
11. Franceschi S, Dal Maso L, Augustin L et al. Dietary glycemic load and colorectal cancer risk. *Ann Oncol* Feb 2001;12(2):173–178.
12. Augustin LS, Gallus S, Bosetti C et al. Glycemic index and glycemic load in endometrial cancer. *Int J Cancer*. June 20 2003;105(3):404–407.
13. Higginbotham S, Zhang ZF, Lee IM et al. Dietary glycemic load and risk of colorectal cancer in the Women's Health Study. *J Natl Cancer Inst* 2004;96:229–233.
14. Flood A, Peters U, Jenkins DJ et al. Carbohydrate, glycemic index, and glycemic load and colorectal adenomas in the Prostate, Lung, Colorectal, and Ovarian Screening Study. *Am J Clin Nutr* 2006;84:1184–1192.
15. Ray KK, Seshasai SR, Erqou S et al. Statins and all-cause mortality in high-risk primary prevention: A meta-analysis of 11 randomized controlled trials involving 65,229 participants. *Arch Intern Med* 2010;170:1024–1031.
16. Mills EJ, Wu P, Chong G et al. Efficacy and safety of statin treatment for cardiovascular disease: A network meta-analysis of 170,255 patients from 76 randomized trials. *QJM* 2011;104:109–124.
17. Duckworth W, Abraira C, Moritz T et al. Glucose control and vascular complications in veterans with type 2 diabetes. *N Engl J Med* 2009;360:129–139.
18. Gerstein HC, Miller ME, Byington RP et al. Effects of intensive glucose lowering in type 2 diabetes. *N Engl J Med* 2008;358:2545–2559.
19. Patel A, MacMahon S, Chalmers J et al. Intensive blood glucose control and vascular outcomes in patients with type 2 diabetes. *N Engl J Med* 2008;358:2560–2572.
20. Currie CJ, Poole CD, and Gale EA. The influence of glucose-lowering therapies on cancer risk in type 2 diabetes. *Diabetologia* 2009;52:1766–1777.
21. Siri-Tarino PW, Sun Q, Hu FB, and Krauss RM. Meta-analysis of prospective cohort studies evaluating the association of saturated fat with cardiovascular disease. *Am J Clin Nutr* 2010;91:535–546.
22. Rauch B, Schiele R, Schneider S et al. OMEGA, a randomized, placebo-controlled trial to test the effect of highly purified omega-3 fatty acids on top of modern guideline-adjusted therapy after myocardial infarction. *Circulation* 2010;122:2152–2159.
23. Kromhout D, Giltay EJ, and Geleijnse JM. n-3 fatty acids and cardiovascular events after myocardial infarction. *N Engl J Med* 2010;363:2015–2026.
24. Trowell H, Burkitt D, and Heaton K. *Dietary Fiber-Depleted Foods and Disease.* London, U.K.: Academic Press, 1985.
25. National Academy of Sciences. Institute of Medicine. Food and Nutrition Board. *Dietary Reference Intakes for Energy, Carbohydrate, Fiber, Fat, Fatty Acids, Cholesterol, Protein, and Amino Acids (Macronutrients).* Washington, DC: The National Academies Press, 2005.
26. Thorne MJ, Thompson LU, and Jenkins DJ. Factors affecting starch digestibility and the glycemic response with special reference to legumes. *Am J Clin Nutr* 1983;38:481–488.

27. Jenkins DJ, Wolever TM, Taylor RH et al. Glycemic index of foods: A physiological basis for carbohydrate exchange. *Am J Clin Nutr* 1981;34:362–366.
28. Jenkins D, Wolever T, Thorne M et al. The relationship between glycemic response, digestibility, and factors influencing the dietary habits of diabetics. *Am J Clin Nutr* 1984;40:1175–1191.
29. Salmeron J, Manson JE, Stampfer MJ, Colditz GA, Wing AL, and Willett WC. Dietary fiber, glycemic load, and risk of non-insulin-dependent diabetes mellitus in women. *JAMA* 1997;277:472–477.
30. Salmeron J, Ascherio A, Rimm EB et al. Dietary fiber, glycemic load, and risk of NIDDM in men. *Diabetes Care* 1997;20:545–550.
31. Jenkins DJ, Kendall CW, McKeown-Eyssen G et al. Effect of a low-glycemic index or a high-cereal fiber diet on type 2 diabetes: A randomized trial. *JAMA* 2008;300:2742–2753.
32. Jenkins DJ, Srichaikul K, Kendall CW et al. The relation of low glycaemic index fruit consumption to glycaemic control and risk factors for coronary heart disease in type 2 diabetes. *Diabetologia* 2011;54:271–279.
33. Wolever TM, Jenkins DJ, Jenkins AL, and Josse RG. The glycemic index: Methodology and clinical implications. *Am J Clin Nutr* 1991;54:846–854.
34. Wolever TM, Brand-Miller JC, Abernethy J et al. Measuring the glycemic index of foods: Interlaboratory study. *Am J Clin Nutr* 2008;87:247S–257S.
35. Brouns F, Bjorck I, Frayn KN et al. Glycaemic index methodology. *Nutr Res Rev* 2005;18:145–171.

35 Chromium (III) in Promoting Weight Loss and Lean Body Mass

Debasis Bagchi, PhD, MACN, CNS, MAIChE,
Manashi Bagchi, PhD, Shirley Zafra-Stone, BS,
and Harry G. Preuss, MD, MACN, CNS

CONTENTS

INTRODUCTION

Chromium (III) has long been known to be essential for proper lipid and carbohydrate metabolism in humans. Numerous studies demonstrated chromium (III) as a micronutrient and its beneficial role in human nutrition by serving as a critical cofactor in the action of insulin.[1–6] Dietary chromium (III) complexes, such as chromium chloride, niacin-bound chromium (NBC), chromium picolinate, chromium dinicocysteinate, and chromium amino acid chelates, are available as stand-alone nutritional supplements or in various formulations which are used for weight loss and weight management, diabetes, and energy. Furthermore, studies have shown chromium (III) chloride, NBC, and chromium picolinate to improve the lipid profile and cardiovascular functions, impaired glucose tolerance, insulin sensitivity, and type 2 diabetes in both animals and humans. NBC and chromium picolinate have been particularly popular, especially with athletes who experience exercise-induced increased urinary chromium loss. In many clinical trials, subjects have been administered an average daily dose in the range of 100–1000 μg elemental chromium (III) and have demonstrated beneficial effects without any adverse events.

Dietary Chromium (III) and Recommended Dietary Intake

A strong association exists between chromium deficiency, high blood glucose, atherosclerosis, and elevated blood cholesterol levels. In rats, chromium deficiency has been reported to increase serum cholesterol levels and formation of aortic plaques.[4] In humans, it has been well demonstrated that chromium deficiency leads to impaired insulin function, obesity, and cardiovascular dysfunction.[4] Research demonstrated that elderly people, diabetics, pregnant women, and athletes suffer from chromium deficiency. Strenuous exercise is another major cause of chromium loss.[1,2] On the positive side, chromium (III) supplementation has been shown to prevent the formation of aortic plaques and the rise of serum cholesterol.[2]

Chromium (III) is available in various food sources including whole-grain products, high-bran breakfast cereals, egg yolks, coffee, nuts, green beans, broccoli, meat, brewers' yeast, and selected brands of beer and wine. Chromium (III) complexes are also found in many mineral or multivitamin supplements. According to the National Research Council (NRC), the Estimated Safe and Adequate Daily Dietary Intake (ESADDI) for chromium (III) is 50–200 μg/day, corresponding to 0.83–3.33 μg/kg/day for an adult weighing 60 kg.[8] The U.S. Food and Drug Administration (FDA) recommends a daily intake (RDI) of 120 μg/day for chromium (III).

Glucose Tolerance Factor

Chromium (III), in the form of the naturally occurring dinicotinic acid-glutathione complex, or glucose tolerance factor (GTF), significantly enhances the effect of exogenous insulin on glucose metabolism.[2,3] GTF influences the action of insulin and potentiates the actions of protein, fat, and carbohydrate metabolism.[2,3] GTF is safe and highly absorbed and known to stabilize blood glucose levels. Furthermore, GTF has easy access to biologically important chromium storage depots in the fetus and placenta.[2–4] The most abundant and naturally occurring form of GTF is found in brewer's yeast.[2–4] The O-coordinated chromium (III)-dinicotinic acid complex is biologically active compound which suggests that a *trans* configuration of pyridine nitrogen atoms resembles that part of the GTF structure that is recognized by the receptors or enzymes and is involved in the expression of the biological effect.[2,3] The body's ability to convert simple chromium (III) compounds into the GTF form declines with advancing age and is impaired in diabetes and probably in hyperlipidemic and atherosclerotic patients as well.[7–9] Unfortunately, naturally occurring GTF has less than 2% of the available chromium in brewer's yeast.[2,3]

Several studies demonstrate that the biologically active form of chromium (III) in brewers' yeast promotes GTF and prevents diabetes in experimental animals by impeding the action of insulin to enhance protein, fat, and carbohydrate metabolism, and significantly reduce plasma glucose levels in diabetic mice.[7–9] Clinical studies on diabetic patients demonstrated highly favorable response to chromium supplementation via brewer's yeast, i.e., increased insulin sensitivity. Twenty-two participants (8 males and 14 females; mean age: 51 year) with fasting values of total cholesterol (TC) and glucose from 3.21 to 6.90 and 4.3 to 6.2 mmol/L, respectively, were evaluated. After a 9 h fast, an oral glucose load (75 g) was administered before chromium (III) supplementation, and blood was drawn before and at 30, 60, 90, and 120 min after the glucose load.[9,10] Subjects were given either brewer's yeast or torula yeast (10 g yeast powder) daily for 12 weeks. Brewer's yeast demonstrated a beneficial effect by decreasing serum triacylglycerol values in subjects. In an oral glucose tolerance test (OGTT), an increment at 0 min and significant decreases at 60 and 90 min were shown. In subjects given torula yeast, glucose values increased at both 0 and 30 min after glucose load and 12 week supplementation. Brewer's yeast and torula yeast significantly altered glucose concentrations at 60 min after glucose dosage. Brewer's yeast had significant decreasing effects on insulin output at both 90 and 120 min after glucose load. Likewise, in subjects given torula yeast, serum insulin contents decreased at 90 min. Brewer's yeast supplementation had beneficial effects both on serum triacylglycerol and on the 60 and 90 min glucose values of OGTT.[9,10]

A complex of chromium (III) and nicotinic acid was demonstrated to facilitate insulin binding similar to the GTF found in brewer's yeast. Urberg et al. have shown that humans' inability to respond to chromium (III) supplementation resulted from suboptimal levels of dietary nicotinic acid to serve as a substrate for GTF synthesis.[9] In a controlled clinical trial, 16 healthy elderly volunteers were given 200 µg chromium (III), 100 mg nicotinic acid, or 200 µg chromium (III) + 100 mg nicotinic acid daily for 28 days and evaluated on days 0 and 28. Fasting glucose and glucose tolerance were unaffected by either chromium (III) or nicotinic acid alone. In contrast, the combined chromium–nicotinic acid supplement caused a 15% decrease in a glucose area integrated total ($p < 0.025$) and a 7% decrease in fasting glucose.[9]

BIOAVAILABILITY OF CHROMIUM (III) COMPLEXES

After absorption in the gastrointestinal tract, chromium is transported to cells bound to the plasma protein transferrin. Insulin initiates chromium (III) transport into the cells where it is bound to the oligopeptide apochromodulin. Apochromodulin, combined in a tetra-nuclear assembly of four chromium (III) atoms, forms the low-molecular-weight oligopeptide chromodulin (MW ~ 1500 Da) which is important in amplifying the insulin signaling effect. After binding to insulin-activated receptor, chromodulin increases tyrosine kinase activity and forms a part of intracellular portion of insulin receptor.[11] In a study conducted by Clodfelder et al., the biomimetic cation $[Cr_3O(O_2CCH_2CH_3)_6(H_2O)_3]^+$ was found to imitate the oligopeptide chromodulin's ability to stimulate the tyrosine kinase activity of insulin receptor, increase insulin sensitivity, and decrease plasma total, LDL, and triglycerides concentrations as shown in healthy and type 2 diabetic rat models.[12] In addition, due to the stability and solubility of the biomimetic cation, a greater magnitude of absorbability is demonstrated.[12]

Olin et al. investigated the absorption and retention of $CrCl_3$, NBC, and chromium picolinate over a 12 h period.[13] Male rats (150–170 g) were gavaged with 44 µCi (1 mL each or 2.7 nmol) chromium as $CrCl_3$, NBC, or chromium picolinate. At 1, 3, 6, and 12 h postgavage, rats were anesthetized and killed. Cardiac blood and urine (at 6 and 12 h) were collected, and liver, kidneys, pancreas, testes, and gastrocnemius were removed, weighed, and assayed to calculate chromium absorbed/retained counts. Results reveal that the highest percent of absorbed/retained counts was observed in urine, followed by the muscle, blood, and liver. The average percent chromium (III) retained in the tissues was higher in NBC-gavaged rats than in $CrCl_3$- or chromium picolinate–gavaged rats in the majority of the time points. One hour postgavage, NBC rats had retention percentages 3.2–8.4-fold higher in tissues collected compared to chromium picolinate and $CrCl_3$ groups. Three hours postgavage, NBC-treated rats had blood, muscle, and pancreatic chromium retentions that were 2.4–8 times higher compared to chromium picolinate–gavaged rats. By 6 and 12 h postgavage, NBC had absorbed/retained Cr in tissues that were 1.8–3.8 times higher compared to rats receiving chromium picolinate. These results demonstrate significant differences in the bioavailability of the different chromium compounds, with NBC exhibiting the superior bioavailability.[13]

CHROMIUM (III) SUPPLEMENTATION, METABOLIC SYNDROME, AND WEIGHT LOSS

Over the last several decades, chromium nutritional supplements became extremely popular for weight loss and muscle development. So popular that sale was second only to calcium among mineral supplements. This is due to the association of existing suboptimal chromium (III) intake and metabolic syndrome, which is characterized by elements of insulin resistance, lipid disturbances and glucose intolerance, obesity, and hypertension.[14–16] However, it is controversial as to trivalent chromium's effects on body composition, including reduction of fat mass and enhancement of lean body mass. In 1989, chromium picolinate was reported to lead to body mass losses and lean muscle mass increases,[17] which was quickly followed by a report of improvement in symptoms associated with type 2 diabetes.[18] The claims of weight loss and muscle development were quickly challenged,[6,19] and changes in body mass and composition in healthy subjects have been refuted.[20,21] Thus, in 1997, the U.S. Federal Trade Commission (FTC) ordered entities associated with the chromium picolinate supplement to stop making representations of body fat reduction, weight loss, and muscle mass increases.[22]

Literature search demonstrates several chromium (III) complexes and its effects on body composition and influences on weight loss. It is important to note that some complexes are in formulation with weight loss ingredients and study subjects had undergone an exercise regimen.

NIACIN-BOUND CHROMIUM

Crawford et al. reported that supplementation of 600 μg per day of elemental chromium (III) as NBC over a period of 2 months by African American women with a moderate diet and exercise regimen favorably influences weight loss and body composition.[23] In a randomized, double-blind, placebo-controlled, crossover study, 20 overweight African American women received placebo t.i.d. during the control period and 200 μg NBC t.i.d. during the verum period and engaged in a modest diet-exercise regimen for 2 months. Group 1 subjects ($n = 10$) received placebo first and then NBC, while Group 2 subjects ($n = 10$) received NBC first and then placebo later. Body weights and blood chemistries were measured by routine clinical methodology. Fat and nonfat body masses were estimated using bioelectrical impedance (electrolipography).[23] In women receiving NBC after the placebo period (Group 1), body weight loss was essentially the same, but fat loss was significantly greater and nonfat body mass loss significantly less with chromium (III) intake. There was a significantly greater loss of fat in the placebo period compared to the verum period of Group 1. However, the ability of Cr supplementation to augment fat loss and decrease lean body mass loss was carried over into the placebo period even after a 1 month washout period. No changes in blood chemistries were observed in either group. To summarize, results confirmed that NBC given to African American women in conjunction with moderate diet and exercise caused a significant loss of fat and sparing muscle compared to placebo and that this effect can be carried over for months.[23]

NBC in combination with HCA-SX and a standardized *Gymnema sylvestre* extract was evaluated in a weight loss study of moderately obese subjects.[24–26] A randomized, double-blind, placebo-controlled human study was conducted in 60 moderately obese subjects (aged 21–50 years, BMI > 26 kg/m^2) for 8 weeks. One group was administered a combination of 4 mg NBC, 4667 mg HCA-SX, and 400 mg *Gymnema sylvestre* extract, while another group was given placebo daily in three equally divided doses 30–60 min before meals.[25,26] All subjects received a 2000 kcal diet/day and participated in supervised walking program. At the end of 8 weeks, body weight and BMI decreased by 5%–6%. Food intake, as well as TC, LDL, triglycerides, and serum leptin levels, was significantly reduced, while HDL levels and excretion of urinary fat metabolites increased.[25,26] In another related study, 30 moderately obese subjects received the same combination of NBC, *Gymnema sylvestre* extract, and HCA-SX or placebo daily in three equally divided doses 30–60 min before each meal for 8 weeks.[25,26] Subjects also received 2000 kcal diet/day and underwent a 30 min/day supervised walking program, 5 days/week, as in the previous study. Results demonstrated that at the end of 8 weeks, chromium combination–supplemented group reduced body weight and BMI by 7.8% and 7.9%, respectively. Food intake was reduced by 14.1%. TC, LDL, and triglyceride levels were reduced by 9.1%, 17.9%, and 18.1%, respectively, while HDL and serotonin levels increased by 20.7% and 50%, respectively. Serum leptin levels decreased by 40.5%, and enhanced excretion of urinary fat metabolites increased by 146%–281%. No significant changes were observed in the placebo group.[25,26]

Grant et al. studied the effects of two chromium (III) supplementation (400 μg elemental chromium/day), as NBC and chromium picolinate, with or without exercise training, in young, obese women.[27] Exercise training combined with NBC supplementation resulted in significant weight loss and lowered the insulin response to an oral glucose load. In contrast, chromium picolinate supplementation was associated with a significant weight gain. Accordingly, exercise training with NBC supplementation is beneficial for weight loss and lowers the risk of diabetes.[27]

CHROMIUM PICOLINATE

A clinical trial assessed the effects of chromium picolinate supplementation, alone and combined with nutritional education, on weight loss in apparently healthy overweight adults.[28] A randomized, double-blind, placebo-controlled trial of 80 otherwise healthy, overweight adults was assessed at baseline for central adiposity measured by computerized tomography. Subjects were randomly assigned to daily ingestion of 1000 μg of chromium picolinate or placebo for 24 weeks. All subjects received passive nutritional education at the 12 week point in both the intervention and control groups. At baseline, both the chromium and placebo groups had similar mean BMI (chromium = 36 ± 6.7 kg/m(2) vs. placebo = 36.1 ± 7.6 kg/m(2); $p = 0.98$). After 12 weeks, no change was seen in BMI in the intervention as compared to placebo (chromium = 0.3 ± 0.8 kg/m(2) vs. placebo = 0.0 ± 0.4 kg/m(2); $p = 0.07$). No change was seen in BMI after 24 weeks in the intervention as compared to placebo (chromium = 0.1 ± 0.2 kg/m(2) vs. placebo = 0.0 ± 0.5 kg/m(2); $p = 0.81$). Variation in central adiposity did not affect any outcome measures. Overall, supplementation of 1000 μg of chromium picolinate alone, and in combination with nutritional education, did not affect weight loss in this population of overweight adults. Response to chromium did not vary with central adiposity.[28]

In another clinical study, moderately obese women participated in a 12 week exercise program, which investigated the effect of chromium picolinate supplementation on body composition, resting metabolic rate, and selected biochemical parameters.[29] In this double-blind study, 44 women (aged 27–51 years) received either 400 μg/day of elemental chromium (III) as chromium picolinate or a placebo and participated in a supervised weight training and walking program 2 days per week for 12 weeks. Body composition and resting metabolic rate were measured at baseline, 6, and 12 weeks. Body composition and resting metabolic rate were not significantly changed by chromium picolinate supplementation. Overall results demonstrated that 12 weeks of chromium picolinate supplementation [400 μg elemental chromium (III)/day] did not significantly affect body composition, resting metabolic rate, plasma glucose, serum insulin, plasma glucagon, serum C-peptide, and serum lipid concentrations.[29]

In another study, the effects of daily chromium supplementation (200 μg elemental chromium as chromium picolinate) were investigated in football players during spring training for 9 weeks in a double-blind study.[30] Subjects receiving chromium picolinate demonstrated urinary chromium losses five times greater than those in the placebo group. However, chromium picolinate supplementation was ineffective in bringing about changes in body composition or strength during a program of intensive weight-lifting training.[30] In a double-blind, randomized, placebo-controlled study, the effects of 14 weeks of chromium picolinate supplementation during preseason resistance and conditioning program on body composition and neuromuscular performance in NCAA Division I wrestlers were assessed.[31] Twenty wrestlers from the University of Oklahoma were assigned to either a treatment group ($n = 7$; 20.4 year ± 0.1) receiving 200 μg elemental chromium (III) as chromium picolinate daily, a placebo group ($n = 7$; 19.9 year ± 0.2), or a control group ($n = 6$; 20.2 year ± 0.1) using a stratified random sampling technique based on weight classification. Body composition, neuromuscular performance, metabolic performance, and serum insulin and glucose were measured before and immediately following the supplementation and training period.[31] Repeat measures by ANOVA indicated no significant changes in body composition for any of the groups. Aerobic power increased significantly ($p < 0.002$) in all groups, independent of supplementation. The results from the two studies mentioned earlier demonstrated that chromium picolinate supplementation coupled with typical preseason training programs did not enhance body composition or performance variables beyond improvements seen with training alone, at least at the relatively low doses used.[31]

In another double-blind, placebo-controlled study, the efficacy of chromium picolinate as a fat-reduction aid for obese individuals enrolled in a physical exercise program was investigated for 16 weeks.[32] Participants were healthy, active-duty Navy personnel (79 men, 16 women) who exceeded the Navy's percent body fat standards of 22% fat for men and 30% for women. Mean age was 30.3 years, and comparisons between the subjects who completed the study ($n = 95$) and dropouts ($n = 109$) revealed no significant differences in demographics or baseline percent body fat. The physical conditioning programs met a minimum of three times per week for at least 30 min of aerobic exercise. On a daily basis, subjects were given either 400 µg elemental chromium (III) as chromium picolinate or a placebo.[32] At the end of 16 weeks, the group as a whole had lost a small amount of weight and body fat. However, the chromium picolinate–supplemented group failed to show a significantly greater reduction in either percent body fat or body weight, or a greater increase in lean body mass, than did the placebo group.[32]

Livolsi et al. examined the effect of chromium picolinate supplementation on muscular strength, body composition, and urinary excretion in women softball athletes.[33] Fifteen women softball athletes were randomly divided into two groups, the chromium picolinate (500 µg elemental chromium/day) treatment group ($n = 8$) and the placebo control group ($n = 7$). Results demonstrated that no significant ($p < 0.05$) differences in muscular strength or body composition were found after 6 weeks of resistance training.[33] In a longitudinal, double-blind, randomly assigned intervention study in 33 female obese subjects for 16 months with supplementation of 200 µg elemental chromium (III) as chromium picolinate along with a very-low-energy diet (VLED) during the first 2 months. Results show that chromium picolinate intake did not result in significant changes in blood parameters and body composition.[34]

CHROMIUM HISTIDINATE

In a recent study, researchers investigated the effects of chromium histidinate (CrHis) on glucose transporter-2 (GLUT-2), nuclear factor erythroid 2–related factor 2 (Nrf2), heme oxygenase-1 (HO-1), nuclear factor-kappa B (NF-κB p65), and the oxidative stress marker 4-hydroxynonenal adducts (HNE) expressions in liver of rats fed high-fat diet (HFD).[35] Male Wistar rats ($n = 40$, 8 weeks old) were divided into four groups. Group I was fed a standard diet (12% of calories as fat), Group II was fed a standard diet and supplemented with 110 µg CrHis/kg BW/d, Group III was fed HFD (40% of calories as fat), and Group IV was fed HFD and supplemented with 110 µg CrHis/kg BW/d. Rats fed HFD possessed greater serum insulin (40 vs. 33 pmol/L) and glucose (158 vs. 143 mg/dL) concentration and less liver Cr (44 vs. 82 µg/g) concentration than rats fed the control diet. However, rats supplemented with CrHis had greater liver Cr and serum insulin and lower glucose concentration in rats fed HFD ($p < 0.05$). The hepatic NF-κβ p65 and HNE were increased in high-fat group compared to control group, but reduced by the CrHis administration ($p < 0.05$). The levels of hepatic Nrf2 and HO-1 were increased by supplementation of CrHis ($p < 0.05$). These findings demonstrate that supplementation of CrHis is protective against obesity, at least in part, through Nrf2-mediated induction of HO-1 in rats fed HFD.[35]

CHROMIUM (III)–GENE INTERACTION

The genomic approach to nutritional research has paved the way for future investigations to unravel the molecular basis of chromium–gene interactions. Although numerous animal and human clinical studies have established the safety and efficacy of chromium (III) supplementation in combating insulin resistance, and potentially reducing body fat and increasing lean body mass,[36] the underlying molecular mechanism for the observed beneficial effects of chromium (III) is unclear. In contrast, the structure, function, and mode of action of the majority of other essential trace elements such as copper and zinc have been well characterized. Even though there have been several attempts to identify the specific organic chromium (III) complex that exhibits biological functions, the results have generally been controversial at best.[3,37–39] In order to decipher the mechanism modulating the genetic response to NBC supplementation, a recent study utilized the high-throughput screening (HTS) technology to examine NBC-induced alteration in gene expression profiles (transcriptome).[40] This study investigated the effect of oral NBC supplementation on the physiological parameters of obese mice homozygous for type 2 diabetes spontaneous mutation (Leprdb) and the alteration in transcriptome of subcutaneous adipose tissues in these obese mice.[40] Supplementation regimen was carried for 10 weeks in male Leprdb mice which were randomly divided into the NBC ($n = 7$, NBC) or placebo ($n = 7$, PBO) group. Blood samples were drawn from the mice before (baseline) and after 6 weeks of supplementation. Blood glucose level as well as lipid profile parameters such as TC, HDL cholesterol (HDLC), triglycerides, LDL, and the TC-to-HDLC ratio were assessed at week 6 and compared to baseline data collected before any supplementation. After 8 weeks of supplementation, OGTT was performed by challenging the mice with 1.5 mg/g body weight of glucose solution and measuring blood glucose levels at 30, 60, and 120 min after glucose challenge.[40] At 10 weeks postsupplementation, mice were euthanized and subcutaneous fat was removed for isolation of RNA. The quality of RNA was verified before the synthesis of targets from RNA for hybridization to probes (41,101 probe sets) on the mouse genome microarrays (430 v2.0). The results of biochemical tests showed that NBC supplementation significantly attenuated the levels of triglycerides, TC, LDL cholesterol, and TC-to-HDLC ratio in the plasma of the obese diabetic mice. The plasma level of HDLC in these mice was significantly increased by NBC supplementation. OGTT findings indicated a significant enhancement by NBC supplementation in the rate of blood glucose clearance from 60 to 120 min after glucose challenge.[40] The observations from this study agreed with the previous findings in other human and animal studies that NBC supplementation play a beneficial role in glucose and lipid metabolism.[40]

COMPARISONS OF BLOOD LIPID PROFILES BETWEEN PLACEBO CONTROL AND NIACIN-BOUND CHROMIUM–TREATED OBESE TYPE 2 DIABETIC RATS

NBC-induced changes in the transcriptome of subcutaneous adipose tissues of these obese diabetic mice were interrogated by an unbiased genome-wide microarray approach in an attempt to identify candidate genes whose expressions were sensitive to NBC supplementation.[40] In a data-mining scheme, among the 45,101 probe sets interrogated, only a small subset of genes was found to be influenced by NBC supplementation. The overall effect of NBC supplementation on the genome of the adipose tissues was positive since it stimulated more genes than it inhibited them. The NBC induced genes are known to be involved in glycolysis, muscle metabolism, and muscle development. The expression of muscle-specific genes in fat tissue over time has been shown to reduce fat content in the adipose tissues.[41] The NBC-suppressed genes in the adipose tissues are known to play important roles in thermogenic process of brown fat tissue. On the whole, the microarray data indicated that NBC supplementation did not induce a genome-wide perturbation; rather, NBC supplementation specifically influenced a small subset of genes that are biologically relevant to adipocyte maintenance.

Bioinformatic analyses of the microarray data resulted in 161 upregulated and 91 downregulated genes by NBC supplementation in obese diabetic mice. The expression of several biologically relevant candidate genes was further verified by real-time PCR. Enolase 3 (ENO3) showed the highest upregulation (7.6-fold) compared to controls in the fat tissues, in response to NBC supplementation.[42] Enolase is a dimeric glycolytic enzyme that catalyzes the interconversion of 2-phosphoglycerate and phosphoenolpyruvate. Beta-enolase subunit is encoded by ENO3 gene and is responsible for more than 90% of the enolase activity in adult human muscle.[42] It has been shown that mutations in ENO3 led to β-enolase deficiency that resulted in defects in glycolysis and metabolic myopathies.[42] Another glycolytic gene, encoding the enzyme glucose phosphate isomerase (GPI), was also upregulated in the NBC-supplemented obese diabetic mice. It has been documented that glycolytic genes such as ENO3 and GPI are downregulated in the visceral adipose tissues of morbidly obese patients as compared to nonobese individuals.[43] Calsequestrin, the most abundant calcium-binding protein in the sarcoplasmic reticulum of skeletal and cardiac muscle, was upregulated by NBC supplementation. Since chromium has been demonstrated to enhance the expression of plasmalemmal calcium-ATPase in smooth muscle cells, it is possible that chromium may influence calcium homeostasis by increasing the calcium storage capacity through upregulation of calsequestrin.[44,45] Tropomyosin-1 (TPM1) gene, which encodes for the α-subunit (α-tropomyosin) of the tropomyosin family of proteins, was upregulated in response to NBC supplementation. TPM1 protein plays an important role in calcium-dependent regulation of striated muscle contraction.[46–48] Expression of these upregulated genes in fat tissue over time has been shown to attenuate the fat content of the tissue.[41]

Candidate Genes in Response to NBC Supplementation

The NBC-induced downregulated genes included adipocyte-specific genes such as the cell death–induced DNA fragmentation factor (CIDEA), mitochondrial uncoupling protein 1 (UCP1), and tocopherol transfer protein (TTP). TTP is involved in the transport of α-tocopherol from hepatocytes into peripheral tissues including adipose tissue.[49] Since α-tocopherol serves as a potent antioxidant, downregulation of TTP may decrease the lipid-phase antioxidant defense in the adipose tissue, thus promoting the breakdown of adipose tissues.[40] In addition, because α-tocopherol readily interconverts into lipoproteins and TTP is likely to facilitate the incorporation of α-tocopherol into LDL,[50,51] downregulation of TTP in the adipose tissues is expected to lower the levels of LDL. Interestingly, the physiological findings indicated that the plasma levels of LDL were indeed reduced. Both CIDEA and UCP1 proteins are highly expressed in brown adipose tissue (BAT), and they play important roles in the thermogenesis and energy expenditure of BAT.[52,53] CIDEA-knockout mice exhibited resistance to diet-induced obesity and diabetes.[53] Thus, downregulation of CIDEA by NBC may exhibit similar effects, i.e., weight loss and resistance to diet-induced obesity. Taken together, the data suggest that NBC exerts its beneficial effects of weight loss through regulation of specific genes in the fat cells of obese diabetic mice.[53]

CONCLUSION

Human and animal studies have shown that chromium (III) complexes are efficacious in maintaining proper carbohydrate and lipid metabolism in both humans and animals. Furthermore, some chromium (III) complexes may play a role in regulating appetite, reducing sugar cravings, and increasing lean body mass.[1–5,53] However, it is controversial as to trivalent chromium's effects on body composition, including reduction of fat mass and enhancement of lean body mass. Additional clinical research on selected chromium (III) complexes, such as chromium nicotinate, chromium picolinate, and CrHis, and their effects on lean body mass and obesity is warranted.

REFERENCES

1. Preuss HG, Bagchi D, and Bagchi M. Protective effects of a novel niacin-bound chromium complex and a grape seed proanthocyanidin extract on advancing age and various aspects of syndrome X. *Ann NY Acad Sci* 2002;957:250–259.
2. Mertz W. Chromium research from a distance: From 1959 to 1980. *J Am Coll Nutr* 1998;17(6):544–547.
3. Mertz W. Effects and metabolism of glucose tolerance factor. In: Nutrition Foundation (Ed.), *Nutrition Reviews: Present Knowledge in Nutrition*. Nutrition Foundation, Washington, DC, 1976, pp. 365–372.
4. Shapcott D and Hubert J. *Chromium in Nutrition and Metabolism*. Elsevier North Holland Biomedical Press, Amsterdam, the Netherlands, 1979.
5. Anderson RA and Kozlovsky AS. Chromium intake, absorption and excretion of subjects consuming self-selected diets. *Am J Clin Nutr* 1985;41(6):1177–1183.
6. Lefavi RG, Anderson RA, Keith RE, Wilson D, McMillan JL, and Stone MH. Efficacy of chromium supplementation in athletes: Emphasis on anabolism. *Int J Sport Nutr* 1992;2(2):111–122.
7. Cooper JA, Anderson BF, and Buckley PD. Structure and biological activity of nitrogen and oxygen coordinated nicotinic acid complexes of chromium. *Inorg Chim Acta* 1984;91:1–9.
8. Glinsmann WH and Mertz W. Effect of trivalent chromium on glucose tolerance. *Metabolism* 1966;15(6):510–520.

9. Urberg M and Zemel MB. Evidence for synergism between chromium and nicotinic acid in the control of glucose tolerance in elderly humans. *Metabolism* 1987;36(9):896–899.

10. Li YC. Effects of brewer's yeast on glucose tolerance and serum lipids in Chinese adults. *Biol Trace Elem Res* 1994;41(3):341–347.

11. Clodfelder BJ, Emamaullee J, Hepburn DD, Chakov NE, Nettles HS, and Vincent JB. The trail of chromium (III) in vivo from the blood to the urine: The roles of transferrin and chromodulin. *J Biol Inorg Chem* 2001;6(5–6):608–617.

12. Clodfelder BJ, Chang C, and Vincent JB. Absorption of the biomimetic chromium cation triaqua-mu3-oxo-mu-hexapropionatotrichromium(III) in rats. *Biol Trace Elem Res* 2004;98(2):159–169.

13. Olin KL, Stearns DM, Armstrong WH, and Keen CL. Comparative retention/absorption of ^{51}chromium (^{51}Cr) from ^{51}Cr chloride, ^{51}Cr nicotinate and ^{51}Cr picolinate in a rat model. *Trace Elem Electrolytes* 1994;11(4):182–186.

14. Reaven GM. Syndrome X. *Curr Treat Options Cardiovasc Med* 2001;3:323–332.

15. Behn A and Ur E. The obesity epidemic and its cardiovascular consequences. *Curr Opin Cardiol* 2006;21(4):353–360.

16. Reaven GM. The metabolic syndrome: Is this diagnosis necessary? *Am J Clin Nutr* 2006;83(6):1237–1247.

17. Evans GW. The effect of chromium picolinate on insulin controlled parameters in humans. *Int J Biosocial Med Res* 1989;11(6):163–167.

18. Lefavi RG. Response to Evans—Chromium picolinate. *Int J Sport Nutr* 1993;3(2):120–122.

19. Press RI, Geller J, and Evans GW. The effect of chromium picolinate on serum cholesterol and apolipoprotein fractions in human subjects. *West J Med* 1990;152(1):41–45.

20. Vincent JB. Quest for the molecular mechanism of chromium action and its relationship to diabetes. *Nutr Rev* 2000;58(3 Pt 1):67–72.

21. Nielsen FH. How should dietary guidance be given for mineral elements with beneficial actions or suspected of being essential? *J Nutr* 1996;126(9 Suppl):2377S–2385S.

22. Federal Trade Commission, Docket No. C-3758 Decision and order. http://www.ftc.gov/os/1997/07/nutritid.pdf (accessed April 1, 2011), 1997.

23. Crawford V, Scheckenbach R, and Preuss HG. Effects of niacin-bound chromium supplementation on body composition in overweight African-American women. *Diab Obes Metab* 1999;1(6):331–337.

24. Talpur N, Echard BW, Yasmin T, Bagchi D, and Preuss HG. Effects of niacin-bound chromium, Maitake mushroom fraction SX and (-)-hydroxycitric acid on the metabolic syndrome in aged diabetic Zucker fatty rats. *Mol Cell Biochem* 2003;252(1–2):369–377.

25. Preuss HG, Bagchi D, Bagchi M, Rao CV, Dey DK, and Satyanarayana S. Effects of a natural extract of (-)-hydroxycitric acid (HCA-SX) and a combination of HCA-SX plus niacin-bound chromium and Gymnema sylvestre extract on weight loss. *Diab Obes Metab* 2004;6(3):171–180.

26. Preuss HG, Bagchi D, Bagchi M, Sanyasi Rao CV, Satyanarayana S, and Dey DK. Efficacy of a novel, natural extract of (-)-hydroxycitric acid (HCA-SX) and a combination of HCA-SX, niacin-bound chromium and Gymnema sylvestre extract in weight management in human volunteers. *Nutr Res* 2004;24:45–58.

27. Grant KE, Chandler RM, Castle AL, and Ivy JL. Chromium and exercise training: Effect on obese women. *Med Sci Sports Exerc* 1997;29(8):992–998.

28. Yazaki Y, Faridi Z, Ma Y, Ali A, Northrup V, Njike VY, Liberti L, and Katz DL. A pilot study of chromium picolinate for weight loss. *J Altern Complement Med* 2010;16(3):291–299.

29. Volpe SL, Huang HW, Larpadisorn K, and Lesser II. Effect of chromium supplementation and exercise on body composition, resting metabolic rate and selected biochemical parameters in moderately obese women following an exercise program. *J Am Coll Nutr* 2001;20(4):293–306.

30. Clancy SP, Clarkson PM, DeCheke ME, Nosaka K, Freedson PS, Cunningham JJ, and Valentine B. Effects of chromium picolinate supplementation on body composition, strength, and urinary chromium loss in football players. *Int J Sport Nutr* 1994;4(2):142–153.

31. Walker LS, Bemben MG, Bemben DA, and Knehans AW. Chromium picolinate effects on body composition and muscular performance in wrestlers. *Med Sci Sports Exerc* 1998;30(12):1730–1737.

32. Trent LK and Thieding-Cancel D. Effects of chromium picolinate on body composition. *J Sports Med Phys Fitness* 1995;35(4):273–280.

33. Livolsi JM, Adams GM, and Laguna PL. The effect of chromium picolinate on muscular strength and body composition in women athletes. *J Strength Cond Res* 2001;15(2):161–166.

34. Pasman WJ, Westerterp-Plantenga MS, and Saris WH. The effectiveness of long-term supplementation of carbohydrate, chromium, fibre, and caffeine on weight maintenance. *Int J Obes Relat Metab Disord* 1997;21(12):1143–1151.

35. Tuzcu M, Sahin N, Orhan C, Agca CA, Akdemir F, Tuzcu Z, Komorowski J, and Sahin K. Impact of chromium histidinate on high fat diet induced obesity in rats. *Nutr Metab* 2011;8:28–35.
36. Zafra-Stone S, Bagchi M, Preuss HG, and Bagchi D. Benefits of chromium (III) complexes in animal and human health. In: Vincent JB (Ed.), *The Nutritional Biochemistry of Chromium (III)*, Elsevier, Amsterdam, the Netherlands, 2007, pp. 183–206.
37. Haylock SJ, Buckley PD, and Blackwell LF. The relationship of chromium to the glucose tolerance factor. II. *J Inorg Biochem* 1983;19(2):105–117.
38. Mirsky N, Weiss A, and Dori Z. Chromium in biological systems, I. Some observations on glucose tolerance factor in yeast. *J Inorg Biochem* 1980;13(1):11–21.
39. Yamamoto A, Wada O, and Ono T. A low-molecular-weight, chromium-binding substance in mammals. *Toxicol Appl Pharmacol* 1981;59(3):515–523.
40. Rink C, Roy S, Khanna S, Rink T, Bagchi D, and Sen CK. Transcriptome of the subcutaneous adipose tissue in response to oral supplementation of type 2 Leprdb obese diabetic mice with niacin-bound chromium. *Physiol Genomics* 2006;27(3):370–379.
41. Kocaefe YC, Israeli D, Ozguc M, Danos O, and Garcia L. Myogenic program induction in mature fat tissue (with MyoD expression). *Exp Cell Res* 2005;308(2):300–308.
42. Comi GP, Fortunato F, Lucchiari S, Bordoni A, Prelle A, Jann S, Keller A, Ciscato P, Galbiati S, Chiveri L, Torrente Y, Scarlato G, and Bresolin N. Beta-enolase deficiency, a new metabolic myopathy of distal glycolysis. *Ann Neurol* 2001;50(2):202–207.
43. Baranova A, Collantes R, Gowder SJ, Elariny H, Schlauch K, Younoszai A, King S, Randhawa M, Pusulury S, Alsheddi T, Ong JP, Martin LM, Chandhoke V, and Younossi ZM. Obesity-related differential gene expression in the visceral adipose tissue. *Obes Surg* 2005;15(6):758–765.
44. Moore JW, Maher MA, Banz WJ, and Zemel MB. Chromium picolinate modulates rat vascular smooth muscle cell intracellular calcium metabolism. *J Nutr* 1998;128(2):180–184.
45. McCarty MF. PKC-mediated modulation of L-type calcium channels may contribute to fat-induced insulin resistance. *Med Hypotheses* 2006;66(4):824–831.
46. Eyre H, Akkari PA, Wilton SD, Callen DC, Baker E, and Laing NG. Assignment of the human skeletal muscle alphatropomyosin gene (TPM1) to band 15q22 by fluorescence in situ hybridization. *Cytogenet Cell Genet* 1995;69(1–2):15–17.
47. Ruiz-Opazo N, Weinberger J, and Nadal-Ginard B. Comparison of alpha-tropomyosin sequences from smooth and striated muscle. *Nature* 1985;315(6014):67–70.
48. Gordon AM, Homsher E, and Regnier M. Regulation of contraction in striated muscle. *Physiol Rev* 2000;80(2):853–924.
49. Stocker A. Molecular mechanisms of vitamin E transport. *Ann NY Acad Sci* 2004;1031:44–59.
50. Bjornson LK, Gniewkowski C, and Kayden HJ. Comparison of exchange of alpha-tocopherol and free cholesterol between rat plasma lipoproteins and erythrocytes. *J Lipid Res* 1975;16(1):39–53.
51. Traber MG, Burton GW, and Hamilton RL. Vitamin E trafficking. *Ann NY Acad Sci* 2004;1031:1–12.
52. Cinti S. Adipocyte differentiation and transdifferentiation: Plasticity of the adipose organ. *J Endocrinol Invest* 2002;25(10):823–835.
53. Zhou Z, Yon Toh S, Chen Z, Guo K, Ng CP, Ponniah S, Lin SC, Hong W, and Li P. Cidea-deficient mice have lean phenotype and are resistant to obesity. *Nat Genet* 2003;35(1):49–56.

36 Overview on (−)-Hydroxycitric Acid in Weight Management

Debasis Bagchi, PhD, MACN, CNS, MAIChE,
Shirley Zafra-Stone, BS, Manashi Bagchi, PhD,
and Harry G. Preuss, MD, MACN, CNS

CONTENTS

INTRODUCTION

Obesity rates worldwide have steadily increased in the last three decades. The World Health Organization's (WHO) latest projections indicate that globally in 2008, approximately 1.5 billion adults (age: 20+) were overweight; of these, more than 200 million men and nearly 300 million women were obese. WHO further projects that by 2015, approximately 2.3 billion adults will be overweight and more than 700 million will be obese.[1] Nearly 43 million children under the age of 5 years were overweight globally in 2010.[1] In the United States, about 34% of adults—almost 73 million people—were obese (roughly 30 or more pounds over a healthy weight) in 2008, up from 31% in 1999.[2] Thirty-three states had a prevalence of obesity to be equal to or greater than 25%; nine of these states (Alabama, Arkansas, Kentucky, Louisiana, Mississippi, Missouri, Oklahoma, Tennessee, and West Virginia) had a prevalence of obesity equal to or greater than 30%. In 2009, only Colorado and the District of Columbia had a prevalence of obesity less than 20%.[2]

Overweight and obesity lead to serious health consequences. Raised body mass index (BMI) is a major risk factor for chronic diseases. Cardiovascular disease, the world's number one cause of death, kills 17 million people each year.[1] Diabetes deaths are projected to increase by more than 50% worldwide in the next 10 years.[1] Other risks for disease include musculoskeletal disorders (osteoarthritis) and cancers (endometrial, breast, and colon). Childhood obesity is associated with a higher chance of premature death and disability in adulthood.

The outcome of *globesity* has generated an unlimited array of weight loss strategies. Fundamental changes to the Food Guide Pyramid are imminent, and new strategies to readdress the consequences of excessive refined carbohydrate consumption are emerging. In addition to drug therapy, numerous procedures suggested to promote weight loss include reduced caloric intake (such as meal replacement products), special weight loss diets (i.e., grapefruit diet or cabbage soup diet), increased caloric expenditure (*via* exercise and/or stimulants), reduced fat diets, increased water consumption, increased fiber consumption, reduced carbohydrate consumption, glycemic indexing (i.e., Atkins' Diet, The South Beach Diet, The Zone Diet, The Cave Man Diet, etc.), appetite suppression, fat blockers, fat burners, starch/sugar blockers, bariatric and other surgeries (i.e., liposuction or stomach reduction), acupuncture, hypnotism, support groups, and body wraps, all supported by products, programs, and/or services designed to help the consumer achieve desired results. Rapid weight loss products and programs dominate the focus of marketers and consumers alike. However, rapid weight loss is potentially unhealthy and disturbs metabolic set point homeostasis, inducing undesirable rebound weight gain consequences.

A number of synthetic drugs and phytopharmaceuticals have demonstrated to help in weight management. However, concerns about exaggerated unsubstantiated benefit claims without scientific evidence, undesirable side effects, and federal regulatory intervention regarding dietary supplements are increasing. Consequently, the search intensifies for products backed by credible scientific research that promote healthy body composition and body mass redistribution but do not stimulate the central nervous system, elevate blood pressure, cause nervousness, interfere with sleep, and/or block nutrient absorption (i.e., fats, starches, and sugar blockers). Outside of significant and permanent lifestyle changes, previously acceptable conventional methods alone, or in combination, have not resulted in sustained success. In some cases, these regimens resulted in undesirable side effects and/or serious consequences, such as the use of ephedrine and phenylpropanolamine (PPA), which have prompted regulatory scrutiny and intervention. At the same time, adverse side effects have been demonstrated for synthetic drugs. Thus, it is very important to develop a strategic therapeutic intervention using safe, novel, natural supplements supported by credible research. This chapter will demonstrate the role of (−)-hydroxycitric acid (HCA) derived from the fruit rind of *Garcinia cambogia* in weight loss.

(−)-HYDROXYCITRIC ACID, A NATURAL EXTRACT FROM *GARCINIA CAMBOGIA* (FAMILY GUTTIFERAE)

(−)-HCA is derived from *G. cambogia* (family Guttiferae), also known as citrin, gambooge, brindal berry, gorikapuli, and malabar tamarind. The fruits of *G. cambogia* are valued for their dried rinds and employed for culinary purposes extensively in Southeast Asia, West and Central Africa, and southern India. In southern India, *G. cambogia* fruit has a distinct sour taste and is used as a condiment in place of tamarind or lemon for flavoring curries, meats, and seafood dishes as well as a unique flavor enhancer for beverages. Dried rind of *G. cambogia* is also made in use of pickling fish,[3,4] a technique commercially known as Colombo curing.[3,5] The organic acids present in the fruit are responsible for the bacteriostatic effect of the pickling medium by a simple lowering of the pH. The fruit has also been used for centuries to make meals more filling and satisfying.[6,7]

In the traditional system of herbal medicine in India or Ayurveda, *Garcinia* is considered to be a prime herb beneficial for health. A decoction of the fruit rind is given for rheumatism, colic, and bowel complaints. *G. cambogia* may decrease acidity and increase the mucosal defense in the gastric areas, thereby justifying its use as an antiulcerogenic agent.[8,9] *Garcinia* also contains significant amounts of vitamin C and has been used as a heart tonic. In veterinary medicine, the extract is employed as a rinse for some diseases of the mouth in cattle.[10]

HCA, the organoleptically characterizing ingredient of *G. cambogia*, is a popular component of several dietary supplements marketed under various trade names. It has been reported that calcium salts of HCA, which are typically less than 50% soluble, are less bioavailable compared to readily soluble calcium-potassium salts of HCA. As a dietary supplement in the United States, HCA is regulated under the Dietary Supplement Health and Education Act (DSHEA) of 1994.[11]

PHARMACOGNOSY

Garcinia is a large genus of approximately 180 species of polygamous trees or shrubs, distributed in tropical Asia, Africa, and Polynesia. Approximately 30 different species of *Garcinia* are found in India and Southeast Asia. *G. cambogia*, commonly found in Southwest India, is a small or medium-sized evergreen tree with a rounded crown and horizontal or drooping branches. The tree flowers during the hot season, and fruits ripen during the rainy season. The flowers are unisexual, sessile, and axillary; and the leaves are dark green and shiny, elliptic to obovate, 5–12 cm long, and 2–7 cm broad. The fruit is ovoid, 5 cm in diameter, and may resemble a small pumpkin, yellow, orange, or red when ripe, with six to eight grooves. The fruit has six to eight seeds surrounded by a succulent aril.

G. cambogia fruit is included in the USDA's inventory of perennial edible fruits of the tropics.[12] The fruit contains approximately 10%–30% acid calculated as citric acid on a dry weight basis.[5] In some early studies, the organic acids present in the fruits were mistakenly identified as tartaric and citric acids. In subsequent studies, the major acid in the fruit of *G. cambogia* was identified as HCA.[13,14] HCA-SX, derived by a novel patented process, from the dried fruit rind of *G. cambogia*, contains approximately 95% calcium–potassium salt of (–)-HCA. The calcium–potassium salt contains approximately 60% HCA, as characterized by high-performance liquid chromatography (HPLC).

CHEMISTRY

HCA (1,2-dihydroxypropane 1,2,3 tricarboxylic acid) has two asymmetric centers; hence, two pairs of diastereoisomers or four different isomers are possible (Figure 36.1a through d). All four isomers, (–)-HCA, (+)-HCA, (–)-allo-HCA, and (+)-allo-HCA, have been chemically synthesized starting from *trans*-aconitic acid.[15] One of these isomers, the principal constituent of HCA-SX, occurs in *Garcinia* (Figure 36.1a) and another in *Hibiscus* species (Figure 36.1b).[14] (–)-HCA is the principal acid in the highly acidic fruit of *G. cambogia*. The absolute configuration

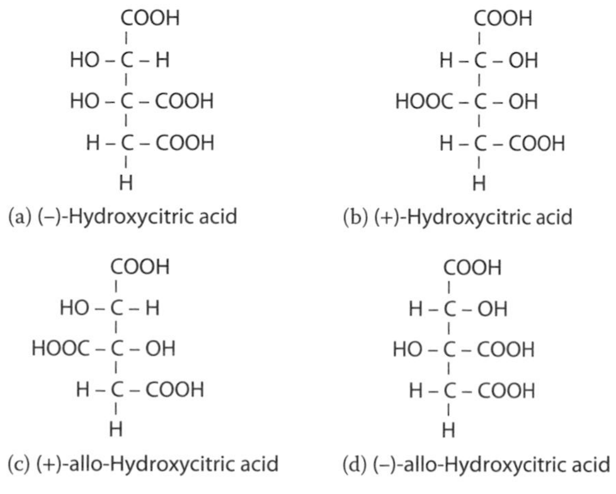

FIGURE 36.1 (a–d) Chemical structures of the stereoisomers of HCA.

of (–)-HCA was determined from Hudson's lactone rule, optical rotatory dispersion curves, circular dichromism curves, and calculation of partial molar rotations.[16] By employing x-ray crystallography, Glusker et al.[17,18] reported the structure and absolute configuration of the calcium hydroxycitrate and HCA lactone. The acid is present at a level of 10%–30% in the dried fruit rind of *G. cambogia*. The acid can be isolated in its free form, as a mineral salt (i.e., Ca^{2+} salt, Na^+ salt, K^+ salt, Mg^{2+} salt, Ca^{2+}/K^+ double salt, Mg^{2+}/K^+ double salt, and others, formed postextraction) or as a lactone by various methods. Lowenstein and Brunengraber[19] have estimated the hydroxycitrate content of the fruit of *G. cambogia* by gas chromatography (GC). During concentration and evaporation, free HCA leads to the formation of HCA lactone. Based on the information submitted to the U.S. Patent Office, several investigators have reported the preparation of HCA concentrate from *Garcinia* rinds with 23%–54% HCA and 6%–20% lactone.[20,21] Recently, Jayaprakasha and Sakariah[22,23] developed HPLC methods for the estimation of organic acids in the fruits of *G. cambogia* and commercial samples of *G. cambogia* extracts (GCEs). Using these methods, dilute extracts can be quantified without concentration, drying, or derivatization. An additional advantage of these methods is that the HCA and its lactone can be quantified separately. Loe et al.[25] reported a gas chromatography/mass spectrophotometry (GC/MS) method for quantitative determination of blood hydroxycitrate levels.

Isolation Techniques and Physicochemical Properties

Lewis and Neelakantan[13] reported a method on isolation of large-scale HCA from the dried rinds of *G. cambogia*. In this method, the acid is extracted by heating the raw material with water under pressure. Subsequently, the extract was concentrated, and pectin was removed by precipitation with alcohol. The clear filtrate was neutralized, and the acid was recovered after passing through cation exchange resin. The recovered acid was concentrated, dried, and recrystallized to small needle-shaped crystals of lactone. In another method, Lewis[14] reported isolation of HCA from dried *Garcinia* fruit rinds using acetone. The acetone (ACON) extract was concentrated, and the acid was extracted in water. The water extract was evaporated to yield lactone. In yet another process, aqueous extract of HCA was passed through anion exchange column for adsorption of HCA. The adsorbed HCA was eluted with sodium–potassium hydroxide. The free acid was prepared by passing through a cation exchange column. In recent years, several manufacturers have employed different procedures (patented) to prepare single and double salts of HCA with improved solubility and bioavailability.

A number of HCA salts are available in the marketplace, which includes Ca^{2+} salt, Na^+ salt, K^+ salt, Mg^{2+} salt, Ca^{2+}/K^+ double salt, Mg^{2+}/K^+ double salt, and others. The solubility of these HCA salts, which can affect bioavailability, ranges from less than 50%–100%. Furthermore, different salts have different physicochemical characteristics including color, taste, and odor.

Extensive research has been conducted on a novel, patented calcium–potassium salt of 60% HCA extract (HCA-SX, commercially known as Super CitriMax), which is tasteless and odorless, as well as 100% water soluble.

Structural Characterization of HCA-SX

A typical compositional analysis of HCA-SX contains 60% (–)-HCA in its free form, 1.0% (–)-HCA in its lactone form, 10% calcium, 15% potassium, 0.5% sodium, 0.05% total phytosterols, 0.3% total protein, 4.5% moisture, and 8.5% soluble dietary fiber (by difference). It also contains 0.1% magnesium, 0.03% iron, and trace amounts of manganese, copper, zinc, selenium, total fat, and total sugar. HCA-SX provides approximately 150 calories per 100 g and exhibits an optical rotation $[\alpha]_D^{20} = -17.55$ (c = 1.0 H_2O), as measured in a Rudolph Autopol II Polarimeter (Hackettstown, NJ) using a 10 cm cell at 589 nm.

Using HPLC, HCA-SX was detected by injecting a 20 µL solution of HCA-SX (sample concentration 1.6 mg/mL) in water (pH 2.1, adjusted with sulfuric acid) on a Shimadzu HPLC (Tokyo, Japan) equipped with LC-10AT pumps, SCL-10A system controller, SIL-10A auto injector, SPD-M10AVP detector (detector was set at 210 nm) and CLASS-M10A software, and a 5 µ Altima C18 column (250 mm × 4.6 mm) (Alltech Associates, Inc., Deerfield, IL, USA) at a flow rate of 1 mL/min in an isocratic mode using a mobile phase of 0.05 M sodium sulfate in water (pH 2.3, adjusted with sulfuric acid) at 25°C ± 2°C. The retention time for HCA was noted at 4.78 min, which was reconfirmed by spiking with an authentic standard of HCA (Wako, Japan).

Ultraviolet (UV) spectra of HCA-SX were recorded on a Varian Cary 50 UV-VIS spectrometer (Mulgrave, Victoria, Australia). UV spectra (H$_2$O) exhibited a shoulder at λ_{max} 210 nm. Infrared spectra (IR) of HCA-SX were recorded on a Perkin Elmer Spectrum BX FT-IR spectrometer (Norwalk, CT, USA). IR (KBr pellet, cm^{-1}) 3403.20 (OH), 1599.39 (asymmetric C=O stretching band), 1397 (symmetric C=O stretching band), 1295.93 (C–O stretch), 1099.74, 1061.98 (alcoholic C–O absorption), 905.99, 837.40 (C–C stretching), and 627.11 (C–C bending). Proton NMR spectrum (300 MHz, D$_2$O) was recorded on a JEOL JNM-LA (Lambda) NMR spectrometer (Tokyo, Japan), and the chemical shift values were expressed in ppm. ^{1}H NMR data of HCA-SX showed H-2 at δ 3.98 s, H-4a at δ 2.53 d (J = 16.5 Hz), and H-4b at δ 2.69 d (J = 16.5 Hz). ^{13}C NMR spectrum (75 MHz, D2O) was recorded on a JEOL JNM-LA (Lambda) NMR spectrometer (Tokyo, Japan), and the chemical shift values were expressed in ppm. ^{13}C NMR spectrum of HCA-SX exhibited C-1, C-5, and C-6 at δ 181.0, 179.7, and 178.7 ppm, and C-2, C-3, and C-4 at δ 42.4, 79.8, and 77.1, respectively. Mass spectrum was recorded on an Agilent 1100 Series LC/MSD (Palo Alto, CA) under electrospray ionization (ESI), negative ion mode conditions. In ESI, the mass spectrum contains abundant pseudomolecular ions (M + 1, M + 23, etc., in positive ion mode and M − 1 in negative ion mode). These ions were used to confirm the molecular weight of the compounds. The peak at m/z 207 (M − 1) in the mass spectrum of HCA-SX corresponds the pseudomolecular ion of HCA (molecular weight 208).[24]

BIOAVAILABILITY OF (–)-HYDROXYCITRIC ACID

Improving bioavailability and reducing dosage frequency is crucial in improvement in subject compliance of chronic treatment regimes. Loe et al.[25] conducted a study utilizing a simple method requiring minimal sample preparation is able to measure trace amounts of HCA with accuracy and precision, using [U-(13)C] citrate (CA*) as internal standard to account for losses associated with the isolation, derivatization, and measurement of HCA. These authors developed a new GC/MS method to measure HCA levels in blood HCA and CA* which were derivatized with BSTFA + 10% TMCS and analyzed using PCI/GC/MS (CA*, m/z 471; and HCA, m/z 553). Plasma HCA concentration was measured over a 3.5 h period in four subjects having ingested 2 g of HCA-SX. Their plasma HCA concentration ranged from 0.8 to 8.4 µg/mL 30 min and 2 h after ingestion, respectively. These results demonstrated that when taken acutely, HCA is absorbed, yet present in small quantities in human plasma. In separate study, these authors assessed the bioavailability of HCA-SX in both fasting and fed states in humans. HCA-SX concentration peaked 2 h postadministration and was not completely cleared after 9 h (Figure 36.2). Feeding appeared to hinder HCA-SX absorption with the peak concentration of approximately 60% lower than that absorbed in the fasting state. HCA-SX absorption was detectable in the urine and used to determine relative HCA-SX absorption.[25,26]

A pharmacokinetics study was conducted on HCA-SX in Sprague-Dawley rats. HCA-SX was given orally at 912 mg/kg by gavage. Blood samples were collected at 0.25, 0.5, 1, 2, 4, 6, 8, and 24 h, and plasma concentrations of HCA-SX were measured. HCA-SX was absorbed in a time-dependent manner, and the T_{max} value (1 h) suggests fairly rapid absorption of HCA-SX. After achieving C_{max}, the HCA-SX levels rapidly declined suggesting that this compound is rapidly metabolized and, by 8–24 h, disappeared from the plasma. Plasma half-life was between 1 and 2 h. Key pharmacokinetic profiles are shown in Table 36.1.

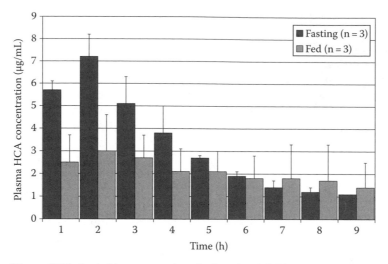

FIGURE 36.2 Plasma HCA (μg/mL) concentrations in fasted and fed human subjects over a period of 9 h following a single oral administration of HCA-SX (2.0 g).

TABLE 36.1
Key Pharmacokinetic Values
for HCA-SX in Rats

Pharmacokinetic Estimates

Half-life (h)	1.3
T_{max} (h)	1
C_{max} (μg/mL)	384.0
AUC 0-T (h × μg/mL)	1336
Volume of distribution (mL/kg)	1286
Clearance (mL/h/kg)	683

TABLE 36.2
Bioavailability of Two Different Salts of HCA
in Albino Wistar Rats

	Serum HCA Concentration (μg/mL)	
Time (h)	HCA-SX (1000 mg/kg)	HCA-Ca (1000 mg/kg)
0	0.00 ± 0.00	0.00 ± 0.00
0.5	9.06 ± 2.23	2.11 ± 0.328
1	18.10 ± 0.94	10.41 ± 1.45
1.5	37.30 ± 5.14	12.93 ± 4.11
2	13.26 ± 1.01	10.88 ± 0.747
3	9.73 ± 1.09	5.83 ± 1.37
5	8.78 ± 0.766	4.17 ± 1.57

Serum concentration (mean ± SEM) of HCA at various time points after oral administration.

In a recent comparative study, we evaluated the oral bioavailability of HCA-SX and calcium salt (HCA-Ca) in healthy albino Wistar rats. Rats were divided randomly into two groups (n = 8) and supplemented orally with a single dose (1000 mg/kg) of each HCA salt. Blood samples were collected before administration followed by 0.5, 1, 1.5, 2, 3, and 5 h after administration. Oral administration of HCA-SX resulted in significantly better bioavailability compared to HCA-Ca. Peak plasma concentration of HCA-SX (37.3 µg/mL) is significantly (p = 0.031) higher than HCA-Ca (12.93 µg/mL). HCA-SX at 93.93% exhibited better bioavailability (AUC 65.55) compared to HCA-Ca (AUC 33.80). Statistically significant improvement in peak plasma concentration was also observed in HCA-SX compared to HCA-Ca. In summary, this study provided strong evidence to prove superior oral bioavailability of HCA-SX compared to HCA-Ca (Table 36.2).

SAFETY OF (–)-HYDROXYCITRIC ACID

An increasing number of well-designed and appropriately controlled weight management studies in animals and humans have indicated that HCA is both safe and efficacious in weight management. Safety studies in experimental animals at up to 25 times the human equivalency doses did not produce hepatotoxicity or other significant adverse effects.

SAFETY STUDIES ON HCA-SX

An extensive safety evaluation was conducted on HCA-SX. Acute oral, acute dermal, primary dermal irritation, and primary eye irritation toxicity studies have demonstrated the safety of HCA-SX.[27] LD_{50} of HCA-SX was found to be greater than 5000 mg/kg body weight when administered once orally *via* gastric intubation to fasted male and female albino rats. No gross adverse toxicological findings were observed under the experimental conditions. The dermal LD_{50} of HCA-SX was found to be greater than 2000 mg/kg body weight when applied once for 24 h to the shaved, intact skin of male and female albino rabbits. There was no evidence of acute systemic toxicity among rabbits that were dermally administered HCA-SX at 2000 mg/kg body weight. In the dermal irritation study, no deaths or significant body weight changes were observed during the study period. HCA-SX induced very slight erythema on one animal.[27] No edema or other dermal findings were noted, and all irritation was reversible and completely subsided by the end of day 1. The primary dermal irritation index (PDII) was calculated to be 0.0. Based on these observations, HCA-SX received a descriptive rating classification of nonirritating. In the eye irritation study, no deaths or remarkable changes in body weights occurred during the study period. The results indicate that HCA-SX causes ocular irritation with production of inflammatory exudate in some animals. Positive iridal and conjictival reactions were present in all animals, which subsided within 48 h. A total maximum score of 110 is possible. A score of 15 was obtained in the study, indicating mild irritation.[27]

The dose- and time-dependent effects of HCA-SX were assessed in Sprague-Dawley rats on body weight, selected organ weights, hepatic lipid peroxidation and DNA fragmentation, hematology, and clinical chemistry over a period of 90 days (subchronic study).[28,29] Furthermore, a 90 day histopathological evaluation was conducted. The animals were treated with 0%, 0.2%, 2.0%, and 5.0% HCA-SX of feed intake and were sacrificed on 30, 60, or 90 days of treatment. The body weight and selected organ weights were assessed and correlated as a percent of body weight and brain weight at 90 days of treatment. A significant reduction in body weight was observed in treated rats as compared to control animals. An advancing age-induced marginal increase in hepatic lipid peroxidation was observed in both male and female rats, while no such difference in hepatic DNA fragmentation was observed as compared to the control animals. Furthermore, selected organ weights individually and as a percent of body and brain weights at 90 days of treatment exhibited no significant difference between the groups. No difference was observed in hematology and clinical chemistry or the histopathological evaluation. Taken together, these results show that 90 day treatment of HCA-SX results in a reduction in body weight and do not cause any changes in major organs or in hematology, clinical chemistry, and histopathology.[28,29]

Ames' bacterial reverse mutation studies and mouse lymphoma tests have shown that HCA-SX does not induce mutagenicity.[29] Five histidine-dependent strains of *Salmonella typhimurium* (TA98, TA100, TA1535, TA 1537, and TA102) were used to evaluate the mutagenic potential of HCA-SX (up to 5000 μg/plate), both in the presence and in the absence of metabolic activation (±S9). No mutagenic potential of HCA-SX was observed. The mutagenic potential of HCA-SX (up to the recommended dose level of 5000 μg/plate) was assessed in the mouse lymphoma assay using L5178Y mouse lymphoma cells, clone −3.7.2C (ATCC #CRL-9518, American Type Culture Collection, Virginia). HCA-SX did not induce mutagenic effects in the mammalian cell gene mutation test on L5178Y mouse lymphoma cells TK+/−, either with or without metabolic activation.[29]

In an independent study, Saito et al.[30] have demonstrated that diets containing 51 mmol HCA/kg diet (389 mg HCA/kg body weight/day) or less did not cause any adverse effects. Accordingly, 51 mmol HCA/kg diet (389 mg HCA/kg body weight/day) was deemed to be the no observed adverse effect level (NOAEL).[30]

The structure, mechanism of action, long history of use of HCA, and other toxicity studies indicate that HCA-SX is unlikely to cause reproductive or developmental effects.

In a study, the effects of HCA-SX on the reproductive systems of male and female rats were evaluated, including the postnatal maturation and reproductive capacity of their offspring and possible cumulative effects through multiple generations.[31] Sprague-Dawley rats (30/sex/group) were maintained on feed containing HCA-SX at dose levels of 0, 1,000, 3,000, or 10,000 ppm for 10 weeks prior to mating, during mating, and, for females, through gestation and lactation, across two generations. During the period of study, animals were examined daily for signs of clinical toxicity, and their body weight and feed consumption were recorded twice a week. For the parents (F0 and F1) and the offspring (F1 and F2a), reproductive parameters such as fertility and mating, gestation, parturition, litters, lactation, sexual maturity, and development of offspring were assessed. At termination, necropsy and histopathological examinations were performed on all animals. Dietary exposure of HCA-SX to parental male and female rats of both (F0 and F1) the generations during the premating and mating periods, for both sexes, and during gestation and lactation in the case of female rats did not reveal any remarkable incidence of mortality or abnormal clinical signs. Compared to respective controls, HCA-SX exposure did not affect feed consumption or body weight at any of the exposure levels. HCA-SX exposure did not affect reproductive performance as evaluated by sexual maturity, fertility and mating, gestation, parturition, litter properties, lactation, and development of the offspring. Based on these results, the parental as well as the offspring NOAEL for HCA-SX was determined to be greater than 10,000 ppm in diet or equivalent to 1018 and 1524 mg/kg body weight/day in male and female rats, respectively.[31]

In continuation of a two-generation reproductive toxicity study, the teratogenic potential of HCA-SX was evaluated in Sprague-Dawley rats.[32] Due to its potential to affect fat continuous synthesis and reduce food intake, processes that are often crucial in normal fetal development, this teratology study was undertaken as part of a multigeneration reproductive investigation. The animals in this study were selected randomly after weaning from each F2b litter of the F1 generation from the two-generation reproductive toxicity study. To start the teratology study, Sprague-Dawley rat pups (~30/sex/group) from the F2b generation were allowed to grow up to 10–12 weeks of age before mating. The rats in the treatment group were exposed directly to HCA-SX through feed, while prior to their weaning, they had indirect exposure to the test material during lactation. The dietary exposure levels were the same as those employed for the two-generation reproductive toxicity study, viz., 1,000, 3,000, or 10,000 ppm. Following mating at maturity, the pregnant rats were observed daily for clinical signs of adverse effects, and body weight and feed consumption were recorded. On day 20 of gestation, animals were subjected to a necropsy and cesarean section to examine the uterus, ovaries, and fetuses for assessment of different parameters of pregnancy and embryo-fetal defects. Despite a slight (13%) lowering of maternal body weight gain during gestation period in the group receiving 10,000 ppm HCA-SX, no evidence of maternal toxicity, adverse effects on the parameters evaluated for the gravid uteri, external abnormalities in the fetuses, soft tissue abnormalities in the fetuses, or skeletal abnormalities in the fetuses were noted. Based on the results of this developmental toxicity study, conducted in continuation of a two-generation reproductive toxicity study, HCA-SX was not found to be teratogenic in the Sprague-Dawley rats at the dietary exposure levels of 1,000, 3,000, and 10,000 ppm, equivalent to the dose levels of 103, 352, or 1240 mg/kg/day, respectively.[32]

In several, placebo-controlled, double-blind trials employing up to 2800 mg/day HCA, no treatment-related adverse effects were reported. There is sufficient qualitative and quantitative scientific evidence, including animal and human data suggesting that intake of HCA at levels up to 2800 mg/day is safe for human consumption.[33]

ANIMAL STUDIES

Since 1970, a number of animal studies conducted with hydroxycitrate, singly and in combination with other ingredients, have demonstrated beneficial effects for weight and fat loss. Early studies shown that (–)-hydroxycitrate is a potent competitive inhibitor of ATP citrate lyase, the extra-mitochondrial enzyme that supplies most of the acetyl coenzyme A for lipid synthesis.[34,35] Hydroxycitrate inhibited the conversion of carbohydrate and its metabolites into lipid by reducing the acetyl coenzyme A pool, the substrate for fatty acids and cholesterol. Studies on HCA supplementation in rats demonstrated evidence of decreased lipogenesis levels and appetite suppression. Lowenstein[36] demonstrated that (–)-hydroxycitrate is a highly effective inhibitor of fatty acid synthesis by rat liver *in vivo*. Hepatic fatty acid synthesis was inhibited strongly by sodium (–)-hydroxycitrate. An i.p. dose of as little as 0.1 mmol/kg body weight inhibited fatty acid synthesis by 25%–30% (equivalent to about 2.9 mg of (–)-hydroxycitrate per 150 g rat). 50% and 75% inhibition was obtained with an i.p. dose of 0.28 and 1 mmol/kg of body weight, respectively. Results also demonstrated that inhibition of fatty acid synthesis remain strong between 50 and 95 min after administration of hydroxycitrate. Additional experiments exhibited that inhibition of fatty acid synthesis remain strong up to 2–3 h after administration of hydroxycitrate.[36]

Sullivan et al. (1972)[37] determined the effect of the hydroxycitrate stereoisomers on the rate of lipogenesis in rat liver. Inhibition of lipogenesis by administration of (–)-hydroxycitrate, (+)-hydroxycitrate, (–)-allo-hydroxycitrate, and (+)-allo-hydroxycitrate stereoisomers i.v. or i.p. demonstrated that only (–)-hydroxycitrate significantly decreased the rates of lipid synthesis in both studies. The *in vivo* rate of lipogenesis was markedly decreased for 150 min following the administration of (–)-hydroxycitrate. Fatty acid and cholesterol synthesis were also significantly inhibited by the oral administration of (–)-hydroxycitrate when the compound was given before the feeding period.[37] In another *in vivo* study, oral administration of (–)-hydroxycitrate in female rats was shown to depress the *in vivo* lipogenic rates in a dose-dependent manner in the liver, adipose tissue, and small intestine.[37] Hepatic lipogenesis was significantly inhibited during the 8 h period in the (–)-hydroxycitrate-treated animals and was 11% less than controls. Rats receiving (–)-hydroxycitrate also consumed less food than the untreated controls.[38] Although this decreased caloric intake was not responsible for the supplement-induced depression of hepatic lipogenesis (as shown by studies in pair-fed rats), a separate pair-feeding study demonstrated that the reduction in food intake accounted for a decrease in weight gain and body lipid observed with (–)-hydroxycitrate treatment.[38,39] In this study, a significant reduction in body weight gain, food consumption, and total body lipid was observed in female rats with a chronic oral administration of (–)-hydroxycitrate for a period of 11–30 days. An equal amount of citrate administration did not have any effects on weight loss. Pair-feeding studies demonstrated that these effects upon weight loss and body lipids were due to the decreased caloric intake produced by (–)-hydroxycitrate.[39]

In another *in vivo* study, Sullivan et al. (1977)[40] examined the influence of (–)-hydroxycitrate on weight gain, appetite suppression, and body composition in several obese rodent model systems: mature normal rat, the gold thioglucose obese mouse, and the ventromedial hypothalamic lesioned obese rat. In all models, food intake and body weight gain were reduced significantly by the chronic oral administration of (–)-hydroxycitrate (52.6 mmol/kg of diet, a dose approximately equivalent to 2.74 mmol/kg body weight) as dietary admixture. Dietary admixture was a G-70 diet, which consisted of 70% glucose, 23% vitamin-free casein, 5% Phillips and Hart salt mixture, and 40 g/kg of cellulose.[40]

Hamilton et al.[41] investigated the influence of (–)-hydroxycitrate on serum triglyceride and cholesterol levels and *in vitro* and *in vivo* rates of hepatic fatty acid and cholesterol synthesis in normal and hyperlipidemic rat model systems. (–)-Hydroxycitrate reduced equivalently the biosynthesis of triglycerides, phospholipids, cholesterol, diglycerides, cholesteryl esters, and free fatty acids in isolated liver cells. *In vivo* hepatic rates of fatty acid and cholesterol synthesis determined in meal-fed normolipidemic rats were suppressed significantly by the oral administration of (–)-hydroxycitrate for 6 h, when control animals exhibited maximal rates of lipid synthesis. Results also demonstrated that serum triglyceride and cholesterol levels were significantly reduced. In two hypertriglyceridemic models—the genetically obese Zucker rat and the fructose-treated rat—elevated triglyceride levels were due, in part, to enhanced hepatic rates of fatty acid synthesis. (–)-Hydroxycitrate significantly reduced the hypertriglyceridemia and hyperlipogenesis in both models. The marked hypertriglyceridemia exhibited by the triton-treated rat was only minimally due to increased hepatic lipogenesis. This study showed that (–)-hydroxycitrate significantly inhibited both serum triglyceride levels and lipogenesis in this model.[41]

In another *in vivo* study conducted by Greenwood et al.[42] (–)-hydroxycitrate treatment in growing lean Zucker rats resulted a decrease in the percent of body fat in the carcass and a significant decrease in fat cell size. Young Zucker lean (Fa/-) and obese (fa/fa) female rats were fed fatty acid synthesis inhibitor (–)-hydroxycitrate as a dietary admixture for 39 days. In the lean rats, (–)-hydroxycitrate treatment decreased body weight, food intake, percent of body fat, and fat cell size. In the obese rat, food intake and body weight were reduced, but the percent of body fat remained unchanged. Throughout the treatment period, obese rats maintained a fat cell size equivalent to their obese controls. Although a reduction in fat cell number in the obese rats occurred during the treatment period, marked hyperplasia was observed during the posttreatment period. The results of this study indicate that the obese rat, despite a substantial reduction in body weight produced by (–)-hydroxycitrate, still defends its obese body composition.[42]

Rao et al.[43] evaluated the effects of (–)-HCA in male albino Wistar rats fed a lipogenic diet for a period of 15 days. A control group was fed a lipogenic diet without HCA. Analysis results from blood, liver, and epididymal fat demonstrated that inclusion of (–)-hydroxycitrate in the diet significantly reduced food intake, body weight, epididymal fat, and serum triglyceride in animals. A decrease in the food intake was also observed. The effect of HCA was dose dependent.[43]

In another study, a decrease in body weight gain and fat deposition were inhibited by (–)-hydroxycitrate while no difference in cumulative food intake was observed.[44] In a study conducted by Vasselli et al.[44] growing male Sprague-Dawley rats (n = 5) were fed (–)-hydroxycitrate *ad libitum* as a dietary admix for 28 days. In a separate experiment, the ability of same dose of (–)-hydroxycitrate was tested to alter 24 h energy expenditure (EE) in rats (n = 6) fed a mixed high-carbohydrate diet (75% CHO, 3.90 kcal/g) known to stimulate lipogenesis in humans. EE was measured in whole body respirometers during days 1–5 of a 28 day test period, and final weight of three fat depositions was determined. Results of the first experiment demonstrated that (–)-hydroxycitrate inhibited body weight gain (−48.9 g, $p < 0.01$) and cumulative food intake (control: 675.7 ± 23.5 g; (–)-hydroxycitrate: 622.5 ± 44.6 g, $p < 0.05$). The second experiment demonstrated that (–)-hydroxycitrate increased 24 h EE by 12.6% (no change in respiratory quotient [RQ] was observed). Results indicated that in the (–)-hydroxycitrate group, body weight gain is 73.8 ± 7.1 g ($p < 0.02$), EE kcal/24 h is 62.59 ± 5.41 ($p < 0.02$), cumulative food intake is 614.7 ± 27.8 g, and total pad weight is 16.04 ± 1.28 g ($p < 0.01$); and in the control group, change in body weight gain is 91.5 ± 12.7 g, EE kcal/24 h is 55.67 ± 2.43, cumulative food intake is 629.1 ± 8.8 g, and total pad weight is 21.45 ± 2.57 g.[44]

Ishihara et al.[45] conducted a study on hydroxycitrate and male Std ddY mice. Mice were divided into three groups (n = 60, 54, and 12) of equal body weights. Mice (n = 60) were placed in metabolic chambers to measure respiratory gas. Diet and water was prohibited from 0930h. At 1000h, they were administered orally 10 or 30mg of a 0.48mol/L hydroxycitrate solution or water, and the respiratory gas was analyzed. The same procedures were applied in a separate mice group (n = 54). Blood was collected 30 or 100min after administrated hydroxycitrate to measure serum variables. The effect of hydroxycitrate on glycogen accumulation was evaluated in the gastrocnemius muscle and liver tissue in the treated mice group (n = 12). In a separate experiment, mice (n = 18) were forced to swim to exhaustion at a flow rate of 8L/min twice a day for a preliminary period of 1 week. They were divided into three groups and were orally administered 10 or 30mg of 0.48mol/L hydroxycitrate or 10mg water (control) and free access to commercial diet and water. Following the treatment, mice swam until fatigue every day at same flow rate and maximum swimming time was measured. Mice were administered hydroxycitrate orally every day after swimming. In another experiment, mice (n = 18) were divided into two groups of equal mean body weights. Animals were orally administered 10mg of 0.48mol/L hydroxycitrate or water (control) twice a day for 25 days. At day 26, each mouse was placed into a treadmill chamber allowed to rest for 1h, followed by 1h run at the speed of 15m/min while respiratory gas was monitored. Body weight and food intake was taken every day until termination. The research demonstrated that oral administration of 10mg hydroxycitrate elevated serum-free fatty acid concentration and increased muscle glycogen concentration in mice at rest. Mice that were chronically (twice daily for 25 days) administered hydroxycitrate had a significantly reduced respiratory exchange ratio (RER) at rest and during running exercise. Lipid oxidation was increased and carbohydrate utilization was less in the early stage of running exercise. These results indicate that the enhancement of endurance exercise occurred due to oral administration of hydroxycitrate in mice and might have occurred by the attenuation of glycogen consumption caused by the promotion of lipid oxidation during running exercise.[45]

In a series of experiments, 24 male rats were fed restrictively (10g/day) for 10 days and then given *ad libitum* access to one of four different diets: high sucrose (HI-Suc), high glucose (HI-Glu), grounded standard rat chow (Chow), high glucose+fat (HI-Glu+fat) varying in the content of fat and low molecular carbohydrates for the following 10 days. In the other rats (n = 12), the *ad libitum* diet was supplemented with 3% (w/w) HCA. HCA reduced body weight regain with all diets except Chow. HCA also reduced food intake temporarily with three of the four tested diets. The suppressive effect of HCA on food intake was particularly strong in the HI-Glu+fat diet group (fat = 24% of energy). With diets HI-Glu and HI-Glu+fat, HCA reduced the feed conversion efficiency (cumulative body weight regain [g]/cumulative food intake [MJ]) during the 10 *ad libitum* days, suggesting that it also increased EE. This effect seemed to be positively related to the glucose content of the diet.[45] Two experiments were performed in 23 and 24 adult male Sprague-Dawley rats.[46,47] Initial body weights for experiment 1 and 2 were 663 ± 12g and 616 ± 7g, respectively. Both groups were fed only 10g powdered standard rodent chow for 10 days before divided into groups. Rats were divided into two groups (n = 11 or 12) for each experiment and matched for body weight loss and given one of two diets *ad libitum* for 22 days. The diet of one group was always supplemented with 3g/100g hydroxycitrate (85mmol/kg) diet. In experiment 1, rats in both groups were given diet of 1% (g/100g) fat diet = 81% carbohydrate, 10% protein, and 1% fat. In experiment 2, rats in both groups were given diet of 12% (g/100g) fat diet = 76% carbohydrate, 9% protein, and 12% fat. Rats lost 72 ± 3g and 75 ± 2g body weight during the 10 day restrictive feeding in experiments 1 and 2. Hydroxycitrate reduced body weight regain in rats fed both diets throughout the period of *ad libitum* consumption. In experiment 1 (1% fat diet group), the cumulative body weight regain in rats fed hydroxycitrate was significantly less than in controls from *ad libitum* in day 2 (control: 17 ± 1g, hydroxycitrate: 12 ± 1g). On day 22, control rats had regained 70 ± 6g body weight and hydroxycitrate rats regained 48 ± 3g body weight, respectively (overall p < 0.01). Thus, hydroxycitrate-fed rats regained only 68% ± 4% of the control group's body weight regain. HCA did not affect any metabolic variables examined. In experiment 2 (12% fat diet group), after day 22 the control group had regained 81 ± 7g while the hydroxycitrate group had regained 49 ± 6g (overall p < 0.01). The latter was 61% ± 8% of the control group's body weight regain. As in experiment 1, the control group had compensated the body weight loss on *ad libitum* day 22: body weight loss 75 ± 3 g and body weight regain 81 ± 3 g; whereas the hydroxycitrate group had not: body weight loss 75 ± 3 g and body weight regain 49 ± 6 g (p < 0.01). Hydroxycitrate had no effect on plasma β-hydroxybutyrate but reduced plasma triacylglycerol and increased liver fat concentration. The suppressive effect of hydroxycitrate on body weight regain, which was maintained for at least 3 weeks, appears to be independent of the dietary fat content. Yet the fat content of the diet seemed to be important for the long-term suppressive effect of hydroxycitrate on feeding.[46,47]

Hayamizu et al.[48] evaluated the effects of 3.3% GCE on 10% sucrose loading and treatment effect was examined in mice for 4 weeks. The authors demonstrated that GCE efficiently improved glucose metabolism and displayed leptin-like activity.[48]

Dose- and time-dependent effects of HCA-SX (Super CitriMax®, 60% calcium-potassium salt of HCA) was evaluated in rats on body weight, selected organ weights, hepatic lipid peroxidation and DNA fragmentation, hematology and clinical chemistry, and histopathological evaluation.[49] Male and female Sprague-Dawley rats (male rats, 251–320 g and female rats, 154–241 g) were treated with 0%, 0.2%, 2.0%, and 5.0% HCA-SX of feed intake and were sacrificed on 30, 60, or 90 days of treatment. The body weight and selected organ weights were assessed and correlated as a percent of body weight and brain weight at 90 days of treatment. A 90 day histopathological evaluation was also conducted. A significant reduction in body weight was observed in treated rats as compared to control animals. An advancing age-induced marginal increase in hepatic lipid peroxidation was observed in both male and female rats, while no such difference in hepatic DNA fragmentation was observed as compared to the control animals. Selected organ weights individually and as a percent of body weight and brain weight at 90 days of treatment exhibited no significant difference between the groups. No difference was observed in hematology and clinical chemistry or the histopathological evaluation. Taken together, these results show that 90 day treatment of HCA-SX results in a reduction in body weight and do not cause any changes in major organs or in hematology, clinical chemistry, and histopathology.[28,29]

Roy et al.[49] determined the effects of low-dose oral HCA-SX on the body weight and abdominal fat gene expression profile of Sprague-Dawley rats. At doses relevant for human consumption, dietary HCA-SX significantly reduced body weight growth. This response was associated with lowered abdominal fat leptin expression. Other genes, including vital genes transcribing for mitochondrial or nuclear proteins, which are necessary for fundamental support of the tissue, were not affected by HCA-SX. Under the current experimental conditions, HCA-SX proved to be effective in restricting body weight gain in adult rats. Functional characterization of HCA-SX-sensitive genes revealed that upregulation of genes encoding serotonin receptors, as well as fat and carbohydrate metabolism, represent a distinct effect of dietary HCA-SX supplementation.[49]

In another study, 24 male Sprague-Dawley rats were fed restrictively (10 g/day) for 10 days and then given *ad libitum* access to a high-glucose diet supplemented with 3% hydroxycitrate for 6 days.[50] Controls received the same diet without the supplement. RQ and EE were measured during *ad libitum* days 1, 2, and 6. An oral glucose tolerance test was performed on *ad libitum* day 4 or 5. Hydroxycitrate decreased RQ and EE during *ad libitum* days 1 and 2. In all probability, these findings reflect a decrease in *de novo* lipogenesis. On *ad libitum* day 6, RQ and EE did not differ between treatment groups. Hydroxycitrate suppressed food intake during the first 3 days *ad libitum*, but overall body weight regain was not decreased in the hydroxycitrate group. The oral glucose tolerance test showed that hydroxycitrate significantly decreased the increase in plasma glucose from baseline and tended to decrease the area under the curve for glucose. Area under the curve for insulin did not differ between groups. These results indicate that, in this animal model, hydroxycitrate suppressed *de novo* lipogenesis and may improve glucose tolerance.[46,50]

Leonhardt et al. conducted a study in which a total of 63 male Sprague-Dawley rats were fed restrictively for 10 days.[51] Animals were then divided into seven groups (n = 9 per group) and switched to *ad libitum* consumption of food and water. The diet contained 70% (w/w) carbohydrates, 9% protein, and 12% fat. Results demonstrated that hydroxycitrate (3%) significantly suppressed food intake and body weight regain, and neither conjugated linoleic acid (CLA) (1%) nor guar gum (3%) increased the effect of hydroxycitrate on these parameters. Also, CLA and guar alone had no effect on food intake and body weight regain. The liver fat content of the combined hydroxycitrate + CLA groups was significantly lower compared to that of the control group. This study confirms the effectiveness of hydroxycitrate to reduce food intake and body weight regain after a period of restrictive feeding.[51]

Wielinga et al. investigated whether HCA reduces the postprandial glucose response by affecting gastric emptying or intestinal glucose absorption in rats.[52] Researchers compared the effect of regulator HCA (310 mg/kg) and vehicle (control) on the glucose response after an intragastric or intraduodenal glucose load to investigate the role of altered gastric emptying. Hydroxycitrate treatment delays the intestinal absorption of enterally administered glucose at the level of the small intestinal mucosa in rats. Hydroxycitrate strongly attenuated postprandial blood glucose levels after both intragastric ($p < 0.01$) and intraduodenal ($p < 0.001$) glucose administration, excluding a major effect of hydroxycitrate on gastric emptying. Hydroxycitrate delayed the systemic appearance of exogenous glucose but did not affect the total fraction of glucose absorbed over the study period of 150 min. This study supports a possible role for hydroxycitrate as food supplement in lowering postprandial glucose profiles.[52]

Another study by Ono et al. shows that calcium salt of HCA does not induce chromosomal aberration.[53] Chromosomal aberration and micronucleus test were investigated in cultured Chinese hamster lung cells and in mice. The extract did not increase the number of cells with structural aberration and/or numerical aberrations, nor did it increase the frequency of micronucleated polychromatic erythrocytes.[53]

CLINICAL STUDIES

Numerous clinical trials were performed to assess the weight management potential of different (–)-HCA preparations. Following are the summaries of the human clinical studies conducted on different forms of HCA and formulations.

A randomized, placebo-controlled, double-blind study was conducted in 54 male and female subjects (age: 21–55 years; degree of obesity: 15%–45% overweight).[54] This 8 week study consisted of group A (n = 30) given Lipodex-2™ (500 mg rind of *Garcinia indica* and 100 μg elemental chromium as chromium nicotinate) three times a day and group B (n = 24) who received placebo. All subjects were given same dietary instructions consisting of a low-fat, low-sugar, low-sodium, and high-fiber diet plan (1200 kcal diet/day) and were encouraged to drink 64 oz of water/day. Twenty two subjects in group A and 17 subjects in group B completed the study. The average weight loss per subject (n = 23) in group A was 5.06 kg (11.14 lb), while under the identical clinical conditions, group B subjects (n = 17) incurred an average weight loss of 1.91 kg (4.2 lb). One subject with multiple allergies experienced itching around the mouth and was advised to discontinue the study.[54]

Ramos et al. conducted a randomized, double-blind, placebo-controlled trial on 35 healthy subjects for 8 weeks.[55] Forty subjects started the program, while 35 completed the study. Three subjects dropped out due to influenza, and two subjects in the placebo group due to lack of positive results. The subjects were randomly divided into placebo group (n = 17, 4 males and 13 females, age: 38.7 ± 12.3 years, % overweight: 52.4 ± 20.5, BMI: 33.2 ± 4.4 kg/m²) and *G. cambogia* extract group (n = 18, 5 males and 13 females, age: 35.3 ± 11.8 years, % overweight: 50.7 ± 20.8, BMI: 32.6 ± 4.3 kg/m²). The placebo group received 500 mg capsule of placebo before each meal, while the second group received 500 mg lyophilized GCE in a similar form daily for 8 weeks. At the beginning of study and every 2 weeks throughout the study, all subjects underwent a physical examination and blood chemistry analysis. Both groups were placed on recommended diets providing 1000, 1200, or 1500 kcal depending on their theoretical ideal weight (TIW). At the end of the study, total cholesterol significantly decreased by 18%, triglyceride levels significantly decreased by 26% in the GCE group as compared to the control group. Average weight loss after 8 weeks was 1.3 ± 0.9 kg in the placebo group and 4.1 ± 1.8 kg (p < 0.001) in the GCE group. The GCE group also experienced reduced appetite starting from the first day of administration. Two subjects treated with GCE stated that they experienced slight headaches and nausea, while one subject in the control group experienced similar symptoms. No other adverse reactions were observed.[55]

Another randomized, placebo-controlled, double-blind study was conducted in 60 obese subjects (44 females and 16 males).[56] All subjects were on a low-fat diet of 1200 kcal/day and were instructed to exercise three times a week for 8 weeks. Subjects were given either placebo (n = 30) or HCA (n = 30) t.i.d. 30 min before meals. The daily dose of HCA was 1320 mg/day. The HCA group significantly lost an average body weight of 6.4 kg (p < 0.001), while the placebo group lost an average body weight of 3.8 kg. The difference in weight reduction is highly significant (p < 0.001). The composition of the weight loss, determined with near infrared (NIR) technique, shows that 87% of the weight loss in the HCA group is due to fat loss, while 80% weight loss was observed in the placebo group. Blood pressure, total cholesterol, and hip and waist circumferences were significantly reduced in both groups. A statistically significant difference between the groups in favor of the HCA group was seen in all these parameters (p < 0.001). Appetite scores during the study, using visual analog scales, were significantly reduced in the HCA group, but not in the placebo group (p < 0.001). The tolerability of the treatments was excellent. Two subjects stopped the treatment due to stomach pain, one in the HCA group and one in the placebo group.[56]

Girola et al. conducted a randomized, double-blind, placebo-controlled trial in 150 obese subjects for 4 weeks.[57] Group 1 (n = 50) received a hypocaloric diet plus one capsule/day of dietary integrator (capsules containing chitosan 240 mg, GCE 55 mg, and chromium 19 µg), group 2 (n = 50) received a hypocaloric diet and two capsules/day, and group 3 (n = 50) received a hypocaloric diet and a placebo. Following completion of the study, group 1 demonstrated a weight loss of 7.9%, total cholesterol reduction of 19.8%, LDL cholesterol reduction of 22.9%, triglycerides reduction of 18.3%, and HDL cholesterol augmentation of 9.0%. Group 2 exhibited a weight loss of 12.5%, total cholesterol reduction of 28.7%, LDL cholesterol reduction of 35.1%, triglycerides reduction of 26.6%, and HDL cholesterol augmentation by 14.1%. In the placebo group (group 3), weight reduction was 4.3%, total cholesterol reduction was 10.7%, LDL cholesterol reduction was 15.2%, triglycerides reduction was 13.2%, and HDL cholesterol augmentation was 6.3%. Adverse events were reported in 6.4% of subjects in the placebo group (nausea and/or constipation), in 6.1% of subjects in group 1 (nausea), and 2.1% of subjects in group 2 (headache) without any statistically significant difference between these three groups. No pathologic or clinically significant changes in blood chemistry or hematological assay were observed.[57]

Rothacker and Waitman evaluated the effectiveness of an HCA and natural caffeine combination in weight loss in a randomized, placebo-controlled, double-blind study for 6 weeks.[58] Fifty obese subjects (BMI: 27–33) enrolled in the study, while 48 completed the study. Subjects were randomized to treatment with a proprietary combination containing 400 mg GCE (≈50% HCA), 25 mg natural caffeine (guarana and green tea), 20 µg elemental chromium as chromium polynicotinate, or identically appearing placebo caplet. Subjects (mostly females) were instructed to take two caplets three times per day, 30–60 min before meals. All subjects were instructed to follow the same 1200 kcal high-fiber diet. Herbal supplement group (n = 25) exhibited a mean weight change of -4.0 ± 3.5 kg while the placebo group (n = 23) exhibited -3.0 ± 3.1 kg. End point revealed directional differences between treatment groups in favor of the HCA group (p = 0.30). No serious adverse events were reported.[58]

Heymsfield et al. conducted a randomized, placebo-controlled, double-blind study to evaluate the antiobesity potential of GCE.[59] One hundred thirty-five overweight men and women (BMI: approximately 32 kg/m^2) enrolled in the study while 84 subjects completed the study. Subjects were randomized or receive either GCE (n = 66; 1500 mg of HCA/day) or placebo (n = 69), and both groups were prescribed a high-fiber, low-energy (1200 kcal) diet. The treatment period was 12 weeks. Body weight was evaluated every other week and fat mass was measured at week 0 and 12. Both the placebo and GCE groups lost weight. However, no significant differences were observed. No significant adverse effects were reported.[59] Unfortunately, the source or physicochemical characteristics of the HCA used in this study[59] was not identified, leading to the questions such as the proper dosing and bioavailability of the HCA in the test substance.

Kriketos et al. conducted a double-blind, placebo-controlled, randomized, crossover study involving 3 days of HCA (3.0 g/day) or placebo supplementation in sedentary adult male subjects (n = 10, age: 22–38 years, BMI: 22.4–37.6 kg/m^2).[60] The effect of HCA supplementation on metabolic parameters with or without moderately intense exercise was studied over four laboratory visits. Two of the four visits involved no exercise (protocol A) with and without HCA treatment, while the remaining two visits included a moderately intense exercise regimen (protocol B; 30 min at 40% maximal aerobic fitness [VO_{2max}] and 15 min at 60% VO_{2max}) with and without HCA treatment. EE (by indirect calorimetry) and RQ were measured for 150 min following an overnight fast. Blood samples were collected for the determination of glucose, insulin, glucagon, lactate, and β-hydroxybutyrate concentrations. In a fasted state and following 3 days of HCA treatment, RQ was not significantly lowered during rest (protocol A), nor during exercise (protocol B) compared with the placebo treatment. Treatment with HCA did not affect EE, either during rest or during moderately intense exercise. Furthermore, the blood substrates measured were not significantly different between treatment groups under the fasting conditions of this study. These results do not support the hypothesis that HCA alters the short-term rate of fat oxidation in the fasting state during rest or moderate exercise, with doses likely to be achieved in humans while subjects maintain a typical Western diet (approximately 30%–35% total calories as fat).[60]

Mattes and Bormann assessed the effects of HCA on appetitive variables in a randomized, placebo-controlled, double-blind, parallel group study in 89 mildly overweight female subjects (age: 18–65 years).[7] Forty-two subjects were given 400 mg caplets of GCE 30–60 min before each meal three times a day (total dose: 2.4 g/day; total dose of HCA: 1.2 g/day); 47 subjects were given placebo for 12 weeks. Weight and body composition were assessed at baseline and every other week. Participants were counseled to adhere to a 1200 kcal exchange diet that contained 30% of energy from fat. Although both groups lost body weight, the active group (*G. cambogia* group) achieved a significantly greater reduction (7.0 ± 3.1 kg vs. 2.4 ± 2.9 kg). No adverse events were reported. No effects of the HCA were observed on appetitive variables.[7]

In a study conducted by van Loon et al., the effects of acute HCA supplementation on substrate metabolism was assessed at rest and during exercise in a randomized, controlled trial in humans.[61] Ten cyclists (age: 24 ± 2 years, weight: 73 ± 2 kg, VO_{2max}: 4.95 ± 0.11 L/min, maximal work output [W:max]: 408 ± 8 W) were studied at rest and during 2 h of exercise at 50% W:max on two occasions. Both 45 and 15 min before exercise and 30 and 60 min after the start of exercise, 3.1 mL/kg body weight of an HCA solution (19 g/L) or placebo was ingested. Total fat and carbohydrate oxidation rates were assessed. Blood samples were collected at 15 min intervals at rest and every 30 min during exercise. Plasma HCA concentrations increased after HCA ingestion up to 0.39 ± 0.02 mmol/L (82.0 ± 4.8 mg/L). However, no significant differences in total fat and carbohydrate oxidation rates were observed between trials. Accordingly, plasma glucose, glycerol, and fatty acid concentrations did not differ between trials. Plasma lactate concentrations were significantly lower in the HCA than in the placebo trial after 30 min of exercise, but at the end of the exercise period, they did not differ between trials. In conclusion, HCA, even when provided in large quantities, did not increase total fat oxidation *in vivo* in endurance-trained humans.[61]

Kovacs et al. assessed the effects of 2 week ingestion of HCA combined with medium-chain triglycerides (MCT) on satiety and food intake in 21 normal to moderately obese subjects (7 males and 14 females; age: 43 ±10 years; BMI: 27.6 ± 2.0 kg/m^2).[62] This study consisted of three intervention periods of 2 weeks separated by washout periods of 2 or 6 weeks in a randomized, crossover, placebo-controlled, double-blind study. Subjects consumed three self-selected meals and four isoenergetic snacks daily with either no supplementation (placebo), with 500 mg HCA, or 500 mg HCA plus 3 g MCT. Each intervention period ended with a test day, consisting of a standardized breakfast and *ad libitum* lunch and dinner. There was significant body weight loss during the 2 weeks of intervention (placebo: -0.5 ± 0.3 kg, $p < 0.05$; HCA: -0.4 ± 0.2 kg, $p < 0.05$; HCA+MCT: -0.7 ± 0.2 kg, $p < 0.01$), but the reduction was not significantly different between the groups. No adverse events were reported.[62]

Hayamizu et al. assessed the effects of long-term administration of GCE on visceral fat accumulation in humans.[63] A randomized, double-blind, placebo-controlled trial was conducted in 40 subjects (BMI: 25–35 kg/m^2) for 8 weeks. Subjects were randomized to either a GCE (n = 20, 1000 mg HCA per day) or a placebo group (n = 20). Each was subjected to a computed tomography (CT) scan at the umbilical level before and after the treatment period, and blood samples were taken to measure the clinical laboratory data every 4 weeks. As for a higher visceral fat area (VFA) in the subjects (with an initial VFA over 90 cm^2), both the VFA and VFA/SFA (subcutaneous fat area) ratio was measured. In the GCE group, both the VFA and VFA/SFA significantly decreased, compared to the placebo group ($p < 0.01$ and $p < 0.05$, respectively). Triacylglycerol was also reduced significantly in higher VFA subjects in the GCE group, compared to the initial levels ($p < 0.05$), but there were no significant difference between the groups in loss of body weight and the waist-hip ratio. Thus, GCE is useful in reducing body fat accumulation, especially visceral fat accumulation. No adverse effects were noted.[63]

Westerterp-Plantenga and Kovacs evaluated the effect of HCA on energy intake and satiety in a randomized, placebo-controlled, single-blind study in 24 overweight, healthy, dietary unrestrained subjects (12 males and 12 females; BMI: 27.5 ± 2.0 kg/m^2; age: 37 ± 10 years).[64] In this 6 week trial, subjects consumed three times for 2 weeks 100 mL tomato juice (placebo) and, separated by a 2 week washout period, 100 mL tomato juice with 300 mg HCA (HCA-SX). After 2 weeks, 24 h energy intake, appetite profile, hedonics, mood, and possible change in dietary restraint were assessed. Prevention of degradation and bio-availability was documented. Twenty-four hour energy intake was decreased by 15%–30% ($p < 0.05$) with HCA treatment compared to placebo. There were no changes observed in the appetite profile, dietary restraint, mood, and taste perception, while body weight tended to decrease and satiety was sustained.[64]

Lim et al. conducted a randomized, placebo-controlled study to determine whether short-term HCA ingestion increases fat oxidation during exercise in athletic human volunteers.[65] Subjects were administered 250 mg of HCA or placebo for 5 days, after each time performing cycle ergometer exercise at 60% VO$_{2max}$ for 60 min followed by 80% VO$_{2max}$ until exhaustion. Blood samples were collected and analyzed at rest and every 15 min. The RER was significantly lower in HCA trial than in the control trial ($p < 0.05$). Fat oxidation was significantly increased by short-term administration of HCA, and carbohydrate oxidation was significantly decreased ($p < 0.05$) during exercise, presumably resulting in increasing the cycle ergometer exercise time to exhaustion after 1 h of 60% VO$_{2max}$ performance with increasing fat oxidation, which spares glycogen utilization during moderate-intensity exercise in athletes.[65]

In another randomized, double-blind, placebo-controlled study, Lim et al. assessed whether HCA ingestion increases fat utilization during exercise in six untrained female subjects.[66] Subjects ingested 250 mg HCA or placebo capsule for 5 days and then participated in a cycle ergometer exercise. Subjects cycled at 40% VO$_{2max}$ for 1 h and then the exercise intensity was increased to 60% VO$_{2max}$ until exhaustion on day 5 of each experiment. HCA decreased the RER and carbohydrate oxidation during 1 h of exercise. In addition, exercise time to exhaustion was significantly enhanced ($p < 0.05$). These results suggest that HCA increases fat metabolism, which may be associated with a decrease in glycogen utilization during the same intensity exercise and enhanced exercise performance.[66]

Preuss et al. conducted a randomized, placebo-controlled, double-blind pilot study to determine the efficacy of HCA-SX and a combination of HCA-SX, niacin-bound chromium (NBC), and *Gymnema sylvestre* extract (GSE) in weight management in 30 obese subjects (age: 21–50 years; BMI > 26 kg/m^2).[67] Subjects were randomly divided into three groups (10 subjects/group): Group A was given 4667 mg HCA-SX (60% Ca^{2+}/K$^+$ salt of HCA as HCA-SX); group B was given a combination of HCA-SX 4667 mg, 400 μg elemental chromium as NBC, and 400 mg GSE; and group C was given a placebo daily in three equally divided doses 30–60 min before meals. In addition, subjects received 2000 kcal/day diet and underwent a 30 min/day supervised walking program, 5 days/week for 8 weeks. In group A, body weight and BMI decreased by 6.3%, food intake was reduced by 4%, and total cholesterol, LDL, and triglycerides levels were reduced by 6.3%, 12.3%, and 8.3%, respectively, while HDL and serotonin levels increased by 10.7% and 40%, respectively. Serum leptin levels were decreased by 36.6%, and the enhanced excretion of urinary fat metabolites, including malondialdehyde (MDA), acetaldehyde (ACT), formaldehyde (FA), and ACON, increased by 125%–258%. Under identical conditions, group B reduced body weight and BMI by 7.8% and 7.9%, respectively, food intake was reduced by 14.1%, and total cholesterol, LDL, and triglyceride levels were reduced by 9.1%, 17.9%, and 18.1%, respectively, while HDL and serotonin levels increased by 20.7% and 50%, respectively. Serum leptin levels decreased by 40.5%, and enhanced excretion of urinary fat metabolites increased by 146%–281%. Group C (placebo) reduced body weight and BMI by only 1.6% and 1.7%, respectively. No other significant changes were observed in the placebo group.[67]

In a following subsequent randomized, placebo-controlled, double-blind study, Preuss et al. evaluated the effects of HCA-SX and a combination of HCA-SX plus NBC and GSE in 60 obese subjects (age: 21–50 years, BMI > 26 kg/m²).[68] Subjects were randomly divided into three groups. Group A was administered 4667 mg HCA-SX; group B was administered a combination of 4667 mg HCA-SX, 400 µg elemental chromium as NBC, and 400 mg GSE; and group C was given placebo daily in three equally divided doses 30–60 min before meals. All subjects received a 2000 kcal diet/ day and participated in a supervised 30 min walking program for 8 weeks. At the end of 8 weeks, body weight and BMI decreased by 5%–6% in both treatment groups A and B. Food intake, total cholesterol, LDL, triglyceride, and serum leptin levels were significantly reduced in both groups, while HDL levels and excretion of urinary fat metabolites increased in both groups. A marginal or nonsignificant effect was observed in all parameters in group C (placebo). Results demonstrate that HCA-SX, and to a greater degree the combination of HCA-SX, NBC, and GSE, is effective in reducing body weight and promoting healthy cholesterol levels. No adverse effects were observed.[68]

BENEFITS OF CA²⁺ AND K⁺ IN HCA-SX IN WEIGHT MANAGEMENT

Potassium (K⁺) and calcium (Ca²⁺) are important cations for regulating a number of metabolic pathways influencing EE, leptin metabolism, and weight control. K⁺ is a major mineral in the body and the recommended daily intake is 3500 mg. Severe K⁺ deficiency causes cardiac arrhythmias, muscle weakness, and glucose intolerance, while moderate deficiency leads to increased blood pressure and salt sensitivity, an increased risk of kidney stones, and increased bone turnover. Inadequate K⁺ intake may also increase the risk of cardiovascular disease, particularly stroke, and may disturb intracellular pH homeostasis. K⁺ and Ca²⁺ flux may play important roles in coupling intracellular energy production to leptin secretion.[69,70] Restriction of Na⁺ intake is a common dietary recommendation in the treatment of syndrome X disorders. However, meta-analyses indicate that increased Ca²⁺ and K⁺ intake should be the focus of dietary recommendations, rather than restriction of Na⁺, in the management of such disorders as hypertension. Evidence demonstrates that diets rich in Ca⁺ and K⁺ produce a potent antihypertensive effect.[69] Angelos et al. reported that rat hearts perfused with glucose, insulin, and K⁺ had significantly higher ATP, creatine phosphate, and NADP(+), and lower AMP and inosine levels compared to controls after 30 min of reperfusion.[70] Reperfusion improved postischemic recovery of contractile function and the myocardial bioenergetic state.[70]

Dietary Ca²⁺ also plays a crucial role in regulating energy metabolism. High-Ca²⁺ diets have been shown to inhibit fat synthesis and storage in adipocytes and reduce weight gain during overconsumption of an energy-rich diet. High Ca²⁺ intake was shown to increase lipolysis and preserve thermogenesis during caloric restriction, accelerating weight loss. In contrast, low-Ca²⁺ diets have been shown to inhibit body fat loss.[71,72] Several clinical studies of Ca²⁺ intake were found to be associated with reduced weight in all groups. The Ca²⁺-treated subjects in a controlled trial exhibited

significant weight loss across nearly 4 years of observation.[73] In addition, other data from six observational studies and three controlled trials were evaluated to determine the relationship between
Ca^{2+} intake and body fat. Analysis reveals that higher intake of Ca^{2+} is consistently associated with
body weight loss and reduced weight gain. Heaney et al. demonstrated that a 300 mg increment
of regular Ca^{2+} intake is associated with 1 kg less body fat loss in children and 2.5–3.0 kg lower
body weight in adults.[74] Furthermore, Heaney et al. estimated that while Ca^{2+} intake explains only
a fraction of the variability in weight gains, increased Ca^{2+} intake could reduce the prevalence of
overweight and obesity significantly.[74,75] A related review by Teegarden reports that Ca^{2+} may play
a key role in reducing the incidence of obesity and prevalence of insulin resistance syndrome.[76]
The most obvious reason for adequate Ca^{2+} intake by postmenopausal women during a weight loss
regimen is to reduce the risk of bone demineralization disorders, like osteoporosis.[77] This evidence
supports the notion that adequate intake of dietary K^+ and Ca^{2+} enhances energy production and
leptin and insulin metabolism and satisfies particular nutrient needs of important pathways required
for healthy sustained weight loss and maintenance.

In addition to 60% HCA, 4500 mg of HCA-SX supplies approximately 495 mg of Ca^{2+} (49.5% of
RDI) and 720 mg of K^+ (15% of RDI) bound to HCA. The Ca^{2+} and K^+ ions in this novel formulation
contribute an important role in achieving significant improvements in body composition and the
weight maintenance effects by multiple synergistic pathways.

MOLECULAR MECHANISMS OF SEROTONIN
AND NPY IN APPETITE SUPPRESSION

Earlier *in vitro* studies have demonstrated that HCA-SX can induce increased serotonin release and
serve as a mild serotonin receptor reuptake inhibitor (SRRI).[27,78] The effect of HCA on basal and
potassium chloride-depolarization-evoked increase in radiolabeled serotonin ([³H]-5-HT) release
from rat brain cortex slices *in vitro* was studied. Results demonstrated that HCA (10 microM-1 mM)
altered the baseline of spontaneous tritium efflux reaching a maximum at 300 μM but had no significant effect on potassium-evoked release of [³H]-5-HT. HCA-SX can inhibit [³H]-5-HT uptake
(and also increase 5-HT availability) in isolated rat brain cortical slices in a manner similar to that
of SRRIs and thus may prove beneficial in controlling appetite, as well as treatment of depression,
insomnia, migraine headaches, and other serotonin-deficient conditions. In subsequent *in vivo*
studies, we found elevated serotonin levels in the brain tissues of male and female rats.

These findings were further corroborated in the human clinical trials and cDNA oligonucleotide microarray study conducted by Preuss et al.[67,68] and Roy et al.,[49] respectively. Thus, serotonin
regulation may be a major mechanism of appetite suppression by HCA-SX. In a very recent study,
HCA-SX caused a significant reduction of basal neuropeptide Y (NPY) concentrations in the
hypothalamic tissues, further establishing a role for HCA-SX as an appetite suppressant.

REGULATION OF GENES BY HCA-SX

Obesity is an energy-balance disorder in which certain genes that are programmed to resist loss of
body fat prevail.[79,80] This programmed genetic predisposition is responsible for downregulating the
resting metabolic rate in response to dietary and caloric restriction, which is significantly disrupted
following rapid weight loss regimens.[81] Overconsumption of food (excess energy intake) is a normal consequence contributing to weight gain and obesity. A resistance to the hormone leptin also
characterizes common obesity. Insulin has been shown to increase leptin secretion by 25%.[82] Ample
evidence demonstrates that insulin resistance is also a primary contributor to obesity, suggesting
that insulin-resistance-induced hyperinsulinemia can provoke leptin-resistant hyperleptinemia
with a consequential increase in fat synthesis and storage in adipocytes, a characteristic sequel of
syndrome X. Furthermore, adipocytes from fatter animals secrete more leptin, and a correlation
between intracellular ATP concentration and the rate of leptin secretion appears to exist.[82] As such,

leptin concentration correlates positively with percent body fat. A low-resting metabolic rate for a given body size and composition, a low rate of fat oxidation, and low levels of physical activity are risk factors for weight gain and common traits of obese individuals.[83]

The effects of low-dose oral HCA-SX was investigated on the body weight and abdominal fat transcriptome in rats.[49] HCA-SX restricted body weight gain in rats and lowered abdominal fat leptin expression. High-density microarray analysis of 9960 genes and ESTs present in the fat tissue identified a specific set of genes sensitive to dietary HCA-SX.[49]

Functional characterization of HCA-SX sensitive genes revealed that upregulation of genes encoding serotonin receptors represents a distinct effect of HCA-SX on appetite suppression.[49] HCA-SX upregulated a significant number of genes associated with serotonin receptor and neuro-peptide signaling, which demonstrate its ability in appetite suppression.[49] Serotonin is believed to be a mood-enhancing chemical in the brain. High levels of serotonin are important for emotional well-being by giving the feeling of satiety and calming effect. It also plays a role in appetite suppression and reduces cravings for carbohydrates and high glycemic index foods.[81] Appetite control involves an integration of the drive signals arising from energy stores in the body with the satiety signals generated by periodic episodes of food consumption. Serotonin (5-hydroxytryptamine, 5-HT) has been implicated in the processes of within-meal satiation and postmeal satiety (5-HT1B and 5-HT2C postsynaptic receptors), which are concerned with the signals arising from the pattern of food intake. Stimulation of serotonergic receptors reduces feeding and perhaps enhances the satiating effect of food. Furthermore, regulation of 5-HT2A gene plays an essential role in body weight management through the regulation of cortisol secretion.[82] Also, polymorphism of the 5-HT2A genes causes abdominal obesity in humans.[82] These findings corroborate with our previously conducted *in vitro* and *in vivo* studies demonstrating HCA-SX's ability to enhance serotonin release and availability in the brain vicinity and act as a mild SRRI.[27,60,61,78]

HCA-SX has also been shown to modulate a significant number of genes including prostaglandin D synthase (PGDS), aldolase B, lipocalin 2, fructose-1,6-biphosphatase 1, and LDL-receptor related protein 2, which play a prominent role in are in lipid metabolism, carbohydrate metabolism, glycolysis, and cell communication.[49] It is worthwhile to mention that PGDS serves as a ligand for the nuclear receptor peroxisome proliferator-activated receptor (PPAR-γ), and PPAR-γ signaling causes metabolic changes ultimately leading to obesity.[84,85] These findings corroborate with our clinical studies, demonstrating HCA-SX's influence on the reduction on LDL, triglycerides, and total cholesterol; enhanced excretion of urinary fat metabolites, including MDA, ACT, FA, and ACON, in conjunction with body weight loss and BMI reduction; and marginal increase in the HDL level.[60,61] Mitochondrial or nuclear proteins necessary for fundamental support of the tissue were not affected by HCA-SX, which demonstrated the safety of HCA-SX.[49] These findings further demonstrate that HCA-SX is safe, efficacious, and capable of regulating a significant number of obesity regulatory genes.

CONCLUSION

G. cambogia preparations are quite popular and have been used in India and Southeast Asia for the last several centuries. In *Ayurveda,* several preparations of *G. cambogia* have been recommended for diverse therapeutic applications. In the Western world, a significant number of scientists have conducted *in vitro, in vivo,* and mechanistic research on *G. cambogia* since the late 1960s. A number of patents and manufacturing process have been developed, and a number of (–)-HCA preparations are commercially available in the marketplace. Extensive safety, mechanistic, and efficacy studies were conducted on a novel calcium–potassium salt of HCA (HCA-SX). Literature shows that solubility, taste, and odor of HCA salts, as well as the structural integrity, bioavailability, and stability of the HCA preparations, depend largely on the binding cation(s) and novel manufacturing technology. It is worthwhile to mention that these physicochemical characteristics are very important to demonstrate the safety and efficacy of HCA salts in weight management. A significant number of studies have shown that HCA-SX is safe and efficacious in obesity management as evidenced by lowering of body weight and BMI in clinical studies. HCA-SX also exhibited discrete mechanisms for appetite suppression through serotonin and hypothalamic NPY regulation. HCA-SX has also been shown to promote fat oxidation as demonstrated by enhanced excretion of urinary fat metabolites and reduce serum leptin levels in human subjects. HCA-SX also promoted healthy blood lipid profile in the clinical study, and no significant adverse effects were observed. Effective dose, bioavailability, balanced diet, and moderate exercise coupled with synergistic influences of calcium and potassium can significantly enhance the therapeutic efficacy of HCA-SX in obesity regulation. These studies were further substantiated by the unbiased cDNA oligonucleotide microarray study, which demonstrated the regulatory role of HCA-SX on obesity genes, without compromising the levels of mitochondrial and nuclear proteins essential for optimal biochemical and physiological functions in cellular system.

REFERENCES

1. World Health Organization. 2011. Media centre. Obesity and overweight. http://www.who.int/mediacentre/factsheets/fs311/en/ (accessed February 4, 2011).
2. Centers for Disease Control and Prevention. 2011. U.S. obesity trends: Trends by state 1985–2009. http://www.cdc.gov/obesity/data/trends.html (accessed February 4, 2011).
3. Sergio, W. 1988. A natural food, the Malabar Tamarind, may be effective in the treatment of obesity. *Medical Hypotheses* 27:39–40.
4. Mattes, R.D. and L. Bormann. 2000. Effects of (−)-hydroxycitric acid on appetitive variables. *Physiology & Behavior* 71:87–94.
5. Sreenivasan, A. and R. Venkataraman. 1959. Chromatographic detection of the organic constituents of Gorikapuli (*Garcinia cambogia* Desr.) used in pickling fish. *Current Science* 28:151–152.
6. Clouatre, D. and M. Rosenbaum. 1994. *The Diet and Health Benefits of HCA (Hydroxycitric Acid)*. Keats Publishing Co., New Canaan, CT, p. 9.
7. Lewis, Y.S., S. Neelakantan, and C. Murthy. 1964. Acids in *Garcinia cambogia*. *Current Science* 33:82–83.
8. Mahendran, P., K.E. Sabitha, and C.S. Devi. 2002. Prevention of HCl-ethanol induced gastric mucosal injury in rats by *Garcinia cambogia* extract and its possible mechanism of action. *Indian Journal of Experimental Biology* 40(1):58–62.
9. Mahendran, P., A.J. Vanisree, and C.S. Shyamala Devi. 2002. The antiulcer activity of *Garcinia cambogia* extract against indomethacin-induced gastric ulcer in rats. *Phytotherapy Research* 16(1):80–83.
10. Jena, B.S., G.K. Jayaprakasha, R.P. Singh, and K.K. Sakariah. 2002. Chemistry and biochemistry of (−)-hydroxycitric acid from Garcinia. *Journal of Agricultural and Food Chemistry* 50(1):10–22.
11. U.S. Food and Drug Administration. 2011. Dietary Supplements Health and Education Act of 1994. (DSHEA 1994). Washington, DC. http://www.fda.gov/food/dietarysupplements/default.htm (accessed February 4, 2011).
12. Martin, F.W., C.W. Campbell, and R.M. Ruberte. 1987. Perennial edible fruits of the tropics: An inventory. United States Department of Agriculture, Agricultural Research Service, Washington, DC, p. 212.
13. Lewis, Y.S. and S. Neelakantan. 1965. (−)-Hydroxycitric acid—The principal acid in the fruits of *Garcinia cambogia* desr. *Phytochemistry* 4:619–625.
14. Lewis, Y.S. 1969. Isolation and properties of hydroxycitric acid. In *Methods in Enzymology, Citric Acid Cycle*, Vol. 13, ed. J.M. Lowenstein, pp. 613–619. Academic Press, New York.
15. Martius, C. and R. Maue. 1941. Preparation, physiological behavior, and importance of hydroxycitric acid and its isomers. *Zeitschrift fur Physiological Chemistry* 269:33–39.
16. Boll, P.M., E. Sorensen, and E. Balieu. 1969. Naturally occurring lactones and lactames. The absolute configuration of the hydroxycitric acid lactones: Hibiscus acid and garcinia acid. *Acta Chemica Scandinavia* 23:286–293.
17. Glusker, J.P., J.A. Minkin, C.A. Casciato, and F.B. Soule. 1969. Absolute configuration of the naturally occurring hydroxycitric acids. *Archives of Biochemistry and Biophysics* 13:573–577.
18. Glusker, J.P., J.A. Minkin, and C.A. Casciato. 1971. The structure and absolute configuration of the calcium salt of garcinia acid, the lactone of (−)-hydroxycitric acid. *Acta Crystallography* B27:1284–1293.
19. Lowenstein, J. and H. Brunengraber. 1981. Hydroxycitrate. In *Methods in Enzymology, Lipids*, Vol. 72, ed. J. Lownestein, pp. 486–497. Academic Press, New York.

20. Guthrie, R.W. and R.W. Kierstead. 1977. Hydroxycitric acid derivatives. U.S. Patent 4005086 and 4006166.

21. Moffett, S.A., A.K. Bhandari, B. Ravindranath, and K. Balasubra-Manvam. 1977. Hydroxycitric acid concentrate and food products prepared there from. U.S. Patent 5656314.

22. Jayaprakasha, G.K. and K.K. Sakariah. 1998. Determination of organic acids in *Garcinia cambogia* (desr.) by HPLC. *Journal of Chromatography* 806:337–339.

23. Jayaprakasha, G.K. and K.K. Sakariah. 2000. Determination of (–)-hydroxycitric acid in commercial samples of *Garcinia cambogia* extracts by liquid chromatography using ultraviolet detection. *Journal of Liquid Chromatography Related Technology* 23:915–923.

24. Downs, B.W., M. Bagchi, G.V. Subbaraju, M.A. Shara, H.G. Preuss, and D. Bagchi. 2005. Bioefficacy of a novel calcium-potassium salt of (–)-hydroxycitric acid. *Mutation Research* 579(1–2):149–162.

25. Loe, Y.C., N. Bergeron, N. Rodriguez, and J.M. Schwarz. 2001. Gas chromatography/mass spectrometry method to quantify blood hydroxycitrate concentration. *Analytical Biochemistry* 292:148–154.

26. Loe, Y.C., N. Bergeron, J. Phan, M. Wen, J. Lee, and J.M. Schwarz. 2001. Time course of hydroxycitrate clearance in fasting and fed humans. *FASEB Journal* 15(4):632, Abs. 501.1

27. Ohia, S.E., C.A. Opere, A.M. LeDay, M. Bagchi, D. Bagchi, and S.J. Stohs. 2002. Safety and mechanism of appetite suppression by a novel hydroxycitric acid extract (HCA-SX). *Molecular and Cellular Biochemistry* 238:89–103.

28. Shara, M., S.E. Ohia, T. Yasmin, A. Zardetto-Smith, A. Kincaid, M. Bagchi, A. Chatterjee, D. Bagchi, and S.J. Stohs. 2003. Dose- and time-dependent effects of a novel (–)-hydroxycitric acid extract on hepatic and testicular lipid peroxidation, DNA fragmentation and histopathological data over a period of 90 days in rats. *Molecular and Cellular Biochemistry* 254:339–346.

29. Shara, M., S.E. Ohio, R.E. Schmidt, T. Yasmin, A. Zardetto-Smith, A. Kincaid, M. Bagchi, A. Chatterjee, D. Bagchi, and S.J. Stohs. 2004. Physico-chemical properties of a novel (–)-hydroxycitric acid extract and its effect on body weight, selected organ weights, hepatic lipid peroxidation and DNA fragmentation, hematology and clinical chemistry, and histopathological changes over a period of 90 days. *Molecular and Cellular Biochemistry* 260:171–186.

30. Saito, M., M. Ueno, S. Ogino, K. Kubo, J. Nagata, and M. Takeuchi. 2005. High dose of *Garcinia cambogia* is effective in suppressing fat accumulation in developing male Zucker obese rats, but highly toxic to the testis. *Food and Chemical Toxicology* 43:411–419.

31. Deshmukh, N.S., M. Bagchi, T. Yasmin, and D. Bagchi. 2008. Safety of a novel calcium/potassium salt of hydroxycitric acid (HCA-SX): I. Two-generation reproduction toxicity study. *Toxicology Mechanisms and Methods* 18:433–442.

32. Deshmukh, N.S., M. Bagchi, T. Yasmin, and D. Bagchi. 2008. Safety of a novel calcium/potassium salt of (–)-hydroxycitric acid (HCA-SX): II. Developmental toxicity study in rats. *Toxicology Mechanisms and Methods* 18:443–451.

33. Soni, M.G., G.A. Burdock, H.G. Preuss, S.J. Stohs, S.E. Ohia, and D. Bagchi. 2004. Safety assessment of (–)-hydroxycitric acid and Super CitriMax, a novel calcium/potassium salt. *Food Chemical Toxicology* 42:1513–1529.

34. Watson, J.A., M. Fang, and J.M. Lowenstein. 1969. Tricarballylate and hydroxycitrate: Substrate and inhibitor of ATP: Citrate oxaloacetate lyase. *Archives of Biochemistry and Biophysics* 135:209–217.

35. Lowenstein, J.M. 1970. Experiments with (–)-hydroxycitrate. In *Essays in cell metabolism*, eds. W. Bartely, H.L. Kornberg, and J.R. Quayle, pp. 153–166. London, U.K.: John Wiley & Sons.

36. Lowenstein, J.M. 1971. Effect of (–)-hydroxycitrate on fatty acid synthesis by rat liver *in vivo*. *Journal of Biological Chemistry* 246:629–632.

37. Sullivan, A.C., J. Triscari, J.G. Hamilton, O.N. Miller, and V.R. Wheatley. 1972. Inhibition of lipogenesis in rat liver by (–)-hydroxycitrate. *Lipids* 150:183–186.

38. Sullivan, A.C., J. Triscari, J.G. Hamilton, O.N. Miller, and V.R. Wheatley. 1974. Effect of (–)-hydroxycitrate upon the accumulation of lipid in the rat: I. Lipogenesis. *Lipids* 9:121–128.

39. Sullivan, A.C., J. Triscari, J.G. Hamilton, O.N. Miller, and V.R. Wheatley. 1974. Effect of (–)-hydroxycitrate upon the accumulation of lipid in the rat: II. Appetite. *Lipids* 9:129–134.

40. Sullivan, A.C., J. Triscari, and J.E. Spiegel. 1977. Metabolic regulation as a control for lipid disorders. II. Influence of (–)-hydroxycitrate on genetically and experimentally induced hypertriglyceridemia in the rat. *American Journal of Clinical Nutrition* 30:777–784.

41. Hamilton, J.G., A.C. Sullivan, and D. Kritchevsky. 1977. Hypolipidemic activity of (–)-hydroxycitrate. *Lipids* 12:1–9.

42. Greenwood, M.R., M.P. Cleary, R. Gruen, D. Blasé, J.S. Stern, J. Triscari, and A.C. Sullivan. 1981. Effect of (–)-hydroxycitrate on development of obesity in the Zucker obese rat. *American Journal of Physiology* 240:E72–E78.

43. Rao, R.N. and K.K. Sakariah. 1988. Lipid-lowering and antiobesity effect of (−)-hydroxycitric acid. *Nutrition Research* 8:209–212.

44. Vasselli, J.R., E. Shane, C.N. Boozer, and S.B. Heymsfield. 1998. *Garcinia cambogia* extract inhibits body weight gain via increased energy expenditure (EE) in rats. *FASEB Journal* 12:A505.

45. Ishihara, K., S. Oyaizu, K. Onuki, K. Lim, and T. Fushiki. 2000. Chronic (−)-hydroxycitrate administration spares carbohydrate utilization and promotes lipid oxidation during exercise in mice. *Journal of Nutrition* 130:2990–2995.

46. Leonhardt, M., B. Hrupka, and W. Langhans. 2001. Effect of hydroxycitrate on food intake and body weight regain after a period of restrictive feeding in male rats. *Physiology & Behavior* 74:191–196.

47. Leonhardt, M. and W. Langhans. 2002. Hydroxycitrate has long-term effects on feeding behavior, body weight regain, and metabolism after body weight loss in male rats. *Journal of Nutrition* 132:1977–1982.

48. Hayamizu, K., H. Hirakawa, D. Oikawa, T. Nakanishi, T. Takagi, T. Tachiban, and M. Furuse. 2003. Effect of *Garcinia cambogia* extract on serum leptin and insulin in mice. *Fitoterapia* 74:267–273.

49. Roy, S., C. Rink, S. Khanna, C. Phillips, D. Bagchi, M. Bagchi, and C. K. Sen. 2004. Body weight and abdominal fat gene expression profile in response to a novel hydroxycitric acid-based dietary supplement. *Gene Expression* 11:251–262.

50. Leonhardt, M., B. Balkan, and W. Langhans. 2004. Effect of hydroxycitrate on respiratory quotient, energy expenditure, and glucose tolerance in male rats after a period of restrictive feeding. *Nutrition* 20:911–915.

51. Leonhardt, M., S. Munch, M. Westerterp-Plantenga, and W. Langhans. 2004. Effects of hydroxycitrate, conjugated linoleic acid, and guar gum on food intake, body weight regain, and metabolism after body weight loss in male rats. *Nutrition Research* 24:659–669.

52. Wielinga, P.Y., R.E. Wachters-Hagedoorn, B. Bouter, T.H. van Dijk, F. Stellaard, A. G. Nieuw enhuizen, H.J. Verkade, and A.J. Scheurink. 2005. Hydroxycitric acid delays intestinal glucose absorption in rats. *American Journal of Physiology—Gastrointestinal & Liver Physiology* 288:G1144–G1149.

53. Ono, H., H. Tamura, Y. Yamashita, K. Tamura, and K. Iwakura. 2006. *In vitro* chromosome aberration test and *in vivo* micronucleus test of Ca-type Garcinia extract. *Shokuhin Eiseigaku Zasshi* 47:80–84.

54. Conte, A.A. 1993. A non-prescription alternative in weight reduction therapy. *American Journal of Bariatric Medicine* Summer:17–19.

55. Ramos, R.R., J.L. Saenz, and C.F. Aguilar. 1995. Extract of *Garcinia cambogia* in controlling obesity. *Investigacion Medica Internacional* 22:97–100.

56. Thom, E. 1996. Hydroxycitrate (HCA) in the treatment of obesity. *International Journal of Obesity Related Metabolic Disorders* 20:75.

57. Girola, M., M. De Bernardi, and S. Contos. 1996. Dose effect in lipid-lowering activity of a new dietary integrator (chitosan, *Garcinia cambogia* extract and chromium). *Acta Toxicologica et Therapeutica* 17:25–40.

58. Rothacker, D.A. and B.E. Waitman. 1997. Effectiveness of a *Garcinia cambogia* and natural caffeine combination in weight loss: A double-blind placebo-controlled pilot study. *International Journal of Obesity* 21:S53.

59. Heymsfield, S.B., D.B. Allison, J.R. Vasselli, A. Pietrobelli, D. Greenfield, and C. Nunez. 1998. *Garcinia cambogia* (hydroxycitric acid) as a potential antiobesity agent: A randomized controlled trial. *JAMA* 280:1596–1600.

60. Kriketos, A.D., H.R. Thompson, H. Greene, and J.O. Hill. 1999. (−)-Hydroxycitric acid does not affect energy expenditure and substrate oxidation in adult males in a post-absorptive state. *International Journal of Obesity and Related Metabolic Disorders* 23:867–873.

61. van Loon, L.J., J.J. van Rooijen, B. Niesen, H. Verhagen, W.H. Saris, and A.J. Wagenmakers. 2000. Effects of acute (−)-hydroxycitrate supplementation on substrate metabolism at rest and during exercise in humans. *American Journal of Clinical Nutrition* 72:1445–1450.

62. Kovacs, E.M., M.S. Westerterp-Plantenga, M. de Vries, F. Brouns, and W.H. Saris. 2001. Effects of 2 week ingestion of (−)-hydroxycitrate and (−)-hydroxycitrate combined with medium-chain-triglycerides on satiety and food intake. *Physiology & Behavior* 74:543–549.

63. Hayamizu, K., Y. Ishii, I. Kaneko, M. Shen, H. Sakaguchi, Y. Okuhara, N. Shigematsu, S. Miyazaki, and H. Shimasaki. 2001. Effects of long-term administration of *Garcinia cambogia* extract on visceral fat accumulation in humans: A placebo-controlled double-blind trial. *Journal of Oleo Science* 50:805–812.

64. Westerterp-Plantenga, M.S. and E.M. Kovacs. 2002. The effect of (−)-hydroxycitric acid on energy intake and satiety in overweight humans. *International Journal of Obesity and Metabolic Disorders* 26:870–872.

65. Lim, K., S. Ryu, Y. Ohishi, I. Watanabe, H. Tomi, H. Suh, W.K. Lee, and T. Kwon. 2002. Short-term (–)-hydroxycitrate ingestion increases fat oxidation during exercise in athletes. *Journal of Nutrition & Science Vitaminology (Tokyo)* 48:128–133.

66. Lim, K., S. Ryu, H.S. Nho, S.K. Choi, T. Kwon, H. Suh, J. So, K. Tomita, Y. Okuhara, and N. Shigematsu. 2003. (–)-Hydroxycitric acid ingestion increases fat utilization during exercise in untrained women. *Journal of Nutrition & Science Vitaminology (Tokyo)* 49:163–167.

67. Preuss, H.G., D. Bagchi, M. Bagchi, C.V.S. Rao, S. Satyanarayana, and D.K. Dey. 2004. Efficacy of a novel, natural extract of (–)-hydroxycitric acid (HCA-SX) and a combination of HCA-SX, niacin bound chromium and *Gymnema sylvestre* extract in weight management in human volunteers: A pilot study. *Nutrition Research* 24:45–58.

68. Preuss, H.G., D. Bagchi, M. Bagchi, C.V.S. Rao, D.K. Dey, and S. Satyanarayana. 2004. Effects of a natural extract of (–)-hydroxycitric acid (HCA-SX) and a combination of HCA-SX plus niacin-bound chromium and *Gymnema sylvestre* extract in weight loss. *Diabetes Obesity Metabolism* 6:171–180.

69. Hermansen, K. 2000. Diet, blood pressure and hypertension. *British Journal of Nutrition* 83 (Suppl 1):S113–S119.

70. Angelos, M.G., H.N. Murray, R.T. Gorsline, and P.F. Klawitter. 2002. Glucose, insulin and potassium (GIK) during reperfusion mediates improved myocardial bioenergetics. *Resuscitation* 55:329–336.

71. Zemel, M.B. 2003. Role of dietary calcium and dairy products in modulating adiposity. *Lipids* 38:139–146.

72. Zemel, M.B. 2003. Mechanisms of dairy modulation of adiposity. *Journal of Nutrition* 133:252S–256S.

73. Davies, K.M., R.P. Heaney, R.R. Recker, J.M. Lappe, M.J. Barger-Lux, K. Rafferty, and S. Hinders. 2000. Calcium intake and body weight. *Journal of Clinical Endocrinology Metabolism* 85:4635–4638.

74. Heaney, R.P., K.M. Davies, and M.J. Barger-Lux. 2002. Calcium and weight: Clinical studies. *Journal of American College of Nutrition* 21:152S–155S.

75. Heaney, R.P. 2003. Normalizing calcium intake: Projected population effects for body weight. *Journal of Nutrition* 133:268S–270S.

76. Teegarden, D. 2003. Calcium intake and reduction in weight or fat mass. *Journal of Nutrition* 133:249S–251S.

77. Shapses, S.A., N.L. von Thun, S.B. Heymsfield, T.A. Ricci, M. Ospina, R.N. Pierson Jr., and T. Stahl. 2001. Bone turnover and density in obese premenopausal women during moderate weight loss and calcium supplementation. *Journal of Bone Mineral Research* 16:1329–1336.

78. Ohia, S.E., S.O. Awe, A.M. LeDay, C.A. Opere, and D. Bagchi. 2001. Effect of hydroxycitric acid on serotonin release from isolated rat brain cortex. *Research Communication Molecular Pathology Pharmacology* 109:210–216.

79. Steinbeck, K. 2002. Obesity: The science behind the management. *Internal Medicine Journal* 32:237–241.

80. Levy, J.R., J. Gyarmati, J.M. Lesko, R.A. Adler, and W. Stevens. 2000. Dual regulation of leptin secretion: Intracellular energy and calcium dependence of regulated pathway. *American Journal of Physiology & Endocrinology Metabolism* 278:E892–E901.

81. Filozof, C.M., C. Murua, M.P. Sanchez, C. Brailovsky, M. Perman, C.D. Gonzalez, and E. Ravussin. 2000. Low plasma leptin concentration and low rates of fat oxidation in weight-stable post-obese subjects. *Obesity Research* 8:205–210.

82. Halford, J.C. and J.E. Blundell. 2000. Separate systems for serotonin and leptin in appetite control. *Annals of Medicine* 32:222–232.

83. Rosmond, R., C. Bouchard, and P. Bjorntorp. 2002. 5-HT2A receptor gene promoter polymorphism in relation to abdominal obesity and cortisol. *Obesity Research* 10:585–589.

84. Jowsey, I.R., P.R. Murdock, G.B. Moore, G.J. Murphy, S.A. Smith, and J.D. Hayes. 2003. Prostaglandin D2 synthase enzymes and PPARg are co-expressed in mouse 3T3-L1 adipocytes and human tissues. *Prostaglandins Other Lipid Mediators* 70:267–284.

85. Zhang, F., B. Lavan, and F.M. Gregoire. 2004. Peroxisome proliferators-activated receptors as attractive antiobesity targets. *Drug News Perspectives* 17:661–669.

37 Review of the Safety and Efficacy of Bitter Orange (Citrus aurantium) and Its Primary Protoalkaloid, p-Synephrine, in Weight Management

Sidney J. Stohs, PhD, FACN, CNS, ATS, FASAHP, and Mohd Shara, PhD, PharmD, FACN

CONTENTS

INTRODUCTION

Citrus aurantium extract and its primary protoalkaloidal constituent, *p*-synephrine, are widely used in weight management products and as thermogenic agents. *C. aurantium* extract is also known as bitter orange extract, a product that is derived from the immature (green) fruits of the Seville orange. In traditional Chinese medicine, it is known as "*Chih-shi*" or "*Zhi shi*." *p*-Synephrine is a phenylethylamine derivative, also known as oxedrine, which has the hydroxy group in the *para* position on the benzene ring.

In recent years, bitter orange extract has been used in weight management products due to its effects on metabolic processes, including increased lipolysis and thermogenesis, as well as its mild appetite suppression. It is also used in sports performance products to enhance stamina.

Controversy has existed regarding the safety and efficacy of bitter orange extract. This controversy has occurred for a number of reasons. It has been only within the last several years that *p*-synephrine and extracts of bitter orange have been studied without the addition of various other ingredients and herbal products. The issue of safety and efficacy is clearly clouded by the structural similarity of p-synephrine to ephedrine, notwithstanding that the pharmacokinetics of the two compounds and the receptor binding specificities are vastly different due to significant structural differences. Properties associated with ephedrine are frequently and inappropriately ascribed to p-synephrine. Risk–benefit ratios have not been conducted, and much of the information published related to risk has been questionable.

Other issues have also clouded the picture with respect to the safety and efficacy of bitter orange extract. Some of the extracts that are used are either nonstandardized or poorly standardized, making it exceedingly difficult to establish reproducibility. Lack of knowledge of the chemical composition of the extracts being used in some cases precludes meaningful comparisons. Products containing bitter orange extracts almost invariably contain a variety of other herbal extracts, many of which contain caffeine. Warnings are largely ignored by the consuming public about not using multiherbal weight management products if one has a history of various diseases. Furthermore, both the lay and scientific communities have failed to differentiate between p-synephrine and m-synephrine (phenylephrine, hydroxyl group in the *meta* position on the benzene ring), which clearly has cardiovascular effects but is not a constituent of bitter orange. Unfortunately, properties possessed by m-synephrine are frequently and inappropriately attributed to bitter orange extract and p-synephrine.

A final serious issue that has added greatly to the overall confusion by the public and scientific community regarding bitter orange has been the release of erroneous adverse events information by governmental agencies. Statements implying that large numbers of adverse events and even deaths due to the use of products containing bitter orange extract have clearly been shown to be incorrect and misleading but are still widely parroted by the news media.

The question to be asked is what information can be obtained from studies that have been conducted on bitter orange extract to date? Is bitter orange extract safe and effective for weight management when used as directed in appropriate amounts? This review will cover published data associated with animal, human, and mechanistic studies; case reports; and unpublished clinical studies. A large number of studies have been conducted over the past 5 years since this chapter was initially written. These investigations have greatly added to our knowledge of bitter orange extract and p-synephrine and are included in this revision and update.

HISTORICAL PERSPECTIVE

Bitter orange has been used for hundreds of years as a medicament. According to traditional Chinese medicine [1], *Zhi shi* (immature bitter orange) "is one of the best herbs to treat gastrointestinal disorders characterized by stagnation and accumulation" and "is one of the best herbs to relieve distention and hardness of the epigastric area caused by cholecystitis." Pharmacologically, this compendium reports that *Zhi shi* does not affect heart rate or respiration and has minimal toxicity.

Youngken [2] described the collection and preparation of bitter orange peel USP and its uses as an aromatic bitter and flavoring agent with an average dose of 1 g for the dried material and 4 mL for the bitter orange peel tincture USP. Trease and Evans [3] denoted the history of bitter orange trees, indicating that they were first brought to Europe about AD 1200, arriving from Northern India via Africa. At the time this book was published, the peel of the bitter orange was official in the British Pharmacopoeia.

Bitter orange peel has been used in South America in folk medicine for anxiety, insomnia, and epilepsy [4]. These same authors reported that the oil from the peel was shown to possess anxiolytic, sedative, and anticonvulsant properties.

The current-day use of bitter orange can be arguably traced to the work of Arch and Ainsworth [5] who noted that this product had the potential to augment thermogenesis and increase calorie consumption, while at the same time producing fewer cardiovascular perturbations than ephedrine due to its lack of penetration of the central nervous system (CNS). As a result of the ban of ephedrine in 2004, bitter orange extract rapidly replaced ephedra, although the use of bitter orange extract had gradually increased as a thermogenic agent over the past two decades.

The consumption of p-synephrine is much more common than generally recognized. It should be kept in mind that millions of people consume on a daily basis without ill effects various juices and food products such as marmalade from *Citrus* species as Seville orange, grapefruit, mandarin, and other orange-related species that contain p-synephrine. An average sweet orange contains approximately 6 mg p-synephrine [6]. A wide variety of citrus juices contain about 5 mg p-synephrine per 8 oz glass [7], while juice from mandarin oranges may contain more than 20 mg and as much as 40 mg p-synephrine per 8 oz glass [7,8], more than is in the typical dietary supplement per serving.

CHEMISTRY

A number of studies have assessed the chemical components in bitter orange extracts responsible for the effects on weight management as well as other physiological effects, and various analytical techniques have been developed to separate and quantify the various alkaloids [6,9–17]. For example, Hashimoto et al. [9] developed a high-performance liquid chromatographic method for determining p-synephrine content in Chinese medicinal drugs and concluded that p-synephrine was present at levels of 0.174%–0.566% in these crude drug preparations. Pellati et al. [11] determined the alkaloidal content of fresh fruit as well as two dried extracts and three herbal products. The p-synephrine content of fresh fruit was approximately 0.02%, which increased to about 0.35% in dried fruit. Two dried extracts contained about 3% p-synephrine, while three herbal products had yields of 0.25%, 0.66%, and 0.99%. Dried extracts also contained approximately 0.25% and 0.06% octopamine and tyramine, respectively. Avula et al. [13] reported that 21 *Citrus* species contained p-synephrine in the amounts of from 0.11 to 2.0 mg/g dry weight, indicating that p-synephrine is widely distributed.

The question regarding which synephrine protoalkaloids are present in *C. aurantium* has been addressed in recent years by various investigators [6,10–16], using analytical techniques that have enabled them to separate and identify the possible isomers of synephrine as well as other protoalkaloids. p-Synephrine (*para*-hydroxy) can be separated and differentiated from m-synephrine (*meta*-hydroxy), which is also known as phenylephrine. The m-synephrine (phenylephrine) is available as an over-the-counter nasal decongestant and an ophthalmic product for mydriasis [18].

The primary pharmacologically active protoalkaloid in bitter orange is p-synephrine [6,10–16]. It is the only form found in bitter orange products (e.g., the patented bitter orange extract Advantra Z [Nutratech, Inc., West Caldwell, NJ]). When m-synephrine has been reported in weight loss products [19], it is believed to be due to addition of the synthetic ingredient [17,19]. m-Synephrine is not a constituent of nor has it been identified in standardized bitter orange reference materials prepared by the National Institute of Standards and Technology [20]. Contrary to some commentaries, misinformation, and/or a lack of understanding of the differences between m-synephrine and p-synephrine [21–26], m-synephrine is not naturally present in bitter orange extracts nor does it exhibit the same pharmacological properties. To further complicate the picture, m-synephrine (phenylephrine) has been assessed as a potential ingredient in a weight loss product [27].

In addition to p-synephrine, *C. aurantium* contains a family of related phenylethylamines including N-methyltyramine, tyramine, hordenine, and octopamine. For example, a bitter orange product (Advantra Z™) used in a clinical trial by Gougeon et al. [28] was reported to contain 26 mg synephrine, 4 mg octopamine, and 3.5 mg N-methyltyramine and hordenine in each capsule. Unfortunately, the entire alkaloidal profile of extracts is usually not determined (see, e.g., Refs. [9,11,21,29–33]). As long as the chemical composition of any given dietary supplement containing a bitter orange extract is not known, it is difficult to make informed comparisons between different research studies, and it is equally difficult to make generalized statements regarding the safety and efficacy of products containing a bitter orange extract. Furthermore, since bitter orange extract and p-synephrine are routinely combined with other ingredients resulting in poly-herbal and poly-alkaloidal products, cause and effect relationships of specific ingredients as well as combinations of ingredients cannot be easily determined.

MECHANISTIC STUDIES

The question regarding which isomer is present in bitter orange is relevant to the effects and side effects of any given product. Both *meta* and *para* isomers of synephrine are phenylethanolamine derivatives. However, as noted earlier, only the *p*-synephrine occurs in bitter orange, and the *m*-synephrine has never been shown to occur in nature. The *p*-isomer is believed to be a β3-adrenergic receptor agonist responsible for inducing a thermogenic and lipolytic response [14,34–38]. *m*-Synephrine (phenylephrine) is believed to exert more α-receptor activity as well as some β1- and β2-receptor activity, resulting in pressor as well as heart rate effects. Jordan et al. [39] have shown that *m*-synephrine is 100-fold and *p*-synephrine 40,000-fold less potent than norepinephrine with respect to binding to β1- and β2-adrenoreceptors in guinea pig atria and trachea. These binding studies provide clear evidence why the *meta* and *para* isomers of synephrine do not have equivalent or similar actions and why *m*-synephrine has much more profound effects than *p*-synephrine on the cardiovascular system.

p-Synephrine is approximately 50-fold less potent than *m*-synephrine in activating human α1a-adrenoreceptors and has even lower binding affinity for human α2a- and α2c-adrenoreceptor subtypes [40]. All of these α-receptor subtypes are involved in local and systemic vasoconstriction, and stimulation results in increased blood pressure. Brown et al. [41] compared the receptor-binding activities of the *meta* and *para* isomers of synephrine as well as octopamine to rat aorta α1-adrenoreceptors and rabbit saphenous vein α2-adrenoreceptors. The binding of *m*-synephrine was sixfold less than norepinephrine to α1-adrenoreceptors and 150-fold less to α2-adrenoreceptors. Moreover, *p*-synephrine was 1000-fold less active than norepinephrine in binding to α1- and α2-adrenoreceptors.

Hwa and Perez [42] examined the structural features necessary for binding to and activation of the α1a-adrenoreceptor. They concluded that it is the *meta*-hydroxy of endogenous agonists as *m*-synephrine (phenylephrine) that hydrogen bonds to a serine moiety at the receptor site and not the *para*-hydroxy that results in receptor activation. Thus, *m*-synephrine will bind to and activate the receptor resulting in vasoconstriction and an increase in blood pressure, while *p*-synephrine would have little or no effect. As a consequence, *p*-synephrine would be expected to have little effect on blood pressure relative to *m*-synephrine or norepinephrine.

Hibino et al. [43] examined the ability of *p*-synephrine to constrict isolated rat aorta at concentrations of 1×10^{-7} to 3×10^{-5} mol/L. Using various receptor antagonists, the authors concluded that the constrictor effects were exerted via α1-adrenoreceptors and serotonergic (5-HT$_{1D}$ and 5-HT$_{2A}$) receptors. How these results relate to the oral consumption of bitter orange and *p*-synephrine is not clear. The concentrations of *p*-synephrine used to produce aortic constriction were approximately 8–2500 times the peak blood levels (2 ng/mL) observed when 46.9 mg *p*-synephrine was given to human subjects that did not produce an increase in either systolic or diastolic blood pressures [44]. These results suggest that *p*-synephrine may produce vasoconstriction but only at concentrations many times above the blood levels achieved under normal conditions of oral usage for weight management and sports enhancement.

Tsujita and Takaku [14] have shown that a *p*-synephrine-rich segment wall extract from a mandarin orange induced lipolysis in rat fat cells in a concentration-dependent manner. A juice sac extract did not induce lipolysis. Furthermore, the nonselective β-antagonist propranolol completely inhibited lipolysis, whereas the α-antagonist phenoxybenzamine had no effect, providing mechanistic insight into the potential weight management effects of *p*-synephrine-containing products. The authors suggested that the segment wall of mandarin orange may be a useful functional food as a fat reduction material.

As previously noted [14,34–38], *p*-synephrine may exert its thermogenic and weight management effects primarily by acting as a β3-adrenoreceptor agonist. Activation of β3-adrenoreceptors has been shown to reduce food intake and weight gain in rats as well as enhance lipolysis in adipose tissue, while improving insulin resistance, glycemic control, and lipid profiles [38]. Other studies have shown that β3-adrenoreceptors endogenously exist in adipose tissues and increase lipolysis and lipid metabolism [36,37]. Of interest is the fact that β3-adrenoreceptors have been identified in cardio-vascular tissues [45], and evidence suggests that their activation acts as a "brake" in sympathetic overstimulation through regulation of nitric oxide [46]. Thus, one can postulate that stimulation of β3-adrenoreceptors by p-synephrine in the cardiovascular system would not result in an increase in blood pressure or heart rate but in fact may have a protective effect. Furthermore, this receptor response may explain why an increase in heart rate or blood pressure is generally not seen when caffeine is combined with p-synephrine or bitter orange extract (see Clinical Studies), in spite of the fact that caffeine alone is well known to produce an increase in these parameters.

Chemically, although ephedrine is structurally related to p-synephrine, it differs in that it is a phenylpropanolamine derivative rather than a phenylethanolamine, and ephedrine does not contain a *para*-substituted hydroxy group. These chemical differences greatly alter pharmacokinetic properties, particularly the transport across the blood-brain barrier. The *para*-hydroxy group of synephrine can predictably decrease lipophilicity and therefore transport into the CNS [34,35,47]. As a consequence, p-synephrine does not exert the CNS effects observed with ephedrine. However, p-synephrine may act locally on the cardiovascular system.

Arbo et al. [48] examined the antiestrogenic effects of p-synephrine and ephedrine involving a uterotrophic assay in immature female rats at doses of 50 and 5 mg/kg/day, respectively, for 3 consecutive days. Only ephedrine presented a significant antiestrogenic effect. However, all compounds tested exhibited a decrease in relative adrenal mass, which the authors suggest may be due to an effect on the α1-adrenoreceptor.

REVIEW ARTICLES

Preuss et al. [49] reviewed the effects of *C. aurantium* as a thermogenic, weight reduction replacement for ephedra. Based on the literature available at that time, these authors concluded that *C. aurantium* might be a possible thermogenic substitute for ephedra. They also concluded that more studies and widespread use of this natural product would reveal the efficacy and relative safety of *C. aurantium* compared to ephedra, which has indeed occurred.

A review of *C. aurantium* as an ingredient in dietary supplements marketed for weight loss was published by Fugh-Berman and Myers [50]. This study is frequently cited as evidence for the lack of safety of bitter orange extracts and their use in dietary supplements associated with weight management. Much of the evidence cited for the lack of safety related to increased blood pressure by p-synephrine is the result of intravenous administration and not oral consumption of extracts containing p-synephrine.

These authors concluded that although no adverse events have been reported in conjunction with ingestion of *C. aurantium* products orally to date, products containing synephrine have the potential to increase cardiovascular events in humans, disregarding the route of administration. These investigators further concluded that there is little evidence supporting the use of *C. aurantium*–containing products as effective aids to weight loss and weight management [50]. It must be concluded that the warning about safety is hypothetical and not based on scientific evidence or actual data involving oral product use.

The safety and efficacy of *C. aurantium* for weight loss was also reviewed by Bent et al. [21]. These authors identified 157 titles of articles referring to *C. aurantium* (bitter orange), of which seven were randomized controlled trials. Six studies were excluded because the products also contained ephedrine. Only one study satisfied all of the inclusion criteria and was a 6 week, randomized, placebo-controlled trial reported by Colker et al. [51]. This study will be described in greater detail under clinical studies. Although a small but significant weight loss was reported [51], Bent et al. [21] concluded that a systematic review failed to produce evidence that *C. aurantium* was effective for weight loss. These authors also concluded that safety information was extremely limited, and since *C. aurantium* contains synephrine, the use of the herb may pose risks of adverse cardiovascular events. No evidence to support this contention was presented other than an inappropriate reference to m-synephrine.

One of the most comprehensive scientific literature reviews relating to bitter orange was prepared by the National Toxicology Program (NTP) of the National Institute of Environmental Health Sciences which is an institute of the National Institutes of Health [52]. The report was intended as background information and makes no conclusions regarding the safety or efficacy of bitter orange. With respect to the discussion on structure-activity relationships, it does state that it focuses on the *para* isomers of synephrine and octopamine as the biogenic amines found in citrus peel.

Haaz et al. [53] published a review of bitter orange and *p*-synephrine in the treatment of overweight and obesity. These authors concluded that while some promising evidence for the use of bitter orange extract exists, larger and more rigorous clinical trials are required in order to draw appropriate conclusions regarding both the safety and efficacy of bitter orange and *p*-synephrine for weight loss.

Stohs and Shara [54] wrote an extensive review of the safety and efficacy of *C. aurantium* in weight management in the previous edition of this *Obesity* book. The authors concluded that based on currently published and unpublished information at that time, bitter orange extract and *p*-synephrine appear to be exceedingly safe. Although some studies supported the efficacy with respect to weight loss and weight management, further long-term studies in both animals and human subjects were necessary. The current review provides an update from the previous review and includes much additional information that has been published or is in press during the intervening years regarding the safety and efficacy of bitter orange and *p*-synephrine.

In a subsequent review of bitter orange, Haaz et al. [55] note that *m*-synephrine (phenylephrine) is not contained naturally in *C. aurantium*, but these authors then included it in a grouping called "synephrine alkaloids," purportedly due to similar properties with *p*-synephrine and *p*-octopamine. Furthermore, discussions regarding cardiovascular as well as metabolic effects of "synephrine alkaloids" involve a number of studies with *m*-synephrine and not with *p*-synephrine or bitter orange extract. As a consequence, the article does not provide clarification of issues surrounding *p*-synephrine and bitter orange extract.

Rossato et al. [56] reviewed the history and use of *C. aurantium* extract and focused on synephrine and its purported cardiovascular effects, suggesting that oxidative stress was involved. As will be discussed later, several studies have demonstrated that both *p*-synephrine and extracts of bitter orange possess antioxidant and anti-inflammatory properties. These authors also indicated that the presence of *m*-synephrine in *C. aurantium* was controversial when, as previously noted, the data clearly indicate that *m*-synephrine does not occur naturally [6,10–16,20]. As with the review by Haaz et al. [53], the information omits many important studies and does not add clarity to the issue of the safety of *p*-synephrine when used in orally ingested dietary supplements.

Finally, two extensive reviews on the safety of bitter orange and *p*-synephrine have been published by Stohs and Preuss [57] and Stohs et al. [58]. Both reviews concluded that based on the ingestion of bitter orange and *p*-synephrine in the form of dietary supplements as well as juices, fruits, and other *Citrus*-derived food products, these ingredients appear to be exceedingly safe with no serious adverse effects being directly attributable to them.

ANIMAL STUDIES

Relatively few studies have been conducted concerning the efficacy and safety of bitter orange extracts in animals. The most definitive study on the safety of *p*-synephrine and bitter orange was recently conducted by Hansen et al. in association with the U.S. Food and Drug Association (FDA) [59]. The study demonstrated that at doses of up to 100 mg *p*-synephrine/kg body weight, no developmental toxicity was produced in Sprague-Dawley rats. The rats were dosed by gavage with *p*-synephrine or bitter orange, and in some cases also with caffeine, and sacrificed on gestation day 21. No adverse effects were observed with respect to fetal weight, embryolethality, or incidence of gross, visceral, or skeletal abnormalities. Maternal body weight decreased when rats were given 50 mg *p*-synephrine/kg with 25 mg caffeine/kg per day. The results clearly demonstrate the lack of toxicity and the high degree of safety of bitter orange extract and p-synephrine. This study is the benchmark study with respect to the safety of bitter orange and p-synephrine.

One of the most widely cited studies is the work of Calapai et al. [29] who examined the effects of repeatedly administering orally 2.5–20 mg/kg of two *C. aurantium* fruit extracts that had been standardized to 4% and 6% p-synephrine. The effects of these extracts on food intake, body weight gain, arterial blood pressure, electrocardiogram (ECG), and mortality in male rats were examined. Animals were treated for 7 consecutive days, and the various measurements were recorded for 15 consecutive days. Significant dose-dependent decreases in food intake as well as body weight were observed. No significant changes were observed in blood pressure, while the alterations in ECG were significant after 10 days of treatment. Some deaths were noted in the treated animals, although the difference was not statistically significant. Unfortunately, the chemical composition of the bitter orange extract was not reported other than the p-synephrine content. Some of these results must be questioned in light of the previously discussed study of Hansen et al. [59].

Parra et al. [60] have examined the LD_{50} of various plant extracts including *C. aurantium* in mice. Of interest was the observation that their calculated LD_{50} for a bitter orange extract was approximately 477 mg/kg in mice as compared to a maximum of 140 mg/kg in rats in the study of Calapai et al. [29]. Differences in the methods of preparing the respective extracts may have contributed to the discrepancies. The concentration of p-synephrine or other alkaloids was not reported by Parra et al. [60].

The toxicity of a 6% p-synephrine-containing bitter orange extract (Advantra Z®) was evaluated in both male and female Sprague-Dawley rats. The animals received a single oral dose of 10,000 mg/kg body weight of the bitter orange extract [61]. All animals were sacrificed at the end of 14 days. No animals died and no gross pathological findings were observed. The acute oral LD_{50} of the product was estimated to be greater than 10,000 mg/kg in these rats. This equates to an LD_{50} of greater than 600 mg p-synephrine/kg body weight in these animals. The reasons for the large differences in the results of the studies mentioned earlier are not clear. Toxicities associated with the products used by Parra et al. [60] and Calapai et al. [29] may have been due to constituents in the extracts other than p-synephrine.

In an earlier study, Huang et al. [62] investigated the effects of a bitter orange extract on portal hypertensive rats. *In vitro* contractile studies as well as hemodynamic effects were performed after partial portal vein ligation. The bitter orange extract was infused into the femoral vein. p-Synephrine at up to 0.38 mg/kg/min was similarly infused. The results demonstrated a dose-dependent decrease in portal venous pressure and heart rate with a dose-dependent increase in mean arterial pressure. Most notable is the fact that the extract and p-synephrine were administered intravenously as opposed to orally and at very high doses. As a consequence, it is difficult to meaningfully extrapolate the data obtained to the typical situation whereby bitter orange extract is used orally in dietary supplements for appetite control and weight management. The concentrations of p-synephrine and related alkaloids used in dietary supplements would not be expected to achieve the blood levels produced following intravenous administration. Unfortunately, this study is frequently cited out of context as evidence for the cardiovascular toxicity of bitter orange extract in orally used preparations.

Titta et al. [63] have conducted an interesting study on inhibition of fat accumulation in mice given juice from either a blood orange (which contains high levels of anthocyanins) or a blond orange. Dietary supplementation with juice from the blood orange but not the blond orange significantly reduced body weight gain and fat accumulation. The antiobesity effect of the blood orange juice could not be explained solely on the basis of the anthocyanin content, and the authors surmised that the anthocyanins may synergize with p-synephrine to produce the observed effect. Unfortunately, this hypothesis was not specifically tested.

Several recent studies have demonstrated that p-synephrine and bitter orange extract can exert antioxidant, anti-inflammatory, and tissue-protective properties. Arbo et al. [64] treated mice daily with bitter orange extract (7.5% p-synephrine) at doses of 400, 2000, or 4000 mg/kg (corresponding to 30, 150, and 300 mg p-synephrine/kg) or 30 or 300 mg p-synephrine/kg. A reduction in body weight gain was observed at all doses relative to controls. No effects were observed on organ weights or biochemical and hematological parameters in the treated mice. However, both doses of *p*-synephrine and the high dose of the bitter orange extract resulted in increases in hepatic-reduced glutathione, while bitter orange extract decreased malondialdehyde content (indicator of lipid peroxidation and lipid damage) levels and *p*-synephrine increased catalase activity by as much as sixfold. High doses of both products produced modest deceases in glutathione peroxidase activity. Taken together, the results demonstrate a beneficial effect with respect to weight loss without adverse effects, while also providing an antioxidant and tissue-protective effect based on the increased glutathione levels and no effect on lipid peroxidation. It should be noted that the doses used were very high compared to a typical human dose. It is not clear why the authors concluded that they were seeing subchronic toxicity when they were observing beneficial effects in terms of weight loss and protection from oxidative stress without cardiac, hepatic, or kidney toxicity.

Tounsi et al. [65] have shown that *C. aurantium* exhibits higher antioxidant activity than other *Citrus* species. Furthermore, a methanolic extract of *C. aurantium* has been shown to have anti-inflammatory properties in a mouse macrophage cell line by modulating the expression of cyclo-oxygenase-2 (COX-2), inducible nitric oxide synthase (iNOS), and proinflammatory cytokines such as tumor necrosis factor-α (TNF-α) and interleukin-6 (IL-6) via the NF-κB pathway [66]. Since inflammation and oxidative tissue damage are associated with obesity, these studies suggest another mechanism for potential beneficial effects of *p*-synephrine and bitter orange extract in weight management and strenuous physical activity.

Several other studies have examined the properties of preparations from *C. aurantium*. Carvalho-Freitas and Costa [4] demonstrated a sedative effect of an essential oil product from peel and a hydroethanolic (70% w/v) extract from leaves. No toxicological studies were conducted, and the product was not known to contain phenylethylamine alkaloids. Hosseinimehr et al. [67] demonstrated that a hydroethanolic extract of the dried peels of ripe fruit provided a radioprotective effect against gamma radiation in mice. The citrus extract was given by intraperitoneal injection at doses up to 1000 mg/kg body weight. No toxicological studies were reported, and the studies were not repeated following oral administration. The authors concluded that flavonoids were responsible for the radioprotective effects, although no chemical analysis data were reported.

Another interesting study not related to weight management involves the effects of an orange peel extract in ameliorating adjuvant arthritis in rats [68]. Arthritis was induced with Freund's complete adjuvant. An orange peel extract inhibited adjuvant arthritis while decreasing production of the inflammatory mediators TNF-α, interleukin-1β (IL-1β), prostaglandin E$_2$, and COX-2. This study again suggests the involvement of constituents in orange peel as antioxidants and anti-inflammatory agents, similar to the results of Tounsi et al. [65].

In general, a limited number of well-defined and definitive studies have been conducted in animals on the safety of *C. aurantium* extracts as related to weight management and thermogenesis. However, the studies do demonstrate that bitter orange extracts can produce weight loss and decrease weight gain with little or no toxicity when given orally at appropriate doses. Furthermore, several studies involving very high doses of bitter orange extract or *p*-synephrine did not produce adverse cardiovascular or developmental toxicological effects when given orally.

CLINICAL STUDIES

As is the case with animal studies, relatively few well-designed, controlled studies have been conducted with bitter orange extracts assessing efficacy and safety. Most studies have been conducted using products that contain not only an extract of *C. aurantium* but also other ingredients such as caffeine, ephedrine, green tea, ginkgo, ginseng, guarana, and St. John's wort. The fact that bitter orange extract is almost invariably incorporated into products containing other potentially active ingredients makes comparative analyses exceedingly difficult. Comparatively few safety and efficacy studies have been conducted on bitter orange extract or *p*-synephrine alone.

Since bitter orange extract is generally incorporated with other ingredients, it is appropriate to conduct studies on these combinations to assess not only their efficacy but also the safety of these diverse preparations. One of the earliest studies to be conducted on the effects of a bitter orange extract–containing product on body fat loss, lipid levels, and mood in overweight adult subjects was conducted by Colker et al. [51]. The product used in this study contained 975 mg *C. aurantium* extract (6% synephrine alkaloids), 528 mg caffeine, and 900 mg St. John's wort on a daily basis. The total daily intake of phenylethylamine-related alkaloids was approximately 58.5 mg. Twenty subjects completed the study. The subjects followed a 1800 kcal/day American Heart Association Step One diet and performed a 3 day/week circuit training exercise program.

After following the protocol for 6 weeks, the treated group lost a small but significant amount of body weight (1.4 kg) and a significant amount of body fat (2.9%). No significant changes in blood pressure, heart rate, electrocardiographic findings, serum chemistry, or urinalysis were noted; and no significant changes were noted in the results of the Profile of Mood States questionnaire for fatigue or vigor. The treated group also experienced a significant increase in basal metabolic rate as compared to the placebo rate, which experienced a significant decrease in this indicator [51].

Several observations can be made regarding this study. St. John's wort (*Hypericum perforatum*) is an antidepressant, and depression is associated with overeating and obesity. However, no change in mood was noted in the study. The amount of caffeine consumed daily in conjunction with the product (528 mg) is equivalent to approximately four cups of coffee and is a well-known thermogenic agent [69]. Whether the weight loss and increase in basal metabolic rate was due to the caffeine, the bitter orange extract, or a combination thereof is not clear. However, the net result is that a small but significant loss in body weight as well as body fat was observed. The authors concluded that this combination of ingredients was effective and safe when used in combination with exercise and mild caloric restriction for promoting fat and body weight loss in healthy, overweight adults.

Kendall-Reed [31] conducted a 10 week study on a system (Ultra Slim Down®) that consisted of two products. One product contained 125 mg hydroxycitric acid (Citrimax™), 125 mg bitter orange extract (Advantra Z™), and 50 mg kola nut extract, while the second product contained 344 mg chitosan. Thirty-two overweight subjects were divided into three groups and either given the two products (one capsule of each in conjunction with each meal), a diet and exercise program, or the products in conjunction with the diet and exercise program. At the end of 10 weeks, the product-only group lost an average of 10.2 lb, the diet and exercise group lost 7.6 lb, and the product plus diet and exercise group lost 14.5 lb. Consumption of the products was more effective than diet and exercise, while the products in combination with diet and exercise were most effective. No adverse side effects were observed or reported.

Kalman et al. [30] reported the results of a 14 day clinical trial using a commercial weight loss product (Xenadrine EFX™) involving 16 overweight/obese healthy subjects in combination with exercise. The product contained a proprietary blend of extracts from *C. aurantium*, yerba mate, grape seed, green tea, and ginger root in conjunction with several vitamins and amino acids. Subjects ingested 6 mg *p*-synephrine, 150 mg caffeine, and 150 mg catechin polyphenols daily. Over the 14 days of the study, no significant effects of the product were noted as compared to the placebo group with respect to blood pressure, heart rate, ECG data, fasting blood glucose, renal function, hepatic function, or complete blood count with differentials. Sleep quality was negatively impacted in the treated group, while this same group experienced a significant reduction in fatigue levels. The treated group experienced a reduction in diastolic blood pressure as compared to the placebo group (−8.0 vs. ± 4.2 mmHg) by the end of the study.

No serious adverse events were reported. Minor effects including headache, sleep disturbance, dry mouth, and "spotting" were reported amount participants of the treated group, while headache, nervousness, and increased sweating were reported by participants of the placebo group. The authors concluded that the product was safe over the course of the study [30]. It should be noted that no weight loss was observed. The study suffers from its short duration and small number of subjects. The lack of physiological effects or loss of weight may have been due to the relatively low doses of the ingredients used in this study.

Sale et al. [70] conducted a study on the metabolic and physiological effects of Xenadrine EFX™ in overweight individuals at rest and during treadmill walking. As noted earlier, this product contained bitter orange, guarana, and green tea extracts. The study was double blinded. Subjects were given the product or placebo and either followed for 7 h or exercised on a treadmill for 60 min. The product had no effect on ATP utilization under resting or exercise conditions relative to control. However, a 30% increase in carbohydrate oxidation was observed. Fatty acid oxidation to ATP decreased, while plasma levels of fatty acids increased in response to the product. The product had no effect on resting heart rate or blood pressure.

Zenk et al. [32] conducted a randomized, double-blind study to evaluate the effect of a proprietary weight management product (Lean Source™) on body composition of overweight men and women. Of the 65 adults enrolled, 54 completed the 8 week study. In addition to bitter orange extract, the product contained extracts of guarana and green tea in conjunction with 7-oxo-dehydroandrostene-dione (DHEA), conjugated linoleic acid, and chromium picolinate. The daily consumption of bitter orange extract was 200 mg. The amount of p-synephrine was not stated.

At the completion of the study, the treated group lost an average of 2.9 kg body weight compared to a 1.5 kg body weight loss by the placebo group. The weight loss experienced by the treated group was not large considering the time frame involved and the fact that the subjects were overweight. No significant differences were noted between the treatment and the placebo groups with respect to systolic and diastolic blood pressures, heart rate, or temperature. Furthermore, there were no significant differences in chemistry profiles and complete blood counts between the two groups. There was also no difference in the reported incidence of adverse events between the two groups, and no serious adverse events were reported. Constipation and back pain were the most prominent adverse events reported among the treated group, while nausea, headache, and peripheral neuropathy were reported by individuals on the placebo [32].

Several conclusions can be drawn. The complex product appeared to be safe when taken as directed. A small but significant amount of weight loss occurred using the product. As with other studies involving complex products, it not possible to determine the contribution of *C. aurantium* to the weight loss, and the net effect may be due to the combination of ingredients.

A study involving the use of another commercial weight loss product (Lean System 7™) on various parameters was assessed by Zenk et al. [33]. The study was a randomized, double-blind, placebo-controlled study involving 47 healthy, overweight adults. A total of 35 subjects completed the 8 week study. Each adult received three capsules of the weight loss product twice daily or an identical placebo in conjunction with a calorie-restricted diet and an exercise program. The product contained 6 mg p-synephrine/capsule (36 mg/day). The product also contained 3-acetyl-7-oxo-dehydroepiandrosterone (17 mg), *Coleus forskohlii* extract (50 mg extract, 10 mg forskolin), yerba mate extract (167 mg), guarana extract (233 mg extract, 51 mg caffeine), piperine (1.67 mg from *Piper nigrum*), and dandelion leaf and root powder (83 mg). The most significant finding of the study was a 7.2% increase in resting metabolic rate in the treated subjects. However, no significant differences were noted between the treated and the placebo-controlled groups with respect to body weight, body fat, or lean tissue [33]. No changes in heart rate or blood pressure were observed and no serious adverse events were reported. In general, the product was well tolerated over the 8 weeks of the study.

The thermic effect of food in conjunction with the phenylethylamine protoalkaloids extracted from *C. aurantium* was investigated in healthy weight-stable male and female subjects [28]. The thermic effect of food on a 1.7 MJ, 30 g protein meal was determined intermittently for 300 min by indirect calorimetry. The *C. aurantium* extract was provided in capsule form. Five capsules provided 26 mg p-synephrine and 4 mg or less each of octopamine, N-methyltyramine, tyramine, and hordenine (Advantra Z™). The thermic effect of food was determined on an initial 30 subjects.

A subset of 11 men and 11 women were studied a second time after ingestion of the bitter orange extract in conjunction with the protein meal, while a subset of 12 women and 8 men were studied a third time following ingestion of the *C. aurantium*–containing capsules alone.

The study demonstrated that the thermic effect of food was 20% lower in women than men following a meal. When the bitter orange extract was used in conjunction with the protein meal, an increase in the thermic effect on food was seen only in women, increasing by 29%. The thermic effect of the bitter orange extract was greater in men than women in the absence of a meal. A significant increase in the respiratory quotient occurred in both sexes in response to the bitter orange extract alone. Following exposure to the bitter orange extract, no significant changes occurred in pulse rates or systolic and diastolic blood pressures when compared with base line values.

The thermogenic effect of a coffee enriched with *C. aurantium* extract, *Garcinia cambogia*, and chromium (JavaFit™) was examined by Hoffman et al. [71] over a 3 h period of time in a randomized, double-blind fashion. Significant increases were observed in responders with respect to resting metabolic rate and respiratory exchange ratio. No significant differences were observed in average heart rate or diastolic blood pressure while a 3 mmHg increase was observed for the systolic blood pressure. The consumed product contained 450 mg caffeine, 21.6 mg *p*-synephrine, 600 mg hydroxycitric acid, and 225 mcg chromium polynicotinate. The lack of effect on heart rate and the modest effect on blood pressure are surprising in light of the amount of caffeine in the product.

Seifert et al. [72] conducted a study on the effects of an herbal blend on energy expenditure in mildly obese subjects. The product contained 13 mg *p*-synephrine (as Advantra Z™), 176 mg caffeine (as guarana), and 55.5 mg of a green tea extract per capsule. The study involved 14 females and 9 males in a placebo-controlled, crossover design. Subjects ingested one capsule with each of three meals on treatment day 1, and one more capsule on the morning of the day 2. Data were collected 60 min after the last administration of the product. The results demonstrated that from pretest on day 1 to posttest on day 2, caloric expenditure increased by 8% following ingestion of the product. Oxygen uptake increased from 230 to 250 mL/min following treatment. No differences were observed following treatment regarding heart rate or blood pressure. The study was an acute study and did not provide information on long-term usage.

Stohs et al. [73] examined the effect of 50 mg *p*-synephrine (Advantra Z™: 60% *p*-synephrine) in 20 human subjects on resting metabolic rate. The study was a randomized, placebo-controlled, double-blind design with the vehicle for the *p*-synephrine being 1 oz of tomato juice. Measurements were taken at baseline prior to consuming the product and at 75 min. At 75 min, a 6.9% increase in resting metabolic rate was observed in response to the *p*-synephrine. No significant effects were noted with respect to heart rate or blood pressure nor were there any significant differences in responses to a 10-item self-report questionnaire which addressed such issues as hunger, energy, nervousness, tension, headache, general discomfort, anxiety, and sleepiness. These results support the previous thermic studies of Gougeon et al. [28] and the caloric expenditure studies of Seifert et al. [72], indicating that *p*-synephrine increases the metabolic rate and may therefore be beneficial with respect to weight management.

Shara et al. [74] conducted a randomized, placebo-controlled, double-blind crossover study involving 16 healthy subjects who consumed a capsule containing 50 mg *p*-synephrine (Advantra Z™) or the placebo daily for 14 days. Over 90% of the protoalkaloidal content of this extract was composed of *p*-synephrine. Baseline ECGs, blood pressures, and heart rates were determined. After the initial dosing, ECGs, blood pressures, and heart rates were determined at 30 min, 60 min, 90 min, 2h, 4h, 6h, and 8h, as well as after 1 and 2 weeks. Blood samples were drawn after 2h after the first dose as well as at 1 and 2 weeks to measure *p*-synephrine levels. A preliminary examination of the data demonstrated that at this dosage level *p*-synephrine had no significant effect on heart rate or blood pressure and caused no cardiovascular abnormalities. This is the first study to investigate cardiovascular effects following oral ingestion of a product containing only bitter orange extract (*p*-synephrine) for longer than a single day and after more than a single dose.

CASE REPORTS

Stohs [75] has reviewed and assessed the 22 FDA adverse event reports (AERs) from April 2004 through October 2009 associated with bitter orange–containing products, as well as 10 clinical case reports published during this time frame regarding the possible involvement of *C. aurantium*–containing weight management products with cardiovascular incidents and other adverse events. Bitter orange extract and/or *p*-synephrine were implicated as the possible causative agent in each case by the authors. In all AERs and cases, the products involved were poly-herbal and poly-alkaloidal.

Adverse events that have been reported in conjunction with the published clinical case reports included acute lateral-wall myocardial infarction [76], exercise-induced syncope associated with QT prolongation [23], ischemic stroke [77], ischemic colitis [78], variant angina [79], coronary vasospasm and thrombosis [25], exercise-induced rhabdomyolysis [80], vasospasm and stroke [81], ST segment myocardial infarction [82], and ventricular fibrillation [26]. In one case report, it was suggested that a bitter orange–containing dietary supplement may have masked bradycardia and hypotension while exacerbating weight loss in an individual with anorexia nervosa [83], although no evidence was provided that an adverse event actually occurred.

Although the products consumed were multi-ingredient, in each case, reference was specifically made to *C. aurantium*, bitter orange, or *p*-synephrine as the most likely causative agent. Unfortunately, a wide range of confounding factors existed among the published case reports including a history of smoking, physical inactivity, obesity, heart murmur, preexisting heart disease, sickle cell trait, dehydration, pneumonia, possible use of anabolic steroids and/or performance enhancing drugs, hypertriglyceridemia, gastroesophageal disease, high caffeine intake, and high alcohol consumption. Products were not always being taken as recommended, and it was not always clear if the subjects were using other unreported dietary supplements and/or drugs. A more probable culprit for these effects may have been the high caffeine intake associated with the products in question. Finally, the possibility exists that the consumption of the product and the adverse event were concurrent but unrelated since millions of individuals use *p*-synephrine and bitter orange-containing dietary supplements and food products on a daily basis while millions of cardiovascular events occur annually.

Therefore, although these case reports should raise the level of consciousness and awareness with regard to the use of complex weight management products, it is not possible to extrapolate the cause of these adverse effects to the *p*-synephrine which may have been present in the products. No evidence showing a direct link between bitter orange extract and the adverse events is provided [75]. Karch [84] has noted that "case reports are incomplete, uncontrolled, retrospective, lack operational criteria for identifying when an adverse event has actually occurred, and resemble nothing so much as hearsay evidence, a type of evidence that is prohibited in all courts of industrialized societies." Several examples of these case reports are presented in the following text with a discussion of inherent issues and questions.

Nykamp et al. [76] reported what they believed to be a possible incidence of myocardial infarction associated with the use of a *C. aurantium*–containing dietary supplement in a patient with previously undetected coronary vascular disease. The product in question contained 200 mg of a bitter orange extract (protoalkaloidal content unknown), an herbal diuretic complex, extracts of guarana and green tea, 250 mg carnitine, 400 µg chromium, and 300 mg of an extract containing hydroxycitric acid.

The authors indicated that the use of *C. aurantium*–containing supplements may pose a risk for cardiovascular toxicity and concluded that the *C. aurantium* "is probably associated with this cardiovascular event." It is truly difficult to determine how this conclusion could be reached in light of the numerous confounding factors present, including preexisting heart disease (undetected), a 37 year history of smoking one and one-half packs of cigarettes per day, overweight, and high caffeine intake. Furthermore, the product in question contained a relatively low (200 mg) amount of *C. aurantium* extract, and if one assumes the synephrine content was as high as 6%, the daily ingestion of this alkaloid would amount to only 12 mg/day. Up to five times this amount of total alkaloids daily has been shown to be without adverse events in healthy adults over a 6 week period of time [51]. The combination of all the confounding factors including the use of this weight management product may have led to the myocardial infarction. However, it is not scientifically or physiologically plausible to assume that the single initiating ingredient or factor was the *C. aurantium* extract.

A case of ischemic stroke associated with the use of a dietary supplement containing synephrine was reported by Bouchard et al. [77]. According to the manufacturer, each capsule contained 6 mg synephrine and 200 mg caffeine alkaloids (kola nut extract). The patient reported having taken one or two capsules per day of the product for 1 week. The individual presented to the emergency room with recent onset of unsteady gait, dizziness, memory loss, and difficulty in concentrating. He had no family history of arteriosclerotic disease. The subject was mildly obese with a moderate history of cigarette smoking.

The authors concluded that the diagnosis could be consistent with stroke of vascular origin based primarily on the patient's symptoms and the coincident ingestion of the synephrine and caffeine-containing weight loss product. However, this conclusion was not supported by laboratory analyses. A magnetic resonance angiography of cervical arteries showed normal course and caliber of all vessels. Transthoracic and transesophageal echocardiography and carotid artery Doppler ultrasonography demonstrated no abnormalities. Furthermore, erythrocyte sedimentation rate, hemoglobin A_1c levels, serum lipid profiles, serum homocysteine, thrombin time and fibrinogen, protein C, protein S, factor II, factor VIII, and factor V were all normal. In addition, no commonly abused drugs were detected in the urine [77]. As a consequence, it is difficult to conclude that the symptoms were related to the *p*-synephrine ingestion at a level of not more than 12 mg/day. The authors did not appear to consider the possibilities that the symptoms might have been related to the ingestion of the kola nut extract or a combination of ingredients, the use of a much higher dose of the product than reported, or other unknown cause.

A case report involving Xenadrine EFX™ was presented by Nasir et al. [23]. Exercise-induced syncope occurred in a healthy 22 year old woman an hour after taking a dose of the weight management product. Electrocardiography indicated a prolongation of the QT interval, which resolved within 24 h. Results of an exercise stress test and an echocardiography were normal, and a 9 month follow-up revealed no arrhythmias.

The cause for the syncope is most probably due to multiple factors. The individual had not run for over 1 month prior to the incident. She also had not used the product regularly for the past month and had taken one dose the previous evening and reported taking one tablet approximately 45 min before running 3 miles. She had not eaten that day prior to the run. As a consequence, the combination of consuming a product with neuroactive ingredients, the failure to have eaten prior to running, the lack of regular exercise, the distance run, possible dehydration, and the consumption of the weight management product a short time before running may have all contributed to the observed outcome. The discussion by the authors is confusing in that they point to *C. aurantium* as the hemodynamically most active component. However, the product was reported to contain only 3 mg of synephrine in addition to caffeine and other ingredients. The authors presumed that the synephrine present was the *meta*-hydroxy isomer, when in reality, the *para*-hydroxy isomer was present, which has little or no cardiovascular activity. Other ingredients in the product including L-tyrosine, caffeine, tyramine, and other methylxanthines may have been contributing factors. This case report is a study in how multiple factors can influence a physiological response and how the inappropriate use of a product may contribute to these consequences.

OTHER SAFETY CONSIDERATIONS

The cardiovascular effects of Seville (sour) orange juice in normotensive adults were determined by Penzak et al. [22]. The study was conducted since extracts of this orange (*C. aurantium*) contain phenylethylamines. Synephrine concentrations were approximately 57 µg/mL, while octopamine was not detected. Twelve subjects consumed 8 oz of orange juice (containing approximately 13 mg *p*-synephrine) and water in a crossover design followed by repeat ingestion 8 h later. Hemodynamic parameters including heart rate and blood pressure did not significantly differ between control and treated groups. The authors, however, concluded that individuals with tachyarrhythmias, severe hypertension, and narrow-angle glaucoma, as well as those taking monoamine oxidase inhibitor receptors, should avoid Seville orange juice.

Gurley et al. [85] conducted a study in human subjects who were given a bitter orange extract for 28 days. The authors concluded that a supplement containing *C. aurantium* extract did not appear to significantly modulate cytochrome P450 enzyme activities in human subjects and, therefore, posed minimal risk for cytochrome P450–mediated herb–drug interactions. The bitter orange extract had no significant effect on CYP1A2, CYP2D6, CYP2E1, or CYP3A4, the major drug-metabolizing cytochromes.

A study was conducted by Min et al. [86] to assess the QTc-prolonging and hemodynamic effects of a single dose of a bitter orange extract (Nature's Way) containing 27 mg *p*-synephrine. The study involved 18 subjects and was randomized, placebo controlled, double blind, and crossover in design. The rate-corrected QT (QTc) interval and blood pressure were measured before dosing and at 1, 3, 5, and 8 h after dosing. The bitter orange extract did not significantly alter the QTc interval or the systolic or diastolic blood pressures at any time point.

Haller et al. [44] have examined the cardiovascular changes associated with a single oral dose of a bitter orange extract (Advantra Z™) (46.9 mg *p*-synephrine) and a multiple-component dietary supplement (Xenedrine EFX™) which contained 5.5 mg *p*-synephrine, caffeine, and other ingredients. The protocol consisted of a randomized, double-blind, placebo-controlled crossover study with a 1 week washout between treatments. The results demonstrated that the dietary supplement but not the *p*-synephrine-containing bitter orange extract increased both systolic and diastolic blood pressures at 2 h posttreatment, while heart rate increased at 6 h by 16.7 beats/min with the dietary supplement and 11.4 beats/min with the bitter orange (*p*-synephrine) extract. The authors concluded that the pressure effects were not likely caused by the *C. aurantium* alone since no blood pressure effect was observed with an eightfold higher dose of *p*-synephrine. The authors also concluded that the increase in blood pressure may be attributable to caffeine and other stimulants in the dietary supplement. The increase in heart rate reported for *p*-synephrine at 6 h is not consistent with its pharmacokinetics, having a half-life of about 2 h, and is not supported by a variety of other studies [28,32,33,51,67,70,71,86,87].

Bui et al. [88] conducted a randomized, double-blind, placebo-controlled, crossover study involving 15 healthy subjects who received a single dose of 900 mg bitter orange extract (Nature's Way) standardized to 6% synephrine (54 mg *p*-synephrine) or the placebo. Heart rate and blood pressure were measured every hour for 6 h. These investigators reported small but significant increases in heart rate, and systolic and diastolic blood pressures for up to 5 h. The difference in the results between this study and the study of Min et al. [86] involved the same product and may be related to the dose which was twice as large in this study by Bui et al. [88]. In addition, these effects on heart rate and blood pressure have not been observed in other studies (see, e.g., Refs. [28,33,51,70,73,74]).

Haller et al. [87] examined the effects of a performance-enhancing dietary supplement under resting and exercise conditions involving 10 subjects. The product (Ripped Fuel Extreme Cut™) contained 21 mg *p*-synephrine and 304 mg caffeine, as well as other ingredients including extracts of green tea, ginger root, cocoa seed, willow bark, and wasabi. The product or placebo was taken 1 h prior to 30 min of moderately intense exercise. There were no significant treatment-related differences in systolic blood pressure, heart rate, or body temperature. Significant, product-related (8.7 mmHg) increases in diastolic blood pressure and blood glucose levels were observed. Exercise was perceived as being less strenuous after consumption of the product. Due to the poly-alkaloidal and poly-protoalkaloidal nature of this product, the effects on blood glucose levels and diastolic blood pressure cannot be ascribed to a single ingredient.

The historical and traditional use of extracts of bitter orange in Chinese medicine as well as the fact that more than millions of doses of products containing *C. aurantium* extracts have been used in this country by several million individuals [89] during the past 20 years without the report of serious incidence must be taken into consideration and should aid in putting the safety issue into context. No serious adverse events have been directly attributable to bitter orange or p-synephrine [21,49,50,54,57,58,75,89,90]. Several minor side effects including nausea, headache, jitters, and dizziness have been reported. However, none of these events is considered serious, and these are common complaints and observations associated with numerous and common over-the-counter drugs as well as with placebos.

A major contributor to the concerns regarding the safety of *C. aurantium* extracts has been the federal government. The FDA anonymously supplied information to a leading newspaper indicating that there had been 85 adverse reactions and seven deaths associated with *C. aurantium*. Subsequently, the purported number of AERs increased to 169 [91]. A dissection of the FDA information upon which the AERS were based indicated that no credible adverse events could be attributed directly to *C. aurantium* extracts [87]. A subsequent review by Stohs [75] of the 22 FDA AERs reported between April 2004 and October 2009 has drawn a similar conclusion. Unfortunately, this reality has not prevented scientifically in-astute and politically misguided individuals and news media from making statements regarding *C. aurantium* that are clearly not based on the facts at hand. Furthermore, the McGuffin [90] review and its conclusions are omitted from discussions in case reports and other articles related to bitter orange extracts (see, e.g., Refs. [55,56,92]).

Are there issues with *C. aurantium* extracts? The answer is clearly yes. Standardization of some products is most assuredly an issue. Furthermore, clear and decisive data regarding the efficacy of bitter orange extracts and/or p-synephrine alone with respect to weight management and weight loss as well as safety issues are needed. Nearly all studies have involved inclusion of bitter orange extract in multicomponent products. Finally, as with anything we ingest, *C. aurantium* can be used inappropriately and misused, and there are individuals for whom it may be contraindicated due to existing sensitivities or physiological conditions.

When comparing the current evidence regarding adverse events for *C. aurantium* with widely and commonly used over-the-counter drugs as well as prescription drugs and many food substances, bitter orange extract appears to be remarkably safe. We tend to forget the high incidence of adverse events and deaths associated with such common household products as ibuprofen, acetaminophen, aspirin, and other nonsteroidal anti-inflammatory agents [93–95], not to mention the anti-inflammatory agents as well as other drugs that have been removed from the market for causing thousands of deaths.

We also tend to ignore the very high incidence of adverse events among the prescription drugs used for weight management. For example, the drug orlistat (Xenical; Alli-Roche), which is used for weight reduction, has a very high incidence of adverse events. One-fifth of users of this drug report abdominal pain and/or flatus with discharge, and as many as 15% of patients report nausea and fecal incontinence (Physicians' Desk Reference, 2010). One can spend much time arguing risk–benefit ratios and risk management. However, to date, literally millions of consumers have used and are using bitter orange–containing products in the form of foods and supplements with no adverse effects being reported.

The widespread advice by federal agencies, politicians, news media, and some health experts to avoid *C. aurantium* (bitter orange)–containing weight loss products does not appear to be based on sound science. Multicomponent products containing bitter orange may be responsible for some adverse events. However, the assumption that these adverse effects are exclusively caused by bitter orange and p-synephrine is not supported by current evidence and usage.

SUMMARY AND CONCLUSIONS

Additional longer-term human research studies are necessary in terms of both safety and efficacy of *C. aurantium* extract. Studies involving the use of standardized products with and without other commonly added ingredients such as caffeine need to be conducted in both animal and human studies based on oral administration. The recent FDA study demonstrating a lack of developmental toxicity even at very high doses of *p*-synephrine and bitter orange extract adds clarity to the safety issue. Although there are few studies involving bitter orange extract or *p*-synephrine alone, a number of studies involving multi-ingredient products that contain bitter orange have demonstrated positive results with respect to weight loss, particularly when used in conjunction with diet and exercise. In addition, several animal studies involving bitter orange and/or *p*-synephrine have also yielded positive results in terms of weight loss and weight management. Both human and animal studies have demonstrated few adverse events associated with the oral consumption of bitter orange extract and *p*-synephrine, contrary to the predictions of many individuals unfamiliar with the structural and pharmacokinetic differences between *p*-synephrine and ephedrine as well as *m*-synephrine.

Current confusion regarding the safety and efficacy is clouded by multiple issues, including the lack of standardization of bitter orange extract with respect to protoalkaloidal constituents, misunderstandings regarding the isomeric forms of synephrine and their differing pharmacological properties, political agendas, and the use of complex mixtures of ingredients including bitter orange extract. Furthermore, much of the projected warnings regarding cardiovascular risks and other adverse effects are extrapolated from studies involving the properties of *m*-synephrine and ephedrine, which are not components of bitter orange and intravenously administered extracts and *p*-synephrine.

Based on the current data presented earlier, what conclusions can be drawn regarding *p*-synephrine-containing extracts of *C. aurantium*? It is clear that many millions of doses of *C. aurantium*-containing extract have been used, and the number of individuals consuming these products may also be in the millions [89]. In spite of the extensive consumption of these products, no serious adverse events (and no deaths) have been directly attributed to bitter orange extract or *p*-synephrine [75,90]. This is truly remarkable in light of the large number of deaths annually due to FDA-approved prescription and over-the-counter drugs, as well as contaminated food products.

A number of case studies have been reported involving adverse events in which *C. aurantium* was present as a component of complex products [75]. In each of these cases, the amount of *p*-synephrine ingested was low relative to amounts used in clinical trials involving healthy but obese subjects. In virtually all of these case reports, a variety of other confounding factors were involved, in addition to the fact that the products in question contained multiple ingredients and relatively low amounts of *p*-synephrine. The high levels of caffeine and other neuroactive ingredients in these products in combination with *p*-synephrine must also be taken into consideration, and the adverse effects which have been infrequently reported are most probably due to a combination of ingredients.

With respect to efficacy in terms of weight loss, the clinical studies that have been conducted to date involve products with multiple ingredients, invariably containing caffeine from various sources in addition to bitter orange extract. Several studies have demonstrated that a *p*-synephrine-containing extract of bitter orange can increase resting energy expenditure and metabolic rate. The majority of studies involving products with *C. aurantium* extract in conjunction with other ingredients have demonstrated modest weight loss after 6–12 weeks of product usage.

In summary, based on currently published information, the dire consequences of using bitter orange extract predicted by some have not materialized, and based on wide product usage, bitter orange extract and *p*-synephrine appear to be exceedingly safe when used orally as directed and in reasonable amounts. As a replacement for ephedrine, the efficacy of *p*-synephrine-containing products has not lived up to the expectations of many with respect to weight loss and weight management due to its structural and pharmacokinetic differences. However, these differences have also precluded the adverse events observed with ephedrine and have thus resulted in products generally devoid of cardiovascular and CNS effects.

As is invariably the case, additional studies in both animals and human subjects are needed to bring greater clarity to issues concerning efficacy as well as the mechanism of action of bitter orange extract and *p*-synephrine. Longer-term studies than those reported to date are essential and should be conducted using bitter orange extract and *p*-synephrine alone as well as in combination with selected ingredients. Finally, the facts should be allowed to speak for themselves.

REFERENCES

1. Chen, J.K. and Chen, T.T., Zhi Shi (Fructus Aurantii Immaturus), in *Chinese Medical Herbology and Pharmacology*, Art of Medicine Press, City of industry, CA, 2004, p. 485.
2. Youngken, A.M., Lemon peel U.S.P. (*Limonis cortex*), in *A Textbook of Pharmacognosy*, 6th edn., McGraw-Hill Book Company, Inc., New York, 1948, p. 503.
3. Trease, G.E. and Evans, W.C., Aurantii amari cortex, in *A Textbook of Pharmacognosy*, 10th edn., Balliere, Tindall and Cassell, London, U.K., 1989, p. 467.
4. Carvalho-Freitas, M.I. and Costa, M., Anxiolytic and sedative effects of extracts and essential oil from *Citrus aurantium L. Biol. Pharm. Bull.*, 25, 1629, 2002.
5. Arch, J.R. and Ainsworth, A.T., Thermogenic and antiobesity activity of a novel beta-adrenoreceptor agonist (BRL26830A) in mice and rats. *Am. J. Clin. Nutr.*, 38, 549, 1983.
6. Mattoli, L. et al., A rapid liquid electrospray ionization mass spectroscopy method for evaluation of *Citrus aurantium L.* samples. *J. Agric. Food Chem.*, 53, 9860, 2005.
7. Blumenthal, M. Bitter orange peel and synephrine. *Whole Foods*, p. 77, March 2004.
8. Dragull, K., Breksa, A.P., and Cain, B., Synephrine content of juice from Satsuma mandarins (*Citrus unshiu* Marcovitch). *J. Agric. Food Chem.*, 56, 8874, 2008.
9. Hashimoto, K., Yasuda, T., and Ohsawa, K., Determination of synephrine from Chinese medicinal drugs originating from citrus species by ion-pair high-performance liquid chromatography. *J. Chromatogr.*, 623, 386, 1992.
10. Pellati, F. et al., Determination of adrenergic agonists from extracts and herbal products of *Citrus aurantium* L. var. *amara* by LC. *J. Pharmaceut. Biomed. Anal.*, 29, 1113, 2002.
11. Pellati, F., Benvenuti, S., and Melegari, M., High-performance liquid chromatography methods for the analysis of adrenergic amines and flavanones in *Citrus aurantium L.var. amara. Phytochem. Anal.*, 15, 220, 2004.
12. Pellati, F., Benvenuti, S., and Melegari, M., Enantioselective LC analysis of synephrine in natural products on a protein-based chiral stationary phase. *J. Pharmaceut. Biomed. Anal.*, 37, 839, 2005.
13. Avula, B. et al., Simultaneous quantification of adrenergic amines and flavonoids in *C. aurantium*, various *Citrus* species, and dietary supplements by liquid chromatography. *J. AOAC Int.*, 88, 1593, 2005.
14. Tsujita, T. and Takaku, T., Lipolysis induced by segment wall extract from Satsuma mandarin orange (*Citrus unshu* Mark). *J. Nutr. Sci. Vitaminol.*, 53, 547, 2007.
15. Arbo, M.D. et al., Concentrations of *p*-synephrine in fruits and leaves of *Citrus* species (Rutaceae) and the acute toxicity testing of *Citrus aurantium* extract and *p*-synephrine. *Food Chem. Toxicol.*, 46, 2770, 2008.
16. Mercolini, L. et al., Fast CE analysis of adrenergic amines in different parts of *Citrus aurantium* fruit and dietary supplements. *J. Sep. Sci.*, 32, 1, 2010.
17. Rossato, L.G, et al., Development and validation of a GC/IT-MS method for simultaneous quantification of the *para* and *meta*-synephrine in biological samples *J. Pharmaceut. Biomed. Anal.*, 52, 721, 2010.
18. USPDI (United States Pharmacopeia Dispensing Information), *Drug Information for the Health Care Professional* (electronic version), Micromedex, Inc., Englewood, CO, 2003, p. 2227.
19. Allison, D.B. et al., Exactly which synephrine alkaloids does *Citrus aurantium* (bitter orange) contain? *Int. J. Obesity*, 29, 443, 2005.
20. Sander, L.C. et al., Certification of standard reference materials containing bitter orange. *Anal. Bioanal. Chem.*, 391, 2023, 2008.
21. Bent, S., Padula, A., and Neuhaus, J., Safety and efficacy of *Citrus aurantium* for weight loss. *Am. J. Cardiol.*, 94, 1359, 2004.
22. Penzak, S.R. et al., Seville (sour) orange juice: Synephrine content and cardiovascular effects in normotensive adults. *J. Clin. Pharmacol.*, 41, 1059, 2001.
23. Nasir, J.M. et al., Exercise-induced syncope associated with QT prolongation and ephedra-free Xenadrine. *Mayo Clin. Proc.*, 79, 1059, 2004.
24. Clauson, K.A. et al., Safety issues associated with commercially available energy drinks. *J. Am. Pharm. Assoc.*, 48, e52, 2008.
25. Smedema, J.P. and Muller, G.J., Coronary spasm and thrombosis in a bodybuilder using a nutritional supplement containing synephrine, octopamine, tyramine and caffeine. *So. African Med. J.*, 98, 372, 2008.
26. Stephensen, T.A. and Sarlay, Jr. R., Ventricular fibrillation associated with use of synephrine containing dietary supplement. *Military Med.*, 174, 1313, 2009.
27. Greenway, F. et al., Dietary herbal supplements with phenylephrine for weight loss. *J. Med. Food*, 9, 572, 2006.

28. Gougeon, R. et al., Increase in the thermic effect of food in women by adrenergic amines extracted from *Citrus aurantium. Obesity Res.*, 13, 1187, 2005.

29. Calapai, G. et al., Antiobesity and cardiovascular toxic effects of Citrus aurantium extracts in the rat: A preliminary report. *Fitoterapia*, 70, 586, 1999.

30. Kalman, D.S., Rubin, S., and Schwartz, H.I., An acute clinical trial to evaluate the safety and efficacy of a popular commercial weight loss supplement when used with exercise. Presented at Federation of American Societies of Experimental Biology, 2003. www.miamiresearch.com.

31. Kendall-Reed, P., Study on the effectiveness of Ultra Slim Down® for the reduction of body weight, unpublished, 2000. http://www.nutratechinc.com/advz/advz.php?p=2 (accessed on June 21, 2011).

32. Zenk, J.L. et al., A prospective, randomized, double blind study to evaluate the effect of Lean Source™ on body composition in overweight adult men and women, on *lean source.com*, unpublished data, 2005. http://www.nutratechinc.com/advz/advz.php?p=2 (accessed on May 23, 2011).

33. Zenk, J.L. et al., Effect of Lean System 7 on metabolic rate and body composition. *Nutrition*, 21, 179, 2005.

34. Dulloo, A.G. et al., Ephedrine, xanthines and prostaglandins inhibitors: Actions and interactions in the stimulation of thermogenesis. *Int. J. Obesity*, 17, S35, 1993.

35. Arch, J.R., β_3-Adrenoceptor agonists: Potential, pitfalls and progress. *Eur. J. Pharmacol.*, 440, 99, 2002.

36. Oana, F. et al., DNA microarray analysis of white adipose tissue from obese (fa/fa) Zucker rats treated with a β3-adrenoreceptor agonist, KTO-7924. *Pharmacol. Res.*, 52, 395, 2005.

37. Hamilton, F. and Doods, H.N., Identification of potent agonists acting at an endogenous atypical β3-adrenoreceptor state that modulate lipolysis in rodent fat cells. *Eur. J. Pharmacol.*, 580, 55, 2008.

38. Alemzadeh, R. et al., Diazoxide enhances basal metabolic rate and fat oxidation in obese Zucker rats. *Metabolism*, 57, 1597, 2008.

39. Jordan, R. et al., Beta-adrenergic activities of octopamine and synephrine stereoisomers on guinea-pig atria and trachea. *J. Pharm. Pharmacol.*, 39, 752, 1987.

40. Ma, G. et al., Effects of synephrine and beta-phenylephrine on human alpha-adrenoreceptor subtypes. *Planta Med.*, 76, 981, 2010.

41. Brown, C.M. et al., Activities of octapamine and synephrine stereoisomers on alpha-adrenoreceptors. *Brit. J. Pharmacol.*, 93, 417, 1988.

42. Hwa, J. and Perez, D.M., The unique nature of the serine interactions for alpha 1-adrenergic receptor agonist binding and activation. *J. Biol. Chem.*, 271, 6322, 1996.

43. Hibino, T. et al., Synephrine, a component of *Evodiae fructus*, constricts isolated aorta via adrenergic and serotonergic receptors. *J. Pharmacol. Sci.*, 111, 73, 2009.

44. Haller, C.A. et al., Hemodynamic effects of ephedra-free weight-loss supplements in humans. *Amer. J. Med.*, 118, 998, 2005.

45. Rozec, B. and Gauther, C., β3-Adrenoreceptors in the cardiovascular system: Putative roles in human pathologies. *Pharmacol. Therap.*, 111, 652, 2006.

46. Moens, A.L. et al., Beta 3-adrenoreceptor regulation of nitric oxide in the cardiovascular system. *J. Mol. Cell. Cardiol.*, 48, 1088, 2010.

47. Jones, D., Citrus and ephedra. *Whole Foods*, p. 40, April 2004.

48. Arbo, M.D. et al., Screening for in vivo (anti)estrogenic activity of ephedrine, *p*-synephrine and their natural sources *Ephedra sinica* Stapf. (Ephedraceae) and *Citrus aurantium* L. (Rutaceae) in rats. *Arch. Toxicol.*, 83, 95, 2009.

49. Preuss, H.G. et al., *Citrus aurantium* as a thermogenic, weight-reduction replacement for ephedra: An overview. *J. Med.*, 33, 247, 2002.

50. Fugh-Berman, A. and Myers, A., Citrus aurantium, an ingredient of dietary supplements marketed for weight loss; Current status of clinical and basic research. *Exptl. Biol. Med.*, 229, 698, 2004.

51. Colker, C.M. et al., Effects of *Citrus aurantium* extract, caffeine, and St. John's wort on body fat loss, lipid levels, and mood states in overweight healthy adults. *Curr. Ther. Res.*, 60, 145, 1999.

52. National Toxicology Program, NIEHS, Bitter orange (*Citrus aurantium* var. amara) extracts and constituents *p*-synephrine [CAS No. 94-07-5] and p-octopamine [CAS No. 104-14-3]. Review of Toxicological Literature. June 2004. Contract No. N01-ES-35515.

53. Haaz, S. et al., Citrus aurantium and synephrine alkaloids in the treatment of overweight and obesity: An update. *Obesity Rev.*, 7, 79, 2006.

54. Stohs, S.J. and Shara, M., A review of the safety and efficacy of *Citrus aurantium* in weight management, in Bagchi, D. and Preuss, H.G., eds. *Obesity: Epidemiology, Pathophysiology, and Prevention*, CRC Press, Boca Raton, FL, 2007, p. 371.

55. Haaz, S. et al., Bitter orange, in Coates, P.M. et al., eds. *Encyclopedia of Dietary Supplements*, 2nd edn., Marcel Dekker, New York, 2010, p. 52.

56. Rossato, L.G. et al., Synephrine: From trace concentration to massive consumption in weight-loss. *Food Chem. Toxicol.*, doi:10.1016/j.fct.2010.11.007, 2010.

57. Stohs, S.J. and Preuss, H.G., The Safety of bitter orange (*Citrus au-rantium*) and its primary protoalkaloid *p*-synephrine. *HerbalGram*, 89, 34, 2011.

58. Stohs, S.J., Preuss, H.G., and Shara, M., The safety of *Citrus aurantium* (bitter orange) and its primary protoalkaloid *p*-synephrine. *Phytother. Res.*, doi: 10.1002/ptr.3490, 2011.

59. Hansen, D.K. et al., Developmental toxicity of *Citrus aurantium* in rats. *Birth Defects Res. Part B. Devel. Reprod. Toxicol.*, doi: 10.1002/bdrb.20308, 2011.

60. Parra, A.L. et al., Comparative study of the assay of *Artemia salina L.* and the estimate of the medium lethal dose (LD50 value) in mice, to determine oral acute toxicity of plant extracts. *Phytomedicine*, 8, 395, 2001.

61. Douds, D.A., An acute oral toxicity study in rats with Advantra Z™. http://www.nutratechinc.com/advz/UploadedFiles/Safety%20Study-Oral%20Toxicity-LD50%20of%20AdvZ%20in%20Rats.pdf (Accessed on March 14, 2011).

62. Huang, Y.T. et al., Fructus aurantii reduced portal pressure in portal hypertensive rats. *Life Sciences*, 57, 2011, 1995.

63. Titta, L. et al., Blood orange juice inhibits fat accumulation in mice. *Int. J. Obesity*, 34, 578, 2010.

64. Arbo, M.D. et al., Subchronic toxicity of *Citrus aurantium* L. (Rutaceae) extract and *p*-synephrine in mice. *Reg. Toxicol. Pharmacol.*, 54, 114, 2009.

65. Tounsi, M.S. et al., Juice components and antioxidant capacity of four Tunisian Citrus varieties. *J. Sci. Food Agric.*, doi 10.1002/jsfa.4164, September 2010.

66. Kang, S.R. et al., Suppressive effect on lipopolysaccharide-induced proinflammatory mediators by *Citrus aurantium* in macrophage RAW 264.7 cells via NF-κB signal pathway. *Evidence-Based Compl. Altern. Med.*, doi: 10.1155/2011/248592, 2011.

67. Hosseinimehr, S.J. et al., Radioprotective effects of citrus extract against γ-irradiation in mouse bone marrow cells. *J. Radiat.*, 44, 237, 2003.

68. Gang, C. et al., Effect and mechanism of total flavonoids of orange peel on rat adjuvant arthritis. *Chin. J. Mater. Med.*, 35, 1298, 2010.

69. Dulloo, A. G. et al., Efficacy of a green tea extract rich in catechin polyphenols and caffeine in increasing 24-h energy expenditure and fat oxidation in humans. *Am. J. Clin. Nutr.*, 70, 1040, 1999.

70. Sale, C. et al., Metabolic and physiological effects of ingesting extracts of bitter orange, green tea and guarana at rest and during treadmill walking in overweight males. *Int. J. Obesity*, 30, 764, 2006.

71. Hoffman, J.R. et al., Thermogenic effect from nutritionally enriched coffee consumption. *J. Int. Soc. Sports Nutr.*, 3, 35, 2006.

72. Seifert, J.G. et al., The effects of acute administration of an herbal preparation in humans. *Int. J. Med. Sci.*, 8, 192, 2011.

73. Stohs, S.J. et al., Effects of *p*-synephrine in the presence and absence of selected flavonoids on resting metabolic rate, heart rate, blood pressure and self-reported mood changes. *Int. J. Med. Sci.*, 8, 295, 2011.

74. Shara, M. et al., The cardiovascular and hemodynamic effects of daily *p*-synephrine administration to healthy human subjects for two weeks. Presented at the annual meeting of the American College of Nutrition. Abstract No. 16. *J Amer Coll Nutr.*, 30, 358, 2012.

75. Stohs, S.J., Assessment of the adverse event reports associated with *Citrus aurantium* (bitter orange) from April 2004 to October 2009. *J. Funct. Foods*, 2, 235, 2010.

76. Nykamp, D.L., Fackih, M.N., and Compton, A.L., Possible association of acute lateral-wall myocardial infarction and bitter orange supplement. *Ann. Pharmacother.*, 38, 812, 2004.

77. Bouchard, N.C. et al., Ischemic stroke associated with use of an ephedra-free dietary supplement containing synephrine. *Mayo Clin. Proc.*, 80, 541, 2005.

78. Sultan, S., Spector, J., and Mitchell, R.M., Ischemic colitis associated with use of a bitter orange-containing dietary weight-loss supplement. *Mayo Clin. Proc.*, 81, 1630, 2006.

79. Gange, C.A. et al., Variant angina associated with bitter orange in a dietary supplement. *Mayo Clin. Proc.*, 81, 545, 2006.

80. Burke, J. et al., A case of severe exercise-induced rhabdomyolysis associated with a weight-loss dietary supplement. *Military Med.*, 172, 656, 2007.

81. Holmes, Jr., R.O. and Tavee, J., Vasospasm and Stroke attributable to ephedra-free Xenadrine: Case study. *Military Med.*, 173, 708, 2008.

82. Thomas, J.E. et al., STEMI in a 24-year-old man after use of a synephrine-containing dietary supplement. A case report and review of the literature. *Texas Heart Inst. J.*, 36, 586, 2009.

83. Gray, S. and Woolf, A.D., *Citrus aurantium* used for weight loss by an adolescent with anorexia nervosa. *J. Adol. Health*, 37, 415, 2005.

84. Karch, S.B., Peer review and the process of publishing of adverse drug event reports. *J. Forensic Legal Med.*, 14, 79, 2007.

85. Gurley, B.J. et al., In vivo assessment of botanical supplementation on human cytochrome P450 phenotypes: *Citrus aurantium*, *Echinacea purpurea*, milk thistle, and saw palmetto. *Clin. Pharmacol. Ther.*, 76, 428, 2004.

86. Min, B. et al., Absence of QTc-interval-prolonging or hemodynamic effects of a single dose of bitter orange extract in healthy subjects. *Pharmacother.*, 25, 1719, 2005.

87. Haller, C.A. et al., Human pharmacology of a performance-enhancing dietary supplement under resting and exercise conditions. *Brit. J. Clin. Pharmacol.*, 65, 833, 2008.

88. Bui, L.T. et al., Blood pressure and heart rate effects following a single dose of bitter orange. *Ann. Pharmacother.*, 40, 53, 2006.

89. Klonz, K.C. et al., Consumption of dietary supplements containing Citrus aurantium (bitter orange)—2004 California behavioral risk factor surveillance survey (BRFSS). *Ann. Pharmacother.*, 40, 1747, 2006.

90. McGuffin, M., Media spins numbers on bitter orange AERs based on erroneous information from FDA. *HerbalGram*, 69, 52, 2006.

91. Anon, The Tan Sheet. F-D-C Reports, Inc., 12, 11, 2004.

92. Anon, Dangerous supplements. What you don't know about these 12 ingredients could hurt you. Consumer Reports, September 16, 2010.

93. Starfield, B., Is U. S. health really the best in the world? *J. Am. Med. Assoc.*, 284, 483, 2000.

94. Lee, W.M., Acetaminophen and the U. S. acute liver failure study group: Lowering the risks of hepatic failure. *Hepatology*, 40, 6, 2004.

95. Anon, CDC's issue brief: Unintentional drug poisoning in the United States. Last updated August 16, 2010. http://cdc.gov/homeandrecreationalsafety/poisoning/brief.htm

38 Antiobesity Effects of Conjugated Linoleic Acid
Fact or Fiction?

Richard Zwe-Ling Kong, PhD

CONTENTS

ABBREVIATIONS

BAT	brown adipose tissue
BMI	body mass index
CLA	conjugated linoleic acid
c9t11-CLA	*cis*-9, *trans*-11 conjugated linoleic acid
t10c12-CLA	*trans*-10, *cis*-12 conjugated linoleic acid
CNF	ciliary neurotrophic factor
CRP	C reactive protein
CVD	cardiovascular disease

DM	diabetes mellitus
ELISA	enzyme-linked immunosorbent assay
FFA	free fatty acid
GADD45	growth arrest and DNA damage–inducible gene
HFD	high-fat diet
IL	interleukin
LA	linoleic acid
LPS	lipopolysaccharide
MCP-1	monocyte chemotactic protein-1
MIF	migration inhibitory factor
MTT	3-(4,5-dimethylthiazol-2-yl)-2,5-diphenyltetrazolium bromide
MS	metabolic syndrome
NFAT	calcineurin/nuclear factor of activated T cells
NGF	nerve growth factor
PAI-1	plasminogen activator inhibitor 1
PPARγ	peroxisome proliferator–activated receptor gamma
PPRE	peroxisome proliferator–responsive element
RA	retinoic acid
RAR	retinoic acid receptor
ROS	reactive oxygen species
RT-PCR	reverse transcriptase polymerase chain reaction
RXR	retinoid X receptor
TG	triglyceride
TNFα	tumor necrosis factor alpha
VEGF	vascular endothelial growth factor
WAT	white adipose tissue

INTRODUCTION

Obesity is the important medical problem worldwide today. It is associated with a number of acute and chronic medical complications, including cardiovascular disease (CVD), diabetes, arthritis, depression, and respiratory and gastrointestinal problems. On the other hand, traditional weight loss treatments, usually involving reduction of fat intake, in fact have generally had very limited success. In this chapter, from the viewpoint of dietary supplement, we will report some of our recent results and review the updated knowledge of the adipocytes regarding CLA effects, focusing on gene expression and cytokines/adipokines in different models, including cultured cell, rodent, and human study. In 1987, Ha et al. [1] found that CLA present in fried ground beef reduced tumor incidence in mice. CLA has also attracted a lot of attention over the past few years for antiobese issue. Earlier research has indicated that intake of CLA might reduce adiposity, providing antioxidant protection to treating diabetes and CVD in humans and could have important other beneficial effects. CLA-enriched diets lead to a rapid and marked decrease in fat stores in several species including pig, rat, hamster, chicken, and mouse [2–6], suggesting that CLA might be useful as a weight loss agent. However, unfortunately, in several recent human subject data of CLA supplementation, in contrast to animal studies, there has been marked variation between reports on the health-related outcomes. Additionally, adverse side effects have been recently reported in mice fed with a commercial CLA mixture. It indicated that the relation between CLA taken as supplements and antiobese could be more complex than initially generally thought. Further, the final administration outcomes will depend on individual genomics, dosage, the form of free fatty acid (FFA) or triacylglycerol, period of duration, and obesity phase.

CHEMICAL PROPERTY, SOURCE, PHARMACOLOGY, AND SAFETY

CHEMICAL PROPERTY, ORIGIN, AND PRODUCTION

The CLA family consists of several different conjugated forms, and many have currently been identified [7–9]. Natural forms of CLA can be found predominantly in ruminant products [10,11], more than 91% of the c9t11-CLA present in milk fat [12–14], also known as rumenic acid [15–19] (see Figure 38.1), and partially hydrogenated vegetable oils. Because the CLA content of dairy products is related to their fat content, CLA levels are greater in higher fat than in lower fat products. The two predominant isomers found in foods and commercial preparations are c9t11-CLA and t10c12-CLA. Commercial dietary supplements contain c9t11-CLA and t10c12-CLA isomers in approximately equal amounts. Measurements of c9t11-CLA in human adipose tissue have found that its presence is highly correlated with milk fat intake [20–24]. Anaerobic ruminant bacteria, such as *Butyrivibrio fibrisolvens* [25], produce predominantly c9t11-CLA through biohydrogenation of linoleic acid and α-linolenic acid obtained from plant material and pathway of linoleic acid by c9t11-octadecadienoate reductase [26]. CLA also identified from fried ground beef, heat-altered derivatives of linoleic acid [1]. In the formation of CLA, a hypothetical mechanism by which oxygen-derived free radicals might induce a double bond of linoleic acid to shift [27].

In addition to dietary sources, some CLA can be produced endogenously by humans [28]. Several methods are currently available to chemically synthesize CLA [29,30], either absorbed or further metabolized to vaccenic acid (trans-11-octadecenoic acid), a predominant trans fatty acid in milk fat, which can be converted to c9t11-CLA by the enzyme Δ9 stearoyl-CoA desaturase, an alternative route in mammals, including in humans [31,32]. Blood levels of CLA in humans may reflect

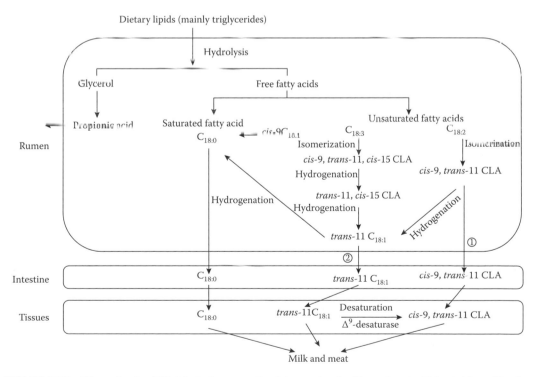

FIGURE 38.1 Biosynthesis of CLA in its incorporation into meat and milk ruminants. (Adapted from Tanaka, K., *Anim. Sci. J.*, 76, 291, 2005. With permission.)

both dietary intake of CLA and endogenous synthesis from *trans*-vaccenic acid. Interestingly, in diabetes, the glycation and subsequent glycoxidation reactions are enhanced by elevated glucose concentrations. Ratios of CLA to LA significantly increased in diabetic erythrocytes compared with control erythrocytes. This indicates that glycation via chronic hyperglycemia links lipid peroxidation in the erythrocytes of both diabetic and healthy subjects [27].

The conjugated trienoic fatty acids produced from α- and γ-linolenic acid were further saturated by *Lactobacillus plantarum* to *trans*-10, *cis*-15–18:2, and *cis*-6, *trans*-10–18:2 [35]. Recently, purified CLA isomers are commercially available and are expected to facilitate the clarification of dietary function paradox and of each isomer's physiological activity.

PHARMACOLOGY AND DOSAGE

In vitro and experimental animal studies found a number of potential health benefits for CLA. CLA inhibits the proliferation of some cancer cells such as mammary, colorectal, prostate, and forestomach cancer cells [36]. Virtually, most studies have used synthetic mixtures of CLA at dose from 10 to 25 µM. In human serum, CLA has been reported to be around 7.1 µM. One report indicates that potent cytotoxic effect on cancer cell line can be exerted at physiological concentration [37,38]. In a study of body composition, intake of CLA reduces body fat and increases lean body mass in several species of growing animals [39] and improves glucose utilization and reverses symptoms of diabetes in laboratory animals. CLA may lower total and LDL cholesterol as well as TG levels and reduce the severity of atherosclerosis in experimental animals [40]. Recent reports also suggest that each CLA isomer has different functions, such as the t10c12-CLA, which has significantly anticarcinogenic, antiobese, and antidiabetic effects, whereas the c9t11-CLA seems to exert an anticancer effect. In addition, CLA enhances select immune responses in experimental animals, as well as increases the rate of bone formation by influencing factors that regulate bone metabolism. Physiological difference between free and triglyceride-type CLA on the immune function of C57BL/6N mice was also investigated [41].

The typical dosage of CLA ranges from 3 to 5 g daily as dietary supplement. CLA was found to induce leptinemia and adiponectinemia, followed by hyperinsulinemia, as determined in C57BL/6J female mice fed with a 1% isomeric mixture of CLA for various periods of time ranging from 2 to 28 days. Additionally, there are still only few reports or weak evidence concerning the anticancer and antiobese effects of CLA in humans study. Therefore, more detailed evaluations of the physiological bioactivities, especially in double-blind and placebo-based research, using pure CLA isomers on lifestyle-/aging-related diseases in humans and animals will be of great interest in future studies.

DIETARY SAFETY AND ADVERSE EFFECTS

The t10c12-CLA isomer is responsible for antiobese effect especially dramatic in the mouse. However, it is noteworthy that a significant impairment of insulin sensitivity has been reported in overweight subjects receiving the purified t10c12-CLA isomer, in which it is associated with severe hyperinsulinemia, insulin resistance, and massive liver steatosis, also called the CLA-mediated lipoatrophic syndrome [42,43]. This finding raises the question of safety of dietary supplements containing CLA. In general, the usual doses of CLA used in animal studies greatly exceed those used in human studies. This is reasonable to explain why animal studies come up with better results than human studies and may also explain the adverse effects of CLA in rats. However, one recent study results show a high intake of CLA unlikely to affect liver or kidney function, at least over a period of weeks [44]. The dosage of CLA is approximately up to 7% of the energy intake a day (subjects were mostly young women). Collectively, evidence for a putative beneficial effect of a CLA supplementation in humans is still inconclusive; maybe the safety of dietary supplements containing CLA needs more concern, and more clearly, further isomer-specific clinical trials are necessary.

CLA ON OBESITY ISSUE: WEIGHT CONTROL AND BODY COMPOSITION IN CULTURED CELL, ANIMAL, AND HUMAN STUDIES

DISEASE RELATED TO OBESITY: ROLE OF INFLAMMATION AND ADIPOKINE

Despite the enormous medical implications of obesity, effective prevention and treatment strategies are still lacking. It is important to distinguish the term obesity, used to describe excess body fat, from other forms of overweight. Obesity results from hypertrophy, and hyperplasia of adipocytes within the organism, later, is generally thought to be the result of both genetic and environmental influences. Being overweight or obese has become highly prevalent in Western countries, and the population is rapidly upgrowing in the developing world [45]. Obesity-related disorders, such as insulin resistance, hypertension, and diabetes, are also dramatically increasing. Obesity is also associated with endothelial dysfunction and arterial stiffness from as early as the first decade of life [46]. This is probably mediated in part by low-grade inflammation associated with cytokine-like molecules, called adipokines. WAT is a major endocrine/secretory organ, which releases a wide range of adipokines. A number of adipokines, including IL-1β, IL-6, MCP-1, MIF, TNFα, leptin, adiponectin, NGF, VEGF, PAI-1, are somehow linked to the inflammatory response. Recent research indicates that those adipose tissue–derived factors influence metabolic and CVD. Leptin is now considered to play a key role in obese, hypertensive patients, and decreased secretion of adiponectin appears to be an important predictor of diabetes [47,48]. A high leptin concentration, in particular, is found in obese individuals and is strongly associated with vascular changes related to early atherosclerosis [49,50].

METABOLIC SYNDROME: ADIPOGENESIS AND NEUROTROPHINS

Obese adipose tissue originating from a long-term process of adipogenesis is characterized by inflammation and progressive infiltration by macrophages as obesity develops [51], which link to metabolic pathways in metabolic disease and immune response, and the signaling pathways at the intersection contribute to diabetes [52]. The elevated production of inflammation-related adipokines is increasingly considered to be important in the development of diseases linked to obesity, particularly thought of as the metabolic syndrome [53]. Metabolic syndrome, such as diabetes, hypertension, dyslipidemia, coronary artery disease, and obesity, is also known as syndrome X, or the insulin resistance syndrome [54–57]. The global epidemic of obesity and DM has led to a marked increase in the number of persons with metabolic syndrome. Both type 2 DM and metabolic syndrome share common features and patients.

An increasing number of researchers of the metabolic syndrome assume that many mechanisms are involved in the impact for complex pathophysiology of neurotrophins, such as disorders of the hypothalamic–pituitary–adrenal axis, an increased sympathetic activity, the chronic subclinical infections, proinflammatory cytokines, the effect of adipocytokines, and/or psychoemotional stress [58]. Scientific research in this field confirms the role of the neurotrophins and mastocytes in the pathogenesis of inflammatory and immune diseases [59]. CNF is another neurocytokine expressed by glial cells in nervous system, generally recognized for its function in survival of nonneuronal and neuronal cell types. It was recently acknowledged for its potential role in the control of obesity [60].

CELL–CELL INTERACTION: INTEGRIN, MATRIX METALLOPROTEINASE

In obesity, changes in fat pad size lead to physical changes in the surrounding area and modifications of the paracrine function of the adipocyte. Such adipocytes begin to secrete TNFα, which will stimulate preadipocytes to produce monocyte chemoattractant [61–65] and contribute to progressive inflammation which occurs later. Noteworthily, the processes of adipogenesis include a process of migration, adhesion, proliferation, and differentiation of preadipocytes into mature adipocytes. Many of these biological functions are related to cell integrins, like the TG content and gene expression of PPARγ, and leptin also decreased in response to the treatment of disintegrin [66].

Moreover, *in vivo* model found that partial inhibition of gelatinolytic activity is associated with moderate effects on adipose tissue development. MMP inhibitor decreases adipose conversion of 3T3-L1, and enhancement of MMP expression counteracts the inhibitor in adipose tissue [67]. These support a role for the MMP system in the control of proteolytic processes and adipogenesis during obesity-mediated fat mass development [68].

CLA ON LIPID METABOLISM: IN CELL, ANIMAL, AND HUMAN STUDY

Antiobesity: this terminology is sometimes ambiguous and very easily misleading by advertising claim. The basic concepts of recovery (like a pharmaceutical drug) and prevention (like a dietary supplement) are totally different. The following are the beneficial effects of CLA on body composition: Potential antiobesity mechanisms of CLA include decrease in preadipocyte proliferation and differentiation into mature adipocytes, decrease in fatty acid and TG accumulation, and increase in energy expenditure, lipolysis, and fatty acid oxidation. CLA intake has been demonstrated consistently to decrease body fat accumulation and increase lean body mass in several experimental animals including mice, rats, hamsters, and pigs. However, CLA's effect on overall body weight appears to be variable [69,70]. CLA was shown to accumulate in the WAT much more than in the serum or liver, and found levels of triglycerides in the WAT and serum nonesterified fatty acid were reduced in a CLA dose-dependent manner [71]. In animal studies, the most dramatic and desirable effects of CLA on body composition are ascribed to the t10c12-isomer rather than the c9t11-isomer.

Recent findings in mice and hamsters indicate that the t10c12-CLA isomer is largely responsible for CLA's effect on body composition, adipocyte morphology, and many of the effects seen in diabetes and obesity [72,73]. As shown in Figure 38.2, we also confirmed the similar result that t10c12-CLA prevents TG accumulation more remarkably. The t10c12-CLA has been reported to inhibit heparin-releasable lipoprotein lipase activity and leptin secretion from 3T3-L1 adipocytes and to suppress delta-9 desaturase activity [74]. Although a lot of mechanisms are presumably involved, how CLA alters body composition is still unclear and remains to be determined. Some metabolic and serum parameters in C57Bl/6J mice fed with CLA isomers and CLA mix [75] are shown in Table 38.1. Results of many published studies in human subjects, such as a randomized crossover study on plasma lipoproteins and body composition in men, found that the CLA-enriched butter induced no significant change in the CVD risk profile and had no effect on the distribution of body fat [76].

Collectively, CLA, from a fundamental viewpoint, as an integral extrapolation of animal data to human seems unrealistic, has only limited effects on immune functions in man. In fact however, dietary CLA is able to be incorporated and metabolized as linoleic acid, to influence linoleic acid desaturation and elongation, and to be beta oxidized finally in peroxisomes, which, via activation of PPARs, increase free retinol levels and link to regulate gene expression [77]. A study was done on 60 abdominally obese men with MS, who were randomly assigned to supplements containing either 3.4 g/day of a CLA isomer mixture or the purified t10c12-CLA isomer. Results found that after

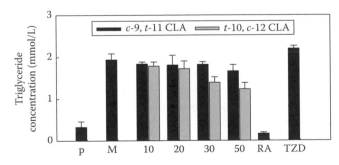

FIGURE 38.2 Effects of c9t11- and t10c12-CLA on triglyceride accumulation in differentiated 3T3-L1 cells (p, preadipocyte; M, MDI; RA, 5 μM retinoic acid; TZD, 10 μM thiazolidine).

TABLE 38.1
Metabolic and Serum Parameters in C57Bl/6J Mice Fed
with CLA Isomers and CLA Mix for 6 Months

Parameter	CO	C9t11	t10c12	CLA Mix
Serum metabolites				
Glucose (mg/dL)	259.6 ± 17.89	228.7 ± 10.98	303.8 ± 20.91*	293.6 ± 18.07*
Insulin (ng/mL)	0.37 ± 0.06	0.43 ± 0.08	0.85 ± 0.14*	0.61 ± 0.14*
Triglycerides (mg/dL)	68.38 ± 3.15	65.67 ± 2.88	43.73 ± 7.11*	37.40 ± 4.09*
NEFA (mEq/L)	0.84 ± 0.06	0.72 ± 0.06*	0.98 ± 0.03	0.92 ± 0.03
HOMA-IR	4.13 ± 0.64	4.51 ± 0.93	10.49 ± 2.35*	7.82 ± 1.10*
R-QUICKI	0.50 ± 0.23	0.54 ± 0.17	0.41 ± 0.37*	0.44 ± 0.26*
Serum hormones and adipocyte cytokines				
Leptin (µg/mL)	6.65 ± 0.87	5.23 ± 0.70	1.65 ± 0.52*	2.30 ± 0.98*
Adiponectin (µg/mL)	2.91 ± 0.06	2.86 ± 0.07	3.16 ± 0.04	2.927 ± 0.05
TNF-α (pg/mL)	50.72 ± 5.16	41.32 ± 3.62	36.51 ± 1.56*	36.83 ± 1.59*
IL-6 (pg/mL)	112.9 ± 8.80	121.0 ± 4.81	91.01 ± 8.92*	54.29 ± 2.49*
IGF-1 (pg/mL)	18.55 ± 0.45	22.90 ± 0.13	24.47 ± 0.15	25.50 ± 0.20*
Organ weights				
Spleen (g)	0.09 ± 0.00	0.11 ± 0.01	0.12 ± 0.00	0.09 ± 0.00
Adipose tissue (g)	2.64 ± 0.25	2.15 ± 0.19	0.98 ± 0.15*	1.17 + 0.16*
Quadriceps (g)	0.14 ± 0.01	0.16 ± 0.01	0.17 ± 0.01	0.16 ± 0.01
Gastrocnemius (g)	0.15 ± 0.02	0.16 ± 0.02	0.16 ± 0.00	0.18 ± 0.01

Source: Adapted from Halade, G.V. et al., *J. Nutr. Biochem.*, 21(4), 332, 2010. With permission.
Effect of CLA isomers on serum metabolites, hormones, and organ weights in C57Bl/6J mice fed with CLA isomers and CLA for 6 months. Data are means ± SEM (n = 8–10 mice/group). Asterisk denotes statistically significant differences compared to CO and c9-CLA groups using Newman–Keuls one-way ANOVA (*P < 05).

12 weeks of supplementation, the t10c12-CLA isomer induced statistically significant deteriorations in insulin resistance, in glycemia, as well as in plasma HDL cholesterol concentrations compared with placebo [76]. CLA supplementation with purified t10c12-CLA isomer decreases fat mass and causes a significant impairment in insulin sensitivity in overweight humans [78].

FUNCTIONAL COMPARISON OF ESTERIFIED AND FREE FORMS CLA

9c11t-CLA concentration was always higher than the 10t12c-CLA concentration following the administration of these compounds in mice and rat model and considered that isomer double bonds structural differences affected absorption in the small intestine [79]. However, the results found that there was no difference in the extent of lymphatic recovery of 9c11t-CLA and 10t12c-CLA after the administration of triacylglycerol-CLA, 9c11t-CLA, and 10t12c-CLA to the rats, suggesting that geometrical and positional isomerism of the conjugated double bonds did not influence the absorption. C57BL/6J mice were fed a control diet, HFD, HFD supplemented with 2% free fatty acid-CLA, or HFD supplemented with 2% triacylglycerol-CLA for 8 weeks. Oral supplementation with both forms of CLA significantly reduced the weights of whole body and adipose tissue (see Figure 38.3) [80]. Nevertheless, no significant increases were found in the levels of expression of β-oxidation-related genes as previous report [81]; triacylglycerol-CLA significantly decreased triacylglycerol accumulation and lipogenic gene expression in the liver as compared to free fatty acid-CLA. This demonstrated that free and esterified forms of CLA actually have differing effects especially on liver and adipose tissue lipogenesis.

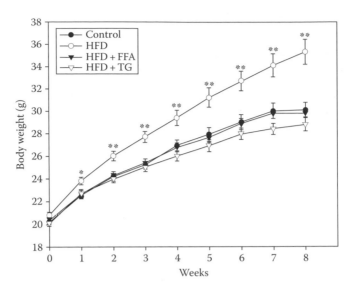

FIGURE 38.3   Effect of dietary supplementation of CLA on body weight. Data represent the mean (SEM of 10 animals; P < 0.05* and P < 0.01**). (Adapted from Kim, J.H. et al., *J. Agric. Food Chem.*, 58(21), 11441, 2010. With permission.)

MECHANISM OF CLA EFFECTS: ON DIFFERENTIATION, ORGANELLES, GENE EXPRESSION, PUTATIVE RECEPTOR, AND IMMUNE RESPONSE

ADIPOCYTE/PREADIPOCYTE DIFFERENTIATION, ACTIVATION

Adipogenesis is a multistage process beginning with mesenchymal cells capable of forming muscle, bone, or adipose tissue. Adipose tissue plays a key role in the pathogenesis of the obesity-related metabolic syndrome. Adipocyte serves as an important source of proinflammatory molecules, including leptin, TNFα, and IL-6, as well as anti-inflammatory molecules, such as adiponectin [82]. Most of these functions are carried out via adipocytokines capable of acting locally or at distant sites [83]. The recent study demonstrates that calcineurin is a critical effector of a calcium-dependent signaling pathway that acts to inhibit adipocyte differentiation [84]. Moreover, a constitutively active NFAT mutant preadipocyte inhibits its differentiation into mature adipocytes. Cell expressing NFAT lose contact-mediated growth inhibition, protected from apoptosis following growth factor deprivation.

The first, and best characterized, model of adipogenesis *in vitro* is the 3T3-L1 mouse fibroblast cell line [85,86]. When confluent/growth-arrested 3T3-L1 cells are subjected to the adipogenic hormones 3-isobutylmethylxanthine (a phosphodiesterase inhibitor), dexamethasone, and insulin, collectively known as MDI, they undergo a defined genetic program of terminal differentiation, giving rise to mature morphologically distinct adipocytes containing large cytoplasmic TG depots [87]. It is dependent on the sequential activation of transcription factors including the C/EBP, PPAR, and SREBP, those leading to changes in gene expression [88]. In addition, 3T3-F442A, at a later stage, requires only insulin to differentiate, as well as AP-18, a new non-embryo-derived preadipocyte cell line established from an adult C3H/HeM mouse provides a useful model for investigating adipocyte differentiation and adipogenesis [89–92].

ORGANELLE FUNCTIONS: MITOCHONDRIA AND ENDOPLASMIC RETICULUM

Increasing evidence show that mitochondrial dysfunction in the prediabetic/insulin-resistant state contributes to a variety of human disorders, ranging from cardiac dysfunction, neurodegenerative diseases, obesity, insulin sensitivity, and cancer, as well as their increasingly acknowledged key role during apoptosis [93–95]. Induction of mitochondrial uncoupling proteins, UCP1, in mouse or human white adipocytes promotes fatty acid oxidation and resistance to obesity. UCP2 and UCP3 do not mediate adaptive thermogenesis physiologically and do not seem to contribute to energy expenditure, but they may be significantly thermogenic under specific pharmacological conditions. Both UCP2 and UCP3 should be considered as potential targets for treatment of aging, degenerative diseases, and perhaps obesity [96,97]. Noteworthily, PPARγ coactivator 1α plays a key role in regulating mitochondrial biogenesis and fuel homeostasis, and overexpression favored a shift from incomplete to complete β-oxidation, enabling muscle mitochondria to better cope with a high lipid load [98]. These possibly reflect a fundamental metabolic benefit of exercise training, and upregulation of PPARγ coactivator 1α may be an effective strategy for preventing or reversing insulin resistance and obesity [99]. On the other hand, obesity-induced endoplasmic reticulum stress recently has been demonstrated to underlie the initiation of inflammatory responses and generation of peripheral insulin resistance [100]. It leads to suppression of insulin receptor signaling through hyperactivation of c-Jun N-terminal kinase and subsequent serine phosphorylation of insulin receptor substrate-1 [101].

In physiology of metabolism, the primary function of WAT is as an energy storage; however, from the immune viewpoint, it is also shown as a big endocrine tissue with the ability to produce a number of proinflammatory cytokines and cause insulin resistance, thereby suppressing lipid synthesis and increasing lipolysis in adipocytes [102]

Many recent results (see Table 38.2) strongly suggest that the principal antiobesity properties of CLA may also rely on other desaturases [103], which may include the isoenzyme SCD2, the stearoyl-CoA desaturase that is required for PPARγ expression and adipogenesis (see Figure 38.4) [104]. CLA may cause insulin resistance through its effects on the insulin-sensitizing hormone adiponectin. Adiponectin mRNA levels were decreased following supplementation with 10, 12-CLA.

The beneficial effects exerted by low amounts of CLA raise the question about their mitochondrial oxidizability. CLA appeared to be both poorly oxidizable and capable of interfering with the oxidation of usual FA at a step close to the beginning of the β-oxidative cycle [99]. It was reported that CLA is more effective than vitamin A in protecting mitochondria from peroxidative damage of 3T3-L1 cells [100]. Our research indicated that CLA-induced apoptosis via mitochondrial pathway through PPARγ signaling reduces mitochondria transmembrane potential, increases mRNA expression of apoptosis regulator Bax and Bcl-2 ratio, and enhances cytochrome c release to cytoplasm and activation of caspase-3 (reversed by pan-caspase inhibitor). CLA reduced mRNA expression of cyclin D and increased mRNA expression of p53 and p21^{waf-1}, but increased mRNA expression of GADD45. In addition, research found that CLA inhibits the elongation and desaturation of 18:2n-6 into 20:4n-6. One might speculate that a diet enriched in CLA would be useful in preventing carcinoma [101].

CLA on Gene Expression: PPARs, Signal Transduction, and Adipokines

Adipocytes act not only as a fuel storage depot but also as a critical endocrine organ that secretes a variety of signaling molecules into the circulation; they play a central role in the maintenance of energy homeostasis by regulating insulin secretion and glucose and lipid metabolism. These secretory factors include enzymes, growth factors, cytokines, and hormones involved in fatty acid and glucose metabolism. For gene expression, the PPARs are ligand-activated transcription factors. PPAR family comprises three closely related gene products—PPARα, PPARγ, and PPARδ/β—and is so named because PPARα is activated that elicits increases in the number and size of peroxisomes. Fatty acids, eicosanoids, and some drugs are PPAR ligands; PPAR-α regulates fatty acid oxidation primarily in liver. PPARγ serves as a key regulator of adipocyte differentiation and lipid storage, while PPARδ is a positive factor for fat burning. PPARs function as important coregulators of energy homeostasis. Moreover, both PPARγ-1 and PPARγ-2 isoforms are generated by alternative splicing; PPARγ 1 isoform is expressed in liver and other

TABLE 38.2

Effect of Δ6-Desaturase Inhibition on Feed Intake, Body Weight, and Tissue Weights

| | Diets[a] | | | | | | | | Significance | | | |
| | INH0 | | INH10 | | INH30 | | INH100 | | | | | |
Criteria[b]	−CLA	+CLA	−CLA	+CLA	−CLA	+CLA	−CLA	+CLA	INH	CLA	INX × CLA	SEM
FI-week 1 (g/day)	5.14	4.81	5.33	4.86	5.30	4.70	4.92	4.71	0.055	**0.001**	0.257	0.101
FI-week 2 (g/day)	5.08	4.47	4.89	4.55	4.01	4.62	4.91	4.40	0.538	**0.001**	0.648	0.116
BW-int. (g)	38.10	37.86	38.36	37.39	37.86	37.29	37.74	38.57	0.626	0.466	0.228	0.453
BW-fin. (g)	39.35	37.18	38.68	37.41	38.36	36.78	39.14	37.43	0.609	**0.001**	0.614	0.555
RP fat (g)	0.35	0.16	0.27	0.12	0.28	0.08	0.20	0.15	0.088	**0.001**	0.123	0.033
EPI fat (g)	0.46	0.26	0.38	0.27	0.41	0.18	0.35	0.28	0.468	**0.001**	0.224	0.043
Liver (g)	1.86	2.03	1.94	2.05	1.99	2.17	2.59	2.59	**0.001**	**0.011**	0.447	0.063
Lean (g)	26.43	26.33	26.27	26.57	25.98	26.57	26.50	26.46	0.924	0.399	0.653	0.309

Source: Adapted from Hargrave-Barnes, K.M. et al., *Obesity*, 16(10), 2245, 2008. With permission.

Main effects or interactions that are significant (P < 0.05) are indicated in boldface.

[a] Diets: AIN-93G diet with 7% soy oil; INH = Δ6-desaturase inhibitor SC-26196 at 0, 10, 30, or 100 mg kg BW^{-1} d^{-1}; CLA (conjugated linoleic acid) = 0% or 0.5% CLA isomers, n = 18–19 per diet.

[b] FI-week 1 = feed intake in week 1 (g/day), FI-week 2 = feed intake in week 2 (g/day), BW-int. = initial body weight (g), BW-fin. = final body weight (g), RP fat = 2 retroperitoneal pads (g), EPI fat = 1 epididymal fat pad (g), liver = whole liver (g), lean = lean mass as determined by dual x-ray densitometry (g).

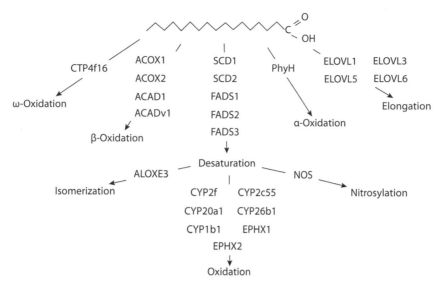

FIGURE 38.4 Diagram showing the multiple pathways of fatty acid metabolism in adipocytes. The double bond in a desaturated fatty acid may then change position through isomerases or be nitrated or oxidized, producing various side groups on the fatty acid. EPHX, epoxide hydrolase; ACOX, acyl-CoA oxidase. (Adapted from Christianson, J.L. et al., *J. Biol. Chem.*, 283(5), 2906, 2008. With permission.)

tissues, whereas PPARγ-2 isoform is expressed exclusively in adipose tissue, where it regulates adipogenesis and lipogenesis. Oxidized LDL regulates macrophage gene expression also through ligand activation of PPARγ [105].

ICR and C57BL/6J mice fed with experimental diets containing CLA greatly decreased weights of WAT and interscapular brown adipose tissue (BAT) in the two strains [106]. It is apparent that dietary CLA's function accompanies changes in the gene expression of proteins regulating energy metabolism in WAT and BAT and skeletal muscle of mice. Inhibition of lipid accumulation induced by t10c12-CLA treatment during adipocyte differentiation is associated with a tight regulatory process between early (PPARγ and C/EBPα) and late (LXRα, aP2, and CD36) adipogenic marker genes [107]. Furthermore, we also confirmed the effects of c9t11- and t10c12-isomers of CLA on the expression of adipogenic genes, results shown in Table 38.3.

TABLE 38.3

Inhibitory Effect of c9t11- and t10c12-CLA in Differentiated 3T3-L1 Cells

Sample	Concentration (ppm)	Inhibitory Activity (%) ($P < 0.05$)		
		SREBP-1	C/EBPα	PPARγ
c9t11-CLA	10	4.14 ± 4.56 a	6.28 ± 1.53 a	0.48 ± 4.28 a
	15	9.99 ± 2.42 a	16.05 ± 2.42 b	7.06 ± 2.09 a
	20	7.09 ± 3.09 a	18.29 ± 1.94 b	7.27 ± 5.67 a
	25	9.87 ± 1.39 a	17.20 ± 1.38 b	19.45 ± 2.99 b
t10c12-CLA	10	2.02 ± 2.15 a	12.46 ± 1.38 a	5.82 ± 2.58 a
	15	1.69 ± 6.10 a	23.79 ± 2.20 b	9.29 ± 4.27 a
	20	13.86 ± 2.46 a	34.09 ± 1.19 c	32.46 ± 3.88 c
	25	35.8 ± 3.87 b	56.06 ± 3.19 d	61.39 ± 5.02 d

The t10c12-CLA at concentration 25 μg/L significantly decreased the mRNA expression of C/EBPα, PPARγ, and SREBP-1, and in a dose-dependent manner. However, c9t11- CLA presents no inhibitive function on the expression of SREBP-1. t10c12-CLA also decreases the triglyceride content of newly differentiated human adipocytes by inducing MEK/ERK signaling through the autocrine/paracrine actions of IL-6 and 8 [108]. Collectively, CLA may impart its effects by increasing expression of genes associated with apoptosis, fatty acid oxidation, lipolysis, and inflammation, as well as decreasing stromal vascular cell differentiation and lipogenesis [72].

Effects of c9t11-CLA on C/EBPα mRNA expression in 3T3-L1 adipocytes: 2 day postconfluent 3T3-L1 cells were differentiated by MDI and treated with CLA. On day 8 after induction of differentiation, total RNA was extracted from 3T3-L1 cells and subjected to RT-PCR with primers specific for C/EBPα.

Serum leptin is correlated to body fat level, acting in the hypothalamus to regulate satiety [109]. Leptin, a cytokine, is the ob gene product from mature adipocytes; its expression is accelerated at obesity state that inhibits food intake and accelerates energy expenditure. Dietary CLA is found to acutely reduce serum leptin level in Sprague–Dawley rats [110].

ANTIADIPOGENESIS OF CLA INVOLVED IN ESTROGEN RECEPTOR? RA RECEPTOR?

Estrogen receptor alpha that plays an important role in mediating estrogen signaling is involved in osteoporosis and obesity [111,112]. Interestingly, obesity is positively associated with breast cancer for postmenopausal women [113]. Estradiol affects the metabolic action of insulin in a concentration-dependent manner such that high concentrations of estradiol inhibit insulin signaling by modulating phosphorylation of IRS-1 via a JNK-dependent pathway [114]. In addition, estrogens and phytoestrogen genistein are also found to regulate adipogenesis and lipogenesis in males and females [115]. CLA compounds possess potent antiestrogenic properties that may partly account for their antitumor activity on breast cancer cells [116,117] caused by inducing the dephosphorylation of estrogen receptor alpha through stimulation of protein phosphatase 2A activity [118]. Nevertheless, at present, no direct evidence to approve the antiestrogenic pathway of CLA contributes to its antiobesity functions.

Retinoids modulate various biological functions, such as cell differentiation, proliferation, and embryonic development, through specific nuclear receptors—RAR and RXR—and their endogenous ligands are all-*trans*-retinoic acid and 9-*cis*-retinoic acid, respectively [119–121]. We and some researcher [122] are convinced that CLA induces apoptosis of 3T3-L1 preadipocyte, through reduced mRNA expression of cyclin D (see Figures 38.5 and 38.6) and increased mRNA expression of p53, GADD45, and p21waf-1, but does not activate RAR in a reporter gene assay.

IMMUNE VIEWPOINT: CLA ON INFLAMMATION AND OXIDATIVE STRESS

Metabolic and immune responses are highly integrated and interdependent. The link between obesity and diabetes is firmly established by inflammatory mediators. Peripheral blood mononuclear cells in obesity are in a proinflammatory state with an increase in intranuclear NFκB binding [123]. NFκB plays a key role in inflammatory and immune responses [124]. TNFα and adiponectin are antagonistic in stimulating NFκB activation. In 3T3-L1 adipocytes model, NGF, a neurotrophin, is shown as an important inflammatory response protein. NGF is secreted in WAT, with synthesis being influenced by TNFα [125].

In response to proinflammatory cytokines such as TNFα, the IκB kinase is activated, further stimulating the formation of additional inflammatory cytokines, along with adhesion molecules which promote endothelial dysfunction and downstream modulation of specific metabolic syndrome. TNFα induces oxidative stress, which leads to oxidized low-density lipoprotein and dyslipidemia, insulin resistance, hypertension, endothelial dysfunction, and atherogenesis [126].

Elevated levels of oxidative stress in obesity correlated with fat accumulation in humans and mice [127], selective increase of ROS, augmented expression of NADPH oxidase and decreased

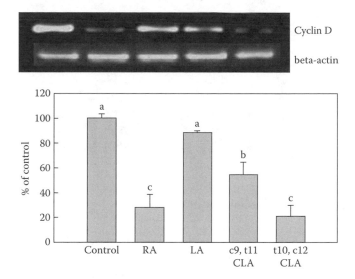

FIGURE 38.5 Effects of 10 μM RA, 200 μM LA, c9t11-CLA, and t10c12-CLA on cyclin D mRNA expression. 3T3-L1 preadipocytes treated for 6 h. Results are expressed as mean ± SD for n = 3 each group (P < 0.05).

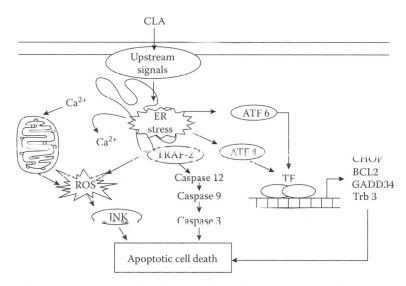

FIGURE 38.6 CLA increases apoptotic cell death of preadipocytes by increasing ER stress. These stress responses increase the levels of intracellular calcium, ROS, and proteins that together induce apoptosis. (Adapted from Kennedy, A. et al., *J. Nutr. Biochem.*, 21(3), 171, 2010. With permission.)

expression of antioxidative enzymes, and dysregulated production of adipocytokines are the important pathogenic mechanisms of obesity-associated metabolic syndrome [128]. Overall, serum concentrations of CRP, TNFα, and IL-6 were significantly correlated with weight, BMI, and visceral adipose tissue [129,130]. Leptin expression is accelerated at obesity state; similar to other proinflammatory cytokines, it promotes Th1 cell differentiation and cytokine production [131]. Leukocyte populations within adipose tissue, which may be involved in the development of elevated inflammation that is characteristic of obesity [132].

Both the innate and acquired immune responses are affected by dietary CLA supplementation. *In vitro* studies of the use of immune cells and animal models demonstrate that CLA modulates immune function and enhances IL-2 production and lymphocyte proliferation but decreases TNFα and IL-6 production [133]. We also confirmed the effect of CLA isoforms on TNFα production in

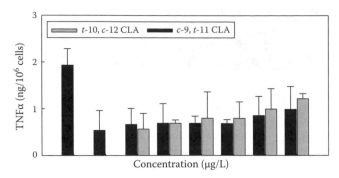

FIGURE 38.7 Production of TNFα by human monocytic THP-1 cells treated with CLA. The concentration of TNFα in the cell supernatant was measured by ELISA.

human monocyte assay, and c9t11-CLA seems to work more effectively (see Figure 38.7). There is a slight but significant difference between the functionalities of triglyceride and free dietary CLA in modulating immunoglobulin and various cytokine productions [41]. In a double-blind, randomized, parallel, reference-controlled intervention study on human immune function, it was found that CLA may beneficially affect the initiation of a specific response to a hepatitis B vaccination [134].

Nitrolinoleic acid, LNO_2, formed via nitric oxide–dependent oxidative inflammatory reactions, is a potent endogenous ligand for PPARγ. NO-mediated cell signaling reactions can be transduced by FA nitration products and PPARs-dependent gene expression [135]. CLA in endotoxin LPS-activated inflammatory events in macrophages (to enhance TNFα production), negatively regulating expression of inflammatory mediators [136], decreases both PGE2 and NO synthesis by suppressing transcription of COX-2 and iNOS [137]. A report reveals that CLA significantly ($P < 0.05$) depressed rat PGF synthesis in placenta, uterus, and liver [138]. On the other hand, results also indicated that the t10c12-CLA supplementation led to a marked increase in human plasma CRP, a marker of inflammation and oxidative stress, compared with the placebo.

The adipokine resistin displays potent proinflammatory properties by strongly upregulating IL-6 and TNFα, which were abrogated by NFκB inhibitor [139]. The t10c12-CLA performing as an antioxidant promotes, at least in part, NFκB activation and subsequent induction of IL-6, which are partly responsible for suppression of PPARγ target gene expression and insulin sensitivity in mature human adipocytes [140]. On the other hand, c9t11-CLA possessed weak antioxidant activity, whereas at 200 μM higher concentration, it acts as a strong prooxidant [141]. Taken together, it is likely that CLA modulates the accumulation of arachidonic acid in phospholipids, resulting in a reduced arachidonic acid pool and reduced production of downstream PGE2, and following anti-inflammation [34].

CONCLUSION

Either aging or hypertrophy is associated with increased body fat and insulin resistance and with a higher risk for CVDs. What happens in obese tissue? Here, we propose that obese tissue may be activated via cell–cell interaction due to sustainable cell proliferation and size enlargement, which trigger progressive inflammation and related adipokine secretion from adipocyte, such as resistin, displaying potent proinflammatory properties and inducing mitochondrial dysfunction as well as metabolic syndrome later. Those complicated mechanisms are involved in immune response, gene expression, and intracellular signal transduction, which CLA or its specific isoform somehow, partly, performs positive biological activity.

However, from the review of updated research data, from *in vitro* to *in vivo* investigation, even in human clinic study, including functions, mechanisms, and safety of dietary CLA, we must conclude that it is still insufficient and ambiguous at present. Despite conflicting results, likely due to large variability in protocols used, the use of CLA for weight management in human should be under medical control. Meanwhile noteworthily, the question of the safety of high dosage dietary CLA supplements is raised. In addition, the development of a commercially available functional food—CLA in soft gelatin capsules—may not be best way to fit the consumer taste demand and to have the best bioavailability of the active form. Finally, a new approach to this problem may be a low glycemic index diet, referring to the effect of food on blood sugar and insulin level after a meal. It may be a practical and safe approach to the prevention and treatment of obesity and related complications.

So, taken together, are antiobesity effects of CLA fact or fiction? Maybe the keypoint that we actually need to be concerned is morbid obesity and NOT obesity itself. Nevertheless, it is somehow vexatious and inconvenient. In this viewpoint, if any bioactive ingredient can prevent or ameliorate (but not cure or recover as a pharmaceutical drug) obesity-induced diseases, for public health benefit, we may suggest it as a dietary supplement.

REFERENCES

1. Ha, Y. L., Grimm, N. K., and Pariza, M. W., Anticarcinogens from fried ground beef: Heat-altered derivatives of linoleic acid, *Carcinogenesis* 8(12), 1881–1887, 1987.
2. Wang, Y. W. and Jones, P. J., Conjugated linoleic acid and obesity control: Efficacy and mechanisms, *Int J Obes Relat Metab Disord* 28(8), 941–955, 2004.
3. Park, Y., Storkson, J. M., Albright, K. J., Liu, W., and Pariza, M. W., Biological activities of conjugated fatty acids: Conjugated eicosadienoic, eicosatrienoic, heneicosadienoic acids and other metabolites of conjugated linoleic acid, *Biochim Biophys Acta* 1687(1–3), 120–129, 2005.
4. Park, Y., Albright, K. J., Storkson, J. M., Liu, W., Cook, M. E., and Pariza, M. W., Changes in body composition in mice during feeding and withdrawal of conjugated linolcic acid, *Lipids* 34(3), 243–248, 1999.
5. Bhattacharya, A., Rahman, M. M., Sun, D., Lawrence, R., Mejia, W., McCarter, R., O'Shea, M., and Fernandes, G., The combination of dietary conjugated linoleic acid and treadmill exercise lowers gain in body fat mass and enhances lean body mass in high fat-fed male Balb/C mice, *J Nutr* 135(5), 1124–1130, 2005.
6. Mirand, P. P., Arnal-Bagnard, M. A., Mosoni, L., Faulconnier, Y., Chardigny, J. M., and Chilliard, Y., Cis-9, trans-11 and trans-10, cis-12 conjugated linoleic acid isomers do not modify body composition in adult sedentary or exercised rats, *J Nutr* 134(9), 2263–2269, 2004.
7. Iacazio, G., Easy access to various natural keto polyunsaturated fatty acids and their corresponding racemic alcohols, *Chem Phys Lipids* 125(2), 115–121, 2003.
8. Hamalainen, T. I., Sundberg, S., Hase, T., and Hopia, A., Stereochemistry of the hydroperoxides formed during autooxidation of CLA methyl ester in the presence of alpha-tocopherol, *Lipids* 37(6), 533–540, 2002.
9. Burger, F., Krieg, P., Marks, F., and Furstenberger, G., Positional- and stereo selectivity of fatty acid oxygenation catalysed by mouse (12S)-lipoxygenase isoenzymes, *Biochem J* 348(Pt 2), 329–335, 2000.
10. Sehat, N., Kramer, J. K., Mossoba, M. M., Yurawecz, M. P., Roach, J. A., Eulitz, K., Morehouse, K. M., and Ku, Y., Identification of conjugated linoleic acid isomers in cheese by gas chromatography, silver ion high performance liquid chromatography and mass spectral reconstructed ion profiles. Comparison of chromatographic elution sequences, *Lipids* 33(10), 963–971, 1998.
11. Parodi, P. W., Cows' milk fat components as potential anticarcinogenic agents, *J Nutr* 127(6), 1055–1060, 1997.
12. Gruffat, D., De La Torre, A., Chardigny, J. M., Durand, D., Loreau, O., and Bauchart, D., Vaccenic acid metabolism in the liver of rat and bovine, *Lipids* 40(3), 295–301, 2005.
13. Lock, A. L. and Bauman, D. E., Modifying milk fat composition of dairy cows to enhance fatty acids beneficial to human health, *Lipids* 39(12), 1197–1206, 2004.
14. Kay, J. K., Mackle, T. R., Auldist, M. J., Thomson, N. A., and Bauman, D. E., Endogenous synthesis of cis-9, trans-11 conjugated linoleic acid in dairy cows fed fresh pasture, *J Dairy Sci* 87(2), 369–378, 2004.
15. Luna, P., Fontecha, J., Juarez, M., and de la Fuente, M. A., Conjugated linoleic acid in ewe milk fat, *J Dairy Res* 72(4), 415–424, 2005.
16. Luna, P., de la Fuente, M. A., and Juarez, M., Conjugated linoleic acid in processed cheeses during the manufacturing stages, *J Agric Food Chem* 53(7), 2690–2695, 2005.
17. Destaillats, F., Trottier, J. P., Galvez, J. M., and Angers, P., Analysis of alpha-linolenic acid biohydrogenation intermediates in milk fat with emphasis on conjugated linolenic acids, *J Dairy Sci* 88(9), 3231–3239, 2005.

18. Destaillats, F., Japiot, C., Chouinard, P. Y., Arul, J., and Angers, P., Short communication: Rearrangement of rumenic acid in ruminant fats: A marker of thermal treatment, *J Dairy Sci* 88(5), 1631–1635, 2005.

19. Ma, D. W., Wierzbicki, A. A., Field, C. J., and Clandinin, M. T., Conjugated linoleic acid in Canadian dairy and beef products, *J Agric Food Chem* 47(5), 1956–1960, 1999.

20. Jiang, J., Wolk, A., and Vessby, B., Relation between the intake of milk fat and the occurrence of conjugated linoleic acid in human adipose tissue, *Am J Clin Nutr* 70(1), 21–27, 1999.

21. Baylin, A., Kabagambe, E. K., Siles, X., and Campos, H., Adipose tissue biomarkers of fatty acid intake, *Am J Clin Nutr* 76(4), 750–757, 2002.

22. Wolk, A., Furuheim, M., and Vessby, B., Fatty acid composition of adipose tissue and serum lipids are valid biological markers of dairy fat intake in men, *J Nutr* 131(3), 828–833, 2001.

23. AbuGhazaleh, A. A., Schingoethe, D. J., Hippen, A. R., and Kalscheur, K. F., Milk conjugated linoleic acid response to fish oil supplementation of diets differing in fatty acid profiles, *J Dairy Sci* 86(3), 944–953, 2003.

24. Boue, C., Combe, N., Billeaud, C., Mignerot, C., Entressangles, B., Thery, G., Geoffrion, H., Brun, J. L., Dallay, D., and Leng, J. J., Trans fatty acids in adipose tissue of French women in relation to their dietary sources, *Lipids* 35(5), 561–566, 2000.

25. Polan, C. E., McNeill, J. J., and Tove, S. B., Biohydrogenation of unsaturated fatty acids by rumen bacteria, *J Bacteriol* 88, 1056–1064, 1964.

26. Hughes, P. E., Hunter, W. J., and Tove, S. B., Biohydrogenation of unsaturated fatty acids. Purification and properties of cis-9,trans-11-octadecadienoate reductase, *J Biol Chem* 257(7), 3643–3649, 1982.

27. Inouye, M., Hashimoto, H., Mio, T., and Sumino, K., Levels of lipid peroxidation product and glycated hemoglobin A1c in the erythrocytes of diabetic patients, *Clin Chim Acta* 276(2), 163–172, 1998.

28. Palmquist, D. L., Lock, A. L., Shingfield, K. J., and Bauman, D. E., Biosynthesis of conjugated linoleic acid in ruminants and humans, *Adv Food Nutr Res* 50, 179–217, 2005.

29. Delmonte, P., Roach, J. A., Mossoba, M. M., Losi, G., and Yurawecz, M. P., Synthesis, isolation, and GC analysis of all the 6,8- to 13,15-cis/trans conjugated linoleic acid isomers, *Lipids* 39(2), 185–191, 2004.

30. Delmonte, P., Kataok, A., Corl, B. A., Bauman, D. E., and Yurawecz, M. P., Relative retention order of all isomers of cis/trans conjugated linoleic acid FAME from the 6,8- to 13,15-positions using silver ion HPLC with two elution systems, *Lipids* 40(5), 509–514, 2005.

31. Turpeinen, A. M., Mutanen, M., Aro, A., Salminen, I., Basu, S., Palmquist, D. L., and Griinari, J. M., Bioconversion of vaccenic acid to conjugated linoleic acid in humans, *Am J Clin Nutr* 76(3), 504–510, 2002.

32. Santora, J. E., Palmquist, D. L., and Roehrig, K. L., Trans-vaccenic acid is desaturated to conjugated linoleic acid in mice, *J Nutr* 130(2), 208–215, 2000.

33. Griinari, J. and Bauman, D., Biosynthesis of conjugated linoleic acid in its incorporation into meat and milk ruminants, *Advances in Conjugated Linoleic Acid Research*, Vol. 1. Champaign, IL: AOCS Press, pp. 180–200, 1999.

34. Tanaka, K., Occurrence of conjugated linoleic acid in ruminant products and its physiological functions, *Anim Sci J* 76, 291–303, 2005.

35. Ogawa, J., Kishino, S., Ando, A., Sugimoto, S., Mihara, K., and Shimizu, S., Production of conjugated fatty acids by lactic acid bacteria, *J Biosci Bioeng* 100(4), 355–364, 2005.

36. Ho, S. S. and Pal, S., Conjugated linoleic acid suppresses the secretion of atherogenic lipoproteins from human HepG2 liver cells, *Asia Pac J Clin Nutr* 13(Suppl), S70, 2004.

37. Yamasaki, M., Nishida, E., Nou, S., Tachibana, H., and Yamada, K., Cytotoxity of the trans10,cis12 isomer of conjugated linoleic acid on rat hepatoma and its modulation by other fatty acids, tocopherol, and tocotrienol, *In Vitro Cell Dev Biol Anim* 41(7), 239–244, 2005.

38. Yamasaki, M., Miyamoto, Y., Chujo, H., Nishiyama, K., Tachibana, H., and Yamada, K., Trans10, cis12-conjugated linoleic acid induces mitochondria-related apoptosis and lysosomal destabilization in rat hepatoma cells, *Biochim Biophys Acta* 1735(3), 176–184, 2005.

39. Blankson, H., Stakkestad, J. A., Fagertun, H., Thom, E., Wadstein, J., and Gudmundsen, O., Conjugated linoleic acid reduces body fat mass in overweight and obese humans, *J Nutr* 130(12), 2943–2948, 2000.

40. Lee, J. H., Cho, K. H., Lee, K. T., and Kim, M. R., Antiatherogenic effects of structured lipid containing conjugated linoleic acid in C57BL/6J mice, *J Agric Food Chem* 53(18), 7295–7301, 2005.

41. Yamasaki, M., Kitagawa, T., Chujo, H., Koyanagi, N., Nishida, E., Nakaya, M., Yoshimi, K., Maeda, H., Nou, S., Iwata, T., Ogita, K., Tachibana, H., and Yamada, K., Physiological difference between free and triglyceride-type conjugated linoleic acid on the immune function of C57BL/6N mice, *J Agric Food Chem* 52(11), 3644–3648, 2004.

42. Poirier, H., Rouault, C., Clement, L., Niot, I., Monnot, M. C., Guerre-Millo, M., and Besnard, P., Hyperinsulinaemia triggered by dietary conjugated linoleic acid is associated with a decrease in leptin and adiponectin plasma levels and pancreatic beta cell hyperplasia in the mouse, *Diabetologia* 48(6), 1059–1065, 2005.

43. Park, Y., Albright, K. J., and Pariza, M. W., Effects of conjugated linoleic acid on long term feeding in Fischer 344 rats, *Food Chem Toxicol* 43(8), 1273–1279, 2005.

44. Wanders, A. J., Leder, L., Banga, J. D., Katan, M. B., and Brouwer, I. A., A high intake of conjugated linoleic acid does not affect liver and kidney function tests in healthy human subjects, *Food Chem Toxicol* 48(2), 587–590, 2010.

45. Sharma, A. M. and Chetty, V. T., Obesity, hypertension and insulin resistance, *Acta Diabetol* 42(Suppl 1), S3–S8, 2005.

46. Singhal, A., Endothelial dysfunction: Role in obesity-related disorders and the early origins of CVD, *Proc Nutr Soc* 64(1), 15–22, 2005.

47. Zhang, F., Chen, Y., Heiman, M., and Dimarchi, R., Leptin: structure, function and biology, *Vitam Horm* 71, 345–372, 2005.

48. Bates, S. H., Kulkarni, R. N., Seifert, M., and Myers, M. G., Jr., Roles for leptin receptor/STAT3-dependent and -independent signals in the regulation of glucose homeostasis, *Cell Metab* 1(3), 169–178, 2005.

49. Park, H. S., Park, J. Y., and Yu, R., Relationship of obesity and visceral adiposity with serum concentrations of CRP, TNF-alpha and IL-6, *Diabetes Res Clin Pract* 69(1), 29–35, 2005.

50. Mandato, C., Lucariello, S., Licenziati, M. R., Franzese, A., Spagnuolo, M. I., Ficarella, R., Pacilio, M., Amitrano, M., Capuano, G., Meli, R., and Vajro, P., Metabolic, hormonal, oxidative, and inflammatory factors in pediatric obesity-related liver disease, *J Pediatr* 147(1), 62–66, 2005.

51. Trayhurn, P., Adipose tissue in obesity—An inflammatory issue, *Endocrinology* 146(3), 1003–1005, 2005.

52. Wellen, K. E. and Hotamisligil, G. S., Inflammation, stress, and diabetes, *J Clin Invest* 115(5), 1111–1119, 2005.

53. Trayhurn, P. and Wood, I. S., Signalling role of adipose tissue: Adipokines and inflammation in obesity, *Biochem Soc Trans* 33(Pt 5), 1078–1081, 2005.

54. Appel, S. J., Harrell, J. S., and Davenport, M. L., Central obesity, the metabolic syndrome, and plasminogen activator inhibitor-1 in young adults, *J Am Acad Nurse Pract* 17(12), 535–541, 2005.

55. Druet, C., Tubiana-Rufi, N., Chevenne, D., Rigal, O., Polak, M., and Levy-Marchal, C., Characterization of insulin secretion and resistance in type 2 diabetes of adolescents, *J Clin Endocrinol Metab* 91(2), 401–404, 2006.

56. Grove, K. L., Grayson, B. E., Glavas, M. M., Xiao, X. Q., and Smith, M. S., Development of metabolic systems, *Physiol Behav* 86, 646–660, 2005.

57. Volek, J. S. und Feinman, R. D., Carbohydrate restriction improves the features of metabolic syndrome. Metabolic syndrome may be defined by the response to carbohydrate restriction, *Nutr Metab (Lond)* 2(1), 31, 2005.

58. Chaldakov, G. N., Fiore, M., Hristova, M. G., and Aloe, L., Metabotrophic potential of neurotrophins: Implication in obesity and related diseases? *Med Sci Monit* 9(10), HY19–HY21, 2003.

59. Hristova, M. and Aloe, L., Metabolic syndrome—Neurotrophic hypothesis, *Med Hypotheses* 66(3), 545–549, 2006.

60. Duff, E. and Baile, C. A., Ciliary neurotrophic factor: a role in obesity? *Nutr Rev* 61(12), 423–426, 2003.

61. Xu, H., Barnes, G. T., Yang, Q., Tan, G., Yang, D., Chou, C. J., Sole, J., Nichols, A., Ross, J. S., Tartaglia, L. A., and Chen, H., Chronic inflammation in fat plays a crucial role in the development of obesity-related insulin resistance, *J Clin Invest* 112(12), 1821–1830, 2003.

62. Trayhurn, P. and Wood, I. S., Adipokines: Inflammation and the pleiotropic role of white adipose tissue, *Br J Nutr* 92(3), 347–355, 2004.

63. Yue, G. P., Du, L. R., Xia, T., He, X. H., Qiu, H., Xu, L. H., Chen, X. D., Feng, S. Q., and Yang, Z. Q., One in vitro model for visceral adipose-derived fibroblasts in chronic inflammation, *Biochem Biophys Res Commun* 333(3), 850–857, 2005.

64. Bouloumie, A., Curat, C. A., Sengenes, C., Lolmede, K., Miranville, A., and Busse, R., Role of macrophage tissue infiltration in metabolic diseases, *Curr Opin Clin Nutr Metab Care* 8(4), 347–354, 2005.

65. Cottam, D. R., Mattar, S. G., Barinas-Mitchell, E., Eid, G., Kuller, L., Kelley, D. E., and Schauer, P. R., The chronic inflammatory hypothesis for the morbidity associated with morbid obesity: Implications and effects of weight loss, *Obes Surg* 14(5), 589–600, 2004.

66. Lin, Y. T., Tang, C. H., Chuang, W. J., Wang, S. M., Huang, T. F., and Fu, W. M., Inhibition of adipogenesis by RGD-dependent disintegrin, *Biochem Pharmacol* 70(10), 1469–1478, 2005.

67. Demeulemeester, D., Collen, D., and Lijnen, H. R., Effect of matrix metalloproteinase inhibition on adipose tissue development, *Biochem Biophys Res Commun* 329(1), 105–110, 2005.

68. Chavey, C., Mari, B., Monthouel, M. N., Bonnafous, S., Anglard, P., Van Obberghen, E., and Tartare-Deckert, S., Matrix metalloproteinases are differentially expressed in adipose tissue during obesity and modulate adipocyte differentiation, *J Biol Chem* 278(14), 11888–11896, 2003.

69. Poulos, S. P., Sisk, M., Hausman, D. B., Azain, M. J., and Hausman, G. J., Pre- and postnatal dietary conjugated linoleic acid alters adipose development, body weight gain and body composition in Sprague-Dawley rats, *J Nutr* 131(10), 2722–2731, 2001.

70. Belury, M. A., Dietary conjugated linoleic acid in health: Physiological effects and mechanisms of action, *Annu Rev Nutr* 22, 505–531, 2002.

71. Yamasaki, M., Mansho, K., Mishima, H., Kimura, G., Sasaki, M., Kasai, M., Tachibana, H., and Yamada, K., Effect of dietary conjugated linoleic acid on lipid peroxidation and histological change in rat liver tissues, *J Agric Food Chem* 48(12), 6367–6371, 2000.

72. House, R. L., Cassady, J. P., Eisen, E. J., Eling, T. E., Collins, J. B., Grissom, S. F., and Odle, J., Functional genomic characterization of delipidation elicited by trans-10, cis-12-conjugated linoleic acid (t10c12-CLA) in a polygenic obese line of mice, *Physiol Genomics* 21(3), 351–361, 2005.

73. House, R. L., Cassady, J. P., Eisen, E. J., McIntosh, M. K., and Odle, J., Conjugated linoleic acid evokes de-lipidation through the regulation of genes controlling lipid metabolism in adipose and liver tissue, *Obes Rev* 6(3), 247–258, 2005.

74. Park, Y., Storkson, J. M., Liu, W., Albright, K. J., Cook, M. E., and Pariza, M. W., Structure-activity relationship of conjugated linoleic acid and its cognates in inhibiting heparin-releasable lipoprotein lipase and glycerol release from fully differentiated 3T3-L1 adipocytes, *J Nutr Biochem* 15(9), 561–568, 2004.

75. Halade, G. V., Rahman, M. M., and Fernandes, G., Differential effects of conjugated linoleic acid isomers in insulin-resistant female C57Bl/6J mice, *J Nutr Biochem* 21(4), 332–337, 2010.

76. Lamarche, B. and Desroches, S., Metabolic syndrome and effects of conjugated linoleic acid in obesity and lipoprotein disorders: The Quebec experience, *Am J Clin Nutr* 79(6 Suppl), 1149S–1152S, 2004.

77. Carta, G., Angioni, E., Murru, E., Melis, M. P., Spada, S., and Banni, S., Modulation of lipid metabolism and vitamin A by conjugated linoleic acid, *Prostaglandins Leukot Essent Fatty Acids* 67(2–3), 187–191, 2002.

78. Poirier, H., Niot, I., Clement, L., Guerre-Millo, M., and Besnard, P., Development of conjugated linoleic acid (CLA)-mediated lipoatrophic syndrome in the mouse, *Biochimie* 87(1), 73–79, 2005.

79. Tsuzuki, T. and Ikeda, I., Slow absorption of conjugated linoleic acid in rat intestines, and similar absorption rates of 9c,11t-conjugated linoleic acid and 10t,12c-conjugated linoleic acid, *Biosci Biotechnol Biochem* 71(8), 2034–2040, 2007.

80. Kim, J. H., Pan, J. H., Park, H. G. et al., Functional comparison of esterified and free forms of conjugated linoleic acid in high-fat-diet-induced obese C57BL/6J mice, *J Agric Food Chem* 58(21), 11441–11447, 2010.

81. Ide, T., Interaction of fish oil and conjugated linoleic acid in affecting hepatic activity of lipogenic enzymes and gene expression in liver and adipose tissue, *Diabetes* 54(2), 412, 2005.

82. Friedman, J. M., Obesity in the new millennium, *Nature* 404(6778), 632–634, 2000.

83. Spiegelman, B. M. and Flier, J. S., Obesity and the regulation of energy balance, *Cell* 104(4), 531–543, 2001.

84. Neal, J. W. and Clipstone, N. A., A constitutively active NFATc1 mutant induces a transformed phenotype in 3T3-L1 fibroblasts, *J Biol Chem* 278(19), 17246–17254, 2003.

85. Russell, T. R. and Ho, R., Conversion of 3T3 fibroblasts into adipose cells: Triggering of differentiation by prostaglandin F2alpha and 1-methyl-3-isobutyl xanthine, *Proc Natl Acad Sci USA* 73(12), 4516–4520, 1976.

86. Toscani, A., Soprano, D. R., and Soprano, K. J., Sodium butyrate in combination with insulin or dexamethasone can terminally differentiate actively proliferating Swiss 3T3 cells into adipocytes, *J Biol Chem* 265(10), 5722–5730, 1990.

87. Rosen, E. D., Hsu, C. H., Wang, X., Sakai, S., Freeman, M. W., Gonzalez, F. J., and Spiegelman, B. M., C/EBPalpha induces adipogenesis through PPARgamma: A unified pathway, *Genes Dev* 16(1), 22–26, 2002.

88. Fu, M., Sun, T., Bookout, A. L., Downes, M., Yu, R. T., Evans, R. M., and Mangelsdorf, D. J., A nuclear receptor atlas: 3T3-L1 adipogenesis, *Mol Endocrinol* 19(10), 2437–2450, 2005.

89. Doi, H., Masaki, N., Takahashi, H., Komatsu, H., Fujimori, K., and Satomi, S., A new preadipocyte cell line, AP-18, established from adult mouse adipose tissue, *Tohoku J Exp Med* 207(3), 209–216, 2005.

90. Boudina, S., Sena, S., O'Neill, B. T., Tathireddy, P., Young, M. E., and Abel, E. D., Reduced mitochondrial oxidative capacity and increased mitochondrial uncoupling impair myocardial energetics in obesity, *Circulation* 112(17), 2686–2695, 2005.

91. Lee, H. K., Park, K. S., Cho, Y. M., Lee, Y. Y., and Pak, Y. K., Mitochondria-based model for fetal origin of adult disease and insulin resistance, *Ann NY Acad Sci* 1042, 1–18, 2005.

92. Parish, R. and Petersen, K. F., Mitochondrial dysfunction and type 2 diabetes, *Curr Diab Rep* 5(3), 177–183, 2005.

93. Brand, M. D. and Esteves, T. C., Physiological functions of the mitochondrial uncoupling proteins UCP2 and UCP3, *Cell Metab* 2(2), 85–93, 2005.

94. Ricquier, D., Respiration uncoupling and metabolism in the control of energy expenditure, *Proc Nutr Soc* 64(1), 47–52, 2005.

95. Koves, T. R., Li, P., An, J., Akimoto, T., Slentz, D., Ilkayeva, O., Dohm, G. L., Yan, Z., Newgard, C. B., and Muoio, D. M., Peroxisome proliferator-activated receptor-gamma co-activator 1alpha-mediated metabolic remodeling of skeletal myocytes mimics exercise training and reverses lipid-induced mitochondrial inefficiency, *J Biol Chem* 280(39), 33588–33598, 2005.

96. McCarty, M. F., Up-regulation of PPARgamma coactivator-1alpha as a strategy for preventing and reversing insulin resistance and obesity, *Med Hypotheses* 64(2), 399–407, 2005.

97. Hotamisligil, G. S., Role of endoplasmic reticulum stress and c-Jun NH2-terminal kinase pathways in inflammation and origin of obesity and diabetes, *Diabetes* 54(suppl_2), S73–S78, 2005.

98. Ozcan, U., Cao, Q., Yilmaz, E., Lee, A. H., Iwakoshi, N. N., Ozdelen, E., Tuncman, G., Gorgun, C., Glimcher, L. H., and Hotamisligil, G. S., Endoplasmic reticulum stress links obesity, insulin action, and type 2 diabetes, *Science* 306(5695), 457–461, 2004.

99. Demizieux, L., Degrace, P., Gresti, J., Loreau, O., Noel, J. P., Chardigny, J. M., Sebedio, J. L., and Clouet, P., Conjugated linoleic acid isomers in mitochondria: Evidence for an alteration of fatty acid oxidation, *J Lipid Res* 43(12), 2112–2122, 2002.

100. Palacios, A., Piergiacomi, V., and Catala, A., Antioxidant effect of conjugated linoleic acid and vitamin A during non enzymatic lipid peroxidation of rat liver microsomes and mitochondria, *Mol Cell Biochem* 250(1–2), 107–113, 2003.

101. Hoffmann, K., Blaudszun, J., Brunken, C., Hopker, W. W., Tauber, R., and Steinhart, H., Distribution of polyunsaturated fatty acids including conjugated linoleic acids in total and subcellular fractions from healthy and cancerous parts of human kidneys, *Lipids* 40(3), 309–315, 2005.

102. Kennedy, A., Martinez, K., Schmidt, S., Mandrup, S., LaPoint, K., and McIntosh, M., Antiobesity mechanisms of action of conjugated linoleic acid, *J Nutr Biochem* 21(3), 171–179, 2010.

103. Hargrave-Barnes, K. M., Azain, M. J., and Miner, J. L., Conjugated linoleic acid-induced fat loss dependence on [delta]6-desaturase or cyclooxygenase, *Obesity* 16(10), 2245–2252, 2008.

104. Christianson, J. L., Nicoloro, S., Straubhaar, J., and Czech, M. P., Stearoyl-CoA desaturase 2 is required for peroxisome proliferator-activated receptor γ expression and adipogenesis in cultured 3T3-L1 cells, *J Biol Chem* 283(5), 2906–2916, 2008.

105. Nagy, L., Tontonoz, P., Alvarez, J. G., Chen, H., and Evans, R. M., Oxidized LDL regulates macrophage gene expression through ligand activation of PPARgamma, *Cell* 93(2), 229–240, 1998.

106. Takahashi, Y., Kushiro, M., Shinohara, K., and Ide, T., Dietary conjugated linoleic acid reduces body fat mass and affects gene expression of proteins regulating energy metabolism in mice, *Comp Biochem Physiol B Biochem Mol Biol* 133(3), 395–404, 2002.

107. Granlund, L., Pedersen, J. I., and Nebb, H. I., Impaired lipid accumulation by trans10, cis12 CLA during adipocyte differentiation is dependent on timing and length of treatment, *Biochim Biophys Acta* 1687(1–3), 11–22, 2005.

108. Brown, J. M., Boysen, M. S., Chung, S., Fabiyi, O., Morrison, R. F., Mandrup, S., and McIntosh, M. K., Conjugated linoleic acid induces human adipocyte delipidation: Autocrine/paracrine regulation of MEK/ERK signaling by adipocytokines, *J Biol Chem* 279(25), 26735–26747, 2004.

109. Mora, S. and Pessin, J. E., An adipocentric view of signaling and intracellular trafficking, *Diabetes Metab Res Rev* 18(5), 345–356, 2002.

110. Yamasaki, M., Mansho, K., Ogino, Y., Kasai, M., Tachibana, H., and Yamada, K., Acute reduction of serum leptin level by dietary conjugated linoleic acid in Sprague-Dawley rats, *J Nutr Biochem* [print] 11(9), 467–471, 2000.

111. Jian, W. X., Yang, Y. J., Long, J. R., Li, Y. N., Deng, F. Y., Jiang, D. K., and Deng, H. W., Estrogen receptor alpha gene relationship with peak bone mass and body mass index in Chinese nuclear families, *J Hum Genet* 50(9), 477–482, 2005.

112. Burris, T. P., Montrose, C., Houck, K. A., Osborne, H. E., Bocchinfuso, W. P., Yaden, B. C., Cheng, C. C., Zink, R. W., Barr, R. J., Hepler, C. D., Krishnan, V., Bullock, H. A., Burris, L. L., Galvin, R. J., Bramlett, K., and Stayrook, K. R., The hypolipidemic natural product guggulsterone is a promiscuous steroid receptor ligand, *Mol Pharmacol* 67(3), 948–954, 2005.

113. Sweeney, C., Blair, C. K., Anderson, K. E., Lazovich, D., and Folsom, A. R., Risk factors for breast cancer in elderly women, *Am J Epidemiol* 160(9), 868–875, 2004.

114. Nagira, K., Saito, S., Wada, T., Fukui, K., Ikubo, M., Hori, S., Tsuneki, H., Kobayashi, M., and Sasaoka, T., Altered subcellular distribution of estrogen receptor {alpha} is implicated in estradiol-induced dual regulation of insulin signaling in 3T3-L1 adipocytes, *Endocrinology* 147(2), 1020–1028, 2006.

115. Cooke, P. S. and Naaz, A., Effects of estrogens and the phytoestrogen genistein on adipogenesis and lipogenesis in males and females, *Birth Defects Res A Clin Mol Teratol* 73(7), 472–473, 2005.

116. Tanmahasamut, P., Liu, J., Hendry, L. B., and Sidell, N., Conjugated linoleic acid blocks estrogen signaling in human breast cancer cells, *J Nutr* 134(3), 674–680, 2004.

117. Durgam, V. R. and Fernandes, G., The growth inhibitory effect of conjugated linoleic acid on MCF-7 cells is related to estrogen response system, *Cancer Lett* 116(2), 121–130, 1997.

118. Liu, J. and Sidell, N., Anti-estrogenic effects of conjugated linoleic acid through modulation of estrogen receptor phosphorylation, *Breast Cancer Res Treat* 94(2), 161–169, 2005.

119. Metzger, D., Imai, T., Jiang, M., Takukawa, R., Desvergne, B., Wahli, W., and Chambon, P., Functional role of RXRs and PPARgamma in mature adipocytes, *Prostaglandins Leukot Essent Fatty Acids* 73(1), 51–58, 2005.

120. Villarroya, F., Iglesias, R., and Giralt, M., Retinoids and retinoid receptors in the control of energy balance: Novel pharmacological strategies in obesity and diabetes, *Curr Med Chem* 11(6), 795–805, 2004.

121. Ogilvie, K. M., Saladin, R., Nagy, T. R., Urcan, M. S., Heyman, R. A., and Leibowitz, M. D., Activation of the retinoid X receptor suppresses appetite in the rat, *Endocrinology* 145(2), 565–573, 2004.

122. Iwaki, M., Matsuda, M., Maeda, N., Funahashi, T., Matsuzawa, Y., Makishima, M., and Shimomura, I., Induction of adiponectin, a fat-derived antidiabetic and antiatherogenic factor, by nuclear receptors, *Diabetes* 52(7), 1655–1663, 2003.

123. Ghanim, H., Aljada, A., Hofmeyer, D., Syed, T., Mohanty, P., and Dandona, P., Circulating mononuclear cells in the obese are in a proinflammatory state, *Circulation* 110(12), 1564–1571, 2004.

124. Sun, Z. and Andersson, R., NF-kappaB activation and inhibition: a review, *Shock* 18(2), 99–106, 2002.

125. Peeraully, M. R., Jenkins, J. R., and Trayhurn, P., NGF gene expression and secretion in white adipose tissue: Regulation in 3T3-L1 adipocytes by hormones and inflammatory cytokines, *Am J Physiol Endocrinol Metab* 287(2), E331–E339, 2004.

126. Sonnenberg, G. E., Krakower, G. R., and Kissebah, A. H., A novel pathway to the manifestations of metabolic syndrome, *Obes Res* 12(2), 180–186, 2004.

127. Vincent, H. K. and Taylor, A. G., Biomarkers and potential mechanisms of obesity-induced oxidant stress in humans, *Int J Obes (Lond)* 30, 400–418, 2005.

128. Furukawa, S., Fujita, T., Shimabukuro, M., Iwaki, M., Yamada, Y., Nakajima, Y., Nakayama, O., Makishima, M., Matsuda, M., and Shimomura, I., Increased oxidative stress in obesity and its impact on metabolic syndrome, *J Clin Invest* 114(12), 1752–1761, 2004.

129. Piche, M. E., Lemieux, S., Weisnagel, S. J., Corneau, L., Nadeau, A., and Bergeron, J., Relation of high-sensitivity C-reactive protein, interleukin-6, tumor necrosis factor-alpha, and fibrinogen to abdominal adipose tissue, blood pressure, and cholesterol and triglyceride levels in healthy postmenopausal women, *Am J Cardiol* 96(1), 92–97, 2005.

130. Behre, C. J., Fagerberg, B., Hulten, L. M., and Hulthe, J., The reciprocal association of adipocytokines with insulin resistance and C-reactive protein in clinically healthy men, *Metabolism* 54(4), 439–444, 2005.

131. Matarese, G., Moschos, S., and Mantzoros, C. S., Leptin in immunology, *J Immunol* 174(6), 3137–3142, 2005.

132. Robker, R. L., Collins, R. G., Beaudet, A. L., Mersmann, H. J., and Smith, C. W., Leukocyte migration in adipose tissue of mice null for ICAM-1 and Mac-1 adhesion receptors, *Obes Res* 12(6), 936–940, 2004.

133. O'Shea, M., Bassaganya-Riera, J., and Mohede, I. C., Immunomodulatory properties of conjugated linoleic acid, *Am J Clin Nutr* 79(6 Suppl), 1199S–1206S, 2004.

134. Albers, R., van der Wielen, R. P., Brink, E. J., Hendriks, H. F., Dorovska-Taran, V. N., and Mohede, I. C., Effects of cis-9, trans-11 and trans-10, cis-12 conjugated linoleic acid (CLA) isomers on immune function in healthy men, *Eur J Clin Nutr* 57(4), 595–603, 2003.

135. Schopfer, F. J., Lin, Y., Baker, P. R., Cui, T., Garcia-Barrio, M., Zhang, J., Chen, K., Chen, Y. E., and Freeman, B. A., Nitrolinoleic acid: An endogenous peroxisome proliferator-activated receptor gamma ligand, *Proc Natl Acad Sci USA* 102(7), 2340–2345, 2005.

136. Cheng, W. L., Lii, C. K., Chen, H. W., Lin, T. H., and Liu, K. L., Contribution of conjugated linoleic acid to the suppression of inflammatory responses through the regulation of the NF-kappaB pathway, *J Agric Food Chem* 52(1), 71–78, 2004.

137. Iwakiri, Y., Sampson, D. A., and Allen, K. G., Suppression of cyclooxygenase-2 and inducible nitric oxide synthase expression by conjugated linoleic acid in murine macrophages, *Prostaglandins Leukot Essent Fatty Acids* 67(6), 435–443, 2002.

138. Harris, M. A., Hansen, R. A., Vidsudhiphan, P., Koslo, J. L., Thomas, J. B., Watkins, B. A., and Allen, K. G., Effects of conjugated linoleic acids and docosahexaenoic acid on rat liver and reproductive tissue fatty acids, prostaglandins and matrix metalloproteinase production, *Prostaglandins Leukot Essent Fatty Acids* 65(1), 23–29, 2001.

139. Bokarewa, M., Nagaev, I., Dahlberg, L., Smith, U., and Tarkowski, A., Resistin, an adipokine with potent proinflammatory properties, *J Immunol* 174(9), 5789–5795, 2005.

140. Chung, S., Brown, J. M., Provo, J. N., Hopkins, R., and McIntosh, M. K., Conjugated linoleic acid promotes human adipocyte insulin resistance through NF{kappa}B-dependent cytokine production, *J Biol Chem* 280(46), 38445–38456, 2005.

141. Leung, Y. H. and Liu, R. H., Trans-10,cis-12-conjugated linoleic acid isomer exhibits stronger oxyradical scavenging capacity than cis-9,trans-11-conjugated linoleic acid isomer, *J Agric Food Chem* 48(11), 5469–5475, 2000.

39 Role of Tea in Weight Management

Chithan Kandaswami, PhD, FACN, CNS

CONTENTS

INTRODUCTION

Biologically active ingredients of dietary origin show a propensity to stimulate energy expenditure (EE) by influencing subtle cellular and metabolic processes linked with energy dissipation. There is immense interest in these naturally occurring substances in view of their potential application in body weight (BW) reduction. Natural ingredients have received particular attention as alternatives to conventional weight management strategies with limited long-term effectiveness. One such natural product–derived ingredient is tea, deemed to possess biological activities relevant to the prevention and treatment of obesity. The potential body fat–suppressive effects of tea have recently drawn attention. The perceived benefits of tea intake have received increased scientific scrutiny. Dietary adjuncts, as exemplified by caffeine and tea-associated constituents, exert a facile effect on metabolic rate and substrate oxidation (Jung et al., 1981; Dulloo et al., 1989, 1999, 2000; Astrup et al., 1990, 2000; Komatsu et al., 2003; Harada et al., 2005).

Tea components exhibit thermogenic properties (Dulloo et al., 1999, 2000; Rumpler et al., 2001), ascribed to their interactions with the sympathoadrenal system (Dulloo et al., 1999, 2000). The activity of the sympathetic nervous system is pivotal in driving energy metabolism and thermogenesis (Landsberg et al., 1984; Blaak et al., 1993; Bray, 1993; Dulloo, 2002). Integral to the process of diet-induced thermogenesis (DIT) is the activation of the sympathetic nervous system by dietary components and the resultant metabolic and cellular processes linked with energy dissipation (Landsberg et al., 1984; Bray, 1993; Cannon and Nedergaard, 2004). Energy metabolism encompasses a complex network of hormonal and neural mechanisms. The sympathoadrenal system plays a marked role in the intricate regulation of thermogenesis and fat oxidation through circulating epinephrine and/or sympathetically released norepinephrine (Landsberg et al., 1984; Bray, 1993; Dulloo 2002; Cannon and Nedergaard, 2004). The stimulation of the sympathetic nervous system ensues increased plasma norepinephrine levels accompanied by postprandial elevation of lipid oxidation (Tappy et al., 1995). Tea components appear to have the potential to elevate endogenous levels of catecholamines (Dulloo et al., 1999). This action could have a pronounced effect on EE and fat oxidation.

Tea, brewed from the dried leaves and buds of the tea plant (*Camellia sinensis* var. *sinensis*, *Camellia sinensis* var. *assamica*), an evergreen shrub of the family Theaceae, is the most popular beverage next to water, consumed by over two-thirds of the world's population (Roberts, 1962; Graham, 1992; Balentine et al., 1997). Tea forms an integral part of the diet in many countries. Tea, touted as a healthful and medicinal beverage for centuries, has been a highly desirable drink. In general, there are three principal types of manufactured tea, namely, green (unfermented), oolong (partially fermented), and black (fully fermented) (Roberts, 1962; Lunder, 1988, Graham, 1992; Balentine et al., 1997). The manufacture of black tea (BT) ensues oxidation due to the activation of polyphenol oxidases, which oxidize susceptible tea leaf polyphenol moieties culminating in the formation of brown pigments, and this process develops the color and aroma of the liquor (Roberts et al., 1959; Roberts and Myers, 1959; Lunder, 1988, 1989).

The term "fermentation" refers to the oxidative transformations undergone by tea phenolics, involving natural browning reactions induced by oxidizing enzymes (polyphenol oxidases) within the plant cell. The production of green tea (GT) comprises the rolling and steaming of tender tea leaves, a process that minimizes the activation of these enzymes and, consequently, oxidation. Oolong tea is a partially fermented product having components common to both green and black teas.

Tea drinking is a very ancient habit. Tea has consistently remained as a choice beverage consumed by some human populations for many generations. A Chinese legend places the introduction of tea at about 2737 BC (Lunder, 1988). Chinese history indicates that emperor Sin-Non declared more than 3000 years ago that the daily consumption of a cup of tea could dissolve many poisons in the body (Liao, 2001). Traditionally, tea consumption was undertaken to improve blood flow, eliminate toxins, and to increase resistance to diseases (Balentine et al., 1997). Tea has been a conventional drink in China to combat obesity (Tian et al., 2004), and traditional medicine has frequently attributed the putative antiobesity effects of herbal medicinal preparations to the inherent properties of tea.

Comprehending the salutary effects of tea constitutes a steadily expanding area of scientific endeavor. Efforts to elucidate and evaluate the therapeutic potential of tea have been very intense during the past 10 years or so, resulting in a spate of information. Key epidemiological studies have highlighted the possible association of tea intake with the attenuation of the incidence of chronic disease prevalence, while laboratory investigations have discerned the ability of tea to impact cellular metabolism and have adduced evidence to support the beneficial effects of tea (Yang and Landau, 2000; Dufresne and Farnworth, 2001). Tea constituents exert profound effects at the cellular and subcellular levels and may subtly influence metabolic processes linked with energy dissipation. The distinctly different and diverse array of components characteristically constituting tea seems to endow it with a plethora of biological properties. While the popularity of tea may be mainly due to its alkaloid content, the potential health-promoting effects of tea have been ascribed to phenolic substances present in tea. Accruing evidence indicates that the pharmacological actions evoked by tea might originate from the intrinsic activities of phenolic and methylxanthine constituents present. This review will deal with the role of tea in weight management with emphasis on thermogenesis and substrate oxidation. It will discuss data garnered from *in vitro* investigations and animal and clinical studies.

COMPOSITION OF TEA

Fresh tea leaves contain upon average (related to dry substance mass) 36% polyphenolic compounds, 25% carbohydrates, 15% proteins, 6.5% lignin, 5% ash, 4% amino acids, 2% lipids, 1.5% organic acids, 0.5% chlorophyll, as well as carotenoids and volatile substances constituting less than 0.1% (Lunder, 1988, 1989; Graham, 1992; Balentine et al., 1997). They contain unusually high concentrations of the polyphenols belonging to the flavanol group denoted as catechins, which may constitute 17%–30% of the dry leaf weight. The flavanols belong to the broad category of flavans and proanthocyanidins, which is a distinct class within the immensely diverse group of plant flavonoids (Harborne 1994; Haslam, 1989, 1998). A flavanol is a 15-carbon (C_6–C_3–C_6 = 6-carbon ring, 3-carbon ring, 6-carbon ring) membered substituted phenylchroman. Fresh tea leaf contains caffeine at an average level of 3% along with smaller amounts of the other common methylxanthines, theobromine, and theophylline.

Tea leaf contains characteristic catechins such as (−)-epigallocatechin-3-gallate (EGCg), (−)-epigallocatechin (EGC), (−)-epicatechin-3-gallate (ECG) and (−)-epicatechin (EC), (+)-catechin, and (−)-gallocatechin (GC) (Roberts and Myers, 1959; Roberts et al., 1959; Roberts, 1962; Lunder, 1988; Graham, 1992; Balentine et al., 1997). EGCg is the most abundant catechin in tea leaves. Flavonols (present as glycosides) and depsides such as chlorogenic acid, coumarylquinic acid, and one unique to tea, theogallin (3-galloylquinic acid) are some of the other polyphenols.

During the manufacture of BT, a major proportion of monomeric-free catechins in the fresh GT leaf undergoes oxidative changes culminating in the generation of a series of compounds, including bisflavanols, theaflavins, epitheaflavic acids, and thearubigins, which impart the characteristic taste and color properties of BT (Roberts and Myers, 1959; Roberts et al., 1959; Sanderson, 1972; Lunder, 1988; Graham, 1992; Haslam, 2003). Unchanged flavanols constitute 3%–10% of the dry weight in BT (Lunder, 1988; Balentine et al., 1997). GT leaf and commercial oolong tea preparations also contain dimeric proanthocyanidins, free and as gallate esters (Nonaka et al., 1983, Hashimoto et al., 1988, 1989a,b). More significantly, Nonaka et al. (1983) detected two novel and distinct dimeric flavan-3-ol gallate esters, theasinensins A and B, in GT leaf, while Hashimoto et al. (1988) noted theasinensins D-G and oolongtheanin in oolong tea. Hashimoto et al. (1989b) isolated 8-C-ascorbyl-(−)-epigallocatechin-3-O-gallate and novel dimeric flavan-3-ols, oolonghomobisflavans A and B, from oolong tea.

Tea leaf contains a unique amino acid, 5-N-ethyl-L-glutamine, named L-theanine, detected by Sakato (1949), which is the γ-ethylamide of L-glutamic acid (γ-glutamylethylamide). L-theanine is a precursor of the nonpeptide antigen ethylamine, an alkylamine (Kamath et al., 2003). Ethylamine is present in brewed tea as an intact molecule and in its precursor form, L-theanine (Sakato, 1949; Cartwright et al., 1954). In addition to catechins, gallic acid, and caffeine, L-theanine (1%–2%, w/w) also contributes to the quality of green and black teas (Aucamp et al., 2000). L-theanine is the predominant amino acid component in tea, constituting between 1% and 2% of the dry weight of the tea leaf. It is as prevalent in tea as all other free amino acids combined. L-theanine content of BT varietals is similar to or higher than that of GTs (Ekborg-Ott et al., 1997). It is present in very high concentrations in certain varietals of BT (Scharbert and Hofmann, 2005).

Green and black teas principally differ in terms of their catechin and oxidized catechin (condensation) contents. Since oolong tea is partially oxidized, it contains both native and oxidized catechins, its composition reflecting an intermediate range between that of green and black teas. In particular, catechins such as EGCg, EGC, ECG, and EC, characteristic of GT, are present in oolong tea, along with catechin oligomers, oligomeric proanthocyanidins, and polymeric polyphenolics, typically constituting BT.

IN VITRO STUDIES: POSSIBLE MECHANISMS OF OBESITY MODERATION BY TEA

Theaflavins, major polyphenol components of BT, were evaluated by Lin et al. (2007) for their potential lipid lowering actions upon administration in fatty acid overloading conditions, both in cell culture (HepG2) and animal experimental models (Wistar rats, 5 weeks old). The authors reported that theaflavins significantly diminished lipid accumulation, depressed fatty acid synthesis, and stimulated fatty acid oxidation. Theaflavins impaired acetyl CoA carboxylase activity by the stimulation of AMPK (AMP-activated protein kinase) through LKB1 and reactive oxygen species pathways. The result indicated the bioavailability of theaflavins both *in vitro* and *in vivo*. Theaflavins might play a role in the prevention of fatty liver and obesity.

Inhibition of AMPK has also been observed with GT polyphenols (reviewed by Moon et al., 2007). Studies employing adipocyte cell lines and animal models have documented that EGCg inhibits extracellular signal-related kinases (ERK), activates AMPK, modulates adipocyte marker proteins, and downregulates lipogenic enzymes as well as other potential targets (Moon et al. 2007).

Glycerol-3-phosphate dehydrogenase (GPDH) mediates NADH-dependent reduction of dihydroxyacetone phosphate (DHAP) to glycerol-3-phosphate, one of the major precursors of triacylglycerols (TGs). Kao et al. (2010) found EGCg dose-dependently inhibited GPDH activity at a concentration of approximately $20\,\mu M$ for 50% inhibition. This finding, along with earlier ones, suggests the potential of EGCg to moderate fat content.

Skrzypczak-Jankun and Jankun (2010) reported the inactivation of plasminogen activator inhibitor type 1 (PAI-1) in plasma by theaflavin digallate [TH(2)], a component of BT, in a concentration-dependent fashion with an IC50 of $18\,\mu M$, which is equal to or better than the IC50 reported for known PAI-1 inhibitor PAI039. Such inactivation may have significance in the moderation of BW in obese individuals. TH(2) appears to be a potential candidate for clinical studies.

While screening for potential inhibitors of tyrosine phosphatase PTP1B, a widely expressed tyrosine phosphatase that is considered as a target for therapeutic drug development for the treatment of diabetes and obesity, Ma et al. (2011) reported that aqueous extracts of teas displayed potent PTP1B inhibitory effects with an IC50 value of 0.4–4 g dry tea leaves per liter of water. BT exhibited the maximal enzyme inhibition, followed by oolong, and then by GT. Biochemical fractionation studies showed that the principal active components in tea corresponded to oxidized polyphenolic compounds. This was further supported by the observation that tea catechins, upon oxidation by tyrosinases (polyphenol oxidizes), became potent inhibitors of PTP1B. Application of tea extracts to cultured cells induced tyrosine phosphorylation of cellular proteins, suggesting that certain potential beneficial effects of tea may be attributed to the inhibition of PTP1B.

ANIMAL STUDIES

Some studies have studied the antiobese effects of GT powder (GTP) and tea extracts by examining their effects in the reduction of BW gain. Studies indicate that GT and EGCg, the major polyphenol of GT, reduce BW in experimental animals (Kao et al., 2000; Sayama et al., 2000), which might be attributed to increased EE.

Oral administration (3 g/100 g of BW) of a BT extract for 15 days resulted in a decrease in body and liver weight gain and food intake in rats (Sugiyama et al., 1999). The administration (1%, w/v) of a BT extract as a drink for 25 days attenuated plasma TG levels and induced a 29% reduction in weight gain in sucrose-fed rats (Yang et al., 2002). There was a 27% decrease in fat pads accompanied by a diminution in food intake. A water extract of oolong tea prevented the obesity and fatty liver induced by a high-fat diet in mice (Han et al., 1999). Further, this extract of oolong tea, in concert with caffeine, accentuated norepinephrine-induced lipolysis in isolated fat cells.

Interestingly, Pu-Erh BT (products of Yunnan District, China) consumption caused a reduction in plasma TG levels in rats ingesting this tea extract (10 g/500 mL for 8–16 weeks) (Sano et al., 1986). There was a significant decrease in the weight of the abdominal tissue. The weight ratio of adipose tissue to whole body was also lower. Lipoprotein lipase activity in the abdominal tissue was low while the activity of epinephrine-induced lipolysis was significantly high in rats fed this tea for 8–16 weeks. These observations suggest that the successive administration of this tea could stimulate lipolysis in the adipose tissue and decrease its weight. Sayama et al. (2000) studied the antiobesity effects of tea in female ICR mice by feeding diets containing 1%, 2%, and 4% GTP for 16 weeks. The administration of diets containing 2% and 4% GTP resulted in BW reduction.

Kao et al. (2000) documented a direct effect of EGCg on BW decrease, independent of caffeine, employing a very high dose of this catechin in acute studies. Parenteral administration (70–92 mg/kg) of EGCg resulted in significant body decrease in both male and female Sprague-Dawley rats. Male rats treated daily with 85 mg EGCg/kg BW lost 15%–21% of their BW relative to their initial weight and 30%–41% relative to the control weight after 7 days of treatment. Administration of 12.5 mg EGCG (92 mg/kg BW) to female Sprague-Dawley rats resulted in a loss of 10% of their BW relative to their initial weight and 29% relative to the control weight after 7 days of treatment. EGCg treatment significantly reduced or prevented an increase in BW in lean and obese male and female Zucker rats. EGCg administration strikingly reduced food (energy) intake in both Sprague-Dawley and Zucker rats and could have contributed to BW reduction. The loss in BW was reversible; the animals regained the lost BW with the withdrawal of EGCg treatment. Structurally related catechins other than EGCg were not effective at the same dose in depressing BW or diminishing food intake. The reduction in food intake and BW observed in both lean (leptin receptor–intact) and obese (leptin receptor–defective) Zucker rats suggested that the effect of EGC was independent of an intact leptin receptor. The loss of appetite might involve neuropeptides(s) other than leptin. Kao et al. (2000) proposed that EGCg might interact specifically with a component of a leptin-independent appetite control pathway.

Zheng et al. (2004) examined the antiobesity effects of three components of GT, namely, catechins, caffeine, and theanine, in female ICR mice fed on diets containing 2% GTP and diets containing 0.3% catechins, 0.05% caffeine, and 0.03% theanine, which correspond, respectively, to their concentrations in a 2% GTP diet, singly and in combination for 16 weeks. There was a significant decrease in the weight of intraperitoneal adipose tissues and in BW increase by diets containing GT, caffeine, theanine, caffeine + catechins, caffeine + theanine, and caffeine + catechins + theanine. In particular, the adipose tissue weight decreased by 76.8% in the caffeine + catechins compared to that from the control group. GT, catechins, and theanine resulted in a diminution of serum concentrations of nonesterified fatty acids (NEFA). These results indicated that caffeine and theanine were possibly responsible for the effect of GTP in suppressing the weight of adipose tissues and BW gain. The authors consider that catechins and caffeine interact synergistically in manifesting antiobesity effects.

Some investigations have evaluated the specific effects of tea and tea-derived polyphenols on EE, respiratory quotient (RQ), the reduction of BW, and the treatment of obesity in experimental animals. Systematic investigations on body composition and regression of obesity in animals are limited.

Dulloo et al. (2000) reported that, in rats, a GTE stimulates brown adipose tissue thermogenesis to a much greater extent than that which can be attributed to its caffeine content *per se*. They suggested that the thermogenic properties of GT are due to an interaction between catechin polyphenols and caffeine, constituents of GT, with sympathetically released catecholamine, norepinephrine, which invoked the following mechanisms. By inhibiting catechol-O-methyl transferase (COMT), catechins would protect NA against inactivation by O-methylation and thereby would sustain the actions of this catecholamine. Tea phenolics competitively inhibit this enzyme (Borchardt and Huber, 1975). The inhibitory action of caffeine on the enzyme, cAMP (adenosine 3′,5′-cyclic monophosphate)-dependent phosphodiesterase, which degrades cAMP, would result in the intracellular accumulation of cAMP, a critical signaling molecule, involved in the direct activation of β-adrenergic receptors (Blaak et al., 1993; Cannon and Nedergaard, 2004). The unimpeded cellular availability of cAMP would endow this intracellular messenger with increased capacity to elicit its intracellular actions on catecholamines in prolonging thermogenesis. At this juncture, mention should be made of the fact that tea contains both the methylxanthines, caffeine, and theophylline, and that the latter is more potent than caffeine in its inhibition of cAMP phosphodiesterase activity (Rall, 1990).

The autonomic nervous system typically modulates carbohydrate and fat metabolism through direct neural stimulation as well as through hormonal effects. Catecholamine hormones such as norepinephrine and epinephrine can increase thermogenesis and lipolysis, leading to increased EE and decreased fat stores. Tappy et al. (1995) reported that the stimulation of the sympathetic nervous system increased plasma norepinephrine levels by 27% and lipid oxidation by 72%, whereas it reduced glucose oxidation by 14% in the postprandial state. Beta-adrenergic receptors of the adipocytes mediate the responses to the catecholamines (Blaak et al., 1993). The potential of tea components to positively impact the pools of endogenous catecholamines (Dulloo et al., 1999) could, therefore, have a pronounced effect on EE and substrate oxidation. Alterations of neurotransmission can markedly change the relative contribution of the catecholamine outflow to the pancreas, liver, adrenal medulla, and adipose tissues, leading to the modulation of carbohydrate and fat metabolism (Nonogaki et al., 2000).

Klaus et al. (2005) examined the acute effects of very high concentrations of orally administered EGCg (500 mg/kg) on body temperature, activity, and EE in male New Zealand black mice by indirect calorimetry. The authors reported no significant changes in any of these parameters. However, there was a decrease in RQ during night (activity phase), supportive of increased fat oxidation. The authors suggest that EGCg attenuates diet-induced obesity in mice by decreasing energy absorption and increasing fat oxidation. In a separate study, the authors (Wolfram et al., 2005) studied the regression of diet-induced obesity by dietary supplementation with EGCg (in a pure form) in Sprague-Dawley rats. Supplemental EGCg reversed established obesity in these rats. *In vitro* studies support the ability of EGCg to enhance adipocyte lipolysis. The incubation of fully differentiated 3T3-L1 cells with EGCg for 4 h strongly stimulated lipolysis (Mochizuki and Hasegawa, 2004). Treatment of mature adipocytes (3T3-L1 cells) with powdered GT in cell culture resulted in enhanced lipolysis (Hasegawa and Mori, 2000).

Theaflavins, major polyphenol components of BT, were evaluated by Lin et al. (2007) for their potential lipid lowering actions upon administration in fatty acid overloading conditions, both in cell culture (HepG2) and animal experimental models (Wistar rats, 5 weeks old). The authors reported that theaflavins significantly diminished lipid accumulation, depressed fatty acid synthesis, and stimulated fatty acid oxidation. Theaflavins impaired acetyl CoA carboxylase activity by the stimulation of AMPK through LKB1 and reactive oxygen species pathways. The result indicated the bioavailability of theaflavins both *in vitro* and *in vivo*. Theaflavins might play a role in the prevention of fatty liver and obesity.

Chen et al. (2009) investigated the effects of long-term (6 months) administration of GT, BT, or isolated EGCg (1 mg/kg/day) on body composition, glucose tolerance, and gene expression relevant to lipid homeostasis and energy metabolism in rats. The results indicated that GT and BT depressed adipocyte differentiation and fatty acid uptake into adipose tissue and elevated fat synthesis and oxidation by the liver, without inducing hepatic fat accumulation. On the other hand, EGCg (1 mg/kg/day) increased markers of thermogenesis and differentiation in adipose tissue, while exerting no effects on liver or muscle tissues. The results highlight novel and separate mechanisms by which tea and EGCg could improve glucose tolerance, indicating the potential of these agents in obesity prevention.

Grove et al. (2011) reported that EGCg supplementation (0.32% EGCg for 6 weeks) lowered final BW and BW gain in obese C57bl/6J mice. EGCg treatment increased fecal lipid content compared to that in the high-fat-fed control. They consider that some of these effects could be owed to the inhibition of pancreatic lipase (PL) by EGCg as EGCg dose-dependently inhibited PL *in vitro*. ECG possessed similar inhibitory potency while the nonester containing EGC did not.

HUMAN STUDIES

In an epidemiological study, Wu et al. (2003) showed an inverse association between the number of cups of tea consumed and body fat content. Tsuchida et al. (2002) reported a reduction of body fat in humans following long-term administration of tea catechins. Consecutive intake of tea catechins (588 mg/day) reduced body fat, especially abdominal fat in humans (Tokimitsu, 2004).

Dulloo et al. (1999) examined whether an extract of GT, by virtue of its high content of both caffeine and catechin polyphenols, could effectively promote thermogenesis in human subjects. They assessed the effect of multiple administrations of capsules containing a GTE (standardized for catechins and caffeine) and caffeine on 24 h EE, RQ, and the urinary excretion of nitrogen and catecholamines in 10 healthy men (mean BMI [body mass index]: in kg/m^2, 25.1) in a respiratory chamber. Inclusion criteria included body fatnesses ranging from lean to mildly obese (8%–30% body fat). Fat contributed 35%–40% of dietary energy intake in these subjects who habitually consumed a typical Western diet, while their estimated intake of methylxanthines (mostly as caffeine-containing beverages) ranged from 100 to 200 mg/day. On three separate occasions, the authors randomly assigned the study subjects among three treatments: GT extract (GTE) (50 mg caffeine and 90 mg EGCg), caffeine (50 mg), and placebo, which they ingested at breakfast, lunch, and dinner. The ingestion of capsules containing the GTE provided total daily intake of 150 mg caffeine and 375 mg catechins, of which 270 mg was EGCg. The amounts of catechin polyphenols consumed with each meal were comparable with the amounts commonly ingested by tea drinkers.

Compared to placebo, treatment with the GTE resulted in a significant increase in 24 h EE (4%) and a significant decrease in 24 h RQ (from 0.88 to 0.85) without any change in urinary nitrogen (Dulloo et al., 1999). None of the subjects experienced any significant differences in heart rates across treatments during the first 8 h that the subjects were assessed in the respiratory chamber. The results indicated that the lower RQ during treatment with the GTE was due to a shift in substrate utilization in favor of fat oxidation. Twenty-four hour urinary norepinephrine excretion was higher during treatment with the GTE than with the placebo (40%). Treatment with caffeine in amounts equivalent to those found in the GTE had no effect on EE, RQ, urinary nitrogen, or catecholamines. Dulloo et al. (1999) concluded that GT has thermogenic properties and promotes fat oxidation beyond that explained by its caffeine content *per se*. The authors believe that caffeine in the dosage (50 mg each treatment, 150 mg total intake/day) employed, although ineffective by itself, might have enabled a synergistic interaction with other bioactive ingredients in the GTE to promote catecholamine-induced thermogenesis and fat oxidation. They perceived that GTE might play a role in the control of body composition via sympathetic activation of thermogenesis, fat oxidation, or both. Dulloo et al. (1999) suggested that interaction between GT (catechin polyphenols) and caffeine to stimulate and prolong thermogenesis could be of value in the management of obesity.

In an open study, Chantre and Lairon (2002) evaluated the effects of a standardized GTE in 70 (63 female, 7 male) moderately obese patients (BMI 25–32 kg/m^2). Each subject received two times per day (i.e., 2 capsules morning, 2 capsules midday) a GTE ingestion of 4 capsules, which provided a daily total of 375 mg catechins, of which 270 mg was EGCg. After 3 months, BW and waist circumference decreased by 4.6% and 4.48%, respectively. The authors did not observe any significant differences in blood pressure during the 3 months of treatment. Martinet et al. (1999) reported that commercial preparations of GT and 11 other plant preparations had no discernible effect on EE or RQ. In view of the comprehended thermogenic activity of defined GTEs in humans (Dulloo et al., 1999) and animals (Dulloo et al., 2000), and oolong tea beverage in human subjects (Chen et al., 1998; Rumpler et al., 2001; Komatsu et al., 2003), the constitution and the standardization of the composition of the tea extract and the dose ranges selected for administration could be critical in evaluating the efficacy of the extract in elevating metabolic rate and fat oxidation.

Chen et al. (1998) evaluated the clinical efficacy of oolong tea in Chinese women. They reported that 102 subjects who consumed four cups of oolong tea per day (the brew from four 2 g tea bags) lost over a kilogram of BW during a 6 week period. The subjects received 125 mg of caffeine per day from the consumption of oolong tea. The data suggested that oolong tea might promote weight loss by increasing EE by 10–20.

Rumpler et al. (2001) evaluated under controlled conditions whether consumption of oolong tea increases EE or modulates substrate oxidation in comparison to that of control beverages. Employing a randomized crossover design, they compared 24 h EE of 12 men consuming each of four treatments: (1) water, (2) full-strength tea (daily allotment brewed from 15 g of tea), (3) half-strength tea (brewed from 7.5 g tea), and (4) water containing 270 mg caffeine, equivalent to the concentration in the full-strength tea treatment. Each treatment consisted of a beverage consumed five times daily containing one of four test beverages, over a period of 6 h (8:30 a.m.–2:30 p.m.). The total caffeine consumption for subjects consuming five servings of the caffeinated water, full-strength tea, and half-strength tea treatments was 270, 270, and 135 mg/day, respectively. The consumption of the full-strength tea and half-strength tea provided a daily total intake of 244 mg of EGCg (662 mg of catechins; 952 mg of polyphenols) and 122 mg of EGCg, (331 mg of catechins; 476 mg of polyphenols), respectively. The subjects refrained from consuming caffeine or flavonoids for 4 days prior to the study. They received each treatment for 3 days; on the third day, EE was determined by indirect calorimetry in a room calorimeter.

The increase in EE for the full-strength tea and caffeinated water treatments in comparison to that from the water treatment was 2.9% and 3.4%, respectively, and was significant (Rumpler et al., 2001). Twenty-four hour fat oxidation was significantly higher (12%) when subjects consumed the full-strength tea beverage rather than water. The elevation in fat oxidation was 12% and 8% for the full-strength tea and the caffeinated water, respectively. These studies indicate that the consumption of oolong tea may promote weight loss by stimulating EE and fat oxidation. The elevation of metabolic rate and fat oxidation by the consumption of tea confirms the results obtained by Dulloo et al. (1999). It is not clear whether one could ascribe the responses mentioned earlier resulting from oolong tea intake exclusively to caffeine.

The intake of EGCg from the full-strength (containing 270 mg of caffeine) oolong tea in the Rumpler (Rumpler et al., 2001) study was similar to that from the GTE employed by Dulloo et al. (1999), even though caffeine levels were nearly twice as high. However, the increases in 24 h EE reported in both investigations were very similar. The administration of oolong tea was as a drink, whereas Dullo et al. (1999) supplied the GTE in capsule form. The elevation in EE associated with the consumption of caffeine (caffeinated water containing 270 mg caffeine) alone was not significantly different from that obtained with the full-strength tea. Rumpler et al. (2001) reasoned that the consumption of the full-strength tea would have elicited a much higher thermic effect in case there had been some synergistic interaction of caffeine with bioactive components in tea as suggested by Dulloo et al. (1999).

The studies of Rumpler et al. (2001) revealed a significant effect of tea on 24 h fat oxidation, which was not evident with caffeinated beverages alone. The observed impact of tea on fat oxidation may reflect the synergistic effect of caffeine and tea catechins, as proposed by Dulloo et al. (1999). However, in the absence of data discriminating the independent effect of noncaffeine components of tea in stimulating fat oxidation, it remains to be determined whether caffeine from tea and extracts is essential to produce this effect.

Komatsu et al. (2003) evaluated the effect of oolong tea on EE in comparison with that of GT. Randomly divided 11 healthy Japanese females consumed one of the following three treatments in a crossover design: (1) water, (2) oolong tea, and (3) GT. The composition of the oolong tea consumed was as follows: caffeine 77 mg, total catechins 206 mg (EGCg 78 mg), and polymerized polyphenols 68 mg. The GT beverage provided the following components: caffeine 161 mg, total catechins 293 mg (EGCg 94 mg), and polymerized polyphenols 17 mg. Resting EE (REE) and EE after the consumption of the test beverage for 120 min were determined using an indirect calorimeter. The cumulative increases of EE for 120 min were 10% and 4% after the consumption of oolong tea and GT, respectively, and were significant. EE at 60 and 90 min were significantly higher after the consumption of oolong tea than that of water. Oolong tea consumed by the subjects contained approximately half the caffeine and EGCg in comparison with the amounts in GT while polymerized polyphenols were double. However, the efficacy of oolong tea was much higher than that of GT. The authors consider that polymerized polyphenols present in oolong promote EE.

Bérubé-Parent (2005) evaluated the effect of ingestion of four mixtures of GT (catechins) and guarana (a plant containing caffeine) extracts (containing a fixed dose of caffeine and different amounts of EGCg) on 24 h EE and fat oxidation in men. Fourteen subjects (25.7 kg/m², mean BMI) participated in this randomized, placebo-controlled, double-blind, crossover study. The subjects consumed a capsule of placebo or capsules containing 200 mg caffeine and a variable dose of EGCg (90, 200, 300, or 400 mg) three times daily, 30 min before standardized meals, between 08.00 h and 18.00 h. Ingestion of the EGCg–caffeine mixtures significantly increased 24 h EE (by 8%) compared with that in the placebo. Increasing the dose of EGCg in the mixtures induced a mild increase in 24 h EE, but these differences were not significant even between the lowest (270 mg/day: 3 × 90 mg) and the highest (1200 mg/day: 3 × 400 mg) doses. EGCg did not evoke a dose-related effect on 24 h EE. The intake of EGCg–caffeine mixtures had no effect on RQ, fat oxidation, or catecholamine excretion. It is surprising that the authors did not find any effect of EGCg–caffeine mixtures on fat oxidation. Their findings are at variance with those of Dulloo et al. (1999) and Rumpler et al. (2001), who demonstrated the elevation of fat oxidation by the ingestion of EGCg-containing green and black teas.

Harada et al. (2005) investigated the effect of the long-term ingestion of tea catechins on post-prandial EE and dietary fat oxidation. Twelve healthy male subjects consumed 350 mL of a test beverage per day that contained either a high dose of catechin (592.9 mg) or a low dose of catechin (77.7 mg) for a period of 12 weeks. The authors conducted respiratory analyses before and at 4, 8, and 12 weeks during the test period, which included oxygen consumption and the excretion of (CO_2)-^{13}C over 8 h after a single ingestion of a test meal containing ^{13}C-labeled triglyceride. There was a significant increase in the excretion of (CO_2)-^{13}C in the high-dose-catechin group (the HC group) at 4 and 12 weeks of the test period compared to that from the low-dose-catechin group (the LC group), and this elevation persisted at 8.9% at week 0 to 12.9% at week 12. DIT, defined as an increase in EE from the fasting baseline for 8 h after the single ingestion of a test meal, was significantly higher in the HC group at 8 and 12 weeks compared to that in the LC group. The results indicate that enhanced dietary fat oxidation and an increased DIT may play an important role in the antiobesity effect of tea catechins.

Kajimoto et al. (2005) assessed the effect of consumption of a catechin-containing drink on body fat levels in healthy adults. The beverage (250 mL/bottle) contained 215.3 mg of tea catechins mostly possessing a galloyl moiety, which included EGCg (74.6 mg), ECG (34.1 mg), (-)-gallocatechin gallate (77.8 mg), and GC (24.5 mg). This double-blind study had three parallel groups. The subjects (98 men and 97 women) received three bottles of placebo drink (control group), two bottles of catechin-containing drink and one bottle of placebo drink (low-dose group), or three bottles of catechin-containing drink (high-dose group) per day at mealtimes for 12 week (daily consumption of catechins was 41.1, 444.3, or 665.9 mg respectively). BW and BMI were significantly lower in both catechin groups than in the control group from 4 to 12 weeks. The authors reported a significant reduction of total fat and visceral fat areas in both catechin groups compared with those from the control group at 12 weeks.

Nagao et al. (2005) performed a 12 week double-blind study to elucidate the effect of catechins on body fat reduction and the relation between oxidized low-density lipoprotein (LDL) and body fat variables. After a 2 week diet run-in period, healthy Japanese males, divided into two groups with similar BMI and waist circumference distributions, ingested one bottle oolong tea per day containing 690 mg catechins (tea extract group; n = 17) or one bottle oolong tea per day containing 22 mg catechins (control group; n = 18). The authors observed that BW, BMI, waist circumference, body fat mass, and subcutaneous fat area were significantly lower in the tea extract group than in the control group. The results showed a positive association of changes in the concentration of malondialdehyde-modified LDL with changes in body fat mass and total fat area in the GTE group.

Kovacs et al. (2004) conducted a randomized, parallel, placebo-controlled study to explore whether GT may improve weight maintenance by preventing or limiting weight regain after weight loss of 5%–10% in overweight and moderately obese subjects. The participants included a total of 104 overweight and moderately obese male and female subjects (BMI, 25–35 kg/m²). The majority of subjects were women. The treatment study consisted of a very-low-energy diet intervention for 4 weeks followed by a weight-maintenance period for 13 weeks, during which the subjects consumed GT or a placebo. The GT capsules used in the study contained caffeine (104 mg/day) and catechins (573 mg/day, of which 323 mg was EGCg). The subjects were in a free-living condition and had their habitual caffeine intake, varying approximately from 0 to 100 mg/day. The results suggested that GT was not effective in weight maintenance after a weight loss of 7.5% in originally overweight and moderately obese subjects. However, there was stronger weight maintenance with GT in the low caffeine users compared with that in the high caffeine consumer.

Kovacs et al. (2004) indicated that the magnitude of habitual caffeine intake might impair the effectiveness of GT administration. The plasma leptin concentration at baseline was lower in high caffeine consumers than in low caffeine consumers, indicating that the habitual use of caffeine may reduce leptin levels. The authors indicate the possibility that supplementation with GT will only be effective under conditions of low habitual caffeine intake and that a much higher dose of GT is required when habitual caffeine intake is high.

The investigations of Westerterp-Plantenga et al. (2005) further corroborated that the magnitude of habitual intake of caffeine was a critical determinant of the effectiveness of GT in maintaining BW. In a randomized, placebo-controlled, double-blind, parallel trial study, these authors evaluated the effect of a GT–caffeine mixture on weight maintenance after BW loss in 76 overweight and moderately obese subjects (BMI, $27.5 \pm 2.7 \, kg/m^2$) matched for sex, age, BMI, height, body mass, and habitual caffeine intake. The treatment comprised a very-low-energy diet intervention for 4 weeks followed by a weight-maintenance period of 13 weeks, during which the subjects consumed a GT–caffeine mixture (270 mg EGCg + 150 mg caffeine per day) or placebo. During weight management, GT reduced BW, waist circumference, RQ, and body fat in the low caffeine consumers, while there was an increase in REE compared with a restoration of these variables with the placebo group. The consumption of the GT–caffeine mixture did not result in any effect on weight management in the high caffeine consumers, whereas it significantly improved weight management in habitual low caffeine consumers, supported by relatively higher thermogenesis and fat oxidation. The authors furnished evidence to suggest that overweight subjects who lose 5–6 kg weight in 4 weeks and who hardly consume coffee or tea or other caffeine-containing products may benefit from a regular intake of GT–caffeine mixture containing 270 mg of EGCg and 150 mg of caffeine per day.

Tea polyphenolics and methylxanthines are known to exhibit strong binding activities. In view of this, the intake of large amounts of tea may be a cause for concern because of the potential consequences of tea drinking on nutritional and other problems. However, the consumption of tea is remarkably safe, and there is no solid evidence concerning the harmful effects of tea consumption.

In a randomized controlled trial, Fukino et al. (2005) examined the effects of dietary GT polyphenol on insulin (Ins) resistance and systemic inflammation. The study involved 66 patients aged 32–73 years (53 males and 13 females) with borderline diabetes or diabetes. Daily supplementation of 500 mg GT polyphenols (catechins) for 2 months did not have discernible effects on blood glucose level, Hb A1c level, Ins resistance, or inflammation markers. The authors opine that further investigations are warranted in order to ascertain potential positive correlation between the levels of polyphenol intake and that of Ins.

In a small, randomized, double-blind, placebo-controlled, crossover pilot study, six overweight men were administered 300 mg EGCg/day for 2 days (Boschmann and Thielecke, 2007). The results suggested that EGCg alone had the potential to increase fat oxidation in men. Further studies are required to ascertain whether this catechin by itself has the capacity to influence substrate oxidation in the absence of caffeine.

Venables et al. (2008) evaluated the effects of acute (total: 890 ± 13 mg polyphenols and 366 ± 5 mg EGCg) ingestion of GTE on glucose tolerance and fat oxidation in 11 healthy men performing a 30 min cycling exercise. The results led the authors to conclude that acute GTE ingestion could enhance fat oxidation during moderate-intensity exercise and improve Ins sensitivity and glucose tolerance in healthy young men.

Hsu et al. (2008) examined the effect of GTE (491 mg catechins containing 302 mg EGCg) on 78 obese women aged between 16 and 60 years with BMI $> 27 \, kg/m^2$ in a randomized, double-blind, placebo-controlled clinical trial. They reported that there was no significant difference in the % reduction in BW, BMI, and waist circumflex (WC) between the GTE and placebo groups after 12 weeks of supplementation.

Within-group comparison showed that the GTE group exhibited significant reductions in LDL-cholesterol and triglyceride and marked increase in the levels of HDL-cholesterol, adiponectin, and ghrelin. In contrast, the placebo group showed significant reduction in triglyceride level only and an appreciable elevation in the level of ghrelin alone.

In an epidemiological study, Polychronopoulos et al. (2008) evaluated the association between tea consumption and blood glucose levels in a sample of elderly adults in Greece (300 men and women from Cyprus, 142 from Mitilini, and 100 from Samothraki islands; aged 65–100 years). Tea consumption is associated with reduced levels of fasting blood glucose only among nonobese elderly people.

He et al. (2009) studied the effect of ingestion of oolong tea (a total of 8 g/day) for 6 weeks in 102 diet-induced overweight or obese subjects. Seventy percent of the severely obese individuals showed a reduction of more than 1 kg in BW, including 22% who lost more than 3 kg; the subcutaneous fat content decreased in 12% of the subjects. The authors reported that BW loss was significantly related to the decrease in waist size in both men and women. The plasma levels of TG and TC (total cholesterol) of the subjects with hyperlipidemia were notably decreased after the ingestion of oolong tea for 6 weeks. *In vitro* studies on the inhibition of PL by oolong tea extract and catechins suggested that the potential of oolong tea to prevent hyperlipidemia might be related to the moderating effect of oolong tea catechins on lipoprotein levels.

In a double-blind controlled study, Nagao et al. (2009) assessed the effects of continuous consumption of a catechin-rich beverage in individuals with type 2 diabetes who were not receiving Ins therapy. The subjects consumed GT containing either 582.8 mg of catechins (catechin group; n = 23) or 96.3 mg of catechins (control group; n = 20) per day for 12 weeks. The diminution in waist circumference at week 12 was more significant in the catechin group than in the control group. Adiponectin, which is negatively correlated with visceral adiposity, was found to be significantly elevated only in the catechin group. Even though the increase in Ins at week 12 was greater in the catechin group than in the control group, no noticeable difference was noted between the two groups with respect to glucose and hemoglobin A1c levels. In subjects treated with insulinotropic agents, the rise in Ins at week 12 was significantly greater in the catechin group than in the control group; the decrease in hemoglobin A1c at week 12 was significantly greater in the catechin group than in the control group.

In a randomized placebo-controlled trial, Wang et al. (2010) assessed the effects of a high-catechin GT on body composition in 182 moderately overweight Chinese subjects. The individuals consumed either two servings of a control drink (C; 30 mg catechins, 10 mg caffeine/day), one serving of the control drink and one serving of an extra-high-catechin GT1 (458 mg catechins, 104 mg caffeine/day), two servings of a high-catechin GT2 (468 mg catechins, 126 mg caffeine/day), or two servings of the extra-high-catechin GT3 (886 mg catechins, 198 mg caffeine/day) for 90 days. The results showed that the ingestion of two servings of an extra-high-catechin GT led to improvements in body composition and reductions in total body fat and abdominal fatness in these subjects.

Lonac et al. (2011) evaluated the effects of short-term consumption of a commercially available EGCg supplement (Teavigo) on RMR (resting metabolic rate) and TEF. Seven placebo or seven EGCg capsules (135 mg/capsule) were administered to 16 adults (9 males, 7 females, aged 25 ± 2 years, BMI 24.6 ± 1.2 kg/m^2 [mean ± s.e.]) over a 48 h period (3 capsules/day). The authors reported that the short-term consumption of the commercially available EGCg supplement did not increase RMR or the thermic effect of feeding (TEF).

In short-term studies, noticeably different outcomes of the effect of catechin–caffeine mixtures and caffeine-only supplementation on EE and fat oxidation have been documented. This prompted Hursel et al. (2011) to conduct a meta-analysis (six articles) to possibly ascertain whether catechin–caffeine mixtures and caffeine-only supplementation increase substrate oxidation and thermogenesis. This meta-analysis indicates that a catechin–caffeine mixture and caffeine-only exerted a dose-dependent stimulating effect on daily EE. Additionally, a catechin–caffeine mixture appeared also to have a stimulating effect on daily fat oxidation compared with placebo. Compared with placebo, daily fat oxidation was only significantly increased after the consumption of catechin–caffeine mixtures.

Certain investigations have raised the potential paradoxical effects of tea components. Park et al. (2009) reported that oral glucose loading 1 h after GTE (GTE ingestion) in humans resulted in higher blood glucose and Ins levels than that in control subjects. Gallated catechins were necessary for these actions to take place. EGCg treatment blocked normal glucose uptake by liver, fat, pancreatic beta-cell, and skeletal muscle cell lines even though gallated catechins have the potential to reduce glucose and cholesterol absorption when they are within the intestinal lumen. Gallated catechin–deficient GTE nullified glucose intolerance. The authors conclude that their findings encourage the development of nonabsorbable derivatives of gallated catechins for the amelioration of type 2 diabetes and obesity as they could selectively exert only the positive luminal effect. Sung et al. (2010) reported that EGCg, at concentrations that are readily achievable in human plasma via GT intake (about 10 mM, Chow et al., 2001), diminished cellular glucose uptake by mouse 3T3-L1 adipocyte cultures. EGCg was also found to enhance the expression and secretion of RBP4 (retinol-binding protein 4) in human adipocyte cultures. The authors contend that EGCg concentrations needed for this inhibition are similar to those required for the inhibition of cellular glucose uptake by cultured mouse 3T3-L1 adipocytes. Therefore, they suggested that the effect of EGCg on the expression and secretion of RBP4 by cultured human adipocytes might be associated with the inhibition of cellular glucose uptake. In view of these observations, the potential impact of circulating EGCg on cellular glucose uptake by various tissues needs to be elucidated.

CONCLUSION

Tea has gained prominence as a functional food and as a repository of pharmacologically active ingredients. Bioactive entities associated with this dietary adjunct could have a propensity to augment EE by influencing subtle cellular and metabolic processes linked with energy dissipation. Conceivably, some of these ingredients may positively influence intracellular energy transduction systems in the mitochondrion and/or promote the mobilization of fat and the catabolic breakdown of TG into free fatty acids. Certain animal and human studies have demonstrated the thermogenic properties of tea. Limited information garnered illustrates that the administration of tea as a beverage or as an extract promotes EE and fat oxidation in human subjects.

Twenty-four hour EE determinations clearly document that both green and oolong teas containing variable amounts of EGCg (and other catechin components) and caffeine promote thermogenesis and fat oxidation, while no specific information exists on the specific contributory role of different tea components and of catechin–caffeine mixtures in these processes (Dulloo et al., 1999; Rumpler et al., 2001). While GT provides native catechins (polyphenol monomers), oolong tea furnishes oxidized catechins and oligomers and polymers derived from catechins, in addition to native catechins. Further studies are necessary to discriminate the exclusive effects of caffeine and noncaffeine components of tea on metabolic rate and fat oxidation in human subjects. Recently accrued evidence suggests that overweight individuals, who underwent BW loss, could substantially benefit from a regular intake of a caffeine and GT mixture in sustaining weight loss (Westerterp-Plantenga et al., 2005). These investigations pinpoint to a promising application of GT components in the maintenance of BW.

Certain encouraging studies have focused on the antiobesity effect of a mixture of EGCg and other tea-derived catechins. These studies document that prolonged (12 weeks) ingestion of a mixture of tea catechins intensifies postprandial EE and fat oxidation in healthy male subjects (Harada et al., 2005). Long-term (12 weeks) administration of a combination of tea-derived catechins significantly diminished BW, body fat mass, and BMI in a large sample of male and female subjects (Kajimoto et al., 2005). The intake of tea catechin mixtures resulted in a significant reduction of total and visceral fat areas. The outcome of these investigations adds a promising new dimension in evaluating the antiobesity effect of tea and tea products. Such investigations provide impetus for spearheading the development of "designer" supplements containing tea components and other thermogenic agents in order to target obesity. The utility of tea as a weight management aid clearly requires further long-term, systematic, and in-depth investigations.

REFERENCES

Astrup, A., Thermogenic drugs as a strategy for treatment of obesity. *Endocrine*, 13, 207–212, 2000.

Astrup, A. et al., Caffeine: A double-blind, placebo-controlled study of its thermogenic, metabolic, and cardio-vascular effects in healthy volunteers, *Am. J. Clin. Nutr.*, 51, 759, 1990.

Aucamp, J.P., Hara, Y., and Apostolides, Z., Simultaneous analysis of tea catechins, caffeine, gallic acid, theanine and ascorbic acid by micellar electrokinetic capillary chromatography, *J. Chromatogr. A*, 876, 235, 2000.

Balentine, D.A., Wiseman, S.A., and Bouwens, L.C.M., The chemistry of tea flavonoids, *Crit. Rev. Food Sci. Nutr.*, 37, 693, 1997.

Bérubé-Parent, S., et al., Effects of encapsulated green tea and Guarana extracts containing a mixture of epigallocat-echin-3-gallate and caffeine on 24 h energy expenditure and fat oxidation in men, *Br. J. Nutr.*, 94, 432, 2005.

Blaak, E.E., Saris, W.H., and van Baak, M.A., Adrenoceptor subtypes mediating catecholamine-induced thermogenesis in man, *Int. J. Obes. Relat. Metab. Disor.*, 17(Suppl 3), S78, 1993.

Borchardt, R.T. and Huber, J.A., Catechol-*O*-methyltransferase: Structure-activity relationships for inhibition by flavonoids, *J. Med. Chem.*, 18, 120, 1975.

Boschmann, M. and Thielecke, F., The effects of epigallocatechin-3-gallate on thermogenesis and fat oxidation in obese men: A pilot study, *J. Am. Coll. Nutr.*, 26, 389S, 2007.

Bray, G.A., Food intake, sympathetic activity, and adrenal steroids, *Brain Res. Bull.*, 32, 537, 1993.

Cannon, B. and Nedergaard, J., Brown adipose tissue: Function and physiological significance, *Physiol. Rev.*, 84, 277, 2004.

Cartwright, R., Roberts, E., and Wood, D., *J. Sci. Food Agric.*, 5, 597, 1954.

Chantre, P. and Lairon, D., Recent findings of green tea extract AR25 (Exolise) and its activity for the treatment of obesity, *Phytomedicine*, 9, 3, 2002.

Chen, W.Y. et al., Clinical efficacy of oolong tea in simple obesity, *Japan. Soc. Clin. Nutr.*, 20, 83, 1998.

Chen, N., Bezzina, R., Hinch, E., Lewandowski, P.A., Cameron-Smith, D., Mathai, M.L., Jois, M., Sinclair, A.J., Begg, D.P., Wark, J.D., Weisinger, H.S., and Weisinger, R.S., Green tea, black tea, and epigallocatechin modify body composition, improve glucose tolerance, and differentially alter metabolic gene expression in rats fed a high-fat diet, *Nutr. Res.*, 29, 784, 2009.

Chow, H.H. et al., Phase I pharmacokinetic study of tea polyphenols following single-dose administration of epigallocatechin gallate and polyphenon E. *Cancer Epidemiol. Biomark. Prev.*, 10, 53, 2001.

Dufresne, C.J. and Farnworth, E.R., A review of latest research findings on the health promotion properties of tea, *J. Nutr. Biochem.*, 12, 404, 2001.

Dulloo, A.G., A sympathetic defense against obesity, *Science*, 297, 780, 2002.

Dulloo, A.G. et al., Normal caffeine consumption: Influence on thermogenesis and daily energy expenditure in lean and postobese human volunteers, *Am. J. Clin. Nutr.*, 49, 44, 1989.

Dulloo, A.G. et al., Efficacy of a green tea extract rich in catechin polyphenols and caffeine in increasing 24 h energy expenditure and fat oxidation in humans, *Am. J. Clin. Nutr.*, 70, 1040, 1999.

Dulloo, A.G. et al., Green tea and thermogenesis: Interactions between catechin-polyphenols, caffeine and sympathetic activity, *Int. J. Obes. Relat. Metab. Disor.*, 24, 252, 2000.

Ekborg-Ott, K.H., Taylor, A., and Armstrong, D.W. Varietal differences in the total and enantiomeric composi-tion of theanine in tea, *J. Agric. Food Chem.*, 45, 353, 1997.

Fukino, Y., Shimbo, M., Aoki, N., Okubo, T., Iso, H., Randomized controlled trial for an effect of green tea consumption on insulin resistance and inflammation markers, *J. Nutr. Sci. Vitaminol. (Tokyo)*, 51, 335, 2005.

Graham, H.N., Green tea composition, consumption and polyphenol chemistry, *Prev. Med.*, 21, 334, 1992.

Grove, K.A., Sae-Tan, S., Kennett, M.J., Lambert, J.D., (−)-Epigallocatechin-3-gallate inhibits pancreatic lipase and reduces body weight gain in high fat-fed obese mice, *Obesity (Silver Spring)*. June 2, 2011. doi:10.1038/oby.2011.139 [Epub ahead of print].

Han, L.K. et al., Anti-obesity action of oolong tea, *Int. J. Obes. Relat. Metab. Disor.*, 23, 98, 1999.

Harada, U. et al., Effects of the long-term ingestion of tea catechins on energy expenditure and dietary fat oxidation in healthy subjects, *J. Health Sci.*, 51, 248, 2005.

Harborne, J.B., *The Flavonoids: Advances in Research Since 1986*, Chapman & Hall/CRC, Boca Raton, FL, 1994, p. 676.

Hasegawa, N. and Mori, M., Effect of powdered green tea and its caffeine content on lipogenesis and lipolysis in 3T3-L1 cells, *J. Health Sci.*, 46, 153, 2000.

Hashimoto, F., Nonaka, G.-I., and Nishioka, I., Tannins and related compounds. LXIX. Isolation and struc-ture determination of B-B′-linked bisflavanoids, theasinensins D-G and oolongtheanin from oolong tea, *Chem. Pharm. Bull.*, 36, 1676, 1988.

Hashimoto, F., Nonaka, G.-I., and Nishioka, I., Tannins and related compounds. LXXVII. Novel chalcan-flavan dimers, assamicains A, B and C, and a new flavan-3-ol and proanthocyanidins from the fresh leaves of *Camellia sinensis* L. var. *assamica* Kitamura, *Chem. Pharm. Bull.*, 37, 77, 1989a.

Hashimoto, F., Nonaka, G.-I., and Nishioka, I., Tannins and related compounds. XC. 8-C-ascorbyl-(−)-epigallocatechin-3-*O*-gallate and novel dimeric flavan-3-ols, oolonghomobisflavans A and B, from oolong tea, *Chem. Pharm. Bull.*, 37, 3255, 1989b.

Haslam, E., *Practical Polyphenolics: From Structure to Molecular Recognition and Physiological Action*, Cambridge University Press, Cambridge, U.K., 1988.

Haslam, E., *Plant Polyphenols: Vegetable Tannins Revisited*, Cambridge University Press, Cambridge, U.K., 1989.

Haslam, E., Thoughts on thearubigins, *Phytochemistry*, 64, 61, 2003.

He, R.-H. et al., Beneficial effects of oolong tea consumption on diet-induced overweight and obese subjects. *Chin. J. Integ. Med.*, 15, 34, 2009.

Hsu, C.H., Tsai, T.H., Kao, Y.H., Hwang, K.C., Tseng, T.Y., Chou, P., Effect of green tea extract on obese women: A randomized, double-blind, placebo-controlled clinical trial, *Clin Nutr.*, 27, 363, 2008.

Hursel, R., et al., The effects of catechin rich teas and caffeine on energy expenditure and fat oxidation: A meta-analysis, *Obes. Rev.*, 12, e573, 2011.

Jung, R.T. et al., Caffeine: Its effect on catecholamines and metabolism in lean and obese humans, *Clin. Sci.*, 60, 527, 1981.

Kajimoto, O. et al., Tea catechins with a galloyl moiety reduce body weight and fat, *J. Health Sci.*, 51, 161, 2005.

Kamath, A.B., Antigens in tea-beverage prime human Vγ2Vδ2 T cells *in vitro* and *in vivo* for memory and nonmemory antibacterial cytokine responses, *Proc. Natl. Acad. Sci. USA.*, 100, 6009, 2003.

Kao, Y. H., Hiipakka, R. A., and Liao, S., Modulation of endocrine systems and food intake by green tea epigallocatechin gallate, *Endocrinology*, 141, 980, 2000.

Kao, C.-C., Wu, B.-T., Tsuei, Y.-W., Shih, L.-J., Kuo, Y.-L., Kao, Y.-H., Green tea catechins: Inhibitors of glycerol-3-phosphate dehydrogenase, *Planta Med.*, 76, 694, 2010.

Klaus, S. et al., Epigallocatechin gallate attenuates diet-induced obesity in mice by decreasing energy absorption and increasing fat oxidation, *Int. J. Obes. Relat. Metab. Disor.*, 29, 615, 2005.

Komatsu, T. et al., Oolong tea increases energy metabolism in Japanese females, *J. Med Invest.*, 50, 170, 2003.

Kovacs, E.M.R. et al., Effects of green tea on weight maintenance after body-weight loss, *Br. J. Nutr.*, 91, 431, 2004.

Landsberg, L., Saville, M.E., and Young, J.B., Sympathoadrenal system and regulation of thermogenesis, *Am. J. Physiol.*, 247, E181, 1984.

Liao, S., The medicinal actions of androgens and green tea epigallocatechin gallate, *Hong Kong Med. J.*, 7, 369, 2001.

Lin, C.-H., Huang, H.-C., and Lin, J.-K. Theaflavins attenuate lipid accumulation through AMPK in human HepG2 cells, *J. Lipid Res.*, 48, 2334, 2007.

Lonac, M.C., Richards, J.C., Schweder, M.M., Johnson, T.K., Bell, C., Influence of short-term consumption of the caffeine-free, epigallocatechin-3-gallate supplement, Teavigo, on resting metabolism and the thermic effect of feeding, *Obesity*, 19, 298, 2011.

Lunder, T.V., *Tea*, Nestec Ltd. Technical Assistance, Nestlé Research Centre, Vevey, Switzerland, 1988, p. 42.

Lunder, T., Tannins of green and black tea: Nutritional value, physiological properties and determination, *Farm. Tijdschr. Belg.*, 66, 34, 1989.

Ma, J., Li, Z., Xing, S., Ho, W.T., Fu, X., Zhao, Z.J., Tea contains potent inhibitors of tyrosine phosphatase PTP1B, *Biochem. Biophys. Res. Commun.*, 407, 98, 2011.

Martinet, A., Hostettman, K., and Schutz, Y., Thermogenic effects of commercially available plant preparations aimed at treating human obesity, *Phytomedicine*, 6, 231, 1999.

Mochizuki, M. and Hasegawa, N., Effects of green tea catechin-induced lipolysis on cytosol glycerol content in differentiated 3T3-L1 cells, *Phytother. Res.*, 18, 945, 2004.

Moon, H.S., Lee, H.G., Choi, Y.J., Kim, T.G., Cho, C.S., Proposed mechanisms of (−)-epigallocatechin-3-gallate for anti-obesity, *Chem. Biol. Interact.*, 167, 85, 2007.

Nagao, T. et al., Ingestion of a tea rich in catechins leads to a reduction in body fat and malondialdehyde-modified LDL in men, *Am. J. Clin. Nutr.*, 81, 122, 2005.

Nagao, T., Meguro, S., Hase, T., Otsuka, K., Komikado, M., Tokimitsu, I., Yamamoto, T., Yamamoto, K., A catechin-rich beverage improves obesity and blood glucose control in patients with type 2 diabetes, *Obesity* (*Silver Spring*), 17, 310, 2009.

Nonogaki, K., New insights into sympathetic regulation of glucose and fat metabolism. *Diabetologia* 43, 533–549, 2000.

Nonaka, G., Kawahara, O., and Nishioka, I., Tannins and Related Compounds. xv. A New Class of Dimeric Flavan-3-ol Gallates, Theasinensins A and B, and Proanthocyanidin Gallates from Green Tea Leaf. (1) Chemical and Pharmaceutical Bulletin, JP, Pharmaceutical Society of Japan, 31, 3906–3914, 1983.

Park, J.H., Jin, J.Y., Baek, W.K., Park, S.H., Sung, H.Y., Kim, Y.K., Lee, J., Song, D.K., Ambivalent role of gallated catechins in glucose tolerance in humans: A novel insight into non-absorbable gallated catechin-derived inhibitors of glucose absorption. *J. Physiol. Pharmacol.*, 60, 101, 2009.

Polychronopoulos, E., Zeimbekis, A., Kastorini, C.M., Papairakleous, N., Vlachou, I., Bountziouka, V., Panagiotakos, D.B., Effects of black and green tea consumption on blood glucose levels in non-obese elderly men and women from Mediterranean Islands (MEDIS epidemiological study), *Eur. J. Nutr.*, 47, 10, 2008.

Rall, T.W., Drugs used in the treatment of asthma. In: Goodman-Gilman, A., Rall, T.W., Nies, A.S., and Taylor, P., eds., *The Pharmacological Basis of Therapeutics*, 8th edn., Pergamon Press, New York, 1990, pp. 618–637.

Roberts, E.A.H., Economic importance of flavonoid substances: Tea fermentation. In: Geissman, T.A., ed., *The Chemistry of Flavonoid Compounds*, Pergamon Press, Oxford, U.K., 1962, pp. 468–512.

Roberts, E.A.H., Cartwright, R.A., and Oldschool, M., The phenolic substances of manufactured tea. I. Fractionation and paper chromatography of water-soluble substances, *J. Sci. Food Agric.*, 8, 72, 1959.

Roberts, E.A.H. and Myers, M., The phenolic substances of manufactured tea. IV. Enzymic oxidations of individual substrates, *J. Sci. Food Agric.*, 10, 167, 1959.

Rumpler, W., Seale, J., Clevidence, B., Judd, J., Wiley, E., Yamamoto, S., Komatsu, T., Sawaki, T., Ishikura, Y., and Hosoda, K., Oolong tea increases metabolic rate and fat oxidation in men. *J Nutr* 131, 2848–2852, 2001.

Sakato, Y., Studies on the chemical constituents of tea. Part III. On a new amide theanine, *Nippon Nogeikagaku Kaishi*, 23, 262, 1949 (in Japanese).

Sanderson, G.W., The chemistry of tea and tea manufacturing, *Recent Adv. Phytochem.*, 5, 247, 1972.

Sano, M. et al., Effects of Pu-Erh tea on lipid metabolism in rats, *Chem. Pharm. Bull.*, 34, 221, 1986.

Sayama, K., Lin, S., and Oguni, I., Effects of green tea on growth, food utilization and lipid metabolism in mice, *In vivo*, 14, 481, 2000.

Scharbert, S. and Hofmann, T., Molecular definition of black tea taste by means of quantitative studies, taste reconstitution, and omission experiments, *J. Agric. Food Chem.*, 53, 5377, 2005.

Skrzypczak-Jankun, E. and Jankun, J., Theaflavin digallate inactivates plasminogen activator inhibitor: Could tea help in Alzheimer's disease and obesity? *J. Int. J. Mol. Med.*, 26, 45, 2010.

Sugiyama, K., et al., Teas and other beverages suppress D-galactosamine-induced liver injury in rats, *J. Nutr.*, 129, 1361, 1999.

Sung, H.Y., Hong, C.G., Suh, Y.S., Cho, H.C., Park, J.H., Bae, J.H., Park, W.K., Han, J., Song, D.K., Role of (−)-epigallocatechin-3-gallate in cell viability, lipogenesis, and retinol-binding protein 4 expression in adipocytes, *Naunyn Schmiedebergs Arch Pharmacol*, 382, 303, 2010.

Tappy, L. et al., Metabolic effects of an increase in sympathetic activity in healthy humans, *Int. J. Obes. Relat. Metab. Disord.*, 19, 419, 1995.

Tian, W.-X. et al., Weight reduction by Chinese medicinal herbs may be related to inhibition of fatty acid synthase, *Life Sci.*, 74, 2389, 2004.

Tokimitsu, I., Effects of tea catechins on lipid metabolism and body fat accumulation, *Biofactors*, 22, 141, 2004.

Tsuchida, T., Itakura, H., and Nakamura, H., Reduction of body fat in humans by long-term ingestion of catechins, *Prog. Med.*, 22, 2189, 2002.

Venables, M.C., Hulston, C.J., Cox, H.R., Jeukendrup, A.E., Green tea extract ingestion, fat oxidation, and glucose tolerance in healthy humans, *Am. J. Clin. Nutr.*, 87, 778, 2008.

Wang, H., Wen, Y., Du, Y., Yan, X., Guo, H., Rycroft, J.A., Boon, N., Kovacs, E.M., Mela, D.J., Effects of catechin enriched green tea on body composition, *Obesity (Silver Spring)*, 18, 773, 2010.

Westerterp-Plantenga, M.S., Lejeune, M.P.G.M., and Kovacs, E.M.R., Body weight loss and weight maintenance in relation to habitual caffeine intake and green tea supplementation, *Obes. Res.*, 13, 1195, 2005.

Wolfram, S. et al., TEAVIGO (epigallocatechin gallate) supplementation prevents obesity in rodents by reducing adipose tissue mass, *Ann. Nutr. Metab.*, 49, 54, 2005.

Wu, C.H. et al., Relationship among habitual tea consumption, percent body fat, and body fat distribution, *Obes. Res.*, 11, 1088, 2003.

Yang, C.S. and Landau, J.M., Effects of tea consumption on nutrition and health, *J. Nutr.*, 130, 2409, 2000.

Yang, M.-H., Wang, C.-H., and Chen, H.-L., Green, oolong and black tea extracts modulate lipid metabolism in hyperlipidemia in rats fed high sucrose-diet, *J. Nutr. Biochem.*, 12, 14, 2002.

Zheng, G. et al., Anti-obesity effects of three major components of green tea, catechins, caffeine and theanine, in mice, *In Vivo*, 18, 55, 2004.

40 Laboratory and Clinical Studies of Chitosan

Harry G. Preuss, MD, MACN, CNS, Debasis Bagchi, PhD, MACN, CNS, MAIChE, and Gilbert R. Kaats, PhD, FACN

CONTENTS

INTRODUCTION

Because public attention was largely focused on avoiding dietary saturated fats with the hope of preventing or ameliorating cardiovascular maladies such as atherosclerosis, less emphasis had been placed on limiting overall caloric intake from all sources to prevent obesity. This strategic error is no longer present, because many are now aware that the aforementioned early strategy may account for some part of the so-called obesity epidemic and even the increasing prevalence of diabetes [1,2]. It is hard to understand how this neglect of caloric consumption became so prolonged time wise, because it has long been held that overweight and obesity are responsible for thousands of deaths each year via heart disease, stroke, and diabetes. To add to the problem, it is common knowledge that most individuals who work so hard to lose fat weight regain it subsequently. Americans are not alone in this dilemma. The World Health Organization (WHO) acknowledged the global spread of overweight and obesity [3]. Accordingly, strategies to prevent the further widening of America and the world are necessary [2].

Largely due to safety considerations, many individuals have turned to dietary supplements in preference to drugs to aid in various "weight loss" regimens. Among a multitude of choices, increased dietary fiber consumption has offered one solution. In this chapter, we will concentrate on one fiber, chitosan. It has been proposed that oral intake of chitosan, a soluble fiber with reputed special properties that prevent gastrointestinal absorption fat calories, offers a possible partial solution to the problem [4,5]. What do we know about chitosan?

Pulverized powders from the exoskeleton of crustaceans were originally noted for their ability to soak up oils after environmental spills [4,5]. Based upon this ability, it was hypothesized that chitosan powder might also soak up fats in the human gastrointestinal tract—limiting the consumption of calories from them. Indeed, animal studies demonstrate that chitosan does bind neutral fats under a variety of conditions.

PROPOSED MECHANISMS OF ACTION BEHIND USE OF CHITOSAN FOR BODY WEIGHT LOSS

Chitin is a "cellulose-like" polymer found principally in exoskeletons of marine invertebrates and arthropods such as shrimp, crabs, and lobsters [4,5]. Chitin is composed of long chains of acetylated glucosamine, and chitosan results from the deacetylation of chitin. Theoretically, weight loss associated with chitosan consumption could occur through a number of physiological mechanisms that are not mutually exclusive. For example, a most popular concept is that positively charged chitosan might bind to negatively charged fat molecules and prevent absorption of calorie-containing fat [4]. In a similar vein, the positive charges of chitosan appear to bind bile acids and thus could indirectly increase fecal fat excretion [6,7]. Also, the ability of other viscous fibers such as guar and psyllium to augment fecal fat loss suggests that chitosan may work like many uncharged soluble fibers in general. What is the mechanism(s) behind the latter?

In an acid stomach, chitosan is a soluble fiber, readily dispersed among the digestive secretions and food particles [8–10]. Binding several times its weight in water, the chitosan fiber begins to swell, entrapping and encapsulating dietary fats and oils [8–10]. As chitosan fiber passes along into the small intestines, it encounters an environment that is no longer acidic. In a nonacid environment, chitosan fiber becomes insoluble and forms a gel-like complex that binds fats and bile acids. This insoluble complex passes undigested through the large intestine and is naturally eliminated.

Another possibility to explain weight loss is that the bulk of ingested chitosan could act to suppress appetite.

TOXICOLOGY OF CHITOSAN

Although chitosan appears quite safe when investigating data from animal and human studies [11–13], theoretically, it can be detrimental like all substances taken improperly or in gross excess. Although minerals and electrolytes could be depleted, evidence for such is rare [12]. Dietary chitosan reportedly affects calcium metabolism in animals [14]. In a large clinical trial [15], allergic reactions were seen in 2%–3% of subjects, mainly in those with an allergy to seafood, while constipation was reported in 20% of the subjects. For the most part, constipation passed over time, especially when the intake of fluids was increased [15]. Problems encountered with extremely high doses of chitosan are caused by gastric dehydration and impaction due to the expansion of the fiber [13,15].

FIBERS IN GENERAL ON FECAL FAT EXCRETION AND BODY WEIGHT LOSS

Based on previous experiences with other fibers, there is a precedent for chitosan to augment fecal fat loss and hasten body fat loss. Bran, resins, pectin, etc., have been used successfully in the past for weight loss and cholesterol reduction [10]. Krotkiewski examined the viscous fiber guar and noted reduced hunger and positive effects on lipid and carbohydrate metabolism in obese individuals [16]. Pectin increased fecal fat excretion by 44% (p < 0.001), neutral steroids by 17% (p < 0.001), and fecal bile acids by 33% (p < 0.02) [17]. In African green monkeys, psyllium husk was associated with increased volatile fatty acid output in [18]. Ganji and Kies, investigating the effects of psyllium fiber supplementation on fat digestibility and fecal fatty acid excretion in healthy humans, reported increased fecal fat loss, decreased fat digestibility, and increased fecal palmitic acid excretion with psyllium supplementation [19]. They hypothesized that these associations played a prominent role in the cholesterol-lowering action of psyllium fiber.

INFLUENCE OF CHITOSAN ON GASTROINTESTINAL ABSORPTION OF FATS

The original rationale for using chitosan in weight loss regimens is based upon the belief that this natural substance could trap calorie-loaded fat in the gastrointestinal tract—preventing absorption of this caloric-rich macronutrient.

In Vitro Studies Examining Fat Trapping

Many *in vitro* studies have corroborated previous environmental studies showing that chitosan can trap neutral fats [4,15].

Animal Studies Examining Lipid Binding and Weight Loss

Animal studies, usually performed on rats, have consistently demonstrated the ability of chitosan to trap fat in the gastrointestinal tract [20]. In one study, a low-molecular-weight chitosan hydrolysate inhibited cholesterol absorption in the intestine and increased fecal neutral steroid excretion similar to highly viscous chitosan [21]. The mechanism for the inhibition of fat digestion by chitosan and also a synergistic effect in the presence of ascorbate was examined extensively in animal models [22]. Chitosan dissolves in the stomach and then changes to a gel in the intestines that entraps fat. The mechanisms behind the synergistic effect of ascorbate are considered to be (a) viscosity reduction in the stomach, (b) an increase in the oil-holding capacity of the chitosan gel, and/or (c) the chitosan-fat gel being more flexible and less likely to leak entrapped fat in the intestinal tract.

One study examined 23 different fibers added to a purified diet containing 20% (w/w) corn oil at 5% (w/w) [23]. After 2 weeks of this regimen, feces were collected from each animal during a 3 day period. Ten of the tested fibers significantly increased fecal lipid excretion compared with the cellulose control. Chitosan reduced the fat digestion to one-half of control and did not influence protein digestibility. Since it was noted that the fatty acid composition of the fecal lipids closely resembled that of dietary fat, these results strongly suggest that chitosan has the potential for interfering with fat digestion and absorption in the intestinal tract.

In an excellent experimental design, rats had their lymphatics cannulated and were subsequently gavaged with a test emulsion containing (a) 25 mg of [^{14}C] cholesterol; (b) 50 mg of either guar gum, cellulose, or chitosan; and (c) 200 mg of either safflower, high-oleic safflower, or palm oil [24]. Both the type of dietary fibers ($p < 0.001$) and fats ($p < 0.05$) examined significantly influenced cholesterol absorption, for example, chitosan effectively lowered cholesterol absorption more than guar gum or cellulose. In addition, the effect of chitosan was more significant when given with safflower or high-oleic safflower oil than with palm oil. Dietary fiber also significantly lowered triglyceride absorption ($p < 0.05$). Absorption tended to be low with chitosan, high with cellulose, and intermediate with guar gum. The results show that the type of dietary fat significantly influences the effect that dietary fiber exerted on lipid absorption.

Two polyglucosamines with similar characteristics and molecular weights were compared in male rats as to their effects on various parameters [25]. Fifteen young male rats were fed a standard diet or the same diet containing 2% of each polyglucosamines for 4 weeks. Both fibers showed less expected weight gain compared to control ($p < 0.05$) despite a greater increase in food intake. Fecal lipid and water concentrations were increased in the polyglucosamine-treated groups ($p < 0.05$).

CLINICAL STUDIES EXAMINING LIPID ABSORPTION

The first reported clinical study on chitosan was performed in Norway [26], where the resultant weight loss found in the test subjects was attributed to the fat-binding abilities of chitosan. In five ensuing studies, all performed in Italy by different principal investigators, many included the observation that stools in weight-losing treatment subjects were larger and softer than placebo-receiving subjects [27–33]. In 30 subjects, Macchi reports that "fecal excretion of fats was observed only in those taking chitosan" [29]. Girola et al. conducted a clinical study on 150 subjects of both sexes, and noted that the administration of the dietary integrator containing 240 mg chitosan per capsule caused significant weight loss [27]. The subjects were also evaluated for changes in circulating triglycerides on the 28th day of study. The placebo group showed a 13.2% reduction, whereas the treatment groups showed a greater 26.6% decrease. The most likely explanation for the exaggerated decrease in triglyceride concentrations in the presence of chitosan is decreased fat absorption. In support of this assumption, Hoffman La Roche investigators found that the triglyceride levels in their animals were lower after chitosan per os and believed that the reduced blood triglycerides were directly correlated with reduced fat availability via digestive processes [34]. While some observers believe the appearance of stools is a good indicator of the presence of fat, still direct measurements are necessary for corroboration.

Many studies have measured fat in the feces directly to gauge absorption. These measurements, mostly performed using a gravimetric procedure, have shown varying results. A group from UC Davis performed direct measurements of fecal fat on healthy subjects in three similar studies [35–37]. In these studies, subjects consumed extraordinary amounts of fat after oral intake of chitosan—no placebo controls were followed. Fecal fat excretion was increased by chitosan under some circumstances but not others. Nevertheless, the investigators questioned the clinical significance of the small differences [37]. In a different study, 12 healthy adult volunteers within 20% of ideal body weight entered a 7 day run-in diet period before one-half were randomized to the drug orlistat (120 mg) and the other one-half to chitosan (890 mg) three times daily for 7 days [38]. Subjects were then crossed over for the other treatment regimen. Fecal fat excretion increased markedly with orlistat, but the 20% average increase with chitosan did not achieve statistical significance. It was concluded that chitosan had no significant effect on fecal fat excretion.

Not all studies have been negative, however. Nesbitt et al. [39] examined a formula containing chitosan. Nineteen female subjects received 2.0 g of formula containing chitosan (40% w/w), psyllium (51% w/w), apple pectin (4% w/w), and glucomannan (4% w/w) twice a day preceding lunch and dinner. Eighteen female subjects were simultaneously given a placebo under similar conditions. After 30 days, the treatment group showed a statistically significantly greater increase in fecal fat content: the supplement group experienced an average of 2.48% increase in fecal fat content over baseline, whereas the placebo group had an average decrease of 3.73% in fecal fat content (p = 0.0002). In another weight loss study examining chitosan, total fecal fat was analyzed at baseline and week 8 in a small set of subjects, three in the placebo group and four in the treatment group [40]. In this small population, there was a statistical trend for chitosan to increase fecal fat excretion. Total fecal fat excretion increased on an average +6.0 g ± 2.7 (SEM) over baseline in the treatment group and decreased −2.3 g ± 2.4 (SEM) under baseline in the placebo group (p < .07). Barroso-Aranda et al. [41] measured fecal fat directly after chitosan administration. While the increase in fecal fat was statistically significant, it could account for only 30–40 kcal/day saving in calories. A paper from Japan discussed the use of chitosan to treat Crohn's disease [42]. The investigators found that a chitosan (1.05 g/d) and ascorbic acid mixture significantly increased the fat concentrations in the feces during treatment (average 60 mg/g dry weight before vs. 79 mg/day after 8 weeks) (p < 0.035).

None of the studies mentioned earlier that made direct measurements of fecal fat reported the accuracy of the methodology. This is particularly important because the presence of chitosan could affect such measurements. Therefore, it is necessary to examine findings utilizing other methods to estimate fecal fat excretion.

Terada et al. reported that levels of total fecal volatile fatty acid increased significantly from 14.3 ± 3.2 to 20.3 ± 2.4 mg/g on day 14 of chitosan intake (p < 0.01), with a significant increase of acetic (p < 0.05) and propionic (p < 0.01) acids [43]. Utilizing a breath test involving radioactive materials, Swedish investigators reported that subjects receiving chitosan showed reduced fat uptake compared to placebo [14]. In the whole group, the reduction in animal fat uptake with the chitosan compound was approximately 13% after 6 h. The results were statistically significant (p < 0.05) at the 5 h mark. Four volunteers did not react at all, but the rest showed an average reduced fat uptake of approximately 25%.

Blum believed as mentioned previously [34] that the amount of fat absorbed from a fat-containing meal is proportional to the incremental increase in plasma triglycerides [44]. Therefore, the effects of chitosan after fat challenge were estimated by examining multiple triglyceride levels over the time necessary for the triglyceride levels to return to baseline. One gram of chitosan was taken 5–10 min before a fatty meal purchased at a local restaurant. Nine out of 13 subjects, roughly two-third, responded favorably. The investigators estimated that chitosan inhibited the absorption of dietary fat in the range of 20–28 g of fat for every gram of chitosan in five of the subjects.

The overall weight of evidence favors the long-held assumption that chitosan fiber taken properly under proper conditions increases fecal fat loss, but whether the trapped fecal fat could account for significant weight loss remains open to question at this time. However, an even more important question is whether chitosan can decrease body fat mass by any means.

CLINICAL STUDIES ON THE ROLE OF CHITOSAN IN BODY FAT LOSS

Results may differ among studies, because conditions are rarely the same. To give examples, (a) the quality of chitosan material often fluctuates [45,46], (b) the quantity of material used (dosage) frequently varies [46], (c) the timing of the dosing may also be an important variable, (d) the diet offered with chitosan (e.g., low or high fat and/or low or high caloric content) can influence outcome, (e) the different methodologies used for assessing end points, for example, weight loss rather than fat loss, may affect interpretations, (f) the individual biological responses may be dissimilar, and finally (g) compliance of subjects may differ markedly. Accordingly, a broad and complete picture emanating from many studies must be used to assess effectiveness of chitosan as a weight loss agent.

The initial weight loss investigation using chitosan, performed over 10 years ago, was a double-blind, placebo-controlled study on 18 subjects ingesting a low caloric diet and consuming 1.92 g of chitosan per day [26]. Weight loss in test subjects compared to controls was significant after 14 and 28 days. The next studies, performed in Italy, were very similar in format—randomized, double-blind, and placebo-controlled [27–29,33]. In these particular studies, subjects consumed a 1000 kcal diet and received four tablets of chitosan or placebo per day for 28 days. Unfortunately, the amount of chitosan in each tablet was never revealed. In addition, other ingredients, such as guar and psyllium, were added to a formula, although the authors tended to attribute benefits principally to chitosan.

Giustini and Ventura reported that weight loss of the chitosan group significantly exceeded the placebo group in 100 subjects [30,31]. Sciutto and Columbo wrote that the chitosan weight loss significantly exceeded placebo in 90 subjects [32]. Girola et al. [27] in 150 subjects noted that weight loss on an integrator containing chitosan significantly exceeded placebo. Veneroni et al. [28] similarly showed that weight loss in the chitosan group significantly exceeded placebo in 80 subjects. Colombo and Sciutto studied 86 subjects: the weight loss in the chitosan group significantly exceeded placebo [33]. Macchi [29] found that the weight loss in the chitosan group also significantly exceeded placebo in 30 subjects.

The earliest studies were performed on subjects consuming very caloric restricted diets. Therefore, the question was raised concerning the influences of chitosan on individuals consuming more normal levels of calories. Wuolijoki et al. [47] showed an effect of chitosan on lipid lowering but discovered no significant change in body weight. However, they raised the possibility of poor compliance in their report. The authors hypothesized that reduced lipid absorption from the gastrointestinal tract decreased energy intake stimulating hunger. Pittler et al. [48], in a double-blind, placebo-controlled study on 34 subjects, reported that weight loss in the chitosan group did not exceed placebo. The subjects ate regular diets and were supposed to consume 1.2 g of chitosan per day for 28 days. Unfortunately, the amount of chitosan given was lower than expected, i.e., 60% of the designated amount. Thus, the treatment group, eating regular amounts of fat, received a relatively small dose. In an open-label study composed of 332 subjects [12], 221 of the subjects responded to chitosan per os by losing a significant amount of weight (−4.1 kg). Nesbitt et al. [38] provided 1.6 g of chitosan per day for 30 days in a formulation comprised mainly of chitosan to 37 mildly to moderately obese subjects and saw a significant decrease in body weight (placebo gained +2.3 lb and treatment lost −3.6 lb). Unfortunately, the average body weight of the treatment group at the initiation of the study was 192 lb compared to the average weight of the placebo group, 172 lb. Obviously, this discrepancy makes interpretation more difficult, even though this weight loss was accompanied by a corresponding significant increase in fecal fat content in the treatment group versus the placebo group. Likewise, total cholesterol and LDL decreased, and HDL increased in the treatment group compared to the placebo group. All differences were statistically significant.

Schiller et al. performed a randomized, double-blind, placebo-controlled study in overweight and mildly obese individuals [40]. Subjects took either three capsules of a rapidly soluble chitosan (1.5 g b.i.d.) or matched placebo twice daily for 8 weeks. Interestingly, the study overlapped a holiday period when increased caloric intake might be expected, because subjects continued to consume their regular diet. To back this assumption, the placebo group showed a mean weight gain of +1.5 kg over the holiday period. Differently, the mean weight loss was −1.0 kg within the treatment group over the 8 week period. Chi-square analysis for weight loss between groups indicated significantly more subjects lost weight within the treatment group than within the placebo group (63% and 17%, respectively, p < 0.001).

Zahorska-Markiewicz et al. reported that their treatment subjects (50 obese women, 22–59 years, BMI > 30) received a low caloric diet (1000 kcal/day during 6 months) along with chitosan in a randomized, placebo-controlled, double-blind study [49]. The 6 month project consisted of 2 h meetings with a physician, psychologist, and dietitian, in a group of about 20 persons every 2 weeks. The chitosan group received 1.5 g three times daily. Significantly greater body weight losses and decreased systolic blood pressure were noted compared to the placebo group. The chitosan-supplemented group lost an average of 15.9 kg compared to the placebo groups' 10.9 kg.

Ho et al. [50] examining 68 subjects who were overweight and hypercholesterolemic found no significant changes in the measured parameters and no severe side effects in chitosan-treated subjects. However, the investigators stated, "We believe that subjects could have inadvertently increased their caloric intake under the false belief that chitosan would bind all fat that was consumed." Further, it was noted that the patients took approximately 80% of the correct dose of chitosan. The authors postulated that this might represent "underdosing."

A 24 week randomized, double-blind, placebo-controlled trial, conducted at the University of Auckland, examined 250 participants (82% women) with a mean body mass index of 35.5 kg/m² [51]. Participants in the treatment group, who were given advice on diet and lifestyle, received 3 g of chitosan per day. In an intention to treat analysis with the last observation carried forward, the chitosan group lost more body weight than the placebo group (−0.4 ± 0.2 kg vs. +0.2 ± 0.2 kg, p = 0.03). The investigators did not deem these differences to be clinically significant. Unfortunately, the report did not give the information on a singled-out group of compliant individuals. Similar small changes occurred in the circulating total and LDL cholesterol and glucose (p < 0.01).

Two authors of this report (GRK, HGP) examined the effects of chitosan on fat loss using DEXA, the state-of-the-art means to estimate body fat [52]. One hundred fifty subjects were examined over an 8 week study period in order to evaluate the effects of a novel chitosan formulation on body weight, body composition (lean-to-fat ratios), bone density, and blood chemistries under real-life conditions. Subjects were randomly assigned to one of three 50-subject groups: a treatment group that was provided with a behavior modification program and consumed a dietary supplement containing principally chitosan, a placebo group that was provided with the same behavior modification program but consumed a placebo supplement, and a control group that was asked to follow any program of their choosing but who also completed the same beginning and ending tests as the treatment and placebo groups. A total of 131 (87%) subjects completed the study. For those completing the study, there were highly statistically significant differences between the treatment group compared to placebo and control in body weight loss. The treatment group lost in body weight −3.4 lb ± 5.9 (SEM) compared to placebo −0.9 lb ± 4.2 (SEM) (p = 0.028) and control +0.6 lb ± 4.4 (SEM) (p = 0.001). In addition, there were highly significant differences between treatment and placebo in reduced percent fat [−1.1% ± 2.0 (SEM) vs. 0.4% ± 1.7 (SEM), p = 0.001] and fat mass [−3.2 lb ± 4.7 (SEM) vs. +0.5 lb ± 4.1 (SEM), p = 0.001]. Comparing treatment to control, there was a significant reduced loss of fat mass [control = −0.1 lb ± 4.4 (SEM), p = 0.002], but only trends in lowering percent fat. These data provide compelling evidence for the efficacy of the novel chitosan product to facilitate the depletion of excess body weight via fat loss under free-living conditions very similar to those in which these products are most likely to be used.

A double-blind study was carried out by Cornelli et al. [53] in two groups of 30 subjects (M/F from 25 to 59 years). Tablets containing the low-molecular-weight chitosan at 2 g/day or a placebo were given for a 4 month period to those undergoing a physical training regimen. In the treated group compared to control, there was a statistically significant reduction in body weight [6.9 kg ± 1.9 (SEM) vs. 3.0 kg + 1.6 (SEM)] and waist circumference [7.3 cm ± 2.5 (SEM) vs. 3.1 cm ± 4.2 (SEM)]. LDL cholesterol and triglycerides decreased more while HDL cholesterol increased more in the chitosan group compared to control. The investigators concluded, "Results indicate that PG (chitosan) may improve the effect of the physical training in moderately overweight patients with dyslipidemia and may be of some help in the treatment of the metabolic syndrome."

CHITOSAN AS A WEIGHT MANAGEMENT OPTION: CONCLUSION

Since the original chapter on chitosan was written approximately 4 years ago, little direct research concerning chitosan and body composition has been carried out. Two exceptions have been mentioned [25,53]. Some reviews that include information on chitosan have been written [54,55].

After examining a myriad of data presented on chitosan as a weight-loss supplement, some could question its importance for a number of reasons. First, only a limited number of human clinical trials have been conducted on chitosan for the purposes of weight management, and with few exceptions, these dealt only with scale weight, not a direct measure of fat mass. As a second point, the results among studies are not as consistent as one would like probably due to the multiple differences in protocols—different varieties of chitosan, different doses, different timing of the doses, different diets, different end points, and different populations.

As a third point, so-called weight loss studies in general, even randomized, double-blind, placebo-controlled ones, present problems. First, odds are stacked against showing significant weight loss in most clinical studies using the randomized, double-blind, placebo-controlled protocol. We base this on the following realities. Regimens that simultaneously increase muscle mass may mask any fat loss when only scale weight is assessed [56]; when in reality, fat loss rather than overall scale weight loss is important.

As a final point, most subjects invariably weigh themselves and subsequently believe they are "on placebo" whether true or not. This leads to poor compliance. Noncompliance will adversely cloud the positive results in the treatment group, especially when an intention-to-treat analysis is used [57]. It is our opinion that merely counting pills is not sufficient to judge compliance. Since we believe that even in randomized, placebo-controlled, double-blind studies on weight loss, the odds are stacked against positive results, when such studies are positive, those consumers willing to comply with directions may have even better success.

REFERENCES

1. Bray GA. Obesity. In: Ziegler EE, Filer, Jr., LJ eds., *Present Knowledge in Nutrition*. ILSI Press, Washington, DC, 1996; pp. 19–32.
2. Farag YM, Gaballa MR. Diabesity: An overview of a rising epidemic. *Nephrol Dial Transpl* 2011;26:28–35.
3. World Health Organization (WHO), *Consultation on Obesity*. WHO, Geneva, Switzerland, 1997.
4. Hennen WJ. *Chitosan*. Woodland Publishing, Inc., Pleasant Grove, VT, 1996, pp. 3–31.
5. Duarte A. *Chitosan Plus: The Fat Magnet*. DMI, Des Moines, IA, 1998, pp. 1–32.
6. Muzzarelli RA. Recent results in the oral administration of chitosan. In: Muzzarelli RA ed., *Chitosan per OS: From Dietary Supplement to Drug Carrier*. Atec, Inc., Grottammare, Italy, 2000; pp. 3–40.
7. Enig MG. Lets get physical with fats. In: *Know Your Fats*. M.G. Enig (ed.), Bethesda Press, Bethesda, MD, 2000; pp. 51–88.

8. Furda I. Non absorbable lipid binder. US Patent, No: 4,223,023.

9. Furda I. Reduction of absorption of dietary lipids and cholesterol by chitosan and its derivatives and special formulations. In: Muzzarelli RA ed., *Chitosan Per OS: From Dietary Supplement to Drug Carrier.* Atec, Inc., Grottammare, Italy, 2000; pp. 41–63.

10. Furda I, Brine CJ. Interaction of dietary fiber with lipids. Mechanistic theories and their limitations. In: Furda I, Brine CJ eds., *New Developments in Dietary Fiber.* Plenum Press, New York, 1990; pp. 67–82.

11. Anderson MA, Slater MR, Hammad TA. Result of a survey of small animal practitioners on the perceived clinical efficacy and safety of an oral nutraceutical. *Prev Veter Med* 1999;38:65–73.

12. Deuchi K, Kanauchi O, Shizukuishi M, Kobayashi E. Continuous and massive intake of chitosan affects mineral and fat-soluble vitamin status in rats fed on a high-fat diet. *Biosci Biotech Biochem* 1995;59:1211–1216.

13. Ylitalo R, Lehtinen S, Wuolijoki E, Ylitalo P, Lehtimaki T. Cholesterol-lowering properties and safety of chitosan. *Arzneim Forsch* 2002;52:1–7.

14. Wada M, Nishimura Y, Watanabe Y, Takita T, Innami S. Accelerating effect of chitosan intake on urinary calcium excretion by rats. *Biosci Biotechnol Biochem* 1997;61:1206–1208.

15. Wadstein J, Thom E, Heldman E, Gudmunsson S, Lilja B. Biopolymer L112, a chitosan with fat binding properties and potential as a weight reducing agent. In: Muzzarelli RA ed., *Chitosan Per OS: From Dietary Supplement to Drug Carrier.*, Atec, Inc., Grottammare, Italy, 2000; pp. 65–76.

16. Krotkiewski M. Effect of guar gum on body-weight, hunger ratings and metabolism in obese subjects. *Br J Nutr* 1984;52:97–105.

17. Kay RM, Truswell AS. Effect of citrus on blood lipids and fecal steroid excretion in man. *Am J Clin Nutr* 1977;30:171–175.

18. Costa MA, Mehta T, Males JR. Effects of dietary cellulose, psyllium husk and cholesterol level on fecal and colonic microbial metabolism in monkeys. *J Nutr* 1989;119:986–992.

19. Ganji V, Kies CV. Psyllium husk fiber supplementation to soybean and coconut oil diets of humans: Effect of fat digestibility and faecal fatty acid excretion. *Eur J Clin Nutr* 1994;48:595–597.

20. Nagyvary JJ, Falk JD, Schmidt ML, Wilkins AK, Bradbury EL. The hypolipidemic activity of chitosan and other polysaccharides in rats. *Nutr Rep Int.* 1979;30:677–685.

21. Ikeda I, Sugano M, Yoshida K, Sasaki E, Iwamoto Y, Hatano K. Hydrolysates with cholesterol and fatty acid absorption and metabolic consequences in rat. *J Agric Food Chem* 1993;41:431–435.

22. Kanauchi O, Deuchi K, Imasato Y, Shizukuishi M, Kobayashi E. Mechanism for the inhibition of fat digestion by chitosan and for the synergistic effect of ascorbate. *Biosci Biotech Biochem* 1995;59:786–790.

23. Deuchi K, Kanauchi O, Imasato Y, Kobayashi E. Decreasing effect of chitosan on the apparent fat digestibility by rats fed on a high-fat diet. *Biosci Biotech Biochem* 1994;58:1613–1616.

24. Ikeda I, Tomari Y, Sugano M. Interrelated effects of dietary fiber and fat on lymphatic cholesterol and triglyceride absorption in rats. *J Nutr* 1989;119:1383–1387.

25. Bondiolotti G, Bareggi SR, Frega NG, Strabioli S, Cornelli U. Activity of two different polyglucosamines, L112 and FF 45, on body weights in male rats. *Eur J Pharmacol* 2007;567:155–158.

26. Abelin J, Lassus A. The Helsinki Report, L-112 Biopolymer fat binder. ARS Medicina, Helsinki, Finland, 1994.

27. Girola M, De Bernardi M, Contos S, Tripodi S, Ventura P, Guarino C, Marletta M. Dose effect in lipid-lowering activity of a new dietary integrator (chitosan), *Garcinia cambogia* extract and chrome. *Acta Toxicol Ther* 1996;17:25–40.

28. Veneroni G, Veneroni F, Contos S, Tripodi S, De Bernardi M, Guarino C, Marletta M. Effect of a new chitosan dietary integrator and hypocaloric diet on hyperlipidemia and overweight in obese patients. *Acta Toxicol Ther* 1996;17:53–70.

29. Macchi G. A new approach to the treatment of obesity: Chitosan's effects on body weight reduction and plasma cholesterol levels. *Acta Toxicol Ther* 1996;17:303–320.

30. Giustini A, Ventura P. Weight-reducing regimens in obese subjects; effects of a new dietary fiber integrator. *Acta Toxicol Ther* 1995;16:199–214.

31. Ventura P. Lipid lowering activity of chitosan, a new dietary integrator. *Chitin Enz* 1996;2:55–62.

32. Sciutto AM, Colombo P. Lipid-lowering effect of chitosan dietary integrator and hypocaloric diet in obese subjects. *Acta Toxicol Ther* 1995;16:215–230.

33. Colombo P, Sciutto AM. Nutritional aspects of chitosan employment in hypocaloric diet. *Acta Toxicol Ther* 1996;17:287–302.

34. Angerer JD, Cyron DM, Iyer S, Jerrell TA. Dry acid-chitosan complexes, Patent No: 6,326,475, December 4, 2001.

35. Gades MD, Stern JS. Chitosan supplementation does not affect fat absorption in healthy males fed a high-fat diet, a pilot study. *Int J Obes Relat Metab Disord* 2002;26:119–122.

36. Gades MD, Stern JS. Chitosan supplementation and fecal fat excretion in men. *Obes Res* 2003;11:683–688.

37. Gades MD, Stern JS. Chitosan supplementation and fat absorption in men and women. *J Am Diet Assoc* 2005;105:72–77.

38. Guercolini R, Radu-Radulescu L, Boldrin M, Dallas J, Moore R. Comparative evaluation of fecal fat excretion induced by orlistat and chitosan. *Obes Res* 2001;9:364–367.

39. Nesbitt L, Ricart CM, Miranda-Massari J, Gonzales MJ. Long term effect of a high fiber dietary supplement on total body weight, fecal fat, lipid profile and blood pressure in female human subjects. *Biomedicina* 1999;2:S9–S12.

40. Schiller RN, Barrager E, Schauss AG, Nichols EJ. A randomized, double-blind, placebo-controlled study examining effects of a rapidly soluble chitosan dietary supplement on weight loss and body composition in overweight and mildly obese individuals. *JANA* 2001;4:34–41.

41. Borosso-Arranda J, Contreras F, Bagchi D, Preuss HG. Efficacy of a novel chitosan formulation on fecal fat excretion: A double-blind, crossover, placebo-controlled study. *J Med* 2002;33:209–225.

42. Tsujikawa T, Kanauchi O, Andoh A, Saotome T, Sasaki M, Fujiyama Y, Bamba T. Supplement of a chitosan and ascorbic acid mixture for Crohn's disease: A pilot study. *Nutrition* 2003;19:137–139.

43. Terada A, Hara H, Sato D et al. Effect of dietary chitosan on faecal microbiota and faecal metabolites of humans. *Microb Ecol Health Dis* 1995;8:15–21.

44. Blum JM. Executive Summary: Chitosol Triglyceride Testing, Technical Report, February 2000.

45. Muzzarelli RA, Tanfani F, Emanuelli M, Muzzarelli MG, Celia G. The production of chitosans of superior quality. *J Appl Biochem* 1981;3:316–321.

46. Bough WA, Salter WL, Wu ACM, Perkins BE. Influence of manufacturing variables on the characteristics and effectiveness of chitosan products. 1. Chemical composition, viscosity, and molecular-weight distribution of chitosan products. *Biotechnol Bioeng* 1978;20:1931–1940.

47. Wuolijoki E, Hirveld T, Yulizalo P. Decrease in serum LDL cholesterol with microcrystalline chitosan. *Methods Find Exp Clin Pharmacol* 1999;21:357–361.

48. Pittler MH, Abbot NC, Harkness EF, Ernst E. Randomized, double-blind trial of chitosan for body weight reduction. *Eur J Clin Nutr* 1999;53:379–381.

49. Zahorska-Markiewicz B, Krotkiewski M, Olszanecka-Glinanowicz M, Zurakowski A. Effect of chitosan in complex management of obesity. *Pol Merkuriusz Lek* 2002;13:129–132.

50. Ho SC, Tai ES, Eng PH-K, Tan EC, Fok ACK. In the absence of dietary surveillance, chitosan does not reduce plasma lipids or obesity in hypercholesterolemic obese Asian subjects. *Singapore Med J* 2001;42:006–010.

51. Mhurchu CN, Poppitt SD, McGill AT, Leahy FE, Bennett DA, Lin RB, Ormrod D, Ward L, Strik C, Rodgers A. The effect of the dietary supplement, chitosan, on body weight: A randomized controlled trial in 250 overweight and obese adults. *Int J Obes Relat Metab Disord* 2004;28:1149–1156.

52. Kaats GR, Michelak JE, Preuss HG. An evaluation of the efficacy and safety of a chitosan fiber product. *J Am Coll Nutr* 2006;25:389–394.

53. Cornelli U, Belcaro G, Cesarone MR, Cornelli M. Use of polyglucosamine and physical activity to reduce body weight and dyslipidemia in moderately overweight subjects. *Minerva Cardioangiol* 2008;56:71–78.

54. Preuss HG, Kaats GR. Chitosan as a dietary supplement for weight loss: A review. *Curr Nutr Rev*, 2006;2:297–311.

55. Cherniack EP. Potential applications for alternative medicine to treat obesity in an aging population. *Altern Med Rev* 2008;13:34–42.

56. Crawford V, Scheckenbach R, Preuss HG. Effects of niacin-bound chromium supplementation on body composition of overweight African-American women. *Diabetes Obes Metab* 1999;1:331–337.

57. Feinman RD. Intention-to-treat. What is the question? *Nutr Metab* 2009;6:1–8.

41 Role of Curcumin, the Golden Spice, in Obesity and Associated Chronic Diseases

Sahdeo Prasad, PhD, Sridevi Patchva, PhD, and Bharat B. Aggarwal, PhD

CONTENTS

INTRODUCTION

Obesity is a medical condition in which excess fat is accumulated in the body, which further results in an adverse health effect (Haslam and James 2005). Measurement of obesity is determined by body mass index (BMI), which compares weight and height. A person is considered to be overweight (or preobese) if BMI is between 25 and 29.9 and obese with BMI over 30. In the United States, obesity is a serious problem. About one-third of the U.S. adults (33.8%) and approximately 17% (or 12.5 million) of children and adolescents aged 2–19 years are obese. The obesity is dramatically increased in the United States during the last 20 years, and the trend is still the same. In 2010, all states had a prevalence of obesity over 20%. In the United States, cost for obesity-related health problems is also high—about $168 billion costs every year, amounting to 17% of all medical bills. Obesity is not a sole disorder; rather it increases the risk of development of many other common diseases including heart disease, hypertension, diabetes, osteoarthritis, cancer, sleep apnea, abdominal hernias, varicose veins, gout, gall bladder disease, respiratory problems, and liver malfunction. Thus, the reduction of obesity could prevent the onset of several chronic diseases.

Obesity is a preventable disease. It needs strong intellectual strategies such as physical activity, lifestyle modification, and behavioral routine. Since diet is one of the major contributors to obesity, the dietary lifestyle modification would minimize excessive accumulation of unwanted fat. It is necessary to understand that certain kinds of diet (proinflammatory) can promote obesity, whereas other kinds (anti-inflammatory) can reduce it (Aggarwal and Shishodia 2006; Ghanim et al. 2001; Lamas et al. 2003; Navab et al. 2008; Rajala and Scherer 2003). A high-calorie, high-fat, and low-fiber diet usually promotes obesity, whereas caloric restriction, exercise, and wholesome foods have been shown to reverse it (Fontana et al. 2010; Reeds 2009; Varady and Hellerstein 2008). It is generally believed that highly processed, packaged, and refined foods loaded with sugar and hydrogenated oils are likely to promote obesity. For centuries, traditional medicines, which include natural compounds from plant sources, are considered to be the remedy for several diseases and disorders.

CURCUMIN: SOURCE, STRUCTURE, AND BIOAVAILABILITY

Curcumin (CCM) is the principal active curcuminoid present in the rhizome of the popular Indian spice turmeric (*Curcuma longa*) (Figure 41.1). It is a member of the ginger family (Zingiberaceae). The curcuminoids are natural phenols and are responsible for the yellow color of turmeric. Naturally, less than 3% of the content of the roots are CCM. CCM can exist in at least two tautomeric forms, keto and enol. The enol form is comparatively more stable in the solid phase as well as in solutions (Kolev 2005). CCM incorporates several functional groups in the structure. The aromatic rings, which are polyphenols, are connected by two α,β-unsaturated carbonyl groups. The diketones of CCM either form stable enols or deprotonated to form enolates, while α,β-unsaturated carbonyl is a good Michael acceptor and undergoes nucleophilic addition.

CCM has shown to have low bioavailability, which means most of ingested CCM goes directly into our gastrointestinal area and is expelled. However, some amount of ingested CCM remains in the bloodstream. The ingested CCM metabolized in the intestine involves sulfation, glucuronidation, and reduction reactions, which result in poor systemic absorption (Baum et al. 2008; Ireson et al. 2002). These metabolites have a very short half-life and poor cell permeability. Whether they are as bioactive as their parent compound is not yet well established (Gonzales and Orlando 2008). However, it is possible that either parent or metabolized CCM gets absorbed and would be enough to function in the body cells.

To improve the systemic absorption of CCM, several challenging efforts have been undertaken. These challenging efforts include the use of adjuvant, liposomal formulation, nanoparticles preparation, and structural modification of CCM. Piperine (an alkaloid in black pepper) has shown to interfere with

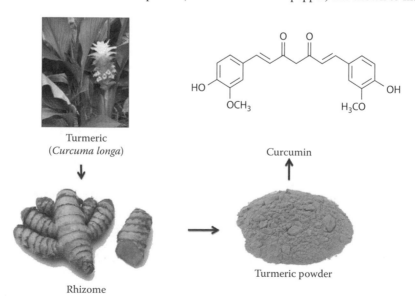

Turmeric
(*Curcuma longa*)

Rhizome

Curcumin

Turmeric powder

FIGURE 41.1 Source CCM and its chemical structure.

glucuronidation of CCM and enhances its bioavailability. In a study, 20 mg of piperine increases 2000% absorption of CCM (Shoba et al. 1998). Nanoparticles of CCM (nanocurcumin) have been developed to improve the solubility and bioavailability of CCM. *In vitro* study showed that nanocurcumin is effective for retrogressing inflammatory responses and promoting apoptosis in human pancreatic cancer cell lines (Bisht et al. 2007). The formulated liposomal CCM also showed *in vitro* and *in vivo* antitumor activity and improved bioavailability. Another study showed that when administered with olive oil, stearic acid, or phosphatidyl choline, the level of CCM in blood increased (Baum et al. 2008). It was also found that turmeric spice added to a food matrix containing oil increased the bioavailability of CCM (Lim et al. 2001). In an *in vivo* experiment performed with murine models, an administration of a combination of CCM and lipids resulted in 50 times higher CCM serum levels, which was found to be effective for ameliorating neuroinflammatory and Alzheimer's diseases (Begum et al. 2008).

ROLE OF CURCUMIN IN OBESITY

Obesity is a major obstacle in the maintenance of the human health system and causes various chronic diseases (Shehzad et al. 2011). Recent evidence has shown that some dietary components such as spices may play a key role in the protection against and/or treatment of obesity and related metabolic disorders. Among these spices, turmeric has received considerable research interest because of its active ingredient, CCM. CCM interacts with specific proteins in adipocytes, pancreatic cells, hepatic stellate cells (HSC), macrophages, and muscle cells, where it suppresses several cellular proteins such as transcription factor nuclear factor-kappaB (NF-κB), signal transducer and activator of transcription (STAT)-3, and Wnt/β-catenin and activates peroxisome proliferator-activated receptor (PPAR)-γ and nuclear factor-erythroid 2 p45-related factor 2 (Nrf2) cell signaling pathway. In addition, CCM downregulates the inflammatory cytokines, resistin and leptin, and upregulates adiponectin as well as other associated proteins (Figure 41.2). The interactions of CCM with several signal transduction pathways

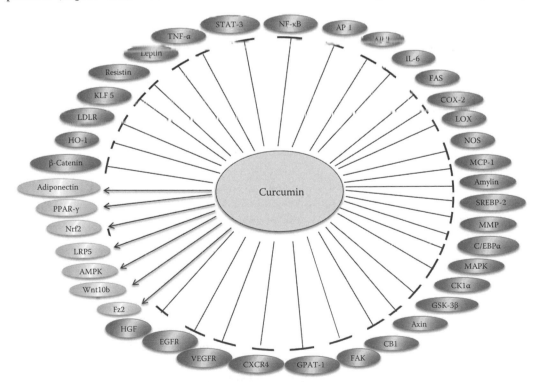

FIGURE 41.2 Multiple targets of CCM involved in development of obesity and associated diseases.

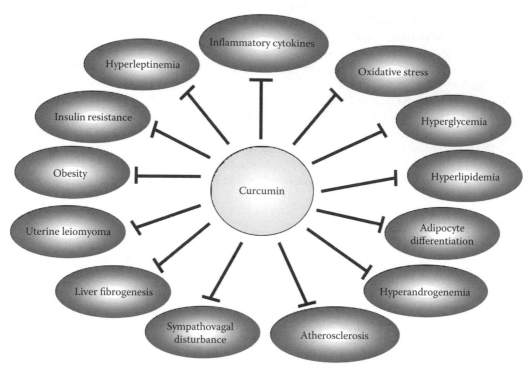

FIGURE 41.3 Role of CCM against obesity.

reverse insulin resistance, hyperglycemia, hyperlipidemia, and other inflammatory symptoms associated with obesity and metabolic diseases (Figure 41.3).

CURCUMIN IN WEIGHT LOSS

CCM has shown to prevent or reduce body weight gain. Experimental study showed that supplementation of CCM with high-fat diet to mice did not affect food intake but reduced high-fat-diet-induced body weight gain, adiposity, and microvessel density in adipose tissue. CCM increased metabolic rate indicated by increase in 5′AMΠ-activated protein kinase (AMPK) phosphorylation, reduction in glycerol-3-phosphate acyl transferase-1, and increase in carnitine palmitoyltransferase-1 expression, which led to increased oxidation and decreased fatty acid esterification (Ejaz et al. 2009). The cannabinoid (CB) receptor, CB-1, which is expressed in the brain, smooth muscle cells, and colon cells, has been linked with food intake and body weight in mice (Pavon et al. 2008). Study showed that CCM is an antagonist of CB-1 receptor, and it selectively binds to CB-1 with nanomolar affinity. This binding affinity of CCM to CB-1 could be the probable reason for weight loss in the mice treated with CCM (Seely et al. 2009). Thus, these studies indicate that CCM could work against obesity by reducing food intake and body weight.

CURCUMIN IN LIPID METABOLISM

CCM is shown to affect the fat metabolism and storage. When CCM (0.05 g/100 g diet) is supplemented to hamsters, which were fed with high-fat diet, it significantly lowered the levels of free fatty acid (FFA), total cholesterol, triglycerides, and leptin and improved homeostasis compared to only high-fat-diet-fed animals. It has also been observed that fatty acid beta-oxidation activity was significantly higher in the liver of CCM-treated group than in the control group, whereas fatty acid synthase (FAS), 3-hydroxy-3-methylglutaryl-coenzyme A (CoA) reductase, and acyl-CoA:cholesterol acyltransferase activities were significantly lower (Jang 2008). This study indicates CCM has hypolipidemic effect. It has been proposed that CCM and its metabolites activate PPAR-γ, which functions in the lowering of lipid level (Asai and Miyazawa 2001). Oxidation of low-density lipid (LDL) resulted in inflammation, which is a substantial factor for obesity. CCM is shown to prevent oxidation and lipid modification of LDL. LDL oxidized in the presence of CCM caused a significant decrease in its by-products like conjugated diene, lipid peroxides, and lysoPC and a significant increase in polyunsaturated fatty acid (PUFA) (Mahfouz et al. 2009). These studies indicate that CCM is effective in the metabolism of lipid, which shows its hypolipidemic properties.

In a clinical study, CCM improved the lipid profile in human subjects. Administration of CCM (500 mg per day for 7 days) in 10 healthy human volunteers reduced the serum levels of total cholesterol (11.63%) and lipid peroxides (33%) and increased the high-density lipoprotein (HDL) cholesterol (HDL-C) (29%) (Soni and Kuttan 1992). In another clinical trial on 75 acute coronary syndrome patients, administration of low-dose CCM showed a trend of reduction in total cholesterol level and LDL-cholesterol (LDL-C) level (Alwi 2008). In an animal study, feeding of high-cholesterol diet resulted in marked hypercholesterolemia, an increase in serum level of LDL-C but a decrease in serum HDL-C). However, CCM admixed diet decreased the serum total cholesterol by 21% and LDL-C by 42.5%, but it increased serum HDL by 50% (Arafa 2005). Another study showed that treatment of 50 mg/L oxidized low-density lipoprotein (ox-LDL) increased cellular lipid contents in rat vascular smooth muscle cells (VSMC). However, ox-LDL-treated cells when exposed to CCM significantly diminished the number and area of cellular lipid droplets, total cholesterol, cholesterol ester, and free cholesterol through the elevation of the caveolin-1 and suppression of nuclear translocation of sterol response element-binding protein-1 (SREBP-1) (Yuan 2008). These studies indicate that CCM improves lipid profile not only in animals but also in human beings.

Curcumin in Lipid Biosynthesis

Turmeric extract and CCM have the ability to prevent the deposition and storage of lipid. In a study, dietary supplementation of turmeric extracts to mice decreased the liver triacylglycerol concentration to one-half of the level in the control mice (Asai et al. 1999). CCM has also been shown to inhibit lipid biosynthesis. CCM specifically downregulates FAS enzyme, leading to an effective decrease in fat storage and adipocyte differentiation (Zhao et al. 2011). In a study, it has been observed that CCM inhibits FAS with an IC50 value of 26.8 μM, noncompetitively with respect to NADPH, and partially competitively against both substrates acetyl-CoA and malonyl-CoA. This suggests that the malonyl/acetyl transferase domain of FAS possibly is one of the main targets of CCM (Zhao et al. 2011). In addition, CCM modulates expression of key transcription factors such as PPAR-γ and CCAAT/enhancer binding protein (C/EBP)-alpha, which are involved in adipogenesis and lipogenesis, and also it significantly lowered serum cholesterol level in obese mice (Ejaz et al. 2009). CCM also acts as antiadipogenic and suppresses adipocyte differentiation. CCM inhibited adipocyte differentiation associated proteins mitogen-activated protein kinase (MAPK) phosphorylation and nuclear translocation of Wnt/β-catenin in 3T3-L1 cells. In parallel, CCM reduced differentiation-stimulated expression of CK1α, glycogen synthase kinase-3beta (GSK-3β), Axin, and components of the destruction complex targeting β-catenin (Ahn et al. 2010), indicating its antilipogenic properties.

Curcumin in Glucose Level

An excess amount of blood glucose is converted into lipid (Day and Fidge 1965; Miras et al. 1967). Thus, the lowering of blood glucose level could help in prevention of fat deposition. Several lines of evidence suggested that CCM might play a beneficial role in lowering blood glucose levels. Administration of CCM showed an antihyperglycemic effect and also improved insulin sensitivity in high-fat-diet-fed rats. It also exhibited antilipolytic effect as evidenced by attenuating plasma FFAs (El-Moselhy et al. 2011). Besides this, CCM also sustained normoglycemia and normal glucose clearance and maintained pancreatic glucose transporter (GLUT)-2 enzyme level (Kanitkar et al. 2008). CCM effectively suppressed the enzymes involved in glucose metabolism such as phosphoenol pyruvate carboxy kinase and glucose6-phosphatase (G6Pase) induced by dexamethasone in H4IIE rat hepatoma and Hep3B human hepatoma cells. It also increased the phosphorylation of AMPK and its downstream target acetyl-CoA carboxylase in H4IIE and Hep3B cells. This study suggested that CCM-induced suppression of hepatic gluconeogenesis could be mediated through AMPK (Kim et al. 2009). In another study, CCM lowered blood glucose and HbA 1c levels in diabetic mice. They found that supplementation of CCM resulted in increase in hepatic glucokinase activity and decrease in G6Pase and phosphoenolpyruvate carboxykinase activities in mice. In addition to increase in hepatic glycogen and skeletal muscle lipoprotein lipase, CCM also lowered plasma FFA, cholesterol, and triglyceride concentrations in mice (Seo et al. 2008). The aqueous extract of turmeric also showed reduction in blood glucose and an increase in total hemoglobin in streptozotocin (STZ)-induced diabetic rats (Hussain 2002).

CURCUMIN IN INSULIN RESISTANCE

Obesity, type 2 diabetes, hypertension, and dyslipidemia are closely linked to insulin resistance. Energy metabolism is primarily controlled by insulin, a hormone that promotes the synthesis and storage of proteins, carbohydrates, and lipids. Thus, insulin resistance is commonly associated with obesity. High levels of proinflammatory cytokines in the blood can be seen in insulin resistance associated with obesity (Muller et al. 2002; Pitsavos et al. 2007). Overproduction of tumor necrosis factor alpha (TNF-α) and interleukin (IL)-6 by activation of NF-κB pathway can disturb the transcriptional activity of insulin receptors (insulin receptor substrate-1, IRS-1) and protein transporters, such as GLUT-4 (Wang et al. 2009; Liang et al. 2008; Rotter et al. 2003).

Experimental studies showed that administration of CCM and thiohydrocurcumin (THC) to diabetic rats resulted in increased levels of plasma insulin, in addition to level of hemoglobin, and erythrocyte antioxidants. It also decreased the level of blood glucose, glycosylated hemoglobin, and erythrocyte TBARS in diabetic rats (Murugan and Pari 2007). In diabetic mice, CCM also improved insulin resistance, glucose tolerance, and elevated the plasma insulin level (Jang 2008; Seo et al. 2008). Adiponectin is shown to positively correlate with insulin sensitivity, and it has been found that CCM markedly enhanced the adiponectin secretion in 3T3-L1 adipocytes (Ohara et al. 2009), indicating its insulin resistance improving property. Best et al. (2007) reported that CCM induces electrical activity in rat pancreatic beta cells by activating volume-regulated anion channel. This effect led to the depolarization of cell membrane potential, generation of electrical activity, and enhancement of insulin release. CCM also decreased the beta cell volume, suggesting its another novel target. CCM has also been shown to protect islets against STZ-induced oxidative stress by scavenging free radicals (Meghana et al. 2007). Meghana et al. (2007) showed that viability and insulin secretion from CCM-pretreated islets were significantly higher than in islets exposed to STZ alone. Nonalcoholic steatohepatitis (NASH) occurs most commonly in patients with insulin resistance. Evidence suggests that CCM may improve insulin sensitivity in diabetes and inflammatory states through the regulation of NASH (Shapiro and Bruck 2005).

Increased phosphorylation of IRS-1 is found in insulin-resistant tissues from diabetics. Ma et al. (2009) showed that beta-amyloid oligomers significantly increased the activation of JNK and phosphorylation of IRS-1 (Ser616) and tau (Ser422) in cultured hippocampal neurons. They also showed that treatment of the 3xTg-AD mice on high-fat diet with fish oil or CCM or a combination of both for 4 months reduced phosphorylated JNK, IRS-1, and tau and prevented the degradation of total IRS-1, which indicate that CCM improved insulin signaling (Ma et al. 2009). CCM also downregulates the secretion of insulin-like growth factor-1 but induces the expression of insulin-like growth factor binding protein-3 (Xia et al. 2007), which is associated with obesity and obesity linked metabolic diseases. The effect of CCM in improvement of muscular insulin resistance was observed in diabetic rats and in L6 myotubes. CCM treatment upregulated the expression of phosphorylated AMPK, CD36, and carnitine palmitoyl transferase 1, but it downregulated expression of pyruvate dehydrogenase 4 and phosphorylated glycogen synthase in both *in vivo* and *in vitro* studies. Thus, it improves insulin resistance by increasing oxidation of fatty acid and glucose mediated through AMPK pathway (Na et al. 2011).

CCM also suppressed the expression of plasminogen activator inhibitor type-1 through the inhibition of the transcription factor early growth response (Egr)-1 gene product (Pendurthi and Rao 2000) that has been closely linked with insulin resistance and obesity. The insulin sensitivity and antihyperglycemic effect of CCM were also found to be attributed to its anti-inflammatory properties as evidenced by attenuating TNF-α levels in high-fat-diet-fed rats (El-Moselhy et al. 2011). The role of the inflammatory cytokine monocyte chemotactic protein (MCP)-1 in obesity is known from several studies in which MCP-1-deficient or MCP-1-receptor-deficient mice were associated with insulin resistance (Kanda et al. 2006). Woo et al. (2007) showed that CCM inhibits the release of MCP-1 from 3T3-L1 adipocytes. They also showed that CCM suppresses obesity-induced inflammatory responses by suppressing macrophage accumulation in adipose tissue and by suppressing expression of adipocytokines including TNF-α, MCP-1, and nitrite. Suppression of MCP-1 expression from adipocytes by CCM should thus have beneficial effects on obesity-related pathologies such as insulin resistance.

Curcumin in Preadipocyte Differentiation

Obesity is characterized by an excess amount of adipose tissue. This tissue is known to release proinflammatory cytokines, which leads to inflammation and subsequently several chronic diseases such as cardiovascular, type 2 diabetes mellitus, hypertension, and others (Wellman and Friedberg 2002; Naderali 2009). Adipocyte differentiation is a tightly controlled process regulated by PPAR-γ and C/EBP-α. PPAR belong to the super family of nuclear receptors. Among all the PPARs, PPAR-γ is a major molecular target for all insulin-sensitizing drugs.

Experimental studies have shown that CCM regulates differentiation of adipocytes. In 3T3-L1 mouse embryonic fibroblasts, Ejaz et al. (2009) showed that CCM suppressed the differentiation of preadipocytes to adipocytes and induced apoptosis; it also inhibited adipokine-induced angiogenesis of human endothelial cells through suppression of expression of vascular endothelial growth factor-α. CCM increased the activation of AMPK in adipocytes by phosphorylating the α-subunit of AMPK and suppressed the expression of aminocyclopropane carboxylic acid by phosphorylation. Treatment of cells with CCM increased the fatty acid oxidation in adipocytes (Ejaz et al. 2009). Recently, CCM was shown to suppress the differentiation of adipocytes through activation of the Wnt/β-catenin pathway. In addition to Wnt signaling, CCM inhibited the expression of other markers of adipocyte differentiation, including Ap2, but it induced Wnt 10β and Lrp 5. In sum, CCM could affect adipocytes through the Wnt/β-catenin pathway (Ahn et al. 2010). Lee et al. (2009) also showed that CCM stimulates AMPK in 3T3-L1 adipocytes, which leads to downregulation of PPAR-γ and thus inhibition of differentiation. Another potential mechanism of suppression of adipocyte differentiation was through inhibition of NF-κB activation in adipocytes. CCM enhanced the expression of adiponectin in adipocytes, which linked to suppression of NF-κB activation (Ohara et al. 2009). Recently, it has been observed that CCM suppressed adipocyte differentiation and lipid accumulation through the inhibition of FAS. CCM was found to decrease the expression of FAS and downregulate the mRNA level of PPAR-γ and CD36 during adipocyte differentiation (Zhao 2011).

Upregulation of PIKfyve protein expression was documented in the early stages of differentiation of cultured 3T3-L1 fibroblasts into adipocytes. However, Ikonomov et al. (2002) showed that CCM at a very low concentration (ID(50) = 6μM) significantly inhibited expression of PIKfyve. When introduced into 3T3-L1 adipocytes, CCM also markedly inhibited insulin-induced GLUT4 translocation and glucose transport. Another study showed that the inhibitory action of CCM was largely limited to the early stage of adipocyte differentiation, where CCM was found to inhibit mitotic clonal expansion (MCE) process. This was evident from impaired proliferation, cell-cycle arrest, and levels of cell-cycle-regulating proteins. CCM also inhibited mRNA levels of early adipogenic transcription factors, particularly Krüppel-like factor 5 (KLF5), C/EBPα, and PPAR-γ in the early stage of adipocyte differentiation (Kim et al. 2011a). Recently, Kim et al. (2011b) showed that conjugation of CCM by polyethylene glycol (PEG) improved the inhibition of adipocyte differentiation in 3T3-L1 cells with no toxic effect. Hence, CCM is considered to be having potential application in the prevention of obesity.

CURCUMIN IN OXIDATIVE STRESS

Oxidative stress is a condition in which either reactive oxygen species (ROS) production is increased and/or antioxidant defenses are reduced, creating an imbalance and allowing oxidative injury (Vincent et al. 2007). In cross-sectional studies, obese subjects have higher levels of oxidative stress biomarkers compared to their leaner counterparts (Keaney et al. 2003). There are several reasons for oxidative stress in relation to obesity. Some of them are inherently related to increased adiposity and fat distribution that correlated with systemic levels of oxidative stress biomarkers, whereas others are the result of behavioral changes associated with being obese (Couillard et al. 2005; Fujita et al. 2006; Steffes 2006). Oxidative stress also resulted due to hypertension, insulin resistance, diabetes, and hyperlipidemia; each of these is common in obese condition. Study showed that obesity-mediated adipokine imbalance, which is characterized by having greater leptin and lower adiponectin levels, has been associated with increased systemic oxidative stress (Holguin et al. 2007).

As a potent antioxidant, CCM inhibited the production of ROS and abolished the oxidative stress in human hepatoma G2 cells (Chan 2005). Exposure of bovine aortic endothelial cells to CCM (5–15 μM) resulted in increase in heme oxygenase-1 (HO-1 or HSP32, an inducible stress protein that degrades heme to the vasoactive molecule carbon monoxide and the antioxidant biliverdin mRNA), protein expression, and activity that mediates cytoprotection against oxidative stress (Motterlini et al. 2000). In rat as well as in mouse liver, CCM ameliorates the cadmium-induced oxidative stress. It suppressed the level of cadmium-induced lipid peroxidation, which was accompanied by significant increase in glutathione (GSH) level (Eybl et al. 2004). CCM and its analogue also suppressed PUFA-induced oxidative stress. It exerts its protective effect by decreasing the lipid peroxidation and improving antioxidant status, thus proving itself as an effective antioxidant (Rukkumani et al. 2004).

In diabetic mice, associated with obesity, CCM treatment normalized erythrocyte and hepatic antioxidant enzyme activities (superoxide dismutase, catalase, glutathione peroxidase) that resulted in a significant reduction in lipid peroxidation (Seo et al. 2008). As leptin induces oxidative stress in many pathological conditions including obesity, CCM dose dependently attenuated leptin-caused oxidative stress by reducing the levels of ROS and lipid peroxidation in cultured HSC. In addition, CCM also increased the contents of cellular GSH and improved the ratio of reduced to oxidized GSH (Tang et al. 2009). Thus, the decrease in ROS and increase in antioxidant enzymes by CCM may therefore contribute to an antiobesogenic environment.

ROLE OF CURCUMIN IN OBESITY-INDUCED INFLAMMATION

In obesity, as in most other chronic diseases, inflammation appears to play a major role. Fat tissue is not a simple energy storage organ but rather exerts important endocrine and immune functions. It also produces inflammatory cytokines such as TNF, IL-6, MCP-1, and IL-1. These cytokines and chemokines are critically involved in insulin resistance and chronic inflammation. Experimental study from our laboratory showed that adipocytes express TNF receptors and mediate catabolic effects (Patton et al. 1986). Adipose tissue of obese animals has also been shown to overexpress TNF-α. Study on obese human subjects also showed that TNF-α was over-expressed in adipocytes and was decreased by weight loss. It has also been observed that high-fat diet can elevate TNF activity in adipose tissue but not the secreted TNF levels (Morin et al. 1997). Further, TNF was found to induce insulin resistance through serine phosphorylation of IRS-1, which then inhibits the tyrosine kinase activity of the insulin receptor in adipocytes (Hotamisligil et al. 1996). In addition, TNF can also induce the secretion of leptin, a fat-specific energy balance hormone, through posttranscriptional mechanism in adipocytes (Kirchgessner 1997). However, it has been reported that blockade of the TNF receptor-1 reverse diet-induced obesity and insulin resistance (Liang et al. 2008). In a TNF-α-lacking mice, obesity-induced insulin resistance was also not observed (Uysal et al. 1997).

Other than TNF-α, activated NF-κB was also observed in adipocytes, and the expression of TNF-α itself is regulated by NF-κB (Ahn et al. 2008; Ruan et al. 2002). The activation of NF-κB is also shown to induce insulin resistance (Gonzalez et al. 2006). Overnutrition, one of associated factor for obesity, activates hypothalamic NF-κB in part through elevated endoplasmic reticulum stress, which interrupts central insulin/leptin signaling and actions (Zhang et al. 2008). Thus, all these studies indicate that regulation of adipocytokines is directly linked to obesity-induced inflammation and insulin resistance, and targeting this pathway may allow the treatment of metabolic diseases such as obesity.

Several reports suggest that CCM has potential in the prevention and treatment of obesity, diabetes, atherosclerosis, and metabolic syndrome. CCM has been reported to modulate numerous inflammatory targets that have been linked to obesity. Recently, CCM is shown to decrease LPS-stimulated secretion of IL-6, and it also affects the leptin release after co-incubation with LPS from cultured adipocytes (Ciardi 2011). CCM has been shown to downregulate the expression of TNF in various tissues (Chan 1995). CCM was also reported to inhibit TNF and other inflammatory agents-induced NF-κB activation through inhibition of IκBα degradation (Singh and Aggarwal 1995). Weisberg et al. found that oral ingestion of CCM significantly reduced macrophage infiltration of white adipose tissue, increased adipose tissue adiponectin production, and decreased NF-κB activity and markers of hepatic inflammation (Weisberg et al. 2008). The expression of various NF-κB-regulated proinflammatory adipocytokines including chemokines such as MCP-1, MCP-4, and eotaxin (Woo et al. 2007) and interleukins (IL-1, IL-6, and IL-8) (Wang et al. 2009) was also reported to be inhibited by CCM treatment. Thus, these studies indicate that CCM reverses many of the inflammatory and metabolic derangements associated with obesity and improves insulin resistance.

ROLE OF CURCUMIN IN OBESITY-ASSOCIATED CHRONIC DISEASES

Obesity is not a single disease; rather it is the root of several other metabolic diseases such as coronary heart disease, hypertension, dyslipidemia, and type 2 diabetes (Figure 41.4). Experimental study showed that CCM ameliorated cardiac sympathovagal disturbance in high-fat-induced obese rats. When Wistar rats were fed with high-fat diet to induce obesity, an elevated plasma FFA level, which is associated with an increased low-frequency/high-frequency (LF/HF) ratio, and an expression of sympathovagal disturbance were observed. However, CCM supplementation with high-fat diet ameliorated the cardiac autonomic imbalance in rats by lowering the FFA plasma concentration (Pongchaidecha et al. 2009).

CCM inhibited the DNA-binding ability of hypertrophy-responsive transcription factor GATA binding protein 4 (GATA4) in rat cardiomyocytes. In addition, CCM prevented the deterioration of systolic function and heart-failure-induced increase in myocardial wall thickness and diameter when examined in *in vivo* heart failure models (Morimoto et al. 2008). LDL oxidation plays an important role in the development of atherosclerosis (a disease characterized by oxidative damage), and inhibition of LDL oxidation can reduce the risk of atherosclerosis. CCM's effects were evaluated based on the development of experimental atherosclerosis in rabbits and its interaction with

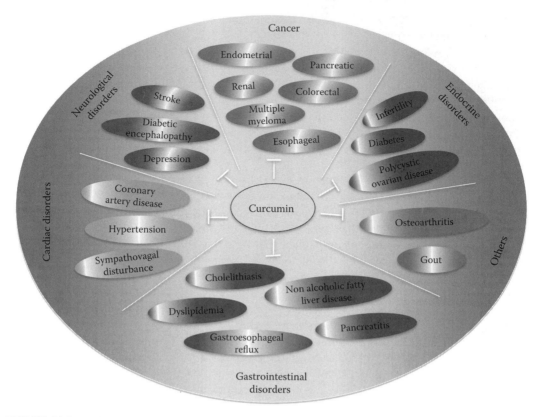

FIGURE 41.4   Role of CCM in prevention and treatment of obesity associated metabolic diseases.

other plasmatic antioxidants. Rabbits were fed an atherogenic diet for 30 days, and histological results for the fatty streak lesions revealed damage in the thoracic and abdominal aorta that was significantly lower in the CCM-fed group than in the control group (Quiles 2002), indicating its antiatherosclerotic properties.

Diabetes is also the most common consequence of obesity, which is further linked to insulin resistance. In a diabetic patient, nephropathic symptoms are most common. This is characterized by increase in production of extracellular matrix (ECM) proteins including fibronectin and extra-domain B containing fibronectin that are regulated by TGF-β1, NF-κB, and p300 in the kidneys. CCM treatment inhibited the neuropathic symptoms by suppressing the p300, activation of NF-κB, and decreasing TGF-β, vasoactive factors (endothelial nitric oxide synthase and endothelin-1), and ECM proteins (Chiu et al. 2009). CCM has also shown to ameliorate diabetes and inflammation in murine models of insulin-resistant obesity. Dietary CCM admixture treatment ameliorated diabetes in high-fat-diet-induced obese and leptin-deficient ob/ob male C57BL/6J mice as determined by glucose and insulin tolerance (Weisberg et al. 2008). In another study, a decrease in the blood glucose level in diabetic models has been reported. Study showed that when diabetic albino rats were fed with CCM (0.08 g/kg body weight), a decrease in blood glucose levels was observed compared to control group (Arun and Nalini 2002). It has also been observed that CCM supplementation in diabetic mice decreased the blood glucose, plasma insulin, and glucose homeostasis-related enzyme activities (Seo et al. 2008). In addition, CCM lowered plasma FFA, cholesterol, and triglyceride concentrations and increased the hepatic glycogen and skeletal muscle lipoprotein lipase in db/db mice (Seo et al. 2008). Besides these, CCM treatment significantly attenuated encephalopathic factors including cognitive deficit, cholinergic dysfunction, oxidative stress, and inflammation in diabetic rats (Kuhad and Chopra 2007).

Obesity is also a significant risk factor for certain forms of cancer including gastrointestinal, ovary, breast, uterus, cervical, pancreatic, hepatic, kidney, multiple myeloma, and lymphoma (Aggarwal 2010; Anand et al. 2008). According to International Agency for Research on Cancer (IARC), obesity is a cause for 11% of colon cancer, 9% of postmenopausal breast cancer, 39% of endometrial cancer, 25% of kidney cancer, and 37% of esophageal cancer cases (IARC 2002). Obesity resulted in inflammation and dysregulation of certain transcription factors, which cause development of cancer. CCM inhibits inflammation by interacting directly with cyclooxygenase-2 (COX-2), lipoxygenase (LOX), GSK-3β, and cytokines (TNF-α) (Shehzad and Lee 2010). It also interacts indirectly with several transcription factors, including NF-κB, activator protein 1 (AP-1), β-catenin, STATs proteins, and PPAR-γ (Shehzad et al., 2010). These multitargeted properties of CCM might contribute to its therapeutic role in obesity and obesity-related cancer.

Obesity is also a major consequence of depression. However, CCM was found to be effective against depression. In experimental study, CCM treatment at 5 and 10 mg/kg (p.o.) significantly reduced the depressive sign as observed in forced swimming tests. In addition, the neurochemical assays showed that CCM produced a marked increase of dopamine, serotonin, and noradrenaline levels at 10 mg/kg in both the frontal cortex and hippocampus and also inhibited monoamine oxidase activity in the mouse brain (Xu et al. 2005). Arora et al. (2011) showed that CCM ameliorates reserpine-induced pain-depression dyad in rats. Administration of reserpine led to a significant decrease in nociceptive threshold and behavioral deficit integrated with decrease in the biogenic amine (dopamine, norepinephrine, and serotonin) levels. However, CCM (100, 200, 300 mg/kg; i.p.) dose dependently ameliorated the depression by restoring behavioral, biochemical, neurochemical, and molecular alterations against reserpine-induced pain-depression dyad in rats. In another study, treatment of the rats with CCM significantly suppressed the depression-like behavior induced by the repeated corticosterone injections. In addition, it also decreased brain-derived neurotrophic factor (BDNF) levels in brain (Huang et al. 2011). CCM has also been shown to inhibit glutamate release in nerve terminals from rat prefrontal cortex, which could be associated to its antidepressant mechanism (Lin et al. 2011). Thus, CCM produces an antidepressant-like effect in animals; however, its antidepressant effects are still not clear in obese experimental models.

CONCLUSION

Obesity is a growing problem worldwide, and treatment potentials are constantly under scrutiny. There is a prevalence of inflammation in obese patients, and this brings with it a cascade of problems including endothelial dysfunction and insulin resistance, ultimately resulting in various metabolic syndromes. The studies summarized in this chapter demonstrate that CCM has a potential role to play in efforts to decrease the incidence of obesity and its associated complications. Because of its relative low cost, safety, and the evidence of their efficacy, it is essential to include CCM as a part of our daily diet. Adding spices, especially turmeric (source of CCM), everyday is likely to help most people in the prevention of obesity, diabetes, and associated diseases. More research, in particular clinical trials, is needed to further strengthen the link between spices like CCM and chronic diseases such as obesity, diabetes, cancer, and other associated metabolic diseases.

ACKNOWLEDGMENTS

Dr. Aggarwal is the Ransom Horne, Jr., Professor of Cancer Research. This work was supported by a core grant from the National Institutes of Health (CA-16672), a program project grant from the National Institutes of Health (NIH CA-124787-01A2), and a grant from the Center for Targeted Therapy of MD Anderson Cancer Center.

REFERENCES

Aggarwal BB. Targeting inflammation-induced obesity and metabolic diseases by curcumin and other nutraceuticals. *Annu Rev Nutr.* 2010 Aug 21;30:173–199.

Aggarwal BB, Shishodia S. Molecular targets of dietary agents for prevention and therapy of cancer. *Biochem Pharmacol.* 2006;71:1397–1421.

Ahn J, Lee H, Kim S, Ha T. Curcumin-induced suppression of adipogenic differentiation is accompanied by activation of Wnt/beta-catenin signaling. *Am J Physiol Cell Physiol.* 2010 Jun;298(6):C1510–C1516.

Ahn KS, Sethi G, Aggarwal BB. Reversal of chemoresistance and enhancement of apoptosis by statins through down-regulation of the NF-kappaB pathway. *Biochem Pharmacol.* 2008;75:907–913.

Alwi I, Santoso T, Suyono S, Sutrisna B, Suyatna FD, Kresno SB, Ernie S. The effect of curcumin on lipid level in patients with acute coronary syndrome. *Acta Med Indones.* 2008 Oct;40(4):201–210.

Anand P, Kunnumakkara AB, Sundaram C, Harikumar KB, Tharakan ST, Lai OS, Sung B, Aggarwal BB. Cancer is a preventable disease that requires major lifestyle changes. *Pharm Res.* 2008;25(9):2097–2116.

Arafa HM. Curcumin attenuates diet-induced hypercholesterolemia in rats. *Med Sci Monit.* 2005 Jul;11(7):BR228–BR234.

Arora V, Kuhad A, Tiwari V, Chopra K. Curcumin ameliorates reserpine-induced pain-depression dyad: Behavioural, biochemical, neurochemical and molecular evidences. *Psychoneuroendocrinology.* 2011;36(10):1570–1581.

Arun N, Nalini N. Efficacy of turmeric on blood sugar and polyol pathway in diabetic albino rats. *Plant Foods Hum Nutr.* 2002;57(1):41–52.

Asai A, Miyazawa T. Dietary curcuminoids prevent high-fat diet-induced lipid accumulation in rat liver and epididymal adipose tissue. *J Nutr.* 2001;131:2932–2935.

Asai A, Nakagawa K, Miyazawa T. Antioxidative effects of turmeric, rosemary and capsicum extracts on membrane phospholipid peroxidation and liver lipid metabolism in mice. *Biosci Biotechnol Biochem.* 1999;63:2118–2122.

Baum L, Lam CW, Cheung SK et al. Six-month randomized, placebo-controlled, double-blind, pilot clinical trial of curcumin in patients with Alzheimer disease. *J Clin Psychopharmacol.* 2008;28:110–113.

Begum AN, Jones MR, Lim GP et al. Curcumin structure-function, bioavailability, and efficacy in models of neuroinflammation and Alzheimer's disease. *J Pharmacol Exp Ther.* 2008;326:196–208.

Best L, Elliott AC, Brown PD. Curcumin induces electrical activity in rat pancreatic beta-cells by activating the volume-regulated anion channel. *Biochem Pharmacol.* 2007;73:1768–1775.

Bisht S, Feldmann G, Soni S, Ravi R, Karikar C, Maitra A. Polymeric nanoparticle-encapsulated curcumin ("nanocurcumin"): A novel strategy for human cancer therapy. *J Nanobiotechnol.* 2007;5:3.

Chan MM. Inhibition of tumor necrosis factor by curcumin, a phytochemical. *Biochem Pharmacol.* 1995;49:1551–1556.

Chan WH, Wu HJ, Hsuuw YD. Curcumin inhibits ROS formation and apoptosis in methylglyoxal-treated human hepatoma G2 cells. *Ann N Y Acad Sci.* 2005;1042:372–378.

Chiu J, Khan ZA, Farhangkhoee H, Chakrabarti S. Curcumin prevents diabetes-associated abnormalities in the kidneys by inhibiting p300 and nuclear factor-kappaB. *Nutrition.* 2009;25(9):964–972.

Ciardi C, Jenny M, Tschoner A, Ueberall F, Patsch J, Pedrini M, Ebenbichler C, Fuchs D. Food additives such as sodium sulphite, sodium benzoate and curcumin inhibit leptin release in lipopolysaccharide-treated murine adipocytes in vitro. *Br J Nutr.* 2011;1:1–8.

Couillard C, Ruel G, Archer WR, Pomerleau S, Bergeron J, Couture P, Lamarche B, Bergeron N. Circulating levels of oxidative stress markers and endothelial adhesion molecules in men with abdominal obesity. *J Clin Endocrinol Metab.* 2005;90:6454–6459.

Day AJ, Fidge NH. Conversion of [1–14C]glucose to lipid by macrophages in vitro. *Biochim Biophys Acta—Lipids Lipid Metab.* 1965 July 7;106(1):19–24.

Ejaz A, Wu D, Kwan P, Meydani M. Curcumin inhibits adipogenesis in 3T3-L1 adipocytes and angiogenesis and obesity in C57/BL mice. *J Nutr.* 2009;139:919–925.

El-Moselhy MA, Taye A, Sharkawi SS, El-Sisi SF, Ahmed AF. The antihyperglycemic effect of curcumin in high fat diet fed rats. Role of TNF-α and free fatty acids. *Food Chem Toxicol.* 2011 May;49(5):1129–1140.

Eybl V, Kotyzová D, Bludovská M. The effect of curcumin on cadmium-induced oxidative damage and trace elements level in the liver of rats and mice. *Toxicol Lett.* 2004 Jun 15;151(1):79–85.

Fontana L, Klein S, Holloszy JO. Effects of long-term calorie restriction and endurance exercise on glucose tolerance, insulin action, and adipokine production. Age (Dordr.) 2010;32(1):97–108.

Fujita K, Nishizawa H, Funahashi T, Shimomura I, Shimabukuro M. Systemic oxidative stress is associated with visceral fat accumulation and the metabolic syndrome. *Circ J.* 2006;70:1437–1442.

Ghanim H, Garg R, Aljada A, Mohanty P, Kumbkarni Y et al. Suppression of nuclear factor-kappaB and stimulation of inhibitor kappaB by troglitazone: Evidence for an anti-inflammatory effect and a potential antiatherosclerotic effect in the obese. *J Clin Endocrinol Metab.* 2001;86:1306–1312.

Gonzales AM, Orlando RA. Curcumin and resveratrol inhibit nuclear factor-kappaB-mediated cytokine expression in adipocytes. *Nutr Metab (Lond).* 2008;5:17.

Gonzalez F, Rote NS, Minium J, Kirwan JP. Increased activation of nuclear factor kappaB triggers inflammation and insulin resistance in polycystic ovary syndrome. *J Clin Endocrinol Metab.* 2006;91:1508–1512.

Haslam DW, James WP. Obesity. *Lancet.* 2005;366(9492):1197–209.

Holguin F, Rojas M, Hart CM. The peroxisome proliferator activated receptor gamma (PPAR gamma) ligand rosiglitazone modulates bronchoalveolar lavage levels of leptin, adiponectin, and inflammatory cytokines in lean and obese mice. *Lung.* 2007;185:367–372.

Hotamisligil GS, Peraldi P, Budavari A, Ellis R, White MF, Spiegelman BM. IRS-1-mediated inhibition of insulin receptor tyrosine kinase activity in TNF-alpha- and obesity-induced insulin resistance. *Science.* 1996;271:665–668.

Huang Z, Zhong XM, Li ZY, Feng CR, Pan AJ, Mao QQ. Curcumin reverses corticosterone-induced depressive-like behavior and decrease in brain BDNF levels in rats. *Neurosci Lett.* 2011 Apr 15;493(3):145–148.

Hussain HE. Hypoglycemic, hypolipidemic and antioxidant properties of combination of curcumin from *Curcuma longa*, Linn. and partially purified product from *Abroma augusta*, Linn. in streptozotocin induced diabetes. *Ind J Clin Biochem.* 2002;17:33–43.

IARC Handbooks of Cancer Prevention. Weight control and physical activity, In: Vainio H and Bianchini F., (eds.), international agency for research on cancer, Lyon. France 2002;6:1–315.

Ikonomov OC, Sbrissa D, Mlak K, Shisheva A. Requirement for PIKfyve enzymatic activity in acute and long-term insulin cellular effects. *Endocrinology.* 2002 Dec;143(12):4742–4754.

Ireson CR, Jones DJ, Orr S et al. Metabolism of the cancer chemopreventive agent curcumin in human and rat intestine. *Cancer Epidemiol Biomarkers Prev.* 2002;11:105–111.

Jang EM, Choi MS, Jung UJ, Kim MJ, Kim HJ, Jeon SM, Shin SK, Seong CN, Lee MK. Beneficial effects of curcumin on hyperlipidemia and insulin resistance in high-fat-fed hamsters. *Metabolism.* 2008;57(11):1576–1583.

Kanda H, Tateya S, Tamori Y, Kotani K, Hiasa K et al. MCP 1 contributes to macrophage infiltration into adipose tissue, insulin resistance, and hepatic steatosis in obesity. *J Clin Invest.* 2006;116:1494–1505.

Kanitkar M, Gokhale K, Galande S, Bhonde RR. Novel role of curcumin in the prevention of cytokine-induced islet death in vitro and diabetogenesis in vivo. *Br J Pharmacol.* 2008 Nov;155(5):702–713.

Keaney JF, Jr., Larson MG, Vasan RS, Wilson PW, Lipinska I, Corey D, Massaro JM, Sutherland P, Vita JA, Benjamin EJ. Obesity and systemic oxidative stress: Clinical correlates of oxidative stress in the Framingham Study. *Arterioscler Thromb Vasc Biol.* 2003;23:434–439.

Kim CY, Bordenave N, Ferruzzi MG, Safavy A, Kim KH. Modification of curcumin with polyethylene glycol enhances the delivery of curcumin in preadipocytes and its antiadipogenic property. *J Agric Food Chem.* 2011a Feb 9;59(3):1012–1019

Kim T, Davis J, Zhang AJ, He X, Mathews ST. Curcumin activates AMPK and suppresses gluconeogenic gene expression in hepatoma cells. *Biochem Biophys Res Commun.* 2009 Oct 16;388(2):377–382.

Kim CY, Le TT, Chen C, Cheng JX, Kim KH. Curcumin inhibits adipocyte differentiation through modulation of mitotic clonal expansion. *J Nutr Biochem.* 2011b;22(10):910–920.

Kirchgessner TG, Uysal KT, Wiesbrock SM, Marino MW, Hotamisligil GS. Tumor necrosis factor-alpha contributes to obesity-related hyperleptinemia by regulating leptin release from adipocytes. *J Clin Invest* 1997;100:2777–2782.

Kolev TM, Velcheva EA, Stamboliyska BA, Spiteller M. DFT and experimental studies of the structure and vibrational spectra of curcumin. *Int J Quant Chem.* 2005;102:1069–1079.

Kuhad A, Chopra K. Curcumin attenuates diabetic encephalopathy in rats: Behavioral and biochemical evidences. *Eur J Pharmacol.* 2007;576(1–3):34–42.

Lamas O, Moreno-Aliaga MJ, Martinez JA, Marti A. NF-kappa B-binding activity in an animal diet-induced overweightness model and the impact of subsequent energy restriction. *Biochem Biophys Res Commun.* 2003;311:533–539.

Lee YK, Lee WS, Hwang JT, Kwon DY, Surh YJ, Park OJ. Curcumin exerts antidifferentiation effect through AMPKalpha-PPAR-gamma in 3T3-L1 adipocytes and antiproliferatory effect through AMPKalpha-COX-2 in cancer cells. *J Agric Food Chem.* 2009;57:305–310.

Liang H, Yin B, Zhang H, Zhang S, Zeng Q et al. Blockade of tumor necrosis factor (TNF) receptor type 1-mediated TNF-alpha signaling protected Wistar rats from diet-induced obesity and insulin resistance. *Endocrinology.* 2008;149:2943–2951.

Lim GP, Chu T, Yang F, Beech W, Frautschy SA, Cole GM. The curry spice curcumin reduces oxidative damage and amyloid pathology in an Alzheimer transgenic mouse. *J Neurosci.* 2001;21:8370–8377.

Lin TY, Lu CW, Wang CC, Wang YC, Wang SJ. Curcumin inhibits glutamate release in nerve terminals from rat prefrontal cortex: Possible relevance to its antidepressant mechanism. *Prog Neuropsychopharmacol Biol Psychiatry.* 2011 Aug 15;35(7):1785–93.

Ma QL, Yang F, Rosario ER, Ubeda OJ, Beech W, Gant DJ, Chen PP, Hudspeth B, Chen C, Zhao Y, Vinters HV, Frautschy SA, Cole GM. Beta-amyloid oligomers induce phosphorylation of tau and inactivation of insulin receptor substrate via c-Jun N-terminal kinase signaling: Suppression by omega-3 fatty acids and curcumin. *J Neurosci.* 2009 Jul 15;29(28):9078–9089.

Mahfouz MM, Zhou SQ, Kummerow FA. Curcumin prevents the oxidation and lipid modification of LDL and its inhibition of prostacyclin generation by endothelial cells in culture. *Prostaglandins Other Lipid Mediat.* 2009 Nov;90(1–2):13–20.

Meghana K, Sanjeev G, Ramesh B. Curcumin prevents streptozotocin-induced islet damage by scavenging free radicals: A prophylactic and protective role. *Eur J Pharmacol.* 2007;577:183–191.

Miras CJ, Legakis NJ, Levis GM. Conversion of Glucose to Lipids by Normal and Leukemic Leukocytes. *Cancer Res.* 1967 Nov;27(Pt 1):2153–2158.

Morimoto T, Sunagawa Y, Kawamura T, Takaya T, Wada H, Nagasawa A, Komeda M, Fujita M, Shimatsu A, Kita T, Hasegawa K. The dietary compound curcumin inhibits p300 histone acetyltransferase activity and prevents heart failure in rats. *J Clin Invest* 2008;118(3):868–878.

Morin CL, Eckel RH, Marcel T, Pagliassotti MJ. High fat diets elevate adipose tissue-derived tumor necrosis factor-alpha activity. *Endocrinology.* 1997;138:4665–4671.

Motterlini R, Foresti R, Bassi R, Green CJ. Curcumin, an antioxidant and anti-inflammatory agent, induces heme oxygenase-1 and protects endothelial cells against oxidative stress. *Free Radic Biol Med.* 2000 Apr 15;28(8):1303–1312.

Muller S, Martin S, Koenig W et al. Impaired glucose tolerance is associated with increased serum concentrations of interleukin 6 and co-regulated acute-phase proteins but not TNF-alpha or its receptors. *Diabetologia.* 2002;45:805–812.

Murugan P, Pari L. Influence of tetrahydrocurcumin on erythrocyte membrane bound enzymes and antioxidant status in experimental type 2 diabetic rats. *J Ethnopharmacol.* 2007 Sep 25;113(3):479–486.

Na LX, Zhang YL, Li Y, Liu LY, Li R, Kong T, Sun CH. Curcumin improves insulin resistance in skeletal muscle of rats. *Nutr Metab Cardiovasc Dis.* 2011 Jul;21(7):526–533.

Naderali, EK Obesity and cardiovascular dysfunction: A role for resveratrol? *Obes Res Clin Pract.* 2009;3:45–52.

Navab M, Gharavi N, Watson AD. Inflammation and metabolic disorders. *Curr Opin Clin Nutr Metab Care.* 2008;11:459–464.

Ohara K, Uchida A, Nagasaka R, Ushio H, Ohshima T. The effects of hydroxycinnamic acid derivatives on adiponectin secretion. *Phytomedicine.* 2009;16:130–137.

Patton JS, Shepard HM, Wilking H, Lewis G, Aggarwal BB et al. Interferons and tumor necrosis factors have similar catabolic effects on 3T3 L1 cells. *Proc Natl Acad Sci USA.* 1986;83:8313–8317.

Pavon FJ, Serrano A, Perez-Valero V, Jagerovic N, Hernandez-Folgado L et al. Central versus peripheral antagonism of cannabinoid CB1 receptor in obesity: Effects of LH-21, a peripherally acting neutral cannabinoid receptor antagonist, in Zucker rats. *J Neuroendocrinol.* 2008;20(Suppl 1):116–123.

Pendurthi UR, Rao LV. Suppression of transcription factor Egr-1 by curcumin. *Thromb Res.* 2000;97:179–189.

Pitsavos C, Tampourlou M, Panagiotakos DB et al. Association between low-grade systemic inflammation and type 2 diabetes mellitus among men and women from the ATTICA study. *Rev Diabet Stud.* 2007;4:98–104.

Pongchaidecha A, Lailerd N, Boonprasert W, Chattipakorn N. Effects of curcuminoid supplement on cardiac autonomic status in high-fat-induced obese rats. *Nutrition.* 2009;25(7–8):870–878.

Quiles JL, Mesa MD, Ramirez-Tortosa CL, Aguilera CM, Battino M, Gil A, Ramírez-Tortosa MC. Curcuma longa extract supplementation reduces oxidative stress and attenuates aortic fatty streak development in rabbits. *Arterioscler Thromb Vasc Biol.* 2002;22(7):1225–1231.

Rajala MW, Scherer PE. Minireview: The adipocyte—at the crossroads of energy homeostasis, inflammation, and atherosclerosis. *Endocrinology.* 2003;144:3765–3773.

Reeds DN. Nutrition support in the obese, diabetic patient: The role of hypocaloric feeding. *Curr Opin Gastroenterol.* 2009;25:151–154.

Rotter V, Nagaev I, Smith U. Interleukin-6 (IL-6) induces insulin resistance in 3T3-L1 adipocytes and is, like IL-8 and tumor necrosis factor-alpha, overexpressed in human fat cells from insulin-resistant subjects. *J Biol Chem.* 2003;278:45777–45784.

Ruan H, Hacohen N, Golub TR, Van Parijs L, Lodish HF. Tumor necrosis factor-alpha suppresses adipocyte-specific genes and activates expression of preadipocyte genes in 3T3-L1 adipocytes: Nuclear factor-kappaB activation by TNF-alpha is obligatory. *Diabetes*. 2002;51:1319–1336.

Rukkumani R, Aruna K, Varma PS, Rajasekaran KN, Menon VP. Comparative effects of curcumin and an analog of curcumin on alcohol and PUFA induced oxidative stress. *J Pharm Pharm Sci*. 2004 Aug 20;7(2):274–283.

Seely KA, Levi MS, Prather PL. The dietary polyphenols trans-resveratrol and curcumin selectively bind human CB1 cannabinoid receptors with nanomolar affinities and function as antagonists/inverse agonists. *J Pharmacol Exp Ther*. 2009;330:31–39.

Seo KI, Choi MS, Jung UJ, Kim HJ, Yeo J, Jeon SM, Lee MK. Effect of curcumin supplementation on blood glucose, plasma insulin, and glucose homeostasis related enzyme activities in diabetic db/db mice. *Mol Nutr Food Res*. 2008 Sep;52(9):995–1004.

Shapiro H, Bruck R. Therapeutic potential of curcumin in non-alcoholic steatohepatitis. *Nutr Res Rev*. 2005 Dec;18(2):212–221.

Shehzad A, Ha T, Subhan F, Lee YS. New mechanisms and the anti-inflammatory role of curcumin in obesity and obesity-related metabolic diseases. *Eur J Nutr*. 2011 Mar 27;50:151–161.

Shehzad A, Lee YS. Curcumin: Multiple molecular targets mediate multiple pharmacological actions. *Drugs Future*. 2010;35(2):113–119.

Shehzad A, Wahid F, Lee YS. Curcumin in cancer chemoprevention: Molecular targets, pharmacokinetics, bioavailability, and clinical trials. *Arch Pharm Chem Life Sci*. 2010;343(9):489–499.

Shoba G, Joy D, Joseph T, Majeed M, Rajendran R, Srinivas PS. Influence of piperine on the pharmacokinetics of curcumin in animals and human volunteers. *Planta Med*. 1998;64:353–356.

Singh S, Aggarwal BB. Activation of transcription factor NF-kappa B is suppressed by curcumin (diferuloylmethane) [corrected]. *J Biol Chem*. 1995;270:24995–25000.

Soni KB, Kuttan R. Effect of oral curcumin administration on serum peroxides and cholesterol levels in human volunteers. *Indian J Physiol Pharmacol*. 1992 Oct;36(4):273–275.

Steffes MW, Gross MD, Lee DH, Schreiner PJ, Jacobs DR, Jr. Adiponectin, visceral fat, oxidative stress, and early macrovascular disease: The coronary artery risk development in young adults study. *Obesity (Silver Spring)*. 2006;14:319–326.

Tang Y, Zheng S, Chen A. Curcumin eliminates leptin's effects on hepatic stellate cell activation via interrupting leptin signaling. *Endocrinology*. 2009 Jul;150(7):3011–3020.

Uysal KT, Wiesbrock SM, Marino MW, Hotamisligil GS. Protection from obesity-induced insulin resistance in mice lacking TNF-alpha function. *Nature*. 1997;389:610–614.

Varady KA, Hellerstein MK. Do calorie restriction or alternate-day fasting regimens modulate adipose tissue physiology in a way that reduces chronic disease risk? *Nutr Rev*. 2008;66:333–342.

Vincent HK, Innes KE, Vincent KR. Oxidative stress and potential interventions to reduce oxidative stress in overweight and obesity. *Diabetes Obes Metab*. 2007;9:813–839.

Wang SL, Li Y, Wen Y, Chen YF, Na LX et al. Curcumin, a potential inhibitor of up-regulation of TNF-alpha and IL-6 induced by palmitate in 3T3-L1 adipocytes through NF-kappaB and JNK pathway. *Biomed Environ Sci*. 2009;22:32–39.

Weisberg SP, Leibel R, Tortoriello DV. Dietary curcumin significantly improves obesity-associated inflammation and diabetes in mouse models of diabesity. *Endocrinology*. 2008 Jul;149(7):3549–3558.

Wellman NS, Friedberg, B. Causes and consequences of adult obesity: Health, social and economic impacts in the United States. *Asia Pac J Clin Nutr*. 2002;11(Suppl 8):s705–s709.

Woo HM, Kang JH, Kawada T, Yoo H, Sung MK, Yu R. Active spice-derived components can inhibit inflammatory responses of adipose tissue in obesity by suppressing inflammatory actions of macrophages and release of monocyte chemoattractant protein-1 from adipocytes. *Life Sci*. 2007;80:926–931.

Xia Y, Jin L, Zhang B, Xue H, Li Q, Xu Y. The potentiation of curcumin on insulin-like growth factor-1 action in MCF-7 human breast carcinoma cells. *Life Sci*. 2007;80:2161–2169.

Xu Y, Ku BS, Yao HY, Lin YH, Ma X, Zhang YH, Li XJ. The effects of curcumin on depressive-like behaviors in mice. *Eur J Pharmacol*. 2005 Jul 25;518(1):40–46.

Yuan HY, Kuang SY, Zheng X, Ling HY, Yang YB, Yan PK, Li K, Liao DF. Curcumin inhibits cellular cholesterol accumulation by regulating SREBP-1/caveolin-1 signaling pathway in vascular smooth muscle cells. *Acta Pharmacol Sin*. 2008 May;29(5):555–563.

Zhang X, Zhang G, Zhang H, Karin M, Bai H, Cai D. Hypothalamic IKKbeta/NF-kappaB and ER stress link overnutrition to energy imbalance and obesity. *Cell*. 2008;135:61–73.

Zhao J, Sun XB, Ye F, Tian WX. Suppression of fatty acid synthase, differentiation and lipid accumulation in adipocytes by curcumin. *Mol Cell Biochem*. 2011 May;351(1–2):19–28.

42 Role of *Caralluma fimbriata* in Weight Management

Ramasamy V. Venkatesh, BSc, PGDIT
and Ramaswamy Rajendran, MSc

CONTENTS

INTRODUCTION

Caralluma fimbriata (a succulent belonging to the family Asclepiadaceae) is a large group consisting of tender succulents found wild in India, Pakistan, the Canary Islands, Arabia, southern Europe, Sri Lanka, and Afghanistan. The plants of this group vary from thin, recumbent stems (Figures 42.1 and 42.2) from ½ to 1½ in. thick to erect growing clumps up to 8 in. high. The spines that cover the angled stems are actually leaves. The star-shaped, fleshy flowers of these plants are some of the worst smelling of the succulent plants. Ordinarily borne in late summer, the foul-smelling blossoms are usually colored purple, black, yellow, tan, maroon, red, or dark brown. They are from ½ to 2 in. or more across and borne at the base of the plant. In the wild, these blossoms are pollinated by flies, which are greatly attracted to the plant. The succulent also is referred to by synonymous names such as *Caralluma adscendens* and *Caralluma attenuata* [3].

This succulent has several local names in India like *Runshabar, Makad shenguli, Shindala makadi* [1], *Kullee Mooliyan, Karallamu,* and *Yungmaphallottama* [2,3].

HISTORY OF USE

Caralluma fimbriata has been in use for centuries in India. It is commonly used as a vegetable in semiarid regions of India. It is eaten raw or cooked with spices. It is also used in pickles and chutneys. Caralluma is also classified as famine food. In arid and semiarid regions, when no food is available, this is consumed as a substitute for food.

Indians are known to chew chunks of *Caralluma fimbriata* to suppress hunger when on a day's hunt. The cactus is used by the South Indians to suppress appetite and enhance endurance. They make their living as hunters, wood collectors, plant collectors, foragers, etc. They do not eat or carry cooked food with them while they go into the forests for hunting. To ensure that they are not hungry and that they have enough endurance to last them on their forays into the forest, they chop off the stems of this succulent and chew a handful of them. By doing so, they do not feel hungry and thirsty. They can hunt and stay out for hours together without food or water. The tribesmen also state that their energy levels are maintained without food and water and that they do not feel any fatigue or

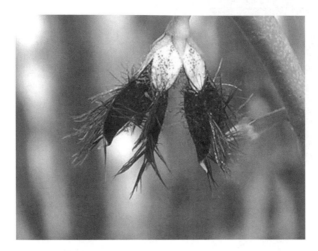

FIGURE 42.1   Flower of *Caralluma fimbriata*.

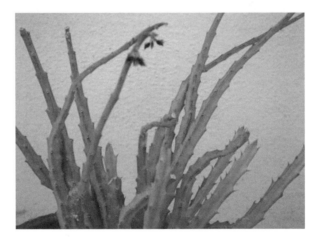

FIGURE 42.2   Stem of *Caralluma fimbriata*.

tiredness. In a day, the consumption of *Caralluma fimbriata* as a vegetable in the manner used by the tribesmen was about 100 g [3].

ACTIVE INGREDIENT, PREPARATION OF EXTRACTS, AND MODE OF ACTION OF *CARALLUMA FIMBRIATA**

The key constituents (Figure 42.3) of *Caralluma fimbriata* are pregnane glycosides, saponin glycosides, and bitter principles.

A standardized extract of *Caralluma fimbriata* (brand name "*Slimaluma*") developed by Gencor Pacific Limited in partnership with Green Chem, India, was designed and developed based upon the traditional usage of the herb. A full spectrum aqueous alcoholic extract of the herb was developed, ensuring that all vital constituents of the whole herb were present in the extract. High pressure liquid chromatography and other techniques were used to validate the profile of the raw herb, dried herb, and the final extract to ensure and verify that consumption of 100 g of the herb traditionally by the tribals was equivalent to consumption of 1 g of the standardized extract. The extract was standardized for pregnane glycosides, saponin glycosides, and bitter principles.

***Source:* Green Chem, Bangalore, India.**

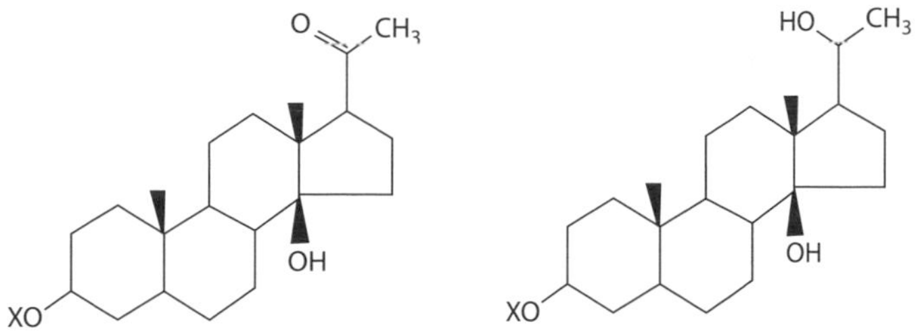

Caratuberside A   Caratuberside B

X = Gal[3-OMe, 6-deoxy](4 → 1)Glu

Pregnane Glycoside	Molecular Formula	Molecular Weight
Caratuberside A	$C_{34}H_{57}O_{12}$	657.819
Caratuberside B	$C_{34}H_{59}O_{12}$	659.835

Pure Caratuberside A is a white crystalline substance.
Melting point is 170°C – 171°C
Rotation is [α] at 20°C D + 60°C (C = 0.66 in methanol)

Pure Caratuberside B is a white crystalline substance.
Melting point is 182°C – 185°C (dec)

FIGURE 42.3 Pregnane glycosides of *Caralluma fimbriata* extract.

When we eat, the nerves from the stomach send a signal to the hypothalamus in the brain. This is the part of the brain that controls appetite. When the stomach is full, the hypothalamus signals the brain to stop eating. When a person is hungry, the hypothalamus sends a signal to the brain that food is needed.

It seems that *Caralluma fimbriata* extract inhibits this hunger sensory mechanism of the hypothalamus. The pregnane glycosides contained in *Caralluma fimbriata*, by interfering with the signaling mechanism and creating a signal on their own seem to fool the brain into thinking that the stomach is full even when the person has not eaten.

The main reason why most weight loss programs fail is because of tiredness and dullness created by the loss of weight, which forces the person to go back to old eating habits, resulting in a rebounding weight gain. *Caralluma fimbriata* extract, however, has demonstrated in controlled clinical trials that it helps participants to feel more energetic and gain lean muscle mass while losing fat.

It appears that this happens because the extract inhibits fat synthesis by blocking the formation of acetyl coenzyme A and malonyl coenzyme A, which are the building blocks of fat synthesis. The extract also seems to increase burning of fat by the body. This makes more energy available to the body and makes the person more active and lively. It is a well-known fact that muscle cells burn more calories than fat cells. So when more energy is available to the body, muscle cells burn energy faster. Muscle cells are heavier than fat cells, but they are also denser than fat cells. So they occupy lesser space and, consequently, the person appears more compact and trimmer compared to before.

SAFETY EVALUATION OF *CARALLUMA FIMBRIATA*

The *Caralluma fimbriata* extract was then put through two human clinical trials to validate its safety and efficacy. The first clinical trial was done in Bangalore, India, at St. John's National Academy of Health Sciences. The full spectrum aqueous alcoholic extract of the herb described earlier was used in the study. The extract dosage was 1 g a day, administered as two doses of 500 mg each, 30–45 min before the two main meals of the day. The participants consisted of 50 overweight/obese subjects (BMI > 26). Around 25 subjects received the active compound and 25 subjects received a placebo (Table 42.1). The study was randomized, double blind, and placebo controlled. Over 8 weeks, the subjects were tested for weight loss, anthropometry, body fat

TABLE 42.1

Results of the Indian Clinical Study

Parameter	Experimental Group (n = 25)
Age (years)	38.6 ± 7.8
Body weight (kg)	79.5 ± 16.9
Height (cm)	160.9 ± 9.1
Body mass index (kg/m²)	30.6 ± 5.5
Waist circumference (cm)	96.9 ± 11.6
Hip circumference (cm)	106.3 ± 11.4
Percent body fat (%)[a]	34.6 ± 5.6

Source: Kuriyan et al., Effect of *Caralluma fimbriata* extract on appetite, food intake and weight control in adult Indian men and women.

Mean ± standard deviation (SD). No significant differences were observed between the physical characteristics of the subjects of the two groups (independent t-test).

[a] Calculated from the sum of four skin fold measurements and applying the formulae of Durnin and Womersley (1974).

TABLE 42.2

Anthropometric Parameters of the Subjects at Baseline, Month 1, and End of the Study

Parameter	Baseline	Month 1	End of the Study
Body weight (kg) experimental	79.5 ± 16.9	78.3 ± 16.5^{b}	$77.5 \pm 16.0^{b,c}$
BMI (kg/m²) experimental	30.6 ± 5.5	30.2 ± 5.6^{b}	$29.9 \pm 5.6^{b,c}$
Waist circumference (cm) experimental	96.9 ± 11.6	95.1 ± 12.0^{b}	$93.9 \pm 11.3^{b,c}$
Hip circumference (cm) experimental	106.3 ± 11.4	105.8 ± 11.5	$105.0 \pm 11.6^{b,c}$
Percent fat (%)[a] experimental	34.6 ± 5.6	34.2 ± 5.3	33.4 ± 5.6^{b}

Source: Kuriyan et al., Effect of *Caralluma fimbriata* extract on appetite, food intake and weight control in adult Indian men and women.

Mean ± SD.

[a] Calculated from the sum of two, three, or four skin fold measurements and applying the formulae of Durnin and Womersley (1974).

[b] Mean value was significantly different from that of baseline (ANOVA for repeated measures with post hoc tests; $p < 0.05$).

[c] Mean value was significantly different from that of Month 1(ANOVA for repeated measures with post hoc tests; $p < 0.05$).

composition, body mass index (BMI), net weight, and systemic functions (Table 42.2). During the study, no changes were made in diet, and all subjects were advised to walk 30 min in the morning and evening. The adverse events were minor and limited to mild upset of the gastrointestinal tract. Importantly, they were present equally in the active and placebo groups. Constipation and flatulence subsided within a week and were attributed to the gelatin capsules more than the ingredients from the cactus present in the capsules. Examination of fasting and postprandial sugar,

TABLE 42.3

Biochemical Parameters of the Subjects at Baseline, Month 1, and End of the Study

Parameter	Baseline	Month 1	End of the Study
Fasting blood sugar (mg/dL) experimental	89.8 ± 16.8	89.3 ± 10.3	88.9 ± 10.4
Postprandial sugar (mg/dL) experimental	110.9 ± 35.3	108.3 ± 25.2	108.6 ± 27.2
Total cholesterol (mg/dL) experimental	192.5 ± 27.1	191.0 ± 25.9	191.8 ± 27.0
High density lipoprotein (HDL) cholesterol (mg/dL) experimental	65.9 ± 11.0	63.6 ± 10.0	64.1 ± 9.95
Low density lipoprotein (LDL) cholesterol (mg/dL) experimental	120.0 ± 39.8	118.0 ± 27.9	115.7 ± 30.3
Serum triglycerides (mg/dL) experimental	111.9 ± 52.0	112.1 ± 55.0	110.3 ± 51.5

Source: Kuriyan et al., Effect of *Caralluma fimbriata* extract on appetite, food intake and weight control in adult Indian men and women.

Mean ± SD. No significant differences in the biochemical parameters at various time points.

total cholesterol, LDL, HDL, triglycerides, serum creatinine, blood urea nitrogen (BUN), total protein, serum albumin, total bilirubin, conjugated bilirubin, aspartate transaminase (AST), alanine transaminase (ALT), alkaline phosphatase, gamma glutamyl transpeptidase (GT), and hemoglobin failed to reveal any overall toxicity from the extract. Blood pressure and ECG also showed no toxic reactions secondary to ingesting *Caralluma fimbriata*.

Statistically significant differences for body weight, BMI, waist circumference, hip circumference, body fat, blood pressure, and hunger levels were seen between time points in the experimental group, while the blood sugars and lipid profile (Table 42.3) did not show any significant results [5].

The second clinical trial was done under the auspices of Western Geriatric Research Institute, Los Angeles, USA. The subjects were taken from two active practices in the Los Angeles area. The subjects were randomly assigned to either the active group or the placebo group. The trial was carried out on 26 patients, 9 of whom were males. They ranged in age from 31 through 73. One patient from each category did not show up for the final visit (dropouts). All patients signed an informed consent. The substance was administered as one capsule to be taken 30 min before each meal. Each subject was weighed before and after completion of the study, height was ascertained at each visit, and the waist and the hips were measured in inches. The hips were measured at the widest girth while the waist was measured at the umbilicus. In addition, the blood pressure was measured in a standard fashion at the brachial artery in the left upper extremity. From the weight and height measurements, BMI of each subject was ascertained. Patients were instructed not to change their daily activity pattern (exercise) or their food intake.

Almost every patient taking the active ingredient lost significant weight. There was almost no weight loss observed in patients on placebo (Table 42.4). Of the patients on actives, 83% lost weight. Patients with a higher BMI lost more weight. Of the patients on the actives, 72% reduced their waist by 0.5–3 in.; 28% felt an increase in energy while on the active substance [6].

These two clinical trials showed that the use of *Caralluma fimbriata* extract along with dietary and physical activity changes may provide an effective method of weight reduction.

In addition to the human studies, which demonstrated safety and efficacy, the following safety studies on animal models were done on the product to evaluate the long-term chronic and mutagenicity studies.

An acute oral toxicity study conducted at St. John's National Academy of Health Sciences, India, on Swiss Wistar rats, as per the organisation for economic cooperation and development (OECD) guidelines, did not exhibit any mortality or toxicity neither in the preliminary study with a lower dose of 2 g per kg body weight nor at a very high dose of 5 g per kg body weight.

TABLE 42.4

Appetite and Food Intake Assessment

Parameter	Baseline (Day 0)	Month 1	End of the Study
Experimental group (n = 25)			
Thoughts of food (%)	34.5 ± 24.3	36.2 ± 21.6	33.2 ± 23.6
Feeling of fullness (%)	33.3 ± 19.3	41.7 ± 20.5	40.5 ± 21.9
Urge to eat (%)	44.0 ± 25.3	39.3 ± 21.5	34.5 ± 21.2
Hunger (%)	47.6 ± 22.6	39.2 ± 21.4	27.9 ± 18.8*
Energy intake (kcal/day)	2276.5 ± 202.3	—	2088.8 ± 183.4*
Fat intake (g/day)	59.0 ± 6.4	—	54.3 ± 3.9*
Carbohydrate intake (g/day)	360.9 ± 26.1	—	340.5 ± 23.7*
Protein intake (g/day)	62.9 ± 6.3	—	59.3 ± 7.2*
Placebo group (n = 25)			
Thoughts of food (%)	33.1 ± 20.3	33.6 ± 15.3	32.0.2 ± 17.5
Feeling of fullness (%)	37.8 ± 26.9	36.6 ± 17.9	38.6.3 ± 21.2
Urge to eat (%)	35.3 ± 25.3	35.2 ± 17.5	33.5 ± 19.71
Hunger (%)	41.9 ± 24.1	41.6 ± 17.3	40.7 ± 18.9
Energy intake (kcals/day)	2303.6 ± 107.9	—	2299.0 ± 10.9.0
Fat intake (g/day)	61.7 ± 2.8	—	60.9 ± 3.9
Carbohydrate intake (g/day)	377.9 ± 21.1	—	376.8 ± 21.3
Protein intake (g/day)	59.1 ± 4.5	—	59.3 ± 4.8

Source: Kuriyan et al., Effect of *Caralluma fimbriata* extract on appetite, food intake, and weight control in adult Indian men and women.

Values are mean values and standard deviation.

The appetite assessment was carried out using Visual Analog Scales and results were expressed as percentage of the scale.

Significant differences between time points were assessed using ANOVA for repeated measures with post hoc corrections.

The food intake assessment was carried out using food frequency questionnaires at baseline and end of the study, and significant differences between time points were assessed using paired t-test with post hoc corrections.

Mean value was significantly different from that of baseline.

* Signifies the p value, p = 0.21, 0.44, 0.18, <0.001.

Body weight and feed and water intake in all the rats were comparable with that of the control [7]. Similarly, a subchronic toxicity study conducted at the Bombay College of Pharmacy, India, on Wistar rats, under OECD guidelines, showed no mortality or chronic effects at 90 mg per kg bodyweight (equivalent to the recommended human dosage of 1 g a day) [8]. Mutagenicity studies (Ames test) by *Salmonella typhimurium* reverse mutation test conducted at Intox Pvt. Ltd., India, as per the OECD guidelines, concluded that the product was nonmutagenic in all the five strains of *Salmonella typhimurium* [9].

CONCLUSION

Obesity is indeed becoming a menace, assuming epidemic proportions. The physiological and psychological problems caused by obesity are enormous. A proper diet and exercise plan with efficacious and safe supplementation seems to be the way to go forward as the first step toward combating obesity. Controlling weight by reducing calorific intake seems to be a vital factor in this whole jigsaw. The extract of *Caralluma fimbriata* could fill the role of being an ideal, clinically tested, safe, and efficacious appetite suppressant in controlling calorific intake, leading to reduction in body weight.

REFERENCES

1. Report of K.S. Laddha, Medicinal Natural Products Research Laboratory, University of Mumbai, Mumbai, India, 2004.
2. Report of K.S. Jayashree, Professor and Head of Department, Department of Post Graduate Studies in Dravyaguna, Government Ayurvedic Medical College, Bangalore, India, 2006.
3. Wealth of India. *A Dictionary of Indian Raw Materials and Industrial Products* 3:266–267, 1992.
4. Report of V. Jayachandran, Lecturer in Botany and Head of the Department of Botany, Tagore Arts College, Pondicherry, India, 2006.
5. Report of S. Aroumougame, Secretary, Society for Health, Environment and Research for Biodiversity, Pondicherry, India, 2005.
6. Kurpad, A.V. et al., *Use of Caralluma fimbriata Extract on Appetite and Weight Control*, St. John's National Academy of Health Sciences, Bangalore, India, 2003.
7. Ronald M. Lawrence and Suneeta Choudhary, *Caralluma fimbriata in the Treatment of Obesity*, Western Geriatric Research Institute, Los Angeles, CA, 2004.
8. Venkataraman, B.V., Suresh, S., and Kurpad, A.V., *Acute Oral Toxicity of Caralluma fimbriata in Rats*, Department of Pharmacology, St. John's Medical College, Bangalore, India (January 9, 2004).
9. Jagtap, A., Mazumdar, A.S., and Rao, V.S.V., *Vadlamudi—Subchronic Oral Toxicity Study of Caralluma fimbriata Extract*, Bombay College of Pharmacy, Mumbai, India (April 2005).
10. Deshmukh, N.S. and Naik, P.Y., *Mutagenicity Study of Caralluma fimbriata Extract by Salmonella typhimurium*, Reverse Mutation Test, Intox Pvt. Ltd., Pune, India (December 27, 2004).
11. Durnin, J. V. G. A., and Womersley, J., Body fat assessed by total body density and its estimation from skinfold thickness: Measurements on 481 men and women aged 16–72 years. *British Journal of Nutrition*, 32:77–97, 1974.
12. Kuriyan, R., Petracchi, C., Ferro-Luzzi, A., Shetty, P.S., and Kurpad, A.V., Validation of expedient methods for measuring body composition in Indian adults. *Indian Journal of Medical Research*, 107:37–45, 1998.

43 Glucomannan in Weight Loss
A Review of the Evidence

Barbara Swanson, PhD, RN, ACRN
and Joyce K. Keithley, DNSc, RN, FAAN

CONTENTS

INTRODUCTION

Treatment of overweight and obesity is exceedingly difficult. Conventional management consists of low-calorie diets, physical activity, behavioral interventions, and/or pharmacological agents. However, long-term adherence to these approaches is problematic and most individuals regain the majority of lost weight within 1 or 2 years.[1] It has been suggested that the addition of novel approaches to conventional treatments may produce sustainable weight loss. One approach is fiber supplements. Glucomannan, a water-soluble dietary fiber supplement, has been associated with reductions in body weight in a few small studies[2–7] and may be an effective adjunct for overweight and obese individuals.

PREVALENCE OF DIETARY SUPPLEMENT USE FOR WEIGHT REDUCTION

Annual global sales of weight-loss supplements are estimated to total 13 billion dollars,[8] likely reflecting the aggressive marketing of these products by their manufacturers. A nationwide cross-sectional telephone survey of adults (N = 9403) found that 15.2% of respondents had used a nonprescription weight-loss supplement and that 8.7% had used them within the past year for an average duration of 3.7 months. Among persons currently trying to lose weight, past year usage increased to 16.1% of respondents. The odds of using a supplement within the past year increased with body mass index (BMI) but did not differ by race, ethnicity, or level of education.[9] Among the many categories of dietary supplements used for weight loss are those containing dietary fiber.

Dietary Fiber and Weight Reduction

Dietary fiber refers to indigestible plant and nonplant dietary substances. Dietary fiber and fiber supplements are postulated to promote weight loss by modulating energy intake and loss. Because of their low energy density, coupled with their bulking and viscosity-producing properties, fiber and fiber supplements can supplant energy dense nutrients, decrease hunger and appetite, and reduce protein, carbohydrate, and fat absorption.[10,11]

Studies examining the association between dietary fiber and weight loss date back to the late 1950s. Epidemiologic studies have generally found that fiber intake is inversely associated with body weight and BMI in individuals consuming self-selected diets.[12–16] With few exceptions, the majority of clinical studies have found that high-fiber diets are associated with reduced energy intake, reduced hunger and increased satiety, and increased weight loss. In a recent systematic review,[11] beneficial effects were seen with both high-fiber diets and fiber supplements. Almost all studies reported decreases in energy intake, increases in satiety or decreases in hunger, and increases in weight loss. Greater reductions in energy intake (82% vs. 94% of baseline intake) and weight (2.4 kg vs. 0.8 kg) were noted in overweight and obese individuals compared to normal weight individuals. In the majority of studies, fiber supplements yielded better results than high-fiber diets, suggesting greater benefits from fiber supplements, as well as easier use and adherence, compared to fiber-rich foods. Fiber supplement dosages ranged from 5 to 40 g/day (mean = 7–10 g/day), and the effects of soluble fiber vs. insoluble fiber vs. mixed fiber supplements were comparable. Other comprehensive reviews provide additional evidence that increased fiber consumption is associated with increases in satiety and reductions in hunger, energy intake, and body weight.[17,18]

The most widely used fiber supplements for achieving weight loss include guar gum, plantago psyllium, and glucomannan. The safety and efficacy of guar gum, a water-soluble fiber, for reducing body weight was evaluated in a meta-analysis.[19] Statistically pooled data from 11 double-blind prospective randomized clinical trials indicated that guar gum was ineffective for promoting weight loss and was associated with numerous adverse events, including diarrhea, flatulence, and other gastrointestinal complaints. Plantago psyllium, another water-soluble fiber, has been evaluated in one prospective randomized clinical trial.[20] No significant changes in weight were reported, although glucose and lipid parameters were significantly improved.

Although fiber is hypothesized to promote weight maintenance following weight loss, few long-term trials have been conducted. Two small studies have shown that mildly obese participants who were given fiber supplements were better able to sustain weight loss over 6 months to 1 year than those given a placebo.[21,22] Limited evidence indicates that glucomannan may be a promising fiber supplement for weight loss.

GLUCOMANNAN

Structure

Glucomannan is a water-soluble, fermentable dietary fiber extracted from the tuber or root of the elephant yam, also known as konjac (*Amorphophallus konjac* or *Amorphophallus rivieri*). Glucomannan consists of a polysaccharide chain of beta-D-glucose and beta-D-mannose with attached acetyl groups in a molar ratio of 1:1.6 with beta 1,4 linkages[23] (Figure 43.1). Human amylase cannot split beta 1,4 linkages; thus, glucomannan passes relatively unchanged into the colon, where it is highly fermented by colonic bacteria. It has a high molecular weight (200–2000 kDa)[23] and can absorb up to

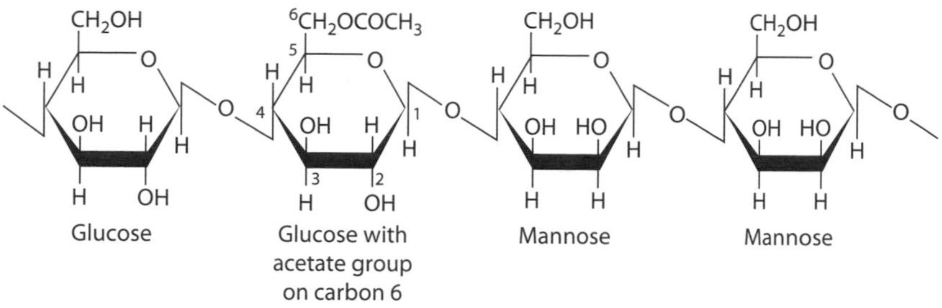

FIGURE 43.1 Structure of a segment of glucomannan with repeating glucose and mannose units.

50 times its weight in water, making it one of the most viscous dietary fibers known.[24] Therefore, much smaller doses of glucomannan are needed compared to other types of fiber supplements.

PROPOSED MECHANISMS OF ACTION (FIGURE 43.2)

Dilution of Energy Density

Fiber has a low calorie content and can lower the energy-to-weight ratio of consumed food.[11] Because studies suggest that eating patterns are driven by the weight of food consumed, rather than caloric intake,[25,26] fiber can displace the energy of other nutrients for a given weight of food and still induce satiety.[10]

Promotion of Satiety

Glucomannan may promote satiety via several mechanisms. Eating fiber requires increased mastication effort that may induce cephalic- and gastric-phase signals that promote satiety.[11] Glucomannan increases the viscosity of the gastrointestinal contents, thus slowing gastric emptying and inducing satiety. Moreover, there is evidence that the short-chain fatty acid by-products of glucomannan fermentation in the gut regulate satiety.[16] Additionally, glucomannan can attenuate postprandial insulin surges by reducing absorption, accelerate the delivery of food to the terminal ileum where satiety signals are transmitted, elevate plasma cholecystokinin levels, a hormone postulated to mediate fat-induced satiety, and decrease ghrelin levels, a hormone that acts centrally to increase appetite and food intake.[10,11,27–30]

Fecal Energy Loss

Soluble fibers have been shown to reduce fat and protein absorption,[31] possibly by reducing their physical contact with intestinal villi. However, it remains unclear whether this mechanism leads to weight loss. Evidence suggests that this energy loss is offset by the energy produced through the fermentation of soluble fibers and trapped nutrients in the colon.[11] There is considerable evidence that soluble fiber inhibits carbohydrate absorption[32] and improves glycemic parameters.[33,34] Recent studies have found that glucomannan supplementation increases colonic contents and motility, although weight loss was not measured.[35,36]

Stomach	Small Bowel	Colon	Feces
Absorption of water → ↑intraluminal viscosity, ↓energy intake, ↑satiety, ↓gastric emptying, ↓insulin secretion	Mechanical barrier to enzymatic digestion	Fermentation → short chain fatty acids → ↓glucose production, ↑insulin sensitivity, ↓insulin secretion	Excretion of most short chain fatty acids and some undigested glucomannan

FIGURE 43.2 Mechanisms by which glucomannan may induce weight loss.

TABLE 43.1
Physiochemical Characteristics of Glucomannan

Characteristic	Property
Molecular weight	Average: 1 million Daltons
Molar ratio	1 glucose:1.6 mannose
Solubility	Highly water soluble; expands up to 50 times its weight in digestive tract
Digestibility	Small intestine: resistant to hydrolysis by digestive enzymes
	Large intestine: fermented by colonic bacteria
Absorption	Minimal from large intestine

PHARMACOKINETICS

The bioavailability of glucomannan is very low; only small amounts are absorbed and reach the plasma (Table 43.1). To date, there are no validated methods to measure plasma concentrations of glucomannan or its metabolites in humans following therapeutic doses, thus limiting investigation of its pharmacokinetic properties. Glucomannan is resistant to hydrolysis by digestive enzymes, so it is only minimally digested in the small intestine. Substantial fermentation by colonic bacteria occurs in the large intestine, producing short-chain fatty acids and several by-products (e.g., formic acid, acetic acid, butyric acid, propanoic acid, glucose, mannose). Although small amounts of some of these products may be absorbed from the large intestine, most are excreted in the feces, along with some undigested glucomannan.[37]

SAFETY

The konjac tuber is widely used in Asia as an ingredient in the manufacture of jelly candies, tofu, and noodles. Konjac flour has been used as a food stabilizer and gelling agent and has been approved by the U.S. Department of Agriculture as a binder for meat products. Because of its water-absorptive properties, konjac jelly candies have been implicated in several choking deaths around the world, leading to its ban in the United States, Europe, and Australia.[38]

Glucomannan is available in capsule form or as a drink mix. It is no longer available in tablet form, as contact with water can cause the tablets to swell before they reach the stomach. There have been at least 10 case reports of esophageal obstruction caused by ingestion of glucomannan tablets.[39,40] There have been no reports of esophageal obstruction associated with ingestion of glucomannan capsules, presumably because the outer casing shields the fiber from water prior to reaching the stomach.[41] Glucomannan is also available in a variety of food products, including noodles and tortillas. Additionally, flour and powder preparations are available that can be used at thickening agents for puddings, pies, sauces, and soups.

There have been few adverse events associated with the use of glucomannan capsules. Most events have involved minor gastrointestinal complaints, such as bloating, gas, and mild diarrhea, and, in clinical studies of glucomannan, the overall rate of adverse effects is less than 0.05%.[42,43] One case report in Spain indicated a possible association between acute hepatitis of cholestatic type and the use of glucomannan in a patient with a previous history of drug use and recent use of several other herbal supplements.[44]

DRUG INTERACTIONS

Glucomannan has been shown to lower blood glucose levels and should not be taken in association with medications or other dietary supplements that have hypoglycemic effects.[33,34,45] Glucomannan reduces the absorption of sulfonylurea medications[46] and may reduce the bioavailability of other oral medications taken concomitantly. Glucomannan also may reduce the absorption of fat-soluble vitamins in supplements or in foods. Therefore, oral medications should be taken 1 h before or 4 h after ingesting glucomannan capsules.[43]

DOSAGE

The recommended dosage for weight loss is 1 g three times/day, 1 h before meals. For managing type 2 diabetes or insulin resistance, 3.6–13 g/day have been administered.[42]

GLUCOMANNAN AND WEIGHT LOSS: REVIEW OF CONTROLLED TRIALS

A few small studies suggest that glucomannan may be well tolerated, promote moderate weight loss in overweight and obese individuals, and have beneficial effects on lipid and glucose parameters. Six studies with weight loss as the primary outcome measure found that daily supplementation with glucomannan (dosage range, 1.24–3.87 g; treatment duration, 5–16 weeks; mean sample size, 38) produced significant (−5.5 to −8.8 lb) or nonsignificant decreases in body weight in overweight and obese individuals[2–7] (Table 43.2). Similar effects were seen whether the participants consumed self-selected, normocaloric, or hypocaloric diets. Other beneficial effects were increased satiety, improved lipid profile, improved diet adherence, and improved glycemic status. Adverse events were minimal and included a few reports of mild bloating/flatulence.

Findings of the two most recent trials[2,7] are consistent with those of the earlier trials.[3–6] Birketvedt et al.[2] examined the use of 1.24 g/day glucomannan supplements in 52 overweight women consuming 1200 kcal diets. Over a 5 week period, a weight loss of approximately 8.8 lb (p < 0.01) occurred; the addition of guar gum and alginate to glucomannan did not confer additional weight loss effects. In 29 obese men, Wood et al.[7] found that adding 3 g/day of glucomannan to a carbohydrate-restricted diet resulted in significant decreases in body weight in both the treatment and placebo groups, but that glucomannan did not provide additional benefits over the diet alone.

TABLE 43.2
Clinical Studies of Glucomannan and Weight Loss

Study	Sample	Design	Glucomannan Intervention	Diet	Duration	Weight Results
Walsh et al.[6]	20 obese women	Parallel	1 g 3 times/day	Customary diet	8 weeks	−5.5 lb, p ≤ 0.005
Livieri et al.[4]	53 obese children	Parallel	2–3 g/day	Balanced diet	16 weeks	Significant reductions[a]
Vido et al.[5]	60 obese children	Parallel	2 g/day	Balanced diet	8 weeks	Significant reductions[a]
Cairella and Marchini[3]	15 obese women	Parallel	3.87 g/day	1200 kcal	8 weeks	Substantial reductions[a]
Birketvedt et al.[2]	52 obese women	Parallel	1.24 g/day	1200 kcal	5 weeks	−8.8 lb, p < 0.01
Wood et al.[7]	29 obese men	Parallel	3 g/day	Carbohydrate restricted	12 weeks	Significant reductions in both groups, p < .01

[a] From English abstract of Italian manuscript.

Limitations of all six studies include the use of sample sizes not supported by power analysis, the use of heterogeneous samples of overweight and obese individuals with lack of appropriate controls for comorbidities and confounders, variable formulations and dosages of glucomannan, and short duration of follow-up. It is also noteworthy that the majority of these studies were conducted 15 or more years ago, and three of the studies were published in Italian,[3-5] limiting the depth and amount of information abstracted.

Combinations of glucomannan and other plant-based products for promoting weight loss recently have been examined in two clinical trials.[47,48] In 200 overweight or obese adults, Salas-Salvado et al.[47] studied a mixture of two soluble fibers, 3 g *Plantago ovata* husk and 1 g glucomannan, given either twice or three times a day over 16 weeks. Weight loss was higher in both the twice and three times daily groups than in the placebo (−4.52, −4.60, −0.79 kg, respectively), but not significantly so. Vasques et al.[48] evaluated the efficacy of *Garcinia cambogia* (a potential inhibitor of fatty acid biosynthesis) and glucomannan in 58 obese adults over a 12 week period. While the combination treatment significantly reduced total and LDL cholesterol, weight and other body composition measures were not significantly affected.

Other recent, uncontrolled studies[49,50] have explored the effects of lifestyle modifications and glucomannan on weight loss. When a novel polysaccharide (glucomannan and other polysaccharides) was combined with a clinical weight-loss program (diet and exercise counseling), significant reductions were noted in weight (−5.79 ± 3.55 kg) and other body composition measures in 29 overweight or obese adults.[49] In contrast, adding exercise to a diet containing glucomannan did not affect weight loss or body composition measures in a sample of 42 overweight adults.[50]

A series of studies have examined the safety and efficacy of glucomannan for modulating lipid and glucose parameters in patients with type 2 diabetes and/or hypercholesterolemia with body weight loss as a secondary outcome measure.[32,33,45,51,52] Lipid profile (total cholesterol, LDL cholesterol, and triglycerides) was significantly improved in these studies.[33,45,52] Similar to the weight loss studies, there were either no adverse events or only a few transient gastrointestinal symptoms (flatulence, soft stools). These findings suggest that glucomannan favorably modulates metabolic parameters.

Supporting these findings is a meta-analysis of 14 clinical trials of subjects with characteristics of metabolic syndrome. Subjects who received glucomannan had significantly lower body weight, fasting blood glucose, total cholesterol, LDL cholesterol, and triglycerides than control subjects.[53] Other endpoints such as HDL cholesterol and blood pressure were not significantly influenced. In contrast to other types of fiber,[54,55] glucomannan appears to be more effective in lowering triglycerides, possibly related to its high viscosity and ability to alter hepatic cholesterol and lipoprotein metabolism.[24]

CLINICAL IMPLICATIONS

Clinicians should encourage patients to use glucomannan supplements from manufacturers that are state-certified as compliant with good manufacturing practices. Additionally, when possible, they should select products whose composition and purity have been tested by an independent laboratory. Such products may contain quality labels, such as USP, ConsumerLab, or TruLabel. Unless purity data are available, supplements imported from foreign countries should be avoided as manufacturing practices may fall short of U.S. standards.

Some glucomannan products contain multiple pharmacologically active ingredients. For example, Glucomannan + ® (Swanson Health Products, Fargo, ND) contains glucomannan, as well as chromium, chitosan, guar gum, gymnema, psyllium, and L-carnitine. Chromium and gymnema both have hypoglycemic properties; thus, the risk of hypoglycemia, as well as pharmacodynamic interactions with oral hypoglycemics or insulin, may be increased. This underscores the need for clinicians to consider the safety profile and potential drug interactions of each ingredient when reviewing multi-ingredient supplements with their patients. The following case study illustrates other clinical implications of glucomannan.

CASE STUDY

BF, a 42-year-old female, presents to the clinic for consultation on weight loss. She mentions that she began taking glucomannan 1 week ago and has lost 2 lb. You have seen BF routinely for several months, and she wonders what you think of glucomannan. She has tried a number of fad diets—Slim Fast, grapefruit diet, Sugar Busters—all without success. You are concerned about her weight (192 lb prior to starting glucomannan), particularly because at her last visit she had an elevated fasting blood glucose (180 mg/dL) and was hypertensive (180/95).

Past medical history
Overweight with history of multiple fad diets and cycles of weight gain/loss

Lifestyle history
Denies use of wine, hard liquor, beer
Denies current use of tobacco products
No structured activity or exercise patterns

Social history
Married, 4 children (ages 3–14)
Homemaker
College educated, degree in English

Family history
Family: tendency to be overweight
Mother: history of diabetes
Father: hypertensive with CAD

Medications
HCTZ 12.5 mg/day
Mavik (ACE inhibitor) 4 mg/day

Over-the-counter
Glucomannan: does not remember type or amount
No other use of dietary supplements/herbal therapies

Physical assessment

Height	61 in.
Weight	190 lb
Pulse	90
BP	145/90
Waist circumference	35.5 in. (90 cm)
BMI	35.9

Comment:
This case highlights the growing use of dietary supplements, such as glucomannan, for weight loss. It also highlights the importance of assessing for CAM use and advising patients about dietary supplements for weight loss. Long-term weight loss and maintenance through lifestyle changes are difficult to attain, and adjunctive therapies have become increasingly popular weight-loss options.

Question: How would you ascertain more about the type and amount of glucomannan that BF is taking?

Comment:
It is laudable that BF mentions that she is taking glucomannan and wants your opinion. An estimated 70% of individuals who use CAM therapies do not report it to their health-care providers because

(a) health-care providers either neglect to ask or are uncomfortable asking about CAM therapies and (b) patients are fearful, embarrassed, or do not see the importance of reporting CAM use. To elicit more specific information about the glucomannan product that BF is using, questions might include the following: (a) where did you learn about glucomannan? (b) what encouraged you to try glucomannan? (c) how often and when do you take it? (d) what form is it in? and (e) where did you obtain the glucomannan? Additionally, arrange to have BF call or e-mail the product brand and ingredients to you.

Question: How would you advise BF about the safety and efficacy of glucomannan?

Comment:
Results from a few, limited studies suggest that glucomannan in doses of 2–4 g/day may be safe and effective in promoting weight loss. Potential advantages of glucomannan are its tolerability and low rate of side effects. However, additional studies of standardized glucomannan products are needed before they are recommended as a weight-loss adjunct. One concern is that many over-the-counter preparations of glucomannan contain a combination of products that may have dangerous side effects. Some examples to review with BF are bitter orange, country mallow, and caffeine from "natural" or "disguised" sources, such as extracts of guarana or tea. A second concern is that glucomannan may reduce the absorption of fat-soluble vitamins and oral medications; therefore, BF should be advised take medications 1 h before or 4 h after taking glucomannan capsules.[41] Another concern is the high solubility of glucomannan capsules; thus, the importance of taking capsules with 8 oz of water and notifying the health-care provider should be discussed if any side effects occur (e.g., difficulty swallowing, abdominal distention). Some reliable sources of information about dietary supplements are the National Center for Complementary and Alternative Therapy at: http://nccam.nih.gov, the Natural Medicines Comprehensive Database (available through many library databases), and the Office of Dietary Supplements at http://dietary-supplements.info.nih.gov/. Additionally, clinicians can keep abreast of new safety information about dietary supplements through the FDA MedWatch program at http://www.fda.gov/medwatch/.

CONCLUSIONS AND FUTURE DIRECTIONS

Studies have shown that dietary fiber is a safe and effective adjunct to weight-reducing diets. Fiber has been shown to promote and prolong satiety,[56–58] to increase long-term adherence to low-calorie diets,[13,59,60] and to be inversely associated with weight gain.[13] However, commonly used dietary fiber supplements, such as guar gum and psyllium, have not been consistently shown to promote weight loss.[61,62]

In contrast to other fiber supplements, glucomannan appears to possess properties that promote weight loss when used in conjunction with either a normocaloric or a hypocaloric diet. The findings of controlled trials[2–7] suggest that doses of 1.24–4 g/day significantly reduce body weight in overweight and obese persons. Moreover, glucomannan is well tolerated and inexpensive and has relatively few side effects. Limited data show that it improves risk factors for cardiovascular disease and diabetes, so it may be an acceptable alternative for overweight individuals who are unable or unwilling to increase their fiber intake through food sources. Yet, before glucomannan can be safely recommended, additional trials using larger numbers of subjects, longer study follow-up periods, and standardized formulations and dosages are needed to further elucidate its safety, efficacy, and weight-reducing mechanisms of action.

REFERENCES

1. Tsai, A.G. and Wadden, T.A. Systematic review: An evaluation of major commercial weight loss programs in the United States. *Ann Intern Med*, 142, 56, 2005.
2. Birketvedt, G.S. et al. Experiences with three different fiber supplements in weight loss. *Med Sci Monit*, 11, P15, 2005.
3. Cairella, M. and Marchini, G. Evaluation of the action of glucomannan on metabolic parameters and on the sensation of satiation in overweight and obese patients. *Clin Ter*, 146, 269, 1995.

4. Livieri, C., Novazi, F., and Lorini, R. The use of highly purified glucomannan-based fibers in childhood obesity. *Pediat Med Chir*, 14, 195, 1992.

5. Vido, L. et al. Childhood obesity treatment: Double blinded trial on dietary fibres (glucomannan) versus placebo. *Padiatr Padol*, 28, 133, 1993.

6. Walsh, D.E., Yaghoubian, V., and Behforooz, A. Effect of glucomannan on obese patients: A clinical study. *Int J Obes*, 8, 289, 1984.

7. Wood, R.J. et al. Effects of a carbohydrate-restricted diet with and without supplemental soluble fiber on plasma low-density lipoprotein cholesterol and other clinical markers of cardiovascular risk. *J Metabol*, 56, 58, 2007.

8. Onakpoya, I. and Ernst, E. Dietary supplements for weight loss. In R.B. Konarek and H.R. Lieberman (eds.), Diet, Brain, Behavior: Practical Implications. 2011, CRC Press, Boca Raton, FL.

9. Blanck, H.M., Serdula, M.K., Gillespie, C. et al. Use of nonprescription dietary supplements for weight loss is common among Americans. *J Am Diet Assoc*, 107, 441, 2007.

10. Burton-Freeman, B. Dietary fiber and energy regulation. *J Nutr*, 130, 272S, 2000.

11. Horwath, N.C., Saltzman, E., and Roberts, S.B. Dietary fiber and weight regulation. *Nutr Rev*, 59, 129, 2001.

12. He, K. et al. Changes in intake of fruits and vegetables in relation to risk of obesity and weight gain among middle-aged women. *Int J Obes*, 28, 1569, 2004.

13. Liu, S. et al. Relation between changes in intakes of dietary fiber and grain products and changes in weight and development of obesity among middle-aged women. *Am J Clin Nutr*, 78, 920, 2003.

14. Ludwig, D.S. et al. Dietary fiber, weight gain, and cardiovascular risk factors in young adults. *JAMA*, 282, 1539, 1999.

15. Newby, P. et al. Dietary patterns and changes in body mass index and waist circumference in adults. *Am J Clin Nutr*, 77, 1417, 2003.

16. Lindstrom, J., Peltonen, M., Eriksson, J.G. et al. High-fibre, low-fat diet predicts long-term weight loss and decreased type 2 diabetes risk: The Finnish Diabetes Prevention Study. *Diabetologia*, 49, 912, 2006.

17. Pereira, M.A. and Ludwig, D.S. Dietary fiber and body-weight regulation. *Ped Clin North Am*, 48, 969, 2001.

18. Rolls, B.J., Ello-Martin, J.A., and Tohill, B.C. What can intervention studies tell us about the relationship between fruit and vegetable consumption and weight management? *Nutr Rev*, 62, 1, 2004.

19. Pittler, M.H. and Ernst, E. Guar gum for body weight reduction. *Am J Med*, 110, 724, 2001.

20. Rodriquez-Moran, M., Guerrero-Romero, F., and Laczano-Burciago, M. Lipid and glucose-lowering efficacy of Plantago Psyllium in type II diabetes. *J Diabet Complications*, 12, 273, 1998.

21. Cairella, G., Cairella, M., and Marchini, G. Effect of dietary fibre on weight correction after modified fasting. *Eur J Clin Nutr*, 49, S325, 1995.

22. Ryttig, K.R. et al. A dietary fibre supplement and weight maintenance after weight loss. A randomized, double-blind, placebo-controlled long-term trial. *Int J Obes*, 13, 165, 1989.

23. Chua, M., Baldwin, T.C., Hocking, T.J., and Chan, K. Traditional uses and potential health benefits of *Amorphophallus konjac* K. Koch ex N.E.Br. *J Ethnopharmacol*, 128, 268, 2010.

24. Doi, K. Effect of konjac fibre (glucomannan) on glucose and lipids. *Eur J Clin Nutr*, 49(suppl), 190S, 1995.

25. Bell, E.A. et al. Energy density of foods affects energy intake in normal weight women. *Am J Clin Nutr*, 68, 412, 1998.

26. Rolls, B.J. et al. Energy density but not fat content of foods affected energy intake in lean and obese women. *Am J Clin Nutr*, 69, 863, 1999.

27. Vuksan, V. et al. Konjac-Mannan and American Ginseng: Emerging alternative therapies for type 2 diabetes mellitus. *J Am Coll Nutr*, 20, 370S, 2001.

28. McCarty, M.F. Glucomannan minimizes the postprandial insulin surge: A potential adjuvant for hepatothermic therapy. *Med Hypotheses*, 58, 487, 2002.

29. Bourden, I. et al. Postprandial lipid, glucose, insulin, and cholecystokinin response in men fed barley pasta enriched with beta-glucan. *Am J Clin Nutr*, 69, 55, 1999.

30. Chearskul, S., Kriengsinyos, W., Kooptiwut, S. et al. Immediate and long-term effects of glucomannan on total ghrelin and leptin in type 2 diabetes mellitus. *Diabetes Res Clin Pract*, 83, e40, 2009.

31. Baer, D.J. et al. Dietary fiber decreases the metabolizable energy content and nutrient digestibility of mixed diets fed to humans. *J Nutr*, 127, 579, 1997.

32. Jenkins, D.L. et al. Low glycemic index: Lente carbohydrates and physiological effects of altered food frequency. *Am J Clin Nutr*, 59, 706S, 1994.

33. Vuksan, V. et al. Konjac-mannan (glucomannan) improves glycemia and other associated risk factors for coronary heart disease in type 2 diabetes. A randomized controlled metabolic trial. *Diabetes Care*, 22, 913, 1999.

34. Vuksan, V. et al. Beneficial effects of viscous dietary fiber from konjac-mannan in subjects with the insulin resistance syndrome: Results of a controlled metabolic trial. *Diabetes Care*, 23, 9, 2000.

35. Chen, H.-L., Cheng, H.-C., Wu, W.-T., Liu, Y.-J., and Liu, S.-Y. Supplementation of Konjac glucomannan into a low-fiber Chinese diet promoted bowel movement and improved colonic ecology in constipated adults: A placebo-controlled, diet-controlled trial. *J Am Coll Nutr*, 27, 102, 2008.

36. Chen, H.-L., Cheng, H.-C., Liu, Y.-J., Liu, S.-Y., and Wu, W.-T. Konjac act as a natural laxative by increasing stool bulk and improving colonic ecology in health adults. *Nutrition*, 22, 1112, 2006.

37. Matsuura, Y. Degradation of konjac glucomannan by enzymes in human feces and formation of short-chain fatty acids by intestinal anaerobic bacteria. *J Nutr Sci Vitaminol*, 44, 423, 1998.

38. FDA. FDA issues a second warning and an import alert about Konjac mini-cup gel candies that pose choking risk, 2001. Retrieved December 8, 2010 from http://www.fda.gov/ICECI/EnforcementActions/EnforcementStory/EnforcementStoryArchive/ucm105953.htm

39. Vanderbeek, P.B., Fasano, C., O'Malley, G., and Hornstein, J. Esophageal obstruction from hygroscopic pharmacobezoar containing glucomannan. *Clin Toxicol*, 45, 80, 2007.

40. Gaudry, P. Glucomannan diet tablets. *Med J Australia*, 142, 204, 1995.

41. Consumerlab.com Glucomannan, 2010. Retrieved December 8, 2010 from http://www.consumerlab.com/tnp.asp?chunkiid=21743&docid=/tnp/pg000631

42. Keithley, J.K. and Swanson, B. Glucomannan and obesity: A critical review. *Alt Ther Health Med*, 11, 30, 2005.

43. Natural Medicines Comprehensive Database (2012). Stockton, CA: Therapeutic Research Center.

44. Villaverde, A.F. et al. Acute hepatitis of cholestatic type possibly associated with the use of glucomannan (amorphophalus konjac) (Letter to the Editor). *J Hepatol*, 41, 1061, 2004.

45. Chen, H.L. et al. Konjac supplement alleviated hypercholesterolemia and hyperglycemia in type 2 diabetic subjects—A randomized double-blind trial. *J Am Coll Nutr*, 22, 36, 2003.

46. Shima, K. et al. Effect of dietary fiber, glucomannan, on absorption of sulfonylurea in man. *Hormone Metab Res*, 15, 1, 1983.

47. Salas-Slavado, J. et al. Effect of two doses of a mixture of soluble fibres on body weight and metabolic variables in overweight or obese patients: A randomized trial. *Brit J Nutr*, 99, 1380, 2008.

48. Vasques, C.A.R. et al. Evaluation of the pharmacotherapeutic efficacy of *Garcinia cambogia* plus *Amorphophallus konjac* for the treatment of obesity. *Phythother Res*, 22, 1135, 2008.

49. Lyon, M.R. and Reichert, R.G. The effect of a novel viscous polysaccharide along with lifestyle changes on short-term weight loss and associated risk factors in overweight and obese adults: An observational retrospective clinical program analysis. *Alt Med Rev*, 15, 68, 2010.

50. Kraemer, W.J. et al. Effect of adding exercise to a diet containing glucomannan. *J Metabol*, 56, 1149, 2007.

51. Arvill, A. and Bodin, L. Effect of short-term ingestion of konjac glucomannan on serum cholesterol in healthy men. *Am J Clin Nutr*, 61, 585, 1995.

52. Gallaher, D.D. et al. A glucomannan and chitosan fiber supplement decreases plasma cholesterol and increases cholesterol excretion in overweight normocholesterolemic humans. *J Am Coll Nutr*, 21, 428, 2002.

53. Sood, N., Baker, W.L., and Coleman, C.I. Effect of glucomannan on plasma lipid and glucose concentrations, body weight, and blood pressure: Systematic review and meta-analysis. *Am J Clin Nutr*, 88, 1167, 2008.

54. Grundy, S.C. et al. Implications of recent clinical trials for the National Cholesterol Education Program Adult Treatment Panel III guidelines. *Circ*, 110, 227, 2004.

55. Anderson, J.M. et al. Cholesterol-lowering effects of psyllium intake adjunctive to diet therapy in men and women with hypercholesterolemia: Meta-analysis of 8 controlled trials. *Am J Clin Nutr*, 71, 472, 2000.

56. Burley, V.J., Paul, A.W., and Blundell JE. Influence of a high-fibre food (myco- protein) on appetite: Effects on satiation (within meals) and satiety (following meals). *Eur J Clin Nutr*, 47, 409, 1993.

57. Hill, A.J. and Blundell, J.E. Macronutrients and satiety: The effects of a high protein for high carbohydrate meal on subjective motivation to eat and food preferences. *Nutr Behav*, 3, 133, 1986.

58. Rigaud, D. et al. Effect of psyllium on gastric emptying, hunger feeling and food intake in normal volunteers: A double blind study. *Eur J Clin Nutr*, 52, 239, 1997.

59. Astrup, A., Vrist, E., and Quaade F. Dietary fibre added to a very low calorie diet reduces hunger and alleviates constipation. *Int J Obes*, 14, 105, 1990.

60. Pasman, W.J. et al. Effect of one week of fibre supplementation on hunger and satiety ratings and energy intake. *Appetite*, 29, 77, 1997.

61. Allison, D.B. et al. Alternative treatments for weight loss: A critical review. *Crit Rev Food Sci Nutr*, 41, 1, 2001.

62. Pittler, M.H. and Ernst, E. Dietary supplements for body-weight reduction: A systematic review. *Am J Clin Nutr*, 79, 529, 2004.

44 Role of Medium-Chain Triglycerides in Weight Management

Mary G. Enig, PhD, FACN, MACN, CNS
and Beverly B. Teter, MACN, CNS

CONTENTS

INTRODUCTION

Human diets are composed of protein, carbohydrate, and fats, the three proximate energy-providing components, as well as minerals, vitamins, and bioactive compounds contained within the proximate components. Of course, water is also essential for good health. Since the early 1900s, the percent of protein in the diet has remained essentially constant at 11% of the calories or about 100 g/day/person in the food supply.[1] Intake surveys indicate about 74 g/day/person in the last quarter of the twentieth century. Since there are only three other proximate calorie-producing components of the diet, and if the protein is constant, if either fat or carbohydrate increases, then the other one *a priori* must decrease. Thus, if a "low-fat diet" is consumed, it could also be called a "high-carbohydrate diet" and *vice versa*. When diets are high in fat calories, that does not mean they are also high in protein as has been claimed in many scientific and almost all articles written for public consumption.

Low-fat diets, which have been promoted by U.S. Government agencies and various health organizations, have not prevented obesity and other health problems.[2–4] In fact, obesity has steadily increased since the early 1980s when the low-fat diet recommendations were introduced. Low-fat diets are *a priori* diets that are high in carbohydrates in the form of simple or complex carbohydrates or as fiber. Any carbohydrate eaten in excess of the body's ability to store glycogen or to immediately burn it for energy is stored as fat either in the liver or the adipose.

In the United States, the food fats that are abundant are high in omega-6 fatty acids and relatively low in omega-3 fatty acids, as well as very low in medium-chain saturated fatty acids such as lauric acid.[2,3] The antisaturated fat rhetoric has been instrumental in most of the changes mentioned earlier, and protective fats have been lost.[2,3] Since trans-fatty acid (tFA) labeling has been in effect, the levels of tFA have decreased substantially in many foods but are still present in some foods. Even the foods labeled "zero" *trans* can have up to 0.49 g/serving of tFA. Multiple servings could still contain substantial amounts of tFA.

MAJOR CLASSES OF LIPIDS

Lipids make up a diverse group of biological moieties known for their solubility primarily in nonpolar solvents such as chloroform, benzene, and hexane.[2] Since human bodies are largely composed of water and water-soluble compounds, the lipids are usually transported associated with lipoproteins or carrier proteins that help solubilize them. Lipids such as cholesterol are carried in the blood on lipoproteins like low-density lipoproteins (LDL) and high-density lipoprotein (HDL) while vitamin D metabolites are associated with a specific binding protein which transports them in solution. Individual fatty acids are often attached to serum albumin (a serum protein) to be transported. Some of the short-chain fatty acids (SCFAs) are water soluble so do not need carriers.

There are basically three major classes of lipids: neutral lipids, phospholipids, and steroids. The lipids soluble in nonpolar medium are typically the triglycerides, which belong to the neutral lipids. Triglycerides are formed from three molecules of fatty acids and one molecule of glycerol. The human body uses fatty acids from food for building tissue, for making phospholipids and steroids, and for the functionality of the lipids.[2–5]

FATTY ACID CATEGORIES FOUND IN FOOD

It is well known that fatty acid categories are widely distributed in natural foods, as well as animal and human tissues. Table 44.1 provides a list of saturated fatty acids that range in length from 3 carbons to 30 carbons, as well as monounsaturated fatty acids and polyunsaturated fatty acids.

DEFINITION OF THE TERM "OMEGA"

One of the major groups of fatty acids is called "essential fatty acids." These fatty acids are either omega-6 or omega-3 fatty acids. The term essential refers to the fact that these two groups of fatty acids are essential to the function and structure of the human body and must be obtained from the diet.[2–5]

Fatty acids are identified by the "families" to which they belong. Families differ from "classes," and the term "families" uses the word omega for its descriptor. Omega-6 fatty acids belong in a family of related polyunsaturated fatty acids (two or more unsaturated double bonds) in which the first fatty acid in the omega-6 family is linoleic acid, which has 18 carbons and two double bonds, one in the omega 6 and one in the omega 9 positions on the carbon chain. The others in the series can be formed from this one if the body is healthy and working properly. If the body cannot desaturate and elongate the carbon chain to form the subsequent fatty acids, then they must be provided by diet or IV. Examples of these omega-6 fatty acids include γ-linolenic acid, dihomo-γ-linolenic acid, and arachidonic acid.[2–4] The first family members are found in abundant amounts in most vegetable oils, such as corn, soy, cottonseed, and canola.

TABLE 44.1

Fatty Acid Categories Found in Food and as Part of Animal/Human Tissues

Fatty Acids	Carbons C=C*	Omega Family
Saturated fatty acids		
Short-chain saturated fatty acids		
Propionic acid	3 : 0	
Butyric acid	4 : 0	
Caproic acid	6 : 0	
Medium-chain saturated fatty acids		
Caprylic acid	8 : 0	
Capric acid	10 : 0	
Lauric acid	12 : 0	
Long-chain saturated fatty acids		
Myristic acid	14 : 0	
Palmitic acid	16 : 0	
Stearic acid	18 : 0	
Very-long-chain saturated fatty acids		
Arachidic acid	20 : 0	
Behenic acid	22 : 0	
Lignoceric acid	24 : 0	
Cerotic acid	26 : 0	
Montanic acid	28 : 0	
Melissic acid	30 : 0	
Unsaturated fatty acids		
Short-chain unsaturated fatty acid		
Crotonic acid	4 : 1	
Long-chain monounsaturated fatty acids		
Palmitoleic acid	16 : 1	omega-9
Oleic acid	18 : 1	omega-9
Long-chain polyunsaturated fatty acids		
Linoleic acid[a]	18 : 2	omega 6
α-Linolenic acid (ALA)	18 : 3	omega-3
γ-Linolenic acid	18 : 3	omega-6
Stearidonic acid (SDA)	18 : 4	omega-6
Very-long-chain poly unsaturated fatty acids		
Arachidonic acid	20 : 4	omega-6
Adrenic acid	22 : 4	omega-6
Eicosapentaenoic acid (EPA)	20 : 5	omega-3
Docosapentaenoic acid	22 : 5	omega-3
Dicosahexaenoic acid (DHA)	22 : 6	omega-3
Nisinic acid	24 : 5	omega-3

[a] C=C represents methylene interrupted double bonds, i.e., linoleic acid contains 18 carbons with 2 double bonds in positions omega 9 and 6. It would be 18:2 omega 6.

Omega-3 fatty acids belong to the family of polyunsaturated fatty acids where the first fatty acid in the metabolic lineup is α-linolenic acid. This fatty acid is an 18-carbon fatty acid found in a number of foods such as green leafs, some oils, and many seeds. It has three double bonds in the omega-3, omega-6, and omega-9 positions. The well-known omega-3 fatty acids are essential because the body needs them in amounts that are not always readily made from the 18-carbon α-linolenic acid. These are 20- and 22-carbon fatty acids called eicosapentaenoic acid (EPA) and docosahexaenoic acid (DHA), respectively.[2,3] One reason that they are not made easily in the body is that our U.S. diet has an excess of linoleic acid (omega-6) and this competes for the same desaturase and elongase enzymes. The proper dietary ratio of omega-6 to omega-3 fatty acids is important to maintain good health—mental and physical.

There are also monounsaturated fatty acids (one double bond) referred to as omega-9 fatty acids, the most common of which is oleic acid, the major fatty acid in olive oil. Monounsaturated fatty acids are not essential in the same way that polyunsaturated fatty acids are essential because they are readily made by the tissues when they are needed. They are, however, necessary fatty acids, and they are elongated when needed for certain tissues and certain functions.[2,3] They are important because they help to modify the fluidity of cell membranes and can be burned for energy by the cells.

Saturated fatty acids are not given a designation of "omega" because they do not have a double bond. Saturated fatty acids come in basic lengths referred to as long-, medium-, and short-chain. The most common of the saturated fatty acids found in foods and made in tissues is palmitic acid. Palmitic acid is a long-chain saturate that is 16 carbons long, and it is the end product of *de novo* fatty acid synthesis. It is a major component of lung surfactant, which is critical for respiratory health, especially in premature infants. It is also a major component of milks, human, cow, etc. Stearic acid, which has 18 carbons, is a long-chain saturate that is common but not found in large amounts in food.[2,3] Stearic acid is readily desaturated to oleic acid (the olive oil acid) in mammalian bodies.

The most important medium-chain fatty acid (MCFA) is the 12-carbon saturate, lauric acid. Lauric acid is found in very small amounts in foods except as a major fatty acid in certain fats and oils called lauric oils, which include coconut oil and palm kernel oil as well as a mother's milk and animal milk.[2,3]

FAT FUNCTIONS AND STRUCTURE

Fat provides energy for immediate use by cells and is stored as adipose fat for later use. Saturated fat is a major fuel for heart, kidney, and skeletal muscle; has protein-sparing action during growth; cushions vital organs; maintains body temperature through thermal regulation (insulation, brown fat); promotes healthy skin; has protective barrier function; is important for reproduction; and carries fat-soluble vitamins and aids in their absorption.[2,3,6] Polyunsaturated fats are precursors to hormones and secretions (essential fatty acids/prostaglandins) and precursors to various hormones (cholesterol/steroid hormones). Fat forms special structures (cellular and subcellular lipid membranes), and it performs special functions (regulates enzyme activity).[2,3,6]

Fat is the major component of brain (white matter), where it forms the covering for nerve tissue as well as cell membranes. Cholesterol is a major fraction of brain lipids comprising 25% of the lipid weight of brain. The myelin which covers and protects the nerves in the brain contains about 70% of the brain cholesterol. Furthermore, the formation of central nervous system (CNS) synapses between neurons is limited by the availability of cholesterol.[7] The rest of the body is composed of about 2% cholesterol where it is used for steroid and sex hormone synthesis, is an intermediate in the synthesis of vitamin D in the skin when exposed to ultraviolet light, and is used for synthesis of bile salts which aid digestion.

Phospholipids are major components of cell membranes in every cell in the body. They also are the lung surfactant molecules to which the palmitic acid is attached. Phospholipids aid in digestion and are used in food preparation as emulsifiers and stabilizers.

There are fatty acids that belong to the neutral lipid category, but most are not natural nor useful except to the food industry. These are commonly known as TFAs, formed by the partial hydrogenation process. They have higher melting points and thus can substitute for the natural fats such as butter, suet, and tallow in baking and frying. They are formed from polyunsaturated fatty acids such as omega-6 oils and from any omega-3 fatty acids when they are present in the original oils. In the United States, most of the TFAs are formed from omega-6 oils because the most common oils in the United States are omega-6 oils such as soybean, corn, canola, and cottonseed oils.[2,3,8–10]

There are small amounts of useful TFAs naturally found in dairy products, which convey definite health benefits, and one can be converted by our bodies into a healthful conjugated fatty acid, 9c,11t-CLA which is very anticarcinogenic.

Fatty acids range from three carbons in length to nearly 30 carbons in length. Generally, the fatty acids are even numbered, except for small numbers of fatty acids of bacterial origin found especially in ruminant fats. These 3-carbon fatty acids are found in dairy foods; 4-carbon fatty acids are also found mostly in animal milk.[2,3]

The saturated fatty acids are almost all even numbers in length, but the saturated fatty acids in dairy foods are commonly seen with small amounts of odd-chain saturated fatty acids.[2,3]

The major saturated fatty acids found in many foods vary and include palmitic acid, which is called the *de novo* fatty acid. The classification of food fats for labeling is saturated, monounsaturated, trans, and polyunsaturated.[2,3]

ESSENTIAL AND NONESSENTIAL FATTY ACIDS

As noted earlier, linoleic acid is the first omega-6 essential fatty acid in the family. In the metabolic lineup, linoleic acid becomes arachidonic acid, and arachidonic acid in turn is important for many functions including certain proinflammatory as well as anti-inflammatory uses. Sometimes linoleic acid is needed by the body for making special prostaglandins that fight certain inflammatory processes. These are from a certain omega-6 fatty acid in the metabolic lineup which starts out as γ-linolenic acid and progresses to a prostaglandin called PGE1. When the metabolic lineup fails to form the γ-linolenic acid or the dihomo-gamma linolenic acid, we need to get this fatty acid as a conditionally essential fatty acid from diet.[2,3]

Omega-6 and omega-3 fatty acids tend to work in opposite directions. The omega-6s tend to be pro-inflammatory, while the omega-3s tend to be anti-inflammatory. Omega-3 fatty acids are essential for building structures and for other functions.[2,3] The first omega-3 essential fatty acid is α-linolenic acid. This fatty acid belongs to the omega-3 family of polyunsaturated fatty acids and is present in soy oil, some nuts, meats, and fish as it is in elongated forms. This fatty acid is not easily converted into DHA or EPA, so it is best to get some "preformed" from cold-water fish.

HISTORY OF FOOD FATS AND OILS IN THE U.S. DIET

There was a time when a cookbook or a treatise on cookery discussed the use of different fats based on the qualities those fats bestowed to the foods of which they were a part. The special flavor imparted to a sauce by olive oil, the superior flavor and texture imparted to a crust or pudding by beef tallow (suet) or lard, the subtle flavor of Chinese foods fried in peanut oil, and the distinctive flavoring of coconut oil in Polynesian cooking were all important to the cook. That emphasis is almost completely gone today. No longer is the cook encouraged to salvage the fat that cooks out of the meat by turning it into gravy to top the potatoes or the rice or the homemade biscuit (and chances are the biscuit is no longer homemade).[2] Table 44.2 exhibits a recommended list of fats and oils, which are most appropriate for domestic/household and commercial use.

Any discussion about fats today, in cookbooks or in magazines devoted to food and cookery, is likely to be negative about fat and additionally to reflect the "anti" saturated fat propaganda, which started about 60 years ago in the United States and spread to most of the world where the United States has influenced the food, nutrition, and biomedical communities. As a result, nearly every article about fats and oils in the diet begins with a faulty premise. That faulty premise is that cholesterol and the saturated fats are the culprits for the myriad of chronic ailments that afflict modern populations. This premise was basically invented in the late 1950s for the purpose of protecting the margarine and shortening industry from the challenges that were newly emerging from some of the scientific critics of hydrogenation who saw this as the cause of the epidemic of heart attacks. This chain of events has been reviewed by Hastert[5] in a 1983 article on hydrogenation.

TABLE 44.2

Recommended List of Fats and Oils, Which Are Most Appropriate for Domestic/Household and Commercial Use

Domestic/household use

For frying: Animal tallows; coconut oil; stable mixtures (blends) of oils such as coconut oil, olive oil,* and sesame oil (1/3 each) (*or sunflower seed oil, or peanut oil instead of olive oil; coconut oil is necessary in the mix for lauric acid, sesame oil is necessary in mix for sesamin)

For baking: Any natural fat or oil that the recipe calls for with the caveat that the recipe should be from a good natural foods cookbook

For salad dressings: Any natural, non-GMO, cold pressed, unrefined liquid oil, e.g., olive oil, mixtures of flaxseed and olive oils, canola oil, or soybean oil

For spreads: Butter and coconut butter

Commercial use

For frying: Coconut oil (if the food is low moisture), palm oil, sunflower oil with added sesame oil, tallow

For bakery goods: Butter, coconut oil, lard, palm oil, tallow

For salad dressings: Any natural, non-GMO, cold pressed, unrefined liquid oil

For spreads: Butter and coconut butter

CHANGES IN THE FOOD FATS USED IN THE UNITED STATES DURING THE PAST CENTURY

The resulting misinformation that was generated has virtually removed the safe and important natural fats from the diets of many people and has replaced these desirable fats with various partially hydrogenated fats and oils or with a myriad of nonfood stabilizers, extenders, and emulsifiers in the low-fat and no-fat versions of traditional foods. Hopefully, with the decrease in the use of partially hydrogenated vegetable oils due to the tFA labeling requirements and emerging studies showing that SCFA and other saturates are not really dangerous, this misinformation may begin to be corrected.[11]

Fats and oils in the U.S. food supply come from several sources. They are either added fats, such as table spreads, shortenings, and salad and cooking oils, or they come from the fat component of the meat and dairy products, from nuts and seeds, or from vegetables and fruit tissues. Added fats in the form of oils, shortenings, spreads (butter and margarine), salad dressing, etc., are listed in government documents such as those published by USDA and/or the Commerce Department as "table and cooking fats."[2] In the late 1800s, commercial shortenings advertised to the housewife were fats such as cottolene (a blend of cottonseed oil and beef tallow), refined leaf lard, or coconut butter (oil). These commercially available fats, as well as fat rendered from beef, poultry, chicken, and pork in the home, were used for frying and as shortening in baking. Butter and cream were valued for table use as well as for cooking and baking. In addition to cottonseed oil and coconut oil, olive oil and poppy seed oil were listed as principal vegetable oils. Table 44.3 shows the major changes in the use of fats and oils in the U.S. food supply chain during the last 120 years.[2,3]

EFFECTS OF THE FOOD SOURCE ON MEDIUM-CHAIN FATTY ACID CONTENT

These profound changes have had a particularly devastating effect on the coconut oil industry, which is the major source of MCFAs in the diet. Coconut oil is one of the most saturated of the natural fats, one of the oldest in use, and one of the most desirable of the natural fats to have in the diets of people. It is considered a lauric fat.[12]

TABLE 44.3

Fats and Oils in the U.S. Food Supply: 1890 versus 2010

1890	2010
Lard/tallow (suet)	Soybean oil (often partially hydrogenated)
Chicken fat	Tallow/grease
Butter fat	Rapeseed oil, e.g., canola oil (often partially hydrogenated)
Olive oil	Palm oil, corn oil
Palm oil	Coconut oil, butter fat
Coconut oil	Lard
Peanut oil	Palm kernel oil, sunflower oil, olive oil, cottonseed oil
Cottonseed oil	Peanut oil

Source: Oil World Statistic Update, No.7, Vol. 54, February 18, 2011.
Listed in descending order of market share.

Thus, we have ended up with a situation where the fats that have been used for centuries are out of our diets, and the fabricated fats that should be out are in our diets. The emphasis is on low fat, but much of the food that is being marketed today is not low fat. Often, this fat is a partially hydrogenated fat that has such a high melting point it is not always noticed by the consumer when the food containing it is eaten. Prepared foods that are actually low in fat are usually high carbohydrate foods. Our bodies make fat from excess carbohydrates that we consume. The fatty acids that result are long-chain saturates.

COMMERCIAL SOURCES OF LAURIC ACID

Coconut (*Cocos nucifera L.*) is one of the most important palms providing food, and it differs from other palms such as oil palms and date palms, with which it should not be confused. Coconut palms grow throughout the world in the wet or humid tropics and have been given the name "the tree of life."[13,14] They spread on the waters from island to island and from coast to coast of the tropical areas of the continents. The trees are grown individually along the coast as well as in groves where they are tended by the owners of the land. Coconut products are shipped to parts of the world where the coconut does not grow and are considered an important food import.[13-16]

The oil palms (*Elaeis guineensis*) originated in the rain forests of Africa and now grow largely in plantations around the world. The fruits of the oil palm provide a stable oil, which differs from the lauric oil of the coconut. However, the seed of the oil palm is a kernel which provides an oil called palm kernel oil. This is a lauric oil similar to coconut oil.[8-15]

There are also palms such as babassu; these grow in the wild in Brazil and have a fruit that provides oil that has a composition similar to coconut. While we are not likely to find babassu oil on the market in North America, there is trade with Brazil, and it is always possible that bakery goods such as crackers could enter the market. It is useful to know that products made with babassu oil would be a source of medium-chain saturates.[13-15]

Date palms should not be mixed up with the oil palms or coconut. They are a useful carbohydrate food that grows in dry areas but does not provide any fat or oil in its fruit and thus is not a source of medium-chain fats.[14,15]

COCONUT STATISTICS

Coconut is grown on approximately 12 million hectares spread over at least 86 countries around the world (Statistics from Asian Pacific Coconut Community as reported by World Bank writer and researcher GJ Persley).[8] There are approximately 86 countries where coconut is an important crop, and Table 44.4 provides a list of largest producers of coconut.

TABLE 44.4

Largest Producers of Coconut

Asia	Africa
Philippines	Benin
Indonesia	Cape Verde
India	Comoros Islands
Sri Lanka	Cote d'Ivoire
Malaysia	Ghana
Thailand	Mozambique
Vietnam	Tanzania
	Kenya
	Somalia
	Oman

The Americas	The Pacific Islands
Mexico	Papua New Guinea
Brazil	Solomon Islands
Jamaica	Vanuatu
Caribbean Islands	Federated States of Micronesia
Dominican Republic	
El Salvador	

Most of the larger countries produce a commercial grade of coconut oil and other coconut products from copra. However, many of the coconut growers are actually raising organic coconut; these growers are small holders and, with some encouragement, have converted their production to organic oils. This is especially true for the small island countries. The coconut oil, coconut milk and cream, and dried coconut products from many of the small countries continue to be available in American and Canadian markets and are of good quality.[13–16]

IMPORTANCE OF LAURIC OIL COMPOSITION (COCONUT OIL, PALM KERNEL OIL)

Most of the people in the United States have been given some unfortunate propaganda regarding the properties of lauric oils and their health effects.[9]

Coconut oil contains 27.5% long-chain saturated fatty acids, 65% medium-chain saturated fatty acids, and the balance unsaturated fatty acids. Of the medium-chain saturated fatty acids, approximately 55% are lauric acid and capric acid, which are antimicrobial fatty acids, especially the 48%–50% which is lauric acid. Lauric acid is a saturated fatty acid that is in mother's milk, and it protects babies from viral and bacterial infections.[9] (Soy, corn, canola, cottonseed, and olive oils contain approximately 20%–32% long-chain saturated fatty acids but virtually no lauric acid [0%–0.3%].)[9,17]

Heart disease is currently considered to be multifactorial and is caused by substances such as oxidized fats, cytomegalovirus virus, *Helicobacter pylori*, homocysteine, and various toxic chemicals, as well as other inflammatory compounds. Increased cholesterol levels in the blood and in atheromas are related to the body's attempt to heal the lesions induced by the substances mentioned earlier. As one of the pathologists who is an expert on atherosclerosis pointed out, the cholesterol does not cause an atheroma any more than the white blood cells cause an abscess; they are both trying to heal. Cholesterol is one of the body's major repair substances.[2,3,9]

Lauric oils (of which coconut is the most widely grown) do not become oxidized (only polyunsaturated fatty acids can become oxidized).[2–4,9] The monoglyceride of lauric acid (which the body makes when lauric oils are eaten) kills cytomegalovirus and *Helicobacter pylori* and thus would be an appropriate treatment and/or preventative substance in heart disease. Also, a number of studies showed that heart disease patients who were fed coconut oil got better, so it is clear that there is no reason to repeat misinformation. Even Harvard medical school researchers have taken out a patent to use lauric oils to treat disease.[2,3,9]

MEDIUM-CHAIN FATS IDENTIFIED AS FUNCTIONAL FOODS

Functional foods were defined at an ILSI North America Special Conference in 1999.[6] Functional foods provide a health benefit over and beyond the basic nutrients they contain. This is exactly what desiccated coconut and coconut oil do. As a functional food, coconut has fatty acids and proteins which provide both energy and nutrients as well as raw material (oil) for antimicrobial monoglycerides (the functional component) when it is eaten. Desiccated coconut is about 65+% coconut fat that contains both lauric (~50%) and capric acids (~8%). Palm kernels are not large enough to provide a usable desiccated component,[5–16] but the oil is rich in lauric acid (~40%) and capric acid (~16%).[22]

Approximately 50% of the fatty acids in coconut fat are lauric acid. Lauric acid is the 12-carbon MCFA, which has additional beneficial functions when it is formed into monolaurin in the human or animal body.[9–20] Monolaurin is the antiviral, antibacterial, and antiprotozoal monoglyceride used by the human or animal to destroy lipid-coated viruses such as HIV, herpes, cytomegalovirus, influenza, various pathogenic bacteria including *Listeria monocytogenes* and *Helicobacter pylori*, and protozoa such as *Giardia lamblia*.[21] Some studies have also shown some antimicrobial effects of the free lauric acid.[21]

Additionally, approximately 6%–8% of the fatty acids in coconut fat are capric acid.[17] Capric acid is another MCFA which has 10 carbons and similar beneficial function when it is formed into monocaprin in the human or animal body.[2,3,9] Monocaprin has also been shown to have antiviral effects against HIV and is being tested for antiviral effects against herpes simplex and antibacterial effects against chlamydia (Reuters, London June 29, 1999).

Dr. Halldor Thormar, the Icelandic scientist, who previously showed that monolaurin, which comes from the fat in coconut, kills lipid-coated DNA and RNA viruses including HIV and herpes viruses as well as other microorganisms including gram-positive bacteria, has identified the potential effectiveness of monocaprin dissolved in a gel in killing HIV. Monocaprin also comes from the fat in coconut.[6,21] Thormar et al. plan to continue the tests with monocaprin against chlamydia and herpes simplex virus.[6,21]

There is a variety of supportive research published in 2003, 2004, and 2005, and it shows the importance of coconut oil.[15,16] Also, information on coconut oil is currently coming into the research literature from numerous countries, for example, India, Norway, Iran, and the United States.[8–15]

A few researchers have known for some time that lipids derived from coconut oil, lauric acid, and monolaurin are safe antimicrobial agents that can either kill completely or stop the growth of some of the most dangerous viruses and bacteria.[9,21] Many bacteria have become resistant to antibiotics but herbal oils such as the oils of oregano and the major fatty acid from coconut oil and lauric acid, which the body turns into the monoglyceride monolaurin, are capable of killing them or inhibiting their growth.[9,21] Monolaurin is being shown to be useful in the prevention and treatment of severe bacterial infections, especially those that are difficult to treat or are antibiotic resistant. Difficult bacteria such as *Staphylococcus aureus* as well as other bacteria have been studied here in the United States in research groups such as Dr. H.G. Preuss's group at Georgetown University Medical Center.[21]

It could possibly be effective against the increasingly prevalent MRSA (methicillin-resistant *Staphylococcus aureus*) bacteria.

MEDIUM-CHAIN FATTY ACIDS AND THERMOGENESIS

Animal studies show a diet containing medium-chain triacylglycerols (MCTs) results in diet-induced thermogenesis and leads to less body fat accumulation compared to a diet containing long-chain triacylglycerols (LCT).[19,20]

A study in humans using a comparative protocol measured diet-induced thermogenesis by feeding 5–10 g/day of either MCT or LCT to healthy humans. The results suggested that the intake of MCT caused larger diet-induced thermogenesis than that of LCT regardless of the rest of the meal containing the MCT.[19]

Using a double-blind crossover protocol to test the different effects of MCT versus LCT in overfed males of ages 22–44, it was found that excess dietary energy as MCT stimulates thermogenesis more than LCT. This increased energy expenditure was considered most likely due to lipogenesis in the liver and provided evidence that excess energy derived from MCT is converted to heat and stored with lesser efficiency than equivalent excess energy derived from dietary LCT.[18]

The thermic effects of MCTs were studied in both lean and obese subjects by evaluating postprandial thermogenesis after ingestion of mixed meals. These studies in lean and obese humans have reported that there is a postprandial thermic effect from a mixed meal with 30 g of MCT plus 8 g of LCT that was significantly greater than the thermic effect of 38 g of LCT.[22]

BIOCHEMICAL FUNCTIONS AND WEIGHT LOSS FROM MEDIUM-CHAIN FATS

Regarding the questions about the biochemical function that produces weight loss, the following research reports are based on the biochemistry. Basically, because MCFAs are oxidized to produce energy and are not stored in adipose as are long-chain fatty acids (LCFA), MCFAs raise the body temperature and effectively use more energy.

Researchers have shown that fatty acids that are more likely to be oxidized are less likely to be stored in adipose tissue. Research from George Bray's group at the Pennington Biomedical Research Center reported that the most highly oxidized fatty acid was the MCFA lauric acid.[3] Coconut oil is almost 50% lauric acid. This research was conducted in humans (males) using labeled fatty acids and showed that the cumulative oxidation of lauric acid was 41% over the 9 h test period, whereas the oxidation of the LCFA stearic acid was 13%.[4]

Research on MCFA metabolism was critically reviewed by Professor P.J. Jones of McGill University.[23–28] They report that the intermediary metabolism (e.g., oxidation) of fatty acids differs depending on their chain length and degree of unsaturation. MCFAs show differences in metabolism from LCFAs that is noted from data in both animals and humans, which show increases in postmeal energy expenditure even after short-term feeding of MCFA. They report that "… differences in metabolic handling of MCFA versus LCFA are considered with the conclusion that MCFA hold potential as weight loss agents."[23–28] Likewise, Moussavi et al. conclude in their review that based on animal and human studies, the MCFAs, compared to LCFAs, appear to promote weight loss.[11] Bray et al. argue that "it may be the types of dietary fats or their dietary interactions that may be a major culprit in the current epidemic of obesity and insulin resistance."[3] They also note that the SCFAs as well as the ketone levels they produce may be signals for satiety, which could easily cross into the brain.

In a review[12] from France, researchers demonstrated that when comparing LCT-fed animals with MCT-fed animals, the final body weight was significantly reduced by all the regimens that provided at least 50% of the fat energy as MCT.[12] According to this research group, the threshold of 50% energy needed to be reached to obtain a reproducible body weight-reducing effect, a threshold which they do not feel is practical in human feeding. However, a recent report indicates that the Atkins diet sample meal contains about 64 cal percent fat in a 1915 calorie meal with 23 cal percent protein compared to a Weight Watcher meal of 1865 cal with 18 cal percent fat and 24 cal percent protein (Consumer Reports June 2011).

IMMUNE-ENHANCING PROPERTIES OF MEDIUM-CHAIN FATTY ACIDS

There are several aspects of fats in our diet that affect our immune systems. A major factor is the presence in our food supply of the tFAs.[29] Another is the extent of processed and incomplete foods in our diets. A third is the amount of viral and bacterial load in our environment and systems. Different aspects of the diet affect different parts of the immune system, for example, helper T cells and proinflammatory cytokines, immunoglobulins (e.g., IgE), immunosuppression, etc.[29]

Many of the good effects from coconut oil and its derivatives such as monoglycerides of medium-chain saturated fatty acids are indirect, and some of the scientific pathways, etc., can only be postulated in general and the actions are different in different people.[9,29]

Coconut in the form of desiccated coconut in foods such as macaroons, and coconut oil as it is added to baked goods or snack foods such as popcorn or used in the home for cooking, is a major source of the *lauric acid* used by the body to make the antimicrobial monoglyceride *monolaurin*. Lauric acid also has its own antimicrobial properties. Humans have need for an antiviral, antibacterial, and antiprotozoal component such as monolaurin, which the human body can make if it receives adequate amounts of lauric acid.[9,29]

Numerous viruses that are pathogenic to humans are known to be inactivated or destroyed in the body by monolaurin. They include the HIV virus, measles virus, herpes viruses, cytomegalovirus, vesicular stomatitis virus, visna virus, influenza virus, pneumonovirus, syncytial virus, and rubeola virus.[9,21] Bacteria that are pathogenic to humans and are known to be inactivated or destroyed in the body by monolaurin include *Listeria monocytogenes*; *Helicobacter pylori*; *Staphylococcus aureus*; numerous Streptococci including groups A, B, F and G; gram-positive organisms; and some gram-negative organisms if pretreated with chelator. Protozoa that are pathogenic to humans and are known to be inactivated or destroyed in the body by monolaurin include *Giardia lamblia*.[9,21]

The scientific backup for this is somewhat complex as it has not been looked at or measured in a homogeneous group all of the time. For example, if one person has a low-grade infection from a virus that is not actually active, that person needs to be evaluated individually for the immune response, but the researchers might have that person in a group where the other individuals are harboring different viruses and the effect on the interleukins (the immune factors) might be the same or different. So basically, most of the research is not set up properly to answer specific questions.

One important paper discusses the potential effect of monolaurin and consequently coconut oil in a rather general manner, for example, monolaurin modulates immune cell proliferation. This paper from the University of Minnesota discusses the mechanism that monolaurin is thought to have on the cell membrane where it exerts inhibition of a variety of toxins being produced by the different group A *Streptococci* and *Staphylococci*.[9,29] Monolaurin has been shown to block toxic shock syndrome, making it especially important to women to have an adequate intake of coconut oil in their diets even if they are not in need of weight loss.[9,29]

BENEFICIAL EFFECTS OF COCONUT OIL ON ATHEROSCLEROSIS RISK FACTORS

Published studies concerning coconut have dealt with coconut oil as a component of human diet where the beneficial effects of consuming virgin coconut oil were shown in laboratory animals (Sprague-Dawley rats).[13–16] In this study, virgin coconut oil, which was obtained by wet process, was beneficial in lowering total cholesterol, triglycerides, phospholipids, and LDL. In serum and tissues, very-low-density lipoprotein (VLDL) cholesterol levels were lowered and HDL cholesterol was increased. The polyphenol fraction of virgin coconut oil was also found to prevent *in vitro* LDL oxidation. The results in this study were interpreted as due to the biologically active polyphenol components present in the oil.[16]

Another study dealt with lipoproteins/cholesterol, etc., and this one done in women showed that coconut oil-based diets lowered postprandial tissue plasminogen activator and lipoprotein[a].[15] The researchers concluded that the serum lipoprotein[a], a heart disease marker said to be important and always thought to be unaffected by various forms of dietary fat intake, was shown to be lowered when the subjects consumed a high saturated fat diet and somewhat lowered when they consumed a slightly lowered saturated fat diet. Both of these diets were based on coconut oil. The third diet was based on a monounsaturated oil.[15]

CONCLUSION

Overall, these studies substantiate that MCTs have significant health benefits and may serve as novel, natural therapeutics in weight management.

REFERENCES

1. Enig, M.G., *Fat, Calories and Tropical Oils in Perspective. Food Product Design*, Weeks Publishing Co., Northbrook, IL, pp.16–17, May 1991.
2. Enig, M.G., *Know Your Fats: The Complete Primer for Understanding the Nutrition of Fats, Oils, and Cholesterol.*, Bethesda Press, Silver Spring, MD, 2000.
3. DeLany, J.P., Windhauser, M.M., Champagne, C.M., and Bray, G.A., Differential oxidation of individual dietary fatty acids in humans. *Am. J. Clin. Nutr.*, 72:905–911, 2000.
4. Hastert, R.C., In: E. Perkins and W. Visek, Eds., *Dietary Fats and Health*, AOCS Press, Champaign, IL, 1983, Chapter 4.
5. Bach, A.C., Ingenbleek, Y., and Frey, A., The usefulness of dietary medium-chain triglycerides in body weight control: Fact or fancy? J. *Lipid Res.*, 37(4), 708–726, 1996.
6. Kaunitz, H. and Dayrit, C.S., Coconut oil consumption and coronary heart disease. *Philippine J. Intern. Med.*, 30, 165–171, 1992.
7. Lim-Sylianco, C.Y., Anticarcinogenic effect of coconut oil. *The Philippine J. Coconut Stud.*, 12, 89–102, 1987.
8. Muller, H., Lindman, A.S., Blomfeldt, A., Seljeflot, I., and Pedersen, J.I., A diet rich in coconut oil reduces diurnal postprandial variations in circulating plasminogen activator antigen and fasting lipoprotein (a) compared with a diet rich in unsaturated fat in women. *J. Nutr.*, 133(11), 3422–3427, 2003.
9. Nevin, K.G. and Rajamohan, T., Beneficial effects of virgin coconut oil on lipid parameters and *in vitro* LDL oxidation. *Clin. Biochem.*, 37(9), 830–835, 2004.
10. Persley, G.J., *Replanting the Tree of Life: Toward an International Agenda for Coconut Palm Research*, C.A.B. International, Oxon, U.K., 1992.
11. Enig, M.G., Lauric oils as antimicrobial agents: Theory of effect, scientific rationale, and dietary application as adjunct nutritional support for HIV-infected individuals. In *Nutrients and Foods in AIDS* (R.R. Watson, Ed.). CRC Press, Boca Raton, FL, 1998, p. 81, Chapter 5.
12. *Functional Foods for Health Promotion: Physiologic Considerations; Experimental Biology '99*, Renaissance Washington Hotel, Washington, DC, Saturday, April 17, 1999; Sponsored by International Life Sciences Institute, ILSI NORTH AMERICA, Technical Committee on Food Components for Health Promotion.
13. Hill, J.O., Peters, J.C., Yang, D., Sharp, T., Kaler, M., Abumrad, N.N., and Greene, H.L., Thermogenesis in humans during overfeeding with medium-chain triglycerides. *Metabolism*, 38(7), 641–648, 1989.
14. Kasai, M., Nosaka, N., Maki, H., Suzuki, Y., Takeuchi, H., Aoyama, T., Ohara, A., Harada, Y., Okazaki, M., and Kondo, K., Comparison of diet-induced thermogenesis of foods containing medium-versus long-chain triacylglycerols. *J. Nutr. Sci. Vitaminol. (Tokyo)*, 48, 5364, 2002.
15. Noguchi, O., Takeuchi, H., Kubota, F.D., Tsuji, H., and Aoyama, T. Larger diet-induced thermogenesis and less body fat accumulation in rats fed medium-chain triacylglycerols than in those fed long-chain triacylglycerols. *J. Nutr. Sci. Vitaminol. (Tokyo)*, 48(6), 524–529, 2002.
16. Preuss, H.G., Echard, B., Enig, M., Brook, I., and Elliott, T.B., Minimum inhibitory concentrations of herbal essential oils and monolaurin for gram-positive and gram-negative bacteria. *Mol. Cell. Biochem.*, 272(1–2), 29–34, 2005.
17. Scalfi, L., Coltorti, A., and Contaldo, F., Postprandial thermogenesis in lean and obese subjects after meals supplemented with medium-chain and long-chain triglycerides. *Am. J. Clin. Nutr.*, 53(5), 1130–1133, 1991.
18. Bourque, C., St-Onge, M.P., Papamandjaris, A.A., Cohn, J.S., and Jones, P.J., Consumption of an oil composed of medium chain triacylglycerols, phytosterols, and N-3 fatty acids improved cardiovascular risk profile in overweight women. *Metabolism*, 52(6), 771–777, 2003.

19. Papamandjaris, A.A., White, M.D., Raeini-Sarjaz, M., and Jones, P.J., Endogenous fat oxidation during medium chain versus long chain triglyceride feeding in healthy women. *Int. J. Obes. Relat. Metab. Disord.*, 24(9), 1158–1166, 2000.
20. Papamandjaris, A.A., MacDougall, D.F., and Jones, P.J., Medium chain fatty acid metabolism and energy expenditure: Obesity treatment implications. *Life Sci.*, 62(14), 1203–1215, 1998.
21. St-Onge, M.P. and Jones, P.J., Greater rise in fat oxidation with medium-chain triglyceride consumption relative to long-chain triglyceride is associated with lower initial body weight and greater loss of subcutaneous adipose tissue. *Int. J. Obes. Relat. Metab. Disord.*, 27(12), 1565–1571, 2003.
22. St-Onge, M.P., Ross, R., Parsons, W.D., and Jones, P.J., Medium-chain triglycerides increase energy expenditure and decrease adiposity in overweight men. *Obes. Res.*, 11(3), 395–402, 2003.
23. St-Onge, M.P. and Jones, P.J.H, Physiological effects of medium-chain triglycerides: Potential agents in the prevention of obesity. *J. Nutr.*, 132, 329, 2002.
24. Witcher, K.J., Novick, R.P., and Schlievert, P.M., Modulation of immune cell proliferation by glycerol monolaurate. *Clin. Diagn. Lab. Immunol.*, 3, 10–13, 1996.
25. Firestone, D., *Physical and Chemical Characteristics of Oils, Fats, and Waxes*, AOCS Press, Champaign, IL, 1999.
26. Huang, Y.S., Yanagita, T., and Knapp, H.R., Eds., *Dietary Fats and Risk of Chronic Disease*, AOCS Press, Champaign, IL, 2006.
27. National Research Council, *DIET and HEALTH, Implications for Reducing Chronic Disease Risk*, National Academy of Sciences, Washington, DC, 1989.
28. Thelen, K.M., Falkai, P., Bayer, T.A., and Lütjohann, D. Cholesterol synthesis rate in human hippocampus declines with aging. *Neurosci. Lett.*, 403, 15–19, 2006.
29. Maussavi, N., Gavino, V., and Receveur, O., Could the quality of dietary fat, and not just its quantity, be related to risk of obesity? *Obesity*, 16, 7–15, 2008.

45 Antiobesity by Marine Lipids

Kazuo Miyashita, PhD and Masashi Hosokawa, PhD

CONTENTS

INTRODUCTION

The rise in the prevalence of obesity has been recognized as a worldwide problem, with ominous implications for public health and health-related costs. It may be a second-most important preventable cause of death, exceeded only by cigarette smoking. The rapid adaptation to the current lifestyle, the reduction in physical exercise, and the increased consumption of tasty, affordable food that has a high energy density are among the causes of the increase in obesity in most industrialized countries, as well as in developing countries that adopt a similar lifestyle.

Humans are generally accepted to have a particular genotype, which is the result of evolution and stores energy in lipid form. Ingestion of either protein or carbohydrate is accompanied by a rapid increase in the oxidation of each. By contrast, consumption of dietary fat does not promote its own oxidation. The fat stored in adipose tissue provides an energy reserve. In evolution, the human body has been compelled to develop regulatory mechanisms that gave higher priority to the control of its carbohydrate economy than to the control of fat metabolism. This genotype has remained unchanged for thousands of years, and the increase in the prevalence of obesity is considered to be the result of the interaction between this genotype and the current lifestyle.

Adipocytes have an important role in energy homeostasis. Adipose tissue stores energy in the form of lipid and releases fatty acids in response to nutritional signals or energy insufficiency.[1] Further, adipocytes have endocrine functions by secreting hormones and factors that regulate physiological functions, such as immune response, insulin sensitivity, and food intake.[2,3] On the other hand, excessive fat accumulation in the body, particularly in abdominal white adipose tissue (WAT), leads to the dysregulation of adipocytokine production in WAT, which is closely involved in the development of metabolic syndrome.[4–6] Metabolic syndrome is a cluster of type-2 diabetes, hypertension, and dyslipidemia. The syndrome markedly increases the risk of cardiovascular disease.[7–12]

Although obesity is a multifunctional condition affected by the combined effects of genes, environment, and their interactions, it may be true that there are only two ways to treat obesity: reduction of energy intake or increase in energy expenditure. However, the simplicity of the energy balance equation has led to an inappropriate focus on obesity. Rapid reduction of total energy intake in a short time has relatively minor impact on energy expenditure and sometimes gives adverse effects. Hard exercise may induce an oxidative damage to biological systems by formation of active oxygen and free radicals.

Several studies that have examined the type of dietary fat have found a negative and positive association with the intake of several kinds of dietary fats and the prevalence of obesity.[13,14] Furthermore, data accumulated from experimental animal and human studies clearly support a beneficial role for several dietary lipids and lipid-related minor compounds in obesity management. Based on nature of fat digestion and absorption, diacylglycerol (DG) with a 1,3-configuration[15,16] and medium-chain triacylglycerol (MCT)[17] have been used for the prevention of obesity. Several studies have demonstrated that conjugated linoleic acids (CLA) reduce body fat accumulation in growing animals, but not all CLA isomers contributed to this effect equally.[18–20] Among CLA isomers, 10*trans*, 12*cis*-CLA induced body fat loss.

Interest in functionality of marine lipids relating to obesity control also continues to grow year by year due to the fact that marine products become familiar to people and prevention of disease through marine dietary means has been better understood by the public at large. Among marine nutraceutical lipids, most extensive research has been documented on eicosapentaenoic acid (EPA; 20:5n-3) and docosahexaenoic acid (DHA; 22:6n-3), two representative omega-3 polyunsaturated fatty acids (PUFAs) from marine origin.[21–23] Another interesting compound from marine origin is brown seaweed carotenoid, fucoxanthin. Antiobesity activity of fucoxanthin has been paid much attention as its effect is based on the specific molecular mechanism. This chapter is concerned with the antiobesity effect of marine nutraceuticals, especially focusing on the effect of fucoxanthin.

EFFECT OF OMEGA-3 PUFA ON LIPID METABOLISM

EPA and DHA are the two typical fatty acids of marine lipids. These two long-chain PUFAs have been shown to cause significant biochemical and physiological changes in the body. Most of these changes exert positive influence on human nutrition and health.[21–23] DHA is an important constituent of the membrane phospholipids of brain and retina, usually occupying the sn-2 position of these phospholipid moiety. Health effects of EPA and DHA are protection of hypertension, cancer, diabetes, neuropsychiatric disorders, and autoimmune diseases. Among the physiological effects of EPA and DHA, the most attention has been paid to their cardioprotective activity.

Substantial epidemiological and case-control study data demonstrate that the risk of coronary heart disease (CHD) is lowest among those with the highest long-chain omega-3 PUFA, such as EPA and DHA, intake.[24,25] The important cardioprotective effect of omega-3 PUFA has been also demonstrated by clinical implications[26] and by genetic and nutrigenetic approach.[27] Thus, American and European heart associations recommend the intake of 1 g/day of EPA and DHA for prevention of sudden cardiac death and other cardiovascular dysfunctions.[28,29] It is apparent that EPA and DHA consumption is of benefits to reduce the risk of CHD. The cardioprotection has been extensively reviewed elsewhere and is thought to occur through various mechanisms, including the reduction of serum triacylglycerol (TG) levels, antiarrhythmic effects, decreasing platelet aggregation, plaque stabilization, and/or reduction of blood pressure.[25–27,30–32]

High TG levels have been shown to be an independent risk factor for cardiovascular diseases in a meta-analysis of 17 large, population-based studies ($N > 56,000$).[33] EPA and DHA can alter the serum lipid profile. The most consistent action is a reduction in TG levels. EPA and DHA also increase high-density lipoprotein cholesterol levels in many studies. However, DHA and EPA supplementation does not affect total cholesterol (TC) levels, and it also reduces the proportion of small dense LDL particles,[34,35] which are potentially more atherogenic.[36] The TG-lowering effect of EPA and DHA is not completely understood, but several potential mechanisms are as follows: reduction of hepatic VLDL-TG synthesis and secretion, and enhancement of TG clearance from chylomicrons and VLDL particles.[37,38]

Effect of EPA and DHA on lipid metabolism would be strongly correlated to antiobesity effect of marine lipids. Former studies described reducing effect of fish oil on abdominal fat pad.[39,40]

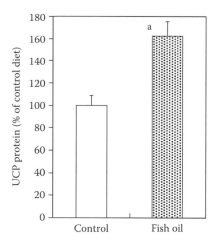

FIGURE 45.1 UCP expression in BAT of control and sardine oil–fed rats. [a]Significantly different from control ($P < 0.05$). The experimental diets contained 10% of either lard (control) or fish oil. Main fatty acids of the fish oil were DHA (27.7%), 16:0 (18.1%), 18:1n-9 (12.0%), and EPA (7.2%). (Adapted from Kawada, T. et al., *J. Agric. Food Chem.*, 46, 1225, 1998.)

Parrish et al. [39] reported that lard-fed rats had 77% more fat in perirenal fat pads and 51% more fat in epididymal fat pads compared with fish oil–fed rats. The same result was obtained by Kawada et al. [41]. They also found that the expression of uncoupling protein (UCP1) in interscapular brown adipose tissue (IBAT) was significantly higher in the fish oil diet–fed rats compared to that in the lard-fed group (Figure 45.1). In IBAT mitochondria, substrate oxidation is poorly coupled to ATP synthesis because of the presence of UCP1, thereby leading to energy dissipation, that is, heat production. Kawada et al. [41] suggested that the intake of PUFA found in fish oil such as EPA and DHA causes UCP induction and enhancement of thermogenesis, resulting in suppression of the excessive growth of abdominal fat pads. PUFA from vegetable oils also suppressed the excessive accumulation of adipose tissue, as compared to animal fats.[42,43] However, the activity of PUFA from vegetable oils was less than EPA and DHA from fish oil.[41] Our study supports these previous results in terms of the higher antiobesity effect of EPA and DHA in fish oils[44] (Figure 45.2).

Recent studies also demonstrated that EPA and DHA improve lipid metabolism and prevent obesity, which partially result from the metabolic action of both PUFAs in adipose and liver tissues.[45–50]

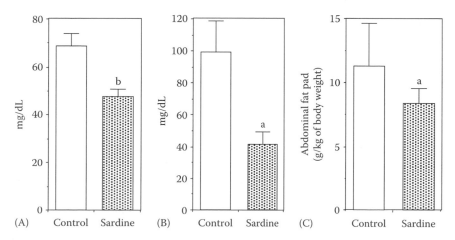

FIGURE 45.2 Plasma lipids and abdominal fat weight of rats fed control (soybean oil) and sardine oil. (A) Plasma TC. (B) Plasma TG. (C) Abdominal fat weight. [a,b]Significantly different from control ([a]$P < 0.05$; [b]$P < 0.01$). (Adapted from Toyoshima, K. et al., *J. Agric. Food Chem.* 52, 2372, 2004.)

EPA and DHA affect fat cells by different mechanisms, including the transcription factors PPARα and PPARγ. Some of the effects of both PUFAs on adipose tissue depend on their active metabolites, especially eicosanoids. Furthermore, EPA and DHA regulate several inflammation molecules including serum amyloid A (SAA), tumor necrosis factor-α (TNF-α), and interleukin-6 (IL-6) in hepatocytes and adipocytes. Actions of both PUFAs are based on the modulation of transcription factors such as PPAR and NF-κB and eicosanoid production, reducing proinflammatory cytokine production from many different cells including the macrophage. EPA and DHA also suppress expressions of perilipin, sterol regulatory element binding protein-1 (SREBP-1), and lipoprotein lipase (LPL) to induce lipolysis and reduce lipogenesis.

ANTIOBESITY THROUGH UCP EXPRESSION

A great deal of interest has been focused on adaptive thermogenesis by UCP families (UCP1, UCP2, and UCP3) as a physiological defense against obesity, hyperlipidemia, and diabetes.[51,52] UCPs are found in BAT (UCP1, UCP2, and UCP3), WAT (UCP2), skeletal muscle (UCP2 and UCP3), and brain (UCP4 and UCP5).[52,53] UCP2 and UCP3 are members of the mitochondrial anion carrier superfamily with high homology to UCP1, a well-characterized UCP playing a key role in facultative thermogenesis in rodents.[54] Interest in UCPs increased with the discovery of proteins similar to UCP1, including UCP2 and UCP3. These proteins are expressed in tissues besides BAT and, thus, are candidates to influence energy efficiency and expenditure.[52,55] Since metabolic rate, metabolic efficiency, and obesity are integrated properties of the whole animal, researchers have produced mice lacking UCP2[56] and UCP3.[57,58] Surprisingly, despite UCP2 or UCP3, no consistent phenotypic abnormality was observed in the knockout mice. They were not obese and had normal thermogenesis. These results suggest that UCP2 and UCP3 are not a major determinant of metabolic rate in normal condition but, rather, have other functions.[52,56,59–64] Indeed, unexpected physiological or pathological implications of the UCP2 and UCP3 function (such as possible UCP2 involvement in diabetes and in apoptosis) could also be implicated.[52] UCP3 has a diminished thermogenic response to the drug 3,4-methylene dioxy methamphetamine or MDMA.[64] Apart from UCP2 and UCP3, it is certain that UCP1 can potentially reduce excess abdominal fat.[65]

Involvement of BAT in cold-induced thermogenesis is well established, and data from rodents have also demonstrated its role in diet-induced thermogenesis.[66,67] Thermogenesis in BAT is due to UCP1. UCP1 is a dimeric protein present in the inner mitochondrial membrane of BAT, and it dissipates the pH gradient generated by oxidative phosphorylation, releasing chemical energy as heat. UCP1 is exclusively expressed in BAT, where the gene expression is increased by cold, adrenergic stimulation, β3-agonists, retinoids, and thyroid hormone.[68] Thermogenic activity of BAT is dependent on UCP1 expression level controlled by the sympathetic nervous system via noradrenaline[65,69–71] (Figure 45.3). As a consequence of noradrenaline binding to the adipocyte plasma membrane, protein kinase (PKA) is expressed, and then, cyclic AMP response element binding protein (CREB) and hormone-sensitive lipase (HSL) are expressed. HSL stimulates lipolysis, and free fatty acids liberated serve as substrate in BAT thermognesis.[71] They also act as cytosolic second messengers which activated UCP1 as PPARγ ligand. The same activity is expected in dietary PUFAs.[72] Antiobesity effect of dietary EPA and DHA may be partly due to their control of PPARγ expression.[41] DHA and EPA inhibit cyclooxygenase, thereby reducing the amount of prostaglandins and increasing the lipoxygenase activity. This in turn results in higher production of hydroxyeicosatetraenoic acids (HETE) and leukotriene B4. Eicosanoids can act as transcriptional regulators of UCP. The antiobesity effect of fish oil may, in part, be correlated to the regulatory effect of both PUFA on eicosanoid formation. Although sympathetic nervous system via noradrenaline is physiologically the most significant, a series of other factors may also influence UCP1 gene expression.[73] Thyroid hormones are essential for regulated UCP1 expression.[68] Also, activators of PPARγ such as pioglitazone[74] and probably essential fatty acids[75] activate UCP1 gene expression, as do retinoids probably through both RXR and RAR receptors.[76,77]

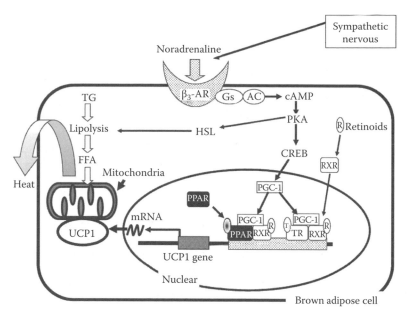

FIGURE 45.3 Possible mechanism for upregulation of BAT UCP1 by food components.

ANTIOBESITY ACTIVITY OF EDIBLE SEAWEED CAROTENOID, FUCOXANTHIN

UCP1 is a key molecule for antiobesity. UCP1 expression is known as a significant component of whole body energy expenditure, and its dysfunction contributes to the development of obesity. However, adult humans have very little BAT and most of fat is stored in WAT. Considered as break-through discoveries for an ideal therapy of obesity, regulation of UCP expression in tissues other than BAT by food constituent would be important. UCP1, usually expressed only in BAT, has also been found in WAT of mice overexpressing Foxc2, a winged helix gene, with a change in steady-state levels of several WAT- and BAT-derived mRNAs.[78] This result suggests the possibility of UCP1 expression in WAT, which would be an increasingly attractive target for the development of antiobesity therapies. As the key molecular components become defined, screening for food con-stituent that increases energy dissipation is becoming a more attainable goal. From this viewpoint, the antiobesity effect of edible seaweed carotenoid, fucoxanthin, is very interesting, as its activity depends on the protein and gene expressions of UCP1 in WAT.[79]

In the study on antiobesity effect of seaweed carotenoid, fucoxanthin, lipids were separated from edible seaweed Wakame (*Undaria pinnatifida*), one of the most popular edible seaweed in Japan and Korea. Undaria lipids, containing 10% fucoxanthin, reduced significantly the weight of WAT (comprising perirenal and epididymal abdominal adipose tissues) of both rats and mice (Figure 45.4). Furthermore, body weight of mice fed 2% Undaria lipid was significantly ($P < 0.05$) lower than that of control, although there was no significant difference in the mean daily intake of diet between both groups. In order to confirm the active component of Undaria lipids, fucoxanthin, and Undaria glyco-lipids, main fraction of the lipids were administered to obese KK-Ay mice. Dietary effects of both fractions on WAT weight of obese mice are shown in Figure 45.5. The WAT weight of fucoxanthin-fed mice was significantly lower than that of control mice. However, there was no difference in WAT weight of mice fed Undaria glycolipids and control diet. This result indicates that fucoxanthin is the active component in the Undaria lipids resulting in the antiobesity effect.

Because of its capacity for uncoupled mitochondrial respiration, BAT has been implicated as an important site of facultative energy expenditure in small rodents. This has led to speculation that BAT normally functions to prevent obesity. In 2.0% Undaria lipids–fed mice, BAT weight was significantly greater than that in control mice. However, there was no significant difference in UCP1 expression

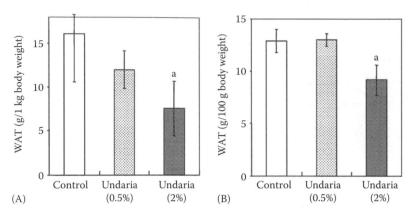

FIGURE 45.4 Weight of WAT of rats (A) and mice (B) fed Undaria lipids and control diet. [a]Significantly different from control ($P < 0.01$). A diet was prepared according to the recommendation of American Institute of Nutrition (AIN-93G). The dietary fats for rats were 7% soybean oil (control), 6.5% soybean oil + 0.5% Undaria lipids, and 5% soybean oil + 2% Undaria lipids. Those for mice were 13% soybean oil (control), 12.5% soybean oil + 0.5% Undaria lipids, and 11% soybean oil + 2% Undaria lipids. (Adapted from Maeda, H. et al., *Biochim. Biophys. Res. Commun.*, 332, 392, 2005.)

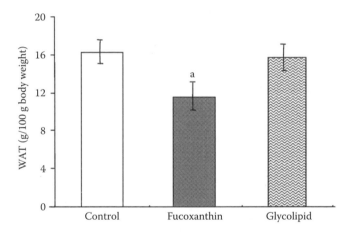

FIGURE 45.5 Weight of WAT of mice fed fucoxanthin, Undaria glycolipids, and control diet. [a]Significantly different from control ($P < 0.01$). The dietary fats were 13% soybean oil (control), 12.6% soybean oil + 0.4% fucoxanthin, and 11.2% soybean oil + 1.8% Undaria glycolipid. (Adapted from Maeda, H. et al., *Biochim. Biophys. Res. Commun.*, 332, 392, 2005.)

among three different dietary groups. Thus, the decrease in abdominal fat pad weight found in Undaria lipids–fed mice could not be explained only by energy expenditure in BAT mitochondria by UCP1. As shown in Figure 45.6, UCP1 expression was found in WAT of Undaria lipids–fed mice, although there was little expression in that of control mice. Expression of UCP1 mRNA was also found in WAT of Undaria lipids–fed mice, but little expression in that of control (Figure 45.6). On the other hand, UCP2 expression in WAT decreased by feeding Undaria lipids as compared with control (Figure 45.6). These results show that the decrease in WAT weight of Undaria lipids–fed mice is partly due to the thermogenesis through UCP1 expression in WAT but also through UCP2 expression. UCP1 expression in WAT was also found in fucoxanthin-fed mice, but little expression of UCP1 was found in WAT of mice fed Undaria glycolipids and control diets (Figure 45.7). This result confirmed the antiobesity activity of seaweed carotenoid, fucoxanthin, through upregulation of UCP1 expression in WAT.

The antiobesity effect of fucoxanthin was confirmed by other *in vivo* studies.[80,81] By feeding with 0.2% fucoxanthin to the obese-diabetes model mice, KK-Ay mice, body weight gain was significantly

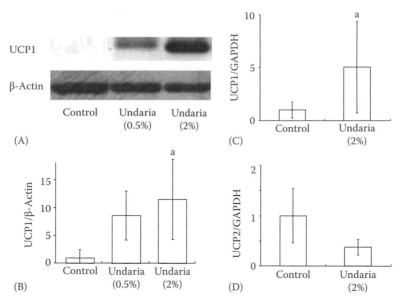

FIGURE 45.6   UCP1 and UCP2 expressions in WAT of mice fed Undaria lipids and control diet. (A) Western blot analysis of UCP1. (B) UCP1 protein expression. (C) UCP1 mRNA expression. (D) UCP2 mRNA expression. [a]Significantly different from control ($P < 0.05$). (Adapted from Maeda, H. et al., *Biochim. Biophys. Res. Commun.*, 332, 392, 2005.)

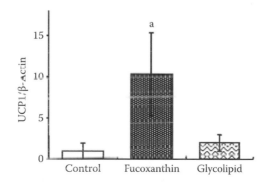

FIGURE 45.7   UCP1 expression in WAT of mice fed fucoxanthin and Undaria glycolipids. [a]Significantly different from control ($P < 0.05$). (Adapted from Maeda, H. et al., *Biochim. Biophys. Res. Commun.*, 332, 392, 2005.)

reduced compared with that of the control, although there was no difference in the amount of food intake. This reduction was consistent with the decrease in the weight of uterine, mesentery, perirenal, and retroperitoneal WAT normalized for body weight in the mice fed 0.2% fucoxanthin, and was significantly lower than in the control group. Further, BAT weight normalized body weight, which is related to energy expenditure, increased in the mice fed 0.1%, 0.2% fucoxanthin compared with the control group.

The antiobesity effect of fucoxanthin was also found in high fat (HF) diet–induced obesity in mice.[82] Fucoxanthin intake significantly suppressed body weight and WAT weight gain induced by the HF diet. Dietary administration of the HF diet resulted in hyperglycemia, hyperinsulinemia, and hyperleptinemia in the mouse model. These perturbations were completely normalized in the fucoxanthin-fed group. In addition, plasma leptin content was significantly lower in fucoxanthin feeding group compared to the control group. Leptin suppresses appetite and controls body weight.[83] However, obese individuals have leptin resistance due to high leptin levels in the blood. Hence, plasma leptin levels can be used as an index of body fat accumulation. Low leptin levels detected in the groups fed a fucoxanthin confirmed the antiobesity effect of fucoxanthin with HF diet–induced obese conditions.

REGULATORY EFFECT OF FUCOXANTHIN ON ADIPOCYTOKINE SECRETIONS

WAT plays an important role as an energy storage organ, as well as an endocrine organ producing adipocytokines such as monocyte chemoattractant protein-1 (MCP-1), TNF-α, IL-6, and adiponectin.[84,85] In obesity, dysregulation of the adipocytokine production in WAT is induced, which promotes glucose intolerance, dyslipidemia, and high blood pressure.[86,87] In the WAT of obese mice such as KK-Ay mice, ob/ob mice, and diet-induced-obesity mice, MCP-1 and TNF-α mRNAs increase compared to normal mice.[88] The overexpressions of MCP-1 and TNF-α mRNAs were markedly attenuated by fucoxanthin in WAT of KK-Ay mice[89] and in WAT of C57BL/6J normal mice fed HF diet.[82] IL-6 mRNA level in the WAT was also reduced by fucoxanthin intake.[89]

MCP-1 induces macrophage infiltration into WAT and promotes the production of inflammatory cytokines such as TNF-α.[90] In addition, MCP-1 inhibits insulin-dependent glucose uptake and leads to insulin resistance.[91] TNF-α and IL-6 levels are increased in obesity and induce insulin resistance.[92,93] Therefore, downregulation of MCP-1, TNF-α, and IL-6 mRNA in the WAT of KK-Ay would be a mechanism that underlies the improvement of hyperglycemia by fucoxanthin.[80,82]

Another remarkable effect of fucoxanthin on adipocytokine secretion was significant decrease in plasminogen activator inhibitor-1 (PAI-1) mRNA expression in the WAT of KK-Ay mice.[89] PAI-1 mRNA level is overexpressed in obese adipose tissue.[94] Recently, increase in PAI-1 has been reported to link not only to thrombosis and fibrosis but also to obesity and insulin resistance.[95] Therefore, the downregulation of PAI-1 mRNA expression in obese WAT would also be a mechanism of the suppressive effects of fucoxanthin on obesity and hyperglycemia.[80,82]

ABSORPTION MECHANISM OF FUCOXANTHIN (FIGURE 45.8)

Absorption and metabolism of fucoxanthin are important to understand its physiological effects. Fucoxanthinol and amarouciaxanthin A are known as major fucoxanthin metabolites (Figure 45.9).[96,97] Dietary fucoxanthin is hydrolyzed to fucoxanthinol in the gastrointestinal tract by digestive enzymes such as lipase and cholesterol esterase[96] and then converted to amarouciaxanthin A in the liver.[97] Fucoxanthinol was detectable at 0.8 pmol/mL in human plasma after a daily intake of cooked edible brown seaweed, *Undaria pinnatifida* (Wakame) (6 g dry weight), including 6.1 mg (9.26 mmol) of fucoxanthin for 1 week.[98] Fucoxanthinol and amarouciaxanthin A have been detected in plasma and

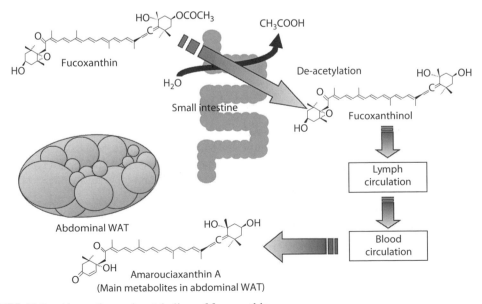

FIGURE 45.8   Absorption and metabolism of fucoxanthin.

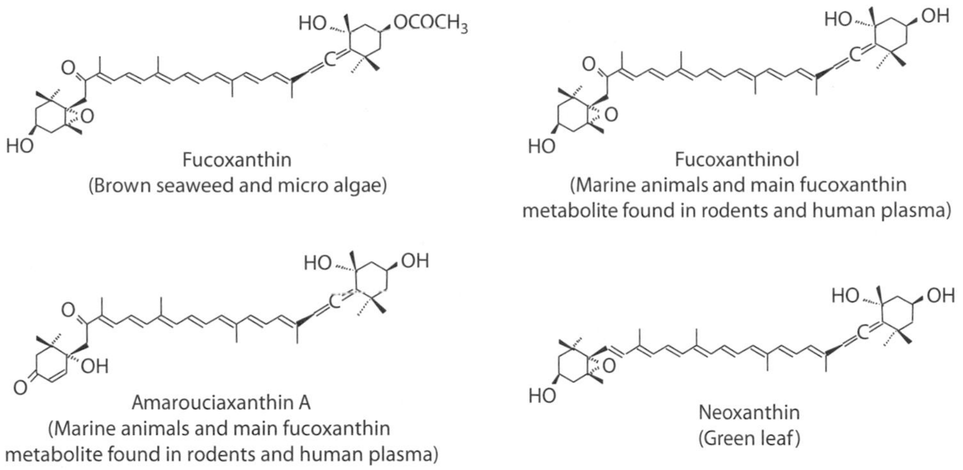

FIGURE 45.9 Structures of allenic carotenoids.

tissues of mouse with different accumulation ratio.[96,97,99–101] Dietary fucoxanthin preferentially accumulates as amarouciaxanthin A in the abdominal WAT and as fucoxanthinol in the other tissues.[100]

Recent study showed that more than 80% of fucoxanthin metabolites accumulated in abdominal WAT.[102] In this study, 0.1% purified fucoxanthin–containing diet (100 mg fucoxanthin/100 g diet) was given to KK-Ay mice, and then fucoxanthin metabolites were analyzed by HPLC, where three peaks appeared in the chromatogram. Two of them were identified as fucoxanthinol and amarouciaxanthin A by nuclear magnetic resonance and mass spectral analyses. The other peak was considered to be a *cis*-isomer of fucoxanthinol or amarouciaxanthin A from its retention time and the UV absorption spectra. Total fucoxanthin metabolites detected as three kinds in the WAT lipids were calculated to be 11.486 μg/mg protein, while those in other tissue lipids were 2.127 μg/mg protein.

When a duodenal infusion of 1 mL of test oil emulsion with 2 mg of fucoxanthin was administered in the lymph duct and the portal-cannulated rats, intact fucoxanthin was not detected in either lymph fluid or portal blood at any time point.[103] On the other hand, fucoxanthinol was detected in the lymph, but not in portal blood, showing a conversion of fucoxanthin to fucoxanthinol during the lymphatic absorption from intestine.

Overall, dietary fucoxanthin is absorbed from small intestine after conversion to fucoxanthinol, and fucoxanthinol enters into a systemic circulation system through lymph. (Figure 45.8) Some of the fucoxanthinols are reduced to amarouciaxanthin A mainly in liver. Although fucoxanthin metabolites are found in plasma and in tissues, the level and the accumulation ratios of fucoxanthinol and amarouciaxanthin A are different from each part. Fucoxanthin metabolites accumulate in abdominal adipose tissue at a higher ratio than plasma and other tissues, suggesting that the adipose tissue will be a main target of fucoxanthin metabolites.

NOVEL BIOLOGICAL ACTIVITY OF FUCOXANTHIN AND OTHER ALLENIC CAROTENOIDS

Fucoxanthin has been reported to be very effective in inducing apoptosis in human leukemia cells[104,105] and colon cancer cells.[106,107] The strong inhibitory effect of fucoxanthin on the growth of cancer cells has been also confirmed using human prostate cancer cells.[108] In their study, the effect of 15 kinds of carotenoids (phytoene, phytofluene, lycopene, β-carotene, β-cryptoxanthin, α-carotene, canthaxanthin, astaxanthin, capsanthin, lutein, zeaxanthin, violaxanthin, neoxanthin, and fucoxanthin) present in food stuffs was evaluated on the growth of the human prostate cancer cell lines (PC-3, DU 145, and LNCap). Among the carotenoids evaluated, they reported two allenic carotenoids, fucoxanthin and neoxanthin (Figure 45.9), to cause a remarkable reduction in the growth of prostate cancer cells.

DNA fragmentation revealed that these two carotenoids apparently reduced the cell viability by inducing apoptosis.[108] Although other acyclic carotenoids such as phytofluene, β-carotene, and lycopene also significantly reduced cell viability, the effect was lower than that of neoxanthin and fucoxanthin. Further, other carotenoids did not affect the growth of the prostate cancer cells. The higher activity of fucoxanthin and neoxanthin will be due to their characteristic chemical structure including allenic bond and other polar groups.

The strong activity of allenic carotenoids has been also found in the inhibition of lipid accumulation in adipose cell. When various carotenoids were screened for potential suppression effects on adipocyte differentiation,[109,110] only fucoxanthin, neoxanthin, and two fucoxanthin metabolites (fucoxanthinol and amarouciaxanthin A) (Figure 45.9) showed an encouraging suppressive effect on the differentiation of 3T3-L1 adipose cells, while other carotenoids did not show such an effect. The previous four allenic carotenoids significantly inhibited intercellular lipid accumulation during adipocyte differentiation of 3T3-L1 cells and significantly decreased glycerol-3-phosphate, an indicator of adipocyte differentiation, as compared with the control cells.[110]

Studies of the uptake and metabolism of fucoxanthin in 3T3-L1 cells indicated that fucoxanthin added into the culture medium was incorporated in cells and further converted to fucoxanthinol by deacetylation within 24 h.[109] Fucoxanthinol, but not fucoxanthin, levels increased in a time-dependent manner. In addition, the carotenoid accumulation in 3T3-L1 cells was greater following treatment with fucoxanthinol than after treatment with fucoxanthin. As described earlier, orally administrated fucoxanthin is converted to fucoxanthinol and amarouciaxanthin A,[97] showing that the active form of fucoxanthin in biological system is fucoxanthinol and/or amarouciaxanthin A. Interestingly, neoxanthin is very similar in structure to fucoxanthinol and amarouciaxanthin A. Thus, it was hypothesized that the specific structure that both carotenoids contain is somewhat responsible for the suppressive effect on the adipocyte differentiation. The relationship between the biological activity of an allenic carotenoid and its chemical structure is very interesting. More research is expected to make clear the active site of allenic carotenoids.

CONCLUSION

In contrast to rodents, humans have only minute amounts of BAT, and thereby, the contribution of BAT to the regulation of energy balance may be less in humans. However, if the expression of UCP1, a key molecule for BAT thermogenesis, can be activated in tissues other than BAT by food constituent, this would be a good antiobesity therapy for humans. From this viewpoint, the activity of fucoxanthin should be paid much attention. Nutrigenomic study reveals that fucoxanthin induces UCP1 expression in WAT mitochondria to lead to oxidation of fatty acids and heat production in WAT. Fucoxanthin improves insulin resistance and decreases blood glucose level through the regulation of cytokine secretions from the WAT. The specific regulation by fucoxanthin on a particular biomolecule is responsible for the characteristic chemical structure which differs depending on the length of the polyene, nature of the end group, and various substituents.

Former studies using animal models indicated that more than 100 mg per kg weight fucoxanthin has been still insufficient to show antiobesity and antidiabetic effects.[79–82,89] On the other hand, recent study demonstrated the significant reduction of abdominal WAT of obese female volunteers by intake of fucoxanthin less than 0.024 mg per kg weight (2.4 mg intake per day for volunteers with 100 kg average weight).[111] This difference in the effectiveness between rodents and human may be due to the different absorption rate and/or to different sensitivity to fucoxanthin.

Although chemical synthesis of fucoxanthin is possible, it costs too much money and its recovery level is very low. Several brown seaweeds contain more than 0.3%–1.0% fucoxanthin.[112] This content is exceptionally high as compared with those of carotenoids in other natural products. Abidov et al. [111] have reported that at most 2.4 mg fucoxanthin intake per day significantly increased energy expenditure of obese female volunteers and decreased body weight, body fat, plasma TG, and liver lipid contents. Judging from the human trial, the fucoxanthin levels of several brown seaweed lipids will be enough to show their physiological activity when these materials are applied to general foods.

REFERENCES

1. Spiegelman, B.M. and Flier, J.S., Adipogenesis and obesity: Rounding out the big picture. *Cell*, 87, 377–389, 1996.
2. Frühbeck, G., Gómez-Ambrosi, J., Muruzábal, F.J., and Burrell, M.A., The adipocyte: A model for integration of endocrine and metabolic signaling in energy metabolism regulation. *Am. J. Physiol. Endocrinol. Metab.*, 280, 827–847, 2001.
3. Gregoire, F.M., Adipocyte differentiation: From fibroblast to endocrine cell. *Exp. Biol. Med.*, 226, 997–1002, 2001.
4. Matsuzawa, Y., The metabolic syndrome and adipocytokines. *FEBS Lett.*, 580, 2917–2922, 2006.
5. Waki, H. and Tontonoz, P., Endocrine functions of adipose tissue. *Annu. Rev. Pathol.*, 2, 31–56, 2007.
6. Guilherme, A., Virbasius, J.V., Puri, V., and Czech, M.P., Adipocyte dysfunctions linking obesity to insulin resistance and type 2 diabetes. *Nat. Rev. Mol. Cell Biol.*, 9, 367–377, 2008.
7. Hotamisligil, G.S., Molecular mechanisms of insulin resistance and the role of the adipocyte. *Int. J. Obes. Relat. Metab. Disord.*, 24, 23–27, 2000.
8. Wong, S.L., Janssen, I., and Ross, R., Abdominal adipose tissue distribution and metabolic risk. *Sports Med.*, 33, 709–726, 2003.
9. Palomo, I., Alarcon, M., Moore-Carrasco, R., and Argiles, J.M., Hemostasis alterations in metabolic syndrome (review). *Int. J. Mol. Med.*, 18, 969–974, 2006.
10. Aguilera, C.M., Gil-Campos, M., Canete, R., and Gil, A., Alterations in plasma and tissue lipids associated with obesity and metabolic syndrome. *Clin. Sci.*, 114, 183–193, 2008.
11. Hollander, J.M. and Mechanick, J.I., Complementary and alternative medicine and the management of the metabolic syndrome. *J. Am. Diet. Assoc.*, 108, 495–509, 2008.
12. Temple, J.L., Caffeine use in children: What we know, what we have left to learn, and why we should worry. *Neurosci. Biobehav. Rev.*, 33, 793–806, 2009.
13. Lissner, L. and Keitmann, B.L., Dietary fat and obesity: Evidence for epidemiology. *Eur. J. Clin. Nutr.*, 49, 79–90, 1995.
14. Bray, G.A. and Popkin, B.M., Dietary fat intake does affect obesity. *Am. J. Clin. Nutr.*, 68, 1157–1173, 1998.
15. Flickinger, B.D. and Matsuo, N., Nutritional characteristics of DAG oil. *Lipids*, 38, 129–132, 2003.
16. Flickinger, B.D., Diacyglycerols (DAGs) and their mode of action, in *Nutraceuticals and Specialty Lipids and Their Co-Products*, Shahidi, F. (Ed.), CRC Press, Boca Raton, FL, 2006, pp. 181–186.
17. Che Man, Y.B. and Manaf, A.A., Medium-chain triacylglycerols, in *Nutraceuticals and Specialty Lipids and Their Co-Products*, Shahidi, F. (Ed.), CRC Press, Boca Raton, FL, 2006, pp. 27–56.
18. Atkinson, R.A., Conjugated linoleic acid for altering body composition and treating obesity, in *Advances in Conjugated Linoleic Acid Research*, Vol. 1, Yurawecz, M.P., Mossoba, M.M., Kramer, J.K.G., Pariza, M.W., and Nelson, G.J. (Eds.), AOCS Press, Champaign, IL, 1999, pp. 348–353.
19. Keim, N.L., Conjugated linoleic acid for altering body composition and treating obesity, in *Advances in Conjugated Linoleic Acid Research*, Vol. 2, Sébédio, J.-L., Christie, W.W. and Adlof, R. (Eds.), AOCS Press, Champaign, IL, 2003, pp. 316–324.
20. Watkins, B.A. and Li, Y., Conjugated linoleic acids (CLAs): Food, nutrition, and health, in *Nutraceuticals and Specialty Lipids and Their Co-Products*, Shahidi, F. (Ed.), CRC Press, Boca Raton, FL, 2006, pp. 187–200.
21. Kris-Etherton, P.M., Harris, W.S., and Appel, L.J., Fish consumption, fish oil, omega-3 fatty acids, and cardiovascular disease. *Circulation*, 106, 2747–2757, 2002.
22. Calder, P.C., N-3 polyunsaturated fatty acids, inflammation, and inflammatory diseases. *Am. J. Clin. Nutr.*, 83, 1505S–1519S, 2006.
23. Narayan, B., Miyashita, K., and Hosokawa, M., Physiological effects of eicosapentaenoic acid (EPA) and docosahexaenoic acid (DHA)—A review. *Food Rev. Int.*, 22, 291–307, 2006.
24. Wang, C., Harris, W.S., Chung, M., Lichtenstein, A.H., Balk, E.M., Kupelnick, B., Jordan, H.S., and Lau, J., Fatty acids from fish or fish-oil supplements, but not alpha-linolenic acid, benefit cardiovascular disease outcomes in primary- and secondary prevention studies: A systematic review. *Am. J. Clin. Nutr.*, 84, 5–17, 2006.
25. Leaf, A., Kang, J.X., and Xiao, Y.-F., Fish oil fatty acids as cardiovascular drugs. *Curr. Vasc. Pharmacol.*, 6, 1–12, 2008.
26. Russo, G.L., Dietary n-6 and n-3 polyunsaturated fatty acids: From biochemistry to clinical implications in cardiovascular prevention. *Biochem. Pharmacol.*, 235, 785–795, 2010.
27. Allayee, H., Roth, N., and Hodis, H.N., Polyunsaturated fatty acids and cardiovascular disease: Implications for nutrigenetics. *J. Nutrigenet. Nutrigenomics*, 2, 140–148, 2009.

28. De Backer, G., Ambrosioni, E., Borch-Johnsen, K., Brotons, C., Cifkova, R., Dallongeville, J., Ebrahim, S., Faergeman, O., Graham, I., Mancia, G., Cats, V.M., Orth-Gomér, K., Joep Perk, J., Pyörälä, K., Rodicio, J.L., Sans, S., Sansoy, V., Sechtem, U., Silber, S., Thomsen, T., and Wood, D., European guidelines on cardiovascular disease prevention in clinical practice. Third joint task force of European and other societies on cardiovascular disease prevention in clinical practice. *Eur. Heart J.*, 24, 1601–1610, 2003.

29. Smith Jr., S.C., Allen, J., Blair, S.N., Bonow, R.O., Brass, L.M., Fonarow, G.C., Grundy, S.M., Loren Hiratzka, L., Daniel Jones, D., Krumholz, H.M., Mosca, L., Pasternak, R.C., Pearson, T., Pfeffer, M.A., and Taubert, K.A., AHA/ACC guidelines for secondary prevention for patients with coronary and other atherosclerotic vascular disease: 2006 Update: Endorsed by the National Heart, Lung, and Blood Institute. *Circulation*, 113, 2363–2372, 2006.

30. Givens, D.I. and Gibbs, R.A., Current intakes of EPA and DHA in European populations and the potential of animal-derived foods to increase them. *Pro. Nutr. Soc.*, 67, 273–280, 2008.

31. Harris, W.S., Miller, M., Tighe, A.P., Davidson, M.H., and Schaefer, E.J., Omega-3 fatty acids and coronary heart disease risk: Clinical and mechanistic perspectives. *Atherosclerosis*, 197, 12–24, 2008.

32. Tziomalos, K., Athyros, V.G., Karagiannis, A., and Mikhailidis, D.P., Omega-3 fatty acids: How can they be used in secondary prevention? *Curr. Atherosclerosis Rep.*, 10, 510–517, 2008.

33. Hokanson, J.E. and Austin, M.A., Plasma triglyceride level is a risk factor for cardiovascular disease independent of high-density lipoprotein cholesterol level: A meta-analysis of population-based prospective studies. *J. Cardiovasc. Risk*, 3, 213–219, 1996.

34. Kelley, D.S., Siegel, D., Vemuri, M., and Mackey, B.E., Docosahexaenoic acid supplementation improves fasting and postprandial lipid profiles in hypertriglyceridemic men. *Am. J. Clin. Nutr.*, 86, 324–333, 2007.

35. Satoh, N., Shimatsu, A., Kotani, K., Sakane, N., Yamada, K., Suganami, T., Kuzuya, H., and Ogawa, Y., Purified eicosapentaenoic acid reduces small dense LDL, remnant lipoprotein particles, and C-reactive protein in metabolic syndrome. *Diabetes Care*, 30, 144–146, 2007.

36. Gazi, I.F., Tsimihodimos, V., Tselepis, A.D., Moses Elisaf, M., and Mikhailidis, D.P., Clinical importance and therapeutic modulation of small dense low density lipoprotein particles. *Expert. Opin. Biol. Ther.*, 7, 53–72, 2007.

37. Davidson, M., Mechanisms for the hypotriglyceridemic effect of marine omega-3 fatty acids. *Am. J. Card.*, 98, 27i–33i, 2006.

38. Harris, W. and Bulchandani, D., Why do omega-3 fatty acids lower serum triglycerides? *Curr. Opin. Lipidol.*, 17, 387–393, 2006.

39. Parrish, C.C., Pathy, D.A., and Angel, A., Dietary fish oils limit adipose tissue hypertrophy in rats. *Metabolism*, 39, 217–219, 1990.

40. Couet, C., Delarue, J., Ritz, P., Antoine, J.-M., and Lamisse, F., Effect of dietary fish oil on body fat mass and basal fat oxidation in healthy adults. *Int, J. Obes.*, 21, 637–643, 1997.

41. Kawada, T., Kayahashi, S., Hida, Y., Koga, K., Nadachi, Y., and Fushiki, T., Fish (bonito) oil supplementation enhances the expression of uncoupling protein in brown adipose tissue of rat. *J. Agric. Food Chem.*, 46, 1225–1227, 1998.

42. Shimomura, Y., Tamura, T., and Suzuki, M., Less body fat accumulation in rats fed a safflower oil diet than in rats fed a beef tallow diet. *J. Nutr.*, 120, 1291–1296, 1990.

43. Okuno, M., Kajiwara, K., Imai, S., Kobayashi, T., Honma, N., Maki, T., Suruga, K., Goda, T., Takase, S., Muto, Y., and Noriwaki, H., Perilla oil prevents the excessive growth of visceral adipose tissue in rats by down-regulating adipocyte differentiation. *J. Nutr.*, 127, 1752–1757, 1997.

44. Toyoshima, K., Noguchi, R., Hosokawa, M., Fukunaga, K., Nishiyama, T., Takahashi, R., and Miyashita, K., Separation of sardine oil without heating from surimi waste and its effect on lipid metabolism in rats. *J. Agric. Food Chem.*, 52, 2372–2375, 2004.

45. Buckley, J.D. and Howe, P.R.C., Anti-obesity effects of long-chain omega-3 polyunsaturated fatty acids. *Obesity Rev.*, 10, 648–659, 2009.

46. Flachs, P., Rossmeisl, M., Bryhn, M., and Kopecky, J., Cellular and molecular effects of n−3 polyunsaturated fatty acids on adipose tissue biology and metabolism. *Clin. Sci.*, 116, 1–16, 2009.

47. Viljoen, A. and Wierzbicki, A.S., Potential options to treat hypertriglyceridaemia. *Curr. Drug Targ.*, 10, 356–362, 2009.

48. Tai, C.C. and Ding, S.T., N-3 polyunsaturated fatty acids regulate lipid metabolism through several inflammation mediators: Mechanisms and implications for obesity prevention. *J. Nutr. Biochem.*, 21, 357–363, 2010.

49. Oliver, E., McGillicuddy, F., Phillips, C., Toomey, S., and Roche, H.M., The role of inflammation and macrophage accumulation in the development of obesity-induced type 2 diabetes mellitus and the possible therapeutic effects of long-chain n-3 PUFA. *Proc. Nutr. Soci.*, 69, 232–243, 2010.

50. Xenoulis, P.G. and Steiner, J.M., Lipid metabolism and hyperlipidemia in dogs. *Veter. J.*, 183, 12–21, 2010.
51. Dulloo, A.G. and Samec, S., Uncoupling proteins: Their roles in adaptive thermogenesis and substrate metabolism reconsidered. *Brit. J. Nutr.*, 86, 123–139, 2001.
52. Ježek, P., Possible physiological roles of mitochondrial uncoupling proteins-UCPn, *Int. J. Biochem. Cell Biol.*, 34, 1190–1206, 2002.
53. Dalgaard, L.T. and Pedersen, O., Uncoupling proteins: Functional characteristics and role in the pathogenesis of obesity and type II diabetes. *Diabetologia*, 44, 946–965, 2001.
54. Lowell, B.B., S-Susullc, V., Hamann, A., Lawitts, J.A., Himma-Hagen, J., Boyer, B.B., Kozak, L.P., and Flier, J.S., Development of obesity in transgenic mice after genetic ablation of brown adipose tissue. *Nature*, 366, 740–742, 1993.
55. Fleury, C., Neverova, M., Collins, S., Raimbault, S., Champigny, O., Levi-Meyrueis, C., Bouilaud, F., Seldin, M.F., Surwit, R.S., Ricquier, D., and Warden, C.H., Uncoupling protein-2: A novel gene linked to obesity and hyperinsulinemia. *Nat. Genetics*, 15, 269–272, 1997.
56. Arsenijevic, D., Onuma, H., Pecqueur, C., Raimbault, S., Manning, B.S., Miroux, B., Couplan, E., Alves-Guerra, M.-C., Goubern, M., Surwit, R., Bouillaud, F., Richard, D., Collins, S., and Ricquier, D., Disruption of the uncoupling protein-2 gene in mice reveals a role in immunity and reactive oxygen species production. *Nat. Genetics*, 26, 435–439, 2000.
57. Gong, D.-W., Monemdjou, S., Garvilova, O., Leon, L.R., Marcus-Samuels, B., Chou, C.J., Everett, C., Kozak, L.P., Li, C., Deng, C., Harper, M.-E., and Reitman, M.L., Lack of obesity and normal response to fasting and thyroid hormone in mice lacking uncoupling protein-3. *J. Biol. Chem.*, 275, 16251–16257, 2000.
58. Vidal-Puig, A.J., Grujic, D., Zhang, C.-Y., Hagen, T., Boss, O., Ido, Y., Szczepanik, A., Wade, J., Mootha, V., Cortright, R., Muoio, D.M., and Lowell, B.B., Energy metabolism in uncoupling protein 3 gene knockout mice. *J. Biol. Chem.*, 275, 16258–16266, 2000.
59. Lowell, B.B. and Spiegelman, B.M., Towards a molecular understanding of adaptive thermogenesis. *Nature*, 404, 652–660, 2000.
60. Harper, M.-E., Dent, R.M., Bezaire, V., Antoniou, A., Gauthier, A., Monemdjou, S., and McPherson, R., UCP3 and its putative function: Consistencies and controversies. *Biochem. Soc. Trans.*, 29, 768–773, 2001.
61. Rodríquez, A.M., Roca, P., and Palou, A., Synergic effect of overweight and cold on uncoupling proteins expression, a role of α2/β3 adrenergic receptor balance? *Euro. J. Phys.*, 444, 484–490, 2002.
62. Schrauwen, P. and Hesselink, M., UCP2 and UCP3 in muscle controlling body metabolism. *J. Exp. Biol.*, 205, 2275–2285, 2002.
63. Ricquier, D., Respiration uncoupling and metabolism in the control of energy expenditure. *Pro. Nutr. Soc.*, 64, 47–52, 2005.
64. Mills, E.M., Banks, M.I.., Sprague, J.E., and Finkel, T., Uncoupling the agony from ecstasy. *Nature*, 426, 403–404, 2003.
65. Nedergaard, J., Golozoubova, V., Matthias, A., Asadi, A., Jacobsson, A., and Cannon, B., UCP1: The only protein able to mediate adaptive non-shivering thermogenosis and metabolic inefficiency. *Biochim. Biophys. Acta*, 1504, 82–106, 2001.
66. Smith, R.E. and Horwitz, B.A., Brown fat and thermogenesis. *Physiol. Rev.*, 49, 330–425, 1969.
67. Rothwell, N.J. and Stock, M.J., A role for brown adipose tissue in diet-induced thermogenesis. *Nature*, 281, 31–35, 1979.
68. Silva, J.E. and Rabelo, R., Regulation of the uncoupling protein gene expression. *Eur. J. Endocrinol.*, 136, 251–264, 1997.
69. Del Mar Gonzalez-Barroso, M., Ricquier, D., and Cassard-Doulcier, A.-M., The human uncoupling protein-1 gene (UCP1): Present status and perspectives in obesity research. *Obesity Rev.*, 1, 61–72, 2000.
70. Argyropoulos, G. and Harper, M.-L., Molecular biology of thermoregulation. Invited review: Uncoupling proteins and thermoregulation. *J. Appl. Physiol.*, 92, 2187–2198, 2002.
71. Mozo, J., Emre, Y., Bouillaud, F., Ricquier, D., and Criscuolo, F., Thermoregulation: What role for UCPs in mammals and birds? *Biosci. Rep.*, 25, 227–249, 2005.
72. Clarke, S.D., Polyunsaturated fatty acid regulation of gene transcription: A mechanism to improve energy balance and insulin resistance. *Brit. J. Nutr.*, 83, 59–66, 2000.
73. Nicholls, D.G. and Locke, R.M., Thermogenic mechanisms in brown fat. *Physiol. Rev.*, 64, 1–64, 1984.
74. Foellmi-Adams, L.A., Wyse, B.M., Herron, D., Nedergaard, J., and Kletzien, R.F., Induction of uncoupling protein in brown adipose tissue. *Biochem. Pharm.*, 52, 693–701, 1996.
75. Sadurskis, A., Dicker, A., Cannon, B., and Nedergaard, J., Polyunsaturated fatty acids recruit brown adipose tissue: Increased UCP content and NST capacity. *Am. J. Physiol. Endocrinol. Metab.*, 269, E351–E360, 1995.

76. Alvarez, R., de Andrés, J., Yubero, P., Viñas, O., Mampel, T., Iglesias, R., Giralt, M., and Villarroya, F., A novel regulatory pathway of brown fat thermogenesis. *J. Biol. Chem.*, 270, 5666–5673, 1995.

77. Alvarez, R., Checa, M.L., Brun, S., Viñas, O., Mampel, T., Iglesias, R., Giralt, M., and Villarroya, F., Both retinoic-acid-receptor- and retinoid-X-receptor-dependent signaling pathways mediate the induction of the brown-sdipose-tissue-uncoupling-protein-1 gene by retinoids. *Biochem. J.*, 345, 91–97, 2000.

78. Cederberg, A., Grønning, L.M., Ahrén, B., Taskén, K., Carlsson, P., and Enerbäck, S., FOXC2 is a winged helix gene that counteracts obesity, hypertriglyceridemia, and diet-induced insulin resistance. *Cell*, 106, 563–573, 2001.

79. Maeda, H., Hosokawa, M., Sashima, T., Funayama, K., and Miyashita, K., Fucoxanthin from edible seaweed, Undaria pinnatifida, shows antiobesity effect through UCP1 expression in white adipose tissues. *Biochim. Biophys. Res. Commun.*, 332, 392–397, 2005.

80. Maeda, H., Hosokawa, M., Sashima, T., and Miyashita, K., Dietary combination of fucoxanthin and fish oil attenuates the weight gain of white adipose tissue and decrease blood glucose in obese/diabetic KK-A^y mice. *J. Agric. Food Chem.*, 55, 7701–7706, 2007.

81. Maeda, H., Hosokawa, M., Sashima, T., Funayama, K., and Miyashita, K., Effect of medium-chain triacylglycerols on anti-obesity effect of fucoxanthin. *J. Oleo Sci.*, 56, 615–621, 2007.

82. Maeda, H., Hosokawa, M., Sashima, T., Murakami-Funayama, K., and Miyashita, K., Anti-obesity and anti-diabetic effects of fucoxanthin on diet-induced obesity conditions in a murine model. *Mol. Med. Rep.*, 2, 897–902, 2009.

83. Watson, P.M., Commins, S.P., Beiler, R.J., Hatcher, H.C., and Gettys, T.W., Differential regulation of leptin expression and function in a/J vs. C57BL/6J mice during diet-induced regulation of leptin expression and function in A/J vs. C57BL/6J mice during diet-induced obesity. *Am. J. Physiol. Endocrinol. Metab.*, 279, E356–E365, 2000.

84. Matsuzawa, Y., Funahashi, T., and Nakamura, T., Molecular mechanism of metabolic syndrome X: Contribution of adipocytokines adipocyte-derived bioactive substances. *Ann. NY Acad. Sci.*, 892, 146–154, 1999.

85. Flier, J.S., Obesity wars: Molecular progress confronts an expanding epidemic. *Cell*, 116, 337–350, 2004.

86. Friedman, J.M., A war on obesity, not the obese. *Science*, 299, 856–858, 2003.

87. Kadowaki, T., Yamauchi, T., Kubota, N., Hara, K., Ueki, K., and Tobe, K., Adiponectin and adiponectin receptors in insulin resistance, diabetes, and the metabolic syndrome. *J. Clin. Invest.*, 116, 1784–1792, 2006.

88. Okada, T., Nishizawa, H., Kurata, A., Tamba, S., Sonoda, M., Yasui, A., Kuroda, Y., Hibuse, T., Maeda, N., Kihara, S., Hadama, T., Tobita, K., Akamatsu, S., Maeda, K., Shimomura, I., and Funahashi, T., URB is abundantly expressed in adipose tissue and dysregulated in obesity. *Biochem. Biophys. Res. Commun.*, 367, 370–376, 2008.

89. Hosokawa, M., Miyashita, T., Nishikawa, S., Emi, S., Tsukui, T., Beppu, F., Okada, T., and Miyashita, K., Fucoxanthin regulates adipocytokine mRNA expression in white adipose tissue of diabetic/obese KK-Ay mice. *Arch. Biochem. Biophys.*, 504, 17–25, 2010.

90. De Taeye, B.M., Novitskaya, T., McGuinness, O.P., Gleaves, L., Medda, M., Covington, J.W., and Vaughan, D.E., Macrophage TNF-α contributes to insulin resistance and hepatic steatosis in diet-induced obesity. *Am. J. Physiol. Endocrinol. Metab.*, 293, E713–E725, 2007.

91. Sartipy, P. and Loskutoff, D.J., Monocyte chemoattractant protein 1 in obesity and insulin resistance. *Proc. Natl. Acad. Sci. USA*, 100, 7265–7270, 2003.

92. Xu, H., Barnes, G.T., Yang, Q., Tan, G., Yang, D., Chou, C.J., Sole, J., Nicols, A., Ross, J.S., Tartaglia, L.A., and Chen, H., Chronic inflammation in fat plays a crucial role in the development of obesity-related insulin resistance. *J. Clin. Invest.*, 112, 1821–1830, 2003.

93. Bastard, J.P., Maachi, M., Van Nhieu, J.T., Jardel, C., Bruckert, E., Grimaldi, A., Robert, J.-J., Capeau, J., and Hainque, B., Adipose tissue IL-6 content correlates with resistance to insulin activation of glucose uptake both *in vivo* and *in vitro*. *J. Clin. Endocrinol. Metab.*, 87, 2084–2089, 2002.

94. Alessi, M.C., Peiretti, F., Morange, P., Henry, M., Nalbone, G., and Juhan-Vague, I., Production of plasminogen activator inhibitor 1 by human adipose tissue. *Diabetes*, 46, 860–867, 1997.

95. Ma, L.J., Mao, S.L., Taylor, K.L., Kanjanabuch, T., Guan, Y.-F., Zhang, Y.-H., Brown, N.J., Swift, L.L., McGuinness, O.P., Wasserman, D.H., Vaughan, D.E., and Fogo, A.B., Prevention of obesity and insulin resistance in mice lacking plasminogen activator inhibitor 1. *Diabetes*, 53, 336–346, 2004.

96. Sugawara, T., Baskaran, V., Tsuzuki, W., and Nagao, A., Brown algae fucoxanthin is hydrolyzed to fucoxanthinol during absorption by Caco-2 human intestinal cells and mice. *J. Nutr.*, 132, 946–951, 2002.

97. Asai, A., Sugawara, T., Ono, H., and Nagao, A., Biotransformation of fucoxanthinol into amarouciaxanthin A in mice and HepG2 cells: Formation and cytotoxicity of fucoxanthin metabolites. *Drug Metab. Dispos.*, 32, 205–211, 2004.

98. Asai, A., Yonekura, L., and Nagao, A., Low bioavailability of dietary epoxyxanthophylls in humans. *Br. J. Nutr.*, 100, 273–277, 2008.
99. Tsukui, T., Baba, T., Hosokawa, M., Sashima, T., and Miyashita, K., Enhancement of hepatic docosahexaenoic acid and arachidonic acid contents in C57BL/6J mice by dietary fucoxanthin. *Fisheries Sci.*, 75, 261–263, 2009.
100. Hashimoto, T., Ozaki, Y., Taminato, M., Das, S.K., Mizuno, M., Yoshimura, K., Maoka, T., and Kanazawa, K., The distribution and accumulation of fucoxanthin and its metabolites after oral administration in mice. *Br. J. Nutr.*, 102, 242–248, 2009.
101. Sangeetha, R.K., Bhaskar, N., Divakar, S., and Baskaran, V., Bioavailability and metabolism of fucoxanthin in rats: Structural characterization of metabolites by LC-MS (APCI). *Mol. Cell Biochem.*, 333, 299–310, 2010.
102. Airanthi, M.K.W.A., Sasaki, N., Iwasaki, S., Baba, N., Abe, M., Hosokawa, M., and Miyashita, K., Effect of brown seaweed lipids on fatty acid composition and lipid hydroperoxide levels of mouse liver. *J. Agic. Food Chem.*, 59, 4156–4163, 2011.
103. Matsumoto, M., Hosokawa, M., Matsukawa, N., Hagio, M., Shinoki, A., Nishimukai, M., Miyashita, K., Yajima, T., and Hara, H., Suppressive effects of the marine carotenoids, fucoxanthin and fucoxanthinol on triglyceride absorption in lymph duct-cannulated rats. *Eur. J. Nutr.*, 49, 243–249, 2010.
104. Hosokawa, M., Wanezaki, S., Miyauchi, K., Kurihara, H., Kohno, H., Kawabata, J., Odashima, S., and Takahashi, K., Apoptosis inducing effect of fucoxanthin on human leukemia cell line HL-60. *Food Sci. Technol. Res.*, 5, 243–246, 1999.
105. Kotake-Nara, E., Asai, A., and Nagao, A., Neoxanthin and fucoxanthin induce apoptosis in PC-3 human prostate cancer cells. *Cancer Lett.*, 220, 75–84, 2005.
106. Das, S.K., Hashimoto, T., Shimizu, K., Yoshida, T., Sakai, T., Sowa, Y., Komoto, A., and Kanazawa, K., Fucoxanthin induces cell cycle arrest at G0/G1 phase in human colon carcinoma cells through up-regulation of p21$^{WAF1/Cip1}$. *Biochim. Biophys. Acta*, 1726, 328–335, 2005.
107. Hosokawa, M., Kudo, M., Maeda, H., Kohno, H., Tanaka, T., and Miyashita, K., Fucoxanthin induces apoptosis and enhances the antiproliferative effect of the PPARγ ligand, troglitazone, on colon cancer cells. *Biochim. Biophys. Acta*, 1675, 113–119, 2004.
108. Kotake-Nara, E., Kushiro, M., Zhang, H., Sugawara, T., Miyashita, K., and Nagao, A., Carotenoids affect proliferation of human prostate cancer cells. *J. Nutr.*, 131, 3303–3306, 2001.
109. Maeda, H., Hosokawa, M., Sashima, T., Takahashi, N., Kawada, T., and Miyashita, K., Fucoxanthin and its metabolite, fucoxanthinol, suppress adipocyte differentiation in 3T3-L1 cells. *Int. J. Mole. Med.*, 18, 147–152, 2006.
110. Okada, T., Nakai, M., Maeda, H., Hosokawa, M., Sashima, T., and Miyashita, K., Suppressive effect of neoxanthin on the differentiation of 3T3-L1 adipose cells. *J. Oleo Sci.*, 57, 345–351, 2008.
111. Abidov, M., Ramazanov, Z., Seifulla, R., and Grachev, S., The effects of Xanthigen™ in the weight management of obese premenopausal women with non-alcoholic fatty liver disease and normal liver fat. *Diab. Obes. Met.*, 12, 72–81, 2010.
112. Terasaki, M., Baba, Y., Yasui, H., Saga, N., Hosokawa, M., and Miyashita, K., Evaluation of recoverable functional lipid components with special reference to fucoxanthin and fucosterol contents of several brown seaweeds of Japan. *J. Phycol.*, 45, 974–980, 2009.

46 Dairy Foods, Calcium, and Weight Management

Antje Bruckbauer, MD, PhD and Michael B. Zemel, PhD

CONTENTS

INTRODUCTION

Thermodynamics and energy balance are clearly the core factors involved in our present obesity epidemic, as modest increases in energy intake coupled with reduced physical activity have resulted in substantial net positive energy balance and progressive weight gain. However, it is equally clear that we operate with varying degrees of energetic efficiency, defined as conversion of food energy to useful work and/or energy storage, and that this variability in energetic efficiency results in corresponding variability in susceptibility to the consequences of chronic imbalance between energy intake and expenditure. The consequence of chronic positive energy balance, obesity, is well understood as a complex genetic trait, with multiple genes interacting to confer relative susceptibility (increased energetic efficiency) or resistance (decreased energetic efficiency) to positive energy balance. However, the metabolic pathways operated by these genetic factors may also be modulated by specific nutrients and/or dietary patterns.

Consequently, although there is no doubt regarding the primacy of energy balance in addressing the obesity epidemic, the additional effects of specific nutrients and foods on modulation of energy efficiency may still have substantial impact on weight gain and obesity incidence. For example, a caloric excess of as little as 1% (or 25 kcal/day) could lead to an annual weight gain of 1 kg. This value is well within the caloric range likely to be influenced by food components. A large number of food components have been proposed to contribute to healthy weight management; these include conjugated linoleic acid, medium-chain triglycerides, green tea, caffeine, and capsaicin [1], but the reported effect for each of these is modest at best, with support limited to a small number of conflicting reports [1]. However, a substantial and largely consistent body of data has emerged over the past years to indicate that both dietary calcium and other components of dairy foods modulate adipocyte lipid metabolism, energy efficiency, and energy partitioning between adipose tissue and muscle, resulting in a meaningful antiobesity effect. This effect is supported by a clear mechanistic framework, retrospective and prospective epidemiological and observational studies, secondary analysis of past clinical trials originally conducted with other primary endpoints (e.g., skeletal, cardiovascular), and prospective clinical trials to be discussed in this chapter. In addition, the role of dairy components in suppressing oxidative and inflammatory stress and thereby reducing the risk of obesity-associated comorbidities and metabolic syndrome will be discussed.

MECHANISMS

A compelling mechanism for the antiobesity effect of dietary calcium was provided by our studies of the mechanism of action of the *agouti* gene in regulating murine and human adipocyte metabolism [2–21]. These studies demonstrated a key role for intracellular Ca^{2+} and calcitrophic hormones in the regulation of adipocyte metabolism, which provides the primary mechanistic basis for the antiobesity effect of dietary calcium. Although it appears to be a paradox, increasing dietary calcium protects against obesity by decreasing intracellular Ca^{2+} levels while increasing intracellular Ca^{2+} increases adipocyte lipid storage. This paradox can be resolved by understanding the role of calcitrophic hormones regulating intracellular Ca^{2+} levels.

Circulating calcium levels are tightly regulated by a complex regulatory system. Key hormones of this system are PTH and calcitriol (1,25-dihydroxyvitamin D), which are increased in response to low calcium intakes to stimulate intestinal calcium absorption, renal calcium reabsorption, and calcium release from the bone. However, in addition to modulating calcium signaling in these tissues, they also stimulate calcium signaling in adipose tissue and thereby modulate adipocyte lipid metabolism. Notably, obesity appears to be associated with an alteration of the vitamin D-endocrine system [22], with increased circulating levels of the active form of the vitamin (1,25-dihydroxyvitamin D) while plasma levels of the precursor (25-hydroxyvitamin D) are decreased [23,24].

We have found both parathyroid hormone (PTH) [4] and $1\alpha,25\text{-}(OH)_2\text{-}D_3$ [25,26] stimulate rapid increases in human adipocyte intracellular Ca^{2+}; accordingly, suppression of these hormones by increasing dietary calcium facilitates repartitioning of dietary energy from lipid storage to lipid oxidation and thermogenesis. Although both PTH and $1\alpha,25\text{-}(OH)_2\text{-}D_3$ modulate adipocyte intracellular Ca^{2+}, a growing body of evidence indicates that $1\alpha,25\text{-}(OH)_2\text{-}D_3$ plays the major role; however, there is insufficient evidence to exclude a significant additional role for PTH.

The action of calcitriol is mediated via genomic and nongenomic processes. Human adipocytes possess nongenomic membrane vitamin D receptors (1,25-D3-MARRS (membrane-associated rapid-response steroid binding) protein), which transduce a rapid intracellular Ca^{2+} response to $1\alpha,25\text{-}(OH)_2\text{-}D_3$ [27–30]. Elevated intracellular Ca^{2+} results in coordinated activation of fatty acid synthase expression and activity, the key regulatory enzyme for lipogenesis, and suppression of lipolysis, leading to an expansion of adipocyte lipid storage [25,28,31]. Consequently, suppression of calcitriol by dietary calcium decreases the intracellular Ca^{2+} concentration and therefore decreases adiposity.

A potential role of $1\alpha,25\text{-}(OH)_2\text{-}D_3$ in human obesity is also suggested by other data. Polymorphisms in the nuclear vitamin D receptor (nVDR) gene are associated with the susceptibility to obesity in humans [32,33], and several lines of evidence demonstrate an alteration of vitamin D-endocrine system in obese humans, with an increase in circulating $1\alpha,25\text{-}(OH)_2\text{-}D_3$ level [22,34]. These observations, coupled with the direct effects of $1\alpha,25\text{-}(OH)_2\text{-}D_3$ on adipocyte lipid metabolism, strongly implicate the increase in $1\alpha,25\text{-}(OH)_2\text{-}D_3$ found on low-calcium diets as a contributory factor to excess adiposity.

In addition to regulating adipocyte metabolism via a nongenomic membrane receptor, $1\alpha,25\text{-}(OH)_2\text{-}D_3$ also acts via the "classical" nVDR in adipocytes to inhibit the expression of uncoupling protein 2 (UCP2) [27]; further, suppression of $1\alpha,25\text{-}(OH)_2\text{-}D_3$ levels by feeding high-calcium diets to mice results in increased adipose tissue UCP2 expression and attenuation of the decline in thermogenesis, which otherwise occurs with energy restriction [31], suggesting that high-calcium diets may also affect energy partitioning by suppressing $1\alpha,25\text{-}(OH)_2\text{-}D_3$-mediated inhibition of adipocyte UCP2 expression. However, the role of UCP2 in thermogenesis is not clear, and the observed thermogenic effect may be mediated by other, as of yet unidentified mechanisms. Moreover, thermogenic effects of dietary calcium and/or dairy products have not yet been demonstrated in humans. Nonetheless, in addition to inducing a mitochondrial proton leak, UCP2 serves to mediate mitochondrial fatty acid transport and oxidation, suggesting that $1\alpha,25\text{-}(OH)_2\text{-}D_3$ suppression of UCP2 expression may still contribute to decreased fat oxidation and increased lipid accumulation on low-calcium diets [27].

Limited human data support these proposed mechanisms. We have found that increasing dietary calcium via isocaloric substitution of three daily servings of dairy (without changing dietary macronutrient composition) results in significant increases in circulating glycerol, reflecting an increase in net lipolysis, compared to low-dairy diets under both eucaloric and hypocaloric conditions [35,36]. Melanson et al. [37] conducted a randomized controlled crossover study of the effects of low- and high-dairy diets on substrate oxidation in a room calorimeter under conditions of both energy balance and acute energy deficit. The high-dairy diets significantly suppressed circulating $1\alpha,25\text{-}(OH)_2\text{-}D_3$ levels without affecting substrate oxidation under zero energy balance conditions. However, under energy-deficit conditions, the high-dairy diet resulted in a significant increase in 24 hour fat oxidation, from 106 to 136 g/day without significantly affecting protein or carbohydrate oxidation. This suggests that high-dairy diets may augment the effects of energy restriction on fat mobilization and oxidation and thereby increase the effectiveness of energy-restricted diets in successful weight management. Similarly, Teegarden et al. [38] found increased fat oxidation in response to calcium supplementation in a randomized, placebo-controlled trial of overweight women undergoing weight loss; however, this effect was not seen with dairy supplementation, possibly due to the small group size and differences in baseline body composition. Interestingly, the baseline 25-hydroxyvitamin-D serum level was positively correlated with the thermic effect of a meal independent of group assignment, suggesting either effects of $1\alpha,25\text{-}(OH)_2\text{-}D_3$ on calcium absorption or direct effects on thermogenesis. Consistent with these findings, Gunther et al. [39] demonstrated that chronic consumption (1 year) of a dairy-rich high-calcium diet resulted in a substantially greater increase in postprandial fat oxidation following either a low- or high-calcium liquid meal challenge. Interestingly, they noted that the 1 year change in fasting levels of serum PTH was significantly correlated with the 1 year change of postprandial fat oxidation, suggesting that dietary calcium suppression of PTH may have permitted increased levels of fat oxidation [39]. Although this evidence is suggestive of a role for PTH, $1\alpha,25\text{-}(OH)_2\text{-}D_3$ levels were not measured, and it is possible that the observed correlation may have resulted from PTH modulation of $1\alpha,25\text{-}(OH)_2\text{-}D_3$ levels. In contrast, Bortolotti et al. [24] reported no significant effect of calcium supplementation on fat oxidation rate and energy expenditure in a double blind placebo-controlled crossover study conducted in 10 obese and overweight subjects with habitual low calcium intakes over 5 weeks. However, this lack of significant effect is likely attributable to the low level of calcium supplementation (400 mg supplements). Overall, Soares et al. [40] recently analyzed nine randomized studies measuring macronutrient oxidation, and six of these demonstrated an increase in fatty acid oxidation by high-calcium diets.

$1\alpha,25\text{-}(OH)_2\text{-}D_3$ modulation of adipocyte apoptosis may also contribute to the antiobesity effect of dietary calcium [40]. This effect is mediated, in part, via inhibition of UCP2 expression and a consequent increase in mitochondrial potential, a key regulator of apoptosis, and in part via $1\alpha,25\text{-}(OH)_2\text{-}D_3$ regulation of cytosolic Ca^{2+} and of Ca^{2+} flux between endoplasmic reticulum and mitochondria ([41] and unpublished data). Consequently, adipocyte apoptosis is significantly impaired in association with increased $1\alpha,25\text{-}(OH)_2\text{-}D_3$ levels in mice fed low-calcium diets, while there is a marked increase in adipocyte apoptosis in mice fed high-calcium and/or high-dairy diets [41]. Although this appears contrary to multiple published reports which indicate a pro-apoptotic effect of $1\alpha,25\text{-}(OH)_2\text{-}D_3$ in other tissues, this apparent discrepancy is the result of dosing differences. The literature which supports a pro-apoptotic effect of $1\alpha,25\text{-}(OH)_2\text{-}D_3$ utilizes supra-physiological concentrations ($\geq 100\,nM$), and we are also able to demonstrate a similar pro-apoptotic effect (resulting from mitochondrial Ca^{2+} overload) in adipocytes at these very high levels of $1\alpha,25\text{-}(OH)_2\text{-}D_3$. In contrast, physiological concentrations exert an anti-apoptotic effect in human adipocytes, primarily due to suppression of UCP2 expression ([41] and unpublished data). Figure 46.1 depicts the role of $1\alpha,25\text{-}(OH)_2\text{-}D_3$ in regulating adipocyte apoptosis, and Figure 46.2 provides an integrated summary of $1\alpha,25\text{-}(OH)_2\text{-}D_3$ modulation of adipocyte lipid metabolism.

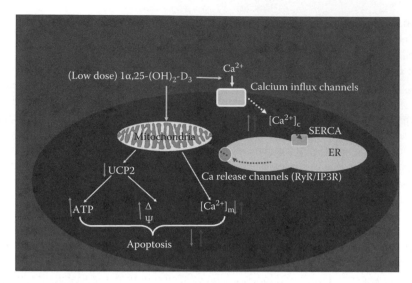

FIGURE 46.1 1α,25-(OH)$_2$-D$_3$ modulation of apoptosis: Low (physiological) doses of 1α,25-(OH)$_2$-D$_3$ inhibit apoptosis by inhibiting UCP2 and thereby restore UCP2-induced loss of mitochondrial potential and ATP reduction, protecting adipocytes from apoptotic death. The reduction in mitochondrial Ca levels found with lower doses of 1α,25-(OH)$_2$-D$_3$ may further contribute to this anti-apoptotic effect. In contrast, high levels of 1α,25-(OH)$_2$-D$_3$ cause markedly greater increases in cytosolic[Ca^{2+}]$_c$, probably resulting in increased [Ca^{2+}]$_{er}$. Since ER can open their Ca^{2+} release channels in response to elevations in [Ca^{2+}]$_c$ and contribute to Ca^{2+}-induced Ca^{2+} release (CICR), the high Ca^{2+} levels achieved at these contact sites favor Ca^{2+} uptake into mitochondria, which is usually located nearby ER. Calcium overloads in mitochondria and in turn triggers apoptosis. *Note:* RyR = ryanodine receptor; IP3R = inositol trisphosphate receptor; SERCA = sarco/endoplasmic reticulum Ca-ATPase.

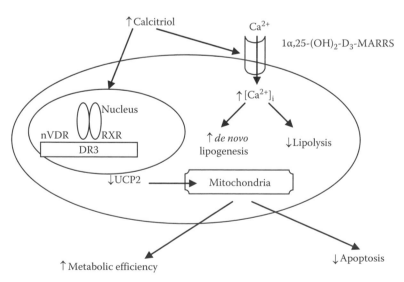

FIGURE 46.2 Role of 1α,25-(OH)$_2$-D$_3$ and dietary calcium in modulating adipocyte lipid metabolism. Calcitriol (1α,25-(OH)$_2$-D$_3$) acts via the membrane vitamin D receptor (MARRS protein) to stimulate Ca^{2+} influx. Increased Ca^{2+} influx exerts lipogenic and anti-lipolytic effects. Calcitriol also acts via the nVDR to suppress the expression of UCP2. Reduced UCP2 levels lead to increased mitochondrial potential, increased metabolic efficiency, and reduced adipocyte apoptosis. Dietary calcium inhibits each of these mechanisms by suppressing 1α,25-(OH)$_2$-D$_3$ levels. *Note:* RXR = retinoic X receptor.

Increasing dietary calcium may also result in increased fecal fatty acid excretion, and accordingly, it is possible that the resultant increase in fecal energy loss also contributes to the antiobesity effects of dietary calcium. In support of this concept, Papakonstantinou et al. [42] demonstrated that feeding a high-calcium diet to rats produced a substantial increase in fecal fat and energy excretion and attributed the observed reduction in adiposity to fecal energy loss, although a marked decrease in circulating $1\alpha,25\text{-}(OH)_2\text{-}D_3$ was found as well. Furthermore, Jacobsen et al. [43] reported that a short-term increase in calcium intake from 500 to 1800 mg/day increased fecal fat excretion ~2.5-fold, from 5.9 to 14.2 g/day. However, while such an increase in fecal fat loss will clearly contribute to a reduction in energy balance, it required a larger level of calcium (1800 vs. 1200 mg used in clinical trials of calcium and obesity) to produce a quantitatively small effect (8.3 g additional fecal fat, representing a 75 kcal/day loss), which is insufficient to explain the magnitude of the effects observed in clinical trials (discussed later in this chapter). Nonetheless, the modest reduction in net energy balance resulting from this mechanism may have a pronounced effect in maintaining healthy weights and promoting weight loss over an extended period of time, and the contributory role of increased fecal fat loss should not be overlooked. Indeed, we have found high-calcium and high-dairy diets to exert a substantial greater antiobesity effect in obese mice on a high-fat diet compared to those on a low-fat diet and attributed the additional effect to increased fecal energy loss in the mice on the high-fat diets [44]. Earlier human studies also demonstrated that large increases in dietary calcium (2–4 g/day) result in statistically significant, but modest, increases in fecal fat loss [45–47]. For example, a supplement of 2 g calcium increased fecal fat excretion from 6.8% to 7.4% of total fat intake [46]. In contrast, in order to achieve a clinically meaningful (albeit modest) contribution to weight loss, the pancreatic lipase inhibitor orlistat must produce approximately a 30% inhibition of total dietary fat absorption versus the approximately 1%–2% found with dietary calcium. Thus, while calcium inhibition of fat absorption appears to contribute to an antiobesity effect, this effect is too small to solely explain the observed effects.

Dairy products have also been proposed to impact energy balance and obesity risk by affecting satiety, and whey-derived peptides do appear to exert a satiety effect [48]. However, increased satiety with milk or dairy-based meals has not been consistently found [48–51]. Increased satiety of dairy products has also been attributed to the satiating effect of protein. However, clinical trials which have demonstrated the effects of calcium and dairy on adiposity and weight loss have been primarily conducted at a fixed level of protein intake. Moreover, the animal studies which have demonstrated these effects have not found measurable differences in energy intake between low- and high-calcium diets or between low- and high-dairy diets (discussed in a subsequent section of this chapter).

OTHER DAIRY COMPONENTS

While the aforementioned mechanisms explain dietary calcium inhibition of adiposity, data from clinical trials, rodent studies, and population studies all indicate a substantially (~twofold) greater effect of dairy versus supplemental sources of calcium in attenuating adiposity. Accordingly, it is important to identify the additional component(s) of dairy that may be responsible for this augmentation. Our studies indicate that the majority of this additional dairy-derived bioactivity resides in the whey fraction [52], a rich source of branched-chain amino acids (BCAAs) and other specific bioactive peptides.

Dairy contains a number of bioactive compounds, which may act either independently or synergistically with calcium to affect lipogenesis, lipolysis, lipid oxidation, and/or energy partitioning. Among these, proline-rich peptides in the whey fraction with angiotensin converting enzyme (ACE)–inhibitory activity may be relevant to adipocyte lipid metabolism. Angiotensin II, a potent vasoconstrictor and key player in hypertension, also upregulates adipocyte fatty acid synthase expression (as reviewed in [53]), and ACE inhibition mildly attenuates obesity in both mice and in hypertensive patients. In addition, angiotensin II plays an important role in adipogenesis and differentiation of pre-adipocytes to mature adipocytes [54,55], and pharmacological blockade of renin-angiotensin system (RAS) reduces adipocyte size and increases the number of smaller and more functional adipocytes [54,56,57]. Consequently, since adipose tissue has an autocrine RAS, it is possible that a whey-derived ACE inhibitor may contribute to the antiobesity effects of dairy.

In support of these concepts, Hammé et al. [58] demonstrated that incubation of immortalized human adipocytes at different stages of development with a goat whey hydrolysate containing lactokinins with ACE-inhibitory activity reduced the lipid content of mature adipocytes by 8% and decreased the proliferation of pre-adipocytes. Further, a whey-derived ACE inhibitor significantly augmented the effects of dietary calcium on weight and fat loss in energy-restricted mice [52]. However, the combination of the calcium and ACE inhibitor was markedly less potent than either milk or whey in reducing body fat; moreover, milk and whey both substantially preserved skeletal muscle mass during energy restriction while calcium and the calcium/ACE inhibitor combination were without effect. Consequently, although calcium plays a significant role in weight management, and this effect is enhanced by whey-derived ACE inhibition, these factors are not sufficient to fully explain the effects of dairy. An evaluation of whey-derived mineral mix versus calcium carbonate indicates that the other minerals contained in whey do not contribute to the antiobesity effects of whey, as milk-derived mineral mix exerted a comparable effect to that of calcium carbonate ([52] and unpublished data).

Although it may be tempting to speculate that the protein content of dairy may play a role in mediating the antiobesity effect, studies demonstrating an antiobesity effect of dairy products in both rodents and humans have maintained constant levels of protein intake. Accordingly, the protein content of dairy and whey *per se* cannot be responsible for the additional bioactivity. However, the amino acid composition of dairy protein may play a role. Dairy proteins have a high protein quality score and contain a high proportion (~26%) of BCAAs [59,60]. In addition to supporting protein synthesis, the BCAAs (leucine, isoleucine, and valine) play specific metabolic roles as energy substrates and in the regulation of muscle protein synthesis, and their potential to participate in these additional metabolic processes is limited by their availability, with first priority provided to new protein synthesis (as reviewed by Layman, [60]). Accordingly, only diets that provide leucine at levels which exceed the requirements for protein synthesis can fully support the intracellular leucine levels required to support additional signaling pathways [60]. The abundance of leucine in both casein and whey is of particular interest because it plays a distinct role in protein metabolism and a pivotal role in translation initiation of protein synthesis [61]. These effects are mediated by both mTOR-dependent and mTOR-independent pathways [62]). In addition, leucine has been shown to stimulate hypothalamic mTOR signaling, resulting in decreases in food intake and body weight and, therefore, also playing a role in satiety [63].

Leucine also appears be an important factor in the repartitioning of dietary energy from adipose tissue to skeletal muscle [64–66]. This suggests an interaction between the high levels of calcium in dairy and the high BCAA content of dairy protein, possibly in concert with other dairy-derived bioactive compounds, which may work in synergy to minimize adiposity and maximize lean mass. We have demonstrated that calcium-depleted milk retains approximately one-half of the antiobesity bioactivity of intact milk, and that most of the non-calcium/non-ACE-inhibitory bioactivity can be recapitulated by increasing the BCAA content of the low-calcium/non-dairy diet to the level found in milk [67]. Moreover, there is evidence that leucine regulates lipid metabolism and energy partitioning between adipocytes and skeletal muscle cells by inhibiting energy storage in adipocytes and instead stimulates skeletal muscle fatty acid oxidation [68]. Accordingly, the energetic requirements of leucine-stimulated protein synthesis appears to create a metabolic demand for increased fatty acid oxidation, and the adipose tissue represents the source for these additional metabolic energy costs [68]. In further support of this concept, we have found leucine to stimulate mitochondrial biogenesis in both adipocytes and skeletal muscle cells, thereby providing increased capacity for fatty acid oxidation in both cell types [69]. The calcium-dependent and calcium-independent effects of dairy diets based on our microarray analysis study are summarized in Figure 46.3.

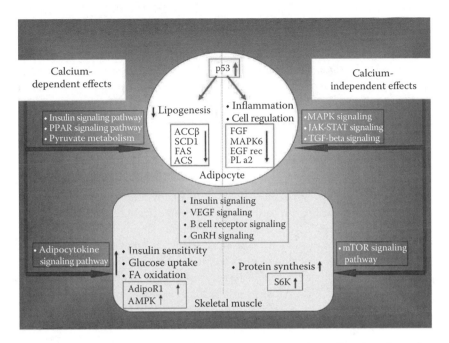

FIGURE 46.3 Summary of calcium-dependent and calcium-independent effects based on microarray analysis results. Calcium-dependent effects involved the modulation of insulin and PPAR signaling pathways and pyruvate metabolism, resulting in suppression of lipogenic genes in adipose tissue, while in skeletal muscle, MAPK and adiponectin receptor 1 were upregulated, leading to increased insulin sensitivity, glucose uptake, and fatty acid oxidation. Calcium-independent effects in adipose tissue included MAPK signaling, JAK-STAT, and TGF-beta signaling, modulating inflammation and cell regulation, whereas in muscle, protein synthesis was stimulated. Common effects of all three diet groups included p53 upregulation in adipose tissue and insulin, VEGF, B cell receptor, and GnRH signaling in skeletal muscle. *Abbreviations*: FGF 18, Fibroblast growth factor; MAPK6, Mitogen-activated protein kinase 6; EGF rec, Epidermal growth factor receptor; PL a2, Phospholipase a2; S6K, Ribosomal protein s6 kinase; ACC beta, Acetyl coenzyme A carboxylase beta; SCD1, Stearoyl-coenzyme A desaturase; FAS, Fatty acid synthase; ACS, Acyl-coenzyme A synthetase; AdipoR1, Adiponectin receptor 1.

MODULATION OF CENTRAL ADIPOSITY

Both rodent and human studies demonstrate a shift in the distribution of body fat loss on high-versus low-calcium diets during energy restriction. In rodents, high-calcium and high-dairy diets produce a preferential loss of visceral adipose tissue [25,31], while clinical trials demonstrate a preferential loss of fat from the trunk region (i.e., an increase in trunk fat loss as a percentage of total fat loss) [36,37,70,71]. This effect may be explained by the greater capacity of visceral adipose tissue to produce active glucocorticoids.

Human adipose tissue expresses significant amounts of 11β-hydroxysteroid dehydrogenase-1 (11β-HSD-1), which can generate active cortisol from cortisone, leading to increased intracellular levels of glucocorticoids in adipocytes. However, the expression of 11β-HSD-1 is greater in visceral than in subcutaneous adipose tissue [72,73]. Further, selective overexpression of 11β-HSD-1 in white adipose tissue of mice results in central obesity [74,75], while homozygous 11β-HSD-1 knockout mice exhibit protection from features of the metabolic syndrome [76]. We have found 1α,25-(OH)$_2$-D$_3$ to exert both short-term and long-term regulation of 11β-HSD-1 and cortisol release in human adipocytes, resulting in approximately twofold increases in 11β-HSD-1 expression and up to sixfold increases in net cortisol production [77]. In addition, data analysis from our microarray study in human adipocytes demonstrated an additional upregulation of 11β-HSD expression by cortisol when combined with calcitriol [78], which may result from an indirect positive feedback loop of cortisol on its own production. Cortisol increases the expression of the nVDR in adipocytes, leading to augmented action of calcitriol on 11β-HSD expression and thereby to increased cortisol production and release [79]. Consequently, using high-calcium diets to suppress calcitriol levels results in a corresponding decrease in adipose tissue cortisol production and thereby contributes to reduced visceral adipose tissue mass; this concept is supported by several animal and clinical studies as discussed in the following.

ANIMAL STUDIES

We have confirmed the antiobesity effect of dietary calcium and dairy products in a series of studies conducted in transgenic mice, which express the *agouti* gene in adipose tissue under the control of the aP2 promoter, similar to the human pattern of expression of *agouti* and other obesity-associated genes [25,31,45,53,80,81]. These mice are not obese when fed standard chow diets but are susceptible to adult-onset diet-induced obesity. They respond to low-calcium diets with accelerated weight gain and fat accretion, while high-calcium diets markedly inhibit lipogenesis, accelerate lipolysis, increase thermogenesis and adipocyte apoptosis, and suppress fat accretion and weight gain in animals maintained at identical caloric intakes [25]. Further, low-calcium diets impede body fat loss while high-calcium diets markedly accelerate weight and fat loss in transgenic mice subjected to identical levels of caloric restriction [31,45,53,80,81]. However, there is one report indicating lack of effect of increasing calcium intake on body weight and body fat in rats and mice [82]. The reason for this difference is not apparent but may be related to the use of older animals with more fully established obesity, as well as the lack of an energy restriction protocol. However, studies in other animal models (Zucker lean and obese rats, Wistar rats, and spontaneously hypertensive rats) confirm the observation that increased calcium intake lowers body weight and fat content [42,83,84].

Dietary calcium and dairy also alter the partitioning of dietary energy during refeeding following weight loss in aP2-agouti transgenic mouse model [85]. Although postobese mice fed a low-calcium diet rapidly regained all of the weight and fat that had been lost, refeeding high-calcium diets prevented the suppression of adipose tissue lipolysis and fat oxidation that otherwise accompanies postdieting repletion and markedly increased indices of skeletal muscle fat oxidation [85]. Consequently, although animals refed low-calcium diets rapidly regained all of the weight and fat that had been lost, animals fed high-calcium diets exhibited a 50%–85% reduction in weight and fat gain. Moreover, dairy exerted markedly greater effects than supplemental calcium on fat oxidation and fat gain [85]. These data are supported by both clinical trials and observational data, as described in the next sections.

CLINICAL DATA

The original concept of calcium and dairy modulation of body composition and weight management emerged from data from a hypertension clinical trial, with subsequent corroboration via secondary analysis of other clinical trials originally conducted with skeletal outcomes and finally prospective clinical trials to evaluate the effects of calcium and dairy on adiposity. In the hypertension study, dietary calcium was increased from ~400 to ~1000 mg/day in obese African Americans without altering dietary energy or macronutrient content. Although body weight did not change, there was a 4.9 kg reduction in body fat [25], which led to the subsequent mechanistic investigations already described.

Heaney and colleagues subsequently reanalyzed a series of calcium intervention studies originally designed with primary skeletal endpoints supporting a calcium-body weight linkage [86–88]. In an analysis of nine studies, including three controlled trials and six observational studies, a significant negative association between calcium intake and body weight was noted for all age groups studied (third, fifth, and eighth decades of life). The odds ratio for being overweight was 2.25 for young women below median calcium intake compared to those above median calcium intake [86], and the controlled trials supported this relationship [86–88]. Overall, increased calcium intake was consistently associated with reduced indices of adiposity (body weight, body fat, and/or weight gain); the aggregate effect was that each 300 mg increase in daily calcium intake was associated with a 3 kg lower weight in adults and a 1 kg decrease in body fat in children.

In contrast, a secondary analysis of three 25 week randomized clinical trials originally conducted to evaluate skeletal outcomes during weight loss did not demonstrate an effect of increased calcium intake on body weight or fat loss in subjects counseled to follow an energy-restricted diet; however, the authors noted that the calcium groups consistently lost more weight and fat and suggested that these studies did not have sufficient statistical power to detect these small effects [89]. Similarly, Reid et al. [90] assessed the results of a study originally designed to assess the effects of calcium on fracture incidence and found no effect of supplementary calcium on body weight or body composition, although there was a trend toward greater weight loss with calcium supplementation in those with the lowest baseline calcium intakes (<600 mg/day).

Notably, both of the aforementioned secondary analyses [89,90] evaluated the effects of supplementary calcium. In contrast, Lin et al. [91] conducted a retrospective analysis of a 2 year prospective study of 54 normal-weight Caucasian women originally conducted to assess the impact of exercise on skeletal outcomes. They found the dietary calcium:energy ratio and the dairy calcium:energy ratio to be significant negative predictors of changes in both body weight and body fat [91]. However, the reported effects appeared to be specific to dairy sources, as dairy calcium predicted changes in body weight and body fat, while nondairy calcium did not [91]. Thus, the failure to find a significant effect in retrospective analysis of calcium supplementation trials may result, in part, from the use of calcium supplements rather than dairy sources. Indeed, we have found dairy sources of calcium to be substantially more effective than supplementary sources in controlling adiposity in prospective studies of both mice and humans, as discussed earlier in this chapter. Lin et al. [91] also noted an important interaction between dietary calcium and energy intake in predicting changes in body fat, as calcium, but not energy, intake predicted changes in body weight and body fat for women below the median energy intake (1876 kcal/day), while energy intake alone predicted changes in weight and fat in women at higher levels of energy intake. This is consistent with the concept that energy balance is the predominant predictor of adiposity, with calcium and dairy effects being evident primarily when energy balance is controlled; clinical trial data (discussed in the next section) further support this concept.

An inverse relationship between energy-adjusted dietary calcium intake and body mass index (BMI) was also reported in lactose-tolerant, but not lactose-intolerant, African American women [92]. Although the reason for the lack of effect in the lactose-intolerant group cannot be definitively inferred from this cross-sectional study, the lactose-intolerant group exhibited a uniformly low calcium intake, presumably due to aversion to dairy products, and the lack of women with adequate calcium intakes in this group therefore precluded a clear relationship emerging as it did for the lactose-tolerant women.

In a recent study [93], the association of dietary calcium intake and changes in body composition and fat distribution was assessed in 119 healthy premenopausal women over a 1 year follow-up. All of these women were normal weight at the beginning of the study; however, half of them had followed a weight loss intervention before. Average dietary calcium intake was retrospectively determined from 4 day food records. Although calcium intake was not significantly associated with change in weight, total fat, or subcutaneous fat, there was as significant inverse relationship to intra-abdominal adipose tissue gain, as determined via computed tomography, after adjusting for confounding variables. Regression slope analysis showed that for every 100 mg/day increase in calcium intake, there was a reduction of intra-abdominal adipose tissue by 2.7 cm^2.

RANDOMIZED CLINICAL TRIALS

We have conducted several clinical trials to evaluate the effects of dietary calcium and/or dairy on adiposity; to date, all available randomized clinical trial data are from adults. In the first trial [71], 32 obese adults were maintained on balanced calorie-deficit diets (500 kcal/day deficit) and

Finally, high-dairy diets markedly attenuate weight regain following successful weight loss compared to a low-dairy diet under eucaloric conditions (3.03 kg vs. 1.02 kg weight regain on low- vs. high-dairy diet, p < 0.05) [101]. Similarly, the high-dairy diet attenuated regain of body fat (1.959 vs. 0.773 kg on low- vs. high-dairy diet, p < 0.01), and trunk fat (1.546 vs. 0.218 kg on low- vs. high-dairy diet, p < 0.01), indicating that dairy-rich diets attenuate short-term (12 week) weight, fat, and trunk fat regain following weight loss. Also longer-term assessment over 5 months showed that adequate levels of dairy food intake increases fat oxidation and permits significantly higher energy consumption without corresponding weight regain during weight maintenance compared to low-dairy foods intake [102], and 18 months follow-up of a weight loss diet in 183 overweight or obese women was associated with an inverse correlation between dietary calcium and weight regain when holding energy intake constant, suggesting a positive role of dietary calcium in weight maintenance [103]. Long-term calcium supplementation also confers beneficial effects on body composition and prevention of age-related weight gain under eucaloric conditions, as recently reported by Zhou et al. [104]. In this large-scale, placebo-controlled longitudinal study, 1179 postmenopausal women were randomly assigned to a calcium-only group with 1400 mg/day of supplemental calcium, a supplemental calcium plus vitamin D group (1400 mg/day calcium, 1100 IU/day vitamin D), or a placebo group, and their change in body weight and composition was assessed over a 4 year period. Although the calcium supplementation only exerted nonsignificant trends on body weight and BMI, long-term supplemental calcium intake had significant effects on body composition, with lower trunk fat mass and higher lean mass. There were no differences detected between the calcium-only and the calcium plus vitamin supplemental groups, suggesting that the observed effects are mainly caused by calcium.

OBSERVATIONAL AND EPIDEMIOLOGICAL STUDIES

Although there have been a limited number of clinical trials to date, these clinical data are supported by multiple lines of evidence, including observational data, noting an inverse relationship between dietary calcium and/or dairy and body weight and/or body fat in children and adolescents [105–109], younger and older women [91,92,110], African American women [92], as well as by epidemiological data from NHANES I [110], NHANES III [25], NHANES 1999–2000 [111], the Continuing Study of Food Intake of Individuals [111], the HERITAGE Study [112], the Quebec Family Study [113], the CARDIA Study [114], the Tehran Lipid and Glucose Study [115], the Dietary Intervention Randomized Controlled Trial (DIRECT) [116], and the Health Survey of São Paulo [117].

While most studies reporting the relationship between dietary calcium and/or dairy and indices of adiposity are in adults, there have been a few studies in children and adolescents [105–109,118–120]. Although one study recently reported no relationship between dietary calcium or dairy consumption in a longitudinal assessment of adolescent females [118], the authors noted that dairy consumption was significantly higher for their study cohort compared to that reported by CSFII for a nationally representative survey of the same age group (428 vs. 269 g/day of milk and milk products). Moreover, overall reported median dairy intake was 2.9 servings of dairy and 827 mg of dairy-derived calcium per day. Accordingly, it is possible that this cohort represented a relatively high-dairy-consuming population and therefore was sufficiently above a yet-to-be determined threshold of dairy intake to observe an effect on indices of adiposity. In contrast, several other studies of children and adolescents suggest a protective effect of dairy [105–109,119].

A significant inverse relationship between dietary calcium and body fat was reported in a 5 year longitudinal study of preschool children studied from 2 months of age ($R^2 = 0.51$) [105]. The group subsequently extended these longitudinal findings to 8 years of age [106]. Overall, in predictive equations that explain 26%–34% of the variability in body fat, variations in dietary calcium explained 7%–9% of the variability in adiposity [106]. Notably, these longitudinal data strongly suggest that dairy and calcium intakes within the first year of life are significant inverse determinants of body fat levels at age 8 [105,106]. Consistent with these findings, longitudinal data from the

Framingham Children's Study indicate that higher intakes of calcium early in life (ages 3–5) were associated with decreased gain of body fat over time (early adolescence), with dairy servings being more strongly correlated to reduced body fat than dietary calcium *per se* [119]. However, it is important to interpret such findings within the context of overall energy balance. For example, Berkey et al. [120] reported that adolescents who consume excess calories from milk exhibit higher gains in BMI than those who do not; however, when adjusted for energy intake, this effect was not evident.

The associations between dairy intake and incidence of the major components of the insulin resistance syndrome (IRS), including obesity, were evaluated in a 10 year population-based prospective study of 3157 black and white adults [114]. Overweight individuals who consumed the most dairy products had a 72% lower incidence of IRS compared to those with the lowest dairy intakes. Moreover, the cumulative incidence of obesity in those who started the study in the overweight category was significantly reduced from 64.8% in those consuming the least amount of dairy foods to 45.1% in the highest-dairy-food-consuming group. Notably, the inverse relationship between dietary calcium and either IRS or obesity incidence in the CARDIA study was explained solely by dairy intake and was not altered by adjustment for dietary calcium, indicating the presence of an additional effect of dairy beyond the mechanisms already cited for dietary calcium in modulating adiposity and obesity risk; this is consistent with both the experimental animal and clinical trial data, which also suggest that other dairy components, in addition to calcium, contribute to an antiobesity effect.

DAIRY AND DIETARY CALCIUM MODULATION OF OBESITY-INDUCED OXIDATIVE AND INFLAMMATORY STRESS AND CHRONIC DISEASE RISK

The view of the adipose tissue as a simple fuel reservoir to supply nonesterified fatty acids (NEFA) to meet the energy requirements of peripheral organs has changed with the discovery of hormones secreted from the adipose tissue. Our current understanding of adipose tissue is that it functions as a major endocrine organ, produces a variety of bioactive proteins (adipokines), and is also a significant source of reactive oxygen species (ROS). ROS and systemic oxidative stress are implicated as causative factors in systemic inflammation and in tissue damage resulting from obesity, diabetes, and atherosclerosis, and are recognized as key factors that contribute to the physiological processes of aging. Indeed, there is a substantial body of evidence indicating that obesity is associated with increased ROS production and a subclinical chronic inflammatory state [121–124].

We have shown adipocyte ROS production to be modulated by mitochondrial uncoupling status and cytosol Ca^{2+} signaling, and $1\alpha,25\text{-}(OH)_2\text{-}D_3$ regulates ROS production *in vitro* and *in vivo* [125,126]. Consequently, we have proposed that increased $1\alpha,25\text{-}(OH)_2\text{-}D_3$ contributes to systemic oxidative stress by inhibiting adipocyte UCP2 expression and increasing cytosolic Ca^{2+} signaling, thereby increasing ROS production. Accordingly, since dietary calcium suppresses $1\alpha,25\text{-}(OH)_2\text{-}D_3$, high-calcium diets would be anticipated to correspondingly decrease adipose tissue ROS production and systemic oxidative stress (Figure 46.4). In support of this concept, we have recently reported that high-calcium diets inhibited adipose tissue NADPH oxidase expression (a key source of intracellular ROS) and resulted in a striking 64% reduction in visceral adipose tissue ROS production in mice [94]. A similar pattern was evident in skeletal muscle, which exhibited a significant increase in UCP3 expression and a corresponding decrease in NADPH oxidase expression [94]. Moreover, visceral fat was associated with a higher ROS production than subcutaneous fat [94]. Accordingly, suppression of calcitriol by dietary calcium resulted in a greater reduction of ROS in visceral fat than in subcutaneous fat.

Overnutrition and obesity are also associated with an imbalance between pro- and anti-inflammatory cytokines, resulting in inflammatory stress, which also plays an important role in the pathogenesis of chronic obesity–related metabolic diseases. Enlarged adipocytes produce more pro-inflammatory cytokines, such as TNF-α and interleukin-6 (IL-6), while the secretion of anti-inflammatory factors such as adiponectin is reduced. In addition, adipose tissue contains a stromal/vascular fraction that consists of endothelial cells with characteristics of progenitor and leukocytes and is infiltrated

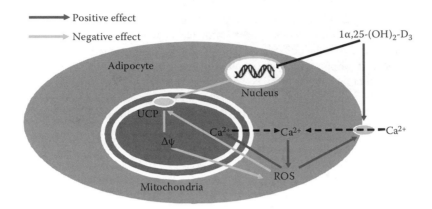

FIGURE 46.4 Schematic illustration of effects and mechanisms of calcitriol (1α,25-(OH)$_2$-D$_3$) on ROS production and adipocyte proliferation. Physiological doses of calcitriol increase ROS production by inhibiting UCP2 expression and stimulating intracellular calcium influx. Dietary calcium inhibits ROS via suppression of calcitriol.

by macrophages, which increase in number with increasing degree of adiposity [127–130]. These macrophages are a major source of additional cytokines, augmenting the inflammatory state [127]. Moreover, oxidative stress contributes to activation of pro-inflammatory cytokine expression including TNF-α [131], and this bidirectional interaction may act as a vicious cycle under conditions of either enhanced ROS or cytokine production as seen in obesity.

Dietary calcium attenuates obesity-associated inflammatory stress in mouse models of obesity by inhibiting the expression of pro-inflammatory factors, such as TNF-α and IL-6, in visceral fat and stimulating the expression of the anti-inflammatory factors such as IL-15 and adiponectin. Notably, dairy foods result in significantly greater suppression of systemic oxidative and inflammatory stress in mice than supplemental calcium, suggesting additional effects from other dairy components such as ACE-inhibitory peptides and leucine [125]. Conversely, calcitriol stimulated the expression of TNF-α, IL-6, and IL-8 in differentiated adipocytes [132]. Calcitriol also induced the production of an array of other inflammatory cytokines in adipocytes and/or adipose tissue–derived macrophages, which include macrophage surface-specific protein CD14, macrophage inhibitory factor (MIF), macrophage colony-stimulating factor (M-CSF), macrophage inflammatory protein (MIP), and monocyte chemoattractant protein-1 (MCP-1). In addition, it regulated the cross talk between adipocytes and macrophages, resulting in an augmentation of inflammatory cytokine production [133]. Both the calcium-channel antagonist nifedipine and the mitochondrial uncoupler dinitrophenol were able to block these effects, suggesting that the calcitriol-induced inflammatory cytokine production involves both calcium-dependent and mitochondrial uncoupling–dependent mechanisms.

Recent human data also support this concept. Increasing dairy foods resulted in substantial suppression of key clinical marker of oxidative (plasma malondialdehyde, 8-isoprostane-F2α) and inflammatory stress (C-reactive protein, TNF-α, IL6, MCP-1) in overweight and obese subjects during both weight loss and weight maintenance [125,134]. These effects were already seen within 7 days of initiation and increased with the duration of supplementation. Moreover, our recent results of dairy feeding in metabolic syndrome patients with elevated oxidative and inflammatory stress markers showed significant improvements of their metabolic state (25%–35% decrease in biomarkers of oxidative stress and 35%–55% decrease in biomarkers of inflammatory stress), which were independent of dairy-induced adiposity changes [135].

In contrast, van Meijl et al. [136] found only a reduction of TNF-α and an increase of soluble TNF-α-receptor-1 (S-TNFR-1) but no effects on other markers of chronic inflammation and endothelial function (such as IL-6, MCP-1, ICAM-1, and VCAM-1) in obese and overweight subjects fed a low-fat-dairy diet for 8 weeks compared to control subjects. However, the estimated calcium intake of their control subjects was 931 mg on average, which is much higher than the calcium intake of our control groups (500–600 mg/day); thus, they were already consuming sufficient levels of calcium and there was little opportunity for the dairy to exert significant effects.

Overall, these findings indicate a potentially important role of dietary calcium/dairy in attenuating obesity-induced oxidative and inflammatory stress and suggest that, in addition to exerting an antiobesity effect, dairy may play a significant role in suppressing key mediators of obesity-induced disease and morbidity, including cardiovascular disease (CVD) and type II diabetes, and consecutively early mortality. In support of this concept, our recent results indicate that calcitriol increases while leucine and calcium decreases vascular infiltration by monocytes, the initial step of atherosclerosis [137]. Monolayers of human endothelial cells were perfused with fluorescently labeled human monocytic cells, which were incubated with conditioned media from adipocytes treated either with vehicle, calcitriol, leucine, or both for 48 h; adherence was quantified by microscopy and image analysis. Calcitriol significantly increased monocyte adherence while leucine not only decreased the adherence but also abolished the effects of calcitriol when treated together. Consistent with these findings, supplementation with whey protein over 12 weeks statistically improved blood pressure and vascular function in overweight and obese individuals [138]. Pilvi et al. [139] found that feeding whey and calcium in addition to an energy-restricted diet to diet-induced obese mice not only resulted in increased loss of body weight and fat but also significantly decreased blood glucose and serum insulin levels. In addition, metabolomic analysis of hepatic lipid profile revealed that whey and calcium reversed the obesity-induced increase in the levels of potentially diabetogenic ceramides and diacylglycerols to the level observed in lean animals. These changes were accompanied by a decrease in glycolytic metabolites and an upregulated pentose phosphate pathway and TCA cycle. Further, lifelong feeding of a eucaloric milk diet not only attenuated adiposity and protected against age-related muscle loss but also decreased oxidative and inflammatory stress in aP2-agouti and wild-type mice and suppressed early mortality [140].

Many observational and epidemiological studies support a beneficial role for dietary calcium and dairy foods in protecting against obesity-related chronic disease; however, the association between full-fat dairy consumption and CVD is controversial. Consequently, Warensjö et al. [141] investigated the association of serum milk fat biomarkers such as pentadecanoic acid (15:0) and heptadecanoic acid (17:0) and a first myocardial infarction (MI) in a prospective, matched case-control study in Sweden with 444 cases and 556 controls. Both fatty acids were negatively associated with biomarkers for metabolic syndrome and inversely related to first MI event. This association was found for both sexes; however, it only reached statistical significance in women. It was also suggested that the concomitant high calcium intake with dairy consumption counteracts the effects of dairy fat on the lipid profile [142]. As expected, full-fat dairy increased total and LDL-cholesterol due to its high concentration of saturated fatty acids such as palmitic acid; however, it also increased the HDL fraction. Moreover, the addition of calcium to the high-fat diet decreased total:HDL-cholesterol and increased HDL:LDL-cholesterol ratios, partly explaining the inverse relationship between dairy intake and CVD despite the high fat content of dairy. Similarly, Bonthuis et al. [143] reported that intake of cheese and fermented milk products was inversely related to first MI. They carried out a 16 year prospective study among a community-based sample in Australia grouped by habitual intakes of dairy products, calcium, and vitamin D validated by food frequency questionnaires. The authors did not find any consistent association between total dairy intake and total or cause-specific mortality; however, the highest intake of full-fat dairy (but not low-fat dairy) was significantly associated with lower cardiovascular mortality compared to lowest intake of full-fat dairy. Goldbohm et al. reported a slightly increased risk of all-cause and ischemic heart disease mortality only for consumption of high-fat dairy such as butter in womens while a statistically significant inverse association was observed for fermented full-fat milk in both men and women [144].

Because of concerns of long-term effects of dairy consumption in childhood on CVD and mortality, Van der Pols et al. [145] investigated this association in a 65 year follow-up study of children in Britain. Their results showed that a family diet with calcium intakes above ~400 mg was associated with 40%–60% lower mortality due to stroke compared to those with lower than 400 mg daily calcium. Although there was no clear linear trend, coronary heart disease mortality was lowest in the group with highest calcium intake. Further, dairy intake during childhood was statistically inversely correlated to all-cause mortality in adulthood.

Kaluza et al. [146] investigated the association of dietary calcium and magnesium intake with all-cause mortality, CVD, and cancer mortality in a prospective study among 23,366 Swedish men who did not use dietary supplements. Dietary calcium (but not magnesium) in the highest intake tertile was associated with statistically significant lower rate of all-cause mortality and with a nonsignificant trend of lower rate of CVD. Further, a meta-analysis of prospective cohort studies of vascular disease and diabetes provided evidence of an overall survival advantage from the consumption of milk and dairy food with lower incidence and death rate of vascular disease, stroke, diabetes, and cancer [147].

SUMMARY AND CONCLUSIONS

An antiobesity effect of dietary calcium and dairy foods is evident from animal studies, observational and population studies, and randomized clinical trials. Moreover, there is a strong theoretical framework in place to explain the effects of dietary calcium on energy metabolism. The supporting mechanisms include dietary calcium correcting suboptimal calcium intakes and thereby preventing the endocrine response (PTH and $1\alpha,25\text{-}(OH)_2\text{ D}$), which favors adipocyte energy storage and inhibits adipocyte loss via apoptosis; dietary calcium appears to further promote energy

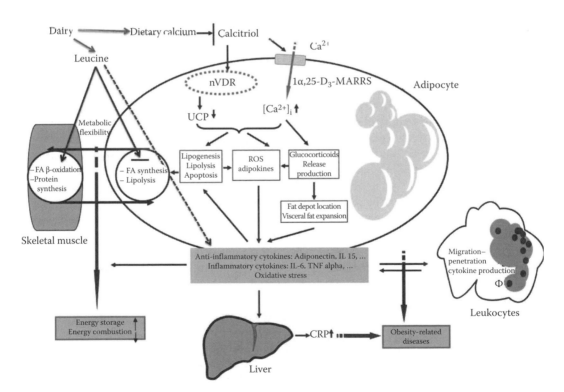

FIGURE 46.5 Schematic illustration of effects of dairy components on adipocyte-skeletal muscle cross talk, energy metabolism, and oxidative and inflammatory stress. Dietary calcium in dairy foods suppresses action of calcitriol in adipocytes, thereby reducing adiposity, and oxidative and inflammatory stress. Additional dairy components such as leucine stimulate adipocyte-muscle cross talk, thereby increasing energy combustion and metabolic flexibility. Together, these effects result in protection against obesity-related disease.

loss via formation of calcium soaps in the gastrointestinal tract and thereby reducing net energy absorption. Dietary calcium appears to be responsible for ~50% of the antiobesity bioactivity of dairy. The additional dairy bioactivity has not been fully identified, but major components are the ACE-inhibitory activity of dairy and the high concentration of BCAAs in dairy; animal studies indicate that the BCAA content of dairy is largely responsible for the repartitioning of dietary energy from adipose tissue to skeletal muscle during weight loss, resulting in greater preservation of skeletal muscle and accelerated loss of adipose tissue during negative energy balance. Finally, high-calcium diets suppress obesity-induced oxidative and inflammatory stress and may thereby contribute to a reduction in obesity comorbidity independent of the direct antiobesity effect (summarized in Figure 46.5).

REFERENCES

1. Kovacs EM, Mela DJ. Metabolically active functional food ingredients for weight control. *Obes Rev*. 2006 Feb;7:59–78.
2. Jones B, Kim J, Zemel M, Woychik R, Michaud E, Wilkison W, Moustaid N. Upregulation of adipocyte metabolism by agouti protein: Possible paracrine actions in yellow mouse obesity. *Am J Physiol*. 1996 Jan;270:E192–E196.
3. Zemel MB, Kim JH, Woychik RP, Michaud EJ, Kadwell SH, Patel IR, Wilkison WO. Agouti regulation of intracellular calcium: Role in the insulin resistance of viable yellow mice. *Proc Natl Acad Sci USA*. 1995 May;92:4733–4737.
4. Xue B. The agouti gene product inhibits lipolysis in human adipocytes via a Ca2+-dependent mechanism. *FASEB J*. 1998 Oct;12:1391–1396.
5. Xue B, Greenberg A, Kraemer F, Zemel M. Mechanism of intracellular calcium ([Ca2+]i) inhibition of lipolysis in human adipocytes. *FASEB J*. 2001 Nov;15:2527–2529.
6. Kim J, Mynatt R, Moore J, Woychik R, Moustaid N, Zemel M. The effects of calcium channel blockade on agouti-induced obesity. *FASEB J*. 1996 Dec;10:1646–1652.
7. Claycombe K, Wang Y, Jones B, Kim S, Wilkison W, Zemel M, Chun J, Moustaid-Moussa N. Transcriptional regulation of the adipocyte fatty acid synthase gene by agouti: Interaction with insulin. *Physiol Genomics*. 2000 Sep;3:157–162.
8. Shi H, Moustaid-Moussa N, Wilkison W, Zemel M. Role of the sulfonylurea receptor in regulating human adipocyte metabolism. *FASEB J*. 1999 Oct;13:1833–1838.
9. Xue B, Zemel M. Relationship between human adipose tissue agouti and fatty acid synthase (FAS). *J Nutr*. 2000 Oct;130:2478–2481.
10. Voisey J, Imbeault P, Hutley L, Prins JB, van Daal A. Body mass index-related human adipocyte agouti expression is sex-specific but not depot-specific. *Obes Res*. 2002 Jun;10:447–452.
11. Zemel M. Agouti/melanocortin interactions with leptin pathways in obesity. *Nutr Rev*. 1998 Sep;56:271–274.
12. Tebar F, Soley M, Ramirez I. The antilipolytic effects of insulin and epidermal growth factor in rat adipocytes are mediated by different mechanisms. *Endocrinology*. 1996 Oct;137:4181–4188.
13. Xue B, Wilkison W, Mynatt R, Moustaid N, Goldman M, Zemel M. The agouti gene product stimulates pancreatic [beta]-cell Ca2+ signaling and insulin release. *Physiol Genomics*. 1999 Jul;1:11–19.
14. Mynatt R, Miltenberger R, Klebig M, Zemel M, Wilkinson J, Wilkinson W, Woychik R. Combined effects of insulin treatment and adipose tissue-specific agouti expression on the development of obesity. *Proc Natl Acad Sci USA*. 1997 Feb;94:919–922.
15. Mynatt RL, Truett GE. Influence of agouti protein on gene expression in mouse adipose tissue. *FASEB J*. 2000;14:A733 (abstract).
16. Zemel MB, Mynatt RL, Dibling D. Synergism between diet-induced hyperinsulinemia and adipocyte-specific agouti expression. *FASEB J*. 1999;13:660.3 (abstract).
17. Kwon HY, Bultman SJ, Loffler C, Chen WJ, Furdon PJ, Powell JG, Usala AL, Wilkison W, Hansmann I, Woychik RP. Molecular structure and chromosomal mapping of the human homolog of the agouti gene. *Proc Natl Acad Sci USA*. 1994 Oct;91:9760–9674.
18. Standridge M, Alemzadeh R, Zemel M, Koontz J, Moustaid-Moussa N. Diazoxide down-regulates leptin and lipid metabolizing enzymes in adipose tissue of Zucker rats. *FASEB J*. 2000 Mar;14:455–460.
19. Alemzadeh R, Slonim AE, Zdanowicz MM, Maturo J. Modification of insulin resistance by diazoxide in obese Zucker rats. *Endocrinology*. 1993 Aug;133:705–712.

20. Alemzadeh R, Jacobs W, Pitukcheewanont P. Antiobesity effect of diazoxide in obese Zucker rats. *Metabolism*. 1996 Mar;45:334–341.

21. Alemzadeh R, Langley G, Upchurch L, Smith P, Slonim AE. Beneficial effect of diazoxide in obese hyperinsulinemic adults. *J Clin Endocrinol Metab*. 1998 Jun;83:1911–1915.

22. Bell NH, Epstein S, Greene A, Shary J, Oexmann MJ, Shaw S. Evidence for alteration of the vitamin D-endocrine system in obese subjects. *J Clin Invest*. 1985 Jul;76:370–373.

23. Wortsman J, Matsuoka LY, Chen TC, Lu Z, Holick MF. Decreased bioavailability of vitamin D in obesity. *Am J Clin Nutr*. 2000 Sep;72:690–693.

24. Bortolotti M, Rudelle S, Schneiter P, Vidal H, Loizon E, Tappy L, Acheson KJ. Dairy calcium supplementation in overweight or obese persons: Its effect on markers of fat metabolism. *Am J Clin Nutr*. 2008 Oct;88:877–885.

25. Zemel M, Shi H, Greer B, Dirienzo D, Zemel P. Regulation of adiposity by dietary calcium. *FASEB J*. 2000 Jun;14:1132–1138.

26. Shi H, Norman A, Okamura W, Sen A, Zemel M. 1alpha,25-Dihydroxyvitamin D3 modulates human adipocyte metabolism via nongenomic action. *FASEB J*. 2001 Dec;15:2751–2753.

27. Shi H, Norman A, Okamura W, Sen A, Zemel M. 1alpha,25-dihydroxyvitamin D3 inhibits uncoupling protein 2 expression in human adipocytes. *FASEB J*. 2002 Nov;16:1808–1810.

28. Zemel M. Role of calcium and dairy products in energy partitioning and weight management. *Am J Clin Nutr*. 2004 May;79:907S–912S.

29. Nemere I, Safford SE, Rohe B, DeSouza MM, Farach-Carson MC. Identification and characterization of 1,25D3-membrane-associated rapid response, steroid (1,25D3-MARRS) binding protein. *J Steroid Biochem Mol Biol*. 2004 May;89–90:281–285.

30. Nemere I, Farach-Carson MC, Rohe B, Sterling TM, Norman AW, Boyan BD, Safford SE. Ribozyme knockdown functionally links a 1,25(OH)2D3 membrane binding protein (1,25D3-MARRS) and phosphate uptake in intestinal cells. *Proc Natl Acad Sci USA*. 2004 May;101:7392–7397.

31. Shi H, Dirienzo D, Zemel M. Effects of dietary calcium on adipocyte lipid metabolism and body weight regulation in energy-restricted aP2-agouti transgenic mice. *FASEB J*. 2001 Feb;15:291–293.

32. Ye WZ, Reis AF, Dubois-Laforgue D, Bellanne-Chantelot C, Timsit J, Velho G. Vitamin D receptor gene polymorphisms are associated with obesity in type 2 diabetic subjects with early age of onset. *Eur J Endocrinol*. 2001 Aug;145:181–186.

33. Barger-Lux MJ, Heaney RP, Hayes J, DeLuca HF, Johnson ML, Gong G. Vitamin D receptor gene polymorphism, bone mass, body size, and vitamin D receptor density. *Calcif Tissue Int*. 1995 Aug;57:161–162.

34. Andersen T, McNair P, Hyldstrup L, Fogh-Andersen N, Nielsen TT, Astrup A, Transbol I. Secondary hyperparathyroidism of morbid obesity regresses during weight reduction. *Metabolism*. 1988 May;37:425–428.

35. Zemel MB, Richards J, Mathis S, Milstead A, Gebhardt L, Silva E. Dairy augmentation of total and central fat loss in obese subjects. *Int J Obes (Lond)*. 2005 Apr;29:391–397.

36. Zemel M, Richards J, Milstead A, Campbell P. Effects of calcium and dairy on body composition and weight loss in African-American adults. *Obes Res*. 2005 Jul;13:1218–1225.

37. Melanson E, Donahoo W, Dong F, Ida T, Zemel M. Effect of low- and high-calcium dairy-based diets on macronutrient oxidation in humans. *Obes Res*. 2005 Dec;13:2102–2112.

38. Teegarden D, White KM, Lyle RM, Zemel MB, Van Loan MD, Matkovic V, Craig BA, Schoeller DA. Calcium and dairy product modulation of lipid utilization and energy expenditure. *Obesity (Silver Spring)*. 2008 Jul;16:1566–1572.

39. Gunther CW, Lyle RM, Legowski PA, James JM, McCabe LD, McCabe GP, Peacock M, Teegarden D. Fat oxidation and its relation to serum parathyroid hormone in young women enrolled in a 1-y dairy calcium intervention. *Am J Clin Nutr*. 2005 Dec;82:1228–1234.

40. Soares MJ, She-Ping-Delfos WLC. Postprandial energy metabolism in the regulation of body weight: Is there a mechanistic role for dietary calcium. *Nutrients*. 2010;2:586–598.

41. Sun X, Zemel M. Role of uncoupling protein 2 (UCP2) expression and 1alpha, 25-dihydroxyvitamin D3 in modulating adipocyte apoptosis. *FASEB J*. 2004 Sep;18:1430–1432.

42. Papakonstantinou E, Flatt WP, Huth PJ, Harris RB. High dietary calcium reduces body fat content, digestibility of fat, and serum vitamin D in rats. *Obes Res*. 2003 Mar;11:387–394.

43. Jacobsen R, Lorenzen JK, Toubro S, Krog-Mikkelsen I, Astrup A. Effect of short-term high dietary calcium intake on 24-h energy expenditure, fat oxidation, and fecal fat excretion. *Int J Obes (Lond)*. 2005 Mar;29:292–301.

44. Zemel MB, Morgan K. Interaction between calcium, dairy and dietary macronutrients in modulating body composition in obese mice. *FASEB J*. 2002;16:301.6 (abstract).

45. Denke MA, Fox MM, Schulte MC. Short-term dietary calcium fortification increases fecal saturated fat content and reduces serum lipids in men. *J Nutr*. 1993 Jun;123:1047–1053.

46. Welberg JW, Monkelbaan JF, de Vries EG, Muskiet FA, Cats A, Oremus ET, Boersma-van Ek W, van Rijsbergen H, van der Meer R, et al. Effects of supplemental dietary calcium on quantitative and qualitative fecal fat excretion in man. *Ann Nutr Metab*. 1994;38:185–191.

47. Shahkhalili Y, Murset C, Meirim I, Duruz E, Guinchard S, Cavadini C, Acheson K. Calcium supplementation of chocolate: Effect on cocoa butter digestibility and blood lipids in humans. *Am J Clin Nutr*. 2001 Feb;73:246–252.

48. Hall WL, Millward DJ, Long SJ, Morgan LM. Casein and whey exert different effects on plasma amino acid profiles, gastrointestinal hormone secretion and appetite. *Br J Nutr*. 2003 Feb;89:239–248.

49. Barr SI, McCarron DA, Heaney RP, Dawson-Hughes B, Berga SL, Stern JS, Oparil S. Effects of increased consumption of fluid milk on energy and nutrient intake, body weight, and cardiovascular risk factors in healthy older adults. *J Am Diet Assoc*. 2000 Jul;100:810–817.

50. Almiron-Roig E, Drewnowski A. Hunger, thirst, and energy intakes following consumption of caloric beverages. *Physiol Behav*. 2003 Sep;79:767–773.

51. Tsuchiya A, Almiron-Roig E, Lluch A, Guyonnet D, Drewnowski A. Higher satiety ratings following yogurt consumption relative to fruit drink or dairy fruit drink. *J Am Diet Assoc*. 2006 Apr;106:550–557.

52. Causey KR, Zemel MB. Dairy augmentation of the anti-obesity effect of Ca in aP2-agouti transgenic mice. *FASEB J*. 2003:A746 (abstract).

53. Morris K, Wang Y, Kim S, Moustaid-Moussa N. Dietary and hormonal regulation of the mammalian FA synthase gene. In: Moustaid-Moussa N, Berdanier CD, eds. *Nutrient-Gene Interactions in Health and Disease*. Boca Raton, FL: CRC Press; 2001.

54. Sharma AM, Janke J, Gorzelniak K, Engeli S, Luft FC. Angiotensin blockade prevents type 2 diabetes by formation of fat cells. *Hypertension*. 2002 Nov;40:609–611.

55. Mogi M, Iwai M, Horiuchi M. Emerging concept of adipogenesis regulation by the renin-angiotensin system. *Hypertension*. 2006 Dec;48:1020–1022.

56. Mori Y, Itoh Y, Tajima N. Angiotensin II receptor blockers downsize adipocytes in spontaneously type 2 diabetic rats with visceral fat obesity. *Am J Hypertens*. 2007 Apr;20:431–436.

57. Furuhashi M, Ura N, Takizawa H, Yoshida D, Moniwa N, Murakami H, Higashiura K, Shimamoto K. Blockade of the renin-angiotensin system decreases adipocyte size with improvement in insulin sensitivity. *J Hypertens*. 2004 Oct;22:1977–1982.

58. Hamme V, Sannier F, Piot J M, Bordenave Juchereau S. Effects of lactokinins from fermented acid goat whey on lipid content and adipogenesis of immortalized human adipocytes. *Int Dairy J*. 2010;20:642–645.

59. Bos C, Gaudichon C, Tome D. Nutritional and physiological criteria in the assessment of milk protein quality for humans. *J Am Coll Nutr*. 2000 Apr;19:191S–205S.

60. Layman DK. The role of leucine in weight loss diets and glucose homeostasis. *J Nutr*. 2003 Jan;133:261S–267S.

61. Anthony JC, Anthony TG, Kimball SR, Jefferson LS. Signaling pathways involved in translational control of protein synthesis in skeletal muscle by leucine. *J Nutr*. 2001 Mar;131:856S–860S.

62. Stipanuk MH. Leucine and protein synthesis: mTOR and beyond. *Nutr Rev*. 2007 Mar;65:122–129.

63. Cota D, Proulx K, Smith KA, Kozma SC, Thomas G, Woods SC, Seeley RJ. Hypothalamic mTOR signaling regulates food intake. *Science*. 2006 May;312:927–930.

64. Garlick PJ, Grant I. Amino acid infusion increases the sensitivity of muscle protein synthesis in vivo to insulin. Effect of branched-chain amino acids. *Biochem J*. 1988 Sep;254:579–584.

65. Ha E, Zemel M. Functional properties of whey, whey components, and essential amino acids: Mechanisms underlying health benefits for active people (review). *J Nutr Biochem*. 2003 May;14:251–258.

66. Fouillet H, Mariotti F, Gaudichon C, Bos C, Tome D. Peripheral and splanchnic metabolism of dietary nitrogen are differently affected by the protein source in humans as assessed by compartmental modeling. *J Nutr*. 2002 Jan;132:125–133.

67. Bruckbauer A, Gouffon J, Rekapalli B, Zemel MB. The effects of dairy components on energy partitioning and metabolic risk in mice: A microarray study. *J Nutrigenet Nutrigenomics*. 2009;2:64–77.

68. Sun X, Zemel M. Leucine and calcium regulate fat metabolism and energy partitioning in murine adipocytes and muscle cells. *Lipids*. 2007 Apr;42:297–305.

69. Sun X, Zemel MB. Leucine modulation of mitochondrial mass and oxygen consumption in skeletal muscle cells and adipocytes. *Nutr Metab (Lond)*. 2009;6:26.

70. Zemel M, Thompson W, Milstead A, Morris K, Campbell P. Calcium and dairy acceleration of weight and fat loss during energy restriction in obese adults. *Obes Res*. 2004 Apr;12:582–590.

71. Zemel MB, Teegarden D, Van Loan M, Schoeller DA, Matkovic V, Lyle M, Craig BA. Role of dairy products in modulating weight and fat loss: A multi-center trial. *FASEB J.* 2004;18:566.5 (abstract).

72. Seckl JR, Walker BR. Minireview: 11beta-hydroxysteroid dehydrogenase type 1- a tissue-specific amplifier of glucocorticoid action. *Endocrinology.* 2001 Apr;142:1371–1376.

73. Rask E, Olsson T, Soderberg S, Andrew R, Livingstone DE, Johnson O, Walker BR. Tissue-specific dysregulation of cortisol metabolism in human obesity. *J Clin Endocrinol Metab.* 2001 Mar;86:1418–1421.

74. Masuzaki H, Paterson J, Shinyama H, Morton NM, Mullins JJ, Seckl JR, Flier JS. A transgenic model of visceral obesity and the metabolic syndrome. *Science.* 2001 Dec;294:2166–2170.

75. Masuzaki H, Yamamoto H, Kenyon CJ, Elmquist JK, Morton NM, Paterson JM, Shinyama H, Sharp MG, Fleming S, et al. Transgenic amplification of glucocorticoid action in adipose tissue causes high blood pressure in mice. *J Clin Invest.* 2003 Jul;112:83–90.

76. Kotelevtsev Y, Holmes MC, Burchell A, Houston PM, Schmoll D, Jamieson P, Best R, Brown R, Edwards CR et al. 11beta-hydroxysteroid dehydrogenase type 1 knockout mice show attenuated glucocorticoid-inducible responses and resist hyperglycemia on obesity or stress. *Proc Natl Acad Sci USA.* 1997 Dec 23;94:14924–14929.

77. Morris K, Zemel M. 1,25-dihydroxyvitamin D3 modulation of adipocyte glucocorticoid function. *Obes Res.* 2005 Apr;13:670–677.

78. Sun XM, Morris KL, Zemel, MB. Role of calcitriol and cortisol on human adipocyte proliferation and oxidative and inflammatory stress: A microarray study. *J Nutrigenet Nutrigenomics.* 2008;1:30–48.

79. Sun X, Zemel MB. 1Alpha, 25-dihydroxyvitamin D and corticosteroid regulate adipocyte nuclear vitamin D receptor. *Int J Obes (Lond).* 2008 Aug;32:1305–1311.

80. Zemel MB, Sun X, Geng X. Effects of a calcium-fortified breakfast cereal on adiposity in a transgenic mouse model of obesity. *FASEB J.* 2001;15:A598 (abstract number 480.7).

81. Zemel MB, Geng X. Dietary calcium and yoghurt accelerate body fat loss secondary to caloric restriction in aP2-agouti transgenic mice. *Obes Res.* 2001;9:146S.

82. Zhang Q, Tordoff MG. No effect of dietary calcium on body weight of lean and obese mice and rats. *Am J Physiol.* 2004;286:R669–R677.

83. Bursey RD, Sharkey T, Miller GD. High calcium intake lowers weight in lean and fatty Zucker rats. *FASEB J.* 1989;3:A265.

84. Metz JA, Karanja N, Torok J, McCarron DA. Modification of total body fat in spontaneously hypertensive rats and Wistar-Kyoto rats by dietary calcium and sodium. *Am J Hypertens.* 1988 Jan;1:58–60.

85. Sun X, Zemel M. Calcium and dairy products inhibit weight and fat regain during ad libitum consumption following energy restriction in Ap2-agouti transgenic mice. *J Nutr.* 2004 Nov;134:3054–3060.

86. Davies KM, Heaney RP, Recker RR, Lappe JM, Barger-Lux MJ, Rafferty K, Hinders S. Calcium intake and body weight. *J Clin Endocrinol Metab.* 2000 Dec;85:4635–4638.

87. Heaney RP, Davies KM, Barger-Lux MJ. Calcium and weight: Clinical studies. *J Am Coll Nutr.* 2002 Apr;21:152S–155S.

88. Heaney RP. Normalizing calcium intake: Projected population effects for body weight. *J Nutr.* 2003 Jan;133:268S–270S.

89. Shapses SA, Heshka S, Heymsfield SB. Effect of calcium supplementation on weight and fat loss in women. *J Clin Endocrinol Metab.* 2004 Feb;89:632–637.

90. Reid IR, Horne A, Mason B, Ames R, Bava U, Gamble GD. Effects of calcium supplementation on body weight and blood pressure in normal older women: A randomized controlled trial. *J Clin Endocrinol Metab.* 2005 Jul;90:3824–3829.

91. Lin YC, Lyle RM, McCabe LD, McCabe GP, Weaver CM, Teegarden D. Dairy calcium is related to changes in body composition during a two-year exercise intervention in young women. *J Am Coll Nutr.* 2000 Nov–Dec;19:754–760.

92. Buchowski MS, Semenya J, Johnson AO. Dietary calcium intake in lactose maldigesting intolerant and tolerant African-American women. *J Am Coll Nutr.* 2002 Feb;21:47–54.

93. Bush NC, Alvarez JA, Choquette SS, Hunter GR, Oster RA, Darnell BE, Gower BA. Dietary calcium intake is associated with less gain in intra-abdominal adipose tissue over 1 year. *Obesity (Silver Spring).* 2010 Nov;18:2101–2104.

94. Sun X, Zemel M. Dietary calcium regulates ROS production in aP2-agouti transgenic mice on high-fat/high-sucrose diets. *Int J Obes (Lond).* 2006 Sep;30:1341–1346.

95. Summerbell CD, Watts C, Higgins JP, Garrow JS. Randomised controlled trial of novel, simple, and well supervised weight reducing diets in outpatients. *BMJ.* 1998 Nov;317:1487–1489.

96. Faghih S, Abadi AR, Hedayati M, Kimiagar SM. Comparison of the effects of cows' milk, fortified soy milk, and calcium supplement on weight and fat loss in premenopausal overweight and obese women. *Nutr Metab Cardiovasc Dis*. 2011 Jul;21:499–503.

97. Torres MR, Francischetti EA, Genelhu V, Sanjuliani AF. Effect of a high-calcium energy-reduced diet on abdominal obesity and cardiometabolic risk factors in obese Brazilian subjects. *Int J Clin Pract*. 2010 Jul;64:1076–1083.

98. Bowen J, Noakes M, Clifton PM. Effect of calcium and dairy foods in high protein, energy-restricted diets on weight loss and metabolic parameters in overweight adults. *Int J Obes (Lond)*. 2005 Aug;29:957–965.

99. Thompson W, Rostad Holdman N, Janzow D, Slezak J, Morris K, Zemel M. Effect of energy-reduced diets high in dairy products and fiber on weight loss in obese adults. *Obes Res*. 2005 Aug;13:1344–1353.

100. Harvey-Berino J, Gold BC, Lauber R, Starinski A. The impact of calcium and dairy product consumption on weight loss. *Obes Res*. 2005 Oct;13:1720–1726.

101. Zemel MB. Role of dairy products in the prevention of weight regain following weight loss. *FASEB J*. 2005:19 (abstract).

102. Zemel MB, Donnelly JE, Smith BK, Sullivan DK, Richards J, Morgan-Hanusa D, Mayo MS, Sun X, Cook-Wiens G, et al. Effects of dairy intake on weight maintenance. *Nutr Metab (Lond)*. 2008;5:28.

103. Ochner CN, Lowe MR. Self-reported changes in dietary calcium and energy intake predict weight regain following a weight loss diet in obese women. *J Nutr*. 2007 Oct;137:2324–2328.

104. Zhou J, Zhao LJ, Watson P, Zhang Q, Lappe JM. The effect of calcium and vitamin D supplementation on obesity in postmenopausal women: Secondary analysis for a large-scale, placebo controlled, double-blind, 4-year longitudinal clinical trial. *Nutr Metab (Lond)*. 2010 Jul;7:62.

105. Carruth BR, Skinner JD. The role of dietary calcium and other nutrients in moderating body fat in pre-school children. *Int J Obes Relat Metab Disord*. 2001 Apr;25:559–566.

106. Skinner JD, Bounds W, Carruth BR, Ziegler P. Longitudinal calcium intake is negatively related to children's body fat indexes. *J Am Diet Assoc*. 2003 Dec;103:1626–1631.

107. Barba G, Troiano E, Russo P, Venezia A, Siani A. Inverse association between body mass and frequency of milk consumption in children. *Br J Nutr*. 2005 Jan;93:15–19.

108. Tanasescu M, Ferris AM, Himmelgreen DA, Rodriguez N, Perez-Escamilla R. Biobehavioral factors are associated with obesity in Puerto Rican children. *J Nutr*. 2000 Jul;130:1734–1742.

109. Novotny R, Daida YG, Acharya S, Grove JS, Vogt TM. Dairy intake is associated with lower body fat and soda intake with greater weight in adolescent girls. *J Nutr*. 2004 Aug;134:1905–1909.

110. McCarron DA. Calcium and magnesium nutrition in human hypertension. *Ann Intern Med*. 1983 May;98:800–805.

111. Albertson AM, Good CK, Holschuh NM, Eldridge EL. The relationship between dietary calcium intake and body mass index in adult women from three National dietary intake databases. *FASEB J*. 2004;18:6259 (abstract).

112. Loos RJ, Rankinen T, Leon AS, Skinner JS, Wilmore JH, Rao DC, Bouchard C. Calcium intake is associated with adiposity in Black and White men and White women of the HERITAGE Family Study. *J Nutr*. 2004 Jul;134:1772–1778.

113. Jacqmain M, Doucet E, Despres JP, Bouchard C, Tremblay A. Calcium intake, body composition, and lipoprotein-lipid concentrations in adults. *Am J Clin Nutr*. 2003 Jun;77:1448–1452.

114. Pereira MA, Jacobs DR, Jr., Van Horn L, Slattery ML, Kartashov AI, Ludwig DS. Dairy consumption, obesity, and the insulin resistance syndrome in young adults: The CARDIA Study. *JAMA*. 2002 Apr;287:2081–2089.

115. Mirmiran P, Esmaillzadeh A, Azizi F. Dairy consumption and body mass index: An inverse relationship. *Int J Obes (Lond)*. 2005 Jan;29:115–121.

116. Shahar DR, Schwarzfuchs D, Fraser D, Vardi H, Thiery J, Fiedler GM, Bluher M, Stumvoll M, Stampfer MJ, Shai I. Dairy calcium intake, serum vitamin D, and successful weight loss. *Am J Clin Nutr*. 2010 Nov;92:1017–1022.

117. Bueno MB, Cesar CL, Martini LA, Fisberg RM. Dietary calcium intake and overweight: An epidemiologic view. *Nutrition*. 2008 Nov–Dec;24:1110–1115.

118. Phillips SM, Bandini LG, Cyr H, Colclough-Douglas S, Naumova E, Must A. Dairy food consumption and body weight and fatness studied longitudinally over the adolescent period. *Int J Obes Relat Metab Disord*. 2003 Sep;27:1106–1113.

119. Moore LL, Singer MR, Bradlee ML, Ellison RC. Dietary predictors of excess body fat acquisition during childhood (abstract). Presented at *44th American Heart Association Annual Conference on Cardiovascular Disease Epidemiology and Prevention*, San Francisco, CA, Mar 2004.

120. Berkey CS, Rockett HR, Willett WC, Colditz GA. Milk, dairy fat, dietary calcium, and weight gain: A longitudinal study of adolescents. *Arch Pediatr Adolesc Med*. 2005 Jun;159:543–550.

121. Furukawa S, Fujita T, Shimabukuro M, Iwaki M, Yamada Y, Nakajima Y, Nakayama O, Makishima M, Matsuda M, Shimomura I. Increased oxidative stress in obesity and its impact on metabolic syndrome. *J Clin Invest*. 2004 Dec;114:1752–1761.

122. Atabek ME, Vatansev H, Erkul I. Oxidative stress in childhood obesity. *J Pediatr Endocrinol Metab*. 2004 Aug;17:1063–1068.

123. Lin TK, Chen SD, Wang PW, Wei YH, Lee CF, Chen TL, Chuang YC, Tan TY, Chang KC, Liou CW. Increased oxidative damage with altered antioxidative status in type 2 diabetic patients harboring the 16189 T to C variant of mitochondrial DNA. *Ann N Y Acad Sci*. 2005 May;1042:64–69.

124. Sonta T, Inoguchi T, Tsubouchi H, Sekiguchi N, Kobayashi K, Matsumoto S, Utsumi H, Nawata H. Evidence for contribution of vascular NAD(P)H oxidase to increased oxidative stress in animal models of diabetes and obesity. *Free Radic Biol Med*. 2004 Jul;37:115–123.

125. Zemel MB, Sun X. Dietary calcium and dairy products modulate oxidative and inflammatory stress in mice and humans. *J Nutr*. 2008 Jun;138:1047–1052.

126. Sun X, Zemel M. 1Alpha,25-dihydroxyvitamin D3 modulation of adipocyte reactive oxygen species production. *Obesity (Silver Spring)*. 2007 Aug;15:1944–1953.

127. Bouloumie A, Curat CA, Sengenes C, Lolmede K, Miranville A, Busse R. Role of macrophage tissue infiltration in metabolic diseases. *Curr Opin Clin Nutr Metab Care*. 2005 Jul;8:347–354.

128. Weisberg SP, McCann D, Desai M, Rosenbaum M, Leibel RL, Ferrante AW, Jr. Obesity is associated with macrophage accumulation in adipose tissue. *J Clin Invest*. 2003 Dec;112:1796–1808.

129. Xu H, Barnes GT, Yang Q, Tan G, Yang D, Chou CJ, Sole J, Nichols A, Ross JS et al. Chronic inflammation in fat plays a crucial role in the development of obesity-related insulin resistance. *J Clin Invest*. 2003 Dec;112:1821–1830.

130. Curat CA, Miranville A, Sengenes C, Diehl M, Tonus C, Busse R, Bouloumie A. From blood monocytes to adipose tissue-resident macrophages: Induction of diapedesis by human mature adipocytes. *Diabetes*. 2004 May;53:1285–1292.

131. Janssen-Heininger YM, Macara I, Mossman BT. Cooperativity between oxidants and tumor necrosis factor in the activation of nuclear factor (NF)-kappaB: Requirement of Ras/mitogen-activated protein kinases in the activation of NF-kappaB by oxidants. *Am J Respir Cell Mol Biol*. 1999 May;20:942–952.

132. Sun X, Zemel MB. Calcium and 1,25-dihydroxyvitamin D3 regulation of adipokine expression. *Obesity (Silver Spring)*. 2007 Feb;15:340–348.

133. Sun X, Zemel MB. Calcitriol and calcium regulate cytokine production and adipocyte-macrophage cross-talk. *J Nutr Biochem*. 2008 Jun;19:392–399.

134. Zemel MB, Sun X, Sobhani T, Wilson B. Effects of dairy compared with soy on oxidative and inflammatory stress in overweight and obese subjects. *Am J Clin Nutr*. 2010 Jan;91:16–22.

135. Zemel MB, Stancliffe R. Dairy attenuation of oxidative and inflammatory stress in metabolic syndrome. *FASEB J*. 2010 Apr;24:105.3 (abstract).

136. van Meijl LE, Mensink RP. Effects of low-fat dairy consumption on markers of low-grade systemic inflammation and endothelial function in overweight and obese subjects: An intervention study. *Br J Nutr*. 2010 Nov;104:1523–1527.

137. Curry B, Biggerstaff J, Zemel MB. Effects of leucine and calcitriol on monocyte-vascular endothelial cell adhesion. *FASEB J*. 2010 Apr;24:230.5 (abstract).

138. Pal S, Ellis V. The chronic effects of whey proteins on blood pressure, vascular function, and inflammatory markers in overweight individuals. *Obesity (Silver Spring)*. 2010 Jul;18:1354–1359.

139. Pilvi TK, Seppanen-Laakso T, Simolin H, Finckenberg P, Huotari A, Herzig KH, Korpela R, Oresic M, Mervaala EM. Metabolomic changes in fatty liver can be modified by dietary protein and calcium during energy restriction. *World J Gastroenterol*. 2008 Jul;14:4462–4472.

140. Bruckbauer A, Zemel MB. Dietary calcium and dairy modulation of oxidative stress and mortality in aP2-Agouti and wild-type mice. *Nutrients*. 2009 Jul;1:50–70.

141. Warensjo E, Jansson JH, Cederholm T, Boman K, Eliasson M, Hallmans G, Johansson I, Sjogren P. Biomarkers of milk fat and the risk of myocardial infarction in men and women: A prospective, matched case-control study. *Am J Clin Nutr*. 2010 Jul;92:194–202.

142. Lorenzen JK, Astrup A. Dairy calcium intake modifies responsiveness of fat metabolism and blood lipids to a high-fat diet. *Br J Nutr.* 2011 Jan;31:1–10.

143. Bonthuis M, Hughes MC, Ibiebele TI, Green AC, van der Pols JC. Dairy consumption and patterns of mortality of Australian adults. *Eur J Clin Nutr.* 2010 Jun;64:569–577.

144. Goldbohm RA, Chorus AM, Galindo Garre F, Schouten LJ, van den Brandt PA. Dairy consumption and 10-y total and cardiovascular mortality: A prospective cohort study in the Netherlands. *Am J Clin Nutr.* 2011 Mar;93:615–627.

145. van der Pols JC, Gunnell D, Williams GM, Holly JM, Bain C, Martin RM. Childhood dairy and calcium intake and cardiovascular mortality in adulthood: 65-year follow-up of the Boyd Orr cohort. *Heart.* 2009 Oct;95:1600–1606.

146. Kaluza J, Orsini N, Levitan EB, Brzozowska A, Roszkowski W, Wolk A. Dietary calcium and magnesium intake and mortality: A prospective study of men. *Am J Epidemiol.* 2010 Apr;171:801–807.

147. Elwood PC, Givens DI, Beswick AD, Fehily AM, Pickering JE, Gallacher J. The survival advantage of milk and dairy consumption: An overview of evidence from cohort studies of vascular diseases, diabetes and cancer. *J Am Coll Nutr.* 2008 Dec;27:723S–734S.

47 Lessons from the Use of Ephedra Products as a Dietary Supplement

Madhusudan G. Soni, PhD, FACN, FATS,
Kantha Shelke, PhD, Rakesh Amin, JD, LLM
and Ashish Talati, JD, MS

CONTENTS

INTRODUCTION

Sales trend of herbal products in the United States suggests a dramatic increase in the use of these products. According to industry reports, consumers spend approximately $14 billion a year on dietary supplements. It has been estimated that as many as 2–3 billion doses of dietary supplements containing ephedrine alkaloids were consumed each year in the United States (GAO, 1999; Andersen, 2000). Among the products containing ephedrine alkaloids, *Ephedra sinica* (ma huang) is the most commonly used plant source. Ephedrine and related alkaloids found in ephedra can also be produced synthetically. Ephedra products have been extensively used for weight loss, weight management, and/or energy enhancement. Dietary supplements containing ephedra extract generally contain 6%–8% ephedrine alkaloids.

Beginning in the 1990s, concerns over the safety of ephedra and products containing ephedra began to be publicly raised in the United States. The FDA received over a thousand reports of adverse effects (including over 100 deaths) related to consumption of ephedra-containing dietary supplements. Because of continued and growing health concerns over the years, on February 6, 2004, the FDA issued a final rule prohibiting the sale of dietary supplements containing ephedrine alkaloids (ephedra), and the rule became effective 60 days from the date of publication. Many advocates for the use of ephedra maintained that it was safe in low doses. The proponents of ephedra use challenged the FDA prohibition, and a federal district judge limited the scope of FDA's ban. However, the FDA argued to restore the ban. In 2006, after a legal challenge by an ephedra manufacturer, the U.S. Court of Appeals for the Tenth Circuit upheld the FDA's ban of ephedra (FDA, 2006). The objective of this chapter is to highlight the controversy surrounding the safety in the use of ephedra as a dietary supplement and lessons learned.

HISTORY OF EPHEDRA

Ephedra sinica is an herb that has been used in traditional Chinese medicine for over 5000 years and is considered the world's oldest medicine. It is used as a stimulant and for the management of bronchial disorders (Anonymous, 1995). Ancient Aryans from India discovered ephedra or *Soma* plant as an energizer-cum-euphoriant. The use of ephedra juice has been mentioned in the Rigveda (the oldest of sacred Sanskrit Vedas) for longevity (Mahdihassan, 1981; Mahdihassan and Mehdi, 1989). Historically, ephedra is recommended for colds and flu, coughing, wheezing, nasal congestion, fever, chills, headaches, edema, hyperhidrosis, and bone pains.

Ephedra, also known as ma huang, is an evergreen perennial herb native to central Asia and now widely distributed and cultivated throughout the temperate and subtropical zones of Asia, Europe, and the Americas. The *Ephedra* genus includes more than 40 species. A majority of these *Ephedra* species contain the alkaloid ephedrine (Chen and Schmidt, 1930; Leung and Foster, 1996). In 1885, the active ingredient ephedrine was isolated from the ephedra plant and was also chemically synthesized. Because of ephedra's pharmacological activity, its active ingredient ephedrine was recommended as the treatment of choice for asthma. Currently, standardized ephedrine/pseudoephedrine preparations are commonly used around the world in the treatment of asthma (Chen and Schmidt, 1930).

CHEMISTRY

The primary compound of interest in commercially cultivated ephedra plant species is the alkaloid, ephedrine. In addition to this, ephedra plants also contain other alkaloids. The yield of alkaloids in ephedra plants ranges from 0.5% to 2.5%, of which 30%–90% is ephedrine. In some ephedra species, pseudoephedrine has also been found. Generally, ephedrine and pseudoephedrine constitute more than 80% of the alkaloid content of the dried herb (Liu et al., 1993). Additional alkaloids found in ephedra include *N*-methylephedrine, *N*-methylpseudoephedrine, norpseudoephedrine, and norephedrine. Ephedrine in its natural form exists as the L isomer (levorotatory), while the synthetic compound is generally a racemic mixture of L and D isomers. Generally, the fruits and roots of the ephedra plant are devoid of alkaloids. The astringent taste of ephedra products is because of the large amounts of tannins present in the plant.

VARIATIONS IN ALKALOID CONTENT

The alkaloid content of the commercially available ephedra products varies considerably and depends on ephedra species, geographical location, parts used (aerial, stem, leaf, or a combination of stem and leaf), harvesting, and extraction techniques. Because of the natural variations in the alkaloid contents of ephedra plant, significant interproduct and intraproduct variability has been reported in the ephedra products (Betz et al., 1997; Gurley et al., 1997a,b, 2000). In a series of studies, Gurley et al. (1997a,b, 1998a,b, 2000) investigated the quantitative variations in alkaloid contents in commercially available ephedra products. The alkaloid content in these products varied by as much as fivefold, with different brands exhibiting lot-to-lot variations of over 44%–260%.

These investigators also noted that several commercially available ephedra products do not report the amount of ephedrine on the label (Gurley et al., 1998b, 2000). Total alkaloid content in ephedra products varied considerably and ranged from 0.0 to 18.5 mg/dosage unit. Gurley et al. (2000) also reported that the ephedrine and pseudoephedrine levels in these products also varied and ranged from 1.1 to 15.3 mg unit dose and from 0.2 to 9.5 mg/unit dose, respectively. Besides variations in alkaloid content, ephedra products may also contain intentionally added ingredients, such as guarana, St. John's wort, chromium picolinate, kola nut, white willow bark, diuretics, or cathartics. Additionally, herbal supplements have been shown to contain undeclared pharmaceuticals, toxic herbs, or heavy metals (Slifman et al., 1998; Gurley et al., 2000). Thus, it is likely that the differences in the alkaloid content, other ingredients, and contaminants found in ephedra products affect the pharmacological and toxicological action of these products.

PHARMACOLOGICAL ACTION OF EPHEDRA

For over 2000 years, ephedra has been used to treat bronchial asthma, cold and flu, chills, fever, lack of perspiration, headache, aching joints and bones, nasal decongestion, and cough and wheezing (Leung and Foster, 1996; Blumenthal et al., 2002). Ephedra is approved by the German Commission E for treatment of respiratory tract diseases with mild bronchospasms (Blumenthal et al., 2002). The use of ephedra preparations in the treatment of nasal decongestion due to hay fever, common cold, rhinitis, and sinusitis and as a bronchodilator in the treatment of asthma is also listed by the World Health Organization (WHO, 1999).

The pharmacological action of ephedra is dependent on its chemical composition and particularly on the levels of ephedrine. As ephedrine is the primary alkaloid present in majority of *Ephedra* species, the effects of ephedrine can represent the expected pharmacological action of ephedra. The pharmacological action of ephedrine has been extensively investigated in human and animal studies. Although the individual alkaloids have similar pharmacological activity, they vary significantly in potency (Cetaruk and Aaron, 1994) and thus alter the net effect. Lee et al. (1999, 2000) reported that the potency of adrenergic activity and cytotoxicity of ephedra extracts correlate with the ephedrine content. However, the cytotoxicity of all ephedra extracts could not be completely accounted for by their ephedrine content alone.

Both ephedrine and pseudoephedrine have been shown to target the adrenergic receptors, the same receptors targeted by adrenaline. The pharmacological action of ephedrine is comparable to amphetamine but at about one-fifth the potency. As a mixed sympathomimetic agent, ephedrine enhances the release of norepinephrine from sympathetic neurons and stimulates α- and β-receptors. Ephedrine stimulates heart rate and thus increases cardiac output. It causes peripheral constriction leading to an increase in peripheral resistance. Ephedrine is known to relax bronchial smooth muscle, and hence, it is used as a decongestant and for temporary relief of shortness of breath caused by asthma. The onsets of pharmacological effects of ephedrine are generally evident within an hour of ingestion. The alkaloids from ephedra are known central nervous system stimulants, and oral administration of a 50 mg dose of ephedrine has been shown to stimulate central nervous system (Bye et al., 1974).

In a number of studies, various cardiovascular effects attributed to ephedrine have been reported. In a double-blind study, Tashkin et al. (1975) reported that in patients with obstructive airway disease, ephedrine at a dose of 25 mg produces a significant increase in specific airway conductance 1 h following the ingestion. The heart rate was significantly increased at 2–5 h, and the bronchodilatory effect lasted for over 4 h. Hoffman and Lefkowitz (1990) reported that ephedrine stimulates the heart rate and cardiac output and variably increases blood pressure. In a double-blind study, Nuotto (1983) investigated psychophysiological effects of ephedrine in healthy volunteers. A single oral dose of ephedrine (25 mg) increased the heart rate and systolic blood pressure and reduced diastolic blood pressure without affecting psychomotor performance. Drew et al. (1978) reported that ingestion of a single dose of 60–90 mg of ephedrine produced a diastolic blood pressure of 90 mmHg and higher in healthy volunteers. A maximum change in heart rate of 12 beats/min was noted after ingestion of 90 mg ephedrine. A significant increase in blood pressure was noted at two to three times the recommended dose of 15–30 mg of ephedrine (Cetaruk and Aaron, 1994). Based on results from several single oral dose studies, Chau and Benrimoj (1988) attributed the discrepancies in cardiovascular effects to the studies' methodology with respect to parameters analyzed and the time intervals assessed.

CONTRAINDICATIONS OF EPHEDRA CONSTITUENTS

Ephedrine, the active ingredient of ephedra, is contraindicated to individuals with heart disease, hypertension, coronary thrombosis, impaired circulation of the cerebrum, glaucoma, diabetes, thyroid disease, autonomic insufficiency, pheochromocytoma, chronic anxiety/psychiatric disorders, or enlarged prostate (Dollery, 1991; Hoffman and Lefkowitz, 1996). Ephedrine is contraindicated for patients treated with monoamine oxidase (MAO) inhibitors as the combination may cause severe, possibly fatal hypertension (Dawson et al., 1995; Hoffman and Lefkowitz, 1996). Special populations such as neonates and breast-fed infants, pregnant women, children, and the elderly may be at increased risk of toxicity from ephedrine and related agents because of increased sensitivity to the effects of sympathomimetic stimulation. Anastario and Haston (1992) reported increased fetal heart rate and beat-to-beat variability following intramuscular administration of ephedrine for the treatment of maternal hypotension.

PHARMACOKINETICS

Ephedrine, the primary active ingredient of ephedra, is completely absorbed from the gastrointestinal tract within 2–2.5 h (Wilkinson and Beckett, 1968a,b). In humans, ephedrine is primarily excreted via urine, and within 24 h of administration, approximately 95% of the ephedrine may be excreted unchanged (55%–75%) or as metabolites (Dollery, 1991). The serum half-life of ephedrine is reported as 2.7–3.6 h (Pentel, 1984). Available studies suggest that the biotransformation of ephedrine takes place through aromatic hydroxylation, N-demethylation, and oxidative deamination pathways. Approximately 8%–20% of the administered ephedrine is metabolized by N-demethylation to norephedrine, while 4%–13% undergoes oxidative deamination, resulting in the formation of 1-phenylpropan-1,2-diol and further side-chain oxidation to benzoic acid and hippuric acid (Wilkinson and Beckett, 1968a,b; Sever et al., 1975). The pharmacokinetics of other ephedrine-related alkaloids in ephedra, including pseudoephedrine and phenylpropanolamine, are similar to ephedrine. As ephedrine contains ionizable groups, its urinary excretion depends on pH, with excretion increasing in acidic urine and decreasing in alkaline urine (Wilkinson and Beckett, 1968a,b; May et al., 1975).

Following oral ingestion, large interindividual variations in plasma levels of ephedrine have been reported. White et al. (1997) reported that absorption of ephedrine in normotensive subjects is much slower when given as a component of an ephedra product compared to its pure form. Comparative absorption of ephedrine following ingestion of pure ephedrine or ephedra products revealed that ingestion of an ephedra product had approximately twice the T_{max} (time to maximum plasma concentration). In a subsequent study by the same group, pharmacokinetic parameters for botanical ephedrine were found to be similar to those for synthetic ephedrine (Gurley et al., 1998a).

Haller et al. (2002) studied the pharmacokinetics and pharmacodynamics of a dietary supplement containing ephedra and guarana. In this study, 80 healthy adults ingested orally a single dose of a dietary supplement containing 20 mg ephedrine alkaloid and 200 mg caffeine. Following the administration, plasma and urine levels of ephedrine alkaloids and caffeine and heart rate and blood pressure were monitored for 14 h. The T_{max} for ephedrine and pseudoephedrine were similar (2.4 h), while the T_{max} of caffeine was shorter (1.5 h). The half-life of ephedrine was determined as 6.1 h. The plasma clearance and elimination half-lives of ephedrine, pseudoephedrine, and caffeine from this study were similar to values reported for drug formulations. The half-life of ephedrine and pseudoephedrine in one subject with a high urinary pH was prolonged. At 90 min after the ingestion, a significant increase in mean systolic blood pressure was observed, while at 6 h after the ingestion, the heart rate reached a maximum change of 15 beats/min above baseline. The investigators concluded that the disposition characteristics of botanical products are similar to their synthetic pharmaceutical counterparts.

HUMAN OBSERVATIONS

CLINICAL STUDIES

In several clinical studies, ephedrine has been extensively investigated alone or in combination with caffeine, particularly for its effect on body weight reduction. Ephedrine is taken along with caffeine as the combination has been shown to result in greater body weight decrease compared to ephedrine alone. Reduction in body weight following combined intake of ephedrine and caffeine has been attributed to both decreased food intake and increased energy expenditure (Malchow-Moller et al., 1981; Dulloo and Miller, 1986, 1987; Astrup et al., 1991; Daly et al., 1993; Toubro et al., 1993). None of the studies reported any serious, unanticipated toxicity.

In a multicenter, randomized, double-blind, placebo-controlled trial, Boozer et al. (2002) studied the safety and efficacy of an herbal supplement in a double-blind trial. A total of 167 subjects were randomized to placebo (84) or herbal treatment (83). Herbal treatment, ma huang (90 mg/day ephedrine) and kola nut (192 mg/day caffeine), was given to subjects for 6 months for weight loss. Alterations in blood pressure, heart function, body weight, and body composition were monitored. A significant beneficial effect on body weight, body fat, and blood lipids of the herbal supplement was noted. The herbal supplement produced no adverse events, and only minimal side effects consistent with the known pharmacological action of ephedrine and caffeine were noted. In a previous study by these authors, ingestion of a herbal dietary supplement containing 72 mg/day ephedrine alkaloids and 240 mg/day caffeine resulted in short-term weight and fat loss (Boozer et al., 2001). In both the studies, small persistent increases in heart rate without any evidence of cardiac arrhythmias were noted. In other studies, the increase in heart rate was also noted following acute treatment with ephedrine/caffeine (Astrup et al., 1991) or with ephedra (White et al., 1997).

In another 8 week study with an ephedra formulation (dose not specified), Kaats et al. (1994) also reported weight reduction without any significant changes in blood pressure or resting heart rates. However, the details of the study were limited. In a 2 week double-blind trial, Kalman et al. (2002) investigated the cardiovascular effects of an ephedra–caffeine supplement in 27 overweight healthy adults. In this study, the subjects were given ephedra (335 mg standardized for 20 mg ephedrine alkaloid), guarana (910 mg containing 200 mg caffeine), and bitter orange (5 mg synephrine). Ingestion of the supplement did not produce any noticeable cardiovascular adverse effects. Contrary to these observations, but based on adverse event reports, Haller and Benowitz (2000) and Samenuk et al. (2002) speculated a link between consumption of low levels of ephedra alkaloid and arrhythmias.

In a recent report, Shekelle et al. (2003) identified 52 controlled clinical trials of synthetic ephedrine or botanical ephedra used for weight loss or athletic performance. A meta-analysis was performed, in which weight loss clinical trials with at least 8 weeks of follow-up data were included. Studies of athletic performance were not included as these studies used a wide variety of interventions. The use of synthetic ephedrine, ephedrine plus caffeine, or ephedra plus botanicals containing caffeine was found to be associated with two to three times the risk of nausea, vomiting, psychiatric symptoms such as anxiety and change in mood, autonomic hyperactivity, and palpitations compared with placebo.

CASE REPORTS AND ADVERSE EVENT REPORTS

Several case reports on ephedra are available in the published case reports in the literature. Several cases of psychiatric illness are reported following consumption of ephedra (Capwell, 1995; Doyle and Kargin, 1996; Jacobs and Hirsch, 2000; Kockler et al., 2002; Tormey and Bruzzi, 2002). In addition to this, Zaacks et al. (1999) reported hypersensitivity myocarditis associated with ephedra use in a 39-year-old male. Powell et al. (1998) reported nephrolithiasis in a 27-year-old male using an energy supplement containing ephedra extract. Warner and Lee (2002) reported a case of Leber hereditary optic neuropathy in a patient using ephedra alkaloids at the time of onset. Vahedi et al. (2000) reported an ischemic stroke in a 33-year-old male who consumed ephedra extract together with creatinine monohydrate for bodybuilding. A Naval reservist taking high doses of *Ephedra sinica* was found to have high blood pressure (Wettach and Falvey, 2002). Theoharides (1997) reported the sudden death of a 23-year-old male, related to ingestion of an ephedra-containing drink. Autopsy revealed myocardial necrosis and cellular infiltration. Other case reports have described ventricular arrhythmias or myocardial infarction in individuals consuming supplements containing ephedrine (Onuigbo and Alikhan, 1998; Zahn et al., 1999; Pederson et al., 2001).

The case reports in the literature do not allow for determination of the overall incidence of different adverse events possibly associated with the use of ephedrine or for all of the patient populations that might be at risk from the use of these types of products. The available case reports support the notion that the use of ephedrine is contraindicated for individuals with a history of cardiovascular diseases, as ephedrine has been shown to have a pharmacologically stimulatory effect on heart rate and cardiac output. However, few case reports have been published describing serious adverse events in individuals without preexisting medical conditions. As ephedra-containing products may also contain other stimulants or may be consumed with other stimulants, the exact role of ephedra/ephedrine alkaloids in these adverse events has been difficult to determine.

In addition to the published case reports, a thousand of adverse reports were submitted by consumers and health-care workers to FDA or manufacturers of ephedra products. At least four groups independently reviewed the adverse event reports filed with the FDA or the manufacturers related to the use of supplements containing ephedra alkaloids to determine the risk to consumer from products containing ephedra. In an initial investigation, Haller and Benowitz (2000) reviewed 140 reports of adverse events of ephedra, which were submitted to the FDA between 1997 and 1999. Among these reports, 31% were "definitely" or "probably" related to the use of supplements containing ephedra alkaloids, and another 31% were deemed to be "possibly" related. Approximately 47% of the events involved the cardiovascular system and 18% were related to the central nervous system. The adverse events included hypertension, palpitations, tachycardia, or both stroke and seizures. Ten events resulted in death, and 13 events produced permanent disability. The investigators determined that the use of ephedra products might pose a health risk to some individuals.

Samenuk et al. (2002) also assessed adverse event reports filed with the FDA from 1995 to 1997. Of the 926 cases of possible ephedra-related toxicity, these investigators identified 37 serious cardiovascular events. In these cases, the use of ephedra was temporally related to stroke (16 reports), myocardial infarction (10), or sudden death (11). The use of ephedra was reported to be within the manufacturers' dosing guidelines in all serious cardiovascular events but one case. The investigators concluded that the use of ephedra is temporally related to stroke, myocardial infarction, and sudden death.

The Council of Responsible Nutrition (2000) also investigated a total of 1173 adverse events filed with the FDA. The database identified 69 reports of death following ephedra use. From the total of 1173 reports, 121 were selected for further evaluation and 47 were considered to contain serious adverse events that included cases of stroke and stroke-like symptoms (15), seizures (13), cardiac arrest (15), and two individuals who collapsed. Among the 121 cases, 8 were reports of death, 6 were cardiovascular, 1 occurred in an automobile accident, and 1 was a spontaneous abortion. Four of the six subjects were using ephedra with other performance-enhancing products, such as caffeine. Autopsy results revealed one patient had atherosclerotic cardiovascular disease and another had myocardial disease due to chronic catecholamine use. Of the six patients, one individual suffered from asthma. The report concluded that based on the available information, it was not possible to determine if there were any unexpected toxicological effects due to the ephedra-containing dietary supplements.

The Texas Department of Health received reports of over 500 adverse events, including seven deaths due to myocardial infarction or stroke in patients who consumed supplements containing ephedrine (CDC, 1996). One of the makers of ephedra-containing weight loss supplements has turned over nearly 1500 consumer complaints to the FDA. These complaints included 14 alleging serious adverse events of which 10 were strokes, 2 heart attacks, and 2 seizures.

The authors of RAND (2003) report reviewed 1820 case reports provided by FDA, and more than 18,000 consumer complaints reported to a manufacturer of ephedra-containing dietary supplements and 71 cases reported in the published literature. The authors stated that majority of the cases were not well documented, and hence, decisions could not be made about the potential relationship between the use of ephedra-containing dietary supplements or ephedrine and the adverse event. Of the available reports, a total of 241 cases from FDA, 43 cases from a manufacturer, and 65 cases from the published literature were analyzed. From these reports, adverse events with prior ephedra consumption included two deaths, three myocardial infarctions, nine cerebrovascular/stroke events, three seizures, and five psychiatric cases. Adverse events with prior ephedrine consumption included three deaths, two myocardial infarctions, two cerebrovascular/stroke events, one seizure, and three psychiatric cases. Approximately 50% of the events were noted in individuals 30 years of age or younger. Of the remaining cases, 43 cases were identified as possible events with prior ephedra consumption and 7 cases as possible events with prior ephedrine consumption. The findings of this analysis raise concerns about the risks posed by ephedra supplements. However, a majority of the case reports were not documented sufficiently to support an informed judgment about the relationship between the use of dietary supplements containing ephedra or ephedrine and the adverse event in question.

Story and Lessons

As early as 1995, FDA convened a special working group to evaluate the potential health effects associated with dietary supplements containing ephedrine alkaloids (FDA, 1995). Based on the group's recommendations, on June 4, 1997, the FDA proposed a rule to (1) limit the total daily intake of ephedrine alkaloids to 24 mg/day or 8 mg/6 h period, (2) require the label to state that the product should not be used for more than 7 days, (3) prohibit the use of ephedrine alkaloids with substances known to have a stimulant effect, and (4) require a specific warning label (FDA, 1997). The proposed rule was based on "serious illnesses and injuries, including multiple deaths, associated with the use of dietary supplement products that contain ephedrine alkaloids."

The FDA received over 15,000 comments in response to its proposed rule. The quality of scientific information and adverse event reports supporting the rule were challenged by the industry groups and the Small Business Administration's Office of Advocacy. The House Committee on Science asked the General Accounting Office (GAO) to examine (1) the scientific basis for FDA's proposed rule and (2) the agency's adherence to the regulatory analysis requirements for federal rule making (GAO, 1999). Following its investigations, the GAO concluded that although the FDA had justifiable concerns, the legitimacy of the adverse events reports as the basis of the FDA's recommendation was questionable.

Following the criticism, on April 3, 2000, the FDA withdrew certain provision of the proposed rules such as limiting the ingredient level and duration of use for these products (FDA, 2000). However, the FDA did not withdraw the proposed prohibition on the use of other ingredients with stimulant effects with dietary supplements containing ephedra alkaloids. Subsequent to the FDA's withdrawal, additional reports of adverse events and case reports on ephedra safety continued to appear (see "Human observations" section). Bent et al. (2003) reported that the use of products containing ephedra accounts for only 0.82% of herbal product sales; however, it represents for 64% of all adverse reactions to herbs in the United States. The investigators concluded that the use of ephedra poses a greatly increased risk of adverse reactions compared with other herbs. Because of increasing concern that the use of dietary supplements containing ephedrine alkaloids (ephedra) presents an unreasonable risk of illness or injury, on February 6, 2004, the FDA issued a final rule prohibiting the sale of supplements containing ephedra.

The advocates for ephedra challenged the ability of the FDA to ban ephedra completely without conclusively demonstrating danger at low doses. Based on inadequate safety data at lower doses, on April 14, 2005, a federal district court in Utah struck down the FDA ban on ephedra. The court determined that the use of a risk-benefit analysis by FDA was against the intent of Congress in passing the Food, Drug, and Cosmetic Act (Amin and Blumenthal, 2005). In 2006, following a legal challenge by an ephedra manufacturer, the U.S. Court of Appeals for the Tenth Circuit upheld the FDA's ban of ephedra (FDA, 2006). A majority of the evidence of ephedra risks is from higher use levels or combinational use with other stimulants. As FDA placed a universal ban, it would be unethical to conduct human studies of lower doses in order to establish safety.

The clinical trials on ephedra and its principal alkaloid, ephedrine, support the safety of ephedra, while the studies investigating adverse event reports and case studies (described earlier) raise concern about the risks associated with the use of ephedra (Haller and Benowitz, 2000; Samenuk et al., 2002). The adverse event studies do not establish a direct causal relationship between the injuries reported and the intake of ephedra. The adverse event reports are voluntary and anonymous and make the reporting system vulnerable. While some genuine adverse events may be under-reported, false reports can be included, creating erroneous information in the database. The differential conclusions drawn from the results of clinical studies and from the adverse event analysis raise an important question. Given that some of the adverse events probably reflect real problems, it is important to understand the other contributing factors. The adverse events of ephedra may be affected by other factors such as the dosage, duration, underlying sensitivity, simultaneous use of other stimulants, contaminants, inconsistent potency, or a combination of these factors. Some of these factors are discussed in the following.

Dosage, Duration, and User Demographics

The overuse (dosage and duration) of this dietary supplement because of its conceived benefits is quite possible. Thus, ephedra has a potential for abuse. User characteristics such as sex, age, and race/ethnicity can also affect the action of ephedra. Several reports of adverse events suggest the possibility of overusage of ephedra. Gurley et al. (2000) concluded that the increased incidence of ephedra toxicity results from accidental overdose, often prompted by exaggerated off-label claims and a belief that "natural" products are inherently safe (Gurley et al., 2000).

Specifications

Marketed ephedra products are subject to variations because of differences in plant species (strain), growth, harvest, and storage conditions. These variations are likely to yield markedly different quantities of active alkaloids, leading to difficulties for consumers trying to find standardized products. In one study, the total alkaloid content of ephedra products showed the actual levels from 0 to 18.5 mg/dosage unit (Gurley et al., 2000). Available information also demonstrates discrepancies between the label claim for ephedrine and the actual amount of ephedrine, and lot-to-lot variations in ephedrine content. These variables are likely to add to the differential pharmacological effects of ephedra. Recently, the U.S. Pharmacopeia (USP) has initiated a service to test and certify dietary supplements for ingredient contents and concentrations per label claim.

Individual Sensitivity

Interindividual differences in the response to ephedra have been reported. It is likely that some individuals may have inherent sensitivity to ephedra. It is also possible that peoples with special health challenges may react differently to ephedra. White et al. (1997) reported wide variations in the blood pressure of individuals taking ephedra.

Drug and Other Products Interactions

Because of the known pharmacological interactions between ephedra and other products, individuals with a history of a psychiatric illness, especially if treated with MAO inhibitors or other prescription drugs, must consult a qualified health-care provider before taking supplements. People with underlying heart conditions, hypertension, diabetes, or thyroid disease should avoid ephedra use as the combination of ephedra and caffeine or caffeine-containing herbs may lead to an increased heart rate and blood pressure (Tyler, 1994).

In summary, as a result of several well-publicized adverse events and the FDA action, dietary supplements containing ephedra generated a controversy. The sequel that leads FDA to ban the use of ephedra-containing dietary supplements and the challenge by manufacturers have some lessons for the scientific community, regulatory agencies, health-care practitioners, consumer advocates, marketers, and the civil courts. As a plant product, the content of its pharmacologically active constituents may be influenced by differences in species and strain, growth, harvest, and storage conditions. Additional factors, such as its perceived and desirable weight loss and bodybuilding effect, ephedra is also susceptible to a variety of adulterants, both economic and efficacious, are also likely to impact the safety. The simultaneous use of drugs, dietary supplements, alcohol, illicit substances, and certain foods (caffeine-containing products) can also influence the desired physiologic outcome. The adverse events of ephedra appear to be affected by several factors such as overuse, inconsistent potency (specifications), individual sensitivity, interactions with drugs and other products, contaminations, etc.

REFERENCES

Amin, R. and Blumenthal, M. (2005) Ban of dietary supplements containing low doses of ephedrine alkaloids overturned by District Court. *HerbalGram* 67:64–67.

Anastario, G. D. and Haston, P. (1992) Fetal tachycardia associated with maternal use of pseudoephedrine and OTC oral decongestant. *Journal of the American Board of Family Practice* 5:527–528.

Andersen, A. (2000) *Ephedra Survey Results: 1995–1999.* Survey Administered & Results Compiled by Arthur Andersen LLP prepared for the American Herbal Products Association, April 28, 2000.

Anonymous (1995) *The Ephedras,* The Lawrence Review of Natural Products, St. Louis, MO, November 1995, pp. 1–2.

Astrup, A., Toubro, S., Cannon, S., Hein, P., and Madsen, J. (1991) Thermogenic synergism between ephedrine and caffeine in healthy volunteers. A double-blind, placebo-controlled study. *Metabolism: Clinical and Experimental* 40:323–329.

Dent, S., Tiedt, T.N., Odden, M.C., and Shlipak, M.G. (2003) The relative safety of ephedra compared with other herbal products. *Annals of Internal Medicine* 38:468–471.

Betz, J. M., Gay, M. L., Mossoba, M. M., Adams, S., and Portz, B. S. (1997) Chiral gas chromatographic determination of ephedrine-type alkaloids in dietary supplements containing Ma Huang. *Journal of AOAC International* 80:303–315.

Blumenthal, M., Goldberg, A., and Brinckmann, J. (Eds.) (2002) *Ephedra Herbal Medicine,* Expanded Commission E Monographs, Boston, MA, pp. 110–117.

Boozer, C. N., Daly, P. A., Homel, P., Solomon, J. L., Blanchard, D., Nasser, J. A., Strauss, R., and Meredith, T. (2002) Herbal ephedra/caffeine for weight loss: A 6-month randomized safety and efficacy trial. *International Journal of Obesity and Related Metabolic Disorders* 26:593–604.

Boozer, C. N., Nasser, J. A., Heymsfield, S. B., Wang, V., Chen, G., and Solomon, J. L. (2001) An herbal supplement containing Ma Huang-Guarana for weight loss: A randomized, double-blind trial. *International Journal of Obesity and Related Metabolic Disorders* 25:316–324.

Bye, C., Dewsbury, D., and Peck, A. W. (1974) Effects on the human central nervous system of the two isomers of ephedrine and triprolidine and their interaction. *British Journal of Clinical Pharmacology* 1:71–78.

Capwell, R. R. (1995) Ephedrine-induced mania from an herbal diet supplement. *American Journal of Psychiatry* 152:647.

CDC (1996) From the Centers for Disease Control and Prevention. Adverse events associated with ephedrine-containing products—Texas, December 1993–September 1995. *Journal of American Medical Association* 276:1711–1712.

Cetaruk, E. W. and Aaron, C. K. (1994) Hazards of nonprescription medications. *Emergency Medicine Clinics of North America* 12:483–510.

Chau, S. S. and Benrimoj, S. I. (1988) Non-prescription sympathomimetic agents and hypertension. *Medical Toxicology* 3:387–417.

Chen, K. K. and Schmidt, C. F. (1930) Ephedrine and related substances. *Medicine* 9:1–117.

Council of Responsible Nutrition (2000) *Safety Assessment and Determination of a Tolerable Upper Limit for Ephedra*, Prepared by Cantox Health Sciences International, Bridgewater, NJ, pp. 1–169.

Daly, P. A., Krieger, D. R., Dulloo, A. G., Young, J. B., and Landsberg, L. (1993) Ephedrine, caffeine and aspirin: Safety and efficacy for treatment of human obesity. *International Journal of Obesity and Related Metabolic Disorders* 17(Suppl. 1):S73–S78.

Dawson, J. K., Earnshaw, S. M., and Graham, C. S. (1995) Dangerous monoamine oxidase inhibitor interactions are still occurring in the 1990s. *Journal of Accident and Emergency Medicine* 12:49–51.

Dollery, C. (1991) Ephedrine (hydrochloride). In *Therapeutic Drugs*, Vol. 1. (C. E. Dollery, Ed.), Churchill Livingstone, New York, pp. E26–E29.

Doyle, H. and Kargin, M. (1996) Herbal stimulant containing ephedrine has also caused psychosis. *British Medical Journal* 313:756.

Drew, C. D., Knight, G. T., Hughes, D. T., and Bush, M. (1978) Comparison of the effects of D-(−)-ephedrine and L-(+)-pseudoephedrine on the cardiovascular and respiratory systems in man. *British Journal of Clinical Pharmacology* 6:221–225.

Dulloo, A. G. and Miller, D. S. (1986) The thermogenic properties of ephedrine/methylxanthine mixtures: Animal studies. *American Journal of Clinical Nutrition* 43:388–394.

Dulloo, A. G. and Miller, D. S. (1987) Aspirin as a promoter of ephedrine-induced thermogenesis: Potential use in the treatment of obesity. *American Journal of Clinical Nutrition* 45:564–569.

FDA (1995) *Minutes of Special Working Group on Food Products Containing Ephedrine Alkaloids of the FDA Advisory Committee. October 11–12, 1995.* Food and Drug Administration. (Visited on December 12, 2002) http://www.cfsan.fda.gov/~dms/ds-ephe1.html

FDA (1997) Dietary supplements containing ephedrine alkaloids; proposed rule. *Federal Register* 62:30677–30724.

FDA (2000) Dietary supplements containing ephedrine alkaloids: Withdrawal in part. *Federal Register* 65:17474–17477.

FDA (2006) *FDA Statement on Tenth Circuit's Ruling to Uphold FDA Decision Banning Dietary Supplements Containing Ephedrine Alkaloids.* (Visited on August 2, 2011) www.fda.gov/bbs/topics/NEWS/2006/NEW01434.html

GAO (1999) *Dietary Supplements: Uncertainties in Analyses Underlying FDA's Proposed Rule on Ephedrine Alkaloids.* United States General Accounting Office. GAO/HEHS/GGD-99-90. (Visited on December 12, 2002) http://www.gao.gov/archive/1999/h299090.pdf

Gurley, B. J., Gardner, S. F., and Hubbard, M. A. (2000) Content versus label claims in ephedra-containing dietary supplements. *American Journal of Health System Pharmacy* 57:963–969.

Gurley, B. J., Gardner, S. F., White, L. M., and Wang, P. (1997a) Ephedrine Pharmacokinetics after the ingestion of commercially available herbal preparations of *Ephedra sinica* (Ma-huang). *Pharmaceutical Research* 14(Suppl. 11):S519.

Gurley, B. J., Gardner, S. F., White, L. M., and Wang, P. L. (1998a) Ephedrine pharmacokinetics after the ingestion of nutritional supplements containing *Ephedra sinica* (Ma huang). *Therapeutic Drug Monitoring* 20:439–445.

Gurley, B. J., Wang, P., and Gardner, S. F. (1997b) Ephedrine alkaloid content of five commercially available herbal products containing *Ephedra sinica* (Ma-huang). *Pharmaceutical Research* 14(11 Suppl. 1):S582–S583.

Gurley, B. J., Wang, P., and Gardner, S. F. (1998b) Ephedrine-type alkaloid content of nutritional supplements containing *Ephedra sinica* (Ma huang) as determined by high performance liquid chromatography. *Journal of Pharmaceutical Science* 87:1547–1553.

Haller, C. A. and Benowitz, N. L. (2000) Adverse cardiovascular and central nervous system events associated with dietary supplements containing ephedra alkaloids. *New England Journal of Medicine* 343:1833–1838.

Haller, C. A., Jacob, P., and Benowitz, N. L. (2002) Pharmacology of ephedra alkaloids and caffeine after single-dose dietary supplement use. *Clinical Pharmacology and Therapeutics* 71:421–432.

Hoffman, B. B. and Lefkowitz, R. J. (1990) Catecholamines and sympathomimetic drugs. In *Goodman and Gilman's the Pharmacological Basis of Therapeutics* (8th Edn.), (A. G. Gilman et al., Eds.), Pergamon Press, New York, pp. 213–214.

Hoffman, B. B. and Lefkowitz, R. J. (1996) Catecholamines, sympathomimetic drugs, and adrenergic receptors antagonists. In *Goodman and Gilman's the Pharmacological Basis of Therapeutics* (9th Edn.), (J. G. Hardman, L. E. Limbird, P. B. Molinoff, R. W. Ruddon, and A. G. Gilman, Eds.), McGraw Hill., New York, pp. 199–248.

Jacobs, K. M. and Hirsch, K. A. (2000) Psychiatric complications of Ma-huang. *Psychosomatics* 41:58–62.

Kaats, G., Adelman, J., and Blum, K. (1994) Effects of a multiple herbal formulation on body composition, blood chemistry, vital signs and self reported energy levels and appetite control. *International Journal of Obesity and Related Metabolic Disorders* 18:S145.

Kalman, D., Incledon, T., Gaunaurd, I., Schwartz, H., and Krieger, D. (2002) An acute clinical trial evaluating the cardiovascular effects of an herbal ephedra-caffeine weight loss product in healthy overweight adults. *International Journal of Obesity and Related Metabolic Disorders* 26:1363–1366.

Kockler, D. R., McCarthy, M. W., and Lawson, C. L. (2002) Seizure activity and unresponsiveness after Hydroxycut ingestion. *Pharmacotherapy* 21:647–651.

Lee, M. K., Cheng, B. W., Che, C. T., and Hsieh, D. P. (2000) Cytotoxicity assessment of Ma-huang (Ephedra) under different conditions of preparation. *Toxicological Sciences* 56:424–430.

Lee, M. K., Wong, Y. K., Che, C. T., and Hsieh, D. P. H. (1999) Adrenergic agonists effects and cyto-toxicity of Chinese ephedra (Ma-huang) used for weight reduction. *Toxicologist* 48(1S):58.

Leung, A. Y. and Foster, S. (1996) Ephedra. In *Encyclopedia of Common Natural Ingredients Used in Foods, Drugs and Cosmetics*, John Wiley & Sons Inc., New York, p. 227.

Liu, Y. M., Sheu, S. J., Chiou, S. H., Chang, S. C., and Chen, Y. P. (1993) A comparative study on commercial samples of *Ephedrae herba*. *Planta Medica* 59:376–378.

Mahdihassan, S. (1981) The tradition of alchemy in India. *American Journal of Chinese Medicine* 9:23–33.

Mahdihassan, S. and Mehdi, F. S. (1989) Soma of the Rigveda and an attempt to identify it. *American Journal of Chinese Medicine* 17:1–8.

Malchow-Moller, A., Larsen, S., Hey, H., Stokholm, K. H., Juhl, E., and Quaade, F. (1981) Ephedrine as an anorectic: The story of 'Elsinore pill'. *International Journal of Obesity* 5:183–187.

May, C. S., Paterson, J. W., Spiro, S. G., and Johnson, A. J. (1975) Intravenous infusion of salbutamol in the treatment of asthma. *British Journal of Clinical Pharmacology* 2:503–508.

Nuotto, E. (1983) Psychomotor, physiological and cognitive effects of scopolamine and ephedrine in healthy man. *European Journal of Clinical Pharmacology* 24:603–609.

Onuigbo, M. and Alikhan, M. (1998) Over-the-counter sympathomimetics: A risk factor for cardiac arrhythmias in pregnancy. *Southern Medical Journal* 91:1153–1155.

Pederson, K. J., Kuntz, D. H., and Garbe, G. J. (2001) Acute myocardial ischemia associated with ingestion of bupropion and pseudoephedrine in a 21-year-old man. *Canadian Journal of Cardiology* 17:599–601.

Pentel, P. (1984) Toxicity of over-the-counter stimulants. *JAMA* 252:1898–1903.

Powell, T., Hsu, F. F., Turk, J., and Hruska, K. (1998) Ma-huang strikes again: Ephedrine nephrolithiasis. *American Journal of Kidney Diseases* 32:153–159.

RAND (2003) Ephedra and Ephedrine for weight loss and athletic performance enhancement: Clinical efficacy and side effects. Evidence Report/Technology Assessment No. 76 (Prepared by Southern California Evidence-Based Practice Center, RAND, under Contract No 290-97-0001, Task Order No. 9), AHRQ Publication No. 03-E022, Agency for Healthcare Research and Quality, Rockville, MD, February 2003.

Samenuk, D., Link, M. S., Homoud, M. K., Contreras, R., Theohardes, T. C., Wang, P. J., and Estes, N. A. (2002) Adverse cardiovascular events temporally associated with Ma huang, an herbal source of ephedrine. *Mayo Clinic Proceedings* 77:12–16.

Sever, P. S., Dring, L. G., and Williams, R. T. (1975) The metabolism of (–)-ephedrine in man. *European Journal of Clinical Pharmacology* 9:193–198.

Shekelle, P. G., Hardy, M. L., Morton, S. C., Maglione, M., Mojica, W. A., Suttorp, M. J., Rhodes, S. L., Jungvig, L., and Gagne, J. (2003) Efficacy and safety of ephedra and ephedrine for weight loss and athletic performance. A meta-analysis. *Journal of American Medical Association* 289:1537–1545.

Slifman, N. R., Obermeyer, W. R., Aloi, B. K., Musser, S. M., Correll, W. A. J., Cichowicz, S. M., Betz, J. M., and Love, L. A. (1998) Contamination of botanical dietary supplements by *Digitalis lanata*. *New England Journal of Medicine* 339:806–811.

Tashkin, D. P., Meth, R., Simmons, D. H., and Lee, Y. E. (1975) Double-blind comparison of acute bronchial and cardiovascular effects of oral terbutaline and ephedrine. *Chest* 68:155–161.

Theoharides, T. C. (1997) Sudden death of a healthy college student related to ephedrine toxicity from a Ma Huang-containing drink. *Journal of Clinical Psychopharmacology* 17:437–439.

Tormey, W. P. and Bruzzi, A. (2002) Acute psychosis due to the interaction of legal compounds—Ephedra alkaloids in 'vigueur fit' tablets, caffeine in 'Red Bull' and alcohol. *Medicine, Science and the Law* 41:331–336.

Toubro, S., Astrup, A., Breum, L., and Quaade, F. (1993) The acute and chronic effects of ephedrine/caffeine mixtures on energy expenditure and glucose metabolism in humans. *International Journal of Obesity and Related Metabolic Disorders* 17(Suppl. 3):S73–S77.

Tyler, V. E. (1994) *Herbs of Choice: The Therapeutic Use of Phytomedicinals*, Pharmaceutical Press, New York, pp. 88–89.

Vahedi, K., Domigo, V., Amarenco, P., and Bousser, M. G. (2000) Ischaemic stroke in a sportsman who consumed Ma Huang extract and creatine monohydrate for body building. *Journal of Neurology Neurosurgery and Psychiatry* 68:112–113.

Warner, R. B. and Lee, A. G. (2002) Leber hereditary optic neuropathy associated with use of ephedra alkaloids. *American Journal of Ophthalmology* 134:918–920.

Wettach, G. E. and Falvey, S. G. (2002) A mysterious blood pressure increase in a drilling Naval reservist. *Military Medicine* 167:521–523.

White, L. M., Gardner, S. F., Gurley, B. J., Marx, M. A., Wang, P. L., and Estes, M. (1997) Pharmacokinetics and cardiovascular effects of Ma-Huang (*Ephedra sinica*) in normotensive adults. *Journal of Clinical Pharmacology* 37:116–122.

WHO (1999) Herba Ephedrae. *WHO Monographs on Selected Medicinal Plants*, Vol. 1, World Health Organization, Geneva, Switzerland, pp. 145–153.

Wilkinson, G. and Beckett, A. (1968a) Absorption metabolism and excretion of the ephedrine in man: II. Pharmacokinetics. *Journal of Pharmaceutical Sciences* 57:1933–1938.

Wilkinson, G. R. and Beckett, A. H. (1968b) Absorption, metabolism, and excretion of the ephedrine in man: I. The influence of urinary pH and urine volume output. *Journal of Pharmacology and Experimental Therapeutics* 162:139–147.

Zaacks, S. M., Klein, L., Tan, C. D., Rodriguez, E. R., and Leikin, J. B. (1999) Hypersensitivity myocarditis associated with ephedra use. *Journal of Toxicology (Clinical Toxicology)* 37:485–489.

Zahn, K. A., Li, R. L., and Purssell, R. A. (1999) Cardiovascular toxicity after ingestion of "herbal ecstacy". *Journal of Emergency Medicine* 17:289–291.

48 *Coleus forskohlii* Extract in the Management of Obesity

Muhammed Majeed, PhD

CONTENTS

INTRODUCTION

Coleus forskohlii Briq. is an aromatic herb from the family of mints and lavenders, which is indigenous to India. The herb has received a lot of attention over the past 40 years, from medical researchers, as the only significant plant source of forskolin, a bioactive compound with diverse pharmacological benefits. These research efforts helped to scientifically validate the versatile health benefits of this herb that have long been known in folk medicine. Interestingly, the roots of the plant have a long history of food use in India, in the form of a pickle or condiment.

The Sami/Sabinsa group pioneered the natural extracts of *Coleus forskohlii* (CF), for use in nutritional and cosmetic applications, in the early 1990s. These include forskolin-enriched extracts from the roots (trademarked ForsLean®, an award-winning ingredient) as well as extracts featuring an aromatic essential oil composition from the roots. Both types of extracts have clinically validated health benefits and are currently used in a wide range of dietary supplements and cosmetics. In another facet of research on forskolin, the group developed novel delivery systems for forskolin, paving the way for the use of the molecule as a natural drug, for example, in the management of glaucoma (Ocufors®). Earlier efforts by pharmaceutical companies were unsuccessful in this regard, because forskolin is insoluble in water.

To ensure a steady and reliable supply of CF roots, the Sami/Sabinsa group also pioneered cultivation efforts for the plant, based on varieties and techniques, developed through focused research, targeting the promotion of "green" practices and sustainability.

A major breakthrough in research on forskolin was the discovery that ForsLean (CF root extract) is a clinically effective natural ingredient in weight management.

A majority of ingredients available for weight management support are designed to decrease body weight or fat with little regard for, and often at the expense of, lean body mass. It is comprehensible that an increase in muscle mass upregulates the body's metabolism, as muscle requires energy to sustain its mass and in turn helps burn additional body fat throughout the day. This plays a major role in not only optimizing body composition more favorably but helps maintain body fat reduction. Based on preclinical studies, it was hypothesized that forskolin could possibly enhance anabolic (lean body mass–building) functions in the body to increase muscle mass. Subsequent clinical studies supported the positive effects of branded ForsLean in enhancing lean body mass, promoting fat loss, and improving the overall body composition.

COLEUS FORSKOHLII: ORIGIN AND BOTANICAL ASPECTS

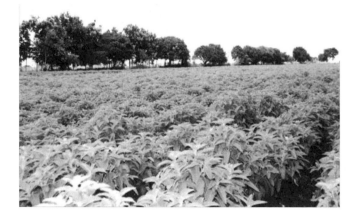

CF is available for centuries as a medicinal herb in India, which is also considered to be the place of origin. It grows in the wild in warm subtropical temperate regions of India, Nepal, Burma, Sri Lanka, and Thailand. Apparently, it has been distributed to Egypt, Arabia, Ethiopia, tropical East Africa, and Brazil as well. In India, wild CF is found mostly on the dry and barren hills. Latitudinal and altitudinal range for the occurrence of the species is between 8°–31°N and 600–800 m, respectively.[1]

TAXONOMIC POSITION

Coleus (genus) was first described by Loureiro in 1790, and the generic name was derived from the Greek word "coleos" meaning sheath.[1] The genus *Coleus* comprises of nearly 200 species distributed in the tropical and subtropical regions. About eight species of *Coleus* are recorded in India. It is classified along with 13 other genera under the subfamily Ocimoideae.[2,3] Of the 13 genera, *Plectranthus* is taxonomically closest to *Coleus*. Among the 200 species of

Coleus, only CF contains the most significant compound forskolin, and, therefore, this herb occupies a unique position in the chemical taxonomy of the family Labiatae (Lamiaceae).[2]

Coleus forskohlii Briq. (synonyms, *C. barbatus* Benth., *Plectranthus forskohlii* Willd., *P. barbatus* Andr.) belongs to the Lamiaceae family, popularly known as the mint or "Tulasi" family. CF is recorded in Ayurvedic *Materia Medica* under the Sanskrit name "Makandi" and "Mayani."[1] The taxonomical classification of *Coleus forskohlii* Briq. syn. *C. barbatus* Benth.[3] is as follows:

Kingdom	Plantae
Division	Magnoliophyta
Class	Magnoliopsida
Order	Lamiales
Family	Lamiaceae
Genus	*Coleus*
Species	*forskohlii*

Description[1,3]

CF is a perennial, branched, aromatic herb and grows to about 45–60 cm (1–2 ft high) tall, with a thick root stalk. It has four angled stems that are branched and nodes are often hairy.

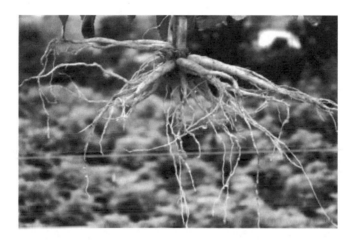

Leaves are 7.5–12.5 cm in length and 3–5 cm in width, usually pubescent, narrowed into petioles. Inflorescence is raceme, 15–30 cm in length; flowers are stout, 2–2.5 cm in size, usually perfect; calyx is hairy inside.

The root is typically golden brown, thick, fibrous, and radially spreading. Roots are tuberous, fasciculate, 20 cm long and 0.5–2.5 cm in diameter, conical fusiform, straight, orangish within.

CF has been used since ancient times in traditional medicine. The root portion of the plant has been used for medicinal purposes and contains the active constituent forskolin. Forskolin, a diterpenoid, was named after the Finnish botanist Forskel.[1]

TRADITIONAL AND ETHNOMEDICINAL USES

Traditional knowledge about medicinal plants remains a very important tool for treating illnesses. According to the World Health Organization (WHO, 2003), it has been estimated that approximately 80% of the world's population is dependent on traditional medicines for their health needs.[1]

Coleus forskohlii Briq. (family Lamiaceae) has several ethnomedicinal uses,[2] which have been transmitted by word of mouth from generation to generation. Historically, it has been used to treat heart diseases, respiratory disorders, insomnia, asthma, bronchitis, intestinal disorders, burning sensation, constipation, and skin diseases.[1]

In the northern parts of India, the paste of fresh roots of the plant is used by local people as topical application on tumors and boils. Ground fresh roots are mixed with mustard oil and are applied on eczema and skin infections.

In south India, the decoction of roots is used as a tonic by the tribals of Trichigadi (Kotas).

The plant is known to pacify vitiated pitta with benefits in supporting the management of fever, burning sensation, inflammation, muscular spasm, hypertension, diabetes, cardiac debility, allergy, anaphylaxis, high cholesterol, and bronchial asthma.[1]

The active phytochemical forskolin in CF was discovered in 1974 and has been the subject of many laboratory studies ever since. The compound has a vast array of effects on the body, working primarily on an enzymatic level, raising the level of cAMP (cyclic adenosine 3'5'monophosphate), a substance that activates a gamut of other cellular enzymes.[2]

CULTIVATION OF *COLEUS FORSKOHLII* FOR FORSKOLIN EXTRACTION

Medicinal plants form the major resource base of our indigenous health-care traditions. They have the additional advantages of simplicity, effectiveness, a broad spectrum of activity, and emphasis on preventive rather than curative drug action. Herbal remedies are fast becoming mainstream consumer products manufactured by multinational corporations among others and sold in supermarket chains and a variety of outlets worldwide. Another parallel development is the incorporation of herbs into an increasing number of health foods and dietary products. Studies have shown that medicinal plants have contributed considerably to economic welfare of people by providing and generating reasonable income.

Moreover, export of value added items requires product development, setting up of processing facilities, and quality assurance. Increasing concerns of unsustainable collection from the wild, disappearance of certain species on one hand, and concerns of quality and standardization on the other make it imperative to promote cultivation of species critical to herbal industry.

Plant tissue culture, touted as the most dynamic discipline of biotechnology, is a versatile cloning technique that offers the benefits of scale, scope, and uniformity. In plant tissue culture, the harvesting of living cells from any plant part (*explants*) facilitates growth of new plants in the sterile laboratory environment under aseptic conditions. It allows exact replication in many locations on a large scale, that is, it can create multiple clones from a single explant. With the objective of becoming a technology-driven, environmentally responsible manufacturer of herbal ingredients and to maintain a sustainable source of herbal raw materials, Sami Labs has adopted tissue culture as an enabling technology for its key raw materials. The adoption of plant tissue culture technology has ensured pathogen-free, disease-resistance, and high-yielding planting material in case of CF, which has helped to increase the yield, productivity, uniformity of produce, and reduced harvesting time and wastage.

Sami Labs has developed premium-quality planting material and established protocols for the micropropagation of *Coleus* by use of tissue culture technology. The "rooted cuttings" of *Coleus* developed through tissue culture technology have been transferred to the farmers and are reaping encouraging results.

The field performances of rooted cuttings and seedlings have been studied extensively. It has been found that vegetatively propagated planting stock had higher field growth performance than seedlings.[4,5] Rooted cuttings had good survival and grew well in the field.[6]

According to Kavitha et al. [1], CF is propagated by seeds as well as vegetatively by terminal stem cuttings.[1] Because seed propagation is difficult and slow, propagation by terminal stem cutting is easy and economical. Terminal cuttings of 10–12 cm length with three to four pairs of leaves are planted in nursery beds to induce rooting. When the 1 month old cuttings have produced sufficient roots, they are transplanted to the main field. The best period of planting in South India is during the month of June and July and during September to October. Rooted cuttings are planted at an interval of 60 cm. Proper irrigation methods, weeding, and plant protection should be adopted.[7]

The forskolin content of the roots obtained from natural habitats ranges from 0.04% to 0.60% of dry cell weight, 0.5% being most common.[8]

CHEMISTRY OF *COLEUS FORSKOHLII* ROOT EXTRACT AND ITS BIOACTIVE CONSTITUENT, FORSKOLIN

Forskolin: identity and nomenclature:

Chemical Abstract Number (CAS No): 66575-29-9.

Synonyms: Colforsin.

Chemical name: (3R, 4aR, 5S, 6S, 6aS, 10S, 10aR, 10bS)-5-(acetyloxy)-3-ethenyldodecahydro-6, 10, 10b trihydroxy-3, 4a, 7, 7, 10a, pentamethyl-1H-naphtho[2,1-b]pyran-1-one. It is also referred by the chemical name 7-β-acetoxy-8, 13-epoxy-1α, 6β, 9γ, trihydroxylabd-14-en-11-one.[9]

Chemical family: Forskolin belongs to the class of labdane diterpenoids. It contains three six-membered rings (one of them being a pyran ring) condensed in the form of a naphthopyran system. It has two secondary hydroxyl groups, one tertiary hydroxyl group, a keto group, and an O-acetyl group. It also has an exocyclic double bond (see Figure 48.1).

Diterpenoids that occur in plants contain 20 carbons from the assembly of four isoprene units (C20 unit). The four isoprene units assemble to form geranylgeranyl pyrophosphate in the plant, which is acted upon by several enzymatic pathways to lead to a variety of diterpenoids. Depending on the biosynthetic pathway, a wide diversity of linear as well as cyclized diterpenoids result in the plant kingdom. This rich structural variety is in turn manifested by a broad spectrum of biological and pharmacological actions of these diterpenoids.

Each structural variety of diterpenoids has yielded some familiar compounds in use today. An example of an acyclic diterpene is phytol, a simple reductive product from geranylgeraniol. The phytyl structural component occurs in chlorophyll and vitamin K and E structures. One of the famous cyclic diterpenoids is paclitaxel, a well-known anticancer agent, with a taxane skeleton. Another well-known diterpene is salvinorin A, active component of traditional medicine of Mexican Indians. Abietic acid is another example of a different diterpenoid skeleton. Forskolin belongs to the class of labdane diterpenoids, presumably arising from the quenching of labdanyl cation with water and further cyclization.

While two rings of forskolin are carbocyclic, the third ring is heterocyclic. Hence, it is usually associated with labdane bicyclic system. Forskolin skeleton is uniquely oxygenated, with each face of the molecule containing two hydroxyl groups, one of them being acetylated.

Unlike triterpenoids (C30 unit), the diterpenoids generally do not occur as glycosides. Thus, their functional groups such as hydroxylic groups especially are not glycosylated. Their occurrence without ligation with carbohydrates makes them generally highly water insoluble in their native form.

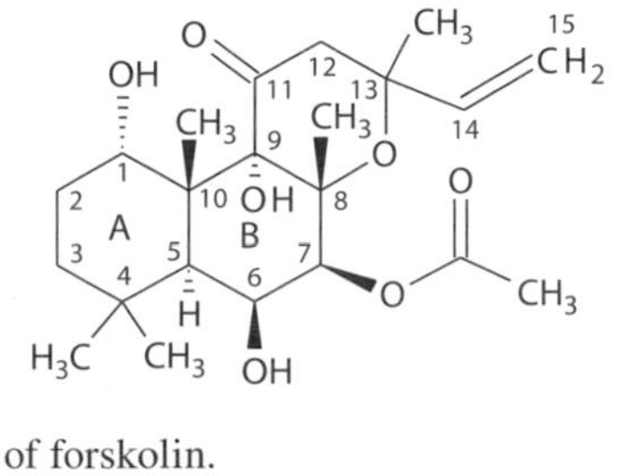

FIGURE 48.1 Chemical structure of forskolin.

Synthetic methods

The total synthesis of forskolin was achieved by starting from an ester aldehyde. Then the development of new carbon–carbon and carbon–oxygen bonds with enduring stereochemistry resulted from several key steps: a stereospecific intramolecular Diels–Alder reaction, a facially selective osmylation, a base-catalyzed intramolecular conjugate addition, a Lewis acid–mediated cuprate addition to a β-substituted dihydropyran-4-one, and a stereo- and regioselective allene photoaddition.[10]

Ester aldehyde Forskolin

Partial synthesis[11] (from 9-deoxyforskolin) and total synthesis[12] of (±) forskolin have been reported.

STEREOCHEMISTRY

The absolute stereochemistry of forskolin was determined by x-ray crystallography.[13] The trans stereochemistry of the A/B ring junction and of the β-configuration at C-10 was obtained from circular dichroism data on 14,15-dihydroforskolin and 1-oxo-analog. The change in cotton effect ($\Delta \Sigma$) values from −0.71, for the former, to −0.76, for the latter, was conclusive. The *cis* orientation of the C-1 and C-9 hydroxy groups was further confirmed by facile formation of the sulfite ester on treatment of forskolin with $SOCl_2$/pyridine.

Formation of the hemiacetal acetate via ozonolysis of 1,6-diacetyl-forskolin, followed by acetylation, provided additional data in support of the 13α-configuration of the vinyl group. Application of Mill's rule to the Δ^5-compound shown, $(M)_D + 347.17°$, derived by thionyl chloride/pyridine treatment of 1-methyl-forskolin, and to the corresponding deacetyl compound, $(M)_D − 32.03°$, established the β-configuration of the 7-acetoxy substituent.

Nuclear Overhauser effect difference spectroscopy (NOEDS) confirms the alpha-orientation of the 7-proton following irradiation at the 8β-CH_3 and the beta-orientation of the 1-proton following irradiation at 10β-CH_3. A two-dimensional correlated spectroscopy spectrum of forskolin has vividly reconfirmed the connectivities of the coupled protons. The absolute configuration of forskolin was finally confirmed by x-ray analysis of forskolin and of its 1-benzyloxy-7-deacetyl-7-bormoisobutyryl derivative.[14–16]

The other most abundantly present diterpene in the plant is 1,9-dideoxy-forskolin.[17] Subsequently, several closely related diterpenes have been isolated from the roots and aerial parts of the plant including stigmasterol.[18,19] Saleem et al. described an isolation procedure that yields 96.9% pure forskolin.[20]

ANALYTICAL METHODS

Many analytical methods have been developed to elucidate the characteristics and attributes of forskolin primarily because of its pharmacological value. A gas–liquid chromatography (GLC) method was developed for quantifying forskolin in plant tissues and in dosage forms.[21] Inamdar et al. [22] have reported the thin layer and high-performance liquid chromatographic (HPLC) methods. The GLC method had better sensitivity, but the HPLC method was found to be more rapid.[22]

SPECTROSCOPIC DETAILS

HPLC data of ForsLean (forskolin 10%) and HPLC, FTIR, mass, and NMR spectroscopic data of pure forskolin are being illustrated in the following section.

HPLC chromatogram of forskolin (pure)

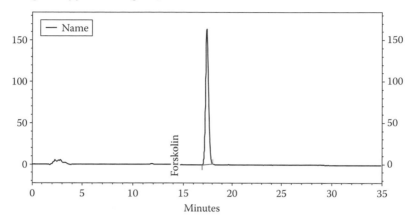

HPLC chromatogram of ForsLean (forskolin 10% extract)

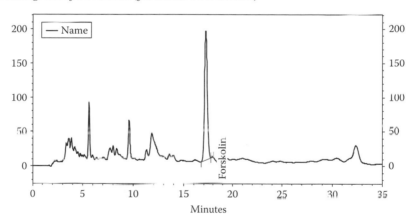

UV spectrum of forskolin (pure)

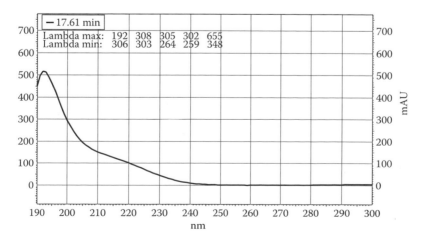

FTIR spectrum of forskolin (pure) in KBr

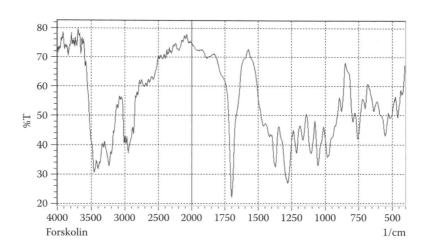

Forskolin

Mass spectrum of forskolin (pure)

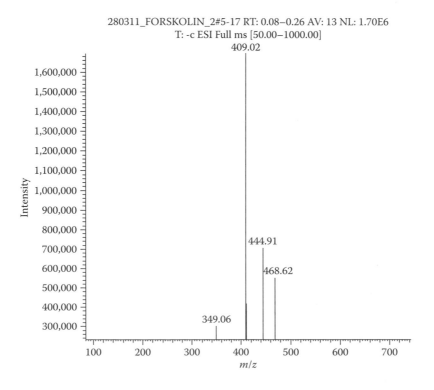

280311_FORSKOLIN_2#5-17 RT: 0.08–0.26 AV: 13 NL: 1.70E6
T: -c ESI Full ms [50.00–1000.00]

¹H NMR spectrum of forskolin (pure) in CDCl₃

Std. proton parameters
Automation directory:
Sample: FORSKOLIN
Pulse sequence: s2pul

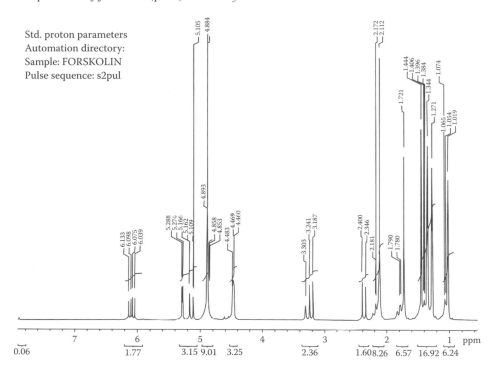

¹³C NMR spectrum of forskolin (pure) in CDCl₃

Std. carbon experiment
Automation directory:
Sample: FORSKOLIN
Pulse sequence: s2pul

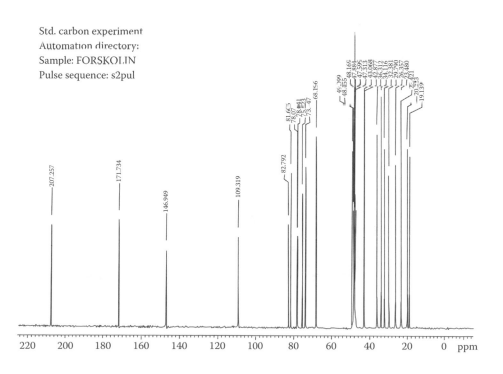

Forskolin, a diterpenoid compound (having a labdane chemical structure), is present in CF roots as the major component, along with isoforskolin, deacetylforskolin, 9-deoxyforskolin, 1,9-dideoxyforskolin, and 1-deoxy deacetyl forskolin.

Conventionally, forskolin is isolated from the roots of CF by hot extraction with solvents like ethyl alcohol, toluene, and similar organic solvents. The pasty oleoresin thus obtained (containing 7%–11% forskolin) is further purified by treatment with mixture of solvents to a brown powder containing 28%–32% forskolin. This powder is then crystallized using organic solvents to upgrade to 95% forskolin and then to an API grade of >98%.

Forskolin can be extracted using the following three processes, all of which have been used by Sami Labs in commercial processes. The current extraction is using continuous extraction technique.

1. Batch-wise solvent extraction
2. Continuous solvent extraction technique
3. Supercritical carbon dioxide extraction

Among these three processes, the continuous extraction process has several advantages over the other two processes, such as the following: (a) large tonnage of roots can be processed in a day, (b) solvent loss is much less, and (c) reduced batch cycle time.

BIOLOGICAL EFFECTS OF FORSKOLIN

Researchers in the early 1970s isolated forskolin from the roots of CF. The unique activity of forskolin as a nonadrenergic stimulator of adenylate cyclase attracted attention of medical researchers to start their work using forskolin in their research. Some of the pharmacological effects of forskolin that have been validated in preclinical and clinical studies are summarized in Figure 48.2.

Research on the *in vivo* effects of forskolin revealed a number of significant biological effects in animal models. Such effects were dose dependent and varied with the route of administration. Some of these researches are summarized here for general information purposes.

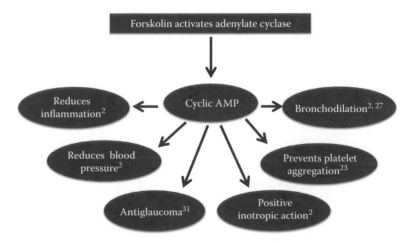

FIGURE 48.2   Spectrum of potential therapeutic activities of forskolin.

Cardiovascular Effects

Forskolin has significant effect on the cardiovascular system. Dohadwalla [2] reported the following:[2]

1. In the preliminary set of acute experiments using anesthetized cats, hypotensive effect was observed on intravenous (i.v.) administration of forskolin. The duration of action was 16 min when the i.v. dose was 50 μg/kg (Table 48.1).

   The cardiovascular responses to bilateral carotid occlusion and vagal and preganglionic sympathetic nerve stimulation to challenges with acetylcholine, epinephrine, norepinephrine, and isoprenaline were not affected by 2 mg/kg of forskolin given i.v. to anesthetized cats. These evidences suggest that the hypotensive action of forskolin may not be due to inhibition of central vasomotor tone or alpha or beta adrenoceptor inhibition.

2. The hypotensive effect of forskolin was studied in detail using normotensive anesthetized dogs.[2] Within 1–5 min of i.v. administration of 0.1 mg/kg of forskolin, a sharp fall in systolic and diastolic blood pressure of about 70 mmHg was recorded. Simultaneously, the left ventricular pressure (dp/dt) was increased from 3100 to 4100 mmHg/s. This steep rise in left ventricular pressure demonstrates its positive inotropic property. There was only marginal increase in heart rate. The duration of action lasted for about 30 min.

3. The hypotensive effect of forskolin was further investigated in conscious spontaneously hypertensive (SH) rats.[2] Forskolin, in doses ranging from 2.5 to 10 mg/kg given intraperitoneally (i.p.) daily for 5 days, showed dose-dependent fall in systolic blood pressure. At a dose of 10 mg/kg, the maximum fall of 48 mmHg in systolic blood pressure was observed on the third day of experiment.

The results obtained from these studies show that forskolin is a potent hypotensive agent in anesthetized cats, dogs, and conscious SH rats. The results also suggest the possibility that the hypotensive property of forskolin is due to its vasodilatory activity on peripheral resistance.

Dohadwalla [2] carried out perfusion studies to find out the underlying mechanism of the hypotensive action of forskolin. Experimental results suggest that the hypotensive action of forskolin may be due to its direct smooth muscle relaxation property. Forskolin stimulates adenylate cyclase, resulting in increase of cAMP levels in smooth muscles of peripheral vessels. This in turn mediates vasodilation and the ensuing hypotension.

Forskolin was also demonstrated to possess strong positive inotropic activity in isolated guinea pig heart (Langendorff) preparation.[2] The compound at a dose of 0.25 μg exhibits positive inotropic activity with marginal increase in the rate of contraction. The rate of coronary blood flow in the guinea pig heart was also increased at a dose of 2 μg of forskolin.

TABLE 48.1
Hypotensive Action of Forskolin in Anesthetized Cats

Dose (μg/kg)	Fall in Mean BP (mm Hg)	Duration (min)
50	49.7 ± 3.2	16.7 ± 2.1
100	63.7 ± 5.5	55.0 ± 3.9
250	72.2 ± 6.2	97.5 ± 5.6

In experiments using isolated guinea pig atrium and electrically driven left atrium and the papillary muscle of cat heart, forskolin produced dose-dependent positive inotropic effect. Results showed that this positive inotropic action is independent of its hypotensive action and is related to its adenylate cyclase stimulation property.

ANTI–PLATELET AGGREGATION ACTIVITY

From the experiments performed in male SH rats, it is evident that forskolin at doses ranging from 2.5 to 10 mg/kg given i.p. caused dose-dependent inhibition of ADP-induced platelet aggregation. A dose-dependent fall in systolic pressure was also observed. Thus, it is apparent that the percentage inhibition of ADP-induced platelet aggregation by forskolin is correlated with the magnitude of fall in systolic blood pressure.[2]

Siegl et al. [23] reported that inhibition of platelet aggregation is due to the elevation of intracellular cAMP.[23] Therefore, it can be reasonably assumed that the hypotensive and anti–platelet aggregation properties of forskolin are due to its ability to stimulate adenylate cyclase.

Forskolin inhibits the binding of platelet-activating factor (PAF) by directly binding to PAF receptor sites. Platelet-activating factor is a key factor in allergic and inflammatory pathways. It also acts on several membrane transport proteins and inhibits glucose transport in erythrocytes, adipocytes, platelets, and other cells.[1,24]

EFFECTS ON THE AIRWAYS/BRONCHODILATION

Forskolin relaxes guinea pig airways, both *in vitro* and *in vivo*.[2] Kreutner et al. [25] reported that forskolin blocked bronchospasms, the chief characteristic of asthma and bronchitis in guinea pigs caused by histamine and leukotriene C4.[25]

Forskolin, when administered i.v. in anesthetized guinea pigs, produced dose dependent abolition of bronchospasms induced by histamine, acetylcholine, and serotonin. It is suggested that the bronchospasmolytic effect may also be brought about through stimulation of adenylate cyclase.[2]

Marone et al. [26] reported that forskolin blocked the release of histamine and leukotriene C4 in human basophils and mast cells,[26] resulting in subsequent bronchodilation.[27]

Studies in dogs suggest that active ion transport across the airways epithelium toward the lumen can be enhanced by β-adrenergic agonists. In amphibian skin and rat colon, forskolin stimulated unidirectional transepithelial transport of sodium and chloride. Therefore, forskolin is likely to have similar effects in the airways. Higher water content of mucus secretion in lumen alters the viscoelastic properties of the mucus and thus facilitates mucociliary clearance.

Bauer et al. [23] reported that in a randomized double-blind placebo-controlled trial, patients with a single inhaled aerosolized dry forskolin powder (10 mg) showed a significant relaxation of bronchial muscles and relief of asthma symptoms compared to the placebo or fenoterol (0.4 mg).[28]

ANTI-INFLAMMATORY EFFECTS

Forskolin exhibits potent anti-inflammatory effect in various animal models. When administered i.p., forskolin significantly inhibited carrageenan-induced paw edema in a dose-dependent manner. Similar effects were also observed in croton oil–induced local inflammation and adjuvant-induced polyarthritis in rats. All these studies are reported in rats. However, the exact mechanism underlying these effects remains unclear.[2]

OCULAR EFFECTS

Neufeld and Sears reported that cAMP plays a pivotal role in mediating the action of catecholamines on aqueous humor dynamics and on the lowering of intraocular pressure (IOP).[29] Since forskolin has a distinctive ability to stimulate adenylate cyclase, the ocular effects of this molecule have attracted the attention of investigators.

ACUTE EYE IRRITATION STUDY

Forskolin ophthalmic solution (Ocufors), containing 1.05% forskolin and manufactured by Sami Labs Limited, was tested for its eye irritation potential in New Zealand white rabbits. A volume of 0.1 mL of the undiluted test item was instilled into the conjunctival sac of the left eye. Similarly, the placebo (blank) preparation was instilled into the conjunctival sac of the right eye. The effects on the conjunctiva, cornea, and iris were scored by Draize's evaluation method at 1, 24, 48, and 72 h postinstillation. Results indicated that Ocufors did not cause any irritation in the eye of the test animals.[30]

ANTIGLAUCOMA/INTRAOCULAR PRESSURE–LOWERING EFFECT

Several studies have demonstrated the effect of forskolin to lower IOP both in animals and humans. Caprioli and Sears [31] reported that forskolin suspension (1% forskolin) lowers the IOP in rabbits, monkeys, and humans by reducing the net aqueous inflow.[31]

The Sami Labs/Sabinsa research groups developed a stable aqueous formulation of forskolin (with patents granted in the United States and several other countries, pending approval in others) for use in the management of ocular hypertension and glaucoma. An Investigational New Drug Application for this product was successfully approved, with the product gone through clinical trials yielding positive results in relation to Timolol, the comparative standard drug. The product has since been approved for marketing in India by Drug Controller General of India (DCGI).

FORSKOLIN IN PROMOTING LEAN BODY MASS: MODE OF ACTION AND SUPPORTING RESEARCH

The primary mode of action of forskolin is by increasing the cellular concentrations of cAMP and cAMP-mediated functions via the activation of the enzyme adenylate cyclase.[2]

Adenylate cyclase is the enzyme involved in the production of cAMP, a very important molecule, known as "second messenger," referring to its broad range of activities in the body's life sustaining reactions. Normally, cAMP is formed when a stimulatory hormone (e.g., epinephrine) binds to a receptor site on the cell membrane and stimulates the activation of adenylate cyclase. The receptors on each cell are specific to the activating hormone. The unique feature of this activation is that the site of action of forskolin is the catalytic subunit of the enzyme or a closely associated protein and not the receptors. Of the nine types of adenylate cyclase in humans, forskolin can activate all except type 9, which is found in spermatozoa. Stimulation of adenylate cyclase is thought to be the mechanism by which forskolin relaxes a variety of smooth muscles.[1]

Forskolin appears to *bypass* the hormone–receptor interactions and activates adenylate cyclase. Adenylate cyclase activation induces a rise in intracellular cAMP levels.[2]

In many hormone-sensitive systems, the hormone itself does not enter the target cell but binds to a receptor and indirectly affects the production of another molecule within the cell, which then diffuses intracellularly to the target enzymes or a receptor inside the cell to produce the response. This intracellular mediator is called the second messenger. cAMP is a "second messenger" hormone signaling system. Therefore, cAMP and forskolin have marked physiological effects through such "second messenger" actions on various biochemical processes in the body.

The biochemical mechanism of maintaining or increasing lean body mass is related to the availability of cAMP. By facilitating hormonal action, cAMP may regulate the body's thermogenic response to food, increase the body's basic metabolic rate, and increase utilization of body fat (since thermogenesis is preferentially fueled by fatty acids derived from body fat and/or food).

Typically, an increase in cAMP levels leads to subsequent activation of protein kinase. Protein kinase has been shown to activate the hormone-sensitive lipase that is involved in the breakdown of triglycerides, known as building blocks of fatty tissue.[32]

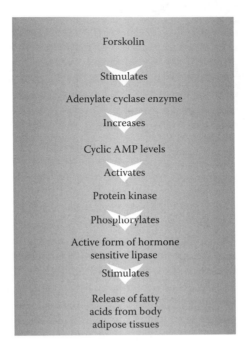

FIGURE 48.3   Mechanism of action of forskolin in promoting a healthy body composition.

The other factor relevant to the weight loss mechanism of forskolin involves its thyroid stimulating action, comparable in strength to thyrotropin or TSH.[33] The thyroid stimulating action of forskolin may also contribute to the increase in the metabolic rate and thermogenesis.

Forskolin may also be involved in regulating insulin secretion.[34] Insulin, although well recognized for its metabolism of carbohydrates, is also involved in the metabolism of fats and proteins that are major contributors to body composition (Figure 48.3).

In summary, forskolin increases cAMP levels, inhibits mast cell degranulation and histamine release, increases force of contraction of heart muscle, relaxes the arteries and other smooth muscles, increases insulin secretion, increases thyroid function, and increases lipolysis (breakdown of fat). The therapeutic implications of CF extract based on the pharmacological effects of forskolin are therefore immense.

SAFETY OF FORSLEAN AS A DIETARY INGREDIENT

Botanicals or phytomedicines have always been a major component of the traditional system of healing in developing countries and have been an integral part of their history and culture. But even though plants have a long history of use in Ayurveda and other traditional medicine, natural products or plant extracts are not altogether exempted from the quintessential safety evaluation. Ideally, rodents in adequate number of cohorts are employed for conducting suitable acute, subacute, and chronic toxicity studies from which toxicological information and data are collated that approve the test sample to be escalated for potential human use.

CF extracts and forskolin have an excellent safety profile and are generally considered safe, nontoxic, and without any side effects at the recommended dosage. Animal studies with forskolin indicate an extremely low order of toxicity for forskolin. Prolonged topical application of forskolin is well tolerated and is not associated with overt toxicity, as judged directly by behavioral observation or by growth and development, and was apparently found to be of no untoward clinical significance.

The safety of ForsLean for use as a dietary supplement was established by means of detailed toxicological evaluation of the product. Tests performed include the following:

- *Acute oral toxicity (LD$_{50}$)*:[35] Acute oral toxicity of CF extract 10% (ForsLean) was done in Sprague Dawley rats. The test substance suspended in 0.1% aqueous carboxymethyl cellulose was administered by oral route, and the experimental animals were observed for 14 days for product-related symptoms. The test substance did not produce any signs of toxicity after the dosing, and all animals survived the study period of 14 days. The LD$_{50}$ value of the test substance in rats by oral route was found to be greater than 2000 mg/kg body weight.

- *Subacute oral toxicity (28 Days)*:[36] Subacute oral toxicity was designed and conducted to determine the toxicity profile of CF extract 10% (ForsLean) when administered daily for 28 days in Sprague Dawley rats. The test substance suspended in 0.1% aqueous carboxymethyl cellulose was administered once daily to animals at various dose levels. Hematological and biochemical analysis were carried out at the end of the experiment. The test substance did not cause any signs of intoxication. Based on these findings, the no observed effect level (NOEL) of this product administered to rats over a period of 28 days was found to be 1000 mg/kg body weight for male and female animals.

- *Chronic oral toxicity (180 days)*:[37] Chronic oral toxicity study with CF extract 10% (ForsLean) was conducted in Wistar rats to examine toxicity and mortality profiles. Groups of 20 male and 20 female rats were subjected to daily administration of 10% forskolin by oral gavage for 180 days at the dose levels of 500 and 1000 mg/kg body weight. Clinical examinations were done daily. The clinical signs that were observed are abdominal breathing, wet perineum, diarrhea, and circling disorder. Results showed that there was no treatment-related mortality in rats treated with the substance at 500 mg/kg and at 1000 mg/kg body weight, and clinical results showed that there were no significant changes in the rats. Ophthalmoscopic and neurological examinations conducted did not show any remarkable changes or neurotoxic effects of the substance. Body weights of the treated rats did not change significantly and had the same level of food intake as the control group of animals.

  At the end of 3 months when the hematological tests were performed, rats treated with ForsLean at doses up to 1000 mg/kg were comparable to normal rats in all parameters. Hematological parameters measured were hemoglobin, packed cell volume, total and differential WBC counts, total RBC count, platelet count, and clotting time. The test substance also did not induce changes in plasma levels of total protein, albumin, alanine aminotransferase, aspartate aminotransferase, cholesterol, alanine phosphatase, glucose, creatinine, urea, urea nitrogen, total bilirubin, calcium, phosphorus, sodium, and potassium. Urine samples examined at the end of the study revealed that there were no significant differences between the treated and nontreated groups. Organ weights were also comparable to control, and the treatment did not induce any gross alterations in the tissues. Based on the findings of this study, it was concluded that the NOEL of ForsLean in Wistar rats, following administration for 180 days, was found to be greater than 1000 mg/kg body weight.

- *Single-dose oral toxicity in rats/LD$_{50}$ in rats*:[38] Single-dose oral toxicity study with CF extract 10% (ForsLean) was conducted in Wistar rats. Groups of five healthy male and five healthy female rats were dosed orally with CF extract at 2000 mg/kg body weight. The rats were observed 1, 2, and 4 h postdose and once daily for 14 days for toxicity, general behavior, and pharmacological effects. The animals were observed for mortality. Body weights were recorded immediately—pretest, weekly, at death, and at termination of the survivors. All animals were examined for gross pathology.

Results:

1. All animals survived the 2000 mg/kg oral dose.
2. Body weight changes were normal in seven tenths of animals. Three females lost weight during the second week of the study.
3. Necropsy results were normal in all animals.

Conclusion: The oral LD_{50} of CF extract 10% was found to be greater than 2000 mg/kg.

- *Coleus forskohlii bacterial reverse mutation assay of extract 10% with an independent repeat assay:*[39] Bacterial reverse mutation assay with CF 10% extract (ForsLean) was conducted using *Salmonella typhimurium* tester strains TA98, TA100, TA1535, and TA1537 and *Escherichia coli* tester strain WP2 *uvr* A in the presence and absence of Aroclor-induced rat liver S9.

The assay was performed in two phases using the plate incorporation method:

1. First phase, the preliminary toxicity assay, was used to establish the dose range for the mutagenicity assay.
2. Second phase, the mutagenicity assay (initial and independent repeat assays), was used to determine the mutagenic potential of the test article.

Dimethyl sulfoxide (DMSO) was selected as the solvent of choice based on compatibility with the target cells and solubility of the test article. Concentrations of 50–75 mg/mL were considered as workable suspensions.

In the preliminary toxicity assay, the maximum dose tested was 5000 μg/plate; this dose was achieved using a concentration of 100 mg/mL and 50 μL plating aliquot. Concentrations from 6.7 to 100 mg/mL were workable suspensions, concentrations from 0.67 to 2.0 mg/mL were soluble but cloudy solutions, and concentrations from 0.13 to 0.20 mg/mL were soluble and clear solutions. Neither precipitation nor appreciable toxicity was observed. Based on the findings of the toxicity assay, the maximum dose plated in the mutagenicity assay was 5000 μg/plate.

In the mutagenicity assay, no positive response was observed. Precipitation was observed beginning at 1800 or 3333 μg/plate in the presence and absence of rat S9 activation. Toxicity was observed in the initial mutagenicity assay at 5000 μg/plate with tester strain TA98 in the absence of S9 activation and beginning at 3333 μg/plate with tester strains TA100 and TA1535 in the absence of S9 activation.

The overall evaluation and dose ranges tested are as follows:

S9 Activation	Overall Evaluation and Dose Range Tested (μg/Plate)									
	TA98		TA100		TA1535		TA1537		WP2 *uvr*A	
	Low	High	Low	High	Low	High	Low	High	Low	High
None	Negative		Negative		Negative		Negative		Negative	
	25	5000	25	5000	25	5000	25	5000	25	5000
Rat	Negative		Negative		Negative		Negative		Negative	
	25	5000	25	5000	25	5000	25	5000	25	5000

Conclusion: CF extract (ForsLean) was concluded to be negative in the bacterial reverse mutation assay with an independent repeat assay (AMES test).

- *Repeated insult patch test:*[40] Repeated insult patch test was done using forskolin 2% w/w solution in wickenol. The study was performed with adherence to ICH Guideline E6 for Good Clinical Practice and requirements provided for in 21 code of federal regulations (CFR) parts 50 and 56 and in accordance to standard operating procedures and applicable protocols.

Fifty-six qualified subjects, male and female ranging in the age from 17 to 75 years, were selected. Forty-five subjects completed the study, and the observations remained within the normal limits throughout the test interval. Hence, forskolin 2% w/w solution in wickenol did not show dermal irritation or allergic contact sensitization.

In this context, topical forskolin has been used with success in the treatment of cellulite. Topical fat reduction in specific areas of the body is a common concern for women.[41] Ronsard popularized the term "cellulite" to describe the dimpling and "orange peel" external appearance of the thighs, the cause of which was attributed to the aging process by later researchers.[42] It has been postulated that the structure of subcutaneous adipose tissue accounts for the development of the "orange peel" appearance. Groups of fat cells are attached to the ventral side of the dermis by fibrous connective tissue. As fat cells enlarge, the fibers are stretched and pull down on the underlying skin. This causes the indentation or dimpling of the skin called cellulite. It has been demonstrated that adipose tissue metabolism varies from one region of the body to another; for example, in severely obese women losing weight after the jejunoileostomy, fat was seen to be absorbed or reduced more slowly in the thigh region than the abdominal region.[43] These differences lead to the hypothesis that localized application of forskolin triggers lipolysis or fat reduction.

Forskolin has been reported to potentiate topical fat reduction in combination with yohimbine and aminophylline.[44] This study proved that topical fat loss for women's thighs can be achieved without diet or exercise.

CLINICAL STUDIES WITH FORSLEAN IN PROMOTING LEAN BODY MASS

Abstracts of several studies are being presented in the following section, encompassing the lean body mass–promoting, antiobesity effects of ForsLean. Readers are reminded that the beneficial effects of forskolin are best obtained when the supplement is used in concurrence with a sensible diet and healthy lifestyle measures.

Study 1: Majced et al. [45]

Diterpene forskolin (Coleus forskohlii, Benth.): A possible new compound for reduction of body weight by increasing lean body mass

An extract of *Coleus forskohlii*, Benth. root standardized for diterpene forskolin (ForsLean) was tested in an open-field study for weight loss and lean body mass increase. The study's hypothesis was based on the recognized role of diterpene forskolin as a plant-derived compound, which stimulates the enzyme adenylate cyclase and subsequently cAMP (3'5'adenosine monophosphate). cAMP may release fatty acids from the adipose tissue depots, which may result in enhanced thermogenesis, loss of body fat, and theoretically increased lean body mass.

Six overweight, but otherwise healthy, women were selected for the trial. Each participant was informed about the purpose of the study and was asked to sign an informed consent before entering the study. Each participant was examined by a physician at the inception and after 4 and 8 weeks of the study. Their body composition was determined by bioelectrical impedance analysis. ForsLean was prepared in the form of two-piece hard-shell capsules. Each capsule contained 250 mg of the extract standardized for 10% forskolin. The participants were instructed to take one capsule in the morning and one in the evening, half an hour before a meal. They were asked to maintain their previous daily physical exercise and eating habits. In addition, physical activity was monitored based on a questionnaire before and during the trial. The study was performed in an outpatient bariatric clinic at Hilton Head, S.C., and supervised by a physician specializing in bariatric medicine for over 30 years.

During the 8 week trial, the mean values for body weight and fat content were significantly decreased, whereas lean body mass was significantly increased as compared to the baseline (Wilcoxon matched pairs test). Weight loss was statistically significant ($p < 0.05$) after 4 and 8 weeks, and the mean amounted to 4.3 and 9.17 lb, respectively. The body fat values expressed as % body fat were as

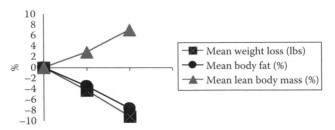

FIGURE 48.4 Open-field study, six overweight women subjects, 500 mg ForsLean corresponding to 50 mg forskolin/day for 8 weeks.

follows: 0 weeks, 33.63 ± 3.02; 4 weeks, 30.10 ± 4.34 (statistically not significant or n.s.); and 8 weeks, 25.88 ± 4.77 ($p < 0.05$). The lean body mass values expressed as % lean body mass were as follows: 0 weeks, 67.07 ± 3.02; 4 weeks, 69.90 ± 4.34 (n.s.); and 8 weeks, 74.13 ± 4.77 ($p < 0.05$) (Figure 48.4).

The 8 week therapy with 50 mg of forskolin per day did not adversely affect the systolic/diastolic blood pressure or the pulse rate. Systolic pressure (mm Hg) values were as follows: 0 weeks, 113.67 ± 14.50; 4 weeks, 110.00 ± 18.93 (n.s.); and 8 weeks, 104.50 ± 17.54 (n.s.). Diastolic pressure (mmHg) values were as follows: 0 weeks, 71.00 ± 12.76; 4 weeks, 69.33 ± 9.93 (n.s.); and 8 weeks, 66.00 ± 8.49 (n.s.). Pulse rates (beats/min) were as follows: 0 weeks, 66.33 ± 8.02; 4 weeks, 69.00 ± 7.97 (n.s.); and 8 weeks, 74.67 ± 11.55 (n.s.). These preliminary data obtained with 250 mg b.i.d. of ForsLean 10% extract indicate that this composition bears promise as a safe and effective weight loss regimen. The effect of ForsLean is particularly valid in the absence of change in frequency and intensity of physical exercise and without diet restrictions during the course of the trial. This study warrants a double-blind clinical trial evaluating the effects of forskolin on body composition and its possible thermogenic mechanism.

Study 2: Tsuguyoshi [46]

Clinical report on root extract of Perilla Plant (Coleus forskohlii) ForsLean® in reducing body fat: Asano Institute, Tokyo, Japan

A standardized extract of CF roots known as ForsLean (10% diterpene forskolin) was evaluated in a 12 week open-field study in overweight volunteers, 1 male and 13 females; average weight, 74.7 ± 11.98 kg; average BMI (body mass index), 29.9 ± 4.31; and average body fat, 38.2% ± 4.87%. ForsLean was administered in a dose of 125 mg twice a day. Total daily intake of ForsLean was calculated as 25 mg of diterpene forskolin. Each patient was examined in the physician's office, and body composition measurements were taken with an infrared analyzer Futurex 6200 on day 0, 1st, 2nd, and 3rd month. Total body weight showed tendency to decrease from an average 74.7 kg at the onset of the study to 73.5 kg on the 3rd month ($p < 0.05$). BMI improved from an initial average value of 29.9–29.4 ($p < 0.05$) at conclusion of the study. The body fat was decreased from an initial average value of 38.2%–37.1% ($p < 0.01$) at conclusion of the study. Lean body mass was preserved in the course of 12 week ForsLean administration (average 45.8 kg vs. 45.9 kg). The 12 week regimen with 25 mg of forskolin per day did not significantly change blood pressure parameters, that is, average systolic blood pressure, 135.7 mmHg versus 128 mmHg; average diastolic blood pressure, 85.3 mmHg versus 83.6 mmHg. This 12 week open-field study of ForsLean on 14 overweight Japanese subjects indicates its usefulness in weight loss management with no apparent subjective and objective side effects of the regimen.

Study 3: Krieder et al. [47]

Effects of Coleus forskohlii extract supplementation on body composition and markers of health in sedentary overweight female

In a double-blind and randomized manner, 23 females were made to supplement their diet with ForsLean 250 mg of 10% CF extract or a placebo group two times per day for 12 weeks. Body composition (dual energy x-ray absorptiometry—DEXA), body weight, and psychometric instruments were obtained at 0, 4, 8, and 12 weeks of supplementation. Fasting blood samples and dietary records (4 days) were obtained at 0 and 12 weeks. Side effects were recorded on a weekly basis. Data were analyzed by repeated measures ANOVA and are presented as mean changes from baseline for the CF and placebo groups, respectively. No significant differences were observed in caloric or macronutrient intake. CF tended to mitigate gains in body mass (-0.7 ± 1.8, 1.0 ± 2.5 kg, $p = 0.10$) and scanned mass (-0.2 ± 1.3, 1.7 ± 2.9 kg, $p = 0.08$) with no significant differences in fat mass (-0.2 ± 0.7, 1.1 ± 2.3 kg, $p = 0.16$), fat-free mass (-0.1 ± 1.3, 0.6 ± 1.2 kg, $p = 0.21$), or body fat ($-0.2\% \pm 1.0\%$, $0.4\% \pm 1.4\%$, $p = 0.40$). Subjects in the CF group tended to report less fatigue ($p = 0.07$), hunger ($p = 0.02$), and fullness ($p = 0.04$). No clinically significant interactions were seen in metabolic markers, blood lipids, muscle and liver enzymes, electrolytes, red cells, white cells, hormones (insulin, TSH, T_3, and T_4), heart rate, blood pressure, or weekly reports of side effects. Results suggest that CF may help mitigate weight gain in overweight females with apparently no clinically significant side effects.

Study 4: Bhagwat et al. [48]

A randomized double-blind clinical trial to investigate the efficacy and safety of ForsLean® in increasing lean body mass

Shri C. B. Patel Research Center for Chemistry and Biological Sciences, Mumbai, India

In a 12 week double-blind and randomized study, 60 overweight male and female volunteers, 25–45 years old with a BMI between 28 and 40 and/or body fat concentration above 30% in males and 40% in females, received 25 mg of diterpene forskolin b.i.d in the form of ForsLean (250 mg of 10% CF root extract) or a matching placebo. The volunteers receiving the ForsLean on average shed 1.73 kg or 4.02% of their total body weight, while the placebo group gained an average of 250 g (0.29%) of the total body weight. The volunteers treated with the placebo gained 0.32% of body fat, while the ForsLean group lost 0.87% of body fat. The difference in the weight and fat reduction was statistically significant between the active and placebo groups. The tests for thyroid function were performed, assessing levels of hormones T_3, T_4, and TSH before and after the completion of the study. It was observed that the levels of all three hormones remained within normal range in both active and placebo-treated groups after 12 weeks of the regimen. The blood lipid profile, performed at the onset and at the conclusion of the study, included triglycerides, total cholesterol, HDL, LDL, and VLDL. Ratio of total cholesterol to HDL was also calculated. At the end of 12 weeks, the placebo-treated volunteers did not show any significant change in any of the lipid parameters recorded. However, those volunteers on the active compound ForsLean showed a significant rise in the concentrations of HDL at the end of the study, while triglycerides, total cholesterol, LDL, and VLDL levels remained unchanged in this group as compared to baseline and placebo group levels (Figure 48.5).

In conclusion, based on this 12 week clinical study, ForsLean may be said to have a weight and fat reduction property. In addition, as compared with the placebo-receiving group, ForsLean may help preserve lean body mass. The 12 week treatment did not produce any subjective or objective side effects in the active compound. The laboratory data indicated that ForsLean regimen did not alter the thyroid hormones and blood lipid profile, with exception of increase in the HDL serum levels and significant decrease of total cholesterol/HDL ratio as compared to the control group.

Study 5: Godard et al. [49]

Body composition and hormonal adaptations associated with forskolin consumption in overweight and obese males

Department of Health Sports and Exercise Sciences, Applied Physiology Laboratory, University of Kansas, Specialized University Center, United States

A study published in the peer-reviewed medical journal, Obesity Research, reports that a dose of 250 mg of ForsLean twice daily significantly increased lean body mass and decreased body fat in obese male subjects (Figure 48.6).

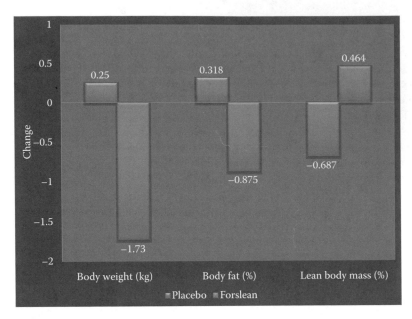

FIGURE 48.5 Change in body weight, body fat, and lean body mass of volunteers treated with ForsLean® and placebo. Change is statistically significant.

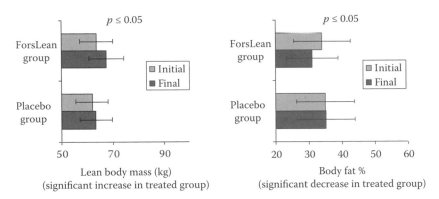

FIGURE 48.6 Changes in lean body mass and body fat ($n = 30$).

This randomized, double-blind, placebo-controlled 12 week study examined the effect of forskolin on body composition, testosterone, metabolic rate, and blood pressure in 30 overweight and obese (BMI $\geq$ 26 kg/m²) men. Fifteen subjects received ForsLean (250 mg twice daily) and 15 subjects received a matching placebo.

ForsLean administration elicited favorable changes in body composition by significantly decreasing body fat percentage and fat mass as determined by DEXA, compared with the placebo group ($p \leq 0.05$). *Additionally, forskolin administration resulted in an increase in bone mass compared with the placebo group* ($p \leq 0.05$). There was a trend toward a significant increase for lean body mass in the forskolin group compared with the placebo group ($p \leq 0.097$).

Serum free testosterone and total testosterone levels were significantly increased in the forskolin group compared to the placebo group ($p \leq 0.05$). The total testosterone increased 16.77% ± 33.77% in the forskolin group compared with a decrease of 1.08% ± 18.35% in the placebo group (Figure 48.7).

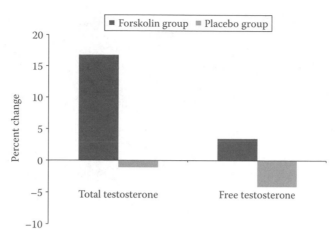

FIGURE 48.7   Percent changes in total testosterone and free testosterone levels.

Study 6: Kamath [50]

Efficacy and Safety of ForsLean® in Increasing Lean Body Mass

Department of Ayurvedic Medicine, Kasturba Medical College, Manipal, India

Fifty subjects, male and female, were randomized to receive 250 mg of ForsLean or placebo capsules twice a day (morning and evening) half an hour before meals for 12 weeks. A significant decrease in body weight and fat content and a significant increase in lean body mass were observed (Figure 48.8).

The mean percentage lean body mass increased by 1.78% in the ForsLean group, while the placebo group showed a mean decrease of 0.2% of LBM from baseline values. No significant changes in blood biochemistry profiles were observed in either ForsLean or placebo-receiving groups.

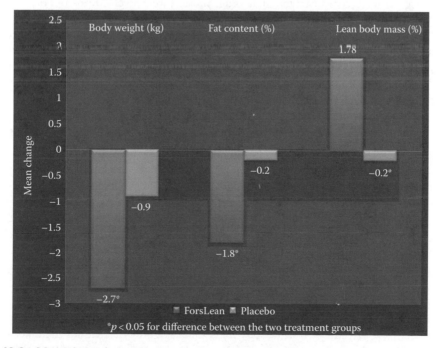

FIGURE 48.8   Mean change in lean body mass, fat content, and body weight ($n = 50$).

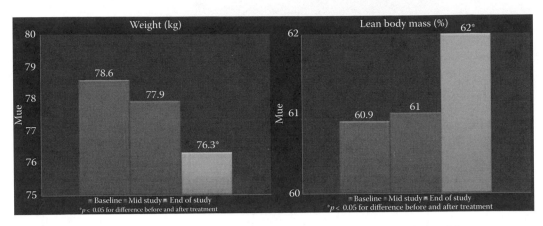

FIGURE 48.9   Effect of forskolin treatment on weight (kg) and lean body mass (%) ($n = 24$).

Study 7: Dr. Pankaj Gandhi and Dr. Parekh [51]

Body composition and hormonal adaptations associated with forskolin consumption in overweight and obese women

This clinical trial evaluated the effect of forskolin on the hormonal levels, particularly testosterone, and the BMD (bone mineral density), along with its effect on lean body mass and weight loss. The study was conducted with compliance to Good Clinical Practice guidelines (Figure 48.9).

Twenty-four obese female subjects, aged 25–35 years, and with BMI ranging from 28 to 45 (I degree to III degree obesity) were enrolled in the study. Subjects were assessed at baseline for demographic and baseline characteristics. Physical examination including blood pressure, weight, BMI, and % body fat measurement (using bioelectrical impedance monitor) were done. Laboratory tests like estrogen, progesterone, testosterone, luteinizing hormone (LH), and BMD were also recorded before the subjects received the study drug. Subjects were given 250 mg of ForsLean capsules twice daily half an hour before breakfast and dinner for 3 months.

The follow-up schedules were fixed at visit 1 (23rd day), visit 2 (46th day), visit 3 (69th day), and visit 4 (92nd day), that is, the final visit. Forskolin demonstrated a significant increase in lean body mass with a corresponding reduction in body weight, BMI, and fat content. There was no effect on hormonal levels or BMD. There were no significant differences across time for daily caloric intake as obtained with the dietary recall. There was no effect on blood pressure or heart rate with forskolin treatment. Neither the systolic nor the diastolic blood pressure showed any significant difference at baseline or during any of the follow-up visits. The good tolerability of ForsLean along with its weight loss efficacy makes it an attractive option in the treatment of obesity.

CONCLUDING REMARKS: FORSKOLIN IN WEIGHT MANAGEMENT

The active ingredient in ForsLean, forskolin, facilitates a cascade of biochemical events in the body that allows fat cells to be used as energy and helps utilize readily available hormones to maintain and/or increase lean body mass.

Specifically, forskolin activates adenylate cyclase, the main enzyme involved in the production of cAMP. cAMP is directly responsible for triggering essential lean body mass–building hormones at the expense of nonessential body fat.

Lean body mass is composed of muscle, vital organs, bone and bone marrow, connective tissue, and body water. The percentage of lean body mass to fat not only determines the body's aesthetic appearance but it is also an index of physical fitness, health status, susceptibility to disease, and premature mortality. Because the body's metabolic rate is directly proportional to the amount of lean body mass, there is substantial interest in products that safely increase lean body mass because they are most likely to work.

Forskolin effectively increases lean body mass and supports fat loss without manifesting the adverse side effects associated with ephedrine and synephrine, which have been used as weight loss agents. Ephedrine and synephrine (bitter orange extract) are sympathomimetics. They stimulate adrenergic receptors, which can increase blood pressure and pulse rate and lead to high blood pressure and anxiety. Ephedrine stimulates adrenergic receptors (which is the primary mechanism for ephedrine, even though this process is not totally accountable for its fat-burning effects) before it reaches cAMP. Unfortunately, many negative side effects can be experienced when some of these adrenergic receptors are stimulated, such as increased blood pressure, anxiety, and cardiovascular distress. Fortunately, forskolin is not a sympathomimetic agent; it bypasses the adrenergic receptors and stimulates the release of fatty acids by increasing cAMP levels directly. As evident from Figure 48.10, both ephedrine and forskolin can reduce adipose tissue. However, in essence, while their final results are similar, the mechanism of action for each differs significantly.

The safety and efficacy of ForsLean are evident from the results in more than seven clinical trials, which showed an overall trend to increase lean body mass and decrease body fat content, weight, and BMI (mean BMI).

ForsLean shifts the proportion between lean body mass and adipose, or fatty, tissue in favor of lean body mass, which improves overall health. The effect can be measured by decreases in the waist–hip ratio and the BMI.

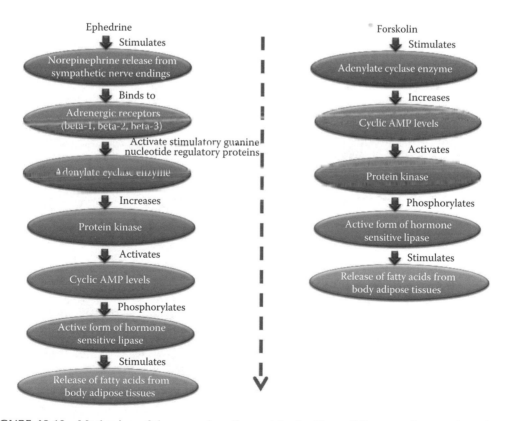

FIGURE 48.10 Mechanism of thermogenic action and its significant differences. Same end result, different pathways. (Adapted from an update on the world's most underestimated supplement for attacking body fat and increasing muscle mass...what is it, is it safe, and should you be taking it?, *Real Solutions Magazine*, Supplement Breakthrough. 2002.)

Although results vary from individual to individual and from study to study, ForsLean helps maintain healthy body weight. Participants in clinical trials shed between 2 and 9 lb over an 8–12 week period or did not gain body weight; more importantly, the participants preserved or increased their lean body mass as compared to the placebo-receiving group.

Based on the results in these studies, it is recommended that individuals desiring maximum benefits take products that contain 250 mg of ForsLean (standardized to 10% forskolin) approximately 30 min before meals twice daily. For best results, Sabinsa recommends integrating ForsLean with a sensible diet along with an exercise regimen lasting 30–45 min, at least 3–5 days a week. Based on effects in clinical studies, perceptible benefits are observed in 3–4 weeks on supplemental ForsLean.

ForsLean can also be used in conjunction with hydroxycitric acid (available in branded GarCitrin), L-carnitine, white kidney bean extract (Fabenol), and BioPerine® (a bioavailability enhancer) in multi-ingredient compositions for weight management support.

The safety of CF has been proved clinically, and so far, it has not been observed to cause any adverse reactions in humans. However, it is not recommended during pregnancy or for nursing/lactating mothers. Those with severe liver or kidney disease should probably avoid it until more research has demonstrated its safety during such conditions. It is contraindicated for ulcers. Those taking blood pressure medications, such as beta-blockers, clonidine, or hydralazine, or blood-thinning drugs, such as coumadin (warfarin), heparin, or Trental (pentoxifylline), should seek medical guidance before starting a forskolin regimen.

REFERENCES

1. Kavitha C, Rajamani K, and Vadivel E. (2010). *Coleus forskohlii*: A comprehensive review on morphology, phytochemistry and pharmacological aspects. *J. Med. Plant. Res.*, 4(4): 278–285.
2. Dohadwalla AN. (1985). Biological activities of forskolin. Edited by Rupp RH; Souza NJ; Dohadwalla AN—Proceedings of the International Symposium on Forskolin: Its Chemical, Biological and Medicinal Potential. Hoechst India Limited, Bombay, India, pp. 19–30.
3. Sastri BN. (Ed.). (1950). *The Wealth of India*, Vol. II. Council of Scientific and Industrial Research, Delhi, India, p. 308.
4. Rockwood DL and Warrag EI. (1994). Field performance of micropropagated, macropropagated, and seed-derived propagules of three Eucalyptus grandis ortets. *Plant Cell Rep.*, 13(11): 628–631.
5. Bergmann BA. (2003). Five years of Paulownia field trials in North Carolina. *New Forests*, 25: 185–189.
6. Emrah Çiçek, Fahrettin Tilki, Ali Kemal Özbayram, and Bilal Çetin. (2010). Three-year growth comparison between rooted cuttings and seedlings of fraxinus angustifolia and ulmus laevis. *J. Appl. Sci. Res.*, 6(3): 199–204.
7. Rajamani K and Vadivel E. (2009). Marunthu Kurkan—Medicinal Coleus. In: *Naveena Mulikai Sagupaddi Thozhil Nuttpangal*, Tamil Nadu Agricultural University, Coimbatore, India, pp. 17–22.
8. Vishwakarma RA, Tyagi BR, Ahmed B, and Hussain A. (1988). Variation in forskolin content in the roots of *Coleus forskohlii*. *Planta Medica*, 54: 471–472.
9. Merck. (2001). *The Merck Index* 13th edn. O'Neil, Ann Smith, Patricia E. Heckelman, and Susan Budavari. (Eds.).Merck & Co., Whitehouse Station, NJ, 2564p. ISBN 0-911910-13-1.
10. The total synthesis of forskolin, unique activator of adenylate cyclase. By Burton Humphrey Jaynes, Yales University (1988).
11. Ziegler FE et al. (1987). A synthetic route to forskolin. *J. Am. Chem. Soc.*, 109: 8115.
12. Hashimoto et al. (1988). Total synthesis of (±)-forskolin. *J. Am. Chem. Soc.*, 110: 3670.
13. Paulus EF. (1980). Molecular and crystal structure of forskolin. *Z. Kristallogr.*, 152: 239; Paulus EF. (1980). Molecular and crystal structure of 1-benzyl-7-desacetyl-7-bromoisobutyryl-forskolin. Absolute configuration of forskolin. *Z. Kristallogr.,* 153: 43.
14. Gross F. (February 4, 1972). In *Proceedings of Scientific*, Hoechst Pharmaceuticals Limited, Bombay, India, pp. 31–46.
15. de Souza NJ, Dohadwalla AN, and Reden J. (1983). Forskolin: A labdane diterpenoid with antihypertensive, positive inotropic, platelet aggregation inhibitory, and adenylate cyclase activating properties. *Med. Res. Rev.*, 3: 201–219.

16. Bhat SV et al. (1977). Structures and stereochemistry of new labdane diterpenoids from Coleus forskohlii Briq. *Tetrahedron Lett.*, 19: 1669.

17. Roy R et al. (1993). Minor diterpenes from Coleus forskohlii. *Phytochemistry*, 34: 1577–1580.

18. Khandelwal Y et al. (1989). Isolation, structure elucidation, and synthesis of 1-deoxyforskolin. *Tetrahedron*, 45: 763–766.

19. Shah VC, D'Sa AS, and de Souza NJ. (1989). Chonemorphine, stigmasterol, and ecdysterone: Steroids isolated through bioassay-directed plant screening programs. *Steroids*, 53: 559–565.

20. Saleem AM, Dhasan PB, and Rafiullah MR. (2006). Simple and rapid method for the isolation of forskolin from Coleus forskohlii by charcoal column chromatography. *J. Chromatograph.*, 1101: 313–314.

21. Inamdar PK, Dornauer H, and de Souza NJ. (1980). GLC method for assay of forskolin, a novel positive inotropic and blood pressure-lowering agent. *J. Pharm. Sci.*, 69: 1449–1451.

22. Inamdar PK, Kanitkar PV, Reden J, and de Souza NJ. (1984). Quantitative determination of forskolin by TLC and HPLC. *Planta. Med.*, 50: 30–34.

23. Siegl AM et al. (1982). Inhibition of aggregation and stimulation of cyclic AMP generation in intact human platelets by the diterpene forskolin. *Mol. Pharmacol.*, 21: 680–687.

24. Patel MB. (2010). Forskolin: A successful therapeutic phytomolecule. *East and Central African J. Pharm. Sci.*, 13: 25–32.

25. Kreutner W, Chapman RW, Gulbenkian A, and Tozzi S. (1985). Bronchodilator and antiallergy activity of forskolin. *Eur. J. Pharmacol.*, 111: 1–8.

26. Marone G, Columbo M, Triggiani M, Cirillo R, Genovese A, and Formisano S. (1987). Inhibition of IgE-mediated release of histamine and peptide leukotriene from human basophils and mast cells by forskolin. *Biochem. Pharmacol.*, 36: 13–20.

27. Lichey I, Friedrich T, Priesnitz M et al. (1984). Effect of forskolin on methacholine-induced bronchoconstriction in extrinsic asthmatics. *Lancet*, 2: 167.

28. Bauer K, Dietersdorfer F, Sertl K et al. (1993). Pharmacodynamic effects of inhaled dry powder formulations of fenoterol and colforsin in asthma. *Clin. Pharmacol. Ther.*, 53: 76–83.

29. Neufeld AH and Sears ML. (1975). Cyclic AMP in ocular tissues of the rabbit, monkey, human. *Invest. Ophthalmol.*, 14, 688–689.

30. Sami Report. (2003). Final report of the study: Acute eye irritation study with Forskolin Ophthalmic Solution in New Zealand white rabbits (study no. 3663/03) sponsored by Sami Labs Ltd., Bangalore 560 058 and conducted at the Toxicology Department of Rallis Research Centre, Bangalore, India.

31. Caprioli J and Sears M. (1983). Forskolin lowers intra ocular pressure in rabbits, monkeys and man *Lancet*, 30: 958–960,

32. Allen DO et al. (1986). Relationships between cyclic AMP levels and lipolysis in fat cells after isoproterenol and forskolin stimulation. *J. Pharmacol. Exp. Therap.*, 238(2): 659–664.

33. Haye B et al. (1985). Chronic and acute effects of forskolin on isolated thyroid cell metabolism. *Mole. Cell. Endocrinol.*, 43: 41–50.

34. Yajima H et al. (1999). cAMP enhances insulin secretion by an action on the ATP-sensitive K+ channel-independent pathway of glucose signaling in rat pancreatic islets. *Diabetes*, 48(5): 1006–1012.

35. Sami Report. (2003). Acute oral toxicity of RD/COL/M-21 (C-F) in Sprague Dawley rats (no. 9577) sponsored by Sami Labs Ltd., Bangalore and conducted at Indian Institute of Toxicology, Pune, India.

36. Sami Report. (2004). Subacute oral toxicity (study no. 9620 of C 31971) in Sprague Dawley rats sponsored by Sami Labs Ltd., Bangalore and conducted at Indian Institute of Toxicology, Pune, India.

37. Sami Report. (2005). Chronic oral toxicity study (180 days) of coleus forskohlii extract (10% forskolin) in wistar rat (study no 4719) sponsored by Sami Labs Ltd., Bangalore and conducted at Intox Pvt. Ltd., Pune, India.

38. Sabinsa Report. (2000). Single dose oral toxicity in rats/LD50 in rats (coleus forskohlii extract) sponsored by Sabinsa Corporation and conducted at MB Research Laboratories, Milford, PA.

39. Sabinsa Report. (2000). Bacterial reverse mutation assay with an independent repeat assay (coleus forskohlii extract) sponsored by Sabinsa Corporation and conducted at BioReliance Corporation, Rockville, MD.

40. Sabinsa Report. (2003). Repeated insult patch test on forskolin 2% w/w solution in wickenol (study no. C02-1103.03) sponsored by Sabinsa Corporation and conducted at Consumer Product Testing Co, Fairfield, NJ.

41. Ronsard N. (1973). *Cellulite: Those Lumps, Bumps and Bulges You Couldn't Lose Before*. Beauty and Health Publishing Co., New York.

42. Bayard E. (1979). *The Thin Game: Dieting, Scams and Dietary Sense*. New York Avon Books, New York.

43. Kral G et al. (1977). Body composition in adipose tissue cellularity before and after jejuno-ileostomy in several obese subjects. *Eur. J. Clin. Invest.,* 7: 414–419.

44. Greenway FL, Bray GA, and Heber D. (1995). Topical fat reduction. *Obes Res.,* 3(Suppl 4): 561S–568S.

45. Majeed M, Badmaev V, Conte AA, and Parker JE. (2002). Diterpene forskolin (coleus forskohlii, Benth.): A possible new compound for reduction of body weight by increasing lean body mass. *NutraCos.,* March/April, 6–7.

46. Tsuguyoshi A. (2001). Clinical report on root extract of Perilla Plant (coleus forskohlii) ForsLean® in reducing body fat. Ansano Institute [for Sabinsa Corporation], Tokyo, Japan.

47. Krieder R, Henderson S, Magu B et al. (2005). Effects of coleus forskohlii supplementation on body composition and hematological profiles in mildly overweight women. *J. Int. Soc. Sports Nutr.,* 2(2): 54–62.

48. Bhagwat AM, Joshi B, Joshi AS et al. (2004). A randomized double-blind clinical trial to investigate the efficacy and safety of ForsLean in increasing lean body mass. Shri C.B. Patel Research Center for Chemistry and Biological Sciences [for Sabinsa Corporation], Mumbai, India.

49. Michael P. Godard, Brad A. Johnson, and Scott R. Richmond. (2005). Body composition and hormonal adaptations associated with forskolin consumption in overweight and obese men. *Obes. Res.,* 13: 1335–1343.

50. Kamath MS Research Report. (2004). Efficacy and safety of ForsLean® in increasing lean body mass in class I obese subjects. Kasturba Medical College, Manipal, India.

51. Dr. Pankaj Gandhi, Dr. Parekh JR, Research Report. (2005). Body composition and hormonal adaptations associated with forskolin consumption in overweight and obese women, ClinWorld (P) Ltd., Mumbai, India.

Curcumin
Potential Role in Obesity and Obesity-Related Metabolic Diseases

Adeeb Shehzad, PhD and Young Sup Lee, PhD

CONTENTS

INTRODUCTION

The worldwide incidence of obesity has been rapidly increasing in the last two decades. According to a World Health Organization (WHO) report, obesity has been classified as a growing epidemic, and if immediate action is not taken, millions will suffer from an array of serious weight-related disorders. Obesity counts as a major health problem and a common chronic disease, affecting more than one in four of all Americans, including children, and its incidence has been steadily increasing in the last two decades. In health surveys conducted in the United States in 2005, 24.2% of men and 23.5% of women or over one-fifth of the respondents were classified as obese (Centers for Disease Control and Prevention 2005). Similarly, in the United Kingdom, a survey conducted in 2009 found that more than a quarter of adults were obese (26 percent of both sexes). In total, 68 percent of men and 58 percent of women were overweight or obese in the year (Health Survey of England 2009). According to German government statistics report, two-thirds of all German men between the ages of 18 and 80 are overweight; almost half of all women have weight problems, and more than 1 million of their youth show symptoms of eating disorders (http://EzineArticles.com/?expert=Vreel_Mistee). Several studies have shown that obesity is associated with an increase in mortality rates. Those persons who suffer from obesity have a 10%–50% increased risk of death from natural causes compared to those of normal healthy-weight individuals. This increased risk of death is due to the obesity-induced cardiovascular diseases, which accounts for about 112,000 deaths per year in the U.S. population, compared with healthy-weight individuals (http://www.cdc.gov/obesity/index.html).

Obesity arises when there is an imbalance between energy intake, principally stored as triglycerides (food consumption), and energy expenditure (basal metabolic rate and biochemical processes). The excess energy is primarily stored in adipose tissue in the form of triglycerides. When adipose tissue function is compromised during obesity, the excessive fat accumulation in adipose tissue, liver, and other organs predisposes the individual to the development of metabolic changes that increase overall morbidity risks (Spiegelman and Flier 2001, Flier 2004). Obesity is a complex trait influenced by diet, developmental stage, age, physical activity, and genes (Friedman 2000). Obesity is also a significant risk factor for major diseases, including type 2 diabetes, coronary heart disease, hypertension, and certain forms of cancer including gastrointestinal, ovary, breast, uterus, cervical, pancreatic, hepatic, kidney, multiple myeloma, and lymphoma (Barsh et al. 2000, Luchsinger 2006, Anand et al. 2008). In addition, the International Agency for Research on Cancer (IARC) used obesity prevalence data from Europe and relative risks from a meta-analysis of published studies had shown that obesity was a cause of 11% of colon cancer, 9% of postmenopausal breast cancer, 39% of endometrial cancer, 25% of kidney cancer, and 37% of esophageal cancer cases (Vainio and Bianchini 2002).

Curcumin [1,7-bis(4-hydroxy-3-methoxyphenyl)-1,6-heptadiene-3,5-dione], the active constituent of turmeric, has been used as a treatment for a wide variety of inflammatory ailments, including obesity and other metabolic diseases. Curcumin interacts directly with cyclooxygenase-2 (COX-2), DNA polymerase, lipoxygenase (LOX), glycogen synthase kinase-3β (GSK-3β), and cytokines (e.g., tumor necrosis factor [TNF]-α) (Shehzad and Lee 2010). It interacts indirectly with several transcription factors, including nuclear factor kappa B (NF-κB), activator protein 1 (AP-1), β-catenin, signal transducer and activator of transcription (STAT) proteins, and PPAR-γ (Shehzad et al. 2010a). Curcumin modulates multiple molecular targets and has potent anti-inflammatory activities, which might contribute to its therapeutic role in obesity and obesity-related metabolic diseases.

After summarizing the background epidemiological observations, this chapter details the evidence behind these various, often overlapping, mechanisms and briefly mentions curcumin's anti-inflammatory role in prevention and treatment of obesity and obesity-related metabolic diseases. It is hoped that this study will add new insights into the molecular pathways that are mediated by curcumin in obesity and may hold promise for future therapeutic intervention.

INFLAMMATION AND OBESITY-RELATED METABOLIC DISEASES

Inflammation is a major component of obesity that is associated with insulin resistance (Figure 49.1). Pharmacological or genetic inhibition of pathways that underlie inflammatory responses has been found to protect experimental animals and human subjects from diet-induced insulin resistance (Schenk et al. 2008). The subclinical or chronic inflammation has been recognized as being involved in the development of obesity, type 2 diabetes, and obesity-related atherosclerosis (Roberts et al. 2010). An important initiator of the inflammatory response to obesity is adipose tissue, which is involved in energy regulation and homeostasis. It is now understood that adipose tissue is not simply a storage depot for excess calories but that it also actively secretes fatty acids and a variety of polypeptides, which can function in an endocrine or paracrine fashion as well as sensitive to insulin. Thus, the mixture of adipokines secreted by adipose tissue in a given pathophysiological state is commonly associated with obesity. The adipose tissue consists of a variety of cell types, including adipocytes, immune cells (macrophages and lymphocytes), preadipocytes, and endothelial cells. Adipocytes uniquely secrete adipokines, such as leptin, adiponectin, and resistin, as well as inflammatory cytokines such as TNF and interleukins 1 and 6 (IL-1 and IL-6) (Scherer 2006, Halberg et al. 2008, Wang et al. 2008). These factors are critically involved in obesity-induced insulin resistance and chronic inflammation. It is proposed that TNF-α and IL-6 expression and secretion increased significantly in adipose tissue of obese subjects and were negatively associated with those of adiponectin. In 3T3-L1 and human adipocyte cultures, insulin strongly enhanced adiponectin expression (twofold) and secretion (threefold). It is believed that insulin upregulates adiponectin expression and that TNF-α opposes the stimulatory effects of insulin (Hajri et al. 2010). Studies have demonstrated the elevated levels of

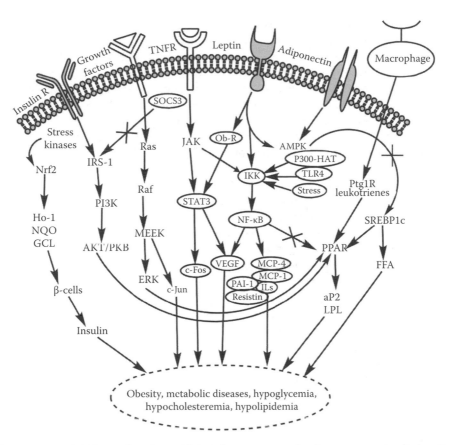

FIGURE 49.1 A model illustrating the multiple inflammatory molecular targets and cell-signaling complexes in obesity and insulin resistance. Cell-signaling intermediates indicated in circles are downregulated, without circles are upregulated, and crosslines indicate inhibition.

adipose IL-6 and TNF-α mRNA in obese subjects, and a decrease was observed in IL-6 and TNF-α with weight loss (Moschen et al. 2010). High TNF secretion from human adipose tissue was associated with decreased [3H] glucose incorporation into lipids (Lofgren et al. 2000). TNF phosphorylate S6K1 (p70S6K) is known to impair insulin resistance through serine phosphorylation of insulin receptor substrate (IRS)-1, which then inhibits the tyrosine kinase activity of the insulin receptor in adipocytes and hepatocytes (Zhang et al. 2008). In addition, dephosphorylation of serine in IRS-1 is also associated with the overexpression of the dual-specificity phosphatase MKP-4/DUSP-9 that was found to protect against stress-induced insulin resistance (Emanuelli et al. 2008). TNF also induces protein tyrosine phosphatase (PTP)-1B, which acts as a negative regulator of TNF signaling, and mice lacking PTP-1B are protected from TNF-induced insulin resistance (Nieto-Vazquez et al. 2008). Numerous studies have shown that a blockade of TNF receptor type 1–mediated TNF-α signaling protected Wistar rats from diet-induced obesity and insulin resistance (Liang et al. 2008). Moreover, circulating concentrations of inflammatory cytokines are considered to be the most important factors in causing and maintaining insulin resistance, although the normal mode of cytokine-mediated insulin resistance involves local paracrine effects and elevated levels of TNF-α, IL-6, and IL-1β. These inflammatory cytokines have been reported in obesity, insulin-resistant states, raising the possibility that tissue cytokines can leak into the circulation and impair insulin sensitivity in distal tissues through endocrine effects (Cai et al. 2005, Tarantino et al. 2010).

NF-κB is a transcription factor that widely acts as a regulator of genes that control cell proliferation and cell survival, as well as promote insulin resistance through inflammation and cytokine production. In adipocytes, inflammatory signals including TNF-α lead to an activation of IKK, which then phosphorylates the inhibitor of NF-κB (IkB). In the resting state, IkB forms a complex with NF-κB, restricting NF-κB to a cytoplasmic location. After phosphorylation, IkB dissociates from NF-κB and undergoes degradation. The released NF-κB translocates to the nucleus, where it binds to its specific DNA response elements, leading to transactivation of inflammatory pathway genes. Several studies have shown that lipid accumulation in the liver leads to hepatic inflammation through NF-κB activation and downstream cytokine production, which leads to insulin resistance hepatically as well as systemically (Shoelson et al. 2003, Ahn et al. 2008). Several studies have also demonstrated that toll-like pattern recognition receptors that play an important role in mediating proinflammatory effects of saturated fatty acids, particularly toll-like receptor 4 (TLR4), which induce insulin resistance through activation of NF-κB. TLR4 expression is increased in obesity, and when this receptor is deleted, saturated fatty acid induces inflammation, which is impaired in adipocytes and skeletal muscle cells (Shi et al. 2006, Reyna et al. 2008). Similarly, the other major intracellular proinflammatory pathways involved in obesity is c-Jun N-terminal protein kinase 1/AP-1 (JNK1/AP1) system (Bennett et al. 2003). In this pathway, external inflammatory signals lead to phosphorylation and activation of JNK, which then phosphorylates the N terminus of c-Jun on target genes. This induces an exchange of c-Jun dimers for c-Jun/c-Fos heterodimers, transactivating a set of inflammatory pathway genes, which substantially overlap with the set of genes transactivated by NF-κB (Ogawa et al. 2004, Huang et al. 2009).

PPARs belong to the super family of nuclear hormone receptors, which antagonize the activities of NF-κB, and have potential role in inflammatory conditions such as obesity. Among PPARs, PPAR-γ is a known molecular target in the treatment of type 2 diabetes, for all insulin-sensitizing drugs (Moller 2001). It has been observed that insulin resistance may be linked with downregulation of PPAR-γ by TNF. In addition, TNF induced NF-κB that blocks the PPAR-γ binding to DNA, by forming complex with PPAR-γ and its AF-1-specific coactivator PGC-2 (Suzawa et al. 2003).

A lot of compelling evidence has suggested that increased infiltration of macrophages in white adipose tissue (WAT) is also an important source of inflammation in obesity. Histological studies indicated that these macrophages are primarily localized to the intramuscular adipose depots, which accumulate within skeletal muscle in obesity. Many inflammatory and macrophage-specific genes are considerably upregulated in WAT in mouse models of genetic and high-fat diet-induced obesity (DIO). The upregulation is progressively increased in WAT of mice with DIO by macrophage-related inflammatory activities and contributes to the pathogenesis of obesity-induced insulin resistance (Xu et al. 2003). In summary, inflammation represents a major role in the progression of obesity toward insulin resistance.

CURCUMIN MOLECULAR TARGETS IN OBESITY AND METABOLIC DISEASES

In the last two decades, a huge amount of research has been published on curcumin, which revealed that it modulates many regulatory proteins, including those of transcription factors, enzymes, cytokines, and growth factors (Table 49.1). Studies have shown that curcumin inhibits a number of signaling pathways and molecular targets involved in inflammation and obesity-related metabolic diseases (Graham 2009). Curcumin can inhibit the IKK signaling complex that is responsible for the phosphorylation of IkB, thereby blocking improper activation of NF-κB induced by various inflammatory agents (Shehzad et al. 2010b). Antiobesity effects of curcumin are also linked with the inhibition of inflammatory and angiogenic biomarkers such as COX-2 and vascular endothelial growth factor (VEGF). Curcumin downregulates the expression of various proinflammatory cytokines including TNF-α, VEGF, IL-1, IL-2, IL-6, IL-8, and IL-12 by inactivation of the NF-κB. Studies have shown that curcumin treatment reduced the tumor-induced overexpression of COX-2 and serum VEGF in HepG2 groups significantly ($p < 0.001$), indicating that curcumin has potential role in angiogenesis (Yoysungnoen et al. 2006). In addition, curcumin has been shown to downregulate the expression of various NF-κB-regulated proinflammatory

TABLE 49.1

Molecular Targets of Curcumin in Obesity and Obesity-Related Metabolic Diseases

		References
Transcription factors	AP-1	Masamune et al. (2006)
	β-Catenin	Jaiswal et al. (2002)
	GATA4	Morimoto et al. (2008)
	NF-κB	Woo et al. (2007)
	Nrf2	Balogun et al. (2003)
	PPAR-γ	Lee et al. (2009)
	STAT	Wang et al. (2009)
	SREBP-2	Kang and Chen (2009)
Adipokines	TNF-α	Wang et al. (2009)
	Interleukins	Yoysungnoen et al. (2006)
	Leptin	Tang et al. (2009)
	Adiponectin	Ejaz et al. (2009)
	Resistin	Graham (2009)
	Monocyte chemotactic proteins	Woo et al. (2007)
Enzymes	Arylamine N-acetyltransferases-1	Seo et al. (2008)
	COX-2	Yoysungnoen et al. (2006)
	Inducible nitric oxide synthase	Chiu et al. (2009)
	LOX	Shehzad and Lee (2010)
	Matrix metalloproteinases	Yoysungnoen et al. (2006)
	NADPH:quinine oxidoreductase	Balamurugan et al. (2009)
	Phospholipase D	Shehzad and Lee (2010)
	HO-1	Zheng and Chen (2006)
Growth factors	Connective tissue growth factor	Zheng and Chen (2006)
	EGF	Pendurthi and Rao (2000)
	Hepatocyte growth factor	Kang and Chen (2009)
	PDGF	Ramirez-Bosca et al. (2000)
	Transforming growth factor-β	Zheng and Chen (2006)
	VEGF	Yoysungnoen et al. (2006)
Kinases	AMPK	Lee et al. (2009)
	Focal adhesion kinase	Zheng and Chen (2006)
	Glycerol-3-phosphate acyltransferase 1	Seo et al. (2008)
	Protein kinases	Ejaz et al. (2009)
	Protein tyrosine kinase	Masamune et al. (2006)
Receptors	Insulin receptors	Seo et al. (2008)
	Chemokine receptor 4	Woo et al. (2007)
	Epidermal growth factor receptor	Pendurthi and Rao (2000)
	Histamine 2 receptor	Graham (2009)
	Integrin receptor	Chiu et al. (2009)
	LDLR	Seo et al. (2008)
Others	Urokinase-type plasminogen activator	Pendurthi and Rao (2000)
	Triglycerides	Alwi et al. (2008)
	Plasma FFAs	Seo et al. (2008)
	Iron regulatory protein	Alwi et al. (2008)
	ARE	Balamurugan et al. (2009)

adipocytokines including chemokines (such as monocyte chemotactic proteins 1 and 4 [MCP-1, MCP-4] and eotaxin) (Woo et al. 2007). Curcumin was reported as an excellent inhibitor of β-catenin/TCF-LEF and hence reduced the β-catenin/TCF signaling, which is closely linked to obesity. This effect is mediated through the inhibition of the GSK-3β, which is responsible for the β-catenin phosphorylation (Jaiswal et al. 2002). Recent studies showed that curcumin-induced suppression of adipogenic differentiation in 3T3-L1 cells is accompanied by activation of Wnt/β-catenin signaling. During differentiation, curcumin restored nuclear translocation of the integral Wnt signaling component β-catenin in a dose-dependent manner. In parallel, curcumin reduced differentiation-stimulated expression of CK1α, GSK-3β, and axin, components of the destruction complex targeting β-catenin (Ahn et al. 2010). Several studies have also demonstrated the antioxidant role of curcumin in obesity. Transcription factors such as AP-1 are activated in response to stress, growth factors, and inflammatory cytokines. Curcumin can inhibit the stress-stimulated activation of AP-1 and has been shown to ameliorate oxidative stress–induced renal injury in mice (Okada et al. 2001). Curcumin in the dose of $10\,\mu M$ prevented the protein glycosylation and lipid peroxidation caused by high glucose levels in erythrocyte cell model. Curcumin inhibited oxygen free radical production caused by high glucose concentrations in a cell-free system and increased glucose utilization in erythrocytes (Jain et al. 2006). Numerous studies have indicated that curcumin reduces serum cholesterol concentrations by increasing the expression of hepatic low density lipoprotein (LDL) receptors; blocks oxidation of LDL, increased bile acid secretion, and metabolic excretion of cholesterol; represses the expression of genes involved in cholesterol biosynthesis; and protects against liver injury and fibrogenesis in animal models (Graham 2009). The hypocholesterolemic effect of curcumin was correlated with increase in LDL-receptor mRNA, whereas mRNAs of the genes encoding the sterol biosynthetic enzymes HMG CoA reductase and farnesyl diphosphate synthase were only slightly increased in human hepatoma cell line (HepG2). Although curcumin strongly inhibited alkaline phosphatase activity, an activation of a retinoic acid response element reporter employing alkaline phosphatase secretion was observed (Peschel et al. 2007). Moreover, curcumin has been identified as a potent inducer of heme oxygenase 1 (HO-1), a redox-sensitive inducible protein via regulation of nuclear factor E2-related factor 2 (Nrf2) and the antioxidant-responsive element (ARE), which provides protection against various forms of stress. Curcumin stimulates HO-1 gene activity through inactivation of the Nrf2-Keap1 complex, leading to increased Nrf2 binding to the resident HO-1 and AREs (Balogun et al. 2003). The early growth response (Egr-1) gene is a transcription factor that modulates the activity of plasminogen activator inhibitor type 1 that has been associated with insulin resistance and obesity. Curcumin inhibits the expression of the plasminogen activator inhibitor type 1 by reducing the activity of Egr-1 in obesity-related diseases (Pendurthi and Rao 2000). Several studies have shown that curcumin blocks the leptin signaling by reducing phosphorylation levels of the leptin receptor (Ob-R) and increases the induction of adiponectin, which improves obesity-associated inflammation (Tang et al. 2009, Weisberg et al. 2009). These findings support the existence of direct and indirect molecular mechanisms by which curcumin inhibits several inflammatory pathways that are responsible for obesity and obesity-related metabolic diseases.

CURCUMIN ROLE IN ADIPOCYTES

Several studies have shown the potential role of curcumin on angiogenesis, adipogenesis, differentiation, and apoptosis in adipocytes. Research evidence narrated that curcumin inhibits the differentiation of preadipocytes to adipocytes and adipokine-induced angiogenesis of human endothelial cell through suppression of VEGF-α. Curcumin treatment in C57/BL mice increased the fatty acid oxidation in adipocytes and also increased the activity of AMP-activated protein kinase (AMPK) by phosphorylating the α-subunit of AMPK, as well as suppressed the expression of amino-cyclopropane carboxylic acid by phosphorylation (Ejaz et al. 2009). Evidence reported the effect of curcumin in cancer and obesity and suggested that activation of AMPK by curcumin was crucial for the inhibition of differentiation or growth in both adipocytes and cancer cells. Curcumin-stimulated AMPK resulted in the downregulation of PPAR-γ in 3T3-L1 adipocytes and decreased the COX-2 expression. Application of a synthetic AMPK activator also supported evidence that AMPK acts as an upstream signal of PPAR-γ in 3T3-L1 adipocytes. It is suggested that regulation of AMPK and its downstream targets such as PPAR-γ, mitogen-activated protein kinase (MAPK), and COX-2 by curcumin appears to be important in controlling adipocytes and cancerous cells (Lee et al. 2009). Curcumin increased the insulin-stimulated glucose uptake in 3T3-L1 cells and suppressed the transcriptional secretion of TNF-α and IL-6 induced by palmitate in a concentration-dependent manner through the inhibition of NF-κB. It is concluded that curcumin reverses palmitate-induced, insulin-resistant state in 3T3-L1 adipocytes through the inhibition of NF-κB and JNK (Wang et al. 2009). In addition, curcumin enhances the expression of adiponectin in adipocytes, which inhibit NF-κB activation and negatively controls obesity (Weisberg et al.). Studies have also shown that curcumin significantly inhibited the cellular production of proinflammatory mediators such as TNF-α and nitric oxide and significantly inhibited the release of MCP-1 from 3T3-L1 adipocytes. Curcumin dose dependently inhibited phorbol myristate acetate (PMA)-induced MCP-1 expression by inhibiting ERK and NF-κB transcriptional activity in U937 cells (Lim and Kwon 2010). These studies suggest that curcumin can suppress obesity-induced inflammatory responses and modulate adipose tissue macrophage accumulation or activation (Woo et al. 2007).

CURCUMIN ROLE IN HEPATIC STELLATE CELLS

Curcumin inhibited HSC activation and intervened in liver fibrogenesis associated with hyperleptinemia in nonalcoholic steatohepatitis (NASH) patients. HSCs are the major effector cells during liver fibrogenesis and could be activated by leptin. Curcumin abrogated the stimulatory effect of leptin on HSC activation *in vitro* by reducing the phosphorylation level of Ob-R, stimulating PPAR-γ activity, and attenuating oxidative stress, which leads to the suppression of Ob-R gene expression and elimination of leptin signaling (Tang et al. 2009). Studies have also shown that curcumin inhibited LDL-induced HSC activation *in vitro* by repressing gene expression of the transcription factor sterol regulatory element binding protein-2 (SREBP-2) by activating PPAR-γ, thus reducing the specificity protein-1 (SP-1) activity, which leads to the repression of LDL receptor (LDLR) expression. Activation of PPAR-γ has been linked to the reduction in the level of intracellular cholesterol in HSCs and to the attenuation of the stimulatory effects of LDL on HSCs activation (Kang and Chen 2009). *In vitro* studies have also shown that activation of PPAR-γ is required for curcumin to induce apoptosis and to inhibit the expression of extracellular matrix (ECM) genes in HSC. Curcumin suppressed the expression of gene products regulated by PPAR-γ including α1 collagen, α-smooth muscle actin (α-SMA), connective tissue growth factor (CTGF), receptors for TGF-β, platelet-derived growth factor (PDGF)-β, and epidermal growth factor (EGF) (Zheng and Chen 2006). Recently, it has been shown that curcumin protected HSCs against leptin-induced activation by accumulating intracellular lipids. Curcumin eliminated the stimulatory effects of leptin on HSCs activation and increased AMPK activity, leading to inducing expression of genes relevant to lipid accumulation and elevating the level of intracellular lipids (Tang and Chen 2010a). The same researcher group also reported that curcumin prevents leptin from raising glucose levels in HSCs by blocking translocation of glucose transporter-4 (GLUT4) and increasing glucokinase. Curcumin prevented leptin from elevating levels of intracellular glucose in rat HSCs and immortalized human hepatocytes by inhibiting the membrane translocation of GLUT4 and inducing the conversion of glucose to glucose-6-phosphate (G-6-P), leading to the inhibition of HSC activation (Tang and Chen 2010b). These observations suggest a novel insight into mechanism of curcumin mediates its effects on HSCs through direct and indirect activation of PPAR-γ as well as by inhibiting leptin-induced HSC activation.

CURCUMIN ROLE IN PANCREATIC CELLS

Activated pancreatic stellate cells (PSCs) play a pivotal role in the pathogenesis of pancreatic fibrosis and inflammation. Curcumin decreased the pancreatic beta cell volume, which could be associated with hypoglycemic/antidiabetic effects of this agent. Curcumin inhibited PDGF-induced proliferation, α-SMA gene expression, IL-1β and TNF-α–induced MCP-1 production, type I collagen production, and activation of AP-1 in activated PSCs. Curcumin also inhibited PDGF-BB-induced cyclin D1 expression and activation of ERK (Masamune et al. 2006). Curcumin has been reported as potent inducers of phase 2 enzyme HO-1, via regulation of nuclear factor Nrf2 and the ARE in mouse beta cells. Curcumin stimulates HO-1 gene activity, which is correlated with the increase in the expression of glutamyl cysteine ligase (GCL) needed for glutathione (GSH) biosynthesis and NADPH2:quinone reductase, which detoxifies quinines (Balogun et al. 2003, Balamurugan et al. 2009). In addition, curcumin protected beta cells from oxidative stress through increased GSH islet content and basal insulin secretions. It has also been observed that curcumin protected islets from cytokine-induced islet death *in vitro* by scavenging ROS and normalized cytokine-induced NF-κB translocation by inhibiting phosphorylation of the inhibitor of kappa B alpha (IkBα). *In vivo*, this group observed that curcumin also prevented the progression of diabetes induced by streptozotocin (STZ), which is associated with the suppression of proinflammatory cytokines (TNF-α and IL-1β). Inflammatory cytokine concentration in the serum and pancreas was raised in STZ-treated animals, but not in animals pretreated with curcumin before STZ (Kanitkar et al. 2008). Currently, it has been shown that combined treatment of tetrahydrocurcumin and chlorogenic acid exerts potential antihyperglycemic effect on streptozotocin-nicotinamide-induced diabetic rats (Karthikesan et al. 2010).

CURCUMIN ROLE IN OBESITY-RELATED DISEASES

CURCUMIN EFFECTS IN ANIMALS

Until recently, the relation between obesity and coronary heart disease was viewed as indirect, that is, through covariates related to both obesity and coronary heart disease risk, including hypertension; dyslipidemia, particularly reductions in high density lipoprotein (HDL) cholesterol; and impaired glucose tolerance or type 2 diabetes. Although most of the comorbidities relating obesity to coronary artery diseases increase as body mass index (BMI), and related to body fat distribution. A lot of compelling evidences have shown that curcumin ameliorated cardiac sympathovagal disturbance in high-fat-induced obese rats. In one study, male Wistar rats were fed with curcumin 30, 60, and 90 mg/kg body weight every day for 12 weeks. The researcher observed an elevated plasma free fatty acid (FFA) level in high-fat-induced obese rats, which is associated with an increased low-frequency/high-frequency (LF/HF) ratio, an expression of sympathovagal disturbance. Curcumin supplementation ameliorated cardiac autonomic imbalance in high-fat-fed rats by lowering the FFA plasma concentration (Pongchaidecha et al. 2009). In addition, Morimoto et al. found that curcumin inhibited the hypertrophy-induced acetylating and DNA-binding abilities of GATA binding protein 4 (GATA4), a hypertrophy-responsive transcription factor, in rat cardiomyocytes. Curcumin also disrupted the p300/GATA4 complex and repressed p300-induced hypertrophic responses in these cells. In addition, the effects of curcumin were examined *in vivo* in two different heart failure models, hypertensive heart disease in salt-sensitive Dahl rats and in surgically induced myocardial infarction rats. In both models, curcumin prevented deterioration of systolic function and heart-failure-induced increase in myocardial wall thickness and diameter (Morimoto et al. 2008). LDL oxidation plays an important role in the development of atherosclerosis (a disease characterized by oxidative damage), and inhibition of LDL oxidation can reduce the risk of atherosclerosis. Curcumin effects were evaluated on the development of experimental atherosclerosis in rabbits and its interaction with other plasmatic antioxidants. Rabbits were fed an atherogenic diet for 30 days, and histological results for the fatty streak lesions revealed damage in the thoracic and abdominal aorta that was significantly lower in the curcumin-fed group than in the control group after 30 days (Quiles et al. 2002).

Diabetes is also the most common cause of kidney failure, and nearly 180,000 people in the United States are living with kidney failure as a result of diabetes (Kutner et al. 2009). Diabetic nephropathy is characterized by increased production of ECM proteins, including fibronectin and extradomain B- containing fibronectin, that are regulated by TGF-β1, NF-κB, and p300 in the kidneys. Curcumin treatment inhibited p300, suppressed the activation of NF-κB, and decreased TGF-β, vasoactive factors (endothelial nitric oxide synthase and endothelin-1), and ECM (Chiu et al. 2009). A decrease in the blood glucose level in diabetic models has been reported in obesity studies regarding the curcumin. Diabetic albino rats were fed with curcumin (0.08 g/kg body weight) and a decrease was observed in blood sugar levels when compared with the control group (Arun and Nalini 2002). In another study, the effect of curcumin supplementation has been investigated on blood glucose, plasma insulin, and glucose homeostasis–related enzyme activities in diabetic db/db mice, which were fed with curcumin (0.02%, wt/wt) for 6 weeks. In db/db mice, curcumin significantly lowered the hepatic activities of fatty acid synthase, beta-oxidation, 3-hydroxy-3-methylglutaryl coenzyme reductase, and acyl-CoA:cholesterol acyltransferase. Curcumin lowered plasma FFA, cholesterol, and triglyceride concentrations and increased the hepatic glycogen and skeletal muscle lipoprotein lipase in db/db mice (Seo et al. 2008). Epidemiological data indicated that diabetes is a potential predisposing factor for neuropsychiatric deficits such as stroke, cerebrovascular diseases, diabetic encephalopathy, depression, and anxiety. Diabetic encephalopathy is characterized by impaired cognitive functions and neurochemical structural abnormalities, which involves direct neuronal damage caused by intracellular glucose. Curcumin (60 mg/kg) treatment significantly attenuated cognitive deficit, cholinergic dysfunction, oxidative stress, and inflammation in diabetic rats (Kuhad and Chopra 2007).

CURCUMIN EFFECTS IN HUMANS

Numerous studies have been carried out in human subjects with curcumin to examine its effect on obesity-related parameters. Cardiovascular complications are common in patients with obesity and to some extent are related with increased FFA level. Curcumin has been observed to lower blood sugar levels in diabetic patients. Curcumin administration also reduced the serum levels of cholesterol and lipid peroxides in 10 healthy human volunteers receiving 500 mg of curcumin daily for 7 days. A significant decrease in the level of serum lipid peroxides (33%), an increase in HDL cholesterol (29%), and a decrease in total serum cholesterol (12%) were noted. Ramirez Bosca et al. found that administration of 10 mg of curcumin per day for 30 days to eight human subjects increased HDL cholesterol and decreased LDL cholesterol. The same research group also investigated the effect of curcumin in human subjects with atherosclerosis, in which 10 mg curcumin was administered twice a day for 15 days to 16 men and 14 women. Curcumin significantly lowered the levels of plasma fibrinogen in both men and women (Ramirez-Bosca et al. 2000a,b). A research group conducted an interventional, randomized, double-blind controlled trial to investigate the effects of curcumin administration at escalating doses (low dose, three times 15 mg/day; moderate dose, three times 30 mg/day; and high dose, three times 60 mg/day) on total cholesterol level, LDL cholesterol level, HDL cholesterol level, and triglyceride level in 75 acute coronary syndrome (ACS) patients. Based on 63 patient's results, it is concluded that the administration of low-dose curcumin showed a trend of reduction in total cholesterol level and LDL cholesterol level in ACS patients (Alwi et al. 2008). However, Baum et al. and his coworkers reported that curcumin consumption does not appear to have a significant effect on the serum lipid profile in 6 months' human study, contrary to the previous reported studies. A 6 month placebo, randomized, double-blinded trial investigated the effects of consuming curcumin (4 g/day and 1 g/day) on the serum lipid profile in both elder genders (n = 36). Plasma curcumin and its metabolites were measured at 1 month, and the serum lipid profile was measured at baseline, 1 month, and 6 months. The plasma curcumin concentration reached a mean of 490 nmol/L, but did not significantly affect triacylglycerols, or total, LDL, and HDL cholesterol over 1 month or 6 months. Moreover, curcumin in physiological concentration of 2 μmol/L was reported to induce expression of ABCG1 in the human hepatoma cell line HepG2, thus increasing HDL-dependent lipid efflux and plasma HDL cholesterol levels (Baum et al. 2007). In addition, hyperglycemia leads to increased oxidative stress resulting in endothelial dysfunction. A randomized, parallel-group, placebo-controlled, 8 week study was performed to evaluate the effects of NCB-02 (a standardized preparation of curcuminoids), atorvastatin, and placebo on endothelial function and its biomarkers in patients with type 2 diabetes mellitus. In this study, 72 patients with type 2 diabetes were randomized to receive NCB-02 (two capsules containing curcumin 150 mg twice daily), atorvastatin 10 mg once daily, or placebo for 8 weeks. NCB-02 had a favorable effect, comparable to that of atorvastatin, on endothelial dysfunction in association with reductions in inflammatory cytokines and markers of oxidative stress. Patients receiving NCB-02 showed significant reductions in the levels of malondialdehyde, endothelin-1 (ET-1), IL-6, and TNFα (Usharani et al. 2008). Recently, the effect of curcumin has been investigated in the activities of drug metabolizing enzymes such as CYP1A2, CYP2A6, N-acetyltransferase (NAT2), and xanthine oxidase (XO) in 16 healthy male Chinese volunteers, using caffeine as a probe drug. After 14 days, in the curcumin (1000 mg/day)-treated group, CYP1A2 activity was decreased by 28.6%, while increase was observed in CYP2A6 by 48.9% (Chen et al. 2010). Curcumin-phosphatidylcholine complex (Meriva®) was evaluated in 50 patients with osteoarthritis at dosages corresponding to 200 mg of curcumin per diem. After 3 months of treatment, C-reactive protein (CRP) levels decreased from 168 ± 18 to 11.3 ± 4.1 mg/L in the subpopulation with high CRP, while the control group experienced only a modest improvement in these parameters (175 ± 12.3 to 112 ± 22.2 mg/L) in the CRP plasma concentration. It has been suggested that Meriva® is clinically effective in the treatment of osteoarthritis and could be taken into consideration for clinical use (Belcaro et al. 2010). In addition, the same curcumin–phosphatidylcholine complex has been investigated among inflammatory conditions such as chronic anterior uveitis relapses in a 12 month follow-up clinical trial. Curcumin–phosphatidylcholine complex, Meriva (Norflo), administered twice a day in 106 patients of recurrent anterior uveitis of different etiologies. The results showed that Norflo was well tolerated and could reduce eye discomfort symptoms and visible effects after a few weeks of treatment in more than 80% of patients (Allegri et al. 2010). Curcumin's ability to lower blood glucose, cholesterol, and antioxidant nature makes it a potential therapeutic for the treatment of obesity-related diseases. Recent evidence has shown that curcumin plays a key role in the protection against various obesity-related cancers including pancreatic cancer. Curcumin (8000 mg/day) in concomitant administration with gemcitabine intravenously (1000 mg/m/week) was observed in 17 patients of advanced pancreatic cancer for 4 weeks. Curcumin has a proven efficacy in patients, with the exception of a few patients (29%), who discontinued curcumin after a few days to 2 weeks due to intractable abdominal fullness or pain, and the dose of curcumin was reduced to 4000 mg/day because of abdominal complaints in two other patients (Epelbaum et al. 2010).

According to a joint report of the Food and Agriculture Organization and the WHO on food additives, the recommended maximum daily intake of curcumin is 0–1 mg/kg body weight, but several clinical studies dealing with its efficacy suggested that it is safe and well tolerated even when intake is as high as 12 g/day (WHO Report 2000, Shehzad and Lee 2010). However, apparent side effects have been reported thus far. Gastrointestinal upset, chest tightness, inflamed skin, and skin rashes are said to occur with high doses. A few cases of allergic contact dermatitis from curcumin have also been reported (Liddle et al. 2006). The chronic use of curcumin can cause liver toxicity; and individuals with hepatic disease, persons misusing alcohol, and those who take prescription medications that are metabolized by liver should probably avoid curcumin. Curcumin is not recommended for persons with biliary tract obstruction, because it stimulates bile secretion (Rasyid et al. 2002). Nevertheless, the multifaceted pharmacological nature of curcumin and its pharmacokinetics in obesity remains unknown and additional research is needed in this field.

FUTURE PROSPECTS

In recent decades, a rapid increase in the costs of health care has increased the importance of naturally occurring phytochemicals in plants for the prevention and treatment of human diseases, including obesity. The modulation of several cellular transduction pathways by curcumin has recently been extended to elucidate the molecular basis for obesity and obesity-related metabolic diseases. Current knowledge suggests that the potential complementary effect of curcumin may occur through several mechanisms including suppression of inflammatory proteins; uptake of glucose; stimulation of catabolic pathways in adipose tissues, liver, and other tissues; inhibition of angiogenesis in adipose tissues; inhibition of differentiation of adipocytes; stimulation of apoptosis of mature adipocytes; and reduction of chronic inflammation associated with adiposity. Numerous studies confirm its potential role *in vitro* and in animals, yet further human studies in particular clinical trials are required to confirm the therapeutic nature of curcumin in obesity and insulin resistance. Expanded use of molecular technologies such as DNA microarrays and proteomics will help to identify newly molecular targets of curcumin and individuals at high risk of obesity-related metabolic diseases. Future trials should also include suitably planned pharmacodynamic studies because the effective dose required for modulating these metabolic responses is unclear at the present. It is important to note that high doses of curcumin in supplement form may have adverse effects. At present, there is not sufficient data to support recommending long-term, safe usage for prevention and treatment of obesity. Future translational and clinical research overlapping metabolism with the aim to unravel the role of curcumin in obesity-related comorbidities is highly warranted. On behalf of such studies, one might be able to gain insights into curcumin mechanisms at a clinical level and assess within a short period the potential success or failure of long-term interventions.

REFERENCES

Ahn, J., Lee, H., Kim, S., and T. Ha. 2010. Curcumin-induced suppression of adipogenic differentiation is accompanied by activation of Wnt/beta-catenin signaling. *Am J Physiol Cell Physiol* 298:C1510–C1516.

Ahn, K.S., Sethi, G., and B.B. Aggarwal. 2008. Reversal of chemoresistance and enhancement of apoptosis by statins through down regulation of the NF-kappaB pathway. *Biochem Pharmacol* 75:907–913.

Allegri, P., Mastromarino, A., and P. Neri. 2010. Management of chronic anterior uveitis relapses: Efficacy of oral phospholipidic curcumin treatment. Long-term follow-up. *Clin Ophthalmol* 4:1201–1206.

Alwi, I., Santoso, T., S. Suyono et al. 2008. The effect of curcumin on lipid level in patients with acute coronary syndrome. *Acta Med Indones* 40:201–210.

Anand, P., Kunnumakkara, A.B., C. Sundaram et al. 2008. Cancer is a preventable disease that requires major lifestyle changes. *Pharm Res* 25:2097–2116.

Arun, N. and N. Nalini. 2002. Efficacy of turmeric on blood sugar and polyol pathway in diabetic albino rats. *Plant Foods Hum Nutr* 57:41–52.

Balamurugan, A.N., Akhov, L., Selvaraj, G., and S. Pugazhenthi. 2009. Induction of antioxidant enzymes by curcumin and its analogues in human islets: Implications in transplantation. *Pancreas* 38:454–460.

Balogun, E., Hoque, M., P. Gong et al. 2003. Curcumin activates the haem oxygenase-1 gene via regulation of Nrf2 and the antioxidant-responsive element. *Biochem J* 371:887–895.

Barsh, G.S., Farooqi, I.S., and S. O'Rahilly. 2000. Genetics of body-weight regulation. *Nature* 404:644–651.

Baum, L., Cheung, S.K., V.C. Mok et al. 2007. Curcumin effects on blood lipid profile in a 6-month human study. *Pharmacol Res* 56:509–514.

Belcaro, G., Cesarone, M.R., M. Dugall et al. 2010. Product-evaluation registry of Meriva®, a curcumin-phosphatidylcholine complex, for the complementary management of osteoarthritis. *Panminerva Med* 52:55–62.

Bennett, B.L., Satoh, Y., and A.J. Lewis. 2003. JNK: A new therapeutic target for diabetes. *Curr Opin Pharmacol* 3:420–425.

Cai, D., Yuan, M., D.F. Frantz et al. 2005. Local and systemic insulin resistance resulting from hepatic activation of IKK-β and NF-κB. *Nat Med* 11:183–190.

Centers for Disease Control and Prevention. 2005. State-specific prevalence of obesity among adults—United States. *MMWR* 55:985–988.

Chen, Y., Liu, W.H., B.L. Chen et al. 2010. Plant polyphenol curcumin significantly affects CYP1A2 and CYP2A6 activity in healthy, male Chinese volunteers. *Ann Pharmacother* 44:1038–1045.

Chiu, J., Khan, Z.A., Farhangkhoee, H., and S. Chakrabarti. 2009. Curcumin prevents diabetes-associated abnormalities in the kidneys by inhibiting p300 and nuclear factor-kappaB. *Nutrition* 25:964–972.

Ejaz, A., Wu, D., Kwan, P., and M. Meydani. 2009. Curcumin inhibits adipogenesis in 3T3-L1 adipocytes and angiogenesis and obesity in C57/BL mice. *J Nutr* 139:919–925.

Emanuelli, B., Eberle, D., Suzuki, R., and C.R. Kahn. 2008. Overexpression of the dual-specificity phosphatase MKP-4/DUSP-9 protects against stress-induced insulin resistance. *Proc Natl Acad Sci USA* 105:3545–3550.

Epelbaum, R., Schaffer, M., Vizel, B., Badmaev, V., and G. Bar-Sela. 2010. Curcumin and gemcitabine in patients with advanced pancreatic cancer. *Nutr Cancer* 62:1137–1141.

Safety Evaluation of Certain Food Additives. 2009. WHO Technical Report Series: 956, WHO Geneva, Switzerland.

Flier, J.S. 2004. Obesity wars: Molecular progress confronts an expanding epidemic. *Cell* 116:337–350.

Friedman, J.M. 2000. Obesity in the new millennium. *Nature* 404:632–634.

Graham, A. 2009. Curcumin adds spice to the debate: Lipid metabolism in liver disease. *Br J Pharmacol* 157:1352–1353.

Hajri, T., Tao, H., Wattacheril, J., Marks-Shulman, P., and N.N. Abumrad. 2011. Regulation of adiponectin production by insulin: Interactions with tumor necrosis factor-alpha and interleukin-6. *Am J Physiol Endocrinol Metab* 300:E350–E360.

Halberg, N., Wernstedt-Asterholm, I., and P.E. Scherer. 2008. The adipocyte as an endocrine cell. *Endocrinol Metab Clin N Am* 37:753–768.

Health Survey for England. 2009. http://www.ic.nhs.uk/statistics-and-data-collections/health-and-lifestyles-related-surveys/health-survey-for-england/health-survey-for-england-2009-health-and-lifestyles.

Huang, W., Ghisletti, S., Perissi, V., Rosenfeld, M.G., and C.K. Glass. 2009. Transcriptional integration of TLR2 and TLR4 signaling at the NCoR depression checkpoint. *Mol Cell* 35:48–57.

Jain, S.K., Rains, J., and K. Jones. 2006. Effect of curcumin on protein glycosylation, lipid peroxidation, and oxygen radical generation in human red blood cells exposed to high glucose levels. *Free Radic Biol Med* 41:92–96.

Jaiswal, A.S., Marlow, B.P., Gupta, N., and S. Narayan. 2002. Beta-catenin-mediated transactivation and cell-cell adhesion pathways are important in curcumin (diferuloylmethane)-induced growth arrest and apoptosis in colon cancer cells. *Oncogene* 21:8414–8427.

Kang, Q. and A. Chen. 2009. Curcumin inhibits srebp-2 expression in activated hepatic stellate cells in vitro by reducing the activity of specificity protein-1. *Endocrinology* 150:5384–5394.

Kanitkar, M., Gokhale, K., Galande, S., and R.R. Bhonde. 2008. Novel role of curcumin in the prevention of cytokine-induced islet death in vitro and diabetogenesis in vivo. *Br J Pharmacol* 155:702–713.

Karthikesan, K., Pari, L., and V.P. Menon. 2010. Combined treatment of tetrahydrocurcumin and chlorogenic acid exerts potential antihyperglycemic effect on streptozotocin-nicotinamide-induced diabetic rats. *Gen Physiol Biophys* 29:23–30.

Kuhad, A. and K. Chopra. 2007. Curcumin attenuates diabetic encephalopathy in rats: Behavioral and biochemical evidences. *Eur J Pharmacol* 576:34–42.

Kutner, N.G., Johansen, K.L., G.A. Kaysen et al. 2009. The Comprehensive Dialysis Study (CDS): A USRDS Special Study. *Clin J Am Soc Nephrol* 4:645–650.

Lee, Y.K., Lee, W.S., Hwang, J.T., Kwon, D.Y., Surh, Y.J., and O.J. Park. 2009. Curcumin exerts antidifferentiation effect through AMPKalpha-PPAR-gamma in 3T3-L1 adipocytes and antiproliferatory effect through AMPKalpha-COX-2 in cancer cells. *J Agric Food Chem* 57:305–310.

Liang, H., Yin, B., Zhang, H., Zhang, S., Zeng, Q., Wang, J., Jiang, X., Yuan, L., Wang, C.Y., and Z. Li. 2008. Blockade of tumor necrosis factor (TNF) receptor type 1-mediated TNF-alpha signaling protected Wistar rats from diet-induced obesity and insulin resistance. *Endocrinology* 149:2943–2951.

Liddle, M., Hull, C., Liu, C., and D. Powell. 2006. Contact urticaria from curcumin. *Dermatitis* 17:196–197.

Lim, J.H. and T.K. Kwon. 2010. Curcumin inhibits phorbol myristate acetate (PMA)-induced MCP-1 expression by inhibiting ERK and NF-kappaB transcriptional activity. *Food Chem Toxicol* 48:47–52.

Lofgren, P., Van, H., V.S. Reynisdottir et al. 2000. Secretion of tumor necrosis factor-alpha shows a strong relationship to insulin-stimulated glucose transport in human adipose tissue. *Diabetes* 49:688–692.

Luchsinger, J.A. 2006. A work in progress: The metabolic syndrome. *Sci Aging Knowl Environ* 10:pe19.

Masamune, A., Suzuki, N., Kikuta, K., Satoh, M., Satoh, K., and T. Shimosegawa. 2006. Curcumin blocks activation of pancreatic stellate cells. *J Cell Biochem* 97:1080–1093.

Moller, D.E. 2001. New drug targets for type 2 diabetes and the metabolic syndrome. *Nature* 414:821–827.

Morimoto, T., Sunagawa, Y., T. Kawamura et al. 2008. The dietary compound curcumin inhibits p300 histone acetyltransferase activity and prevents heart failure in rats. *J Clin Invest* 118:868–878.

Moschen, A.R., Molnar, C., S. Geiger et al. 2010. Anti-inflammatory effects of excessive weight loss: Potent suppression of adipose interleukin 6 and tumour necrosis factor alpha expression. *Gut* 59:1259–1264.

Nieto-Vazquez, I., Fernandez-Veledo, S., Kramer, D.K., Vila-Bedmar, R., Garcia-Guerra, L., and M. Lorenzo. 2008. Insulin resistance associated to obesity: The link TNF-alpha. *Arch Physiol Biochem* 114:183–194.

Ogawa, S., Lozach, J., K. Jepsen et al. 2004. A nuclear receptor corepressor transcriptional checkpoint controlling activator protein 1-dependent gene networks required for macrophage activation. *Proc Natl Acad Sci USA* 101:14461–14466.

Okada, K., Wangpoengtrakul, C., Tanaka, T., Toyokuni, S., Uchida, K., and T. Osawa. 2001. Curcumin and especially tetrahydrocurcumin ameliorate oxidative stress-induced renal injury in mice. *J Nutr* 131:2090–2095.

Pendurthi, U.R. and L.V. Rao. 2000. Suppression of transcription factor Egr-1 by curcumin. *Thromb Res* 97:179–189.

Peschel, D., Koerting, R., and N. Nass. 2007. Curcumin induces changes in expression of genes involved in cholesterol homeostasis. *J Nutr Biochem* 18:113–119.

Pongchaidecha, A., Lailerd, N., Boonprasert, W., and N. Chattipakorn. 2009. Effects of curcuminoid supplement on cardiac autonomic status in high-fat-induced obese rats. *Nutrition* 25:870–878.

Quiles, J.L., Mcsa, M.D., C.L. Ramirez-Tortosa et al. 2002. Curcuma longa extract supplementation reduces oxidative stress and attenuates aortic fatty streak development in rabbits. *Arterioscler Thromb Vasc Biol* 22:1225–1231.

Ramírez-Boscá, A., Soler, A., Carrión, M.A., Díaz-Alperi, J., Bernd, A., Quintanilla, C., Almagro, Q.E., and J. Miquel. 2000a. An hydroalcoholic extract of Curcuma longa lowers the apo B/apo A ratio. Implications for atherogenesis prevention. *Mech Ageing Dev* 119:41–47.

Ramirez Boscá, A., Soler, A., M.A. Carrión-Gutiérrez et al. 2000b. An hydroalcoholic extract of Curcuma longa lowers the abnormally high values of human-plasma fibrinogen. *Mech Ageing Dev* 114:207–210.

Rasyid, A., Rahman, A.R., Jaalam, K., and A. Lelo. 2002. Effect of different curcumin dosages on human gall bladder. *Asia Pac J Clin Nutr* 11:314–318.

Reyna, S.M., Ghosh, S., P. Tantiwong et al. 2008. Elevated toll-like receptor 4 expression and signaling in muscle from insulin-resistant subjects. *Diabetes* 57:2595–2602.

Roberts, D.L., Dive, C., and A.G. Renehan. 2010. Biological mechanisms linking obesity and cancer risk: New perspectives. *Annu Rev Med* 61:301–316.

Schenk, S., Saberi, M., and J.M. Olefsky. 2008. Insulin sensitivity: Modulation by nutrients and inflammation. *J Clin Invest* 118:2992–3002.

Scherer, P.E. 2006. Adipose tissue: From lipid storage compartment to endocrine organ. *Diabetes* 55:1537–1545.

Seo, K.I., Choi, M.S., U.J. Jung et al. 2008. Effect of curcumin supplementation on blood glucose, plasma insulin, and glucose homeostasis related enzyme activities in diabetic db/db mice. *Mol Nutr Food Res* 52:995–1004.

Shehzad, A., Khan, S., Shehzad, O., and Y.S. Lee. 2010a. Curcumin therapeutic promises and bioavailability in colorectal cancer. *Drugs Today* 46:523–532.

Shehzad, A. and Y.S. Lee. 2010. Curcumin: Multiple molecular targets mediate multiple pharmacological actions. *Drugs Future* 35:113–119.

Shehzad, A., Wahid, F., and Y.S. Lee. 2010b. Curcumin in cancer chemoprevention: Molecular targets, pharmacokinetics, bioavailability, and clinical trials. *Arch Pharm Chem Life Sci* 343:489–499.

Shi, H., Kokoeva, M.V., Inouye, K., Tzameli, I., Yin, H., and J.S. Flier. 2006. TLR4 links innate immunity and fatty acid-induced insulin resistance. *J Clin Invest* 116:3015–3025.

Shoelson, S.E., Lee, J., and M. Yuan. 2003. Inflammation and the IKKβ/IκB/NF-κB axis in obesity- and diet-induced insulin resistance. *Int J Obes Relat Metab Disord* 3:S49–S52.

Spiegelman, B.M. and J.S. Flier. 2001. Obesity and the regulation of energy balance. *Cell* 104:531–543.

Suzawa, M., Takada, I., J. Yanagisawa et al. 2003. Cytokines suppress adipogenesis and PPAR-gamma function through the TAK1/TAB1/NIK cascade. *Nat Cell Biol* 5:224–230.

Tang, Y. and A. Chen. 2010a. Curcumin protects hepatic stellate cells against leptin-induced activation in vitro by accumulating intracellular lipids. *Endocrinology* 151:4168–4177.

Tang, Y. and A. Chen. 2010b. Curcumin prevents leptin raising glucose levels in hepatic stellate cells by blocking translocation of glucose transporter-4 and increasing glucokinase. *Br J Pharmacol* 161:1137–1149.

Tang, Y., Zheng, S., and A. Chen. 2009. Curcumin eliminates leptin's effects on hepatic stellate cell activation via interrupting leptin signaling. *Endocrinology* 150:3011–3020.

Tarantino, G., Savastano, S., and A. Colao. 2010. Hepatic steatosis, low-grade chronic inflammation and hormone/growth factor/adipokine imbalance. *World J Gastroenterol* 16:4773–4783.

Usharani, P., Mateen, A.A., Naidu, M.U., Raju, Y.S., and N. Chandra. 2008. Effect of NCB-02, atorvastatin and placebo on endothelial function, oxidative stress and inflammatory markers in patients with type 2 diabetes mellitus: A randomized, parallel-group, placebo-controlled, 8-week study. *Drugs R D* 9:243–250.

Vainio, H. and F. Bianchini. 2002. *Weight Control and Physical Activity*. IARC Handbooks of Cancer Prevention, Vol. 6, Lyon, France: IARC Press.

Wang, S.L., Li, Y., Y. Wen et al. 2009. Curcumin, a potential inhibitor of up-regulation of TNF-alpha and IL-6 induced by palmitate in 3T3-L1 adipocytes through NF-kappaB and JNK pathway. *Biomed Environ Sci* 22:32–39.

Wang, P., Mariman, E., Renes, J., and J. Keijer. 2008. The secretory function of adipocytes in the physiology of white adipose tissue. *J Cell Physiol* 216:3–13.

Weisberg, S.P., Leibel, R., and D.V. Tortoriello. 2009. Dietary curcumin significantly improves obesity associated inflammation and diabetes in mouse models of diabesity. *Endocrinology* 149:3549–3558.

Woo, H.M., Kang, J.H., Kawada, T., Yoo, H., Sung, M.K., and R. Yu. 2007. Active spice-derived components can inhibit inflammatory responses of adipose tissue in obesity by suppressing inflammatory actions of macrophages and release of monocyte chemoattractant protein-1 from adipocytes. *Life Sci* 80:926–931.

Xu, H., Barnes, G.T., Q. Yang et al. 2003. Chronic inflammation in fat plays a crucial role in the development of obesity-related insulin resistance. *J Clin Invest* 112:1821–1830.

Yoysungnoen, P., Wirachwong, P., Bhattarakosol, P., Niimi, H., and S. Patumraj. 2006. Effects of curcumin on tumor angiogenesis and biomarkers, COX-2 and VEGF, in hepatocellular carcinoma cell-implanted nude mice. *Clin Hemorheol Microcirc* 34:109–115.

Zhang, J., Gao, Z., Yin, J., Quon, M.J., and J. Ye. 2008. S6K directly phosphorylates IRS-1 on Ser-270 to promote insulin resistance in response to TNF-(alpha) signaling through IKK2. *J Biol Chem* 283:35375–35382.

Zheng, S. and A. Chen. 2006. Curcumin suppresses the expression of extracellular matrix genes in activated hepatic stellate cells by inhibiting gene expression of connective tissue growth factor. *Am J Physiol Gastrointest Liver Physiol* 290:G883–G893.

50 Review of the Safety and Efficacy of Banaba (*Lagerstroemia speciosa* L.) and Its Major Constituents, Corosolic Acid and Ellagitannins, in the Management of Metabolic Syndrome

Sidney J. Stohs, PhD, FACN, CNS, ATS, FASAHP, Howard Miller, MS, and Gilbert R. Kaats, PhD, FACN

CONTENTS

INTRODUCTION

Banaba (*Lagerstroemia speciosa* L., crepe myrtle) has been used as a folk medicine to treat diabetes in Southeast Asia and various other parts of the world. The hypoglycemic and weight management effects of aqueous (hot water) and methanolic extracts have been demonstrated in a number of human studies as well as several animal models, and mechanistic studies have been conducted in *in vitro* systems. The majority of these studies have focused on corosolic acid (2α-hydroxyursolic acid) which is isolated with an organic solvent as methanol from the leaves of the plant, and corosolic acid is used to standardize banaba extracts [1,2].

Some studies indicate that ellagitannins in water-soluble fractions may be responsible for at least some of the insulin-like activity of banaba, and the antioxidant, anti-inflammatory, and glucose regulatory properties of tannins in general have been reviewed by Klein et al. [3].

Unfortunately, no standardization has occurred with respect to ellagitannins in banaba, and no studies involving banaba extracts standardized to both corosolic acid and ellagitannins have been conducted. Hayashi et al. [4] showed that an ellagitannin preparation from banaba called lagerstroemin exhibits glucose transport stimulation. Subsequent studies by Liu et al. [5] reported that commercial tannic acid was more potent than lagerstroemin from banaba in stimulating glucose transport, and the most active component of tannic acid was penta-O-galloyl-D-glucopyranose [6]. However, this substance has not been directly shown to be present in banaba, although it has been surmised that this is the active constituent in banaba with respect to the stimulation of glucose transport [3].

Corosolic acid also occurs in a number of other plant species including but not limited to *Perilla frutescens* [7], *Campsis grandiflora* [8], *Glechoma longituba* [9], *Potentilla chinensis* [10], *Ugni molinae* [11], *Eriobotrya japonica* [12–15], *Symplocos paniculata* [16], *Weigela subsessilis* [17,18], *Rubus biflorus* [19], *Phlomis umbrosa* [20], and *Vaccinium macrocarpon* (cranberry) [21]. Most of these plants are native to Asia, although corosolic acid has also been isolated from various European and South American plants. A discussion of the pharmacological effects of these various plant species is beyond the scope of this review.

This review summarizes studies that have been conducted in humans, animals, and *in vitro* systems on weight management and antihyperglycemic, antihyperlipidemic, anti-inflammatory, antioxidant, antifungal, antiviral, and antineoplastic activities of banaba extracts, corosolic acid–standardized banaba extracts, and isolated and structurally characterized corosolic acid and ellagitannins. Various safety and mechanistic studies conducted to date on these diverse banaba preparations are also reviewed.

HUMAN STUDIES

Ikeda et al. [22] conducted a human clinical study on banaba involving a proprietary product called Banabamin. The product was an aqueous extract of banaba in tablet form which also contained extracts of green tea, green coffee, and *Garcinia*. Twenty-four human subjects with mild type 2 diabetes were given three tablets three times daily. A significant average decrease (13.5%) in blood glucose levels was reported, and no adverse effects were observed. The active constituents in the product responsible for the antidiabetic effect were not determined.

In a subsequent investigation, Ikeda et al. [23] performed a 1 year open-label safety and efficacy study involving 15 subjects, administering 100 mg tablets daily of a water-soluble banaba extract. As in previous studies, the extract was not standardized, and the specific constituents responsible for the antidiabetic effects were not determined. A significant decrease (16.6%) in fasting blood glucose levels was observed in individuals with fasting blood glucose levels greater than 110 mg/dL. At both 6 months and 1 year, glucose tolerance and glycosylated albumin following treatment with the banaba extract were significantly improved. No hypoglycemia occurred in response to the banaba extract. No adverse effects and no changes in hematological or biochemical characteristics were observed over the 1 year course of the study in response to daily administration of the water-soluble banaba extract preparation.

Judy et al. [24] examined the antidiabetic activity of a banaba extract standardized to 1% corosolic acid in a soft gel capsule formulation has been examined. Ten type 2 diabetic subjects were given 32 or 48 mg of the product (0.32 or 0.48 mg corosolic acid, respectively) daily for 2 weeks. A decrease (30%) in blood glucose levels was observed after the 2 weeks. Whether the observed effect was due to corosolic acid, the tannin components, or a combination thereof is not clear, and the ellagitannins were neither identified nor quantitated.

Lieberman et al. [25] conducted a 12 week lifestyle intervention study involving 56 subjects that included use of dietary supplements, diet, and exercise. The dietary supplements were ingested prior to each meal and contained 16 mg banaba extract, 1500 mg *Garcinia cambogia* extract (60% hydroxycitric acid), 100 mg bitter melon extract, 133 mg *Gymnema* extract, 50 mg elemental magnesium, 10 mg wheat amylase inhibitor, 2.6 mg BioPerine (from black pepper), 167 μg elemental chromium, and 50 μg elemental vanadium. The subjects lost an average of 6.29 kg (13.8 lb), including 3.72 kg (8.2 lb) body fat as determined by a bioelectric impedance body fat analyzer at the end of 12 weeks. Approximately 73% of subjects completed the study. It is not clear what contribution to the weight loss was provided by each constituent in the product, and the amounts of corosolic acid and ellagitannins in the banaba extract were not reported or determined.

In a study published by Tsuchibe et al. [26], 12 subjects were given a soft gel capsule daily for 2 weeks containing 10 mg corosolic acid as a banaba extract standardized to 18% corosolic acid. The subjects started with a baseline blood glucose level of 104 mg/dL. A significant decrease (12%) in fasting as well as 60 min postprandial blood glucose levels was observed after consuming the product daily for 2 weeks. An average 3 lb weight loss after the 2 weeks was also reported, and no adverse effects were observed throughout the trial. In spite of the high level of corosolic acid administered, it is unclear if the weight loss and blood sugar regulation were due entirely to the corosolic acid or a combination of the corosolic acid with possible tannin components.

In an unpublished study by Xu [27] using the same soft gel product containing 10 mg corosolic acid as described by Tsuchibe et al. (2006), 100 subjects were enrolled who were either prediabetic or had type 2 diabetes. Half the subjects consumed one soft gel containing the corosolic acid–standardized banaba extract, and the other half received a placebo soft gel daily for 30 days. Both fasting and 2 h postprandial blood glucose levels in the treated group decreased by 10% relative to the control (placebo) group. An improvement in diabetic symptoms including a decrease in thirst, drowsiness, and hunger was also reported. No changes in blood pressure, liver or kidney function, blood cell count, or hemoglobin were observed, and no adverse effects reported.

Fukushima et al. [28] conducted a study involving 31 subjects in a double-blind crossover design. The subjects were given a capsule containing 10 mg corosolic acid or a placebo 5 min prior to a 75 g oral glucose tolerance test. Blood glucose levels were assessed at 30 min intervals for 2 h. Corosolic acid treatment resulted in lower blood glucose levels from 60 to 120 min as compared to controls with the 90 min time point being statistically significant ($P < 0.05$). The authors noted that the corosolic acid used in the study was 99% pure, thus signifying that the blood sugar lowering effect was due directly to the corosolic acid.

There has been one single report suggesting that corosolic acid may have caused nephrotoxicity and lactic acidosis in a diabetic patient with impaired kidney function who was also taking diclofenac for joint pain [29]. Diclofenac is a nonsteroidal anti-inflammatory drug known to cause renal damage and kidney failure. The role of corosolic acid, if any, is not clear. The use of a drug known for its nephrotoxicity in conjunction with impaired kidney function readily explains the resulting kidney failure. It is theoretically possible that corosolic acid inhibition of gluconeogenesis could favor lactic acid production. If corosolic acid impaired the metabolism of lactic acid, it could possibly exacerbate the known nephrotoxicity of the drug. However, no evidence was provided to specifically demonstrate this possible effect. Furthermore, no controlled clinical studies have ever reported nephrotoxicity in diabetic subjects receiving corosolic acid.

The human clinical studies described earlier demonstrate that unstandardized hot water and methanolic banaba extracts, banaba extract standardized to corosolic acid, and corosolic acid itself decrease fasting as well as postprandial blood glucose levels in humans and support weight loss and weight management. A decrease in blood glucose levels has been observed within 2 h of dosing, and the decrease is typically in the range of 10%–15%, although a decrease of 30% has been reported. No adverse effects have been reported in subjects receiving banaba for up to 1 year. The role of corosolic acid in blood glucose regulation has been shown. Unfortunately, the role of ellagitannins is not well characterized, and no standardization of ellagitannin extracts has occurred.

ANIMAL STUDIES

Garcia [30,31] published the first research on the hypoglycemic, insulin-like activity of banaba. An aqueous extract equivalent to 1–2 g of dried leaves per kg body weight given orally lowered blood sugar for 4–6 h in rabbits. A number of animal studies have subsequently demonstrated that banaba extracts of unknown composition, banaba extracts standardized to corosolic acid, and highly purified corosolic acid exert beneficial effects with respect to blood glucose and lipid regulation as well as inhibition of body weight gain.

Kakuda et al. [32] fed genetically diabetic (KK-AY) mice diets containing 5% of a hot water extract and 2% of a methanol extract of banaba leaves for 5 weeks. The elevation of blood glucose levels was significantly suppressed by feeding either of the two extracts. The levels of serum insulin, plasma total cholesterol, and amount of urinary glucose were all lowered by feeding the extracts, with somewhat greater activity with the water extract that was given at a higher concentration. No determination was made of the specific constituents in the extracts responsible for these effects.

In 1999, Suzuki et al. [33] fed female diabetic KK-AY mice a diet containing 5% of a hot water extract of banaba for 12 weeks. As compared to the control group, the banaba diet group of animals exhibited significantly lower weight gain and adipose tissue. Furthermore, the banaba extract resulted in a suppression of hemoglobin A1C and resulted in a 35% decrease in serum total lipids. The identity of the constituents responsible for these effects was not determined, although subsequent studies assumed that the active constituents were ellagitannins [3].

Suzuki et al. [34] also showed that a hot water extract of banaba leaves suppressed blood glucose elevation following starch administration but not after glucose administration to rats. In addition, they demonstrated that the extract inhibited the activities of various hydrolytic enzymes including α-amylase, glucoamylase, maltase, isomaltase, and sucrase. Again, the specific constituents responsible for these enzyme inhibitory activities in banaba were not determined.

Yamaguchi et al. [35] fed 0.072% corosolic acid in the diet to spontaneously hypertensive rats for 14 weeks. Significant decreases in blood pressure, serum-free fatty acids, and oxidative stress markers relative to the diet containing no corosolic acid were reported. Although the product contained a known amount of corosolic acid, there is no evidence to indicate that the observed effects were due strictly to corosolic acid. No determination of ellagitannin content was made. Furthermore, no effect of the corosolic acid in the diet on body weight gain or blood glucose levels was observed.

Matsuura et al. [36] examined the abilities of various teas (aqueous decoctions), including from banaba leaves, to suppress blood glucose levels in rats from continuous intragastric infusion of sucrose or maltose. Banaba did not significantly alter glucose levels. The reason for the lack of effect of banaba on blood glucose levels in these two rat studies [35,36] is not known. These results are in sharp contrast to the results presented in the following, which primarily involve mouse studies as well as streptozotocin-induced diabetic rats and the human studies reported earlier. As is true for many of these studies, the composition of the banaba extract was not determined.

In a study by Hong and Maeng [37] involving genetically diabetic mice given an extract of banaba (0.8 mg/kg body weight) for 12 weeks orally, no effect was observed on fasting blood sugar levels, hemoglobin 1AC content, body weight, or insulin levels. Kidney glucose-6-phosphatase activity was significantly lower than in control animals. The most plausible explanation for the poor antidiabetic effect is that the dose of the extract that was used appears to be very low. In addition, the extract was not standardized or analyzed with respect to potential active constituents.

Yamada et al. [38] examined the effects of feeding mice a high-fat diet for 9 weeks with and without 0.023% corosolic acid (not a standardized extract of banaba). A 10% decrease in body weight and a 15% loss in fat total mass were also observed relative to animals receiving the diet without the corosolic acid. The diet containing the corosolic acid reduced fasting plasma levels of glucose, insulin, and triglycerides by 23%, 41%, and 22%, respectively. The corosolic acid in the diet increased the expression of peroxisome proliferator-activated receptor-alpha (PPAR-α) in the liver and PPAR-γ in white adipose tissues, thus providing an explanation regarding the mechanism for the loss in body weight and the decrease in hepatic lipids in these mice. The results indicate that corosolic acid may be beneficial in addressing weight management and various aspects of the metabolic syndrome.

In another investigation by Yamada et al. [39], the mechanism of action of corosolic acid on gluconeogenesis in rat liver was assessed using perfused livers and isolated hepatocytes. Corosolic acid ($20-100\,\mu M$) was shown in a dose-dependent manner to decrease gluconeogenesis by increasing production of fructose-2,6 diphosphate by lowering cyclic AMP levels and inhibiting protein kinase A activity. Corosolic acid also increased glucokinase activity without affecting glucose-6-phosphatase activity, suggesting an increase in glycolysis. The results provide additional insight into the antidiabetic actions of corosolic acid.

Deocaris et al. [40] administered various banaba leaf extracts subcutaneously to alloxan-induced diabetic mice. The extracts were prepared with 80% ethanol and of unknown and unstandardized composition. The banaba leaf extract had little effect on blood glucose levels, but when combined with insulin, the hypoglycemic activity was synergistically enhanced. Gamma irradiation of banaba leaves leads to extracts with higher hypoglycemic activity when mixed with insulin than unirradiated extracts, suggesting that irradiation improved extraction efficiency of the active component(s).

Park et al. [2] conducted a study involving genetically diabetic (db/db) mice that were fed a diet containing a water-soluble extract of banaba at a 0.5% concentration. Animals receiving the banaba extract exhibited significantly reduced blood glucose, insulin, triglycerides, and hemoglobin A1c levels at the end of 12 weeks. In addition, increased expressions of liver PPAR-α mRNA and lipoprotein lipase (LPL) mRNA as well as adipose tissue PPAR-γ mRNA were observed. The data indicate that the banaba extract increased insulin sensitivity and blood sugar regulation by regulating PPAR-mediated lipid metabolism. However, the identity of the responsible factor(s) in banaba was not determined, and it is not clear whether the effects were due specifically to corosolic acid, ellagitannins, or a combination thereof.

Miura et al. [41] administered a single dose of corosolic acid (10 mg/kg) to genetically diabetic (KK-AY) mice. The corosolic acid significantly reduced blood sugar levels. This effect was shown to be associated with an increase in the muscle glucose transporter (GLUT4). In a subsequent study, Miura et al. [42] showed that a single dose of 2 mg/kg corosolic acid reduced blood sugar levels for up to 2 weeks, therefore supporting the hypothesis that corosolic acid improves glucose metabolism by reducing insulin resistance.

Takagi et al. [43] demonstrated that an oral dose of 10 mg/kg corosolic acid suspended in water given to mice inhibited the intestinal hydrolysis of sucrose, but not maltose or lactose. The inhibition of sucrase at least in part facilitated the lowering of blood glucose levels since sucrose is a disaccharide composed of glucose plus fructose. In this study, the sugar solutions were administered 30 min orally after the corosolic acid, and blood samples were drawn at 30, 60, and 120 min. The results of this study agree with the observations of Suzuki et al. [34] who showed that an extract of banaba leaves inhibited sucrase activity. Based on other studies, the results indicate that the hypoglycemic effects of banaba extracts and corosolic acid are exerted through multiple mechanisms.

In a follow-up study, Takagi et al. [44] have shown that when genetically diabetic (KK-AY) mice are fed a high-cholesterol diet with and without 0.023% corosolic acid for 10 weeks, the corosolic acid–containing diet significantly decreased blood cholesterol and liver cholesterol content by 32% and 46%, respectively. In addition, diabetic mice were given corosolic acid (10 mg/kg body weight) orally in water followed by the oral administration of a high-cholesterol cocktail 30 min later. Mean blood cholesterol levels were significantly lower 4 h after administration of the cholesterol in animals that received the corosolic acid relative to control animals. The effect was believed to be due to inhibition of cholesterol absorption via inhibition of the enzyme cholesterol acyltransferase by the corosolic acid.

A number of studies have examined the effects of aqueous banaba extracts on streptozotocin-induced diabetic rats. Unfortunately, the active constituents were not determined in any of these studies. Saha et al. [45] showed that a hot water (75°C–90°C) extract of banaba leaves could depress the elevated blood glucose levels in streptozotocin-diabetic rats by about 43%. It also increased the activity of glucose-6-phosphate dehydrogenase as well as the glutathione content and decreased the activity of the gluconeogenic enzymes glucose-6-phosphatase and fructose-1,6-diphosphatase. The dose of the extract used and the duration of the study were not reported. No effect on body weight was reported. However, the data suggest that the hypoglycemic activity of the extract occurs through suppression of gluconeogenesis and stimulation of glucose oxidation via the pentose phosphate pathway.

Thuppia et al. [46] prepared an extract of banaba leaves by boiling for 2 h, which was subsequently freeze-dried. The reconstituted extract was administered orally at doses up to 2000 mg/kg body weight for 12 days to streptozotocin-diabetic rats. A dose of 1000 mg/kg decreased fasting blood glucose levels by approximately 43% on day 12. The blood sugar levels returned to normal pretreatment values by day 3 after treatment ceased. No changes in blood glucose levels were observed in nondiabetic rats in response to the aqueous banaba extract. The high doses of the extract needed to produce a hypoglycemic effect may be reflected in the extraction procedure. Boiling of the banaba for 2 h may have destroyed some of the active constituents.

Saumya and Basha [47] gave an aqueous banaba extract (150 mg/kg body weight) of unknown composition to streptozotocin-induced diabetic mice for up to 15 days. Significant decreases in blood glucose levels and a potent antioxidant effect were observed. The banaba extract reduced streptozotocin-generated reactive oxygen species (superoxide anion, hydrogen peroxide, and nitric acid) by upregulating superoxide dismutase, catalase, and glutathione-S-transferase activities as well as increasing reduced glutathione levels. The possible effects on body weight were not reported.

Administration of a spray-dried extract of banaba of unknown composition (100 mg/kg body weight) for 28 days by gavage to alloxan-induced diabetic mice resulted in significantly lower blood and urine glucose levels [48]. In response to the banaba extract, lower food and fluid intakes as well as lower body weights were also observed.

Oleanolic acid is a pentacyclic terpene acid that is structurally related to corosolic acid. Hou et al. [49] isolated oleanolic acid from banaba leaves and demonstrated that it exhibits α-glucosidase activity. In another study involving oleanolic acid, oleanolic acid and insulin decreased blood glucose levels in control and streptozotocin-induced diabetic rats that had been given a glucose load after an 18 h fast [50]. In addition, daily treatment with oleanolic acid for 5 days significantly decreased blood glucose levels in diabetic animals while restoring hepatic and muscle glycogen stores to near normal level. Furthermore, oleanolic acid in combination with insulin provided even greater antihyperglycemic activity. No effect on body weight was reported. The authors concluded that oleanolic acid may act via a mechanism distinct from insulin including its α-glucosidase activity, and the two may exert a synergistic effect in the regulation of hyperglycemia. Whether oleanolic acid acts via identical mechanisms to corosolic acid is not clear.

Aguirre et al. [11] assessed the anti-inflammatory activity of various pentacyclic triterpene acids including corosolic acid *in vivo* using a mouse ear assay, with arachidonic acid and 12-O-tetradecanoylphorbol-13 acetate as the inflammation-inducing agents. Corosolic acid was shown to be effective against both inflammatory agents.

In summary, a growing number of studies have demonstrated that unstandardized banaba extracts as well as corosolic acid significantly decrease blood glucose levels in genetic as well as streptozotocin- and alloxan-induced diabetic animals. Better responses appear to occur in mice as compared to rats. In general, banaba extracts and corosolic acid have also been shown to facilitate weight loss, improve insulin sensitivity, increase cellular uptake of glucose, decrease serum cholesterol and triglycerides, and improve oxidative stress markers without production of adverse or toxic effects. In addition, the animal studies suggest that banaba extracts and corosolic acid may have additional health-enhancing benefits that extend beyond the effects observed to date in human subjects. The animal studies also support the safety findings reported in human studies and have provided useful information on the mechanisms of action of banaba extract and corosolic acid. The lack of standardization of the aqueous extracts and the lack of quantitation of ellagitannin content are problematic. Reproducibility involving unstandardized preparations is a major issue.

IN VITRO STUDIES

The free radical scavenging and antioxidant activities of an aqueous extract of banaba were demonstrated in *in vitro* free radical generating systems in a concentration-dependent manner [51]. The banaba extract exhibited potent radical scavenging activity and also inhibited lipid peroxidation in a rat liver homogenate system. Although the chemical components in the extract responsible for these observed effects were not determined, the tannin content of the extract was determined to be about 37% of dry weight.

A methanolic extract of banaba demonstrated high inhibitory activity at a concentration of 10 mg/mL against two fungal strains [52]. A hot water extract exhibited lower activity. The banaba extract was one of five extracts from 29 plant species to demonstrate significant antifungal activity. The components responsible for this antifungal activity were not determined.

As previously noted, Lui et al. [53] demonstrated that both water and methanol extracts of banaba stimulated glucose uptake by 3T3- adipocytes. The extracts also inhibited adipocyte differentiation induced by insulin. The active components in these banaba extracts were not identified.

Although no studies have been conducted with standardized ellagitannin preparations of banaba, Tanaka et al. [54] isolated and structurally characterized various ellagitannins from the fruit and leaves of banaba. Lagerstannins A and B together with five known tannins including lagerstroemin were isolated from the fruit, while lagerstannin C was isolated and characterized from banaba leaves. The three lagerstannins possess a gluconic acid core which is rarely found in the plants.

Hayashi et al. [4] isolated three ellagitannins, lagerstroemin, flosin B, and reginin, from banaba and assessed their abilities to increase glucose uptake by isolated rat adipocytes. Lagerstroemin exhibited glucose transport stimulation with a 50% effective concentration (EC50) of 80 μM, with a maximum effect of approximately 54% of that of insulin. However, it is doubtful that this concentration of lagerstroemin can be achieved *in vivo* following oral administration of the doses commonly used for banaba extracts. Furthermore, tannic acid, which is commercially available and widely distributed in plants, was shown to exhibit glucose transport activity with an EC50 of 17 μM, approximately five times more potent than lagerstroemin [6]. Thus, it may not be possible to ascribe the predominant glucose regulatory activity of banaba extract to lagerstroemin, although it may be a contributing factor.

Hattori et al. [55] demonstrated that lagerstroemin exhibited insulin-like activities including increased glucose uptake and decreased isoproterenol-induced glycerol release in rat adipocytes. In a Chinese hamster ovary cell system, lagerstroemin increased extracellular signal–related kinase (Erk) activity. Similar activities have not been demonstrated in animals or humans.

Bai et al. [56] have isolated and structurally characterized seven ellagitannins and four methyl ellagic acid derivatives from banaba leaves. A number of polyphenolic compounds including corosolic acid and quercetin were also isolated. All isolated ellagitannins exhibited the ability to stimulate insulin-like glucose uptake as well as inhibit adipocyte differentiation in 3T3-L1 adipocyte cells in culture, while the methyl ellagic acid derivatives exhibited inhibitory activity with respect to glucose transport. These studies demonstrate the antihyperglycemic activity of well-characterized ellagic acid derivatives from banaba. This activity is not restricted to a single compound and indicates that multiple mechanisms of action are involved in the hypoglycemic activity of banaba and its constituents.

Hosoyama et al. [57] assessed the α-amylase inhibitor activity in aqueous banaba leaf extracts. The extracts were hydrolyzed with hydrochloric acid, extracted with an organic solvent, and subjected to high-performance liquid chromatography (HPLC). Using bioassay-guided analysis of various fractions, the polyphenolic valoneaic acid lactone was isolated and identified as a potent α-amylase inhibitor. The valoneaic acid content of eight banaba leaf decoctions was subsequently determined, and the α-amylase inhibiting activities were shown to correlate with the content of this polyphenolic acid. The α-amylase inhibiting activity of corosolic acid was not determined. Since water was used to make for the initial banaba extractions, corosolic acid may not have been present in large amounts.

Vijaykumar et al. [58] determined the corosolic acid content of banaba leaves, banaba methanolic extracts, and various commercial dosage forms using HPLC as well as high-performance thin-layer chromatography (HPTLC). Several banaba leaf preparations were shown to contain 0.31–0.38 mg corosolic acid/100 mg, while methanol extracts of the leaves contained up to 11.3 mg/100 mg.

Shi et al. [59] demonstrated that corosolic acid stimulated glucose uptake in a Chinese hamster ovary cell system by enhancing insulin receptor phosphorylation. In addition, corosolic acid inhibited several diabetes-related nonreceptor protein tyrosine phosphatase enzymes. These studies provide mechanistic information concerning the ability of corosolic acid to exert a hypoglycemic effect.

Ichikawa et al. [60] demonstrated the ability of an aqueous banaba extract to block the activation of nuclear factor (NF)-κB by tumor necrosis factor (TNF) in a dose- and time-dependent manner using the cardiomyocyte cell line H9c2. This anti-inflammatory action may explain the ability of banaba extract to inhibit diabetes-induced cardiomyocyte hypertrophy. This study may explain the anti-inflammatory activity demonstrated for corosolic acid and other pentacyclic terpene acids in mice [11]. However, a water-soluble extract was used in the studies by Ichikawa et al. [60], and the corosolic acid content was not determined.

Hou et al. [49] isolated six pentacyclic triterpene acids (oleanolic acid, arjunolic acid, asiatic acid, maslinic acid, corosolic acid, and 23-hydroxyursolic acid) from banaba leaves by ethyl acetate extraction, and their abilities to inhibit α-amylase and α-glucosidase activities were determined. Corosolic acid exhibited greatest inhibitory activity against α-glucosidase, while all of the six pentacyclic triterpenes exhibited weak or no inhibitory activity against α-amylase. These results provide additional mechanistic information with respect to the antidiabetic activity of banaba.

Shim et al. [61] examined the anabolic effects of corosolic acid on osteoblastic bone formation. Concentrations of up to 5 μM corosolic acid significantly stimulated differentiation of mouse osteoblasts. This stimulatory effect was shown to be mediated by activation of mitogen-activated protein kinase (MAPK), NF-κB, and activator protein-1. Based on these results, corosolic acid may be a useful therapy in conjunction with bone diseases as osteoporosis and periodontitis as well as the promotion of bone fracture healing.

Several studies have examined the effects of corosolic acid on various human tumor cells. Fujiwara et al. [62] demonstrated corosolic acid inhibited the proliferation of glioblastoma cells by suppressing the activation of signal transducer and activator transcription-3 (STAT3) and NF-κB in both glioblastoma cells and tumor-associated macrophages. These authors concluded that corosolic acid may have potential for tumor prevention and therapy. Xu et al. [63] demonstrated that corosolic acid induced apoptotic cell death in human cervical adenocarcinoma HeLa cells through the activation of caspases via a mitochondrial pathway. They also concluded that corosolic acid had potential for clinical application.

Lee et al. [64,65] conducted two studies on the ability of corosolic acid to induce cell cycle arrest and apoptosis (programmed cell death) in human gastric cancer cells. In a gastric cancer cell line, corosolic acid was shown to produce apoptosis by activation of AMP-activated protein kinase and caspase-3 [64]. In the other report involving a second gastric cancer cell line [65], corosolic acid dramatically inhibited expression of human epidermal growth factor receptor (HER2) oncogene which in turn promotes apoptosis. The results of these studies suggest corosolic acid may exhibit clinical potential with respect to gastric cancers.

Orobol-7-O-ᴅ-glucoside is an isoflavonoid that has been isolated from banaba and has been shown to have broad spectrum antiviral activity against human rhinoviruses [66]. The 50% inhibitory concentration (IC50) ranged from 0.58 to 8.80 μg/mL. Based on these initial results, the authors proposed that this substance may be useful in treating human rhinoviruses that are commonly associated with respiratory infections.

Morshed et al. [67] assessed the antinociceptive activity of a chloroform extract of banaba bark in mice based on folk medicine used for treatment of pain. A dose of 500 mg of the extract/kg body weight produced a 51% reduction in the pain incidence as compared to a 38% reduction when 200 mg aspirin/kg was administered. Identities of the active constituents were not determined, and no information was provided regarding the mechanism of this action.

Corosolic acid isolated from cranberry was tested for its ability to inhibit cytochrome P450 3A, the most prominent drug-metabolizing enzyme system in the body [21]. A human intestinal microsomal system was used. The concentration of corosolic acid needed to provide 50% inhibition (IC50) was about 4.3–8.8 µM, and the authors concluded that corosolic acid could contribute to drug-dietary substance interactions. However, this concentration of corosolic acid cannot be achieved in the blood following an oral dose of corosolic acid as high as 10 mg, although this concentration might be achieved locally in the intestine at lower doses.

Nagai et al. [68] examined the potential of a banaba extract to influence the bioavailability of drugs. The authors examined the abilities of various herbal extracts to inhibit the activity of human sulfotransferase 1A3 (SULT1A3), a prominent detoxifying enzyme in the intestinal epithelium. A banaba extract was shown to inhibit the sulfation of dopamine and ritodrine at IC50 concentrations of 16.0 and 7.5 µg/mL, respectively. The authors concluded that an extract of banaba may increase the bioavailability of drugs when the bioavailabilities are limited by the action of this enzyme in the intestine. The extracts were of unknown composition, and the method of extraction was not described. The factor or factors responsible for the enzyme inhibition are not known, and the affect of corosolic acid on this enzyme was not assessed. As a consequence, the clinical significance of this study is unclear.

In summary, various *in vitro* studies involving cell-free systems and cell cultures have demonstrated antioxidant, antifungal, antiviral, antineoplastic, and osteoblastic activities of banaba extracts and corosolic acid. In addition, various ellagitannins have also been isolated from banaba and shown to exhibit antihyperglycemic activity. Information regarding the mechanisms of action of banaba extracts, corosolic acid, and ellagitannins has also been obtained using these *in vitro* systems.

CONCLUSIONS

A growing body of evidence involving animal and human studies as well as *in vitro* systems indicates that banaba leaf extracts exert antiobesity and antidiabetic effects. There is strong evidence to indicate that corosolic acid is responsible for these effects, with less evidence to date supporting a role for ellagitannins. Other polycyclic terpene acids as oleanolic acid and valoneaic acid may also contribute to the antihyperglycemic effects of banaba. With the development of techniques to purify various components of banaba, studies are now being conducted with more highly purified and structurally characterized materials As a consequence, information is being obtained regarding the specific effects of the various constituents, particularly with respect to corosolic acid.

A number of studies in animals and human subjects using highly purified corosolic acid and corosolic acid–standardized preparations indicate that this component of banaba exhibits properties that are beneficial in addressing various factors involved in glucose regulation and metabolism, including the enhanced cellular uptake of glucose, improved insulin sensitivity, decreased gluconeogenesis, and inhibited intestinal hydrolysis of sucrose. Furthermore, decreased serum cholesterol and triglycerides have been observed in response to corosolic acid. Based on the studies conducted to date, no adverse effects have been reported in animals using either corosolic acid or standardized banaba extracts, nor have adverse events been observed in controlled human clinical studies.

The studies mentioned earlier indicate that corosolic acid and corosolic acid–standardized banaba extracts may be beneficial in addressing issues associated with obesity and elevated blood sugar levels. Furthermore, corosolic acid exhibits anti-inflammatory, antihyperlipidemic, antiviral, and antitumor-promoting effects. Standardized banaba extracts, corosolic acid, and/or ellagitannins in combination with other ingredients may be useful in dealing with obesity and symptoms associated with metabolic syndrome. Patented banaba leaf extracts standardized to 1%, 2%, and 5% corosolic acid are commercially available (Glucolate™; Novel Ingredient Services, West Caldwell, NJ). Corosolic acid and standardized banaba extracts may also be highly effective either as stand-alone products or in combination with other natural products possessing hypoglycemic, antihyperlipidemic, and appetite-suppressant activities.

Additional human efficacy and safety studies are warranted. Additional studies are needed to assess the dose- and time-dependent effects of corosolic acid, corosolic acid–standardized banaba extracts, and ellagitannins alone or in combination with other ingredients with respect to weight loss and weight management, blood lipids (triglyceride and cholesterol), insulin, and glucose levels. A need exists for the development of banaba products standardized to ellagitannins as well as to both corosolic acid and ellagitannins. Finally, additional investigations are needed to clearly define and understand the roles and importance of corosolic acid and related pentacyclic terpene acids relative to the ellagitannins present in banaba.

SUMMARY

Banaba (*Lagerstroemia speciosa* L.) extracts and decoctions have been used for many years in folk medicine to treat diabetes, with the first published research study being reported in 1940. The hypoglycemic effects of banaba have been attributed to both corosolic acid as well as ellagitannins. Studies have been conducted in various animal models, human subjects, and *in vitro* systems using water-soluble banaba leaf extracts, corosolic acid–standardized extracts, and purified corosolic acid and ellagitannins. Pure corosolic acid has been reported to decrease blood sugar levels within 60 min in human subjects. In addition to its insulin-like effects, corosolic acid exhibits antihyperlipidemic, antioxidant, anti-inflammatory, antifungal, antiviral, antineoplastic, and osteoblastic activities. The beneficial effects of banaba and corosolic acid with respect to weight management and various aspects of glucose and lipid metabolism appear to involve multiple mechanisms, including enhanced cellular uptake of glucose, impaired hydrolysis of sucrose and starches, decreased gluconeogenesis, and regulation of PPAR-mediated lipid metabolism. No adverse effects have been reported in animal studies or controlled human clinical trials. Current studies indicate that banaba extract, corosolic acid, and other constituents may be beneficial in promoting weight management and addressing issues associated with metabolic syndrome, as well as offer other health benefits.

CONFLICT OF INTEREST

SJS has served as a consultant for Nutratech Inc., West Caldwell, NJ, a supplier of banaba extracts. HM is an employee of Nutratech, Inc. GRK reported no conflicts of interest.

REFERENCES

1. Ulbricht C, Dam C, Milkin T, Seamon E, Weissner W, and Woods J. 2007. Banaba (*Lagerstroemia speciosa* L.): An evidence-based systematic review by the natural Standard Research Collaboration. *J Herb Pharmacother* 7: 99–113.
2. Park MY, Lee KS, and Sung MK. 2005. Effects of dietary mulberry, Korean red ginseng, and banaba on glucose homeostasis in relation to PPAR-α, PPAR-γ, and LPL mRNA expressions. *Life Sci* 77: 3344–3354.
3. Klein G, Kim J, Himmeldirk K, Cao Y, and Chen X. 2007. Antidiabetes and anti-obesity activity of *Lagerstroemia speciosa. Evidence-Based Comp Alt Med* 4: 401–407.
4. Hayashi T, Maruyama H, Kasai R, Hattori K, Takasuga S, Hazeki O, Yamasaki K, and Tanaka T. 2002. Ellagitannins from *Lagerstroemia speciosa* as activators of glucose transport in fat cells. *Planta Med* 68: 173–175.
5. Liu F, Kim J, Li Y, Liu X, Li J, and Chen X. 2005. Tannic acid stimulates glucose transport and inhibits adipocyte differentiation in 3T3-L1 cells. *J Nutr* 135: 165–171.
6. Li Y, Kim J, Li J, Liu F, Liu X, Himmeldirk K, Ren Y, Wagner TE, and Chen X. 2005. Natural antidiabetic compound 1,2,3,4,6-penta-O-galloyl-D-glucopyranose binds to insulin receptor and activates insulin-mediated glucose transport signaling pathway. *Biochem Biophys Res Commun* 336: 430–437.
7. Banno N, Akihisa T, Tokuda H, Yasukawa K, Higashihara H, Ukiya M, Watanabe K, Kimura Y, Hasegawa J, and Nishino H. 2004. Triterpene acids from the leaves of *Perilla frutescens* and their anti-inflammatory and anti-tumor promoting effects. *Biosci Biotechnol Biochem* 68: 85–90.

8. Kim DH, Han KM, Chung IS, Kim DK, Kim SH, Kwon BM, Jeong TS, Park MH, Ahn EM, and Baek NI. 2005. Triterpenoids from the flower of the *Campsis grandiflora* K. Schum as human acyl CoA: Cholesterol acyltransferase inhibitors. *Arch Pharmacol Res* **28**: 550–556.

9. Yang NY, Duan JA, Li P, and Qian SH. 2006. Chemical constituents of *Glechoma longituba* (In Chinese). *Yao Xue Xue Bao* **41**: 431–434.

10. Shen Y, Wang QH, Lin HW, Shu W, Zhou JB, and Li ZY. 2006. Study on chemical constituents of *Potentilla chinensis* Ser (In Chinese). *Zhong Yao Cai* **29**: 237–239.

11. Aguirre MC, Delporte C, Backhouse N, Erazo S, Letelier ME, Cassels BK, Silva X, Alegria S, and Negrete R. 2006. Topical anti-inflammatory activity of 2-alpha-hydroxy pentacyclic triterpene acids from the leaves of *Ugni molinae*. *Bioorg Med Chem* **14**: 5673–5677.

12. Hu C, Chen L, Xin Y, and Cai Q. 2006. Determination of corosolic acid in *Eriobotrya japonica* leaves by reversed-phase high performance liquid chromatography (In Chinese). *Se Pu* **24**: 492–494.

13. Lu H, Chen J, Li WL, and Zhang HQ. 2008. Studies on the triterpenes from ioquat leaf (Eriobotrya japonica) (In Chinese). *Zhang Yao Cai* **31**: 1351–1354.

14. Lu H, Xi C, Chen J, and Li W. 2009. Determination of triterpenoid acids in leaves of *Eriobotrya japonica* collected at different seasons (In Chinese). *Zhongguo Zhong Yao Za Zhi* **34**: 2353–2355.

15. Rollinger JM, Kratschmar DV, Schuster D, Pfisterer PH, Gumy C, Aubry EM, Brandstotter S, Stuppner H, Wolber G, and Odermatt A. 2010. 11-Beta-Hydroxysteroid dehydrogenase-1 inhibiting constituents from *Eriobotrya japonica* revealed by bioactivity-guided isolation and computational approaches. *Bioorg Med Chem* **18**: 1507–1515.

16. Na M, Yang S, He L, Oh H, Kim BS, Oh WK, Kim BY, and Ahn JS. 2006. Inhibition of protein tyrosine phosphatase 1B by ursane-type triterpenes isolated from *Symplocos paniculata*. *Planta Med* **72**: 261–263.

17. Thuong PT, Min BS, Jin W, Na M, Lee J, Seong R, Lee YM, Song K, Seong Y, Lee HK, Bae K, and Kang SS. 2006. Anti-complementary activity of ursane-type triterpenoids from *Weigela subsessilis*. *Biol Pharm Bull* **29**: 830–833.

18. Lee MS and Thuong PT. 2010. Stimulation of glucose uptake by triterpenoids from *Weigela subsessilis*. *Phytother Res* **24**: 49–53.

19. Kang SH, Shi YQ, and Yang CX. 2008. Terpenoids and steroids of root of *Rubus biflorus* (In Chinese). *Zhong Yao Cai* **31**: 1669–1671.

20. Liu P, Deng R, Duan H, and Yin W. 2009. Chemical constituents from roots of *Phlomis umbrosa* (In Chinese). *Zhongguo Zhong Yao Za Zhi* **34**: 867–870.

21. Kim E, Sy-Cordero A, Graf TN, Brantley SJ, Paine MF, and Oberlies NH. 2011. Isolation and identification of intestinal CYP3A inhibitors from cranberry (*Vaccinium macrocarpon*) using human intestinal microsomes. *Planta Med* **77**: 265–270.

22. Ikeda Y, Chen JT, and Matsuda T. 1999. Effectiveness and safety of banabamin tablet containing extract from banaba in patients with mild type 2 diabetes (In Japanese). *Jap Pharmacol Therap* **27**: 829–035.

23. Ikeda Y, Noguchi M, Kishi S, Masuda K, Kusumoto A, Zeida M, Abe K, and Kiso Y. 2002. Blood glucose controlling effects and safety of single and long-term administration on the extract of banaba leaves (In Japanese). *J Nutr Food* **5**: 41–53.

24. Judy WV, Hari SP, Stogsdill WW, Judy JS, Naguib YMA, and Passwater R. 2003. Antidiabetic activity of a standardized extract (Glucosol™) from *Lagerstroemia speciosa* leaves in type II diabetics: A dose-dependence study. *J Ethnopharmacol* **87**: 115–117.

25. Lieberman S, Spahrs R, Stanton A, Martinez L, and Grinder M. 2005. Weight loss, body measurements, and compliance: A 12-week total lifestyle intervention pilot study. *Alt Compl Therap* December 1, **11**: 307–313.

26. Tsuchibe S, Kataumi S, Mori M, and Mori H. 2006. An inhibitory effect on the increase in the post-prandial glucose by banaba extract capsule enriched corosolic acid. *J Integr Study Diet Habits* **17**: 255–259.

27. Xu H. 2008. Action of helping lower blood glucose level-clinical test. Chinese Center for Disease Control and Prevention, Beijing Hospital (Unpublished study). GlucoHelp™, a technical report. Soft Gel Technologies, Inc. www.soft-gel.com.

28. Fukushima M, Matsuyama F, Ueda N, Egawa K, Takemoto J, Kajimoto Y, Uonaha N, Miura T, Kaneko T, Nishi Y, Mitsui R, Fujita Y, Yamada Y, and Seino Y. 2006. Effects of corosolic acid on post-challenge plasma glucose levels. *Diab Res Clin Pract* **73**: 174–177.

29. Zheng JQ, Zheng CM, and Lu KC. 2010. Corosolic acid-induced acute kidney injury and lactic acidosis in a patient with impaired kidney function. *Amer J Kidney Dis* **56**: 419–420.

30. Garcia F. 1940. On the hypoglycemic effect of a decoction of *Lagerstroemia speciosa* leaves (banaba) administered orally. *J Phil Med Assoc* **20**: 193–201.

31. Garcia F. 1941. Distribution and deterioration of insulin-like principle in *Lagerstroemia speciosa* (banaba). *Acta Med Phil* **3**: 99–104.
32. Kakuda T, Sakane I, Takihara T, Ozaki Y, Takeuchi H, and Kuroyangi M. 1996. Hypoglycemic effect of extracts of Lagerstroemia speciosa L. leaves in genetically diabetic KK-AY mice. *Biosci Biotechnol Biochem* **60**: 204–208.
33. Suzuki Y, Unno T, Hayashi K, and Kakuda T. 1999. Antiobesity activity of extracts of *Lagerstroemia speciosa* L. leaves in female KK-AY mice. *J Nutr Sci Vitaminol* **45**: 791–795.
34. Suzuki Y, Hayashi K, Sukabe I, and Kakuda T. 2001. Effects and mode of action of banaba (Lagerstroemia speciosa L.) leaf extracts on postprandial blood glucose in rats. *J Jap Soc Nutr Food Sci* **54**: 131–137.
35. Yamaguchi Y, Yamada K, Yoshikawa N, Nakamura K, Haginaka J, and Kunitomo M. 2006. Corosolic acid prevents oxidative stress, inflammation and hypertension in SHR/HDmcr-cp rats, a model of metabolic syndrome. *Life Sci* **79**: 2474–2479.
36. MatsuuraT, Yoshikawa Y, Masui H, and Sano M. 2004. Suppression of glucose absorption by various health teas in rats (In Japanese). *Yakugaku Zasshi* **124**: 217–223.
37. Hong H and Maeng WJ. 2004. Effects of malted barley extract and banaba extract on blood glucose levels in genetically diabetic mice. *J Med Food* **7**: 487–490.
38. Yamada K, Hosokawa M, Yamada C, Watanabe R, Fujimoto S, Fujiwara H, Kunitomo M, Muira T, Kaneko T, Tsuda K, Seino Y, and Inagaki N. 2008a. Dietary corosolic acid ameliorates obesity and hepatic steatosis in KK-AY mice. *Biol Pharm Bull* **31**: 651–655.
39. Yamada K, Hogokowa M, Fujimoto S, Fujikawa H, Fujita Y, Harada N, Yamada C, Fukushima M, Ueda N, Kaneko T, Matsuyama F, Yamada Y, Seino Y, and Inagaki N. 2008b. Effect of corosolic acid on gluconeogenesis in rat liver. *Diabetes Res Clin Pract* **80**: 48–55.
40. Deocaris CC, Aguinaldo RR, dela Ysla JL, Asencion AS, and Mojica ERE. 2005. Hypoglycemic activity of irradiated banaba (*Lagerstroemia speciosa* L.) leaves. *J Appl Sci Res* **1**: 95–98.
41. Miura T, Itoh Y, Kaneko T, Ueda N, Ishida T, Fukushima M, Matsuyama F, and Seino Y. 2004. Corosolic acid induces GLUT4 translocation in genetically type 2 diabetic mice. *Biol Pharm Bull* **27**: 1103–1105.
42. Miura T, Ueda N, Yamada K, Fukushima M, Ishida T, Kaneko T, Matsuyama F, and Seino Y. 2006. Antidiabetic effects of corosolic acid in KK-AY diabetic mice. *Biol Pharm Bull* **29**: 585–587.
43. Takagi S, Miura T, Ishibashi C, Kawata T, Ishihara E, Gu Y, and Ishida T. 2008. Effect of corosolic acid on the hydrolysis of disaccharides. *J Nutr Sci Vitaminol* **54**: 266–268.
44. Takagi S, Miura T, Ishihara E, Ishida T, and Chinzei Y. 2010. Effect of corosolic acid on dietary hypercholesterolemia and hepatic steatosis in KK-AY diabetic rats. *Biomed Res* **31**: 213–218.
45. Saha BK, Bhuiyan NH, Mazumder K, and Haque KMF. 2009. Hypoglycemic activity of *Lagerstroemia speciosa* L. extract on streptozotocin-induced diabetic rat: Underlying mechanism of action. *J Bangladesh Pharmacol Soc* **4**: 79–83.
46. Thuppia A, Rabintossaporn P, saenthaweesuk S, Ingkaninan K, and Sireeratawong S. 2009. The hypoglycemic effect of a water extract from leaves of *Lagerstroemia speciosa* L. in streptozotocin-induced diabetic rats. *Songklanakarin J Sci Technol* **31**: 133–137.
47. Saumya SM and Basha PM. 2011. Antioxidant effect of *Lagerstroemia speciosa* Pers (banaba) leaf extract in streptozotocin-induced diabetic mice. *Ind J Exptl Biol* **49**: 125–131.
48. Tanquilut NC, Tanquilut MRC, Estacio MAC, Torres EB, Rosario JC, and Reyes BAS. 2009. Hypoglycemic effect of *Lagerstroemia speciosa* L. Pers. on alloxan-induced diabetic mice. *J Med Plants Res* **3**: 1066–1071.
49. Hou W, Li Y, Zhang Q, Wei X, Peng A, Chen L, and Wei Y. 2009. Triterpene acids isolated from *Lagerstroemia speciosa* leaves as alpha-glucosidase inhibitors. *Phytother Res* **23**: 614–618.
50. Musabayane CT, Tufts MA, and Mapanga RF. 2010. Synergistic antihyperglycemic effects between plant-derived oleanolic acid and insulin in streptozotocin-induced diabetic rats. *Renal Failure* **32**: 832–839.
51. Unno T, Sakane I, Masumizu T, Kohno M, and Kakuda T. 1997. Antioxidant activity of water extracts of Lagerstroemia speciosa leaves. *Biosci Biotech Biochem* **61**: 1772–1774.
52. Sato J, Goto K, Nanjo F, Kawai S, and Murata K. 2000. Antifungal activity of plant extracts against *Arthrinium sacchari* and *Chaetomium funicola*. *J Biosci Bioeng* **90**: 442–446.
53. Liu F, Kim JK, Li Y, Liu XQ, Li J, and Chen X. 2001. An extract of *Lagerstroemia speciosa* L. has insulin-like glucose uptake-stimulatory and adipocyte differentiation-inhibitory activities in 3T3-L1 cells. *J Nutr* **131**: 2242–2247.
54. Tanaka T, Tong HH, Xu YM, Ishimaru K, Nonaka G, and Nisioka I. 1992. Tannins and related compounds. CXVII. Isolation and characterization of three new ellagitannins, Lagerstannins A, B, and C, having a gluconic acid core, from *Lagerstroemia speciosa* (L.) Pers. *Chem Pharm Bull* **40**: 2975–2980.

55. Hattori K, Sukenobu N, Sasaki T, Takasuga S, Hayashi T, Kasi R, Yamasaki K, and Hazeki O. 2003. Activation of insulin receptors by lagerstroemin. *J Pharmacol Sci* **93**: 69–73.

56. Bai N, He K, Roller M, Zheng B, Chen X, Shao Z, Peng T, and Zheng Q. 2008. Active compounds from *Lagerstroemia speciosa*, insulin-like glucose uptake-stimulatory/inhibitory and adipocyte differentiation-inhibitory activities in 3T3L1 cells. *J Agric Food Chem* **56**: 11668–11674.

57. Hosoyama H, Sugimoto A, Suzuki Y, Sakane I, and Kakuda T. 2003. Isolation and quantitative analysis of the α-amylase inhibitor in *Lagerstroemia speciosa* (L.) Pers. (banaba) (In Japanese). *Yakugaku Zasshi* **123**: 599–605.

58. Vijaykumar K, Murthy PB, Kannababu S, Syamasundar B, and Subbaraju GV. 2006. Quantitative determination of corosolic acid in Lagerstroemia speciosa leaves, extracts and dosage forms. *Int J Appl Sci Eng* **4**: 103–114.

59. Shi L, Zhang W, Zhou YY, Zhang YN, Li JY, Hu LH, and Li J. 2008. Corosolic acid stimulates glucose uptake via enhancing insulin receptor phosphorylation. *Eur J Pharmacol* **584**: 21–29.

60. Ichikawa H, Yagi H, Tanaka T, Cyong JC, and Masaki T. 2010. *Lagerstroemia speciosa* extract inhibit TNF-induced activation of nuclear factor-κB in rat cardiomyocyte H9c2 cells. *J Ethnopharmacol* **128**: 254–256.

61. Shim KS, Lee SU, Ryu SY, Min YK, and Kim SH. 2009. Corosolic acid stimulates osteoblast differentiation by activating transcription factors and MAP kinases. *Phytother Res* **23**: 1754–1758.

62. Fujiwara Y, Komohara Y, Ikeda T, and Takeya M. 2011. Corosolic acid inhibits glioblastoma cell proliferation by suppressing the activation of signal transducer and activator of transcription-3 and nuclear-factor kappa B in tumor cells and tumor-associated macrophages. *Cancer Sci* **102**: 206–211.

63. Xu Y, Ge R, Du J, Xin H, Yi T, Sheng J, Wang Y, and Ling C. 2009. Corosolic acid induces apoptosis through mitochondrial pathway and caspase activation in human cervix adenocarcinoma HeLa cells. *Cancer Lett* **284**: 229–237.

64. Lee MS, Lee CM, Cha EY, Thuong PT, Bae K, Song IS, Noh SM, and Sul JY. 2010a. Activation of AMP-activated protein kinase on human gastric cancer cells by apoptosis induced by corosolic acid isolated from *Weigela subsessilis*. *Phytother Res* **24**: 2857–1861.

65. Lee MS, Cha EY, Thuong PT, Kim JY, Ahn MS, and Sul JY. 2010b. Down-regulation of human epidermal growth factor receptor 2/ncu oncogene by corosolic acid induces cell cycle arrest and apoptosis in NCI-N87 human gastric cancer cells. *Biol Pharm Bull* **33**: 931–937.

66. Choi HJ, Bae EY, Song JH, Baek SH, and Kwon DH. 2010. Inhibitory effects of orobol-7-O-D-glucoside from banaba (*Lagerstroemia speciosa* L.) on human rhinoviruses replication. *Lett Appl Microbiol* **51**: 1–5.

67. Morshed A, Hossain MH, Shakil S, Nahar K, Rahman S, Ferdausi D, Hossain T, Ahmad I, Chowdhury MH, and Rahmatullah M. 2010. Evaluation of the antinociceptive activity of two Bangladeshi medicinal plants, *Kalanchoe pinnata* (Lam.) Pers. and *Lagerstroemia speciosa* (L.) Pers. *Adv Nat Appl Sci* **4**: 193–197.

68. Nagai M, Fukamachi T, Tsujimoto M, Ogura K, Hiratsuka A, Ohtani H, Hori S, and Sawada Y. 2009. Inhibitory effects of herbal extracts on the activity of human sulfotransferase isoform sulfotransferase 1A3 (SULT1A3). *Biol Pharm Bull* **32**: 105–109.

51 Appetite, Body Weight, Health Implications of a Low-Glycemic-Load Diet

Stacey J. Bell, DSc, RD

CONTENTS

INTRODUCTION

Overweight and obesity pose a major public health concern in terms of increased mortality and morbidity, which are associated with increased risk of cardiovascular disease (CVD), type 2 diabetes mellitus, and osteoarthritis. Compared to normal-weight individuals, obesity (body mass index [BMI] $\geq 30\,kg/m^2$) was associated with over 110,000 excess deaths per year (Flegal et al., 2005). Inspection of telomere length as a marker of aging showed that obesity corresponded to 8.8 years of aging; this was similar to smoking a pack of cigarettes a day for 40 years (7.4 years) (Valdes et al., 2005). It has been postulated that only about a 10 cal energy gap per day is the cause of obesity, so it would seem that it could be readily treated (Brown et al., 2005). However, few strategies for losing weight have been effective, and new ones are welcome (Pawlak et al., 2002; Bell and Sears, 2003a). In contrast, strategies to get individuals to quit smoking have been more successful, showing that behaviors can be changed to improve health.

Of the numerous strategies that exist for helping individuals lose weight, the most invasive, bariatric surgery is still the most effective at producing weight loss (about 61% per patient) (Buchwald et al., 2004). Pharmacological agents have met with mixed results. One of the most promising nonsurgical, nonpharmacological strategies to promote weight loss was ephedra because it induced weight loss without its users actually having to consciously reduce calorie intake (Coffey et al., 2004). However, in 2004, the Food and Drug Administration banned it from being sold, citing significant side effects, including death.

Equally promising weight loss strategies have been the so-called low-carbohydrate diets popularized by the late Dr. Atkins (Foster et al., 2003; Samaha et al., 2003). It seemed that everyone in America knew someone who had lost weight on the Atkins diet. However, two major clinical studies evaluating the Atkins diet showed that although weight loss after 6 months was greater compared to the conventional heart-healthy, low-fat diet, the difference disappeared by 1 year (Foster et al., 2003). Soon after the publication of these articles, the appeal of the "low-carb" phenomenon waned.

There is a lesser-known weight loss program called the low-glycemic-load (low-GL) or low-glycemic-index (low-GI) diet (Ludwig, 2003; Dickinson and Brand-Miller, 2005). Of the seven leading drivers of health in the Western diet, a diet high in GL was identified as that having the greatest impact (Cordain et al., 2005). The low-GL diet is gaining popularity among clinicians, researchers, and overweight and obese patients because it has been shown to promote satiety, to have a sound physiological basis behind how it works, and to contain all the essential nutrients. In addition, following a low-GL diet for both the short and long terms has been shown to promote weight loss without hunger and reduce the risk of many chronic diseases of aging including obesity, CVD, and type 2 diabetes.

This chapter serves as a review on the subject of the GL of the diet. Beginning with definitions of terms (e.g., GL, GI), this chapter will also explore the physiological effects of GL, including its effects on satiety, as well as the health implications of following a high-GI or high-GL diet. And finally, practical information is given on how to follow a low-GI or low-GL diet.

DEFINITION OF TERMS

The GL and GI are rating systems for evaluating the change in postprandial blood glucose levels after consuming carbohydrate-containing foods (Table 51.1). Each is defined in the following.

TABLE 51.1
GI and GL of Commonly Consumed Food Categories (Expressed as Approximate Values)

Food Category	GI (Compared to Glucose)	GL
Dairy (milk, cheese, yogurt)	20–40	<10
Fruits	20–40	<10
Vegetables (nonstarchy)	Insignificant	Insignificant
Vegetables (starchy)	60–90	10–25
Legumes, nuts	25–45	<5–15
Nonsweetened and sweetened bakery products, cereals, pasta, grains[a]	50–80	10–20
Carbonated beverages (Coca Cola)	63	16
Juices	40–60	15–25
Snack foods	>50	10–25+

Source: Based on Foster-Powell, K. et al., *Am. J. Clin. Nutr.*, 76, 5, 2002.
[a]   White and whole wheat products differ only slightly.

Glycemic Index

The concept of postprandial glucose levels was originally deemed important in the early 1980s when it was thought that setting limits would lead to better daily glucose management in patients with diabetes (Jenkins, 1981; Wolever et al., 1991). The GI relates to the rate at which recently ingested carbohydrates appear in the blood as glucose. The GI is expressed as a percentage:

Integrated increase in blood glucose level during a 2 h period after a known
quantity of carbohydrate is ingested (usually 50 g of available carbohydrate) $\times 100$

Integrated increase in blood glucose level during a 2 h period after a known
quantity of a reference food is ingested (usually 50 g of white bread or glucose)

The values for GIs of foods typically range from 20 to 100. However, some foods that are highly processed may exceed this upper value (e.g., cornflakes have a GI of 120).

Conceptually, a low-GL diet involves limiting the intake of foods that have the greatest impact on postprandial blood glucose concentrations. For example, foods that are composed of mainly protein and fat have virtually no impact on GI or GL. These include all meats, dairy products, and fats and oils. However, too much protein produces an undesirable insulinemic effect, which may promote weight gain and increased hunger (Parcell et al., 2004). Protein from either a bar (29 g) or a shake (15 g) had a 2 h area under the curve (AUC) insulin response of 90% or 88%, respectively, compared to 50 g of glucose. Thus, both postprandial glucose and insulin should be controlled on a low-GL diet.

The procedures for obtaining measurements of GI are described elsewhere (Jenkins, 1981; Wolever et al., 1991). The GI of carbohydrate-containing foods varies widely and cannot be predicted based on chemical analysis of the carbohydrates (i.e., simple vs. complex). In fact, large differences in GIs even exist within foods found in the same food group. For example, wholemeal bread was found to have a GI of 72, while wholemeal spaghetti had only 42. Similarly, for some tubers and root vegetables, parsnips have a GI of 97, while sweet potatoes have one of 48. Ironically, the fiber content of foods had very little effect on GI. Other oddities occur. For example, the GI of sucrose (glucose and fructose)—thought to be diabetogenic—is not among one of the highest food measured, because the GI of fructose is much lower than glucose (Buyken and Liese, 2005). And in addition to all of the other variables, cooking can affect the GI of a food. Precooked Russet potatoes elicited lower AUC glucose responses than those cooked the day that they were consumed (Fernandes et al., 2005). However, this same effect was not seen in boiled white potatoes. All of these variables underscore the importance of measuring the GI of individual foods to determine the true effect that food has on postprandial blood glucose levels.

With so many factors affecting the GI of individual foods, it isn't surprising that the concept of GI has been criticized (Pi-Sunyer, 2005). In response, an international group of researchers recently validated it. Seven different research groups from around the world measured the GI of four foods: instant potato, rice, spaghetti, and barley (Wolever et al., 2003). Locally obtained white bread served as the control. All laboratories followed the protocol established by the FAO/WHO to measure GI. The GI of these foods did not vary significantly in the different centers, nor was there a center and food interaction identified. The mean between-laboratory standard deviation (s.d.) was small (approximately 9), and the measurements of GI were closer to 9 when capillary, rather than venous blood, was sampled. The size of the s.d. confirmed the validity of the GI measurements because most foods have GIs ranging from 20 to 120, and an s.d. of 9 indicates the tightness of the data. Moreover, the ease of using capillary blood compared to venous blood confirmed that this test can easily be conducted at many facilities around the world.

GLYCEMIC LOAD

Ultimately, over 1200 GI measurements of individual carbohydrate-containing foods were conducted (Foster-Powell et al., 2002). Each was measured using the requisite 50 g of available carbohydrate (total carbohydrate minus fiber) in the food. However, these portion sizes do not always match up with actual serving sizes, making GI of limited use in meal planning. This limitation led to the development of a methodology, called GL, which took this portion size into account.

The GL is representative of the GI of a food, but reflective of a usual serving size of a carbohydrate-containing food (Salmeron et al., 1997; Liu et al., 2001; Ebbeling et al., 2005). The GL can be calculated thus as follows:

$$\frac{\text{Glycemic index of a food (\%)} \times \text{Grams of carbohydrate in that food}}{100}$$

The GLs of foods typically range from 2 to 30 (Table 51.1). Each unit of the GL represents the equivalent of 1 g of carbohydrate from white bread (Michaud et al., 2005). White bread is often used as the standard (i.e., equal to a GI of 100). Of the carbohydrate-containing foods, nonstarchy vegetables and legumes have the lowest GLs (<5). Fruit and dairy foods are next (around 10), followed by unsweetened, grain-based foods (10–20) and then sweetened, grain-based foods, candy, and carbonated beverages (>15). Foods that have GLs in excess of 10 are typically considered to have high GLs. Most grain-based snack foods—both salty and sweet—have GLs at or above this value. Such foods only started creeping into the food supply within the past 100 years.

The GLs from all of the foods ingested in a single day can be summed and used to compare dietary regimens among different populations. For example, the sum of all of the GLs of a day when a low-GL diet was followed is about 50–70 (Bell and Sears, 2003b). In contrast, consuming a high-carbohydrate, heart-healthy, low-fat diet, such as that outlined in the U.S. Department of Agriculture's Food Guide Pyramid, yields a total dietary GL for the day of at least 80, but it could be as high as 120. And the typical American diet that also includes numerous servings of sweetened carbonated beverages, salty snacks, candy, and baked goods could have a dietary GL of over 200.

The GL and GI often trend in the same direction, but not always. For example, carrots have a high GI (71), but have a low GL (4) (Bell and Sears, 2003b). The difference comes from the fact that the 50 g of carbohydrate used to compute the GI of carrots is more than a typical single serving of vegetables. To get 50 g of the available carbohydrate in carrots, you would have to consume about four cups of carrots at a sitting. Carrots are high in fiber and water that take up space and weight, and a typical serving does not have an appreciable effect on blood glucose concentrations. Other nonstarchy vegetables and some fruits (e.g., berries) have this unique phenomenon, which explains their low GL. These examples demonstrate that the GL is a better tool than the GI for meal planning because single servings of nonstarchy vegetables and selected fruits have minimal impact on blood glucose levels, which drive GI.

The GL methodology was recently validated (Brand-Miller et al., 2003a). In this two-part study, 10 healthy subjects consumed foods that were thought to have the same GL to confirm that they evoked similar effects on blood glucose levels. In the second part, another group of 10 healthy subjects consumed different foods that were thought to produce a stepwise increase in GL. Both studies yielded predictable results. This was the first report confirming that the GL of foods has the physiological validity to predict glycemic response.

GLYCEMIC LOAD AND THE AMERICAN DIET

One of the reasons that the low-GL-diet concept is gaining in popularity is that the rising obesity rates are coincident with the consumption of foods with extremely high GLs. Never before in our evolution have foods been consumed that have such very high GIs (>100) or GLs (>10) (Foster-Powell et al., 2002). As more individuals eat an appreciable amount of calories from snacks, it is easy to understand why the GL of the diet has increased.

The GL of the diet of women aged 34–59 years rose 22% between 1980 and 1990 (Hu et al., 2000). During the same time, the percentage of women who were overweight increased 38%, which may have been related to the change in the GL of the diet, or the fact that the percentage of women who smoked declined 41%. Other dietary factors improved, such as the consumption of fewer trans fats, the increase in the ratio of polyunsaturated to saturated fat intake, the increase in cereal fiber, and the increase in omega-3 fatty acids. None of these were thought to cause the increase in body weight, except the change in the GL of the diet. Thus, these data provide a compelling relationship between body weight and GL of the diet.

PHYSIOLOGICAL EFFECTS OF A LOW-GLYCEMIC-LOAD DIET

Ludwig et al. (1999) and Ludwig (2002) and others have conducted an elegant series of studies identifying the physiological basis for why a low-GL diet may be effective at promoting satiety, reducing body weight, and lowering the risk of many chronic diseases of aging. Physiological changes were characterized by their sequential effects at three stages postprandially.

EARLY POSTPRANDIAL PERIOD

Within 2 h of ingesting a high-GL carbohydrate-containing food or meal, blood glucose concentrations can be more than double that of a eucaloric meal with a low-GL (Ludwig et al., 1999; Ludwig, 2002). (These data were obtained from measurements from obese adolescents.) These higher blood glucose levels trigger the release of increased amounts of insulin to reduce them. High circulating insulin levels favor anabolism, thereby signaling the storage of all incoming nutrients (mainly lipids and carbohydrates) as fat in the adipocytes (lipogenesis) or as glycogen stored in muscle and the liver (glycogenesis). The disappearance of these substrates from the blood is rapid, and upon their disappearance, hunger sets in.

The constant exposure to high-GL foods and meals may promote the development of insulin resistance mainly because the pancreas is required to regularly secrete high amounts of insulin throughout the day. When circulating insulin levels are elevated, lipolysis is inhibited, thereby making it hard to use body fat stores for energy and to lose weight. Similarly, glycolysis is suppressed because glucose levels are maintained at normal levels, or may even be elevated depending upon how much insulin resistance is already present. Others have argued that habitual consumption of high-GL diets has no effect on the risk of insulin resistance (Lau et al., 2005), but others refute this (Ludwig, 2002). What is particularly problematic is that Americans tend to snack frequently on high-GL foods, which causes hyperinsulinemia and creates a state of anabolism most of the time.

MIDDLE POSTPRANDIAL PERIOD

Two to four hours after the ingestion of a high-GL meal, nutrients are almost completely absorbed from the gastrointestinal tract (Ludwig et al., 1999; Ludwig, 2002). Glucagon is the counterregulatory hormone that is released in response to insulin, and an elevated ratio of insulin/glucagon persists from the early 2 h phase. This skewed ratio may drive blood glucose concentrations down, even to the point of creating a hypoglycemic state. Glucose serves as the primary fuel for the brain, and hunger sets in when the brain senses food deprivation. The other major fuel source of the body is free fatty acids, which are also suppressed by the exaggerated insulin/glucagon ratios. Thus, both of the body's key metabolic hormones are unbalanced, which leads to hunger because the body is without its two major fuel sources.

Late Postprandial Period

Four to six hours after ingestion of a high-GL meal, the low circulating concentrations of glucose and free fatty acids stimulate the release of counterregulatory hormones (i.e., glucagons, epinephrine, cortisol, and growth hormone) (Ludwig et al., 1999; Ludwig, 2002). This is the body's attempt to release the recently stored energy sources. Glucagon and cortisol primarily cause the release of glycogen, thereby increasing blood glucose concentrations. Fat is mobilized from the adipocytes primarily by epinephrine and growth hormone, which restores free fatty acid levels to normal. However, if insulin levels are still elevated at this time, these catabolic processes are blunted, so it is possible that an individual will remain hungry beyond the 4 h after eating a high-GL meal. Thus, high-GL meals and snacks promote the hunger that can lead to obesity by fostering more frequent snacking.

In contrast, a low-GL meal or snack does not induce such dramatic hormonal shifts (Ludwig et al., 1999; Ludwig, 2002). Low-GL foods take longer to digest and absorb, thereby minimizing the impact on hyperglycemia and hyperinsulinemia. In addition, the liver can undergo glycolysis and release glucose, and the adipocytes can undergo lipolysis to release free fatty acids. Thus, hunger is avoided and stored substrates can be mobilized to promote weight loss. And insulin resistance is curtailed, as insulin levels rarely go into superphysiologic range.

These glycemic and insulinemic changes seen in adolescents were confirmed in obese, adult women (Diaz et al., 2005). In a crossover design, the subjects, on separate occasions, consumed low-GL and high-GL test meals (breakfast and lunch). Glucose and insulin AUCs were significantly higher following the high-GL meals compared to the low-GL ones. Serum free fatty acids were suppressed by both meals by 3 h postprandially but then raised significantly more in the low-GL meal group by the fourth and fifth hour ($P < 0.05$). However, glucagon concentrations did not differ significantly between the two test meals as found earlier (Ludwig et al., 1999). Diaz et al. (2005) speculated that carbohydrate oxidation would be favored and fat oxidation reduced, but this did not occur. The short-term period for the changes in insulin concentrations during this feeding study likely explained why no differences were observed in fuel partitioning between the two dietary regimens. In contrast, when insulin is infused in a stepwise manner at nonphysiological levels for a long time (>100 min), such differences in substrate utilization are observed.

EFFECT OF GLYCEMIC LOAD ON HUNGER

Hunger, satiety, and satiation have long been associated with the GI or GL of the diet (Ludwig, 2000; Roberts, 2000). Satiation is the sensation of fullness that develops during the process of a meal and contributes to its termination. Satiety is the sensation of fullness between one meal and the next. Hunger is the degree of appetite suppression between one meal and the next. Looking at the totality of the published studies (reviewed elsewhere), all three sensations are affected by the GL and GI of the diet. The lower the GI or GL of the day's foods consumed, the earlier satiation occurs, the longer satiety is, and the less of a sensation of hunger there is before each meal (Ludwig, 2000; Roberts, 2000).

On average, total daily caloric intake was 20% greater after consumption of a high-GL meal than after a low-GL meal (Roberts, 2000). To emphasize the importance of this relationship between food consumption and GL, one laboratory has developed a validated satiety index of commonly consumed foods (Holt et al., 1995). It can be used by overweight and obese individuals to make better food choices on a weight loss regimen. These investigators found that isoenergetic servings of a variety of foods differed greatly for hunger and satiety, and the predictability of these effects was related to the GI of the individual foods.

Clinical support exists for a low-GL diet in curtailing hunger and promoting satiety (Agus et al., 2000; Ludwig, 2000, 2002; Roberts, 2000; Dumesnil et al., 2001). Two studies have shown that less hunger occurs within 6 days of consuming a low-GL diet compared to a high-GL diet (Agus et al.,

2000; Dumesnil et al., 2001). In both short-term studies, subjects reported that they were less hungry while following a low-GL diet and ate 25% fewer calories compared to when they consumed a high-GL diet.

Another group of investigators measured both hormonal changes and hunger to confirm that the two are related (Ludwig et al., 1999). Twelve obese adolescents were evaluated on three separate occasions using a crossover design protocol. Eucaloric test meals were consumed at breakfast, but each varied by GL (low, medium, and high). Subjects were monitored during the subsequent 5 h, and selected blood chemistries, including hormones, were measured. The voluntary caloric intake after the test meals was 53% higher in the medium-GL meal and 81% higher in the high-GL meal compared to the low-GL meal. The difference in energy intakes was supported by how hungry the subjects felt. Using a 10-point analog hunger scale, subjects were consistently less hungry following consumption of the low-GL meal, intermediate after the medium-GL meal, and most hungry following the high-GL meal.

The researchers demonstrated that serial hormonal changes were responsible for the different degrees of hunger (Ludwig et al., 1999). The measured AUC for plasma insulin levels was 52% higher for the high-GL meal compared to the low-GL meal. The mean plasma glucose nadir was 42% lower after the high-GL meal compared to both the low-GL and medium-GL meals. Thus, the high-GL meal produced the greatest adverse effect on glycemia (i.e., greatest hypoglycemia) and the greatest insulin secretion, further exacerbating falling blood glucose levels. Plasma glucagon levels predictably rose after the low-GL meal but were suppressed about 10% for the medium-GL and high-GL meals. This was likely related to the presence of hyperinsulincmia. Finally, the serum free fatty acids were suppressed the most after ingestion of the high-GL meal compared to the other two diets. To compensate for this, the counterregulatory hormones epinephrine and growth hormone were higher following the high-GL meal compared to the low-GL meal, causing free fatty acids to increase. These results suggest that a single meal can have an immediate and profound metabolic consequence that can last up to 5 h. The degree of hunger was supported by the metabolic changes that occurred postprandially.

A subsequent study, however, did not support the relationship between changes in glycemic and insulinemic responses and hunger (Alfenas and Mattes, 2005). Thirty-nine healthy adults consumed either high-GL foods or low-GL foods for 8 days. Appetite sensation and blood tests were performed before and 2 h following breakfast and lunch on days 1 and 8. The magnitude of the glycemic and insulin responses did not differ between the diets at any time point. Caloric intake between the groups did not differ either. Thus, no close relationship between hunger and blood glucose and insulin levels was observed. However, this study was short term and was conducted in normal-weight volunteers. The randomized prospective studies and epidemiological data would suggest a benefit of the low-GL in controlling appetite and, thus, weight (see following text).

GLYCEMIC LOAD AND WEIGHT LOSS

Several studies have confirmed that low-GL diets promote weight loss (Spieth et al., 2000; Ebbeling et al., 2003; Young et al., 2004; Bell et al., 2005; Armendariz-Anguiano et al., 2011), while others have not found a benefit (Carels, 2004; Raatz et al., 2005; Sichieri et al., 2007).

FAVORABLE STUDIES

Short-term data showed that obese children (n = 64) who consumed a low-GL diet lost more weight than those who followed a high-GL, low-fat, energy-restricted diet (n = 43) (Spieth et al., 2000). After 4 months, the low-GL group experienced a −1.53 kg/m² change in BMI, while the control group had a −0.06 kg/m² change. In contrast to the high-GL group, the low-GL diet group was instructed to eat to satiety and lost more weight.

The same laboratory followed 14 obese adolescents aged 13–21 years for 1 year (Ebbeling et al., 2003). The dietary protocols were the same as mentioned earlier. At 12 months, both BMI ($-1.3 \pm 0.7 \text{kg/m}^2$ vs. $0.7 \pm 0.5 \text{kg/m}^2$; $P = 0.02$) and fat mass ($-3.0 \pm 1.6 \text{kg}$ vs. $1.8 \pm 1.0 \text{kg}$; $P = 0.01$) decreased significantly in the low-GL group compared to the high-GL, energy-restricted, low-fat group, respectively. Insulin resistance, measured by means of homeostasis model assessment (HOMA), increased less in the low-GL group. Despite no energy restriction, the low-GL group ate fewer calories at the 12 month measurement compared to the high-GL group, respectively (1621 ± 159 kcal vs.1439 ± 104 kcal). Although hunger and satiety were not measured, it seemed that those in the low-GL group were more satisfied since they lost more weight while eating fewer calories.

A couple of small pilot studies showed the ease with which a low-GL diet could be followed by free-living overweight children and adults (Young et al., 2004; Bell et al., 2005). Children were recruited from a pediatrician's office (Young et al., 2004). They received a brief description of the diet and a handout categorizing the foods based on their GI value; sample meal plans were also provided (Young et al., 2004). Subjects were monitored for 12 weeks, and calorie counts and food frequency questionnaires were obtained. Although 34 children were enrolled in the study, only 15 completed it. Fourteen children lowered the GI score of their diets and decreased carbohydrate intake by 73 g compared to baseline ($P < 0.02$). Mean caloric intake decreased by 292 kcal/day ($P < 0.02$), leading to 12 of the 15 children losing weight. The participants and their parents described the diet as easy to understand. These promising data provided a protocol to assist busy pediatricians with a tool to help children lose weight.

The effect of a low-GL diet to promote weight loss was assessed in free-living overweight and obese adults living in Grand Rapids, Michigan (Bell et al., 2005). All were recruited from a newspaper advertisement. The study lasted 8 weeks, and the subjects were instructed on the diet at baseline. They were weighed on the same scale at baseline, week 4, and week 8. At these visits, they also had their waist circumference measured. Each in-between week, the subjects were called by the study coordinator to assess compliance. Subjects were instructed on a low-GL diet that included the following information:

- Consume two servings of low-fat dairy each day.
- Eat two servings of fruit per day.
- At lunch and dinner, consume low-GL, low-starch vegetables, eating at least two cups of different kinds at each meal.
- Eat 4 oz of meat protein (beef, pork, veal, poultry, fish, shellfish) at lunch and dinner.
- Limit high-GL, starchy vegetables (potatoes, corn, rice), grain-based foods (breads, pasta, salty snacks), flour-based foods (pastries, cakes, cookies, donuts), candy, and sugar-containing beverages including juices.
- For breakfast, consume a low-GL meal replacement shake made with skim or 1% milk, preferably including one of the day's servings of fruit.
- Low-GL snack bars were provided to be used as in-between-meal snacks at least once a day.
- Appetite suppressant (soluble fiber and chromium) capsules were provided to be used before meals.

Twenty individuals began the study, 17 completed 4 weeks, and 14 completed all 8 weeks. The study included 6 males of which 5 completed the entire study, and 11 females of which 9 completed it. All participants consumed the meal replacement shake at breakfast, and only two participants did not use the snack bars. All used the capsules to control hunger, but most used them only twice a day.

The entire group lost an average of 10 lb after 8 weeks, which is consistent with a good, weight-reducing diet of about 1–2 lb per week (Table 51.2). Males lost more (17 vs. 5 lb) than females primarily because one male lost 37 lb, thereby skewing the average upward. Waist circumference averaged a decrease of 1.75 in., with males and females about even (−1.6 vs. −1.8 in., respectively). This may reflect an improvement in insulin sensitivity (Si). Subjects in this study did not complain of hunger after the first week, and no clinically relevant side effects were reported. The participants

TABLE 51.2
Changes in Weight and Anthropometric Data

Parameter	Males	Females
Weights (lb) Baseline	233 (182–322)	210 (144–318)
Week 4 change	−10 (2–21)	−3 (0–6)
Week 8 change	−17 (1–37)	−5 (0–11)
Waist circumference (in.) Baseline	44 (39–49)	41 (33–48)
Week 8 change	−1.6 (0–3.3)	−1.8 (0.5–3.5)
BMI (kg/m²) Baseline	33 (25–39)	34 (25–51)
Week 8	−2.3 (0–5)	−1 (0–1.8)

Source: Presented as means and ranges. (Bell, S.J. et al., *Nutra World,* 8, 50, 2005.)

reported that the diet was easy to follow. These data are consistent with earlier reports showing that weight loss can be achieved without hunger.

The previous studies supported the notion that a low-GL diet reduces hunger, which led to weight loss. Others have suggested that a low-GL diet may also affect energy metabolism (Agus et al., 2000). Ten moderately overweight subjects participated in two, 8 day feeding regimens. The purpose of the study was to determine if metabolic adaptations to energy restriction differed between eucaloric, energy-restricted high-GL and low-GL diets. The subjects consumed each diet for 6 days and then were followed for 2 more days using the same diet, but without the energy restriction.

Two of the findings from this study helped explain how a low-GL diet may promote weight loss, above and beyond hunger control (Agus et al., 2000). First, serum leptin concentrations decreased to a greater extent between day 0 and day 6 with the low-GL diet than the high-GL diet. This is what would have been expected because serum leptin concentrations and carbohydrate intake are positively associated. The low-GL group consumed a smaller percentage of energy from carbohydrates compared to the high-GL group (43% vs. 67%). In addition, the lower serum leptin concentrations seen in the low-GL group were also predictable because insulin is a leptin secretagogue. The mean AUC for insulin was 50% lower in the low-GL group compared to the high-GL group (478 ± 82.2 pmol h/L vs. 700 ± 98.4 pmol h/L; $P = 0.01$).

Second, resting energy expenditure declined significantly less ($P = 0.04$) in the low-GL (4.6%) compared to the high-GL diet (10.5%) during the energy-restricted phase (Agus et al., 2000). This difference, coupled with the greater decrease in serum leptin concentrations, may help explain how a low-GL diet could promote weight loss.

Long-term (6 months), low-GL diets were shown to be of benefit in overweight and obese subjects (Armendariz-Anguiano et al., 2011). At the end of the study, both groups experienced significant weight loss, but significantly more was lost in the low-GL group compared to the high-GL group (4.5% [$P = 0.006$] vs. 3% [$P = 0.18$]). In addition, those assigned to the low-GL group had significant reductions in body fat, waist circumference, and HOMA. These findings suggested that a low-GL diet may contribute to preventing type 2 diabetes.

UNFAVORABLE STUDIES

Five day food records were examined from over 179 elderly subjects (≥65 years of age) (Davis et al., 2004). Subjects were clustered according to the GL of the diet and by gender. In both sexes, those who followed a low-GL diet, compared to those consuming a high-GL diet, weighed significantly less ($P < 0.001$), ate fewer grams of carbohydrate ($P < 0.06$), and had significantly higher healthy eating index score ($P < 0.001$). However, the BMIs of the groups did not differ. It may be that all that the low-GL regimen offers is better eating habits, with a more nutrient-rich diet. That alone may suggest that the low-GL regimen promotes a lessening of disease risk rather than weight loss.

A couple of laboratories did not find that the low-GI diet promoted weight loss (Carels et al., 2005; Raatz et al., 2005). Fifty-three free-living adults were randomly assigned to receive a behavioral weight loss program (BWLP), which consists of an energy-restricted, low-fat diet, and were encouraged to exercise; another group received all of these plus education about the GI value of foods (BWLP + GI) (Carels et al., 2005). In the BWLP + GI group, despite consuming a lower-GI diet and having more knowledge about how to select low-GI foods, no significant differences in weight, fat loss, or BMI were observed after 1 year. However, the dietary GL for the day dropped in both groups, so that differences would be hard to detect between the two treatment modalities. Besides, the dietary GL for the day in the BWLP + GI group still exceeded 100 (112.2 ± 51.7), which may not have been low enough to control appetite and promote weight loss.

Other investigators similarly found no benefit of a low-GL diet beyond energy restriction (Raatz et al., 2005). Twenty-nine obese subjects were assigned to one of three energy-restricted dietary regimens for 36 weeks—a high-GL diet (dietary GL for the day was 272), a low-GL diet (dietary GL for the day was 172), or a high-fat diet (40% of the calories from fat). During the first 12 weeks, all subjects were provided their meals. During that phase of the study, each group experienced a significant weight loss (around 10 kg) and improvement in Si, which was measured by HOMA. No differences among the groups were detected within these parameters, except that the HOMA values differed between the low-GL and high-fat regimen at week 12 ($P < 0.03$, with the low-GL being significantly better). A subgroup (n = 22) continued on their assigned diet for another 24 weeks. The groups were similar at the end of this period in that the weight loss was maintained and Si continued to improve. But no benefit was observed in the low-GL diet over the high-GL or high-fat diets.

During the free-living phase, the GL of all groups was similar (Raatz et al., 2005). All subjects reduced portion sizes, which lowered the GL of the overall diet. This is an interesting finding in and of itself, in that it may be sufficient to concentrate on portion size rather than GL to achieve weight loss. In addition, dietary fat intake increased in all groups and approximated their prescreening levels. The study was small, and about one-fourth of the subjects dropped out, making it difficult to fully assess the effect of a low-GL diet. Unlike the earlier studies where Si was assessed, these data did not corroborate those findings (Ludwig et al., 1999; Ludwig, 2002).

One long-term study (18 months) conducted on healthy women failed to show a difference in weight loss between a low-GI or high-GI diet (Sichieri et al., 2007). After a 6 week run-in period, subjects were assigned to one of these options with minimal energy restriction. Carbohydrate intake was 60% of energy, and the difference between the diets in GI was 35–40 units (40 for the low-GI compared with 79 in the high-GI). After 2 months, weight loss was greater in the low-GI group; at 1 year, both groups began to regain weight. At the end of the study, there was no difference in weight loss, suggesting that the long-term use of a low-GI diet does not translate into sustained weight loss.

As with most weight loss studies, conflicting data usually appear in the medical literature. The physiological responses to a high-GL diet were not supported in the Raatz et al. (2005) study, which will likely provoke more studies evaluating the effect of a low-GL diet on weight loss. Others who did not find favorable results suggested that the concept of low-GL diets was only effective at breakfast, following an overnight fast (Hui et al., 2005). These investigators found the same variation in blood sugar levels after consuming high-, middle-, and low-GL meals at all times during the day except after breakfast. These similarities throughout the day were likely driven by snacking, which so many individuals do. In addition, cortisol levels are highest in the early morning, so postprandial blood sugar levels responded more predictably at that time (i.e., lower for the low-GL meals). Another group (Pittas et al., 2005) suggested that overweight individuals with relatively greater insulin secretion in response to a glucose tolerance test (GTT) lost more weight than those who responded normally. Thus, patient screening by GTT response may improve the chances of losing weight. Nevertheless, most of the previous studies showed that weight loss could be achieved without hunger and that changes in metabolic parameters supported the change in body weight.

GLYCEMIC LOAD AND DISEASE

Unlike the relatively few studies showing that a low-GL diet promotes weight loss, many more are available showing that following a low-GL diet for a long time (for up to 10 years) leads to risk reduction of a whole host of medical conditions including CVD, type 2 diabetes, and various other conditions.

META-ANALYSES

Two meta-analyses reviewed the effect of low-GL diets on chronic conditions (Brand-Miller et al., 2003b; Opperman et al., 2004). Opperman et al. (2004) included 16 studies in their analysis, which had major outcomes as the change in markers of carbohydrate and lipid metabolism. The low-GL diets significantly reduced fructosamine by -0.1 mmol/L (95% confidence intervals [CI]: 0.20, 0.00; $P = 0.05$), hemoglobin (Hgb) A_{1c} by 0.27% (95% CI: 0.5, -0.03; $P = 0.03$), and total cholesterol by -0.33 mmol/L (95% CI: 0.47, -0.18; $P < 0.0001$), and tended to reduce LDL-cholesterol in patients with type 2 diabetes by -0.15 mmol/L (95% CI: 0.31, 0.00; $P = 0.06$) compared to high-GL diets. No changes were observed in HDL-cholesterol and triglyceride levels. From this study, the use of a low-GL diet appears beneficial at reducing total cholesterol levels and improving the overall metabolic control of diabetes.

Another group of investigators used meta-analysis to evaluate the effect of low-GL diets on improving overall glycemic control in individuals with diabetes as assessed by fructosamine or Hgb A_{1c} (Brand-Miller et al., 2003b). Fourteen studies were identified that included 356 subjects (203 with type 1 and 153 with type 2 diabetes) who were randomly assigned to consume the low-GL or high-GL diets for 12 days to 12 months. The Hgb A_{1c} was reduced by 7.4% more with the low-GL diet than the high-GL diet. Choosing low-GL foods had a clinically useful effect on glycemic control in patients with diabetes.

CARDIOVASCULAR DISEASE

The incidence of CVD has declined since 1980, but dietary strategies like the low-GL diet continue to be explored to reduce the incidence even further (Hu et al., 2000). The effect of a low-GL diet on cardiovascular health is of particular interest because for the past two decades patients with CVD or at risk for it were provided low-fat, high-carbohydrate diets, which had inherently high GLs (Dickinson and Brand-Miller, 2005). Some have expressed a concern that such a diet increases the risk of CVD rather than reducing it because of the high-GL nature of the diet. Epidemiological data and short-term studies exploring the effect of low-GL diets on CVD risk are reviewed separately.

Epidemiological Data

A 10 year study including over 75,000 women aged 38–63 years suggested that regular consumption of a high-GL diet from refined carbohydrates increased the risk of coronary heart disease (CHD), independent of other cardiac risk factors (Liu et al., 2000). Using validated food frequency questionnaires to compute the sum of the GL of all the foods consumed in a day (i.e., dietary GL), those in the lowest quintile (dietary GL = 117) were assigned an RR (relative risk) of 1.0 for CHD risk. The other quintiles had RRs of 1.01 (dietary GL = 145), 1.25 (dietary GL = 161), 1.51 (dietary GL = 177), and 1.98 (dietary GL = 206) (P for trend < 0.0001). These data reflected adjustment of age, smoking status, and other CHD risk factors. Classifying carbohydrate intake merely according to simple or complex did not yield significant outcomes as compared with classifying carbohydrates according to GL.

A subset of the previous population (n = 244) had high-sensitivity C-reactive protein (hs-CRP) concentrations measured; these were compared to the dietary GL (Liu et al., 2002). This measurement is an indicator of CVD risk, especially of ischemic heart disease. A significant and positive relationship was seen between the dietary GL and hs-CRP (P for trend < 0.01). The difference in hs-CRP between the lowest and highest dietary GL was twofold. The association was even more pronounced when the women were segmented by BMI $\geq$ 25 kg/m² or BMI < 25 kg/m². The mean hs-CRPs were higher at each dietary GL quintile, suggesting an added effect of body weight on CVD risk. These data showed that a high-GL diet led to increased body weight, which was positively related to hs-CRP, a risk factor for CVD.

Both of these large-scale studies indicated a significant relationship between the GL of the diet and the risk of CVD.

Short-Term Studies

The effect of a low-GL diet on reducing CVD risk factors was seen in young (Pereira et al., 2004; Ebbeling et al., 2005) and older adult subjects (Dumesnil et al., 2001; Patel et al., 2004; Sloth et al., 2004; Shikany et al., 2005).

During a 12 month study, 23 young adults aged 18–35 years consumed either an *ad libitum* low-GL diet or an energy-restricted, low-fat (<30% of the energy) diet (Ebbeling et al., 2005). Body weight decreased in both groups at 6 months (about 8%) and remained below baseline at 1 year (about 6.5%); no differences were observed between the two groups. Compared to the conventional, low-fat diet, the low-GL diet group experienced a significantly greater mean decline in serum triglycerides (P < 0.005) and a reduction in plasminogen activator inhibitor, which increased in the control group. These markers are associated with CVD events and should be controlled throughout life. As CVD takes many decades to develop, a low-GL diet may be appropriate for young adults to reduce its risk later on.

Others observed similar changes in CVD risk markers (Pereira et al., 2004). After having lost 10% of body weight, young adults who consumed a low-GL diet experienced significant reductions in insulin resistance (P = 0.01), serum triglyceride concentrations (P = 0.01), C-reactive protein levels (P = 0.03), and blood pressure compared to the conventional low-fat diet (as mentioned earlier). This study again confirmed that the low-GL diet reduces CVD risk markers. Interestingly, these investigators determined that energy expenditure reduced less after weight loss in the low-GL diet, which theoretically afforded an 80 kcal/day advantage compared to those consuming the low-fat diet. Whether this caloric difference occurs long term is unknown but worth exploring.

Middle-aged adults (average age = 47 ± 11 years) also experienced improvement in CVD risk factors with a low-GL diet compared to the American Heart Association (AHA)–recommended low-fat diet (Dumesnil et al., 2001). Twelve overweight men (BMI = 33 ± 3.5 kg/m²) consumed each diet *ad libitum* for 6 days, in a crossover design. Significant adverse changes occurred while following the AHA diet: a 28% increase in serum triglycerides and a 10% reduction in HDL-cholesterol levels, which increased the cholesterol/HDL-cholesterol ratio. During the low-GL phase, serum triglycerides decreased 35%, peak particle LDL size increased (1.6%), and plasma insulin levels measured either fasting or during the day were lower compared to the AHA diet. During this part of the study, the subjects consumed 25% fewer calories during the low-GL phase compared to the AHA diet.

These same subjects then consumed the AHA diet, but energy intake was set at the amount consumed while following the low-GL diet in the first part of the study (Dumesnil et al., 2001). There was a trend for the HDL-cholesterol to decrease, leading to a significant increase in the cholesterol/HDL-cholesterol ratio (P < 0.0001). In addition to these unfavorable effects on CVD risk, the subjects reported an increase in hunger (P < 0.0002) and a decrease in satiety (P < 0.007) while on this diet compared to their usual diet. These results support a role for a low-GL diet in reducing CVD risk and question the role of the recommended AHA diet.

Another study in middle-aged adults showed that a low-GL diet reduced risk factors associated with CVD (Sloth et al., 2004). During the 10 week trial, healthy, overweight subjects experienced a 10% decrease in LDL-cholesterol levels ($P < 0.05$) and a trend toward reducing total cholesterol levels ($P < 0.07$). Others were randomized to a high-GL group. However, unlike other studies, no difference in energy intake, body weight, or fat mass was observed between the two dietary regimens. Regardless, the low-GL diet again was shown to be favorable at reducing CVD risk.

Fifty-seven middle-aged subjects (average age was 48 years) with elevated LDL-cholesterol levels consumed either a low-fat, low-GL diet or a low-fat diet only for 12 weeks (Shikany et al., 2005). Despite a reduction in the dietary GI and dietary GL in the low-fat, low-GL group, the blood lipids did not differ between the groups at any time, except for HDL-cholesterol levels, which decreased significantly in the low-fat group ($P = 0.05$). This blood lipid did not change in the low-fat, low-GL group. These findings support the earlier study of Dumesnil et al. (2001), who questioned the wisdom of a low-fat diet for reducing the risk of CVD.

A small, retrospective study suggested that the use of a low-GL diet preoperatively before coronary artery bypass surgery may shorten hospital stay (Patel et al., 2004). During the 4 weeks prior to surgery, patients who were randomized to a low-GL diet, but not those in the high-GL diet group, had improved glucose tolerance and greater adipocyte insulin activity at the time of surgery, which resulted in a significantly shorter length of hospitalization (7.06 ± 0.38 days vs. 9.53 ± 1.44 days; $P < 0.05$). Thus, a low-GL diet may benefit patients who already have CVD.

Type 2 Diabetes

More data exist in support of the use of a low-GL diet for the prevention and management of type 2 diabetes than for CVD. This makes sense because the GI and GL were developed initially to help manage blood sugar control in these patients.

Epidemiological Data

Five large-scale studies assessed the effect of consuming a low-GL diet over extended periods of time and in different age groups (Salmeron et al., 1997; Schulze et al., 2004; Lau et al., 2005; Qi et al., 2005; Sahyoun et al., 2005). Young women, aged 24–44 years, were followed for 8 years during which an assessment of their dietary intake was obtained as it related to fiber and GL of carbohydrates (Schulze et al., 2004). Of the 91,249 women included in the study, 741 developed type 2 diabetes. After adjustment of other factors that could predict the development of diabetes, overall GL of the diet was significantly associated with it (P for trend = 0.001). There was a 59% increase in the diabetes risk between the highest quintile of GI and the lowest. Fiber from cereals and fruits were inversely associated with the risk of diabetes as well. These authors speculated that the reason for this significant association was because high-GI foods produced higher blood glucose concentrations and a greater insulin demand than did low-GI foods. It is possible that chronically increased insulin demand results in pancreatic exhaustion that can result in glucose intolerance. In addition, high-GI diets may directly increase insulin resistance.

An older, healthy group of women (over 120,000) were followed for 6 years to determine the risk of type 2 diabetes (Salmeron et al., 1997). Both the dietary GI and dietary GL were positively associated with the risk of diabetes. Combining a low cereal fiber intake and a high dietary GL resulted in an RR of diabetes of 2.50 (95% CI, 1.14–5.51). Thus, the incidence of diabetes may be reduced with incorporating more cereal fiber into the diet as well as following a low-GL diet.

Older men were also shown to be at increased risk of type 2 diabetes if they regularly consumed a high-GL diet (Qi et al., 2005). In another large-scale study in older men (n = 51,529), aged 40–75 years, the GI and GL of the diet were inversely associated with adiponectin concentrations (P for trend = 0.005). Of this population, 780 developed type 2 diabetes during the 8 year study. There was a 13% difference for GI and 18% difference for GL between the lowest and highest quintile for serum adiponectin. Adiponectin is an adipose-secreted cytokine that is present at low levels in the plasma of patients with type 2 diabetes. In contrast to GI and GL, dietary fiber and magnesium were associated with higher levels of this cytokine. Thus, adiponectin may become a new risk factor for type 2 diabetes, and the GI and GL appear to be positively related to it.

Large-scale, cross-sectional studies conducted in men and women revealed mixed results as to the relationship between the GL of the diet and the risk of type 2 diabetes (Lau et al., 2005; Sahyoun et al., 2005). In a group of over 75,000 nondiabetic men and women, aged 30–60 years, GI and GL were not predictive of developing insulin resistance as estimated by HOMA (Lau et al., 2005). Insulin resistance developed in 5675 subjects. The risk of developing type 2 diabetes was significantly and inversely associated with dietary fiber, which was a confounding variable that reduced the effectiveness of GI and GL on HOMA. The results of this study differ from others but support the recommendation for increasing fiber intake through carbohydrate-rich foods such as cereals, fruits, and vegetables to prevent insulin resistance and reduce the risk of type 2 diabetes.

Others found fiber intake to be a more important predictor of Si than GI or GL (Liese et al., 2005). Participants were selected from an ongoing study (Insulin Resistance Atherosclerosis Study) and were selected based on glucose tolerance status (e.g., normal, impaired). Subjects underwent a dietary assessment that included data on fiber intake and the GI and GL of the diet. In addition, they underwent measurements of Si, fasting insulin, acute insulin response (AIR), disposition index, BMI, and waist circumference. No association was observed between GI and these measurements. Relationships between these measurements and digestible carbohydrate and GL were entirely explained by energy intake. In contrast, fiber intake was associated positively with Si and disposition index, and inversely associated with fasting insulin, BMI, and waist circumference, but not AIR. This was the first report to address the relationship of GI and GL with direct measure of Si. Earlier reports (Salmeron et al., 1997; Schulze et al., 2004) had hinted at a stronger relationship between GI and GL and insulin and blood sugar control, but with these data, it appeared that fiber intake is a more important aspect of the diet. Unfortunately, the type of fiber—soluble or insoluble—was not determined.

In contrast to the aforementioned studies (Lau et al., 2005; Liese et al., 2005), older individuals aged 70–80 years appeared to show a benefit of the low-GL diet in improving markers that predict type 2 diabetes (Sahyoun et al., 2005). From a sample of over 3000, the number of men and women were nearly equal for those who participated in the study. For men, the dietary GI was positively associated with 2h glucose levels after a 75 g challenge (P for trend = 0.04) and fasting insulin concentrations (P for trend = 0.004). It was inversely associated with thigh intramuscular fat (P for trend = 0.02). Dietary GL was inversely associated with visceral abdominal fat (P trend for = 0.02) only. For women, dietary GI and GL were not significant for any markers. This is the only study to identify differences between the genders. One of the problems with this study is that the investigators based the GI (and thus GL) on glucose rather than on the most commonly used standard, white bread. This produced GI and GL values that are lower than those based on white bread and, in this study, may explain the lack of statistical significance for women and for other parameters in men (i.e., fasting blood glucose, glycated Hgb, or visceral abdominal fat). However, in the previous study, the investigators (Lau et al., 2005) used white bread as the standard, and no significant relationships were found between GI and GL and diabetes risk either. Thus, basing the GI and GL on either standard cannot fully explain the discrepancy between these studies.

The risk of type 2 diabetes was not consistently associated with the GI and GL of the diet in a study of 26,000 males (Simila et al., 2011). The multivariant RR between the lowest and highest quintile for GI and GL in the diet was 0.87 for GI and 0.88 for GL. Substitution of lower-GI carbohydrates to higher-GI carbohydrates were not consistently associated with a lower diabetes risk.

From these large-scale cross-sectional and long-term studies, the relationship between GI and GL and the risk of type 2 diabetes cannot be ignored. Not all studies showed a positive result, but those that did were fairly convincing in showing such a relationship.

Short-Term Study

In a 4 week study in middle-aged men (around age 50 years) with type 2 diabetes, those who consumed a low-GL diet improved glycemic control (fasting blood glucose and Hgb A_{1c}) and glucose utilization compared with when they consumed a high-GL diet (Rizkalla et al., 2004). The only difference between the two dietary regimens was the GI of the carbohydrates consumed; the total grams of carbohydrate consumed was the same. Despite the short time span and the small differences between the groups, the study gives support for the long-term use of a low-GL diet for the management of type 2 diabetes.

The effect of dietary GI combined with exercise was assessed in obese, prediabetic individuals over 12 weeks (Solomon et al., 2010). Weight loss and changes in adiposity were similar between the two groups. However, oral glucose-induced insulin secretion was reduced in the low-GI diet and became elevated in the high-GI group. These finding suggest that postprandial hyperinsulinemia can only be attenuated with a low-GI diet and that high-GI diets impair pancreatic beta cell function, even in the presence of weight loss.

Despite the numerous studies showing the positive effects of a low-GL diet on the management of type 2 diabetes, the American Diabetes Association (ADA) had been conspicuously absent in saying anything on the subject until 2004 (Sheard et al., 2004). In a position statement from the ADA, these authors reviewed the available data regarding the type or source of carbohydrate on the prevention and management of diabetes. They asserted that the total grams of carbohydrate consumed was more important that the dietary GL. Thus, in counseling patients with diabetes about their diets, more importance should be placed on the amount rather than the type (low- or high-GI) of carbohydrate. Although, the authors conceded that GI affects blood glucose control and that its consideration can provide benefit beyond managing dietary carbohydrate intake, they went on to state that the data showing that GI or GL can prevent the development of type 2 diabetes are unclear.

Many studies exist that show the benefit of consuming a low-GL diet to prevent and manage type 2 diabetes. Others do not show such relationships. It seems prudent to provide a low-GL diet to reduce body weight because blood glucose control and blood lipid levels will likely improve.

OTHER CONDITIONS

The GL of the diet has been investigated for its possible effects on other diseases (Table 51.3). These include blood pressure (Visvanathan et al., 2004), stroke (Oh et al., 2005), colorectal cancer (Oh et al., 2004; Michaud et al., 2005), pancreatic cancer (Michaud et al., 2002), prostate cancer (Nimptsch et al., 2011), breast cancer (Frazier et al., 2004), cholecystectomy (Tsai et al., 2005), and disease of the eye (Schaumberg et al., 2004; Chiu et al., 2005). Of these, the most promising relationships were seen between women developing breast cancer or needing a cholecystectomy. Other conditions were not related to the GI or GL of the diet (i.e., blood pressure, stroke, age-related cataracts, or early cortical and nuclear lens opacities). The GL of the diet was related to the risk of colorectal cancer in men but not women and the risk of pancreatic cancer in overweight and obese women and in sedentary women but not normal-weight women. Thus, in contrast to the numerous reports showing a relationship between dietary GL in reducing the risk of and in helping to manage CVD and type 2 diabetes, most other conditions do not seem to be affected by it.

HOW TO EAT A LOW-GLYCEMIC-LOAD DIET

Some have argued that all obese patients should be counseled on a low-GL diet (Pawlak et al., 2002; Bell and Sears, 2003a,b; Johnston, 2005). The science behind the diet is complex, and teaching the diet to patients may prove challenging. To meet all nutritional needs for macronutrients, micronutrients, and a low GL, the following basic principles should be followed (Table 51.4). Using this guide, most patients should be able to grasp these concepts and eat a healthier, more nutrient-dense diet. With this diet come enhanced satiety, reduced hunger, weight loss, and a reduced risk of CVD and type 2 diabetes.

TABLE 51.3
Common Medical Conditions Affected by Dietary GI or GL

Medical Condition	Effect of Dietary GI or GL
Blood pressure (Visvanathan et al., 2004)	No change in blood pressure after ingestion of 50 g of carbohydrate in a beverage
Risk of stroke (Oh et al., 2005)	Neither GI nor GL was significantly associated with the risk of stroke in over 78,000 women followed for 18 years
Risk of colorectal cancer (Michaud et al., 2005)	GL was related to risk of colorectal cancer in men (from over 50,000) but not women (from over 120,000) followed over 20 years
Risk of distal colorectal adenoma (Oh et al., 2004)	Neither a high-GI nor high-GL diet was associated with colorectal adenoma in a large group of women (>34,000) followed for 18 years
Risk of pancreatic cancer (Michaud et al., 2002)	GL was associated with an increased risk only in overweight and obese women and those who were sedentary, but not in normal-weight women who were active from a large-scale study (over 88,000) followed 18 years
Risk of prostate cancer (Nimptsch et al., 2011)	Dietary GI and GL were not associated with risk of prostate cancer based on a study including 5000 males, indicating that long-term exposure to a high insulin response does not affect the incidence of this cancer
Risk of breast cancer (Frazier et al., 2004)	GL was associated with the risk of breast cancer in adulthood from data collected about what women ate in their teens
Risk of cholecystectomy (Tsai et al., 2005)	Higher intakes of total carbohydrate and a high-GI and high-GL diet may enhance risk in women (over 120,000) followed for 16 years
Age-related cataracts (Schaumberg et al., 2004)	GL was not related to the risk of cataracts in men (nearly 40,000) and women (over 70,000) followed 12 years and 14 years, respectively
Risk of early cortical and nuclear lens opacities	GI was not associated with either eye condition based on 1717 women followed over 14 years

TABLE 51.4
How to Follow a Low-GL Diet

Food Group	Servings per Day	Comments
Dairy (e.g., milk, cheese)	Two	Use reduced-fat products to reduce energy intake
Meat, fish, poultry, eggs	8–10 oz/day One egg = 1 oz	To reduce energy intake: —Trim visible fat and skins —Cook with minimal added fats, sauces, and breaded coatings
Fruits	Two pieces or two 1/2-cup servings	If using canned or frozen, choose sugar-free to reduce energy intake Avoid dried fruits and fruit juices
Nonstarchy vegetables	Unlimited	Use limited fats and sauces to reduce energy intake
Starchy vegetables and unsweetened grain-based foods	3–5 servings per day A serving is 1/2 cup, 1 slice, 1 whole (e.g., potato)	Use fewer servings during active weight loss than during maintenance
Sweetened grain-based foods, candy, sugary beverages, salty snacks	None to use sparingly	Use none during active weight loss and sparingly during maintenance

REFERENCES

Agus, M.S.D., Swain, J.F., Larson, C.L., Eckert, E.A., and Ludwig, D.S. Dietary composition and physiologic adaptations to energy restriction. *Am J Clin Nutr* 2000; 71:901–907.

Alfenas, R.C.G. and Mattes, R.D. Influence of glycemic index/load on glycemic response, appetite, and food intake in healthy humans. *Diabetes Care* 2005; 28:2123–2129.

Armendariz-Anguiano, A.L., Jimenez-Cruz, A., Bacardi-Gascon, M., and Hurtado-Ayala, L. Effect of a low glycemic load on body composition an Homeostasis Model Assessment (HOMA) in overweight and obese subjects. *Nutr Hosp* 2011; 26:170–175.

Bell, S.J. and Sears, B. A proposal for a new national diet: A low-glycemic load diet with a unique macronutrient composition. *Metab Syndrome Rel Dis* 2003a; 1:199–208.

Bell, S.J. and Sears, B. Low-glycemic-load diets: Impact on obesity and chronic diseases. *Crit Rev Food Sci Nutr* 2003b; 43:357–377.

Bell, S.J., Wolbers, J., and Casterton, W. Use of a low-glycemic load diet to promote weight loss. *Nutra World* 2005; 8:50–51.

Brand-Miller, J.C., Hayne, S., Petocz, P., and Colagiuri, S. Low-glycemic index diets in the management of diabetes: A meta-analysis of randomized controlled trials. *Diabetes Care* 2003b; 26:2261–2267.

Brand-Miller, J.C., Thomas, M., Swan, V., Ahmad, Z.I., Petocz, P., and Colagiuri, S. Physiological validation of the concept of glycemic load in lean young adults. *J Nutr* 2003a; 133:2728–2732.

Brown, W.J., Williams, L., Ford, J.H., Ball, K., and Dobson, H.A. Identifying the energy gap: Magnitude and determinants of 5-year weight gain in midage women. *Obes Res* 2005; 13:1431–1441.

Buchwald, H., Avidor, Y., Braunwald, E., Jensen, M.D., Pories, W., Fahrbach, K., and Schoelles, K. Bariatric surgery: A systemic review and meta-analysis. *JAMA* 2004; 292:1724–1737.

Buyken, A.E. and Liese, A.D. Dietary glycemic index, glycemic load, fiber, simple sugars, and insulin resistance: The Inter99 study. Letter. *Diabetes Care* 2005; 28:2986–2987.

Carels, R.A., Darby, L.A., Douglass, O.M., Cacciapaglia, H.M., and Rydin, S. Education on the glycemic index of foods fails to improve treatment outcomes in a behavioral weight loss program. *Eat Behav* 2005; 6:145–150.

Chiu, C.-J., Morris, M.S., Rogers, G., Jacques, P.F., Chylack, L.T., Tung, W., Hankinson, S.E., Willett, W.C., and Taylor, A. Carbohydrate intake and glycemic index in relation to the odds of early cortical and nuclear lens opacities. *Am J Clin Nutr* 2005; 81:1411–1416.

Coffey C.S., Steiner, D., Baker, B.A., and Allison, D.B. A randomized double-blind placebo-controlled clinical trial of a product containing ephedrine, caffeine, and other ingredients from herbal sources for treatment of overweight and obesity in the absence of lifestyle treatment. *Int J Obes Rel Metab Disord* 2004; 28:1411–1419.

Cordain, L., Eaton, S.B., Sebastian, A., Mann, N., Lindeberg, S., Watkins, B.A., O'Keefe, J.H., and Brand-Miller, J. Origins and evolution of the Western diet: Health implications for the 21st century. *Am J Clin Nutr* 2005; 81:341–354.

Davis, M.S., Miller, C.K., and Mitchell, D.C. More favorable dietary patterns are associated with lower glycemic load in older adults. *J Am Diet Assoc* 2004; 104:1828–1835.

Diaz, E.O., Galgani, J.E., Aguirre, C.A., Atwater, I.J., and Burrows, R. Effect of glycemic index on whole-body substrate oxidation in obese women. *Inter J Obes* 2005; 29:108–114.

Dickinson, S. and Brand-Miller, J. Glycemic index, postprandial glycemia and cardiovascular disease. *Curr Opin Lipidol* 2005; 16:69–75.

Dumesnil, J.G., Turgeon, J., Tremblay, A., Poirier, P., Gilbert, M., Gagnon, L., St-Pierre, S., Garneau, C., Lemieux, I., Pascot, A., Bergeron, J., and Despres, J.-P. Effect of a low-glycemic index-low-fat-high protein diet on the atherogenic metabolic risk profile of abdominally obese men. *Br J Nutr* 2001; 86:557–568.

Ebbeling, C.B., Leidig, M.M., Sinclair, K.B., Hangen, J.P., and Ludwig, D.S. Reduced glycemic load in the treatment of adolescent obesity. *Arch Pediat Adol Med* 2003; 157:773–779.

Ebbeling, C.B., Leidig, M.M., Sinclair, K.B., Seger-Shippee, L.G., Feldman, H.A., and Ludwig, D.S. Effects of an ad libitum low-glycemic load diet on cardiovascular disease risk factors in obese young adults. *Am J Clin Nutr* 2005; 81:976–982.

Fernandes, G., Velangi, A., and Wolever, T.M.S. Glycemic index of potatoes commonly consumed in North America. *J Am Dietet Assoc* 2005; 105:557–562.

Flegal, K.M., Graubard, B.I., Williamson, D.F., and Gail, M.H. Excess deaths associated with underweight, overweight, and obesity. *JAMA* 2005; 293:1861–1867.

Foster, G.D., Wyatt, H.R., Hill, J.O., McGuckin, B.G., Brill, C., Mohammed, B.S., Szapary, P.O., Rader, D.J., Edman, J.S., and Klein, S. A randomized trial of a low-carbohydrate diet for obesity. *N Engl J Med* 2003; 348:2082–2090.

Foster-Powell, K., Holt, S.H.A., and Brand-Miller, J.C. International table of glycemic index and glycemic load values: 2002. *Am J Clin Nutr* 2002; 76:5–56.

Frazier, A.L., Li, L., Cho, E., Willett, W.C., and Colditz, G.A. Adolescent diet and risk of breast cancer. *Cancer Cause Control* 2004; 15:73–82.

Holt, S.H.A., Miller, J.C., Petocz, P., and Farmakalidis, E. A satiety index of common foods. *Eur J Clin Nutr* 1995; 49:675–690.

Hu, F.B., Stampfer, M.J., Manson, J.E., Grodstein, F., Colditz, G.A., Speizer, F.E., and Willett, W.C. Trends in the incidence of coronary heart disease and changes in diet and life style in women. *N Engl J Med* 2000; 343:530–537.

Hui, L.-L., Nelson, E.A., Choi, K.-C., Wong, G.W.K., and Sung, R. Twelve-hour glycemic profiles with meals of high, medium, or low glycemic load. *Diabetes Care* 2005; 28:2081–2083.

Jenkins, D.J., Wolever, T.M., Taylor, R.H. et al. Glycemic index of foods: A physiologic basis for carbohydrate exchange. *Am J Clin Nutr* 1981; 34:363–366.

Johnston, C.S. Strategies for healthy weight loss: From vitamin C to the glycemic response. *J Am Coll Nutr* 2005; 24:158–165.

Lau, C., Faerch, K., Glumer, C., Tetens, I., Pedersen, O., Carstensen, B., Jorgensen, T., and Borch-Johnsen, K. Dietary glycemic index, glycemic load, fiber, simple sugars, and insulin resistance: The Inter99 study. *Diabetes Care* 2005; 28:1397–1403.

Liese, A.D., Schulz, M., Fang, F., Wolever, T.M.S., D'Agostino, R.B., Sparks, K.C., and Mayer-Davis, E.J. Dietary glycemic index and glycemic load, carbohydrate and fiber intake, and measurements of insulin sensitivity, secretion, and adiposity in the Insulin Resistance Atherosclerosis Study. *Diabetes Care* 2005; 28:2832–2838.

Liu, S., Manson, J.E., Buring, J.E., Stampfer, M.J., Willett, W.C., and Ridker, P.M. Relationship between a diet with a high glycemic load and plasma concentrations of high-sensitivity C-reactive protein in middle-aged women. *Am J Clin Nutr* 2002; 75:492–498.

Liu, S., Manson, J.E., Stampfer, M.J., Holmes, M.D., Hu, F.B., Hankinson, S.E., and Willett, W.C. Dietary glycemic load assessed by food-frequency questionnaire in relation to plasma high-density-lipoprotein cholesterol and fasting plasma triacylglycerols in postmenopausal women. *Am J Clin Nutr* 2001; 73:560–566.

Liu, S., Willett, W.C., Stampfer, M.J., Hu, F.B., Franz, M., Sampson, L., Hennekens, C.H., and Manson, J.E. A prospective study of dietary glycemic load, carbohydrate intake, and risk of coronary heart disease in US women. *Am J Clin Nutr* 2000; 71:1455–1461.

Ludwig, D.S. Dietary glycemic index and obesity. *J Nutr* 2000; 130:280S–283S.

Ludwig, D.S. The glycemic index: Physiological mechanisms relating to obesity, diabetes, and cardiovascular disease. *JAMA* 2002; 287:2414–2423.

Ludwig, D.S. Glycemic load comes of age. *J Nutr* 2003; 133:2728–2732.

Ludwig, D.S., Majzoub, J.A., Al-Zahrani, A., Dallal, G.E., Blanco, I., and Roberts, S.B. High glycemic index foods, overeating, and obesity. *Pediatrics* 1999; 103:e26.

Michaud, D.S., Fuchs, C.S., Liu, S., Willett, W.C., Colditz, G.A., and Giovannucci, E. Dietary glycemic load, carbohydrate, sugar, and colorectal cancer risk in men and women. *Cancer Epidem Biomar* 2005; 14:138–143.

Michaud, D.S., Liu, S., Giovannucci, E., Willett, W.C., Colditz, G.A., and Fuchs, C.S. Dietary sugar, glycemic load, and pancreatic cancer risk in a prospective study. *J Natl Cancer I* 2002; 94:1293–1300.

Nimptsch, K., Kenfield, S., Jensen, M.K., Stampfer, M.J., Franz, M., Sampson, L., Brand-Miller, J.C., Willett, W.C., and Giovannucci, E. Dietary glycemic index, glycemic load, insulin index, fiber and whole-grain intake in relation to risk of prostate cancer. *Cancer Cause Control* 2011; 22:51–61.

Oh, K., Hu, F.B., Cho, E., Rexrode, K.M., Stampfer, M.J., Manson, J.E., Liu, S., and Willett, W.C. Carbohydrate intake, glycemic index, glycemic load, and dietary fiber in relation to risk of stroke in women. *Am J Epidemiol* 2005; 161:161–169.

Oh, K., Willett, W.C., Fuchs, C.S., and Giovannucci, E.L. Glycemic index, glycemic load, and carbohydrate intake in relation to risk of distal colorectal adenoma in women. *Cancer Epidem Biomar* 2004; 13:1192–1198.

Opperman, A.M., Venter, C.S., Oosthuizen, W., Thompson, R.L., and Vorster, H.H. Meta-analysis of the health effects of using the glycemic index in meal-planning. *Br J Nutr* 2004; 92:367–381.

Parcell, A.C., Drummond, M.J., Christopherson, E.D., Hoyt, G.L., and Cherry, J.A. Glycemic and insulinemic responses to protein supplements. *J Am Diet Assoc* 2004; 104:1800–1804.

Patel, V.C., Aldridge, R.D., Leeds, A., Dornhorst, A., and Frost, G.S. Retrospective analysis of the impact of a low glycaemic index diet on hospital stay following coronary artery bypass grafting: A hypothesis. *J Hum Nutr Diet* 2004; 17:214–247.

Pawlak, D.B., Ebbeling, C.B., and Ludwig, D.S. Should obese patients be counselled to follow a low-glycaemic index diet? Yes. *Obes Rev* 2002; 3:235–243.

Pereira, M.A., Swain, J., Goldfine, A.B., Rifai, N., and Ludwig, D.S. Effects of a low-glycemic load diet on resting energy expenditure and heart disease risk factors during weight loss. *JAMA* 2004; 292:2482–2490.

Pi-Sunyer, X. Do glycemic index, glycemic load, and fiber play a role in insulin sensitivity, disposition index, and type 2 diabetes? *Diabetes Care* 2005; 28:2978–2979.

Pittas, A.G., Das, S.K., Hajduk, C.L., Golden, J., Saltzman, E., Stark, P.C., Greenberg, A.S., and Roberts, S.B. A low-glycemic load diet facilitates greater weight loss in overweight adults with high insulin secretion but not in overweight adults with low insulin secretion in the CALERIE trial. *Diabetes Care* 2005; 28:2939–2941.

Qi, L., Rimm, E., Liu, S., Rifai, N., and Hu, F.B. Dietary glycemic index, glycemic load, cereal fiber, and plasma adiponectin concentration in diabetic men. *Diabetes Care* 2005; 28:1022–1028.

Raatz, S.K., Torkelson, C.J., Redmon, J.B., Reck, K.P., Kwong, C.A., Swanson, J.E., Liu, C., Thomas, W., and Bantle, J.P. Reduced glycemic index and glycemic load diets do not increase the effects of energy restriction on weight loss and insulin sensitivity in obese men and women. *J Nutr* 2005; 135:2387–2391.

Rizkalla, S.W., Taghrid, L., Laromigeuiere, M., Huet, D., Boillot, J., Rigoir, A., Elgrably, F., and Slama, G. Improved plasma glucose control, whole-body glucose utilization, and lipid profile on a low-glycemic index diet in type 2 diabetic men: A randomized controlled trial. *Diabetes Care* 2004; 27:1866–1872.

Roberts, S.B. High-glycemic index foods, hunger, and obesity: Is there a connection? *Nutr Rev* 2000; 58:163–169.

Sahyoun, N.R., Anderson, A.L., Kanaya, A.M., Koh-Banerjee, P., Kritchevsky, S.B., de Rekeneire, N., Tylavsky, F.A., Schwartz, A.V., Lee, J.S., and Harris, T.B. Dietary glycemic index and load, measures of glucose metabolism, and body fat distribution in older adults. *Am J Clin Nutr* 2005; 82:547–552.

Salmeron, J., Manson J.E., Stamper, M.J., Colditz, G.A., Wing, A.L., and Willett, W.C. Dietary fiber, glycemic load, and risk of non-insulin-dependent diabetes mellitus in women. *JAMA* 1997; 277:472–477.

Samaha, F.F., Iqbal, N., Seshadri, P., Chicano, K.L., Daily, D.A., McGrory, J., Williams, T., Williams, M., Gracely, E.J., and Stern, L. A low-carbohydrate as compared with a low-fat diet in severe obesity. *N Engl J Med* 2003; 348:2074–2081.

Schaumberg, D.A., Liu, S., Seddon, J.M., Willett, W.C., and Hankinson, S.E. Dietary glycemic load and risk of age-related cataract. *Am J Clin Nutr* 2004; 80:489–495.

Schulze, M.B., Liu, S., Rimm, E.B., Manson, J.A.E., Willett, W.C., and Hu, F.B. Glycemic index, glycemic load, and dietary fiber intake and incidence of type 2 diabetes in younger and middle-aged women. *Am J Clin Nutr* 2004; 80:348–356.

Sheard, N.F., Clark, N.G., Brand-Miller, J.C., Franz, M.J., Pi-Sunyer, F.X., Mayer-Davis, E., Kulkarni, K., and Geil, P. Dietary carbohydrate (amount and type) in the prevention and management of diabetes. *Diabetes Care* 2004; 27:2266–2271.

Shikany, J.M., Goudie, A., and Oberman, A. Comparison of a low-fat/low-glycemic index diet to a low-fat only diet in the treatment of adults with hypercholesterolemia. *Nutr Res* 2005; 25:971–981.

Sichieri, R., Moura, A.S., Genelhu, V., Hu, F., and Willett, W.C. An 18-mo randomized trial of a low-glycemic-index diet and weight change in Brazilian women. *Am J Clin Nutr* 2007; 86:707–713.

Simila M.E., Valsta, L.M., Kontto, J.P., Albanes, D., and Virtamo, J. Low-, medium- and high-glycemic index carbohydrates and risk of type 2 diabetes in men. *Br J Nutr* 2011; 105:1258–1264.

Sloth, B., Krog-Mikkelsen, I., Flint, A., Tetens, I., Bjorck, I., Vinoy, S., Elmstahl, H., Astrup, A., Lang, V., and Raben, A. No difference in body weight decrease between a low-glycemic-index and a high-glycemic-index diet but reduced LDL cholesterol after 10-wk ad libitum intake of the low-glycemic-index diet. *Am J Clin Nutr* 2004; 80:337–347.

Solomon, T.P., Haus, J.M., Kelly, K.R., Cook, M.D., Filion, J., Rocco, M., Kashyap, S.R., Watanabe, R.M., Barkoukis, H., and Kirwan, J.P. A low-glycemic index diet combined with exercise reduces insulin resistance, postprandial hyperinsulinemia, and glucose-dependent insulinotropic polypeptide responses in obese, prediabetic humans. *Am J Clin Nutr* 2010; 92:1359–1368.

Spieth, L.E., Harnish, J.D., Lenders, C.M., Raezer, L.B., Pereira, M.A., Hangen, S.J., and Ludwig, D.S. A low-glycemic index diet in the treatment of pediatric obesity. *Arch Pediat Adol Med* 2000; 154:947–951.

Tsai, C.-J., Leitzmann, M.F., Willett, W.C., and Giovannucci, E.L. Glycemic load, glycemic index, and carbohydrate intake in relation to risk of cholecystectomy in women. *Gastroenterology* 2005; 129:105–112.

Valdes, A.M., Andrew, T., Gardner, J.P., Kimura, M., Oelsner, F., Cherkas, L.F., Aviv, A., and Spector, T.D. Obesity, cigarette smoking, and telomere length in women. *The Lancet* 2005; 366:662–664.

Visvanathan, R., Chen, R., Horowitz, M., and Chapman, I. Blood pressure responses in healthy older people to 50 g carbohydrate drinks with differing glycaemic effects. *Br J Nutr* 2004; 92:335–340.

Wolever T.M.S., Jenkins, D.J.A., Jenkins, A.L., and Josse, R.G. The glycemic index: Methodology and clinical implications. *Am J Clin Nutr* 1991; 54:846–854.

Wolever, T.M.S., Vorster, H.H., Bjorck, I., Brand-Miller, J., Brighenti, F., Mann, J.I., Ramdath, D.D., Grandfeldt, Y., Holt, S., Perry, T.L., Venter, C., and Wu, X. Determination of the glycaemic index of foods: interlaboratory study. *Eur J Clin Nutr* 2003; 57:475–482.

Young, P.C., West, S.A., Ortiz, K., and Carlson, J. A pilot study to determine the feasibility of the low glycemic index diet as a treatment of overweight children in primary care practice. *Ambul Pediatr* 2004; 4:28–33.

52 Herbals and Dietary Nutrients Associated with Weight Loss

Akhtar Afshan Ali, PhD, Sherry M. Lewis, PhD, Xi Yang, PhD, William Frederick Salminen, PhD, DABT, and Julian E. Leakey, PhD, DABT

CONTENTS

DISCLAIMER

The opinions expressed in this document should not be considered the official regulatory position of the U.S. Food and Drug Administration (FDA), nor should any views or comments be considered reflective of the current or future position of the FDA regarding any specific botanical mentioned. The mention of trade names does not constitute an endorsement by the FDA.

INTRODUCTION

Obesity is a growing public health problem in the United States and in other developed countries. It has become an epidemic despite efforts to promote healthy eating and physical activity behavior. Obesity is on the rise because food is abundant and physical activity is optional. It is considered a chronic (long-term) disease with many serious long-term consequences for health and is related to metabolic disorders such as cardiovascular disease and Type 2 diabetes. Obesity is defined as having a body mass index (BMI) of greater than 30 [1].

The obesity epidemic has caused many people to focus on weight loss. Millions of people in the United States use nonprescription weight loss products, believing them to be safe and effective. Approximately 38 million U.S. adults use herbal and dietary supplements to achieve these health goals [2]. Dietary supplements used for weight loss can contain purified or synthesized chemicals of natural origin, botanicals and herbal extracts (which can contain several or many ill-defined constituents), and probiotics (microbial derivatives of human microflora or genetic engineering) [3]. Reasons why consumers might use dietary supplements for weight loss include the following: (1) There is a desire for a "magic bullet" due to frustration with previous failed attempts at dieting and/or exercise, since supplement consumption is less demanding than accepting lifestyle changes accompanying exercise and diet. (2) Supplements are easily available without a prescription and without the requirement for a professional consultation with a physician, nurse, or nutritionist. (3) The consumer may respond to inflated advertising claims and testimonials and to the appeal of a "natural" remedy, where the perception is that natural always equals safe [1]. In addition, it must be considered that these supplements are also consumed by the bodybuilding community and by patients with eating disorders such as anorexia nervosa, who do not suffer from obesity. Prevalence of all supplement use is greatest for women, and that use is growing with increasing age of the population [4,5].

Issues of toxicity, inadequate efficacy studies, and lack of regulatory agency premarket assessment are major limitations surrounding herbal and probiotic therapies. These therapies involve heterogeneous modalities which are difficult to define [3]. Systematic reviews and meta-analyses of evidence from multiple, double-blind, randomized clinical trials are available for many of those primary constituents of weight loss dietary supplements that have been in use for some time, while less information is available for newer constituents. These trials and reviews have evaluated efficacy and safety, and while there is some encouraging evidence for efficacy of certain agents, overall these evaluations have provided little convincing evidence that any specific dietary supplement is effective in reducing body weight [3,6–8].

However, an important factor often overlooked in evaluating success of clinical trials for weight loss activity is that obesity is not a primary disease, but rather the endpoint of a number of genetic, epigenetic, pathological, and behavioral conditions [9–12]. If these etiological variables are not controlled for during patient selection, the heterogenicity of subject response will dilute the trial's sensitivity.

The nutraceutical industry's response to the sparsity of positive data from independent clinical trials has been to market new combinations of several ingredients with the rationale that the sum is greater than the parts. Moreover, as ingredients fall out of favor due to safety or efficacy problems, they are sometimes replaced with only minor modifications of the product's trade name so that it is difficult to keep abreast with what a supplement currently contains. This leads to potential problems with both drug–supplement interactions and supplement–supplement interactions as new products arrive on the mass market with little or no prior clinical evaluation [8,13].

This chapter firstly describes the current regulatory organizations in the United States and other nations that have been established to oversee the dietary supplement industry and provide information on the current safety evaluations of supplement constituents. Secondly, the chapter lists the major established and newer weight loss supplement constituents that are currently being marketed and describes the mechanistic rationale behind their selection as weight loss agents.

REGULATORY RESPONSE

In an attempt to remain abreast of rapidly developing herbal and alternative medicine therapies, the U.S. National Institutes of Health (NIH) created a division to address this area, the National Center for Complementary and Alternative Medicine (NCCAM; http://www.nccam.nih.gov/ [accessed February 2012]). The site provides a link to the FDA, which has created an RSS feed to alert consumers rapidly when FDA finds fraudulent or defective products.

In the United States, herbal products are not considered drugs and are not regulated as such by the U.S. federal government. A product with a history of use is generally considered safe with the burden upon the FDA to prove otherwise [7,8]. Herbal products are classified as "dietary supplements" and marketed pursuant to the U.S. Dietary Supplement Health and Education Act of 1994 (DSHEA) and are presumed to be safe and freely available [2,14]. DSHEA authorized the establishment of the Office of Dietary Supplements (ODS) at the NIH (http://www.ods.od.nih.gov).

In 2007, the FDA issued its current "good manufacturing practices" (GMPs) regulations to maintain that dietary supplements are processed consistently and meet quality standards. Issues continue to be reported, and in 2010, the U.S. Government Accountability Office (GAO) released a report finding trace levels of lead and other contaminants and examples of deceptive or suspect marketing claims [15].

As in the United States, herbal products are sold as dietary supplements in the Netherlands. In the United Kingdom, any product not granted a license as a medical product by the Medicines Control Agency is treated as a food, and no health claim or medical advice can be included on the label. In Germany, comprehensive herbal monographs are prepared by an interdisciplinary committee (German Commission E); if a herb has an approved monograph, it can be marketed [16]. In Canada, dietary supplements are regulated by the Natural Health Products Regulations, which became effective January 1, 2004 (http://www.hc-sc.gc.ca/dhp-mps/prodnatur/index_e.html).

In addition, the Canadian Institutes of Health Research funded the CONSORT group, which attempts to improve the quality of reports of randomized trials using an evidence-based approach (http://www.consort-statement.org) [17]. Increased public health concern reports have increased sixfold for weight loss supplements in the past 7 years to the European Rapid Alert System for Food and Feed (RASFF); the United States and China have been the major offenders [18]. Finland and Italy lead in detecting unpermitted substances and contaminants in supplements; however, significant proportions of the supplement market are distributed via the Internet, which makes ensuring and enforcing safety a challenging task.

DIETARY SUPPLEMENTS FOR WEIGHT LOSS

PHENYLETHYLAMINES

Phenylethylamines (Figure 52.1) that possess potent β-adrenergic activity are effective weight loss agents for most obese and normal subjects by virtue of their ability to mimic dopamine, norepinephrine, and epinephrine in stimulating the sympathetic nervous system and peripheral intracellular responses via β-adrenergic receptors [19]. This results in increased metabolism, thermogenesis, hypophagia, and decreased lipogenesis [20]. *In vivo*, norepinephrine and epinephrine concentrations

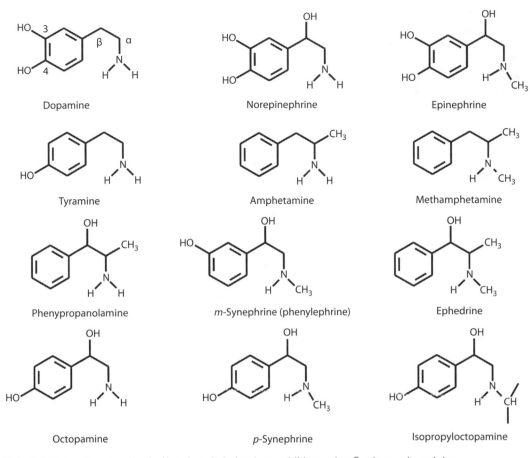

FIGURE 52.1   Structurally similar phenylethylamines exhibit varying β-adrenergic activity.

are tightly controlled via their synthesis, transport, and degradation. The latter is catalyzed by the enzymes monoamine oxidase (which converts their amino groups to inactive aldehydes) and catechol-O-methyltransferase (which alkylates the 4-hydroxy groups of their aromatic rings).

Synthetic and botanically derived phenylethylamines differ in specificity and potency depending upon their substitutions to the basic structure (Figure 52.1). For example, the lack of aromatic hydroxy groups on amphetamine and methamphetamine allow these amines to freely diffuse across the blood–brain barrier, thereby potentiating their central dopaminergic activity as compared to their α- and β-adrenergic activity in adipose and other peripheral tissues. Phenylethylamines with a single hydroxyl group in the aromatic ring are not degraded by catechol-O-methyltransferase, whereas substitutions on the α-carbon block oxidation by monoamine oxidases [21,22]. In addition, substitutions can influence relative binding affinity to α- and β-adrenergic receptors. For example, the shift in the aromatic hydroxylation position from 4 to 3 of the ring is responsible for a higher α-adrenergic activity of m-synephrine when compared with p-synephrine [23]. Alkylation and the larger the size of the alkyl group linked to the amine group of the side chain potentiate affinity for β-adrenergic receptors [22,24]. Stimulation of the β-adrenergic system results in increased lipolysis and mitochondrial uncoupling in adipose tissue [25,26] and activates a satiety response in the hypothalamus [20]. Overstimulation of adrenergic systems results in tachycardia, hypertension, muscle tremor, and hyperthermia.

d-Amphetamine, introduced in the 1930s, was originally developed as a treatment for narcolepsy but was subsequently found to produce weight loss by reducing appetite, thus introducing a new era of pharmacological therapy for obesity [27]. Likewise, methamphetamine, developed in Japan prior to World War II, has also been used to treat obesity [28]. Both amphetamine and methamphetamine are available on prescription in the United States as Adderall and Desoxyn, respectively [28,29], but their use for weight loss is restricted to drugs of last resort due to their side effects and potential for abuse. The less potent phenylethylamines that are available from botanical sources have therefore been developed as "safer" alternatives that can be marketed as dietary supplements.

Ephedra

Plants of the *Ephedra* genus, such as *E. sinica, E. intermedia,* and *E. equisetina*, have been used for over 5000 years in Chinese traditional medicine as the herb *ma huang* to treat asthma and the common cold [30,31]. Modern ephedra preparations have a phenylethylamine content of between 0.5% and 2% consisting of ephedrine and its optical isomer pseudoephedrine with smaller amounts of phenylpropanolamine [31]. Both ephedrine and pseudoephedrine were sold as nonprescription weight loss aids in the 1980s and early 1990s. Following the passage of the DSHEA in1994, which defined ephedra as a dietary supplement, ephedra was a leading component of weight loss supplements [30,32]. A meta-analysis of clinical trials conducted during this time period concluded that ephedra and ephedrine were effective for short-term weight loss with moderate incidence of side effects [33]. However, by 2003, the FDA had received thousands of adverse event reports, including instances of myocardial infarction, stroke, and death, all potentially related to the use of products containing ephedra [30]. Following a high-profile case involving the death of an athlete in 2004, the FDA banned the sale of ephedra products as dietary supplements because they were determined to present an unreasonable risk. Although the ban was contested in court, it was upheld on appeal in 2006 [30]. Ephedra is still available in the United States as a decongestant.

Citrus aurantium

Citrus aurantium is the botanical name for a plant commonly named bitter orange, sour orange, or Seville orange. Components of the fruit are sometimes used as a food, but the plant is more widely used as a medicinal or dietary supplement, and since 2004, it has essentially replaced ephedra as a source of phenylethylamines. It contains *p*-synephrine, *m*-synephrine (phenylephrine), and *p*-octopamine [34]. Although these alkaloids are believed to primarily be α-adrenergic agonists, they also have some β-adrenergic agonist properties. [34]. Recently, the isopropyl derivative of *p* octopamine has been reported to be a potent agonist of the β-adrenergic receptor and is being developed as an antiobesity drug [35].

Like ephedra, *Citrus aurantium* and *p*-synephrine have been associated with adverse reactions such as ischemic stroke, hypertension, tachycardia, and QT prolongation [36,37].

METHYLXANTHINES

The methylxanthines, caffeine and theophylline (Figure 52.2), are major constituents of most weight loss supplements. Methylxanthines have been shown to inhibit phosphodiesterase activity

Caffeine   Theophylline

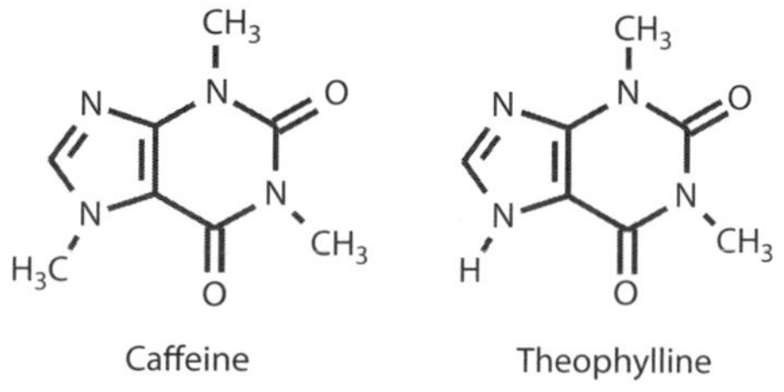

FIGURE 52.2 Methylxanthines, caffeine and theophylline, inhibit intracellular phosphodiesterase activity and antagonize adenosine receptor activity.

in adipocytes [38]. This enzyme degrades intracellular cAMP, which is part of the signal transduction system that links β3-adrenergic response to lipolysis and thermogenesis in these cells. Thus, caffeine and other methylxanthines will potentiate the effects of β3-adrenergic receptor agonists through this mechanism [38]. Methylxanthines are also nonselective antagonists of adenosine receptors in the brain, and their stimulatory and anxiogenic effects are reported to be mediated through inhibition of these receptors [39–41].

Caffeine

Caffeine is extracted from coffee bean (*Coffea arabica*) or kola nut (*Cola acuminate*) and is present in significant concentrations in guarana seeds (*Paullinia* sp.), yerba maté (*Ilex paraguariensis*), and tea leaves (*Camellia sinensis*). Weight loss supplements can either contain purified caffeine or extracts from one or more of these botanicals [42,43]. Extracts generally contain other methylxanthines in addition to caffeine.

Green Tea Extract: [From *Camellia sinensis*] [44]

All teas contain high quantities of several polyphenolic catechin components, such as epicatechin, epicatechin gallate, epigallocatechin, and, the most abundant and probably the most pharmacologically active, epigallocatechin gallate (Figure 52.3). Tea leaves that have been processed the least contain the most catechins. The observation that green tea extract stimulates thermogenesis cannot be completely attributed to its xanthene (caffeine and theophylline) content because the thermogenic effect of green tea extract containing caffeine and catechin polyphenols is greater than that of an equivalent amount of caffeine [45]. Green tea catechins, such as epigallocatechin gallate, inhibit catechol-*O*-methyltransferase which is the rate limiting enzyme in norepinephrine degradation. Animal studies have demonstrated that feeding green tea extract can reduce body weight gain in mice fed a high-fat diet and induce fatty acid oxidation [46], and in rats, green tea extract induced apoptosis in adipose tissue [47]. Human studies suggest that consumption of green tea extract may have some short-term benefit in controlling obesity, but that efficacy is influenced by caffeine consumption and ethnicity [48,49].

In 2003, regulatory agencies in France and Spain suspended market authorization of a weight loss product *Exolise*, which contained a hydroalcoholic extract of green tea (standardized to 25% catechins), because of reports of hepatotoxicity associated with its use [50]. Sporadic cases of hepatotoxicity associated with excessive consumption of green tea extract have been reported in other countries including the United States [50], and epigallocatechin gallate has been reported to be highly toxic to isolated rat hepatocytes *in vitro* [51].

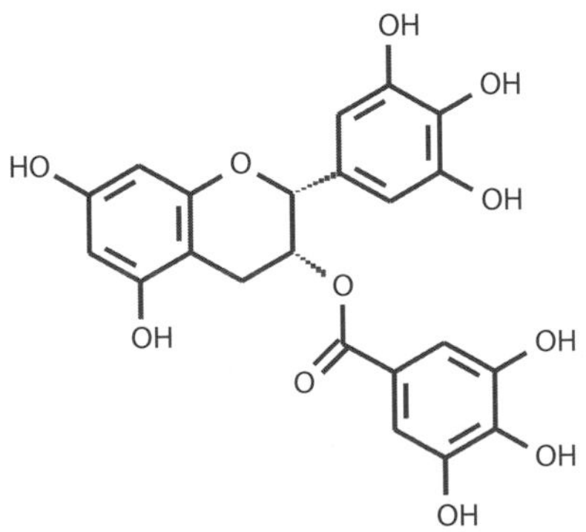

Epigallocatechin gallate

FIGURE 52.3 Epigallocatechin gallate is the major catechin present in green tea but is generally absent from black tea.

Mitochondrial Uncoupling Agents

Mitochondrial uncoupling proteins, (UCP1, UCP2, and UCP3) are expressed in white and brown adipose tissue and induced via the β-adrenergic system [11,52]. Their induction and activation increase energy expenditure and heat production. Mechanistically, these proteins span the inner mitochondrial membrane and, when activated, allow protons to transverse across the membrane, reducing the proton gradient and the membrane potential that drives ATP synthesis (Figure 52.4). Increased calorie consumption and NADH production are then required to maintain the proton gradient, and heat is generated at the expense of ATP synthesis.

Chemicals that are protonophoric uncouplers, such as 2,4-dinitrophenol and usnic acid (Figure 52.5), are functionally similar to uncoupling proteins. They are highly lipophilic in both their neutral and anionic forms because they contain electrophilic groups that absorb the negative charges of their anions by resonance stabilization [53,54]. According to the chemiosmotic theory, such molecules easily diffuse through biological membranes in both their charged and neutral forms which results in the breakdown or uncoupling of ion gradients [53]. For example, usnic acid can pass through the inner mitochondrial membrane by passive diffusion into the matrix where it is ionized, releasing a proton into the matrix. The resulting anion can then diffuse back into

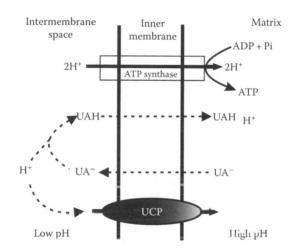

FIGURE 52.4 Protonophoric uncoupling of the inner mitochondrial membrane mediated by usnic acid or by UCP-mediated physiological uncoupling reduces the proton gradient required to maintain ATP synthesis. (Figure based on the work of Mitchell, P., *Biochem. Soc. Trans.*, 4, 399, 1976.)

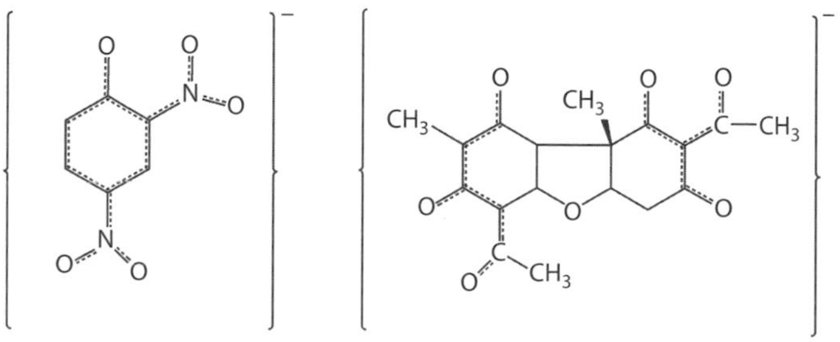

2,4-Dinitrophenol   Usnic acid

FIGURE 52.5 Protonophoric uncouplers: The nitro group of 2,4-dinitrophenol and the α-triketone groups of usnic acid absorb the negative charges of their anionic forms by resonance stabilization, allowing the ions to retain hydrophobicity. (From Guo, L. et al., J. *Environ. Sci. Health C. Environ. Carcinog, Ecotoxicol. Rev.*, 26, 317, 2008.)

the intermembrane space, where it binds to a proton on the acidic side of the inner membrane to re-form usnic acid, which can then diffuse back into the matrix (Figure 52.4). The resulting cycle causes proton leakage that eventually can dissipate the proton gradient across the inner membrane, disrupting the tight coupling between electron transport and adenosine triphosphate (ATP) synthesis. This property of 2,4-dinitrophenol and usnic acid have, therefore, led to both of them being utilized as compounds that increase internal energy use to maintain mitochondrial function (e.g., fat burning).

2,4-Dinitrophenol

It was noticed during World War I that munitions workers who were exposed to 2,4-dinitrophenol tended to lose weight, and in the 1930s, 2,4-dinitrophenol was marketed as an antiobesity drug [55]. However, it was found to have serious side effects such as cataracts. The FDA banned its medical use in 1948 [55], but it is still occasionally used as a weight loss supplement by body builders, and adverse reactions have been reported [56].

Usnic Acid

Usnic acid (2,6-diacetyl-7,9-dihydroxy-8, 9b-dimethyl-dibenzofuran-1,3(2H,9bH)-dione, Figure 52.5) was first isolated as a prominent secondary metabolite of beard lichens of the *Usnea* genus (*U. barbata, U. cavernosa, U. longissima, U. scabrata,* and others) in 1844. These lichen species have been used traditionally in northern Eurasia and the Americas for their antimicrobial properties [57,58]. Usnic acid exists as two bright yellow enantiomers, and in northern Europe, *Usnea* lichen extracts were traditionally used for coloring textiles [57]. Prior to the advent of modern antibiotics, pure usnic acid was used clinically as an antimicrobial in certain countries [59], and recently, interest has reemerged due to the observation that usnic acid is active against methicillin-resistant *Staphylococcus aureus* [60].

In 1996, Abo-Khatwa and coworkers [61] reported that usnic acid exhibited protonophoric uncoupling activity in isolated mitochondria. The minimum concentration of usnic acid ([+]-enantiomer) required to cause complete uncoupling of oxidative phosphorylation was found to be $1\,\mu M$, suggesting that it was up to 50% more potent than 2,4-dinitrophenol in uncoupling oxidative phosphorylation [61]. Subsequently, usnic acid was developed and marketed as a fat burner.

Usnic acid or its sodium salt (sodium usniate) have been marketed as constituents of several dietary supplements for weight reduction, and in some cases, it has been marketed as pure usnic acid [54,62]. Serious hepatotoxicity has been reported in some users, which has limited its use.

In 2000, Favreau et al. [63] reported that seven previously healthy patients developed acute hepatitis after ingesting *LipoKinetix* (Syntrax, Cape Girardeau, MO) and recovered spontaneously after discontinuing its use. Subsequently, two more cases of acute hepatitis were reported after the patients had consumed *LipoKinetix*, with one requiring a liver transplant [64]. *LipoKinetix* was a multi-ingredient product; one capsule contained 25 mg of norephedrine hydrochloride, 100 mg of usnic acid, $100\,\mu g$ of 3,5-diiodothyronine, 3 mg of yohimbine hydrochloride, and 100 mg of caffeine. It was sold as a dietary supplement to promote weight loss. The manufacturer claimed that *LipoKinetix* "affects oxidative phosphorylation in such a way that an incredible amount of fatty acids are burned," therefore promoting weight loss. The recommended dose of *LipoKinetix* was one to two capsules three times per day, which is three to six times greater than the antimicrobial doses of usnic acid that have been used clinically [54].

Other usnic acid–containing supplements included *UCP-1* (BDC Nutrition, Richmond, KY), which was marketed for weight loss as capsules containing 150 mg of usnic acid, 525 mg of L-carnitine, and 1050 mg of calcium pyruvate. The recommended dose of *UCP-1* was three capsules three times per day. Sanchez and coworkers [65] reported the development of severe liver failure in two patients who were taking the recommend dose of *UCP-1*. One resulted in a liver transplant. Druazo and coworkers [62] also reported one case of a healthy woman who, after taking pure usnic acid (Industrial Strength AAA Services, Frazer Park, CA), presented with liver failure requiring a transplant. The recommended dose of pure usnic acid from this manufacturer was 500 mg per day.

Based on the initial adverse events described earlier and first reported by MedWatch in November 2001, the Center for Food Safety and Applied Nutrition of the U.S. FDA issued a warning letter describing the dangers of *LipoKinetix* [66]. This was followed by a strong recommendation to Syntrax Innovation Inc., that their Dietary Supplement *LipoKinetix* be withdrawn from the market [59,67]. Production and sale of *LipoKinetix* was terminated in 2002, but Syntrax continued to produce a product with similar ingredients, but without usnic acid. This was called *AdipoKinetix* [54,67].

As of 2011, the FDA had received at least 22 adverse event reports including 1 death attributed to the weight loss dietary supplements containing usnic acid. However, in 2010, usnic acid was still being marketed in the United States as a constituent of *Lipolyze* (Species, Seaford, NY) which contained a reduced recommended daily dose of 12 mg per day.

Several *in vitro* toxicological studies of usnic acid have been conducted. Pramyothin and coworkers [68] studied hepatotoxic effects of usnic acid in isolated rat hepatocytes. Treatment with 100 or 1000 µM usnic acid in rat primary hepatocytes for 1 h induced the release of hepatic transaminases (aspartate aminotransferase (AST) and alanine aminotransferase (ALT)), decreased the content of reduced glutathione, and caused loss of cell membrane integrity. The study also compared usnic acid toxic effects with a well-known hepatotoxicant, carbon tetrachloride. Treatment with usnic acid and carbon tetrachloride exhibited similar cellular responses, suggesting that usnic acid may have the same hepatotoxic mechanisms as presented by carbon tetrachloride [68]. Another toxicological study was performed in mouse primary hepatocytes [69]. Treatment with 5 µM usnic acid for 16 h in mouse primary hepatocytes resulted in 98% cell death, which appeared to be associated with cell necrosis rather than apoptosis.

In male Swiss mice, usnic acid treatment (15 mg/kg intraperitoneally for 15 days) caused no apparent general toxicity, as evidenced by the negative observations in clinical signs or changes of body weight [70,71]. However, strong hepatotoxicity, including elevated serum transaminase activity and extensive liver necrosis, was observed. No toxicity in other organs such as kidney and spleen was detected in the study. Usnic acid has the potential to attain significant hepatic concentrations at doses used in humans for weight loss and may be subject to variable hepatotoxic risk. Metabolism studies with human and recombinant drug metabolizing enzymes suggest that genetic differences in drug metabolizing enzyme expression may contribute to differential sensitivity to hepatotoxicity among consumers of usnic acid–containing supplements [72].

N-Nitrosofenfluramine

N-Nitrosofenfluramine (Figure 52.6) is a mitochondrial membrane uncoupler that increases mitochondrial permeability transition by opening high-conductance pores in the inner membrane rather than by protonophoric activity [73,74]. It is a derivative and metabolite of fenfluramine, which is a fluorinated amphetamine drug that has been used to treat obesity [75]. *N*-Nitrosofenfluramine has been used as an adulterant in herbal products sold in Asia as weight loss aids. Like usnic acid, exposure to *N*-nitrosofenfluramine through such adulterated supplements has resulted in liver failure and death [76,77].

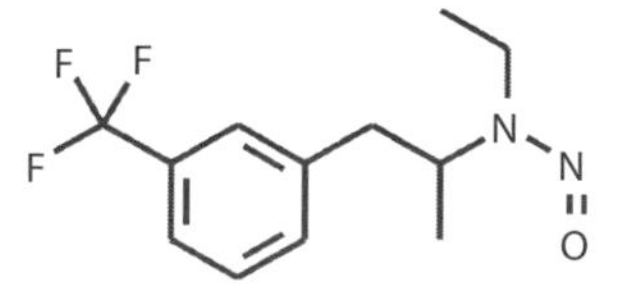

N-nitrosofenfluramine

FIGURE 52.6 *N*-Nitrosofenfluramine, the *N*-oxy derivative and metabolite of fenfluramine, has been illicitly added to herbal weight loss supplements in Asia.

Vanilloid Receptor Agonists

Capsaicin

Capsaicin (8-methyl-*N*-vanillyl-trans-6-nonenamide, Figure 52.7) is the active component of chili peppers, which belong to the genus *Capsicum*. It is an irritant for mammals, including humans, and produces a sensation of burning in any exposed tissue [78]. Capsaicin, as a member of the vanilloid family, binds to a receptor called the vanilloid receptor subtype 1 (VR1) [79]. First cloned in 1997, VR1 is an ion channel-type receptor. VR1, which can also be stimulated with heat and physical abrasion, permits cations to pass through the cell membrane and into the cell when activated. The resulting depolarization of the neuron stimulates it to signal the brain. By binding to the VR1 receptor, the capsaicin molecule produces the same sensation that excessive heat or abrasive damage would cause, explaining why the spiciness of capsaicin is described as a burning sensation [79].

The VR1 ion channel has subsequently been shown to be a member of the superfamily of transient receptor potential (TRP) ion channels and, as such, is now referred to as TRPV1 [80]. There are a number of different TRP ion channels that have been shown to be sensitive to different ranges of temperature and probably are responsible for our ability to distinguish different temperatures. Thus, capsaicin does not actually cause a chemical burn, or indeed any direct tissue damage at all, when chili peppers are the source of exposure. The inflammation caused by the burn or physical abrasion that the body believes it has undergone can potentially cause tissue damage in cases of extreme exposure, as is the case for many substances that trick the body into inflaming itself [79]. Experiments have revealed that dietary capsaicin reduced obesity-induced glucose intolerance and hepatic steatosis by modulating inflammatory responses and fatty acid oxidation in both adipose tissue and liver. Hence, capsaicin may be useful as a dietary additive for reducing obesity-induced metabolic disorders [81].

Hoodia

Hoodia gordonii, a succulent cactus-like plant grown in South Africa, has been used there in traditional medicine [82]. It is used by the Khoi-San (Bushmen) people of South Africa, Botswana, and Namibia as a hunger and thirst suppressant while on long hunting trips. Its use as a dietary supplement to promote weight loss has recently gained popularity, but the commercialization of this plant has been highly controversial due to intellectual property rights and benefit sharing issues, as well as the fact that several prominent pharmaceutical companies involved in its development have withdrawn their interest [82,83]. *H. gordonii* contains an abundance of pregnane glycosides, which comprise of hoodigogenin A, and calogenin as the predominant aglycones [84].

However, the main focus has been on the hoodigogenin A glycoside, P57AS3 (Figure 52.8), which is considered to be the active ingredient responsible for anorexigenic activity, and is used as a marker molecule to determine quality of raw material and products.

Although hoodia has been marketed as a weight loss supplement in North America for over 10 years, a recent literature review concluded that there are currently no peer-reviewed, randomized clinical trials available that evaluate the efficacy of hoodia extracts [85]. Initially, *in vitro* work (reviewed in [82]) suggested that P57AS3 acted directly on neurons in the hypothalamus to produce

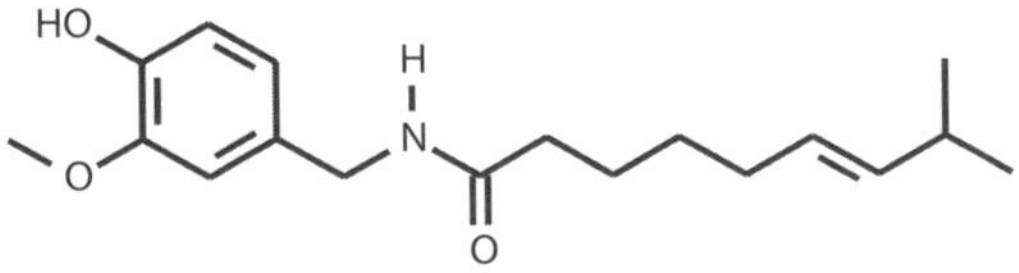

Capsaicin

FIGURE 52.7   Capsaicin (8-methyl-*N*-vanillyl-6-nonenamide) is the major capsaicinoid present in chili peppers and is responsible for their burning taste. It is a natural ligand of the vanilloid receptor, VR1 (TRPV1).

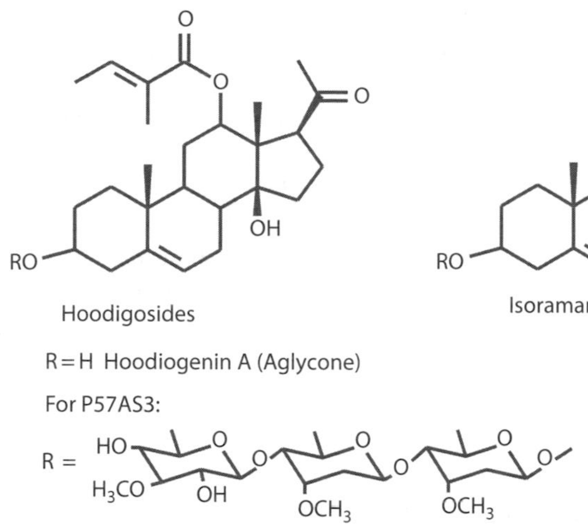

FIGURE 52.8 Pregnane glycosides from *Hoodia gordonii*, such as P57AS3, are reported to be hydrolyzed in the gut prior to absorption of their aglycones. (From Vermaak, I. et al., *Planta. Med.*, 77, 1149, 2011.)

an anorexigenic response by increasing intracellular ATP concentrations, and further *in vivo* studies in rats demonstrated that the direct injection of P57AS3 into the third ventricle of the brain decreased subsequent food intake. Other hoodigogenin A glycosides were not effective. However, pharmacokinetic studies in mice have demonstrated that after oral exposure to hoodia extract or pure P57AS3, only very low concentrations of P57AS3 were isolated from liver and kidney and none was found in brain tissue [86], and *in vitro* studies showed that P57AS3 is rapidly hydrolyzed to hoodigogenin A and isoramanone (Figure 52.8) by simulated gastric fluid and simulated intestinal fluid [82,83]. More recently, an alternative mechanism of action has been proposed [87]. The investigators demonstrated that P57AS3 elicits cholecystokinin secretion both *ex vivo* in rat intestine and *in vitro* in cultured human enteroendocrine cells. This cholecystokinin secretion appeared to be mediated via the intestinal vanilloid receptors, TAS2R7 and TAS2R14, which were selectively activated by P57AS3. In addition, they reported that bitter receptor activation and subsequent satiety hormone secretion *in vitro* were linked to essential structural features of P57AS3.

Evodiamine

Fructus evodiae (*Evodia rutaecarpa* Bentham, Rutaceae) has been used extensively in Chinese traditional medicine [88].The major alkaloidal components of the dried fruits of *E. rutaecarpa*, evodiamine and rutaecarpine (Figure 52.9), are reported to have a wide variety of biological activities, such as antinociceptive effects, inhibition of platelet aggregation, and vasodilatory effects [89]. Studies demonstrated that evodiamine exhibited antitumor and anti-inflammatory bioactivities [90]. These activities are similar to those of capsaicin and are blocked competitively by capsazepine, a specific antagonist of the capsaicin receptor/TRP V1 channel [90]. Evodiamine is, therefore, thought to act as a vanilloid receptor agonist, interacting with TRPV1 or other TRP channels, which are implicated in diverse cellular functions, including pain sensation, temperature, osmolarity, and

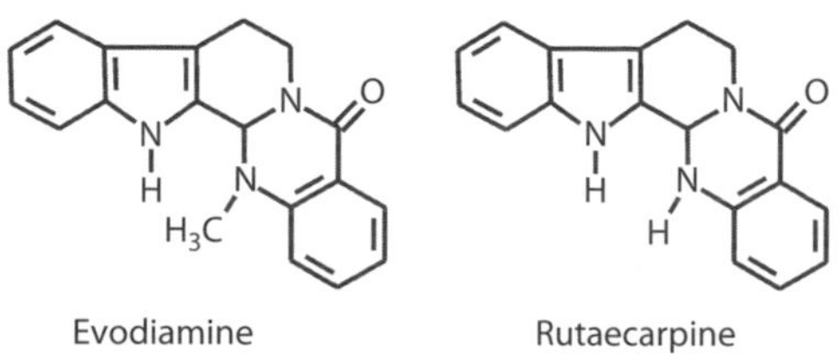

FIGURE 52.9 Major alkaloids from *Evodia rutaecarpa*.

taste sensation [91,92]. Kobayashi and coworkers [93] reported a capsaicin-like antiobese activity of evodiamine, which could be due to serial stimulation of the sympathetic nervous system and UPC1-dependent thermogenesis in brown adipose tissue.

However, it was recently demonstrated [94] that evodiamine improved diet-induced obesity in a UPC1-independent manner, such that evodiamine (but not capsaicin) increased phosphorylation of extracellular signal-regulated kinase/mitogen-activated protein kinase (ERK/MAPK), reduced the expression of transcription factors such as peroxisome proliferator-activated receptor-γ, and strongly inhibited adipocyte differentiation. Further studies reported a novel inhibitory mechanism by which evodiamine stimulates protein kinase Cα via phosphorylation of the epidermal growth factor receptor, leading to ERK activation [90].

OTHER MECHANISMS

L-Carnitine

L-carnitine (3-hydroxy-4-[trimethylazaniumyl]butanoate) (Figure 52.10) is a naturally occurring quaternary ammonium compound biosynthesized in the body from lysine and methionine. It can be easily obtained in a number of foods, including red meat, dairy products, avocados, and pork [95]. About 75% of the body's requirement for carnitine is met by the diet [96], and it is uncommon for a well-nourished individual to be diagnosed as carnitine-deficient. Because L-carnitine is responsible for transport of long-chain fatty acids from the cytosol to mitochondria, it is postulated that carnitine supplementation will enhance lipid oxidation and improve weight loss. Oral L-carnitine supplementation has been reported to increase β-oxidation of lipid acids in healthy volunteers [97]. L-carnitine and its metabolite, acetyl-L-carnitine (ALCAR, Figure 52.10), have been sold as an active ingredient in hundreds of over-the-counter "herbal" diet pills and dietary supplements. For example, ALCAR is currently the primary ingredient of *PrimaForce Alcalean*. L-carnitine is also available as a stand-alone supplement for weight loss.

In a randomized, placebo-controlled study, 18 moderately overweight teenagers (aged 13–17) were assigned into two groups: 2 g of L-carnitine per day or placebo, along with physical training and a diet program. Three months later, weight loss in the treatment group was 5.11 kg, while in the control group it was 0.52 (P < 0.001) [98]. In another randomized, double-blind, placebo-controlled study, 36 moderately overweight premenopausal women were administered L-carnitine (4 g/day) or placebo for 8 weeks; BMIs were matched between the two groups. Thirteen women in the L-carnitine and 15 in the placebo group completed the study; all subjects walked for 30 min 4 days/week. All groups increased the resting energy expenditure, which was related to the aerobic training as opposed to the L-carnitine treatment. Mean total body mass, fat mass, and resting lipid utilization were not affected in both groups after 8 weeks of treatment. Five of the 18 women taking L-carnitine experienced adverse effects such as nausea or diarrhea and did not complete the study. These findings indicated no influence of L-carnitine supplementation on weight loss in moderately obese women [99].

In a third randomized, double-blind, placebo-controlled trial, the effect of L-carnitine was studied in bipolar patients who had gained weight on sodium valproate. Sixty bipolar patients were administered placebo or L-carnitine (15 mg/kg/day) for 26 weeks. All participants were placed on

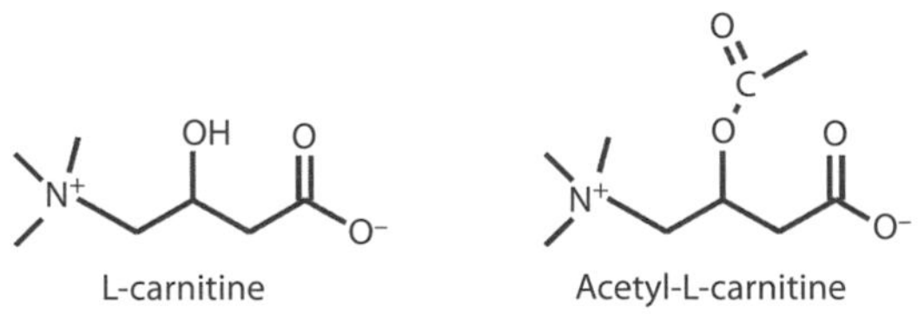

L-carnitine   Acetyl-L-carnitine

FIGURE 52.10   L-carnitine and its acetylated derivative.

an individualized, low-fat, moderately restricted diet (500 kcal/day energy deficit) and were encouraged to accumulate ≥30 min of regular exercise. The researchers found no significant effect of carnitine for individuals who lost weight, but more individuals lost weight in the L-carnitine group than in the control group [100].

In summary, even though L-carnitine plays a vital role in fatty acid metabolism, its beneficial effect on weight loss remains unproven. Research done on L-carnitine shows mixed results in human and animals concerning its weight loss effect [99,101,102]. There are a few small-scale clinical studies which suggested that some individuals experienced increased weight loss [98,103]; however, L-carnitine did not show any effect in the later studies. Larger controlled clinical studies are needed to support that L-carnitine effectively helps weight loss as claimed by some manufacturers. High-dose carnitine has been associated with unpleasant side effects, like vomiting, nausea, diarrhea, body odor, and rash [99].

Chromium

Chromium exists in various oxidation states from Cr^{2+} to Cr^{6+}, with the trivalent Cr^{3+} and hexavalent Cr^{6+} being the predominant forms. While hexavalent chromium is highly toxic and a mutagen and carcinogen, trivalent Cr^{3+} is believed to be an essential trace mineral that forms ion complexes with proteins [104–106]. The rationale behind using chromium as a weight loss supplement is that it is the active component of chromodulin, a peptide complex of four amino acids bound to four Cr^{3+} ions, which interacts with the insulin receptor enhancing the activity of insulin [105]. Thus, the claimed clinical effects of Cr^{3+} include weight loss, increased lean body mass, decreased percentage of body fat, and increased basal metabolic rate resulting from a more efficient insulin response.

Chromium is available in various forms, but the most common is the complex consisting of trivalent chromium with picolinic acid, a naturally occurring derivative of tryptophan (Figure 52.11). This form of chromium is believed to have better bioavailability from the gastrointestinal tract than other common chromium salts; however, the evidence is equivocal and other forms of chromium may have similar bioavailability [106]. A wide array of studies ranging from small pilot to well-controlled clinical trials have been conducted with chromium, primarily chromium picolinate, to assess the effect on weight loss and body composition and on serum lipid profiles and other clinical parameters [107–114]. Collectively, these studies have demonstrated little or no significant effects of chromium on body weight, body composition, or clinical and lipid parameters.

In a meta-analysis of 10 double-blind randomized clinical trials, Pittler and coworkers [115] concluded that chromium picolinate could produce a relatively small reduction in body weight (0.08–0.1 kg/week) when compared to placebo during an intervention period of 10–13 weeks. However, they observed that this was a minimal effect since, by comparison, a moderate caloric restriction of 1200 kcal/day typically results in a weight loss of 0.5–0.6 kg/week. The patients in this analysis were overweight and had an average BMI of 28–33. No adverse events were reported in any of the patients receiving chromium picolinate on these trials [6,115].

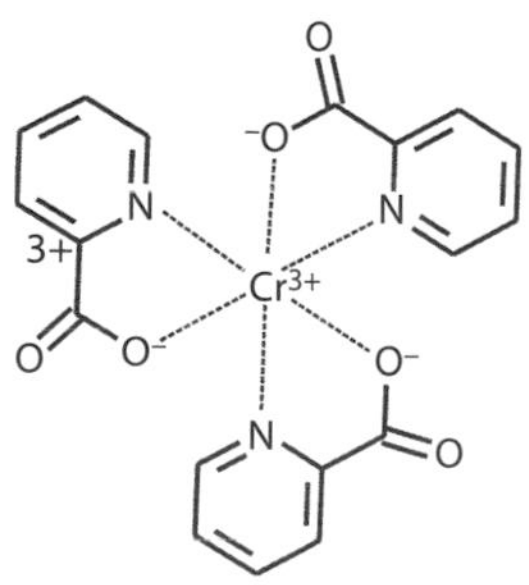

Chromium (III) picolinate

FIGURE 52.11 Chromium picolinate is the chromium salt most frequently used in chromium-containing weight loss supplements.

Although generally regarded as a safe supplement, chromium has the potential to lead to undesired metabolic effects. Large doses of chromium can inhibit iron binding to transferrin and impair iron transport and utilization. The picolinate portion of chromium picolinate may also cause adverse effects. Picolinic acid is a potent metal binding agent and may bind and sequester iron and other essential minerals, preventing their use by the body. Several of the clinical trials reviewed earlier assessed iron status, and no clear adverse effects were noted, indicating that typically used doses of chromium are unlikely to result in clinically relevant adverse effects [104]. Other adverse effects that have been associated with chromium supplementation are anemia, thrombocytopenia, liver dysfunction, dermatitis, hypoglycemia, rhabdomyolysis, renal impairment, and generalized exanthematous pustulosis [104,115,116].

The potential toxicity of chromium picolinate has been evaluated in animal studies by the U.S. National Toxicology Program [117,118]. Exposure in feed up to 50,000 ppm did not induce biologically significant changes in survival, body weight, feed consumption, or nonneoplastic lesions in rats or mice. However, in male rats, a statistically significant increase in the incidence of preputial gland adenoma at 10,000 ppm dose was considered an equivocal finding. Chromium picolinate was not carcinogenic to female rats or to male or female mice. Thus, in these animal studies, there was no evidence of efficacy for chromium picolinate in reducing body weight. Conflicting results have been observed in various genotoxicity (mutagenicity) assays with chromium III salts, whereas chromium VI compounds are highly mutagenic [117].

In summary, the weight of clinical evidence and animal study data suggests that chromium supplementation provides minimal, if any, benefit as a weight loss agent and, if consumed in high doses, may produce some adverse reactions. This suggests that for most individuals, chromium present in food and water is sufficient to provide adequate chromodulin concentrations to maintain functional insulin action and normal homeostasis.

Hydroxycitric Acid

Garcinia cambogia is a subtropical garcinia that is native to Southeast Asia where it is known as Gambooge. It is used in traditional Indian medicine and a flavoring in curries. Hydroxycitric acid (Figure 52.12) is obtained from extracts of *G. cambogia* and has been shown in rodents to competitively inhibit the extramitochondrial enzyme, ATP-citrate-lyase, which catalyzes the cleavage of citrate to acetyl-CoA and oxaloacetate, a key step in lipogenesis. It also suppresses *de novo* fatty acid synthesis and food intake and decreases body weight gain in rodents [119,120]. While animal studies have demonstrated reproducible effects of hydroxycitric acid on weight gain and lipolysis, human clinical trials have been less convincing [121].

Raspberry Ketone

Raspberry ketone (4-(4-hydroxyphenyl)-butan-2-one) is a natural phenolic compound that is the primary aroma compound of red raspberries (*Rubus idaeus*). It is used in perfumery, in cosmetics, and as a food additive to impart a fruity odor. It is one of the most expensive natural flavor components used in the food industry, and it is now generally synthesized from chemical intermediates [122]. Raspberry ketone has a chemical structure (Figure 52.13) that is somewhat similar to that of synephrine and other phenylethylamines (Figure 52.1), and this led to evaluation of its effects on body weight gain in rodents [122]. In this study, raspberry ketone was reported to decrease body weights and hepatic triacylglycerol content of mice fed a high-fat diet. Raspberry ketone also significantly

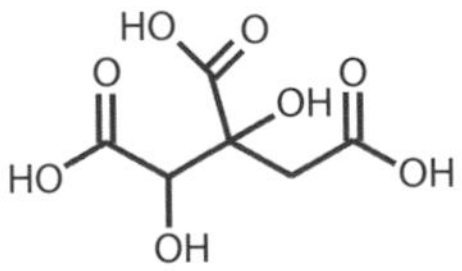

Hydroxycitric acid

FIGURE 52.12 Hydroxycitric acid from *Garcinia cambogia*.

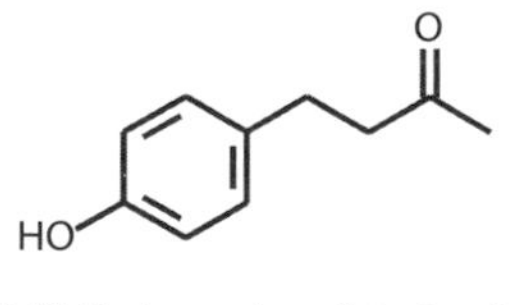

(4-(4-Hydroxyphenyl)-butan-2-one)

FIGURE 52.13 Raspberry ketone (4-(4-hydroxyphenyl)-butan-2-one) is generally produced via chemical synthesis rather than by extraction from red raspberries.

increased norepinephrine-induced lipolysis associated with the translocation of hormone-sensitive lipase from the cytosol to lipid droplets in rat epididymal fat cells, suggesting that raspberry ketone decreased obesity and steatosis by altering the lipid metabolism and increasing norepinephrine-induced lipolysis in white adipocytes [122].

Acai Berry

Acai fruits are obtained from the Amazon River basin where they are manually harvested from wild cabbage palms (*Euterpe oleracea*) native to this area. Traditionally, acai pulp is consumed as a food in the form of a viscous pulp that has been associated with nutritional and medicinal properties including antidiarrheal activity [123,124]. Acai fruit contains high concentrations of antioxidant polyphenolics, primarily the anthocyanins cyanidin 3-rutoside, cyanidin 3-glucoside, cyanidin 3-arabinoside, and cyanidin 3-sambubioside [125] (Figure 52.14), which are structurally

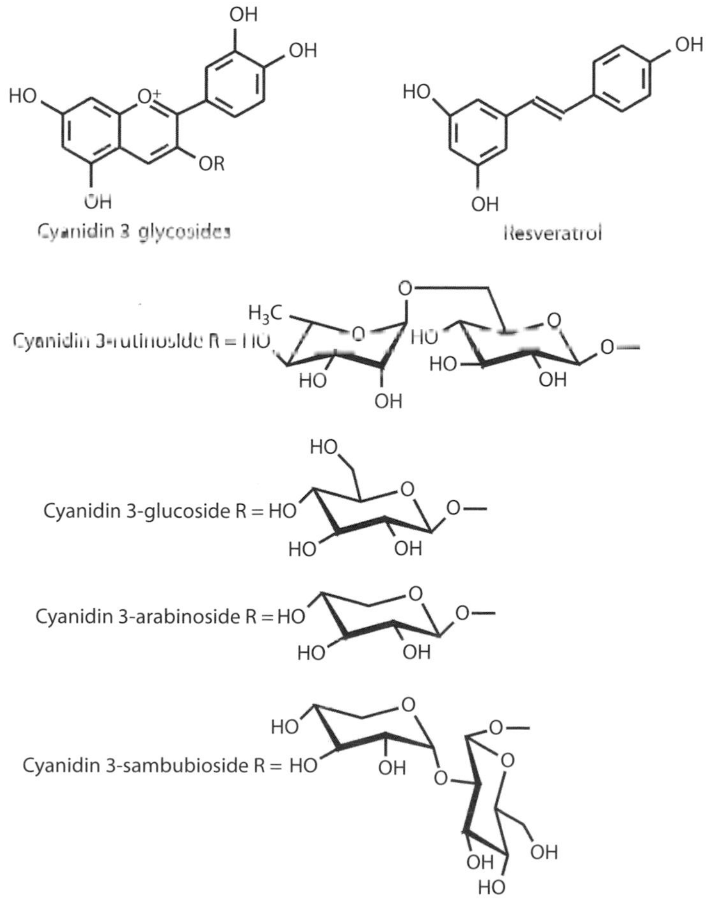

Cyanidin 3 glycosides

Resveratrol

Cyanidin 3-rutinoside R = HO

Cyanidin 3-glucoside R = HO

Cyanidin 3-arabinoside R = HO

Cyanidin 3-sambubioside R = HO

FIGURE 52.14 Cyanidin glycosides from *Euterpe oleracea* are structurally similar to resveratrol glycosides.

related to the well-known herbal antioxidant, resveratrol. Thus, purported antioxidant activity has provided the main rationale for marketing it as a dietary supplement [125]. While acai berry drinks have recently been advertised and marketed as promoting weight loss, the evidence for this claim is not readily available. Paradoxically, when diets containing acai berry extract were fed to rats for 7 weeks, it was associated with not only an improvement of their serum cholesterol profiles and atherogenic index but also an increase in their body weight gain and metabolic efficiency [126].

Fucoxanthin

Fucoxanthin (Figure 52.15) is a carotenoid pigment present in brown algae such as *Eisenia bicyclis* and *Undaria pinnatifida*, which are used in traditional medicine in Japan and Northeast Asia where they have been attributed to possess a number of medicinal functions including anticancer, antihypertensive, anti-inflammatory, antioxidant, and antiobesity effects [127,128]. "Fucoxanthin-rich" ethanol extracts of *U. pinnatifida* have been shown to reduce body weight gain, abdominal white adipose tissue weights, plasma and hepatic triglyceride, and/or cholesterol concentrations in mice fed high-fat diets supplemented with the extract [128], and these changes were associated with increased expression of uncoupling protein, UCP1, mRNA in adipose tissue. Other studies using purified fucoxanthin have produced similar improvements in body weight and serum lipid profile and also demonstrated decreases in serum insulin:glucagon ratios and induction of peroxisome proliferator activated receptor α mRNA expression [129].

3,5-Diiodo-L-Thyronine

3,5-Diiodo-L-thyronine, a naturally occurring iodothyronine (Figure 52.16), is a precursor of 3,3′,5-triodo-L-thyronine and thyroxine but has also been reported to affect lipid metabolism and energy expenditure independently of thyroid hormonal pathways by directly acting upon mitochondria [130]. When tested in rats fed a high-fat diet, treatment with 3,5-diiodo-L-thyronine (250 μg/kg/day, i.p. for 30 days) resulted in 13% lower mean body weight, a 42% higher liver fatty acid oxidation rate, approximately 50% less fat mass, a complete disappearance of fat from the liver, and significant reductions in the serum triglyceride and cholesterol levels (−52% and −18%, respectively). Thyroid hormones and thyroid-stimulating hormone serum levels were not influenced by 3,5-diiodo-L-thyronine administration [130]. The biochemical mechanism underlying the effects of 3,5-diiodo-L-thyronine on liver metabolism is reported to involve the carnitine palmitoyltransferase system and mitochondrial uncoupling, and recent *in vitro* work suggests that thyroid

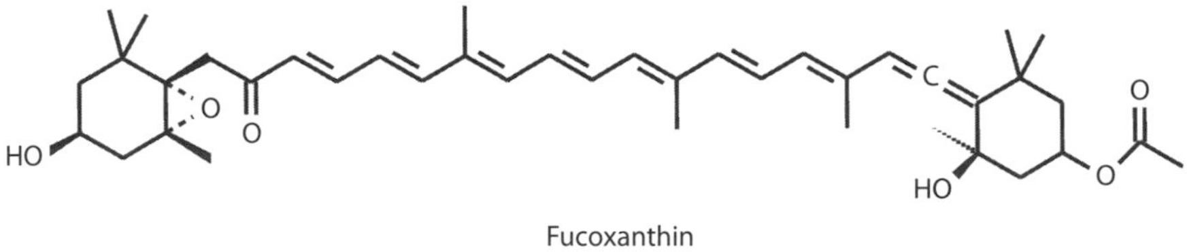

Fucoxanthin

FIGURE 52.15   Fucoxanthin is an accessory pigment of brown algae species that are used in traditional medicine in Northeast Asia.

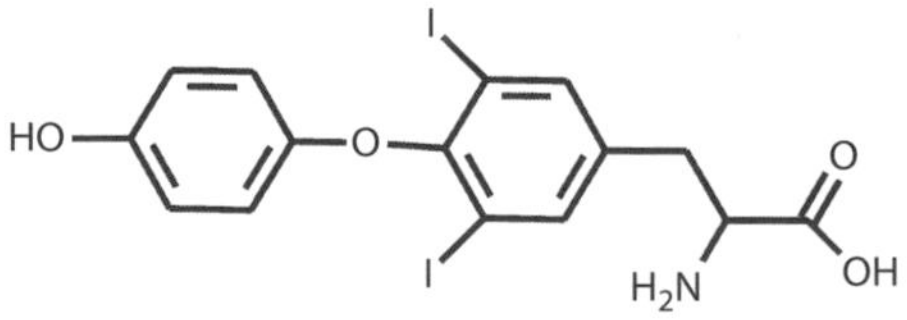

3,5-Diiodo-L-thyronine

FIGURE 52.16   3,5-Diiodo-L-thyronine is reported to stimulate uncoupling activity in mitochondria independently of classical thyroid hormone receptors. (From Lanni, A. et al., *FASEB J.*, 19, 1552, 2005.)

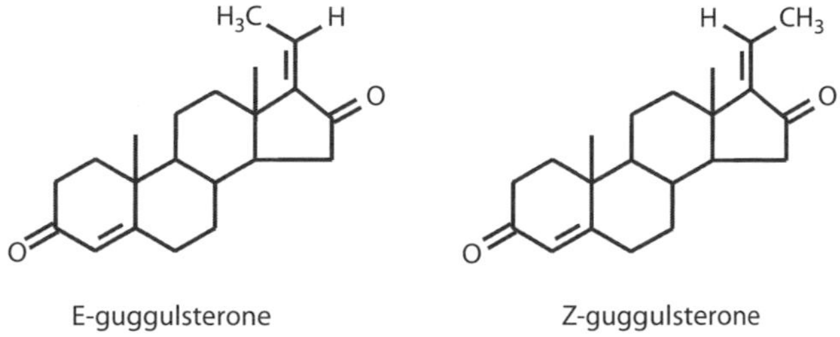

E-guggulsterone   Z-guggulsterone

FIGURE 52.17   Guggulsterones are the major active ingredients of guggul tree (*C. mukul*) lipid extract.

hormone receptors do not mediate these effects of 3,5-diiodo-L-thyronine [131,132]. It is not known whether similar mechanisms occur in human liver after oral exposure to 3,5-diiodo-L-thyronine.

Guggulipids

Guggulipid is an extract of the guggul tree, *Commiphora mukul*, that is native to the Indian subcontinent and is used to treat hyperlipidemia in traditional Ayurvedic medicine. Two plant sterol stereoisomers, Z-guggulsterone and E-guggulsterone (Figure 52.17), have been reported to be responsible for the lipid-lowering activity of guggulipid. The molecular basis for the lipid-lowering action of these guggulsterone isomers has been suggested to be antagonism of the farnesoid X receptor, a member of the nuclear receptor superfamily of ligand-activated transcription factors [133].

Mint, Cumin, Olive, Lady's Mantle

Recently, mixtures of extracts of the herbs *Mentha longifolia* (horse mint), *Cuminum cyminum* (cumin), *Olea europaea* (olive leaf), and *Alchemilla vulgaris* (lady's mantle) have been produced in Israel and Palestine and marketed in Europe as *Weighlevel* and in the United States as part of the current (2011) version of *Pro Clinical Hydroxycut*. These herbal extracts are reported to have been used to treat obesity in traditional Arab and Greek medicine [134], but the active ingredients are currently unknown.

CONCLUDING REMARKS

Supplements marketed as weight loss aids and fat burners usually contain mixtures of several ingredients that can include both herbal extracts and pure chemicals. While the efficacy of certain ingredients may have been demonstrated in clinical trials, in the majority of cases, the actual mixtures being marketed have not been evaluated. Claims of efficacy are merely supported by testimonials and descriptions of the rationale behind each ingredient. Safety is inferred by assurances that the constituents are "natural," but one must remember that nature produces some of the most potent toxins known to man. Rather, the concept of natural being safe is based not on a substance's biological origin but on its association with a "herb lore" derived from many generations of trial and error experience within the traditional culture that developed its use. However, with the globalization of the nutraceutical industry, modern supplements being marketed for weight loss in the United States and elsewhere tend to contain a plethora of ingredients from multiple geographical sources. For example, a product could contain acai extract from Brazil, guarana from Central America, *Citrus aurantium* from Iberia, olive leaf from Lebanon, *Evodia rutaecarpa* from China, fucoxanthin from Japan, and guggulipid extract from India. There is a lack of any traditional experience in the use such combinations.

Moreover, for some cases where a long history of traditional use is available, that use does not include weight loss. It is probably more than coincidence that the traditional uses of usnic acid and ephedra, the two weight loss constituents that have so far caused the greatest problems, are as an antimicrobial and a decongestant, respectively, and not in higher doses as metabolic uncouplers or stimulants. Reputable manufacturers of weight loss supplements should at least attempt to test their combination for safety and efficacy to a standard that approaches what is required for new pharmaceuticals. In particular, they should at least establish that sufficient concentrations of the active ingredient(s) reach the target tissue to evoke the desired effect and determine whether synergistic or adverse interactions occur between all the constituent chemicals that are present in significant amounts in their products. Unfortunately, it is not always economically feasible for small companies to achieve this. It is therefore important for government and academic researchers to help, where possible, by providing mechanistic and toxicity data on potential new weight loss agents to the public domain prior to their commercial development so that adverse effects can be more readily anticipated.

REFERENCES

1. Saper RB, Eisenberg DM, Phillips RS. Common dietary supplements for weight loss. *Am Fam Physician* **70**: 1731–1738. 2004.
2. Anastasi JK, Chang M, Einarson A, Capili B. Herbal supplements: Talking with your patients. *J. Nurse Pract* **7**: 29–35. 2007.
3. Lipman TO. The role of herbs and probiotics in GI wellness for older adults. *Geriatr Aging* **10**: 182–191. 2007.
4. Vitalone A, Menniti-Ippolito F, Moro PA, Firenzuoli F, Raschetti R, Mazzanti G. Suspected adverse reactions associated with herbal products used for weight loss: A case series reported to the Italian National Institute of Health. *Eur J Clin Pharmacol* **67**: 215–224. 2011.
5. Ervin RB, Wright JD, Reed-Gillette D. Prevalence of leading types of dietary supplements used in the Third National Health and Nutrition Examination Survey, 1988–1994. *Adv Data* **349**: 1–7. 2004.
6. Pittler MH, Ernst E. Dietary supplements for body-weight reduction: A systematic review. *Am J Clin Nutr* **79**: 529–536. 2004.
7. Lobb A. Science of weight loss supplements: Compromised by conflicts of interest? *World J Gastroenterol* **16**: 4880–4882. 2010.
8. Tachjian A, Maria V, Jahangir A. Use of herbal products and potential interactions in patients with cardiovascular diseases. *J Am Coll Cardiol* **55**: 515–525. 2010.
9. Clement K, Vaisse C, Manning BS, Basdevant A, Guy-Grand B, Ruiz J, Silver KD, Shuldiner AR, Froguel P, Strosberg AD. Genetic variation in the β3-adrenergic receptor and an increased capacity to gain weight in patients with morbid obesity. *N Engl J Med* **333**: 352–354. 1995.
10. Arner P. Hunting for human obesity genes? Look in the adipose tissue! *Int J Obes Relat Metab Disord* **24** (**Suppl 4**): S57–S62. 2000.
11. Nagai N, Sakane N, Kotani K, Hamada T, Tsuzaki K, Moritani T. Uncoupling protein 1 gene-3826 A/G polymorphism is associated with weight loss on a short-term, controlled-energy diet in young women. *Nutr Res* **31**: 255–261. 2011.
12. Godfrey KM, Sheppard A, Gluckman PD, Lillycrop KA, Burdge GC, McLean C, Rodford J, Slater-Jefferies JL, Garratt E, Crozier SR, Emerald BS, Gale CR, Inskip HM, Cooper C, Hanson MA. Epigenetic gene promoter methylation at birth is associated with child's later adiposity. *Diabetes* **60**: 1528–1534. 2011.
13. Shord SS, Shah K, Lukose A. Drug-botanical interactions: A review of the laboratory, animal, and human data for 8 common botanicals. *Integr Cancer Ther* **8**: 208–227. 2009.
14. Hebert LF, Jr., Daniels MC, Zhou J, Crook ED, Turner RL, Simmons ST, Neidigh JL, Zhu JS, Baron AD, McClain DA. Overexpression of glutamine: Fructose-6-phosphate amidotransferase in transgenic mice leads to insulin resistance. *J Clin Invest* **98**: 930–936. 1996.
15. US Government Accountability Office. Herbal dietary supplements: Examples of deceptive or questionable marketing practices and potentially dangerous advice. 2010. Publication No. GAO-10-662T US GAO, Washington, DC.
16. Dasgupta A. Review of abnormal laboratory test results and toxic effects due to use of herbal medicines. *Am J Clin Pathol* **120**: 127–137. 2003.
17. Gagnier JJ, Boon H, Rochon P, Moher D, Barnes J, Bombardier C. Reporting randomized, controlled trials of herbal interventions: An elaborated CONSORT statement. *Ann Intern Med* **144**: 364–367. 2006.
18. Petroczi A, Taylor G, Naughton DP. Mission impossible? Regulatory and enforcement issues to ensure safety of dietary supplements. *Food Chem Toxicol* **49**: 393–402. 2011.
19. Haddock CK, Poston WS, Dill PL, Foreyt JP, Ericsson M. Pharmacotherapy for obesity: A quantitative analysis of four decades of published randomized clinical trials. *Int J Relat Metab Disord* **26**: 262–273. 2002.

20. Leibowitz SF. Hypothalamic β-adrenergic "satiety" system antagonizes an alpha-adrenergic "hunger" system in the rat. *Nature* **226**: 963–964. 1970.

21. Fugh-Berman A, Myers A. Citrus aurantium, an ingredient of dietary supplements marketed for weight loss: Current status of clinical and basic research. *Exp Biol Med (Maywood)* **229**: 698–704. 2004.

22. Brunton L, Lazo J, Parker K. *Goodman and Gilman's The Pharmacological Basis of Therapeutics 11th Edition*. Goodman, Gilman. P. 11. 2005. New York, McGraw-Hill.

23. Brown CM, McGrath JC, Midgley JM, Muir AG, O'Brien JW, Thonoor CM, Williams CM, Wilson VG. Activities of octopamine and synephrine stereoisomers on alpha-adrenoceptors. *Br J Pharmacol* **93**: 417–429. 1988.

24. Rossato LG, Costa VM, Limberger RP, Bastos ML, Remiao F. Synephrine: From trace concentrations to massive consumption in weight-loss. *Food Chem Toxicol* **49**: 8–16. 2011.

25. Lafontan M, Berlan M. Fat cell adrenergic receptors and the control of white and brown fat cell function. *J Lipid Res* **34**: 1057–1091. 1993.

26. Skeberdis VA. Structure and function of β3-adrenergic receptors. *Medicina (Kaunas)* **40**: 407–413. 2004.

27. Bray GA. Use and abuse of appetite-suppressant drugs in the treatment of obesity. *Ann Intern Med* **119**: 707–713. 1993.

28. Anglin MD, Burke C, Perrochet B, Stamper E, wud-Noursi S. History of the methamphetamine problem. *J Psychoactive Drugs* **32**: 137–141. 2000.

29. Schepis TS, Marlowe DB, Forman RF. The availability and portrayal of stimulants over the Internet. *J Adolesc Health* **42**: 458–465. 2008.

30. Palamar J. How ephedrine escaped regulation in the United States: A historical review of misuse and associated policy. *Health Policy* **99**: 1–9. 2011.

31. Hong H, Chen HB, Yang DH, Shang MY, Wang X, Cai SQ, Mikage M. Comparison of contents of five ephedrine alkaloids in three official origins of Ephedra Herb in China by high-performance liquid chromatography. *J Nat Med* **65**: 623–628. 2011.

32. Li MF, Cheung BM. Rise and fall of anti-obesity drugs. *World J Diabetes* **2**: 19–23. 2011.

33. Shekelle PG, Hardy ML, Morton SC, Maglione M, Mojica WA, Suttorp MJ, Rhodes SL, Jungvig L, Gagne J. Efficacy and safety of ephedra and ephedrine for weight loss and athletic performance: A meta-analysis. *JAMA* **289**: 1537–1545. 2003.

34. Haaz S, Fontaine KR, Cutter G, Limdi N, Perumean-Chaney S, Allison DB. Citrus aurantium and synephrine alkaloids in the treatment of overweight and obesity: An update. *Obes Rev* **7**: 79–88. 2006.

35. Mercader J, Wanecq E, Chen J, Carpene C. Isopropylnorsynephrine is a stronger lipolytic agent in human adipocytes than synephrine and other amines present in Citrus aurantium. *J Physiol Biochem* **67**: 443–452. 2011.

36. Bouchard NC, Howland MA, Greller HA, Hoffman RS, Nelson LS. Ischemic stroke associated with use of an ephedra-free dietary supplement containing synephrine. *Mayo Clin Proc* **80**: 541–545. 2005.

37. Bui LT, Nguyen DT, Ambrose PJ. Blood pressure and heart rate effects following a single dose of bitter orange. *Ann Pharmacother* **40**: 53–57. 2006.

38. Beavo JA, Rogers NL, Crofford OD, Baird CE, Hardman JG, Sutherland EW, Newman EV. Effects of phosphodiesterase inhibitors on cyclic AMP levels and on lipolysis. *Ann NY Acad Sci* **185**: 129–136. 1971.

39. Snyder SH, Katims JJ, Annau Z, Bruns RF, Daly JW. Adenosine receptors and behavioral actions of methylxanthines. *Proc Natl Acad Sci USA* **78**: 3260–3264. 1981.

40. Baldwin HA, File SE. Caffeine-induced anxiogenesis: The role of adenosine, benzodiazepine and noradrenergic receptors. *Pharmacol Biochem Behav* **32**: 181–186. 1989.

41. Nehlig A, Daval JL, Debry G. Caffeine and the central nervous system: Mechanisms of action, biochemical, metabolic and psychostimulant effects. *Brain Res Brain Res Rev* **17**: 139–170. 1992.

42. Glade MJ. Caffeine-not just a stimulant. *Nutr* **26**: 932–938. 2010.

43. Duchan E, Patel ND, Feucht C. Energy drinks: A review of use and safety for athletes. *Phys Sportsmed* **38**: 171–179. 2010.

44. Hursel R, Westerterp-Plantenga MS. Thermogenic ingredients and body weight regulation. *Int J Obes (Lond)* **34**: 659–669. 2010.

45. Dulloo AG, Duret C, Rohrer D, Girardier L, Mensi N, Fathi M, Chantre P, Vandermander J. Efficacy of a green tea extract rich in catechin polyphenols and caffeine in increasing 24-h energy expenditure and fat oxidation in humans. *Am J Clin Nutr* **70**: 1040–1045. 1999.

46. Murase T, Nagasawa A, Suzuki J, Hase T, Tokimitsu I. Beneficial effects of tea catechins on diet-induced obesity: Stimulation of lipid catabolism in the liver. *Int J Obes Relat Metab Disord* **26**: 1459–1464. 2002.

47. Monteiro R, Assuncao M, Andrade JP, Neves D, Calhau C, Azevedo I. Chronic green tea consumption decreases body mass, induces aromatase expression, and changes proliferation and apoptosis in adult male rat adipose tissue. *J Nutr* **138**: 2156–2163. 2008.

48. Westerterp-Plantenga MS, Lejeune MP, Kovacs EM. Body weight loss and weight maintenance in relation to habitual caffeine intake and green tea supplementation. *Obes Res* **13**: 1195–1204. 2005.

49. Diepvens K, Kovacs EM, Vogels N, Westerterp-Plantenga MS. Metabolic effects of green tea and of phases of weight loss. *Physiol Behav* **87**: 185–191. 2006.

50. Sarma DN, Barrett ML, Chavez ML, Gardiner P, Ko R, Mahady GB, Marles RJ, Pellicore LS, Giancaspro GI, Low DT. Safety of green tea extracts: A systematic review by the US Pharmacopeia. *Drug Saf* **31**: 469–484. 2008.

51. Galati G, Lin A, Sultan AM, O'Brien PJ. Cellular and in vivo hepatotoxicity caused by green tea phenolic acids and catechins. *Free Radic Biol Med* **40**: 570–580. 2006.

52. Nedergaard J, Bengtsson T, Cannon B. Three years with adult human brown adipose tissue. *Ann NY Acad Sci* **1212**: E20–E36. 2010.

53. Mitchell P. Vectorial chemistry and the molecular mechanics of chemiosmotic coupling: Power transmission by proticity. *Biochem Soc Trans* **4**: 399–430. 1976.

54. Guo L, Shi Q, Fang JL, Mei N, Ali AA, Lewis SM, Leakey JE, Frankos VH. Review of usnic acid and Usnea barbata toxicity. *J Environ Sci Health C Environ Carcinog Ecotoxicol Rev* **26**: 317–338. 2008.

55. Colman E. Dinitrophenol and obesity: An early twentieth-century regulatory dilemma. *Regul Toxicol Pharmacol* **48**: 115–117. 2007.

56. Hsiao AL, Santucci KA, Seo-Mayer P, Mariappan MR, Hodsdon ME, Banasiak KJ, Baum CR. Pediatric fatality following ingestion of dinitrophenol: Postmortem identification of a "dietary supplement". *Clin Toxicol (Phila)* **43**: 281–285. 2005.

57. Ingolfsdottir K. Usnic acid. *Phytochemistry* **61**: 729–736. 2002.

58. Cocchietto M, Skert N, Nimis PL, Sava G. A review on usnic acid, an interesting natural compound. *Naturwissenschaften* **89**: 137–146. 2002.

59. Frankos VH. NTP nomination for usnic acid and *Usnea barbata*. 2004. NCI, Available at: http://ntp-server.niehs.nih.gov/ntp/htdocs/Chem_Background/ExSumPdf/UsnicAcid.pdf (accessed February 2012).

60. Elo H, Matikainen J, Pelttari E. Potent activity of the lichen antibiotic (+)-usnic acid against clinical isolates of vancomycin-resistant enterococci and methicillin resistant Staphylococcus aureus. *Naturwissenschaften* **94**: 465–468. 2007.

61. Abo-Khatwa AN, al Robai AA, al Jawhari DA. Lichen acids as uncouplers of oxidative phosphorylation of mouse-liver mitochondria. *Nat Toxins* **4**: 96–102. 1996.

62. Durazo FA, Lassman C, Han SH, Saab S, Lee NP, Kawano M, Saggi B, Gordon S, Farmer DG, Yersiz H, Goldstein RL, Ghobrial M, Busuttil RW. Fulminant liver failure due to usnic acid for weight loss. *Am J Gastroenterol* **99**: 950–952. 2004.

63. Favreau JT, Ryu ML, Braunstein G, Orshansky G, Park SS, Coody GL, Love LA, Fong TL. Severe hepatotoxicity associated with the dietary supplement LipoKinetix. *Ann Intern Med* **136**: 590–595. 2002.

64. Neff GW, Reddy KR, Durazo FA, Meyer D, Marrero R, Kaplowitz N. Severe hepatotoxicity associated with the use of weight loss diet supplements containing ma huang or usnic acid. *J Hepatol* **41**: 1062–1064. 2004.

65. Sanchez W, Maple JT, Burgart LJ, Kamath PS. Severe hepatotoxicity associated with use of a dietary supplement containing usnic acid. *Mayo Clin Proc* **81**: 541–544. 2006.

66. FDA Medwatch announcement on *LipoKinetix*. (Updated 07/30/2009). USFDA, Silver Spring, MD. http://www.fda.gov/Safety/MedWatch/SafetyInformation/SafetyAlertsforHumanMedicalProducts/ucm172824.htm (accessed February 2012).

67. OBGYN-NET, FDA warns against dietary supplement. 2001, http://www.obgyn.net/newsrx/general_health-Nutriceuticals-20011217-11.asp (accessed February 2012).

68. Pramyothin P, Janthasoot W, Pongnimitprasert N, Phrukudom S, Ruangrungsi N. Hepatotoxic effect of (+)usnic acid from Usnea siamensis Wainio in rats, isolated rat hepatocytes and isolated rat liver mitochondria. *J Ethnopharmacol* **90**: 381–387. 2004.

69. Han D, Matsumaru K, Rettori D, Kaplowitz N. Usnic acid-induced necrosis of cultured mouse hepatocytes: Inhibition of mitochondrial function and oxidative stress. *Biochem Pharmacol* **67**: 439–451. 2004.

70. Ribeiro-Costa RM, Alves AJ, Santos NP, Nascimento SC, Goncalves EC, Silva NH, Honda NK, Santos-Magalhaes NS. *In vitro* and *in vivo* properties of usnic acid encapsulated into PLGA-microspheres. *J Microencapsul* **21**: 371–384. 2004.

71. da Silva Santos NP, Nascimento SC, Wanderley MS, Pontes-Filho NT, da Silva JF, de Castro CM, Pereira EC, da Silva NH, Honda NK, Santos-Magalhaes NS. Nanoencapsulation of usnic acid: An attempt to improve antitumour activity and reduce hepatotoxicity. *Eur J Pharm Biopharm* **64**: 154–160. 2006.

72. Foti RS, Dickmann LJ, Davis JA, Greene RJ, Hill JJ, Howard ML, Pearson JT, Rock DA, Tay JC, Wahlstrom JL, Slatter JG. Metabolism and related human risk factors for hepatic damage by usnic acid containing nutritional supplements. *Xenobiotica* **38**: 264–280. 2008.

73. Nakagawa Y, Suzuki T, Kamimura H, Nagai F. Role of mitochondrial membrane permeability transition in N-nitrosofenfluramine-induced cell injury in rat hepatocytes. *Eur J Pharmacol* **529**: 33–39. 2006.

74. Samartsev VN, Polishchuk LS, Paydyganov AP, Zeldi IP. Features of the uncoupling effect of fatty acids in liver mitochondria of mammals with different body weight. *Biochemistry (Mosc)* **69**: 678–686. 2004.

75. Satoh K, Nonaka R, Tada Y, Fukumori N, Ogata A, Yamada A, Satoh T, Nagai F. Effects of N-nitrosofenfluramine, a component of Chinese dietary supplement for weight loss, on CD-1 mice. *Arch Toxicol* **80**: 605–613. 2006.

76. Lau G, Lo DS, Yao YJ, Leong HT, Chan CL, Chu SS. A fatal case of hepatic failure possibly induced by nitrosofenfluramine: A case report. *Med Sci Law* **44**: 252–263. 2004.

77. Kawaguchi T, Harada M, Arimatsu H, Nagata S, Koga Y, Kuwahara R, Hisamochi A, Hino T, Taniguchi E, Kumemura H, Hanada S, Maeyama M, Koga H, Tomiyasu N, Toyomasu H, Kawaguchi M, Kage M, Kumashiro R, Tanikawa K, Sata M. Severe hepatotoxicity associated with a N-nitrosofenfluramine-containing weight-loss supplement: Report of three cases. *J Gastroenterol Hepatol* **19**: 349–350. 2004.

78. Johnson W. Final report on the safety assessment of capsicum annuum extract, capsicum annuum fruit extract, capsicum annuum resin, capsicum annuum fruit powder, capsicum frutescens fruit, capsicum frutescens fruit extract, capsicum frutescens resin, and capsaicin. *Int J Toxicol* **26 (Suppl 1)**: 3–106. 2007.

79. Luo XJ, Peng J, Li YJ. Recent advances in the study on capsaicinoids and capsinoids. *Eur J Pharmacol* **650**: 1–7. 2011.

80. Zhu Z, Luo Z, Ma S, Liu D. TRP channels and their implications in metabolic diseases. *Pflugers Arch* **461**: 211–223. 2011.

81. Kang JH, Goto T, Han IS, Kawada T, Kim YM, Yu R. Dietary capsaicin reduces obesity-induced insulin resistance and hepatic steatosis in obese mice fed a high-fat diet. *Obesity (Silver Spring)* **18**: 780–787. 2010.

82. Vermaak I, Hamman JH, Viljoen AM. Hoodia gordonii: An up-to-date review of a commercially important anti-obesity plant. *Planta Med* **77**: 1149–1160. 2011.

83. Madgula VL, Avula B, Pawar RS, Shukla YJ, Khan IA, Walker LA, Khan SI. In vitro metabolic stability and intestinal transport of P57AS3 (P57) from Hoodia gordonii and its interaction with drug metabolizing enzymes. *Planta Med* **74**: 1269–1275. 2008.

84. Shukla YJ, Pawar RS, Ding Y, Li XC, Ferreira D, Khan IA. Pregnane glycosides from Hoodia gordonii. *Phytochemistry* **70**: 675–683. 2009.

85. Whelan AM, Jurgens TM, Szeto V. Case report. Efficacy of Hoodia for weight loss: Is there evidence to support the efficacy claims? *J Clin Pharm Ther* **35**: 609–612. 2010.

86. Madgula VL, Ashfaq MK, Wang YH, Avula B, Khan IA, Walker LA, Khan SI. Bioavailability, pharmacokinetics, and tissue distribution of the oxypregnane steroidal glycoside P57AS3 (P57) from Hoodia gordonii in mouse model. *Planta Med* **76**: 1582–1586. 2010.

87. Le NB, Foltz M, Daniel H, Gouka R. The steroid glycoside H.g.-12 from Hoodia gordonii activates the human bitter receptor TAS2R14 and induces CCK release from HuTu-80 cells. *Am J Physiol Gastrointest Liver Physiol* **299**: G1368–G1375. 2010.

88. Jiang J, Hu C. Evodiamine: A novel anti-cancer alkaloid from Evodia rutaecarpa. *Molecules* **14**: 1852–1859. 2009.

89. Kobayashi Y, Hoshikuma K, Nakano Y, Yokoo Y, Kamiya T. The positive inotropic and chronotropic effects of evodiamine and rutaecarpine, indoloquinazoline alkaloids isolated from the fruits of Evodia rutaecarpa, on the guinea-pig isolated right atria: Possible involvement of vanilloid receptors. *Planta Med* **67**: 244–248. 2001.

90. Wang T, Wang Y, Yamashita H. Evodiamine inhibits adipogenesis via the EGFR-PKCα-ERK signaling pathway. *FEBS Lett* **583**: 3655–3659. 2009.

91. Borrelli F, Izzo AA. Role of acylethanolamides in the gastrointestinal tract with special reference to food intake and energy balance. *Best Pract Res Clin Endocrinol Metab* **23**: 33–49. 2009.

92. Liu D, Zhu Z, Tepel M. The role of transient receptor potential channels in metabolic syndrome. *Hypertens Res* **31**: 1989–1995. 2008.

93. Kobayashi Y, Nakano Y, Kizaki M, Hoshikuma K, Yokoo Y, Kamiya T. Capsaicin-like anti-obese activities of evodiamine from fruits of *Evodia rutaecarpa*, a vanilloid receptor agonist. *Planta Med* **67**: 628–633. 2001.

94. Wang T, Wang Y, Kontani Y, Kobayashi Y, Sato Y, Mori N, Yamashita H. Evodiamine improves diet-induced obesity in a uncoupling protein-1-independent manner: Involvement of antiadipogenic mechanism and extracellularly regulated kinase/mitogen-activated protein kinase signaling. *Endocrinology* **149**: 358–366. 2008.

95. Kanter MM, Williams MH. Antioxidants, carnitine, and choline as putative ergogenic aids. *Int J Sport Nutr* **5 (Suppl)**: S120–S131. 1995.

96. Vaz FM, Wanders RJ. Carnitine biosynthesis in mammals. *Biochem J* **361**: 417–429. 2002.

97. Muller DM, Seim H, Kiess W, Loster H, Richter T. Effects of oral L-carnitine supplementation on in vivo long-chain fatty acid oxidation in healthy adults. *Metabolism* **51**: 1389–1391. 2002.

98. Zhou S, He Z, Liu J, Se H. L-Carnitine's effect on comprehensive weight loss program in obese adolescents. *Acta Nutrimenta Sinica* **19**: 146–150. 1997.

99. Villani RG, Gannon J, Self M, Rich PA. L-Carnitine supplementation combined with aerobic training does not promote weight loss in moderately obese women. *Int J Sport Nutr Exerc Metab* **10**: 199–207. 2000.

100. Elmslie JL, Porter RJ, Joyce PR, Hunt PJ, Mann JI. Carnitine does not improve weight loss outcomes in valproate-treated bipolar patients consuming an energy-restricted, low-fat diet. *Bipolar Disord* **8**: 503–507. 2006.

101. Center SA, Harte J, Watrous D, Reynolds A, Watson TD, Markwell PJ, Millington DS, Wood PA, Yeager AE, Erb HN. The clinical and metabolic effects of rapid weight loss in obese pet cats and the influence of supplemental oral L-carnitine. *J Vet Intern Med* **14**: 598–608. 2000.

102. Melton SA, Keenan MJ, Stanciu CE, Hegsted M, Zablah-Pimentel EM, O'Neil CE, Gaynor P, Schaffhauser A, Owen K, Prisby RD, LaMotte LL, Fernandez JM. L-carnitine supplementation does not promote weight loss in ovariectomized rats despite endurance exercise. *Int J Vitam Nutr Res* **75**: 156–160. 2005.

103. Lurz R, Fischer R. Carnitine as supporting agent in weight loss in adiposity. *Aerztezeitschrift für Naturheilverfahren* **39**: 12–15. 1998.

104. Vincent JB. The potential value and toxicity of chromium picolinate as a nutritional supplement, weight loss agent and muscle development agent. *Sports Med* **33**: 213–230. 2003.

105. Viera M, vis-McGibony CM. Isolation and characterization of low-molecular-weight chromium-binding substance (LMWCr) from chicken liver. *Protein J* **27**: 371–375. 2008.

106. Vincent JB. Chromium: Celebrating 50 years as an essential element? *Dalton Trans* **39**: 3787–3794. 2010.

107. Kaats GR, Keith SC, Pullin D, Squires WG, Jr., Wise JA, Hesslink R, Jr., Morin RJ. Safety and efficacy evaluation of a fitness club weight-loss program. *Adv Ther* **15**: 345–361. 1998.

108. Lukaski HC, Siders WA, Penland JG. Chromium picolinate supplementation in women: Effects on body weight, composition, and iron status. *Nutr* **23**: 187–195. 2007.

109. Yazaki Y, Faridi Z, Ma Y, Ali A, Northrup V, Njike VY, Liberti L, Katz DL. A pilot study of chromium picolinate for weight loss. *J Altern Complement Med* **16**: 291–299. 2010.

110. Volpe SL, Huang HW, Larpadisorn K, Lesser II. Effect of chromium supplementation and exercise on body composition, resting metabolic rate and selected biochemical parameters in moderately obese women following an exercise program. *J Am Coll Nutr* **20**: 293–306. 2001.

111. Pasman WJ, Westerterp-Plantenga MS, Saris WH. The effectiveness of long-term supplementation of carbohydrate, chromium, fibre and caffeine on weight maintenance. *Int J Obes Relat Metab Disord* **21**: 1143–1151. 1997.

112. Martin J, Wang ZQ, Zhang XH, Wachtel D, Volaufova J, Matthews DE, Cefalu WT. Chromium picolinate supplementation attenuates body weight gain and increases insulin sensitivity in subjects with type 2 diabetes. *Diabetes Care* **29**: 1826–1832. 2006.

113. Grant KE, Chandler RM, Castle AL, Ivy JL. Chromium and exercise training: Effect on obese women. *Med Sci Sports Exerc* **29**: 992–998. 1997.

114. Diaz ML, Watkins BA, Li Y, Anderson RA, Campbell WW. Chromium picolinate and conjugated linoleic acid do not synergistically influence diet- and exercise-induced changes in body composition and health indexes in overweight women. *J Nutr Biochem* **19**: 61–68. 2008.

115. Pittler MH, Stevinson C, Ernst E. Chromium picolinate for reducing body weight: Meta-analysis of randomized trials. *Int J Obes Relat Metab Disord* **27**: 522–529. 2003.

116. Lukaski HC. Chromium as a supplement. *Ann Rev Nutr* **19**: 279–302. 1999.

117. NTP. NTP Technical Report on the Toxicology and Carcinogenesis Studies of Chromium Picolinate Monohydrate (Cas No. 27882-76-4) in F344/n Rats and B6C3F1 Mice (Feed Studies). 2010. Research Triangle Park, NC, National Toxicology Program, USDHHS, PHS, NIH.

118. Stout MD, Nyska A, Collins BJ, Witt KL, Kissling GE, Malarkey DE, Hooth MJ. Chronic toxicity and carcinogenicity studies of chromium picolinate monohydrate administered in feed to F344/N rats and B6C3F1 mice for 2 years. *Food Chem Toxicol* **47**: 729–733. 2009.

119. Sullivan AC, Triscari J, Spiegel JE. Metabolic regulation as a control for lipid disorders. II. Influence of (−)-hydroxycitrate on genetically and experimentally induced hypertriglyceridemia in the rat. *Am J Clin Nutr* **30**: 777–784. 1977.

120. Leonhardt M, Hrupka B, Langhans W. Effect of hydroxycitrate on food intake and body weight regain after a period of restrictive feeding in male rats. *Physiol Behav* **74**: 191–196. 2001.

121. Onakpoya I, Hung SK, Perry R, Wider B, Ernst E. The use of garcinia extract (Hydroxycitric acid) as a weight loss supplement: A systematic review and meta-analysis of randomised clinical trials. *J Obes* 2012 (In Press, Epub. ID 509038, pp. 1–9).

122. Morimoto C, Satoh Y, Hara M, Inoue S, Tsujita T, Okuda H. Anti-obese action of raspberry ketone. *Life Sci* **77**: 194–204. 2005.

123. Mertens-Talcott SU, Rios J, Jilma-Stohlawetz P, Pacheco-Palencia LA, Meibohm B, Talcott ST, Derendorf H. Pharmacokinetics of anthocyanins and antioxidant effects after the consumption of anthocyanin-rich acai juice and pulp (*Euterpe oleracea Mart.*) in human healthy volunteers. *J Agric Food Chem* **56**: 7796–7802. 2008.

124. Schauss AG, Wu X, Prior RL, Ou B, Patel D, Huang D, Kababick JP. Phytochemical and nutrient composition of the freeze-dried amazonian palm berry, *Euterpe oleraceae mart.* (acai). *J Agric Food Chem* **54**: 8598–8603. 2006.

125. Jensen GS, Wu X, Patterson KM, Barnes J, Carter SG, Scherwitz L, Beaman R, Endres JR, Schauss AG. In vitro and in vivo antioxidant and anti-inflammatory capacities of an antioxidant-rich fruit and berry juice blend. Results of a pilot and randomized, double-blinded, placebo-controlled, crossover study. *J Agric Food Chem* **56**: 8326–8333. 2008.

126. de Souza MO, Silva M, Silva ME, Oliveira RP, Pedrosa ML. Diet supplementation with acai (*Euterpe oleracea Mart*) pulp improves biomarkers of oxidative stress and the serum lipid profile in rats. *Nutr* **26**: 804–810. 2010.

127. Shang YF, Kim SM, Lee WJ, Um BH. Pressurized liquid method for fucoxanthin extraction from Eisenia bicyclis (Kjellman) Setchell. *J Biosci Bioeng* **111**: 237–241. 2011.

128. Jeon SM, Kim HJ, Woo MN, Lee MK, Shin YC, Park YB, Choi MS. Fucoxanthin-rich seaweed extract suppresses body weight gain and improves lipid metabolism in high-fat-fed C57BL/6J mice. *Biotechnol J* **5**: 961–969. 2010.

129. Woo MN, Jeon SM, Kim HJ, Lee MK, Shin SK, Shin YC, Park YB, Choi MS. Fucoxanthin supplementation improves plasma and hepatic lipid metabolism and blood glucose concentration in high-fat fed C57BL/6N mice. *Chem Biol Interact* **186**: 316–322. 2010.

130. Lanni A, Moreno M, Lombardi A, de LP, Silvestri E, Ragni M, Farina P, Baccari GC, Fallahi P, Antonelli A, Goglia F. 3,5-Diiodo-L-thyronine powerfully reduces adiposity in rats by increasing the burning of fats. *FASEB J* **19**: 1552–1554. 2005.

131. Grasselli E, Voci A, Canesi L, Goglia F, Ravera S, Panfoli I, Gallo G, Vergani L. Non-receptor mediated actions are responsible for the lipid-lowering effects of iodothyronines in FaO rat hepatoma cells. *J Endocrinol* **210**: 59–69. 2011.

132. Grasselli E, Voci A, Canesi L, De MR, Goglia F, Cioffi F, Fugassa E, Gallo G, Vergani L. Direct effects of iodothyronines on excess fat storage in rat hepatocytes. *J Hepatol* **54**: 1230–1236. 2011.

133. Brobst DE, Ding X, Creech KL, Goodwin B, Kelley B, Staudinger JL. Guggulsterone activates multiple nuclear receptors and induces CYP3A gene expression through the pregnane X receptor. *J Pharmacol Exp Ther* **310**: 528–535. 2004.

134. Said O, Saad B, Fulder S, Khalil K, Kassis E. Weight Loss in Animals and Humans Treated with 'Weighlevel', a Combination of Four Medicinal Plants Used In Traditional Arabic and Islamic Medicine. *Evid Based Complement Alternat Med* published online June 16, 2011, Article ID 874538, doi:10.1093/ecam/nen067.

53 Calcium and Obesity
A Microcosm of the Nutrient Problem

Robert P. Heaney, MD

CONTENTS

INTRODUCTION

A connection between calcium intake and body weight was first made by McCarron, from the NHANES-I data, and published in 1984 [1]. This observation was widely ignored, probably for three reasons: (1) it did not make sense in terms of what was generally understood with regard to how calcium functioned in the body; (2) there was sufficient nutritional charlatanry prevalent in modern times to make it easy to place this effect in precisely such a category; and (3) understanding of nutritional biology was not sufficiently nuanced to allow integration of the nontraditional effects, not just of calcium, but of most other nutrients as well.

Nevertheless, the issue kept reasserting itself. In 1998, Summerbell et al. showed that an all-milk diet produced better weight loss in a weight-reducing context than alternative dietary regimens [2], and in 2000, Zemel et al. showed not only that dairy products augmented weight loss in a randomized controlled design, but that one of the consequences of low calcium intake, that is, high parathyroid hormone production, produced effects on adipocytes which changed their metabolism in such a way as to lead to increased fat storage and decreased fat release [3]. The latter finding, while intriguing in its own right, failed to address the question of energy imbalance, which had to occur for either weight gain or weight loss to develop. Further, attempts to reproduce Zemel's clinical observations were generally less successful [4,5] than he had originally reported.

As a result, the skepticism that followed McCarron's original observation once again dominated the scientific landscape. Nevertheless, in the past 10 years, well over 100 clinical studies have been published, evaluating the association between calcium intake, body composition, weight loss, and related variables. Two years ago, Heaney and Rafferty [6] reviewed this body of evidence and suggested a framework within which the evidence should be interpreted. In brief, they found that the preponderance of the evidence, both from observational studies and from randomized clinical trials and controlled metabolic experiments, indicated that there was a beneficial effect of high calcium intake on body composition, body weight, and weight loss. In this chapter, I bring that prior review up to date, quantify the effect, and review the evidence with respect to mechanisms by which calcium may be operative. But, in order to interpret this now large body of evidence, it is necessary, first, to review certain of the advances in nutritional biology which provide the theoretical framework in which nontraditional effects of nutrients can best be situated and understood.

ADVANCES IN NUTRITIONAL BIOLOGY

PANSYSTEMIC EFFECTS OF NUTRIENT

Following the discovery of the association of beriberi with thiamine deficiency slightly more than a century ago, clinical nutrition adopted a paradigm in which each nutrient had a specific effect and prevented a specific disease. Thus, very low intakes of thiamine produced beriberi; of ascorbic acid, scurvy; of vitamin D, rickets; etc. This paradigm has long dominated the determination of nutrient intake recommendations (which, in simplest terms, boiled down to the lowest intake of a given nutrient that prevents the univocally associated disease). Its continuing hold on the thinking of the nutrition community is dramatically exemplified in the curious designation "insufficiency" for vitamin D status when serum 25(OH)D values fall between 10 and 30 ng/mL. (Values below 10 were designated "deficient" and values above 30 are commonly considered "normal" or "adequate.") Individuals in the "insufficiency" range have been shown to have preventable fractures, preventable falls, a greater incidence of high blood pressure, and many other adverse health outcomes, all of which could be reduced by vitamin D supplementation that moved their 25(OH)D values up into the "normal" range. In any other situation, disease preventable by physiological intakes of a given nutrient would be considered "deficiency," but that could not have been the case with vitamin D, because the patients did not have rickets or osteomalacia. Thus, they could not be "deficient."

It is necessary to abandon this century-old paradigm and to recognize that nutrients do not act in single systems, need not act through single mechanisms, and need not produce a single disease when their intake is inadequate [7]. For all practical purposes, most tissues need most nutrients, and to that extent, their functioning will be impaired if the intake of a given nutrient is suboptimal. Seen from this perspective, McCarron's observation of an inverse association between calcium intake and body weight—while needing confirmation of course—no longer seems outlandish.

SUBTLETY OF NUTRIENT EFFECTS

Simple life forms are able to make most of the biochemicals they need from simple precursors plus a source of energy and minerals, but complex higher organisms, such as humans, have come to depend upon the environment to provide a wide variety of the chemical agents needed for cell function, which simpler organisms make for themselves. There are now more than 50 nutrients essential for humans, and the inevitable consequence of this multiplicity is that, if each contributes to tissue function, then the discernible effect of only one of them will usually be relatively small. If we take a given instance of tissue functioning, such as phagocytic response to a foreign particle, or tissue response to an inflammatory signal, or any number of other end points, and if we mount a series of experiments quantifying that response, there will inevitably be a certain amount of variation distributed around a central or typical value for the response concerned. If we then manipulate the concentration (or intake) of nutrient X, there will be some shift in that distribution of responses. In short, nutrient X explains some fraction of the variance in tissue, organ, or organism response. The relatively dramatic changes produced in the early days of nutrition by thiamine in beriberi, vitamin D in rickets, and vitamin C in scurvy have, in a sense, misled us. Rather than being typical, such responses need to be seen as exceptions to the rule which is simply stated: nutrient effects are generally small and subtle. And if this general rule applies to the issue of calcium intake and body weight, then one should expect the calcium effects to be, likewise, small and subtle. That does not mean that they are unimportant, as the next section attempts to make clear.

INDIVIDUALS VS. POPULATIONS

When one evaluates any given variable (such as bone mineral density, body weight, or systolic blood pressure) across a population, one finds a distribution of values, which often follows the normal or Gaussian curve. The concern of public health with such distributions is generally focused on the tails, the high end for blood pressure and body weight, the low end for bone mineral density, and so forth. By contrast, the concern of health practitioners is focused on the individual members of that cohort. This distinction is crucial, but is often lost sight of.

In the 20 years from 1988 to 2008, age-adjusted obesity prevalence in the United States rose from 22.9% to 33.8%, an increase of nearly 50%. What that increase means is simply that the number of individuals in a population who exceed a certain value (i.e., a BMI of 30 kg/m²) has increased by about 50%. It does not mean that everyone has had a 50% increase in weight. The actual mean change in weight across the population as a whole has been much smaller. For example, over the same time period, mean weight of midlife women increased from 74.3 to 78.0 kg, an increase of only 5%.

The same is true, for other such variables, for example, blood pressure. Figure 53.1A shows a distribution of systolic blood pressure values in a cohort of women at midlife, locating the cutoff between normal and high blood pressure at 140 mmHg. About 8% of this cohort exceeds that value and would, therefore, be labeled hypertensive. In Panel B of Figure 53.1, the entire distribution has been shifted downward by 5 mmHg. Notice that the fraction above 140 mmHg has dropped to just under 4%, or a 50% reduction in prevalence of hypertension, for a mere 4% drop in average blood pressure.

In both examples, there is a striking contrast between the responses of individuals and of populations. For a person weighing 300 lb, a weight reduction of 3–4 kg would seem to be trivial,

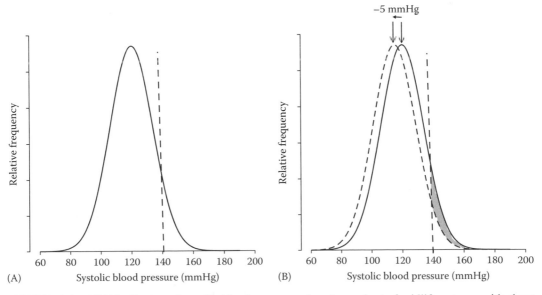

FIGURE 53.1   (A) Distribution of systolic blood pressure values in a cohort of midlife women, with about 8% of them exhibiting values above 140 mmHg, that is, hypertensive. (B) The same distribution as in (A), but shifted down by 5 mmHg. Note that the percentage above 140 mmHg has shifted downward from 8% to 4%, a 50% drop. (Copyright Robert P. Heaney, 2010. Used with permission.)

just as would a reduction of 4 mmHg in systolic blood pressure in an individual with a value of 180. But at a population level, the impact on disease prevalence of such seemingly small changes can be profound.

NUTRIENTS ARE NOT DRUGS

Although nutrients are sometimes touted for their ostensible curative powers, they are much more accurately conceptualized as preventive maintenance measures, needed for the body to deal with the myriad assaults and injuries to which it is subject every day [7]. If I fail to maintain a good diet, the immediately perceptible effects are usually negligible, just as my automobile continues to run perfectly well if I fail to change the oil—for a while. But the end result is premature breakdown—of my body and my machines.

Nevertheless, when health-related claims for nutrients are evaluated, nutritional policymakers seem to slip almost automatically into the drug evaluation mode. We somehow expect to see large effects and, when they are not found, as is often the case, the hypothesis seems unsupported. Or when in meta-analyses, an effect is found, but it is considered too small to be of much interest, once again, the health claim seems to be unsupported. My thesis is that large effects are atypical and should not be expected, and, when evaluating claims, the focus must be at a population, not an individual, level. There with populations, as I have just shown, small individual effects have large population significance.

There are many additional problems [7,8] with using the drug evaluation model for testing nutrient-health hypotheses, not least of which is the fact that there is no true analog of the placebo control in a nutrient study, that is, one cannot feasibly or ethically place a control group on an intake low enough to permit estimating the effect of an adequate intake (whatever its value may be). In observational studies, it is common to find segments of the population with intakes of a given nutrient that are truly low (though not, of course, zero). And, if one could mount a trial confining the study to individuals with such low intakes (leaving half of them at their prevailing intake and augmenting the intakes of the other half), sufficient contrast could be created to allow an adequate test of the relevant health claim. But it is nearly impossible to do that, as a healthy volunteer effect enters into the context, and ethical considerations almost always preclude such an approach even if technically feasible.

Classical examples of each difficulty are found in two U.S. government-sponsored studies, the Women's Health Initiative (WHI) [9] and the Calcium Preeclampsia Prevention Trial (CPEP) [10]. In the first, it was anticipated from NHANES data that women in the target age range would have a median calcium intake under 600 mg/day, substantially below current intake recommendations. Randomly assigning half of them to a calcium supplement regimen would, thereby, produce the contrast needed to determine if additional calcium made a difference. As it turned out, when enrollment was completed, median calcium intake was approximately 1100 mg/day, a value actually above the recommended intake, suggesting selective recruitment of health-conscious women, and destroying the intended contrast. Similarly, in CPEP, it would have been untenable for a government-sponsored study to place pregnant women on a calcium intake below that recommended, even though such a diet would have been comparable to what many of them might spontaneously have chosen for themselves. Hence, the control group was given sufficient supplementation to bring their calcium intake above the minimum recommended for pregnancy. Thus, in both studies (though for different reasons), there was no low-calcium-intake group, and therefore, it was not possible to test the cognate hypothesis.

It is sometimes argued that one can, of course, test the hypothesis that "more is better," which is correct, but that does not address the actual underlying question.

What, in the final analysis, is that research question? Is it that calcium reduces age-related bone loss and fractures or that calcium reduces the incidence of preeclampsia? No. That, once again, is thinking of a nutrient—calcium—as a drug. The actual hypothesis is that low calcium intake *causes* (or predisposes to) preeclampsia in pregnant women or that low calcium intake causes (or augments) age-related bone loss and fracture risk in older women. At a deeper level, the question is not even: Does a low intake cause harm? That question has been answered. All nutrients, as noted earlier, are essential. Without one or more of them, health is impaired. Rather it is, how low an intake? and what harm? Note that always it is *harm* that is the outcome measure, and in contrast with drugs, where reversal of harm is the expected outcome, it is never ethically permissible to use an investigational design (i.e., the randomized clinical trial) in which the control group is expected to be harmed.

PREPONDERANCE OF THE EVIDENCE

When Heaney and Rafferty [6] reviewed the issue of calcium and weight through 2007, they noted that most of the published reports were not sufficiently powered to find the small effects on energy balance that would underlie the kinds of changes in weight or body composition at issue. They identified 31 randomized controlled trials or controlled metabolic experiments and 61 observational studies, and noted that, for both categories, the preponderance of the evidence clearly favored a beneficial effect of calcium intake on such variables as percent body fat, age-related bone gain, rate of rebound after weight loss, potentiation of weight loss regimens, and similar outcomes. Since that earlier review, at least 19 further studies have been published [11–29], for a total of 42 RCTs and 70 observational studies. With this expanded study set, as had been noted earlier by Heaney and Rafferty [6], the preponderance of the evidence clearly points to a beneficial effect of high-calcium diets. Figure 53.2 shows the distribution of the RCTs and metabolic studies, and Figure 53.3, the distribution of the observational studies. This analysis uses the convention adopted by Heaney and Rafferty, characterizing each individual study as significantly negative (SN), negative but not statistically significant (N), no difference (Z), positive but not statistically significantly so (P), and finally significantly positive (SP). ("Negative" in this sense indicates that the study showed that calcium *increased* the weight-related outcome variable rather than decreased it, whereas "positive" designates studies that found a beneficial effect of calcium on the weight-related outcome variable.) Superimposed on the respective distributions in Figures 53.2 and 53.3 is the expected distribution for a null-effect interventional relationship. As noted by Heaney and Rafferty, a truly null intervention would be expected to produce as many negative studies as positive, barring publication bias. As is visually evident, the actual distributions for the 112 calcium studies included in the analysis

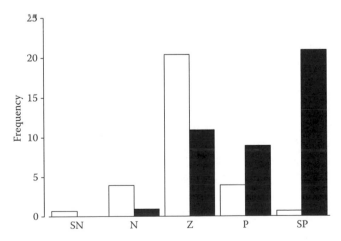

FIGURE 53.2 Distribution of randomized controlled trials and metabolic experiments (solid bars) testing the relationship of calcium intake to various body fat measures. The horizontal axis categories are "SN," significantly negative; "N," negative but not statistically significant; "Z," no difference; "P," positive but not statistically significant; and "SP," significantly positive. The open bars are the expected distribution of studies under the null hypothesis. (Copyright Robert P. Heaney, 2010. Used with permission.)

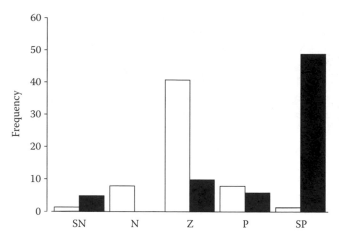

FIGURE 53.3 Distribution of observational studies (solid bars) testing the relationship of calcium intake to various body fat measures. See legend for Figure 53.2 for other details. (Copyright Robert P. Heaney, 2010. Used with permission.)

differ markedly from what would have been expected under the null hypothesis. Hence, it can be reasonably concluded that high calcium intakes do, overall, have a beneficial effect on various body compositional and weight-related outcome variables.

MAGNITUDE OF THE EFFECT

Randomized controlled trials are most useful in confirming a causal connection, in this case between calcium intake and weight control, and seldom permit quantification of the effect that they may confirm. That is partly because they rarely test a range of intakes and partly because the size of the effect is heavily dependent upon the control group intake. As noted earlier for bone mass and preeclampsia, if the control group intake is high, the effect size will necessarily appear to be small and will often be statistically nonsignificant. Hence, for estimates of the magnitude of the effect, we necessarily turn to observational studies which can, and frequently do, encompass a broad range of intakes.

This was precisely the case in the longitudinal cohort analyzed by Davies et al. [30]. Two hundred sixteen women at midlife, followed for periods of up to more than 20 years, had an observed mean rate of weight gain of just under 0.5 kg/year. However, those with the lowest calcium intake gained the most ($P < 0.01$), and analysis of the regression of weight change on calcium intake showed that the average weight gain was zero at a calcium intake of approximately 1500 mg/day. This value was roughly double the mean calcium intake for the group and was associated with an effective blocking of the mean weight change for the group (i.e., ~0.5 kg/year). It is worth noting, moreover, that the zero gain calcium intake is exactly what had been recommended for bone health in postmenopausal women by two NIH Consensus Development Conferences [31,32]. This strongly suggests that optimal weight control, as related to calcium intake, is achievable at the same calcium intake that is judged to ensure optimal bone status.

MECHANISMS OF THE EFFECT

It is hardly necessary to stress in this volume that weight maintenance (i.e., the prevention of unwanted weight gain) requires a balance between energy in and energy out. Similarly, weight loss (i.e., from the status of weight excess) requires an energy imbalance, with calories in being less than calories out. Thus, the effect of a high calcium intake must be sought either in a reduction of energy input or an increase in energy output. As noted earlier, the effect is likely to be subtle and hence hard

TABLE 53.1
Mechanisms of a Calcium Effect

Mechanism		Status of Evidence
Input	Satiety/adherence	+
	Absorption	++++
Output	Metabolic rate	+
	Physical activity	NA

to find. An imbalance of as little as 50–70 kcal/day (equivalent to about one-half serving of a sugar-sweetened soft drink) is sufficient to account for weight gain or loss on the order of 2.7 kg (6 lb)/year, and the weight gain in the cohort analyzed by Davies et al. [30], that is, 0.5 kg/year (i.e., only 1.4 g/day), requires an energy imbalance which, if mainly fat, would be less than 15 kcal/day.

Table 53.1 lists the logical possibilities and indicates the status of the evidence with regard to the role of calcium in each. On the input side, the only alternatives are eating less or absorbing less. The principal mechanism whereby a nutrient may lead to less consumption is satiety. Satiety is a plausible mechanism in this context, particularly for food sources of calcium, since proteins are known to be more satiating than, for example, most carbohydrates, and the principal food source of calcium in modern diets will be dairy products, which are typically high-protein foods. A satiating effect of dairy is suggested also by the weight loss experiment of Summerbell et al. [2] in which an all-milk, weight reduction regimen produced substantially greater weight loss than did a standard energy-deficit weight reduction regimen. However, there is little to no actual evidence with respect to satiety itself, either from dairy or from calcium *per se*, and it is unlikely that such evidence will be forthcoming, pro or con. This is simply because our means of assessing satiety are not sufficiently sensitive to detect a 1%–3% reduction in energy intake, which is all that is required to explain commonly experienced weight gain or loss.

Decreased energy absorption, on the other hand, is easier to measure. Denke, for example, showed that high-calcium diets increased fecal fat content [33], a finding that was subsequently confirmed by Astrup and his colleagues [34,35], who showed that fecal fat content was doubled in individuals receiving calcium supplements. The increase in fecal fat was equivalent to ~50 kcal and is, thus, by itself, of the approximate magnitude needed to explain commonly observed rates of weight gain and loss. Incidentally, it should be clear that a 100% increase in fecal fat is much easier to detect in small sample sizes than is a 1%–3% reduction in energy intake.

On the output side, the only alternative mechanisms are decreased metabolic efficiency (i.e., burning more calories for the same amount of physical work) or increased physical activity, with its concomitant energy cost. There is some hint that there might be an increase in respiratory quotient associated with a high calcium intake [36], and, in inbred mice, it has been shown that high calcium intakes increase the activity of the uncoupling enzyme [37], increasing fuel consumption for heat rather than work. However, the human respiratory quotient experiments have not been confirmed in subsequent work [38,39], and as for satiety, mentioned earlier, the methods for measuring the efficiency of energy utilization are not sufficiently sensitive to detect the 1%–3% change in energy balance that is involved. The same must be said for the issue of increased physical activity, for which there is no hint of a calcium effect.

SPECIAL CONSIDERATIONS: DAIRY

Calcium is an alkaline earth element, but does not enter the body as such. Rather, it does so as a divalent cation associated with a wide array of anions, such as phosphate, bicarbonate, as well as a number of protein complexes. And these salts and complexes are, in turn, embedded in foods that themselves contain multiple nutrients which may be expected to influence calcium's effect on many of its measurable end points. In brief, as nutritionists have long recognized, humans do not eat nutrients; we eat foods, and a one-nutrient-at-a-time, reductionist approach can sometimes obscure as much as it reveals.

For calcium, the principal modern dietary source is dairy, which accounts for 65%–75% of total calcium intake in the North American diet. Dairy, manifestly, is a rich source of many essential nutrients and is the principal dietary source not only of calcium but of branched-chain amino acids which are necessary not just for nitrogen balance but for muscle metabolism and the protection of lean body mass [40]. Most of the observational studies of calcium intake contrasted not so much low and high calcium intakes, but low and high *dairy* intakes, and it is thus difficult to disentangle the effect of calcium from the effects of other dairy nutrients and, perhaps of more salience, the effects of calcium consumed as a component of a dairy matrix. Both Dawson-Hughes and Harris [41] and Heaney [42] have shown that calcium's effects on bone are substantially augmented on high-protein diets, which, of course, is what a high-dairy diet often is. This same sort of interaction for calcium and weight has been reported by Zemel et al. [3], who found not only better fat loss on a high-dairy, energy-deficit reducing diet, but also better preservation of lean body mass.

In any case, it seems clear that weight loss diets need to be protein rich in order to protect lean mass, and when that protein source is dairy, the regimen adds the calcium effect as well. So, how much of the effect in such circumstances is due to the energy deficit, or to the high protein intake, or to calcium, will likely remain uncertain beyond the fact that they each contribute to the effect and that the total effect is very likely more than the sum of its parts.

SUMMARY

The preponderance of the evidence clearly indicates that, other things being equal, high calcium intakes help to sustain lean body mass, reduce adipose tissue gain, reduce weight regain after weight reduction, and augment weight loss on energy-restricted diets. However, when computed on a daily basis, the effect is relatively small, as is typical of most nutrient effects. In the aggregate, the effect amounts to a favorable energy balance shift on the order of 50–150 kcal/day. This effect, though seemingly small, is nevertheless often enough to eliminate midlife gain in weight.

Because of the smallness of the measurable effect size, studies of the mechanisms of calcium's effects have for the most part produced ambiguous results. The sole exception is the well-attested binding of ingested fat in the gut by calcium, thereby reducing effective energy intake, without affecting satiety.

Calcium's role in obesity is an illustration of the principle that all body systems need all nutrients. However, high calcium intake, alone, will not be sufficient to produce the needed weight loss in already obese individuals. Nevertheless, a high calcium intake, preferably in the form of dairy foods, will augment the effect of the energy deficit of weight loss regimens and at the same time help to preserve lean body mass. In that sense alone, calcium plays a key role in weight loss.

REFERENCES

1. McCarron, D. A., Morris, C. D., Henry, H. J., and Stanton, J. L. 1984. Blood pressure and nutrient intake in the United States. *Science* 224:1392–1398.
2. Summerbell, C. D., Watts, C., Higgins, J. P. T., and Garrow, J. S. 1998. Randomised controlled trial of novel, simple, and well supervised weight reducing diets in outpatients. *Br Med J* 317:1487–1489.
3. Zemel, M. B., Shi, H., Greer, B., DiRienzo, D., and Zemel, P. C. 2000. Regulation of adiposity by dietary calcium. *FASEB J* 14:1132–1138.
4. Barr, S. I. 2003. Increased dairy product or calcium intake: Is body weight or composition affected in humans? *J Nutr* 133:245S–248S.
5. Gunther, C. W., Legowski, P. A., Lyle, R. M. et al. 2005. Dairy products do not lead to alterations in body weight or fat mass in young women in a 1-y intervention. *Am J Clin Nutr* 81:751–756.

6. Heaney, R. P. and Rafferty, K. 2008. Preponderance of the evidence: An example from the issue of calcium intake and body composition. *Nutr Rev* 67:32–39.

7. Heaney, R. P. 2008. 2008 W.O. Atwater Memorial Lecture: Nutrients, endpoints, and the problem of proof. *J Nutr* 138:1591–1595.

8. Blumberg, J., Heaney, R. P., Huncharek, M. et al. 2010. Evidence-based criteria in the nutritional context. [Appendix: Amplification on certain of the points discussed in the paper (online only).] *Nutr Rev* 68:478–484.

9. Jackson, R. D., LaCroix, A. Z., Gass, M. et al. 2006. Calcium plus vitamin D supplementation and the risk of fractures. *N Engl J Med* 354:669–683.

10. Levine, R. J., Hauth, J. C., Curet, L. B. et al. 1997. Trial of calcium to prevent preeclampsia. *N Engl J Med* 337:69–76.

11. Torres, M. R. S. G., da Silva, T., Carvalho, D. C., and Sanjuliani, A. F. 2011. Dietary calcium intake and its relationship with adiposity and metabolic profile in hypertensive patients. *Nutrition* 27:666–671.

12. Kelishadi, R., Zemel, M. B., Hashemipour, M., Hosseini, M., Mohammadifard, N., and Poursafa, P. 2009. Can a dairy-rich diet be effective in long-term weight control of young children? *J Am Coll Nutr* 28:601–610.

13. O'Neil, C. E., Nicklas, T. A., Liu, Y., and Franklin, F. A. 2009. The impact of dairy product consumption on nutrient adequacy and weight of Head Start mothers. *Pub Health Nutr* 12:1693–1701.

14. Wyatt, H. R., Jortberg, B. T., Babbel, C. et al. 2008. Weight loss in a community initiative that promotes decreased energy intake and increased physical activity and dairy consumption: Calcium weighs-in. *J Phys Act Health* 5:28–44.

15. Foo, L. H., Zhang, Q., Zhu, K., Ma, G., Greenfield, H., and Fraser, D. R. 2007. Influence of body composition, muscle strength, diet and physical activity on total body and forearm bone mass in Chinese adolescent girls. *Br J Nutr* 98:1281–1287.

16. Saelens, B. E., Couch, S. C., Wosje, K. S., Stark, L. J., and Daniels, S. R. 2006. Relations among milk and non-milk beverage consumption, calcium, and relative weight in high-weight status children. *J Clin Psychol Med Settings* 13:121–129.

17. Moore, L. L., Bradlee, M. L., Gao, D., and Singer, M. R. 2006. Low dairy intake in early childhood predicts excess body fat gain. *Obesity* 14:1010–1018.

18. Berkey, C. S., Rockett, H. R. H., Willett, W. C., and Colditz, G. A. 2005. Milk, dairy fat, dietary calcium, and weight gain. *Arch Pediatr Adolesc Med* 159:543–550.

19. Zhou, J., Zhao, L.-J., Watson, P., Zhang, Q., and Lappe, J. M. 2010. The effect of calcium and vitamin D supplementation on obesity in postmenopausal women: Secondary analysis for a large-scale, placebo controlled, double-blind, 4-year longitudinal clinical trial. *Nutr Metab* 7:62–70.

20. Angeles-Agdeppa, I., Capanzana, M. V., Li-Yu, J., Schollum, L. M., and Kruger, M. C. 2010. High-calcium milk prevents overweight and obesity among postmenopausal women. *Food Nutr Bull* 31:381–390.

21. Shahar, D. R., Schwarzfuchs, D., Fraser, R. et al. 2010. Dairy calcium intake, serum vitamin D, and successful weight loss. *Am J Clin Nutr* 92:1017–1022.

22. Phillips, S. M., Bandini, L. G., Cyr, H., Colclough-Douglas, S., Naumova, E., and Must, A. 2003. Dairy food consumption and body weight and fatness studied longitudinally over the adolescent period. *Int J Obes Relat Metab Disord* 27:1106–1113.

23. Reidt, C. S., Schlussel, Y., von Thun, N., Ambia-Sobhan, H., Stahl, T., Field, M. P. et al. 2007. Premenopausal overweight women do not lose bone during moderate weight loss with adequate or higher calcium intake. *Am J Clin Nutr* 85:972–980.

24. Reidt, C. S., Cifuentes, M., Stahl, T., Chowdhury, H. A., Schlussel, Y., and Shapses, S. A. 2005. Overweight postmenopausal women lose bone with moderate weight reduction and 1 g/day calcium intake. *J Bone Miner Res* 20:455–463.

25. Ricci, T. A., Chowdhury, H. A., Heymsfield, S. B., Stahl, T., Pierson, J. N. Jr., and Shapses, S. A. 1998. Calcium supplementation suppresses bone turnover during weight reduction in postmenopausal women. *J Bone Miner Res* 13:1045–1050.

26. Shalileh, M., Shidfar, F., Haghani, H., Eghtesadi, S., and Heydan, I. 2010. The influence of calcium supplement on body composition, weight loss and insulin resistance in obese adults receiving low calorie diet. *JRMS* 15:191–201.

27. Shapses, S. A., Heshka, S., and Heymsfield, S. B. 2004. Effect of calcium supplementation on weight and fat loss in women. *J Clin Endocrinol Metab* 89:632–637.

28. Shapses, S. A., von Thun, Z. L., Heymsfield, S. B., Ricci, T. A., Ospina, M., Pierson, F. N. Jr. et al. 2001. Bone turnover and density in obese premenopausal women during moderate weight loss and calcium supplementation. *J Bone Miner Res* 16:1329–1336.

29. Yanovski, J. A., Parikh, S. J., Yanoff, L. B., Denkinger, B. I., Calis, K. A., Reynolds, J. C. et al. 2009. Effects of calcium supplementation on body weight and adiposity in overweight and obese adults. *Ann Intern Med* 150:821–829.

30. Davies, K. M., Heaney, R. P., Recker, R. R. et al. 2000. Calcium intake and body weight. *J Clin Endocrinol Metab* 85:4635–4638.

31. NIH Consensus Development Conference Statement 1984. Osteoporosis. *JAMA* 252:799–802.

32. NIH Consensus Development Panel 1994. Optimal calcium intake. *JAMA* 272:1942–1948.

33. Denke, M. A., Fox, M. M., and Schulte, M. C. 2003. Short-term dietary calcium fortification increases fecal saturated fat content and reduces serum lipids in men. *J Nutr* 123:1047–1053.

34. Bendsen, N. T., Hother, A.-L., Jensen, S. K., Lorenzen, K. J., and Astrup, A. 2008. Effect of dairy calcium on fecal fat excretion: A randomized crossover trial. *Int J Obesity* 32:1816–1824.

35. Christensen, R., Lorenzen, J. K., Svith, C. R. et al. 2009. Effect of calcium from dairy and dietary supplements on faecal fat excretion: A meta-analysis of randomized controlled trials. *Obes Rev* 10:475–486.

36. Melanson, E. L., Sharp, T. A., Schneider, J., Donahoo, W. T., Grunwald, G. K., and Hill, J. O. 2003. Relation between calcium intake and fat oxidation in adult humans. *Int J Obesity* 27:196–203.

37. Shi, H., Norman, A. W., Okamura, W. H., Sen, A., and Zemel, M. B. 2002. 1α,25-dihydroxyvitamin D3 inhibits uncoupling protein 2 expression in human adipocytes. *FASEB J* 16:1808–1810.

38. Melanson, E. L., Donahoo, W. T., Dong, F., Ida, T., and Zemel, M. B. 2005. Effect of low- and high-calcium dairy-based diets on macronutrient oxidation in humans. *Obesity Res* 13:2102–2112.

39. Jacobsen, R., Lorenzen, J. K., Toubro, S., Krog-Mikkelsen, I., and Astrup, A. 2005. Effect of short-term high dietary calcium intake on 24-h energy expenditure, fat oxidation, and fecal fat excretion. *Int J Obesity* 29:292–301.

40. Layman, D. K. 2003. The role of leucine in weight loss diets and glucose homeostasis. *J Nutr* 133:261S–267S.

41. Dawson-Hughes, B. and Harris, S. S. 2002. Calcium intake influences the association of protein intake with rates of bone loss in elderly men and women. *Am J Clin Nutr* 75:773–779.

42. Heaney, R. P. 2007. Effects of protein on the calcium economy. In *Nutritional Aspects of Osteoporosis 2006*, eds. P. Burckhardt, R. P. Heaney, and B. Dawson-Hughes, pp. 191–197. Amsterdam, the Netherlands: Elsevier Inc.

54 Dietary Supplementation in Weight Loss

A Dietitian's Perspective

Betty Wedman-St. Louis, PhD, RD, LD

CONTENTS

The Centers for Disease Control and Prevention in 2009 estimated that 68% of American adults were overweight, and 38% of them could be classified as obese. Thirty-three states were indentified where more than 25% of the population is obese. A report from the George Washington University School of Public Health and the Health Services' Department of Health Policy calculated the individual cost of being obese as $4879 for women and $2646 for men. These calculations put a price tag on the obesity epidemic that includes lost productivity and obesity-related medical expenditures, in addition to other indirect and direct costs [1].

As health-care costs continue to escalate from an estimated $147 billion annually, we cannot continue to focus on a health-care system that treats individuals after they get diagnosed with a disease. Instead, the focus needs to be on a wellness system that can reduce absenteeism, workmen's compensation, and medical expenses. Treating overweight and obesity with diet, dietary supplements, and lifestyle modification can provide a positive return on investment.

FOOD AND DIETARY SUPPLEMENTS

During the past 35 years in dietetics practice, many diets and weight-loss schemes have come and gone. The cornerstone of any successful weight-loss program is reduced food intake. A reduction in food intake due to inactive lifestyle and greater abundances of food choices makes dietary supplements an important adjunct in a world full of less than perfect food choices.

Food is not the sole source of nutrients that the human body can use to meet its dietary requirements, as schools of dietetics have taught for the past 50 years. Science has provided structure and function data on vitamins, minerals, and numerous phytonutrients so they can be produced to supplement diets when individuals cannot eat or do not choose food wisely. As a dietitian with over 40 years of experience, I have yet to plan a perfect diet for a person that meets all the daily nutrient requirements modified for that individual's health needs and food preferences. Randolph [2] stated it best when he described the difference between analytical vs. biological dietetics. Foods can be analyzed for nutrient content and organized into a meal plan, but that does not mean that the same food meets the biological needs of the person consuming it. Food storage, food preparation, drug–food interactions, and individual genetic differences mean the menu and food choices must be customized to the individual. Dietary supplements can be added to ensure adequacy until dietetics research can provide more definitive answers.

RDA AND WEIGHT LOSS

Dietetics has relied on the recommended dietary allowance (RDA) and government guidelines for assessing nutritional adequacy of diets. Using the RDA is not good science for an individual weight-loss regime. As Williams [3] pointed out, "Nutrition is for real people. Statistical humans are of little interest." The "average" person on which the RDA is based does not exist in weight-loss clinics.

Overweight does not mean well nourished. Optimum nutrition support needs to be provided to everyone planning a weight management regime, especially those undergoing bariatric surgery.

MAKING WISE FOOD CHOICES

Inadequate research has been done on whether most individuals can routinely select a healthy diet. Dietetics training emphasizes cultural and lifestyle practices as determinants of food selection. If wise food choices are learned from example at the family dinner table, then what happens when families do not sit down to dinner or lunch or breakfast? Eating habits learned as children affect eating patterns throughout life. As children have become less active, obesity has resulted from their selection of highly processed foods mass produced from white flour and sugar which, according to Haas [4], provide useless calories with few nutrients. Haas also believes that, "We require more food on this kind of diet to obtain all our needed nutrients." The selection of foods in the standard American diet (SAD) generates "a diet rich in refined sugars such as high-fructose corn syrup, saturated fat, and trans-fatty acids and low in fiber, legumes, nuts, fruits and vegetables, essential fatty acids, essential nutrients, and phytonutrients" [5]. Unfortunately, many individuals in weight-loss programs are unable to significantly or permanently change their eating habits or alter their dependence on convenience foods. The self-selection of foods was studied in the 1940s before the days of television and mass media advertising. At that time, most people ate because they were hungry; they selected what they liked and stopped eating when they were full [3]. That is not the case today for the thousands of weight-loss clients I have counseled.

Alcohol and sugar calories are a major factor in many obesity cases. Williams [3] reported several examples of rat studies and their desires for alcohol with and without diets supplemented with vitamins. Rats supplemented with vitamins did not consume alcohol like the depleted animals. In other experiments by Williams, rats on nutrient-depleted diets consumed more sugar than when their nutritional needs were better met. How much we can infer in human nutrition from these rat studies is subject to debate, but when trying to establish dietary supplement protocols for individuals, it is worth keeping the animal studies in mind.

BIOCHEMICAL INDIVIDUALITY

Williams [3] broadened the perspective of nutrition requirements with his simple thesis that all human beings are biochemically unique; therefore, we metabolize nutrients differently. Recent scientific advances in the study of individual genetic variations have confirmed Williams' hypothesis of many years ago. We now know that individual nutrient needs are a function of not only genetic differences but also differences in genetic expression, as influenced by many environmental and lifestyle factors. Such variations may also be contributors to weight management issues, as no two humans have the same genes—not even identical twins. Williams emphasized that chemical reactions in the body and in specific organ systems vary in efficiency from person to person, and these reactions are influenced by the nutritional status of every cell in the body [3]. A personalized diet and nutrition supplementation program is needed for each individual based on that person's genetics, environment, and lifestyle.

CREATING NUTRITION PLAN IN WEIGHT LOSS

Dietary assessment through a 24 h food recall or a food frequency questionnaire can provide insight into cultural, religious, and caloric practices. Estimating activity level and realistic weight-loss goals can be more challenging.

A body mass index (BMI) is the objective tool used by many clinicians to assess degree of overweight/obesity. Since being overweight is related to the development of chronic diseases like hypertension, osteoarthritis, sleep apnea, stroke, dyslipidemia, heart disease, and some cancers, an early intervention in weight management is encouraged.

BMI goal values increase with age. A 65 year old or older with a BMI = 27 is considered acceptable despite the values in this table.

BMI	Implications	Health Risk
<18.5	Underweight	May be nutrient deficient/insufficient
18.5–24.9	Normal weight	Minimum risk
25.0–29.9	Overweight	Moderate risk
30.0+	Obesity	High risk

A waist circumference or waist-to-hip ratio may also be used to help set realistic weight management goals. The waist circumference for women >35 in. or men >40 in. can be a risk guide for serious health problems. Waist-to-hip ratio is used to measure distribution of adipose tissue. A waist-to-hip ratio of 1.0 or greater in men or 0.8 or greater in women is a risk for obesity-related diseases.

Calorie and protein recommendations in a weight-loss program are determined by considering activity or illness as defined in this chart.

Activity or Illness	Calorie/kg/Day	Protein g/kg/Day
No apparent illness	30 cal/kg	1.0–1.2 g/kg
Chronic kidney disease	35 cal/kg	1.2 g/kg
Diabetes	30 cal/kg	0.8–1.0 g/kg
Geriatrics (>55 years old)	25 cal/kg	1.0–1.1 g/kg

Once the daily calorie determination is calculated, then the daily total needs to be reduced by 500 cal (1 lb per week weight loss) or 1000 cal (2 lb per week weight loss). If an individual calculates a need for 2000 cal per day and a 1 lb weight loss per week is the goal, then 1500 cal can be consumed daily (2000–500 cal). A 2 lb per week weight loss means that a daily total of 1000 cal in carefully selected foods needs to be maintained. At the 1000 cal level, dietary supplements are important to maintain adequate nutrition.

Fluid needs are also estimated since numerous myths abound regarding hydration status. Fluid needs for overweight/obese individuals are calculated at 30–35 cc/kg body weight. Excess fluids and overhydration are not recommended.

MEDICATIONS AND WEIGHT LOSS

Individuals usually eat when they are hungry and usually choose foods that taste good. But medications (prescription and over the counter) can override their metabolic utilization of food components. Diuretics, calcium channel blockers, beta blockers, and alpha-adrenergic blockers can promote weight gain by increasing appetite or reducing exercise tolerance [6]. Diabetes medication drugs may also influence weight gain as described in this case history.

JE is a 53 year old male weighing 292 lb. As a type II diabetic, he uses insulin and sulfonylurea medications to control his diabetes. During the nutrition counseling appointment in preparation for bariatric surgery, he stated that he felt hungry "all the time" and was "too tired to do anything physical."

Medication, diet, and lifestyle changes allowed JE to achieve weight loss without surgery.

Insulin and sulfonylurea increase appetite so the first step was a modification to the diet to eliminate refined carbohydrate foods (high glycemic foods). Refined carbohydrates rapidly raise blood glucose which induces insulin production. When blood glucose falls too fast, the insulin can stimulate appetite which stimulated his weight gain.

JE reported that his weight increased "overnight" when exogenous insulin was started to improve his blood glucose management. After explaining how exogenous insulin has a greater effect on appetite than endogenous insulin, a goal of reducing the need for exogenous insulin allowed JE to lower his BMI over a 3 month period.

Other modifications have similar effects on appetite management. Sulfonylureas increase appetite by stimulating insulin secretion from the pancreas. Steroid hormones like corticosteroids have been known to increase appetite and produce undesirable effects in body composition. The most obvious effect is a decrease in muscle mass, leading an individual to gain weight.

NUTRITION PROTOCOLS

As a registered dietitian, I lacked the nutrition protocols for counseling weight-loss patients until I met Dr. Jeffry Bland, founder and board chairman of the Institute for Functional Medicine (IFM). Bland provided the nutrition guidelines necessary for identifying and following biomarkers in weight management cases. In addition to helping me recognize the extent to which chronic symptoms (i.e., inflammation, food sensitivity, and metabolic syndrome) can effect weight management, IFM provided a framework for understanding the importance of the mind–body relationship in promoting healthy weight loss [5]. Protocols are important in guiding the nutrition counselor in making assessments with appropriate treatment plans. It has been my experience that individuals seeking weight-loss counseling do not care about how many scientific studies promoting or not promoting dietary supplements have been done and the outcomes. They just want to know if they can be helped. They do not care to read the science. They only want to know that their health-care provider has read it and what the treatment plan involves.

Functional medicine testing can provide significant insight into nutrition insufficiencies/deficiencies. Standard laboratory tests like the comprehensive metabolic panel (CMP) and complete blood count (CBC) can identify protein malnutrition (albumin < 3.5 g/L) and iron and anemia problems. Vitamin D status can also be requested from many laboratories. But the complete nutrition overview is best achieved from urine organic acid testing, gastrointestinal function profiles, fatty acid profiles, amino acid analysis, and food antibody panels. Without these tests, nutrient needs are a guessing game that costs the individual dearly in loss of productivity and quality of life.

The United States can no longer afford a disease-care system. Keeping individuals healthy instead of sick can improve quality of life, productivity, and more personal responsibility for lifestyle choices. Vitamins and minerals are important to enhance visual acuity, immune function, cell proliferation and differentiation, and protect against free radical oxidation. As energy needs in our lifestyles decrease, dietary supplement needs are increased to maintain adequate nutritional status.

NUTRITIONAL SUPPLEMENTS

Traditional clinical nutrition and dietetics resources fail to provide nutrition supplementation protocol, but Functional Medicine symposiums provide needed resources to develop nutrition protocols in assisting weight-loss clients. Weight issues are usually a factor in cases of rheumatoid arthritis, systemic lupus erythematosus, multiple sclerosis, and fibromyalgia, as well as hyperlipidemia, metabolic syndrome, and premenstrual syndrome. All of these conditions, and numerous others, need to be evaluated for possible nutrient deficiencies that could assist in the clinical management of these patients [7]. As examples, when obesity was a major nutritional factor for two multiple sclerosis cases, high doses of linoleic acid (almost 10 times the Dietary Reference Intake) were recommended [8]. A lupus patient who wanted to lead a normal life without dialysis challenged all the nutritional biochemistry available in standard dietetics manuals until a librarian found a journal article describing high levels of pantothenic acid and vitamin E being used for the treatment of lupus erythematosus [9]. Nutritional supplementation is not the standard of care, despite increasing medical literature citations.

Vanadium (vanadyl sulfate) has rarely been mentioned as an adjunct to weight loss in syndrome X. As a result of a study by Boden et al. [10] of the effect of vanadyl sulfate on carbohydrate and lipid metabolism, its use has become a standard in my practice for non-insulin-dependent diabetes mellitus (NIDDM) cases with elevated triglycerides.

These are only a few examples of how dietary supplements have been used to assist weight-loss clients. As one individual boldly stated during a counseling session, "I came here to get your professional opinion on what dietary supplements to take and how much. I'm not interested in what the FDA or pharmaceutical studies say. I am paying you for your expertise because I don't have 10 or 20 years until they decide nutrition may be helpful."

WHY DIETARY SUPPLEMENTS

Five key reasons given to clients for recommending dietary supplements as part of their weight-loss regime are the following:

- Food intake in the SAD does not meet dietary recommendations for numerous nutrients.
- Dietary supplements are safe within a broad range of doses.
- Science has demonstrated the health benefits of high levels of some nutrient such as folic acid, vitamin D, and vitamin B12.
- Criticism of supplement doses in excess of the RDA is overstated; "expensive" urine and feces may result, but that is of little relevance in disease management.
- Herbs and botanicals were the original sources of pharmaceutical drugs, and they generate many orders of magnitude fewer unplanned effects.

A healthy diet is the keystone of good health because food provides many substances not yet identified or available as dietary supplements. In weight-loss regimes, however, individuals may need the placebo effect of dietary supplements [11], in addition to the enhanced nutrient benefits.

GUIDELINES FOR SUPPLEMENTS IN WEIGHT LOSS

Individualization of meal plans and nutrient supplements regimes is helpful for many tackling body fat issues. Many people need a handy guide to selecting dietary supplements so that they can evaluate whether they are getting too high a dose when they combine different capsules, bars, and drinks. A general guideline offered in our weight-loss clinic is provided in the following.

Dietary Supplements for Weight Loss			
Ingredient	Amount	Ingredient	Amount
Vitamin A	2,000–5,000 IU	Biotin	500–1,000 µg
Beta-carotene	10,000–20,000 IU	Vitamin C	2,000–5,000 mg
Vitamin D	1,000–2,000 IU	Bioflavonoid	250–500 mg
Vitamin E	400–800 IU	Calcium	800–1,200 mg
Vitamin K	200–300 µg	Chromium (III)	400–500 µg
Thiamine (B1)	75–150 mg	Copper	2–3 mg
Riboflavin (B2)	50–100 mg	Iron (women)	15–25 mg
Niacinamide (B3)	75–150 mg	Magnesium	400–800 mg
Pantothenic acid	250–500 mg	Manganese	5–10 mg
Pyridoxine (B6)	50–100 mg	Selenium	200–400 µg
Pyridoxal 5 phosphate	100–200 mg	Zinc	20–50 mg
Cobalamin (B12)	500–1,000 µg	CoQ10	30–100 mg
Folic acid	800–1,000 µg	Omega-3 fatty acids (EPA and DHA)	1,000–1,200 mg

Health-care professionals intuitively understand the benefits of dietary supplements but are not adequately trained on dosage and formulation needed to appropriately recommend nutrients outside of food. This lack of knowledge needs to be addressed immediately if Americans are to improve their quality of life and manage chronic diseases better, especially those undergoing weight-loss surgery.

Weight-Loss Surgery

Weight-loss surgery for obesity is often an option for those with BMI >40 or BMI >35 with comorbid complications. The FDA has sanctioned the use of gastric banding for those with BMI >30 according to Med Page Today [12]. A recent study in BMJ 2010 described the national trends in bariatric surgery in England. Of the 6953 bariatric procedures performed during the period April 2000 to March 2008, 3649 were band procedures, 3191 were gastric bypass procedures, and 113 were sleeve gastrectomy procedures. A significant increase in procedures was noted—238 in 2000 to 2543 in 2007 [13]. The dramatic increase in bariatric surgery in the United States from 63,000 in 2002 to 103,000 in 2003 and over 150,000 in 2004 suggests that overnutrition in Americans has reached epidemic proportions.

Micronutrient deficiencies in overweight and obese individuals prior to surgery means excess calorie intake but not excess nutrient intake. Of the hundreds of bariatric surgery cases I have counseled, most have no fruits and vegetables in their presurgical diet and rely on highly processed, convenience, high-calorie, low-quality nutrition foods to satisfy their need to eat. Numerous studies have currently begun to discuss the nutritional deficiencies in bariatric surgery [14–17].

Presurgery nutritional supplementation reduces mortality rates. Flum et al. [18] studied gastric bypass surgery patients for 15 years and found that 88.2% were more likely to be alive if they had the surgery compared to 83.7% of those who did not have the surgery; thus, gastric bypass surgery can be a cost-effective means of reducing overall mortality among the obese [19]. Nutrition assessment of gastric surgery patients should be individualized and not based solely on weight loss. Alterations in anatomy may create significant potential for nutrient deficiencies and metabolic complications.

Malabsorption, food intolerance, nausea, and vomiting are complications that can interfere with nutrient adequacy. Thiamine insufficiency/deficiency can be noted in 3–4 weeks postsurgery as skeletal muscle storage is depleted. Zinc, iron, calcium, and fat-soluble vitamins A, D, E, and K insufficiency have also been reported [20–22] postsurgery.

After bariatric surgery, patients consume a liquid diet for the first week, and liquid dietary supplements are recommended to maintain lean muscle mass and improve immune function [23]. By week two, they are taking chewable dietary supplements and eating soft protein foods. Crushed prenatal supplements can be used as an inexpensive dietary supplement which is readily available. Too many bariatric surgery patients get more interested in losing weight than taking their dietary supplements and learning healthy food choice habits. Unfortunately, insurance companies require or encourage presurgery nutrition counseling but no emphasis is made on postsurgery diet consultation. Within 6 months of surgery, many individuals begin to consume high-calorie, low-nutrient foods again which causes weight rebound.

Bariatric surgery patients need absorbable nutrients to promote not only long-term health following surgery but also long-term nutrition status monitoring. Lifelong dietary supplementation is critical in these individuals since the surgery sets up a state of malnutrition with B vitamin insufficiency/deficiencies reported by Dr. Dyck, Associate Professor of Neurology, May Clinic, Rochester, Minnesota [24].

EVIDENCE-BASED DIETETICS PRACTICE

As Dr. Sidney Baker stated in 1993 at the Symposium on Man and His Environment in Health and Disease, each health-care practitioner must determine whether "you see what you believe or you believe what you see" [25]. Nutrition counseling has given me the opportunity to believe what I see, and dietary supplements really can make a difference in weight loss, as well as in other chronic disease management. Dr. Mark Hyman described nutrition as being a young science: "The view of nutrition as simply a source of energy or calories to prevent malnutrition and micronutrients to prevent deficiency diseases is being supplanted by a new conception of nutrition in health and disease" [4].

The calories-in vs. calories-out model of weight management is too simplistic to explain the obesity crisis. Both macro- and micronutrient components of the diet need to be evaluated with regard to their influence on thermodynamics because calorie counting is obsolete as far as changing eating habits. Science has shown that dietary supplements can help upgrade the metabolic processes of detoxification and toxic overload found in many chronic diseases such as obesity [5]. The food industry and researchers need to focus more on these uses of nutrients rather than on reducing calories through sugar substitutes and fat replacers.

Evidence-based guidelines for additional nutrient use among Americans who spend more than $20 billion annually on herbal and dietary supplements [26] are greatly lacking. The argument that dietary supplements lack safety and efficacy data does not make a difference to those individuals in weight-loss programs who seek increased energy to get physically active plus the enhanced health and sense of well-being that they believe comes from using them. Choosing quality manufacturers with outstanding safety and efficacy records is essential when recommending nutritional supplements in weight-loss programs [27].

Nutrition is eating healthy foods, using appropriate dietary supplements, and modifying a lifestyle to improve health. The new paradigm of health requires more than swallowing a one-a-day multinutrient supplement or a bowl of cereal advertised as a "totally complete" source of daily nutrition needs. Food habits are ingrained early, and choices are determined more by marketing than nutrition labels. Dietary supplements can help in weight management when food choices are less than ideal.

REFERENCES

1. Dor, A., Ferguson, C., Tan, E., and Langwith, C., A Heavy Burden: The individual cost of being over-weight and obese in the United States. September 21, 2010, George Washington University Medical Center. www.gwumc.edu/sphhs/departments/healthpolicy
2. Randolph, T.G., *Human Ecology and Susceptibility to the Chemical Environment.* Charles C Thomas, Springfield, IL, 1962.
3. Williams, R.J., *Biochemical Individuality: The Basis for the Genetotropic Concept.* Keats Publishing, New Canaan, CT, 1998.
4. Haas, E.M., *Staying Healthy with Nutrition: The Complete Guide to Diet and Nutritional Medicine.* Celestial Arts, Berkeley, CA, 1992, pp. 375–383.
5. Jones, D.S., Ed., *Textbook of Functional Medicine, Institute for Functional Medicine.* Gig Harbor, WA, 2005.
6. Kohlstadt, I., Ed., *Food and Nutrients in Disease Management.* CRC Press, Boca Raton, FL, 2009.
7. Levin, B., *Environmental Nutrition: Understanding the Link between Environment, Food Quality, and Disease.* Hinge Pin, Vashon Island, WA, 1999, pp. 58–61.
8. Bates, D. Fawcett, P.R.W., Shaw, D.A. et al., Polyunsaturated fatty acids in treatment of acute remitting multiple sclerosis. *Br. Med. J.*, 2, 1390–1391, 1978.
9. Welsh, A.L., Lupus erythematosus; treatment by combined use of massive amounts of pantothenic acid and vitamin E. *Arch. Dermotol. Syph.*, 70, 181–198, 1954.
10. Boden, G., Chen, X., Ruiz, J. et al., Effects of vanadyl sulfate on carbohydrate and lipid metabolism in patients with non-insulin dependent diabetes mellitus. *Metabolism*, 45, 1130–1135, 1996.
11. Lipton, B., *The Biology of Belief: Understanding the Power of Consciousness.* Matter and Miracles, Mountain of Love/Elite Books, Santa Rosa, CA, 2005.
12. Peck, P., FDA Expands Gastric Band Indication. Med Page Today, February 16, 2011.
13. Burns, E.M., Naseem, H., Bottle, A., Lazzarino, A.I., Ayline, P., Danzi, A., and Moorthy, K., Introduction of laparoscopic bariatric surgery in England: Observational population cohort study. *BMJ*, 341, c4296, August 26, 2010.
14. Xanthakos, S., Nutritional deficiencies in obesity and after bariatric surgery. *Pediat Clini. North Am.*, 56, 1105–1121, October 2009.
15. Schweitzer, D.H. and Posthuma, E.F., Prevention of vitamin and mineral deficiencies after bariatric surgery: Evidence and algorithms. *Obes. Surg.*, 18, 1485–1488, 2008.
16. Flancbaum, L., Belsley, S., Drake, V. et al., Preoperative nutritional status of patients undergoing Roux-en-Y gastric bypass for morbid obesity. *J. Gastrointest Surg.*, 10, 1033–1037, 2006.
17. Tucker, O.N., Szomstein, S., and Rosenthal, R.J., Nutritional consequences of weight loss surgery. *Med. Clin. North Am.*, 91, 499–514, 2007.
18. Flum, D.R., Salem, L., Elrod, J.A. et al., Early mortality among Medicare beneficiaries undergoing bariatric surgical procedures. *JAMA*, 294, 1903–1908, 2005.
19. Craig, B.M. and Tseng, D.S., Cost effectiveness of gastric bypass for severe obesity. *Am. J. Med.*, 113, 491–490, 2002.
20. Alvarez-Leith, J., Nutrient deficiencies secondary to bariatric surgery. *Curr. Opin. Clin. Nutr. Metab. Care*, 7, 569–575, 2004.
21. O'Donnell, K., Small but Mighty: Selected micronutrient issues in gastric bypass patients. *Pract. Gastroentrol.*, 37–48, 2008.
22. Madan, A.K., Orth, W.S., Tichansky, D.S., and Ternovits, C.A., Vitamin and trace mineral levels after laparoscopic gastric bypass. *Obes. Surg.*, 16, 603–606, 2006.
23. Scheier, L., Bariatric surgery: Life threatening risk or life-saving procedure?. *J. Am. Diet. Assoc.*, 104(9), 1338–1340, 2004.
24. Tucker, M.E., Proper nutrition key following bariatric surgery. *Intern. Med. News*, 37(22), 57, Retrieved October 27, 2010.
25. Baker, S.M., The relationship of chemical interaction on the nutritional chain. In *Proceedings of Symposium on Man and His Environment in Health and Disease*, Human Ecology Research Foundation, Dallas, TX, 1993.
26. Anon, *Natural Supplement: An Evidence-Based Update.* Scripps Center for Integrative Medicine, La Jolla, CA, 2006.
27. Poston, W.S.C. and Haddock, C.K., Eds., Food as a drug. *Drugs Soc.*, 15(1/2), 1, 2000.

Horizons for Long-Term
Weight Management

Corinne Bush, MS, CNS and Dana Reed, MS, CNS, CDN

CONTENTS

INTRODUCTION

Achieving long-term weight management is widely recognized as an important factor in reducing risk of many chronic diseases as well as enhancing quality of life. Short-term weight loss can be achieved by a number of different dietary plans (Dansinger et al., 2005). However, if weight loss cannot be maintained, and in fact is subsequently reversed, this may have adverse effects on health. Studies have shown that losing and regaining weight repeatedly may lead to worse outcomes than simply remaining obese (Jeffery, 1996).

One of the most challenging tasks clinicians face is helping patients to achieve long-term weight loss. The foundation must be a focus on nutrient quality rather than reliance on macronutrient partitioning and calorie restriction. Plans must then be customized to reflect clients' specific health issues and lifestyles as the emphasis shifts away from "diet" to a long-term strategy. Compliance is the key factor (Wing and Phelan, 2005). Limiting glycemic load (GL) through a combination of modulating total carbohydrate and selecting low-glycemic-index (GI) carbohydrate foods is one method of achieving compliance when used as part of an overall weight-loss strategy.

The concepts of GI and GL as a means of qualifying the carbohydrate component of a diet have relevance for the treatment of chronic, insulin-stimulated diseases in addition to obesity (Barclay et al., 2008).

Replacing high-GI foods with low-GI foods has a significant effect on postprandial glucose and insulin responses leading to control of inflammatory processes as measured by high-sensitivity C-reactive protein (Liu et al., 2002; Levitan et al., 2008). This has relevance for the treatment of metabolic syndrome, non-insulin-dependent diabetes mellitus (NIDDM), cardiovascular disease (CVD), and some cancers. This chapter is limited to a discussion of the effects of carbohydrate foods on obesity and weight management including our proposal for an evidence-based clinical strategy.

CARBOHYDRATE CLASSIFICATION SYSTEMS

Carbohydrate foods are important to health and a necessary component of any diet as they are converted to glucose, the body's preferred source of fuel. The historical progression of methods that have been used to classify carbohydrate foods based on their glycemic response is described. The chemical structure method is no longer considered accurate, although it is defined here for background. Although the terms GI and GL are often used interchangeably, they have distinct meanings. Newer methods of classification are also described. (Refer to Table 55.1—Definition of Terms.)

CHEMICAL STRUCTURE: AN OUTDATED CLASSIFICATION SYSTEM

The traditional approach of classifying carbohydrate foods based on saccharide chain length was first proposed in the early twentieth century (Allen, 1920). Starchy foods (complex carbohydrates) with longer chain lengths were thought to be digested and converted to blood glucose at a slower rate than mono- and disaccharides, which were thought to have a faster and sharper rate of uptake. Historically, most calorie-restricted, low-fat diets and diabetic diets have emphasized complex carbohydrates at the expense of simple sugars. This approach has been challenged by more recent research proving that some starches have higher impacts on glycemic response than do some simple sugars. Postprandial responses to carbohydrate foods cannot be accurately predicted based on chain length (Wahlvqvist et al., 1978).

GLYCEMIC INDEX

The GI system was proposed to more accurately describe the physiological basis of glycemic response in order to aid diabetics with blood sugar control (Jenkins et al., 1981). GI provides a way of categorizing carbohydrate foods based on the food's impact on glycemic response and, as such, is considered a measure of the food's quality.

TABLE 55.1
Definition of Terms

Term	Definition
Glycemic response	The change in blood sugar concentration following a meal or snack
GI	Incremental area under the 2 h blood glucose response curve (AUC) of 50 g of available carbohydrate of a given food expressed as a percentage of the area of the 2 h blood glucose response curve as the same amount of carbohydrate as glucose
Available carbohydrate	Total carbohydrate minus fiber
GL	GI multiplied by the amount of carbohydrate in a typical serving of a given food. It is calculated as the quantity in grams of carbohydrate content multiplied by GI and divided by 100
Relative glycemic impact	The weight of glucose that would induce glycemic response equivalent to that of a given amount of food
Satiation	The sensation of fullness that develops during the process of a meal and contributes to meal termination
Hunger	The degree of appetite suppression between one meal and the next

High-GI foods are more rapidly converted to glucose and elicit sharper blood glucose elevations than low-GI foods. GI values generally range from 20 to 100, with some highly processed foods exceeding 100. Using white bread as the standard, foods with a GI under 40 are considered low GI, those that have a GI between 40 and 70 are considered to have a moderate GI, while those over 70 are considered high-GI foods (Bell and Sears, 2003). The vast majority of whole grain breads, breakfast cereals, and processed cereal products have a high GI. By contrast, most fruits, nonstarchy vegetables, nuts, seeds, and legumes tend to have a low GI (Foster-Powell et al., 2002).

GI has been widely used in the treatment of diabetes in many countries. In 1997, the Food and Agriculture Organization (FAO) and the World Health Organization (WHO) recommended the use of GI as a tool for comparing foods of similar macronutrient composition in the treatment of diabetes and glucose intolerance. Major diabetes associations in the United Kingdom, Canada, and Australia now recommend judicious use of the GI diet. However, the American Diabetes Association does not endorse its use. Expanding the use of GI beyond diabetes to weight control, sports performance, treatment of CVD, and cancer prevention is the subject of ongoing research.

GI has a number of other limitations in its practical application (Wolever et al., 1991) and is not effective when used as a stand-alone for making food choices:

- There are two standard values against which GI is calculated (glucose and bread), yielding two sets of indices.
- The values are not necessarily equivalent to typical serving sizes, making it of limited use in meal planning.
- GI values of a given food are inconsistent, as they may be affected by many factors such as degree of processing, cooking method used, when the food is consumed in relation to when it is cooked, soluble fiber content, presence of organic acids, etc.
- GI cannot be estimated based on product ingredients or nutritional composition. For instance, it cannot be assumed that whole grain products and high-fiber foods carry low GI values.
- Large amounts of low-GI foods can have a significant impact on glycemic response.

Subsequent studies have shown that control of the overall blood glucose response to a serving of food is determined not only by the quality based on GI but also by the quantity. To address the limitations, GL was proposed as a measure of overall blood glucose and insulin-raising potential of the diet.

Glycemic Load

In 1997, Walter Willet and researchers from Harvard University addressed these issues when they introduced the concept of GL to describe how portions differing in both quantity and quality of carbohydrate affect glycemic response and risk of diabetes in women (Salmeron et al., 1997).

In general, a food with a GL of 20 or more is high, 11–19 is medium, and 10 or under is low. The GL of 750 foods has been calculated (Foster-Powell et al., 2002). In general, low-GL foods consist of nonstarchy vegetables and legumes; moderate-GL foods are most fruits, dairy foods, and unsweetened, grain-based foods; and high-GL foods are sweetened grain-based foods, candy, and sweetened beverages.

GL can also be used to describe the overall glycemic response to a food, a meal, or a diet. Reducing the GL can be achieved in one of three ways: (1) decreasing the carbohydrate amount without changing carbohydrate sources, (2) maintaining the carbohydrate amount while selecting carbohydrates with lower GI values, and (3) decreasing both the carbohydrate amount and selecting foods with lower GI values (Ebbeling and Ludwig, 2010).

Although GI and GL are commonly independently assessed, GI alone is unable to predict glycemic response when different amounts of carbohydrates are eaten, supporting the concurrent use of GL. A recent study concluded that both GI and GL should be used to characterize the metabolic responses of meals differing in carbohydrate quality. Researchers looked at the effects of five meals differing in both GI and GL. Results varied depending on whether GI, GL, or both were considered. For a given

GL, high GI showed sharper blood glucose elevations 120 min postprandially than low-GI meals and sharper drops during the 120–180 min postprandial period. Low-GL meals showed an improved glycemic response although effects were not significant in the 120–180 min period (Micha and Nelson, 2011).

GL PATTERNS AND INFLUENCES ON OBESITY

A low-GL diet is considered to have a total daily GL of 50–70, whereas a low-fat, high-carbohydrate diet as outlined by the USDA food pyramid yields a GL of at least 80 and up to 120. The standard American diet, high in processed carbohydrates and sugars and low in vegetables, typically has a dietary GL of over 200 (Bell and Sears, 2003).

An investigation of trends in coronary heart disease and diet revealed that the prevalence of overweight women increased by 38% from 1980 to 1994. Diets improved significantly during the same period in all but one of six main criteria, GL, which increased by 22% (Hu et al., 2000). This is suggestive of the influence of carbohydrate quality and quantity on the obesity epidemic.

RELATIVE GLYCEMIC IMPACT AND GLYCEMIC GLUCOSE EQUIVALENTS

Recognizing the limitations of determining glycemic response based solely on the content of available carbohydrate, the American Association of Cereal Chemists established an ad hoc committee in 2004. The objective was to develop a meaningful approach to standardizing glycemic response that would enable consumers to make informed choices. The relative glycemic impact, as measured by glycemic glucose equivalent (GGE), is a simplified concept established for use on food labels that has potential for broader research applications. For example, a sweet muffin has a glycemic impact equivalent to that of 46 g of glucose, expressed as a GGE value of 46, whereas an apple has a glycemic impact equivalent to that of 7.9 g of glucose, expressed as a GGE value of 7.9 (Monro and Shaw, 2008).

FACTORS THAT IMPACT GLYCEMIC RESPONSE TO STARCH-CONTAINING FOODS

Foods and meals show great variation in the extent to which they influence glycemic response. This variation is due to characteristics of the starch content or other components of the meal. These differences appear to relate to the digestibility of the starch, with more slowly digested starches showing less impact on glycemic response.

- *Starch structure.* Starch is a carbohydrate consisting of two types of molecules: amylose and amylopectin. Amylose accounts for about 20%–30% of the starch molecule, and amylopectin constitutes about 70%–80%. The ratio of amylose to amylopectin has been found to influence glycemic response, with higher levels of amylose stimulating lower postprandial glucose and insulin (Behall and Howe, 1995).
- *Physical entrapment.* Physical entrapment refers to the way the starch is encased in the food. For example, bran has a physical barrier that slows down the enzymatic activity of the internal starch layer during digestion.
- *Soluble versus insoluble fiber.* Viscous soluble fiber transforms intestinal contents into a gel-like substance that slows enzymatic activity and increases gastric distention, thereby slowing gastric emptying rate and lowering glycemic response. The impact of insoluble fiber on glycemic response is controversial, with most studies indicating little or no impact on glycemic response.
- *Presence of other macronutrients (fat and protein).* Fats and proteins slow gastric emptying and, consequently, the rate at which foods exit the stomach and enter the duodenum.
- *Acid content.* Organic acids have been shown to reduce postprandial glycemia without altering GL when added to a meal or food. Vinegar reduced the 60 min glucose response to a high-GL meal by approximately 55%. In addition, energy consumption for the remainder

of the day was reduced by approximately 250 cal. The identified mechanism is related to acidity and inhibition of digestive amylases (Johnston and Bulle, 2005).

- *Food processing.* Milling and grinding removes the fiber-rich outer bran and the vitamin- and mineral-rich inner germ, leaving mostly the starchy endosperm. Highly processed foods have a higher GI compared to their unprocessed equivalents.
- *Cooking.* The cooking process swells the starch molecules in food and softens it, speeding up the rate of digestion and resulting in greater glycemic response.
- *Antinutrient content.* GI correlates negatively with antinutrients such as phytic acid. Both added and endogenous phytic acid reduced *in vitro* rate of starch digestion and *in vivo* blood glucose response. This is thought to be due to enzymatic interaction with amylase or another starch protein (Thompson et al., 1987).
- *Resistant starch.* Resistant starch has fiber-like effects in that it reaches the large intestine without being broken down into glucose; therefore, its presence in a food lowers glycemic response. It is fermented by colonic bacteria to short-chain fatty acids (SCFA) contributing to colon health and lessening glycemic response to carbohydrates ingested later in the day (Livesey and Tagami, 2009).

PHYSIOLOGICAL MECHANISMS OF WEIGHT REGULATION

EFFECTS OF A LOW-GLYCEMIC-LOAD DIET

There is increasing evidence that reducing dietary GL by selecting carbohydrate foods of lower GI value, while maintaining or reducing total carbohydrate energy improves the rate of fat loss. Several key mechanisms have been proposed:

1. Reduced postprandial glycemia and insulinemia, resulting in improved insulin sensitivity
2. Increased fat oxidation
3. Slower rates of absorption and digestion in the gut, resulting in greater satiety, reduced hunger, and reduced food intake
4. Minimized decline in metabolic rate during energy restriction (Ludwig, 2000, 2002; Pawlak et al., 2002; Bell and Sears, 2003; McMillan-Price and Brand-Miller, 2006; Brand-Miller et al., 2008)

Modulating quality and quantity of carbohydrate foods affects these mechanisms in profound ways to influence weight loss. The body has complex regulatory systems that carefully control blood sugar concentrations after eating and until the next meal. Low-GL meals and low-GI foods enhance the elegant hormone mechanisms that balance blood sugar and return it to normal levels after a meal. Soon after eating such meals, nutrients stimulate the release of incretins, hormones that trigger the release of insulin from the pancreas. Insulin then delivers glucose to the liver, fat storage cells, or muscle cells for glycogen storage, an anabolic process. In the postabsorptive state, counterregulatory hormones (glucagons, epinephrine, cortisol, growth hormone) counteract insulin action, stimulating release of stored fuels to stabilize blood sugar concentrations and return to normal blood sugar levels. This encourages catabolic reactions, which convert the nutrients previously stored in fat, muscle, or liver to glucose for energy and delay the return of hunger.

Low-GL meals result in optimal function of hormones regulating appetite, fuel sources, and metabolism. These meals reduce the rate at which digestion and absorption take place, resulting in a blunted blood sugar response. Additional catabolic processes, such as lipolysis, augment fuel supplies by releasing fatty acids. This enhances insulin sensitivity and reduces hunger, promoting fat loss and preservation of lean body tissue, which results in higher resting metabolic rates. This metabolic effect is sustained and persists to the next meal, a mechanism that has been termed the "second meal effect" (Wolever et al., 1988). Slower absorption of carbohydrate results in smaller counterregulatory hormone (glucagons, GH, catecholamines, cortisol) response, higher free fatty acids in the postabsorptive phase, and improved glucose disposal after the next meal. The lentils and barley tested in Wolever's study are high in soluble fiber, as are many low-GI foods. Soluble fiber offers the added benefit of stimulating colonic fermentation, an important factor in improving the postprandial glycemic response to the second meal effect evidenced in this study.

Brighenti et al. (2006) found that low-GI foods often increase colonic fermentation due to the presence of soluble fiber and resistant starch. Fermentable carbohydrates have the potential to improve postprandial responses to a second meal by several mechanisms: reducing fatty acid competition for glucose disposal, slowing gastric emptying, and contributing to the production of SCFA in the colon which can be oxidized for energy in preference to glucose. These mechanisms result in more stable glucose patterns over time and may potentially reduce appetite.

The soluble fiber found in most low-GI foods offers additional benefits. The partially digested food particles that result stimulate satiety hormones, such as the glucagon-like peptide-1 in the lower ileum (de Graaf et al., 2004), and greater secretion of cholecystokinin, a gut hormone that acts as a hunger suppressant (Holt et al., 1992). Greater satiety during the meal process results in reduced hunger in between meals and reduced food intake at the next meal.

EFFECT OF A HIGH-GLYCEMIC-LOAD DIET

Contrasted to the elegant mechanisms of normal hormonal response and return to euglycemia that occurs with low-GL meals, high-GL meals cause a cascade of negative metabolic reactions. This impairs blood sugar control, alters the availability of fuel sources, and encourages more food intake and subsequent weight gain. After eating a meal of highly processed carbohydrate foods, there is a sharper and faster rise in blood sugar. This results in higher levels of insulin in relation to glucagon, stimulating greater than normal anabolic response and encouraging greater nutrient storage. Several hours later, nutrient absorption from the gut declines. Rather than oxidizing stored fat, abnormally high insulin levels continue to stimulate glucose uptake from stored liver glycogen. This results in a sharper than normal decline in blood sugar and hypoglycemia, often to lower than premeal levels. These levels are similar to what would be expected in a fasting state, which is normally reached only after many hours without food. Since fuel continues to be stored rather than taken from storage to be burned, fatty acid oxidation and other catabolic processes slow down. Consequently, hunger sets in. In the next part of this cycle, an exaggerated counterregulatory hormone response finally drives blood sugar levels back up by stimulating release of fatty acids from fat cells; however, there is a subsequent sharp insulin spike to handle the sudden heavy glucose load. These elevated glucose levels blunt the normal catabolic processes, causing hunger to remain.

These dietary patterns continue to challenge normal responses and cause the pancreas to secrete much higher than normal amounts of insulin. Over time, this increases the risk of developing Metabolic or Insulin Resistance Syndrome. Anabolism is favored over catabolism, especially lipolysis, making it difficult for the body to use fat stores for energy and weight loss. Greater food intake is encouraged because hunger sets in much sooner, even when energy and nutrient intake is sufficient. Patients report constant hunger.

LOW-GLYCEMIC-INDEX/LOAD DIETS FOR WEIGHT MANAGEMENT: EXPERIMENTAL EVIDENCE

The hypothesis that lowering dietary GI/GL will result in long-term weight loss has yet to be proven, although the trend is promising. Research findings have been mixed for several reasons: (1) most studies are underpowered; (2) there are factors confounding glycemic response other than GI/GL, which have not been addressed; and (3) these parameters are used inconsistently. Based on our review of research, the glucose-modulating effects of specific micronutrients in whole foods and the glycemic response to nonstarch carbohydrate foods are factors that have not been studied in conjunction with GI/GL. In addition, most intervention studies do not address long-term weight management; all but one we reviewed ranged in duration from 5 to 12 months.

Short-term weight-loss studies (12 weeks to 12 months) using various dietary interventions (low fat, low carbohydrate, low GI/GL) usually show across the board weight loss likely due to overall caloric restriction. Among studies that support this premise is Dansinger's comparison of four popular diets for weight loss—Atkins, Ornish, Weight Watchers, and Zone (Dansinger et al., 2005). However, the weight-loss benefits of low-GI/GL diets are clear in *ad libitum* studies where guidance was given about the quality of food choices but participants were not restricted regarding quantity of food intake. This provides a promising outlook for long-term weight management due to relative ease of compliance and the physiological mechanisms outlined.

The recent DIOGENES study reported in the *New England Journal of Medicine* provides intriguing support for the efficacy of low-GI/GL diets for weight loss and weight maintenance (Larsen et al., 2010). Following extreme calorie restriction during which they lost at least 8% of initial body weight, 548 people were assigned to one of four test diets varying in protein content and GL for 26 weeks. Those in the low-protein, high-GI group (a high-GL diet) experienced significant weight gain, and participants assigned to the low-protein/low-GI group (a moderate-GL diet) maintained weight loss. In contrast, participants in the high-protein, low-GI group (a low-GL diet) continued to lose weight after the initial weight loss. This study is meaningful for several reasons: (1) it clearly distinguished the quality/quantity factors, (2) it was based on *ad libitum* diets, (3) it followed a period of extreme calorie deprivation during which weight rebound is expected when returning to an *ad libitum* diet, and (4) the lower-GI diets were associated with a lower rate of dropout.

Another study compared the effects of an *ad libitum* low-GL diet to a calorie-restricted, low-fat diet on weight loss in obese adolescents during a 12 month period. Measure of adiposity fell significantly more in the low-GL group than the calorie-restricted group (Ebbeling et al., 2003).

A short-term, calorie-restricted 12 week study compared the independent effects of carbohydrate quality and quantity in 120 obese or overweight young adults. Subjects were assigned to one of four diets—high carbohydrate/high GI, high carbohydrate/low GI, high protein/high GI, and high protein/low GI. All four diets were calorie-restricted and high fiber. Both low-GI diets resulted in greater weight loss, however the high-carbohydrate, low-GI diet also resulted in enhanced cardiovascular benefits (McMillan-Price and Brand Miller, 2006). Although this study enabled the researchers to evaluate the factors of carbohydrate quality and quantity independently, it did not allow them to separate the effects of calorie restriction. Calorie restriction adds a confounding variable absent from *ad libitum* studies. It is difficult to distinguish whether weight loss is due to calorie restriction, macronutrient quantity or quality, or all of these factors combined. In any case, it is difficult to separate the GI impact from the other potential factors.

Further support for the use of low-GL *ad libitum* diets for weight loss can be gleaned from a meta-analysis of 23 studies, 16 of which found a negative correlation between weight and GI/GL. A statistically significant trend showed body weight falling with reduction in GL and vice versa. This occurred both in studies of *ad libitum* diets and controlled food intake diets. In one study, GL reduction by >17 g glucose equivalents per day was associated with significantly reduced body weight (Livesey et al., 2008). In this study, body weight reduction related more to GL than to GI.

In a 2009 Cochrane Review, six randomly controlled trials were selected to assess the effects of low-GI/GL diets for weight loss on overweight or obese subjects. Interventions ranged from 5 weeks to 6 months and included a total of 202 participants, ranging from 11 to 64 per trial. Primary outcomes of low-GI/GL diets, when compared to high-GI/GL diets, or energy-restricted, conventional diets, included reductions in body weight, decreases in BMI, and decreases in fat mass. In addition, two studies showed no significant change in fat-free mass. The authors concluded that lowering the GL of the diet without changing the carbohydrate content appears to be an effective method of promoting weight loss and can easily be incorporated into a person's lifestyle (Thomas et al., 2009).

In a 2007 Tufts University study, the CALERIE trial, 29 overweight but otherwise healthy men and women aged 24–42 years were assigned to either a high-GL or a low-GL diet for 12 months. Both diets were calorie restricted to 30%. The low-GL diet was achieved by reducing both total carbohydrates and replacing high-GI foods with low-GI foods. Adherence to the low-GI regimen resulted in greater loss of body fat and less loss of fat-free mass for the same amount of overall weight loss (Das et al., 2007). These findings suggest a beneficial effect of low-GL diets for weight control independent of an effect on absolute weight loss.

Research supports our clinical findings that low-GI/GL diets result in better compliance and, therefore, greater weight loss. Four popular diets—Atkins, Ornish, Weight Watchers, and Zone—were compared for weight loss and reduced cardiovascular risk factors. One hundred and sixty overweight or obese participants with known high risk of hypertension, dyslipidemia, and/or hyperglycemia were randomly assigned to one of the four diets for 1 year. All diets resulted in modest but significant weight loss at 1 year, with no significant differences between diets and no difference in cardiac risk factors. However, overall adherence rates were best in the two least stringent approaches, supporting the importance of ease of compliance in long-term weight management (Dansinger et al., 2005).

Additional benefits of low-GI/GL meals and diets are that they have been found to enhance the effects of exercise:

- A breakfast of low-GI foods contributed less carbohydrate to glycogen stores than a breakfast of high-GI foods, with better preservation of glycogen during subsequent exercise, due to higher fat oxidation (Wee et al., 2005). This may have application for the moderate exerciser aiming for weight control.
- During moderate exercise, a low-GI meal resulted in larger amounts of fat being oxidized at the expense of carbohydrates than did a high-GI meal (Stevenson et al., 2006).

PRACTICAL APPLICATIONS FOR LONG-TERM WEIGHT MANAGEMENT: OUR PROPOSED INTERVENTION PLAN

Patients come to us with a wide variety of clinical concerns and issues. Establishing healthy glycemic response is the foundation for restoring health for most, whether the issue is obesity or any of a number of chronic diseases from diabetes to cancer. The concepts of GI/GL provide practitioners with an important tool for designing programs for patients that will improve carbohydrate choices, thus enhancing glycemic response. We do not, however, counsel patients to refer to food lists of GI and GL indices. Rather, we incorporate these concepts into a customized intervention program that includes the healthiest food choices for each individual. In these interventions, we also address other factors that impact glycemic response, such as the quality of fat and protein, the importance of micronutrients, meal timing, and how to combine foods in each meal. When followed, the improvement in diet quality results not only in glycemic balance and weight loss, but also in subsequent control of inflammation, the major underlying factor in chronic disease.

Any successful eating plan must meet the following criteria for long-term compliance:

1. It must be readily incorporated into one's lifestyle—convenient, easy to follow, meals easy to prepare or obtain, easily adaptable to fit tastes and preferences, and able to be viewed as "meal plan" rather than "diet."
2. It must be satisfying—it must enable variety in food and meal options, allow the dieter to feel sated and not deprived, and result in greater satiation during a meal, with less hunger between meals.
3. It must be long-term quantifiable, with measurable results—it must achieve and maintain weight and fat loss as well as favorable clinical markers for reduced risk of chronic disease, with continuing motivation due to these payoffs.
4. It must be nutritious—it must contain all essential nutrients.

TABLE 55.2
Example of Glycemic Balance Diet Plan

Nonstarchy, low-GI vegetables: *Unlimited but a minimum of 4 servings per day*

- Try to make 1/2 raw and 1/2 cooked
- Serving sizes:
  - Raw: 1 cup = 1 serving
  - Steamed, roasted, grilled, or sautéed: 1/2 cup = 1 serving

1. Green, leafy vegetables: spinach, kale, dandelion greens, chard, collard greens, mustard greens, beet greens
2. Cruciferous vegetables: broccoli, cabbage, cauliflower, Brussels sprouts
3. Others: zucchini, spaghetti squash, eggplant, artichoke, asparagus, okra, tomato, green beans, snow peas, leeks, onion, bok choy, garlic, mushrooms
4. Salad: Concentrate on dark colored greens—arugula, red and green leaf lettuce, romaine lettuce, mesclun, etc. The darker and deeper the color, the better. Add parsley, coriander, basil, radicchio, cabbage, endive, mushroom, watercress, peppers, cucumbers, sprouts, tomatoes, etc.
5. Dried ocean vegetables: seaweed, agar, arame, dulse, hijiki, kelp, kombu, nori, sea palm, wakame, spirulina (1 oz. = 1/2 serving) (add as seasoning to salads, soups, vegetables, tofu/tempeh, pastas)

Whole grains and starchy vegetables: *Limit servings to _____ per day*

- Serving size: 1/2 cup cooked or 1 oz. of bread, cracker, cereal

1. Legumes—starchy beans, peas, and lentils (2/3 cup cooked = 1 serving): azuki, black, garbanzo, chickpeas, kidney, lentils, lima, navy, peas, pinto, red, white
2. Cooked whole grains: brown rice, wild rice, basmati rice, barley, millet, quinoa, amaranth, kamut, spelt, buckwheat, rolled oats, steel cut oats, oat bran, wheat bran, wheat germ
3. Tubers/starchy vegetables: sweet potato, yam, corn, winter squash, parsnips, peas, turnip, pumpkin, beets, rhubarb, rutabaga
4. Whole grain breads, whole grain crackers, whole grain pastas and whole grain, high-fiber/low-sugar dry cereals

Fruit: *Limit servings to _____ per day*

- Eat only fresh, frozen, or dried fruits
- Serving sizes:
  - 1 medium piece = 1 serving
  - 1 cup raw or frozen = 1 serving
  - 1/3 cup dried = 1 serving

1. Choose from lower-GI fruits: melons, berries, cherries, peaches, plums, apples, pears, apricots, kiwi, grapes, oranges, grapefruits, tangerines, clementines, etc.
2. *Limit* higher-GI fruits to 1 serving per day: bananas, dates, figs, guava, mango, papaya, pineapple, raisins, and all other dried fruits
3. *Avoid* fruit juices unless using a small amount in a marinade or other recipe

Preferred protein: *Eat just enough to be satisfied*

A. *Plant proteins*
  1. Soy beans and edamame: (2/3 cup cooked = 1 serving)
  2. Tofu or tempeh (4 oz. = 1 serving)
  3. Soy, rice, or whey protein powder (1 scoop = 1 serving)

B. *Animal proteins (serving size: 3 oz. = 1 serving = visually "deck of cards")*
  1. Fish (3 oz. cooked = 1 serving): salmon, tuna, haddock, arctic char, halibut, red snapper, bass, cod, shrimp, scallops, lobster
  2. Fowl (3 oz. cooked = 1 serving): chicken, turkey, hens (white meat without skin)
  3. Wild game (3 oz. cooked = 1 serving)
  4. Lean red meats, lamb, veal (3 oz. cooked = 1 serving)
  5. Eggs (2 eggs = 1 serving): organic with yolk, poached, or boiled

(continued)

TABLE 55.2 (continued)

Example of Glycemic Balance Diet Plan

6. Organic, plain goat, sheep, or cow milk yogurt (8 oz. = 1 serving)
7. Organic nonfat or 1% cow or goat milk (8 oz. = 1 serving)
8. Natural, aged cheeses: Parmesan, cheddar, goat, feta, Jarlsberg, Emmentaler, Gouda (1 oz. = 1 serving)
9. Cottage or farmer cheese (1/2 cup = 1 serving)

Healthy fats and oils: *Limit servings to _____ per day*

1. Cold-pressed oils: extra virgin olive oil, nuts oils, sesame oil, flaxseed oil, grapeseed oil, hemp oil, soybean oil, canola oil (1 Tbs. = 1 serving)
2. Avocado (1/4 = 1 serving)
3. Nuts (2 T. = 1 serving): almonds, hazelnuts, walnuts, soy nuts, cashews, Brazil nuts, pine nuts, macadamia, peanuts, pistachios. Eat raw or lightly toasted
4. Seeds (2 T. = 1 serving): pumpkin, sesame, sunflower, flax, hemp
5. Nut and seed butters made from any of the previous items—nonhydrogenated, unsweetened (1 Tbs. = 1 serving)
6. Olives (8–10 medium sized = 1 serving)

Note: Choose foods from each of the above-mentioned categories. Include the number of servings that your practitioner has indicated is optimal for you every day. Get as much variety as you can.

The uniqueness of each patient dictates that we design nutrition interventions that fit specific health issues, lifestyle, tastes, and preferences. Within that framework, all weight-loss interventions focus on lowering overall glycemic response through a selected combination of the following guidelines:

1. *Focus on food quality first.* We advocate an *ad libitum approach* with portion recommendations for certain foods. Emphasizing quality over quantity of food choices enables patients to view eating plans as lifestyle plans rather than as diets. This results in greater compliance and better long-term results.
2. *Emphasis on low-glycemic-index/load food choices.* (Refer to Table 55.2—Example of Glycemic Balance Diet Plan.)
3. *Overall carbohydrate reduction*, if necessary.
4. *Small, frequent meals* with consistent eating schedule, beginning at breakfast. Establishing a regular eating schedule is key to balancing blood sugar and insulin-regulating mechanisms. This, in turn, helps to manage hunger and cravings. If there is a long gap between two meals (greater than 4 h), we recommend including a snack and outline healthy options.
5. *Mindful eating techniques.* Eating in a relaxed manner without distraction improves the digestibility of all food components and favorably influences glycemic balance and, ultimately, satisfaction. We counsel patients to preplate food and wait for at least 20 min before getting seconds. This often helps them discover that they are satisfied with less.
6. *Awareness of physiological cues of hunger, satiety.* We spend time addressing these important issues.
7. Overall *increase in soluble fiber* through diet and supplements. We explain to our patients the importance of fiber in glycemic balance and appetite control. We explain the effect of adding soluble fiber to a meal and how this slows the rate of digestion and absorption of carbohydrate foods in the meal.
8. *Adequate hydration.* We encourage our patients to favor water as the beverage of choice. Good hydration is important for optimal energy and metabolism.

9. *Balancing starchy carbohydrates* with protein or fat at every meal or snack. We explain the importance of these foods in counteracting the glycemic response of carbohydrate foods in the same meal and that they also remain in the stomach longer, resulting in greater satiety.

10. *Elimination of artificial sweeteners.* Studies suggest that artificially sweetened foods and beverages may stimulate hunger (Lavin, 1997), lead to a greater preference for sweets, and increase risk of weight gain and metabolic syndrome (Dhingra et al., 2007).

CONCLUSION

Clinical results in weight management have been disappointing, partly due to overemphasis on calorie intake ("a calorie is a calorie") and macronutrient partitioning (ratio of calories coming from carbohydrate, fat, and protein). Often overlooked are the quality of the macronutrients and the impact of quality on glycemic response, hormone regulation, and, consequently, weight loss.

Modulating the quality of dietary carbohydrate has a significant impact on weight and body composition. GI and GL are valuable therapeutic tools for measuring carbohydrate quality, controlling glycemic response, and promoting long-term weight management when used as part of a total weight loss and weight maintenance strategy. In addition, new metrics are being developed to further understanding and the ability to manage this complex issue.

Studies on the use of low-GI/GL diets for weight loss show inconsistent and only moderately positive results. The most meaningful long-term interventions showing the effects of *ad libitum* low-GI/GL diets are few (Esfahani et al., 2009, 2010). However, one recent notable study does demonstrate that benefits do accrue over the long term (Larsen et al., 2010). Further research is needed to clarify and confirm the effects of low-GI/GL for continued weight loss and weight maintenance, especially those associated with increased appetite control and metabolism.

REFERENCES

Allen, F. 1920. Experimental studies on diabetes: Production and control of diabetes in the dog: Effects of carbohydrate diets. *Journal of Experimental Medicine* 31:381–402.

Barclay, A., Petocz, P., McMillan-Price, J. et al. 2008. Glycemic index, glycemic load, and chronic disease risk—A meta-analysis of observational studies. *American Journal of Clinical Nutrition* 87:627–637.

Behall, K. and Howe, J. 1995. Contribution of fiber and resistant starch to metabolizable energy. *American Journal of Clinical Nutrition* 62(suppl):1158S–1160S.

Bell, S. and Sears, B. 2003. Low-glycemic-load diets: Impact on obesity and chronic diseases. *Critical Reviews in Food Science and Nutrition* 43(4):357–377.

Brand-Miller, J., McMillan-Price, J., Steinbeck, K. et al. 2008. Carbohydrates—The good, the bad and the wholegrain. *Asia Pacific Journal of Clinical Nutrition* 17(SI):16–19.

Brighenti, F., Benini, L., Del Rio, D. et al. 2006. Colonic fermentation of indigestible carbohydrates contributes to the second-meal effect. *American Journal of Clinical Nutrition* 83:817–822.

Dansinger, M., Gleason, J., Griffith, J. et al. 2005. Comparison of the Atkins, Ornish, weight watchers, and zone diets for weight loss and heart disease risk reduction. *Journal of the American Medical Association* 293:43–53.

Das, S., Gilhooly, C., Golden, J. et al. 2007. Long term effects of energy-restricted diets differing in glycemic load on metabolic adaptation and body composition. *Open Nutrition Journal* 85(4):1023–1030.

De Graaf, C., Blom, W., Smeets, P. et al. 2004. Biomarkers of satiation and satiety. *American Journal of Clinical Nutrition* 79:946–961.

Dhingra, R., Sullivan, L., Jacques, P. et al. 2007. Soft drink consumption and risk of developing cardiometabolic risk factors and thee metabolic syndrome in middle-aged adults in the community. *Circulation* 116:480–488.

Ebbeling, C., Leidig, M., Sinclair, K. et al. 2003. A reduced-glycemic load diet in the treatment of adolescent obesity. *Archives of Pediatrics and Adolescent Medicine* 157:773–779.

Ebbeling, C. and Ludwig, D. 2010. Glycemic index, obesity, and diabetes. In *Treatment of the Obese Patient*, eds. R.F. Kusher and D.H. Bessesen, pp. 281–298. Totowa, NJ: Human Press, Inc.

Esfahani, A., Wong, J., Mirrahimi, A. et al. 2009. Glycemic index: Physiological significance. *Journal of the American College of Nutrition* 28(4):439S–445S.

Esfahani, A., Wong, J., Mirrahimi, A. et al. 2010. The application of the glycemic index and glycemic load in weight loss: A review of the clinical evidence. *Life* 63(1):7–13.

Foster-Powell, K., Holt, S., and Brand-Miller, J. 2002. International table of glycemic index and glycemic load values: 2002. *American Journal of Clinical Nutrition* 76:5–56.

Holt, S., Brand, J., Soveny, C. et al. 1992. Relationship of satiety to postprandial glycaemic, insulin and cholecystokinin responses. *Appetite* 18:129–141.

Hu, F., Stampfer, M., Manson, J. et al. 2000. Trends in the incidence of coronary heart disease and changes in diet and lifestyle in women. *The New England Journal of Medicine* 343:530–537.

Jeffery, R. 1996. Does weight cycling present a health risk? *American Journal of Clinical Nutrition* 63(Suppl):452S–455S.

Jenkins, D., Wolever, T., Taylor, R. et al. 1981. Glycemic index of foods: A physiological basis for carbohydrate exchange. *American Journal of Clinical Nutrition* 34:362–366.

Johnston, C. and Buller, A. 2005. Vinegar and peanut products as complementary foods to reduce postprandial glycemia. *Journal of the American Diabetic Association* 105:1939–1942.

Larsen, T., Dalskov, S., van Baak M. et al. 2010. Diets with high or low protein content and glycemic index for weight-loss maintenance. *The New England Journal of Medicine* 363:2102–2113.

Lavin, J. 1997. The effect of sucrose- and aspartame-sweetened drinks on energy intake, hunger and food choice of female, moderately restrained eaters. *International Journal of Obesity* 21:37–42.

Levitan, E., Cook, N., Stampfer, M. et al. 2008. Dietary glycemic index, dietary glycemic load, blood lipids, and C-reactive protein. *Metabolism—Clinical and Experimental* 57(3):437–443.

Liu, S., Manson, J., Buring, J. et al. 2002. Relation between a diet with a high glycemic load and plasma concentrations of high-sensitivity C-reactive protein in middle-aged women. *American Journal of Clinical Nutrition* 75:492–498.

Livesey, G. and Tagami, H. 2009. Interventions to lower the glycemic response to carbohydrate foods with a low-viscosity fiber (resistant maltodextrim): Meta-analysis of randomized controlled trials. *American Journal of Clinical Nutrition* 89:114–125.

Livesey, G., Taylor, R., Hulshof, T. et al. 2008. Glycemic response and health—A systematic review and meta-analysis: Relations between dietary glycemic properties and health outcomes. *American Journal of Clinical Nutrition* 87(S):258S–268S.

Ludwig, D. 2000. Symposium: Dietary composition and obesity: Do we need to look beyond dietary fat? *Journal of Nutrition* 130:280S–283S.

Ludwig, D. 2002. The glycemic index physiological mechanisms relating to obesity, diabetes, and cardiovascular disease. *Journal of the American Medical Association* 287:2414–2423.

McMillan-Price, J. and Brand-Miller, J. 2006. Review Low-glycaemic index diets and body weight regulation. *International Journal of Obesity* 30:540–546.

Micha, R. and Nelson, M. 2011. Glycemic index and glycemic load used in combination to characterize metabolic responses of mixed meals in healthy lean young adults. *Journal of the American College of Nutrition* 30:113–125.

Monro, J. and Shaw, M. 2008. Glycemic impact, glycemic glucose equivalents, glycemic index, and glycemic load: Definitions, distinctions, and implication. *American Journal of Clinical Nutrition* 87(Suppl):237S–243S.

Pawlak, C., Ebbeling C., and Ludwig, D. 2002. Should obese patients be counseled to follow a low-glycaemic index diet? Yes. *Obesity Reviews* 3:235–243.

Salmeron, J., Manson, J.E., Stampfer, M.J. et al. 1997. Dietary fiber, glycemic load, and risk of non-insulin-dependent diabetes mellitus in women. *Journal of the American Medical Association* 277:472–477.

Stevenson, E., Williams, C., Mash, L. et al. 2006. Influence of high-carbohydrate mixed meals with different glycemic indexes on substrate utilization during subsequent exercise in women. *American Journal of Clinical Nutrition* 84:354–360.

Thomas, D., Elliott, E., and Baur, L. 2009. Low glycaemic index or low glycaemic load diets for overweight and obesity (Review). *The Cochrane Library*, Issue 1, pp. 1–38.

Thompson, L., Button, C., and Jenkins, D. 1987. Phytic acid and calcium affect the in vitro rate of navy bean starch digestion and blood glucose response in humans. *American Journal of Clinical Nutrition* 46:467–473.

Wahlqvist, M., Wilmshurst, E., Murton, C. et al. 1978. The effect of chain length on glucose absorption and the related metabolic response. *American Journal of Clinical Nutrition* 31:1998–2001.

Wee, S., Williams, C., Tsintzas, K. et al. 2005. Ingestion of a high-glycemic index meal increases muscle glycogen storage at rest but augments its utilization during subsequent exercise. *Journal of Applied Physiology* 99:707–714.

Wing, R. and Phelan, S. 2005. Long-term weight loss maintenance. *American Journal of Clinical Nutrition* 82(Suppl):222S–225S.

Wolever, T., Jenkins, D., Jenkins, A. et al. 1991. The glycemic index: Methodology and clinical implications. *American Journal of Clinical Nutrition* 54:846–854.

Wolever, T., Jenkins, D., Ocana, A. et al. 1988. Second-meal effect: Low-glycemic-index foods eaten at dinner improve subsequent breakfast glycemic response. *American Journal of Clinical Nutrition* 48:1041–1047.

56 Challenges to the Conduct and Interpretation of Weight Loss Research

Reflections on 35 Years of Weight Loss Research

Gilbert R. Kaats, PhD, FACN and
Harry G. Preuss, MD, MACN, CNS

CONTENTS

MAGNITUDE OF THE OBESITY/OVERWEIGHT PROBLEM

Of all the debilitating health-related conditions and diseases in America today, perhaps none is as widespread and potentially devastating as overweight/obesity. According to Dr. Richard H. Carmona, MD, a former U.S. surgeon general, "Obesity is the terror within. Unless we do something about it, the magnitude of the dilemma will dwarf 9/11 or any other terrorist attempt" [1]. As Dr. Charles Bennett, past editor of the *Harvard Medical Letter* concluded over two decades ago, "No intervention has been shown to consistently achieve true weight control. Although the precise reason for the high relapse rate is not known, the stunning uniformity of these findings, which now extend over nearly five decades, should give pause to anyone who proposes to treat, much less cure, obesity" [2]. Little has changed since Bennett's observation. It is not only the fact that rates are not declining, but a number of studies have suggested that the rates of obesity and overweight have been steadily increasing for the past five decades and have more than doubled in the past 30 years [3–10]. In June 2010, the Trust for America's Health and the Robert Wood Johnson Foundation concluded that adult obesity rates increased in 28 states in the past year and declined only in the District of Columbia (DC) [11]. The report concluded that more than two-thirds of states have adult obesity rates above 25%, whereas in 1991, no state had an obesity rate above 20%. Another study found similar increases in rates and concluded that the predictions concerning the future of obesity are even more sobering. For example, in 2007, the U.K. Government Office for Science's *Foresight Report* estimated that by 2050, 60% of men and 50% of women will be clinically obese. Other analyses project that obese adults in the United States will increase by 65 million, and in the United Kingdom, by 11 million, resulting in approximately 7 million cases of diabetes, 6 million cases of heart disease and stroke, 492,000–669,000 additional cases of cancer, and 26–55 million quality-adjusted life years forgone for the United States and the United Kingdom combined [12]. Even more troubling, a U.S. researcher extended the current trends into future projections suggesting that by 2015, 75% of all U.S. adults will be overweight or obese; by 2030 that number will be 86.3%, and by 2048 all American adults will be overweight or obese [13].

FINANCIAL BURDEN OF OBESITY/OVERWEIGHT

The previously cited *Foresight Report* estimates that obesity-related diseases will cost the United Kingdom £45–£50 billion a year that "…could develop into a massive problem not just for the UK, but globally" [14]. The combined medical costs associated with treatment of these preventable diseases are estimated to increase by $48–$66 billion a year in the United States and by £1.9–£2 billion a year in the United Kingdom by 2030. An estimate released by the Organization for Economic Cooperation and Development [15] concluded that the annual cost of treating obesity in the U.S. adult noninstitutionalized population is $168.4 billion, which translates into 16.5% of national spending on medical care. They also suggest that their data imply that previous estimates of the medical costs of obesity have significantly underestimated the cost-effectiveness of antiobesity interventions and the economic rationale for government intervention to reduce obesity-related disorders. Their data are consistent with data reported by a number of other researchers [16–28]. These costs come about primarily because obesity is associated with an increased risk of myocardial infarction, stroke, type 2 diabetes, hypertension, osteoarthritis, asthma, and depression [29]. Other studies have found significant associations between obesity and virtually every type of cancer [30] increased mortality [31–35] and quality of life [20]. Conversely, significant improvements in virtually all of these risk factors and quality of life have been associated with fat reduction [36].

PROBLEM IS FAT, NOT WEIGHT

The risk factors associated with obesity and overweight are, more correctly, the results of excess body fat, not excess body weight. It is well established that excess fat accelerates the risk factors for major degenerative diseases such as ischemic heart disease, congestive heart failure, stroke, cancer, respiratory disease, diabetes, hyperlipidemia, hypertension, asthma, sleep apnea, arthritis, degenerative joint disease, gastric reflux, and depression [37–40]. Until recently, accumulation of excess body fat has been attributed to overeating symptomatic of poor discipline, lack of willpower and self-control, or underlying psychological pathologies. From this perspective, the cure for obesity and overweight is to cure these underlying personality issues. In spite of the fact that there has been little evidence to support this view, it nevertheless influenced weight control effort for decades. Contrary to the dearth of evidence to support this psychological view, there is increasing evidence implicating genetic and neurochemical–neuroendocrine factors in the brain. Under this rubric, obesity becomes a chronic disease like hypertension or diabetes.

Another line of research supporting this paradigm shift suggests that stored fat itself produces adverse metabolic effects derived from secretions of fatty acids from enlarged fat cells. These fat cells are believed to be stored in liver and muscle cells and exacerbate insulin resistance by overwhelming the pancreas. This view suggests that body fat acts as an endocrine organ and leads to insulin resistance and type 2 diabetes. One of the clearest statements of this shift is George A. Bray's seminal report, in which he summarizes studies supporting these adverse metabolic effects:

> This concept of the pathogenesis of obesity as a disease allows an easy division of disadvantages of obesity into those produced by the mass of fat and those produced by the metabolic effects of fat cells. In the former category are the social disabilities resulting from the stigma associated with obesity, sleep apnea that results in part from increased parapharyngeal fat deposits, and osteoarthritis resulting from the wear and tear on joints from carrying an increased mass of fat. The second category includes the metabolic factors associated with distant effects of products released from enlarged fat cells. The insulin-resistant state that is so common in obesity probably reflects the effects of increased release of fatty acids from fat cells that are then stored in the liver or muscle. When the secretory capacity of the pancreas is overwhelmed by battling insulin resistance, diabetes develops. The strong association of increased fat, especially visceral fat, with diabetes makes this consequence particularly ominous for health care costs. The release of cytokines, particularly IL-6, from the fat cell may stimulate the proinflammatory state that characterizes obesity. The increased secretion of prothrombin activator inhibitor-1 from fat cells may play a role in the procoagulant state of obesity and, along with changes in endothelial function, may be responsible for the increased risk of cardiovascular disease and hypertension. For cancer, the production of estrogens by the enlarged stromal mass plays a role in the risk for breast cancer. Increased cytokine release may play a role in other forms of proliferative growth. The combined effect of these pathogenetic consequences of increased fat stores is an increased risk of shortened life expectancy [40].

This view places the emphasis on body fat, not body weight, and suggests the need to measure body composition (lean, fat, and bone) as the primary outcome measure of weight loss interventions; it calls into question the value of using scale weight changes or the body mass index (BMI) as appropriate outcome measures. But even depletion of excess body fat does not tell the whole story. The benefits of depleting excess body fat will be attenuated, even negated, if depletion of fat results in a concomitant loss of lean and bone mineral density (BMD). Thus, the litmus test for evaluating the safety and efficacy of weight loss interventions is the extent to which the intervention improved body composition by depleting excess fat while maintaining, or ideally, increasing bone density and metabolically active lean tissue. Unfortunately, use of the BMI does not adequately meet that standard.

BODY MASS INDEX ≠ BODY FAT

Even though there is strong evidence that the risk factors associated with obesity and overweight are due not to excess scale weight but to excess body fat, scale weight and BMI continue to be used as outcome measures. For example, in spite of the fact that the Robert Woods Johnson Foundation's report cited earlier, "F as in Fat: How Obesity Threatens America's Future 2010" [11], it provides no actual data on changes in fat, but rather only on changes in scale weight using the BMI, the most common measure used to define obesity and evaluate the outcome of weight loss interventions. The BMI is not a measure fat; it is only an estimate of fat derived from the relationship between height and weight. Furthermore, as a measure of change, BMI reflects only change in scale weight since height typically remains constant from trial to trial. The deficiencies in using scale weight and/or the BMI as outcome measures have been reported in a number of studies [41–45]. As one researcher concludes,

> Virtually all social science research related to obesity uses body mass index (BMI), usually calculated using self-reported values of weight and height, or clinical weight, classifications based on BMI. Yet there is widespread agreement in the medical literature that such measures are seriously flawed because they do not distinguish fat from fat-free mass such as muscle and bone…. Despite the widespread use of BMI among social scientists, within the medical literature BMI is considered to be a very limited measure of fatness and obesity because it does not distinguish body composition [44].

In our own database of over 24,000 dual energy x-ray absorptiometry (DXA) total body measurements, one of the most reliable measurements of body composition, the BMI correlated 67% with measured fat levels, thus accounting for just 33% of between-individual differences in percent body fat—a figure consistent with other researchers who have reported that it accounted for only 25% of between-individual differences in percent body fat [44]. These and other data prompted an editorial in *Lancet* that concluded "…the current practice with body-mass index as a measure of obesity is obsolete, and results in considerable underestimation of the grave consequences of the overweight epidemic" [46]. BMI and stroke for younger subjects, but not from older subjects, suggesting that the loss of lean body mass with age may lead to a reduction in BMI, but may also result in an increase in percent body fat. In this case, BMI may no longer capture the impact of adiposity on disease risk. Since strokes often occur among the elderly, other measures such as waist circumference or waist-to-hip ratio may provide better assessment of obesity-related risk. This is not to suggest that use of the BMI be abandoned, but rather that when clinical trials are initially being conducted to assess the effects of a weight loss intervention, changes in body composition should be reported as the primary outcome measure.

IMPROVING BODY COMPOSITION: A LITMUS TEST OF SAFETY AND EFFICACY

An often overlooked adverse effect of weight loss is that it typically depletes fat-free mass (FFM) and BMD with or without depletion of excess fat. Even when an intervention reduces excess fat, these benefits will be attenuated if it also depletes lean and BMD, a common outcome from weight loss and one that distorts the safety and efficacy of the outcome. In fact, the weight change may actually mask positive or negative changes in body composition. Thus, it is not the amount but rather the kind of weight that is lost or gained that is a much more accurate measure of the safety and efficacy of a weight loss intervention. It has been our experience that a body composition improvement (BCI) index [47,48] can best capture these changes. The BCI is the net result of scoring gains in lean and decreases in fat as positive outcomes and losses in lean and increases in fat as negative outcomes. Accordingly, a person gaining 2.0 lb of lean and losing 2.0 lb of fat would have no change in scale weight, thus suggesting a lack of effect. However he or she would have a BCI of +4 suggesting a positive outcome since both of the changes in lean and fat are positive outcomes. Conversely, a person losing 2 lb of lean and gaining 2 lb of fat would have no change in scale weight, but would have a −4 BCI since both of these changes are considered negative outcomes. Using only scale weight instead of the BCI would lead one to conclude that both interventions were ineffective, while, in fact, one intervention was effective, and the other was ineffective.

To examine the difference between using changes in scale weight as opposed to using the BCI, we compared changes of over 15,000 body composition measurements in the our database. Differences were based on five possible outcomes:

1. No change in scale weight, but a positive BCI
2. No change in scale weight, but a negative BCI
3. No change in scale weight and no change in body composition with a BCI of 0
4. Gain in scale weight, but a negative BCI
5. Loss of scale weight, but a positive BCI

Different conclusions would be drawn about the success or failure of weight loss interventions in 84% of the 15,000 changes when comparing results using scale weight as the outcome measure as opposed to using the BCI. Furthermore, the average difference between the scale weight changes versus the BCI was 8.1 lb. Thus, not only is this problem widespread, but it can seriously mislead anyone reviewing the safety and efficacy of weight loss interventions.

We have no evidence as to how much muscle it takes to offset gains in body fat or how much fat one has to lose to offset losses in metabolic active lean. But what is clear is that loss of lean and gains of body fat are clearly negative treatment outcomes irrespective of any changes in scale weight and need to be addressed. Thus, as we said earlier, the litmus test of a safe and efficacious weight loss program is the preservation of lean and bone and the depletion of excess body fat. In short, the *kind*, not the *amount*, of weight that is lost or gained is the appropriate measure of positive or negative outcomes. Thus, when using the BCI as a primary outcome measure, the challenge for weight loss interventions is to incorporate components that will not only facilitate the depletion of excess fat but will also support retention or increases in FFM. In our view, two components that are most likely to provide this benefit are increases in physical activity (PA) and health literacy.

PHYSICAL ACTIVITY

While the need to exercise and eat a healthy diet are often stated as requirements for weight loss interventions, few research protocols and marketing campaigns offer realistic plans that are likely to be adopted as a permanent lifestyle change. However, using the BCI as an outcome measure virtually dictates inclusion of PA to facilitate the retention or, ideally, the increases in FFM. While adding dietary supplements may have a positive effect on FFM, their benefit is likely to be minimal, or even nonexistent, unless accompanied by increased PA. Therein lays the challenge for weight loss studies, particularly those with interventions suggesting that taking a supplement or medication will enable the user to lose weight without changing diet or exercise. Use of the BCI counters suggestions that a "magic" pill, potion, or medication will lead to weight loss; it increases the need to provide a weight loss *plan*, not just a weight loss product. Thus, in reality, the product becomes the plan.

In our accompanying chapter on exercise, we review decades of compelling evidence supporting the weight loss and health benefits of exercise. However, in spite of overwhelming evidence and pervasive regulatory, medical, and public exhortations to exercise, there is little evidence that these campaigns have had any noticeable effect on the increasingly sedentary lifestyles of Americans. For many, the definition of exercise is "the art of converting big meals and fattening snacks into back strains and pulled muscles by lifting heavy things that didn't have to be lifted in the first place, or running when no one is chasing you." We suggest that the major resistances (or rationalizations) to exercise are a lack of time, motivation, physical difficulties, and lack of financial resources. Although the medical community has long encouraged physicians to promote exercise to their patients, few actually do, citing lack of time, inadequate reimbursement, unfamiliarity with appropriate techniques, and repeated observations of patient noncompliance. It is also difficult for physicians to ascertain the veracity of patient self-reports since patients typically overestimate the amount of time spent exercising. One study found that most people, particularly those who have sedentary lifestyles, tend to overstate how much they exercise, often by as much as three times.

It is our conclusion that use of a pedometer and tracking of daily step totals can lead to increased PA by capitalizing on a well-established behavior modification principle: "What gets measured, gets managed; what gets measured and tracked, gets managed better; what gets measured, tracked and fed-back, gets managed even better." Pedometer usage is also consistent with a reframing of "exercise" as "physical activity." This reframing is not just a matter of semantics, but rather one of the substances based on growing evidence that encouraging PA, as opposed to exercise, is more likely to facilitate behavior change. This new view of PA is suggested in the U.S. Surgeon General's report on Physical Activity and Health [49] that brings together, for the first time, what has been learned about PA and health from decades of research. Among the report's major findings are that people

TABLE 56.1
Click-Equivalents

Bowling	55
Cycling, 5 mph	55
Dancing (slow)	55
Shopping for groceries	60
Walking, 2 mph (30 min/mile)	60
Canoeing, 2.5 mph	70
Golfing (with a cart)	70
Volleyball (leisurely)	70
Rowing (leisurely)	75
Vacuuming	75
Washing the car	75
Window cleaning	75
Painting	80
Walking, 3 mph (20 min/mile)	80
Mopping	85
Gardening, moderate	90
Housework	90
Ping pong	90
Ice skating (leisurely)	95
Dancing (noncontact)	100
Golfing (walking, without cart)	100
Walking, 4 mph (15 min/mile)	100
Waxing the car	100
Tennis (doubles)	110
Aerobic dancing (low impact)	115
Swimming (25 yards/min)	120
Volleyball (game)	120
Bicycling, 10 mph (6 min/mile)	125
Weight training (90 s between sets)	125
Basketball (leisurely, nongame)	130
Snow skiing, downhill	130
Mowing	135
Scrubbing the floor	140
Stair climbing	140
Aerobics step training, 4″ step (beginner)	145
Badminton	150
Roller skating (moderate)	150
Cross-country snow skiing (leisurely)	155
Gardening (heavy)	155
Hiking, no load	155
Stair climber machine	160
Tennis (singles)	160
Water skiing	160
Ice skating (competitive)	170
Dancing (fast)	175
Backpacking with 10 lb load	180
Hiking with a 10 lb load	180

TABLE 56.1 (continued)
Click-Equivalents

Rowing machine	180
Jogging, 5 mph (12 min/mile)	185
Aerobics (intense)	190
Scuba diving	190
Weight training (60 s between sets)	190
Snow shoveling	195
Soccer (competitive)	195
Cycling, 15 mph (5 min/mile)	200
Elliptical jogger (medium)	200
Racquetball	205
Squash	205
Cross-country snow skiing, moderate	220
Basketball (game)	220
Swimming (50 yards/min)	225
Jogging, 6 mph (10 min/mile)	230
Backpacking with 30 lb load	235
Hiking with a 30 lb load	235
Weight training (40 s between sets)	255
Elliptical jogger (fast)	270
Skipping rope	285
Swimming (75 yards/min)	290
Running, 8 mph (7.5 min/mile)	305
Cross-country snow skiing, intense	330
Running, 10 mph (6 min/mile)	350

---

who are usually inactive can improve their health and well-being by becoming even moderately active, and that PA need not be strenuous in order to achieve significant health benefits. When using a pedometer, people are encouraged to find ways in their daily activities to increase their step totals without taking additional time out of their day, for instance, by pacing or walking while talking on the phone. This is not to suggest that people refrain from exercising, but rather to view it as one of many ways to increase daily step totals. There also are a number of activities where a pedometer cannot be worn (e.g., swimming) or the user simply may not wish to wear it. When analyzing activity levels or incorporating them into treatment plans, these activities can be added to daily step totals as "step-equivalents" by using Table 56.1.

While a plethora of studies and health-care providers have cited the deleterious effects of a sedentary lifestyle, there is no standard definition of sedentary. Additionally, many studies that have drawn conclusions about the effects of sedentary behavior have not actually measured this behavior. Despite frequent claims regarding the harmful health effects of sedentary behavior "… investigators have rarely measured sedentary behavior in direct ways…in the future, investigators should focus as much attention on the lower end of the activity intensity continuum as has traditionally been placed on the higher end of that continuum if valid conclusions … are to be made" [50]. When incorporating step-equivalent data, pedometer data can go a long way in meeting this need and objectifying the health effects of varied levels of PA. In addition to direct measurements of PA, pedometer usage can lead to significant increases in health literacy.

HEALTH LITERACY

The U.S. surgeon general has suggested that "Promoting health literacy is perhaps the most important role of any health professional" [51]. Health literacy is typically defined as the degree to which individuals have the capacity to obtain, process, and understand basic information and services needed to make appropriate decisions about their health. We would add to that definition "and provide motivation to implement these decisions." We think that pedometers can provide some of this motivation by providing users with an objective and a continual stream of feedback throughout the day. For many, this is a "wake-up call" as to how sedentary they actually are, dispelling beliefs that their activity levels are average or above average. Additionally, providing the user with the wealth of research data suggesting the positive effects of realistic and achievable increases in PA can empower the user to make these changes. For example, the DHHS PA guidelines [49] suggest that persons reporting moderate amounts of activity have a 20% lower risk of CHD and CVD morbidity and mortality, and those reporting activity of even higher levels have a 30% lower risk than least active persons. As pointed out in an editorial on the beneficial effects, "To put this benefit in proper perspective, this risk reduction [from increased PA] equals or exceeds that for statins.... The potential impact of increasing physical activity on CHD-associated health care is astounding" [52]. Even more specific, in a study of 416,175 individuals who participated in brisk walking for 92 min a week had a 14% reduced risk of all-cause mortality, a 3 year longer life expectancy, and all-cancer mortality by 1%. Even more dramatic were estimates provided by the Mayo Clinic [53] that compared the effects on major degenerative diseases realized from increasing one's daily activity level by what we estimated was equivalent to 3000 and 6000 steps or step-equivalents from the time a person awakes in the morning until they retire at night. Our bar-graphed interpretation of their data is present in Figure 56.1.

As opposed to focusing on the adverse effects of sedentary lifestyles, we have found it more empowering to provide people with data on how they can reduce their risk factors for disease in conjunction with reducing their excess body fat while retaining metabolically active FFM. The key to validating the effects of weight loss plans is to obtain accurate and reliable measurements of fat and FFM. Total body DXA measurement meets this need.

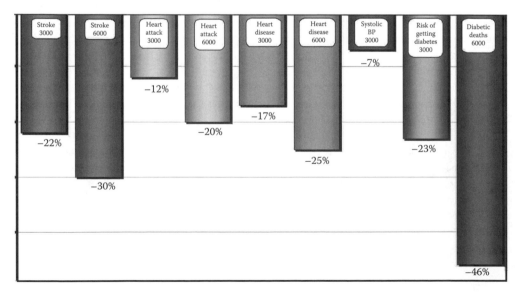

FIGURE 56.1 Health benefits from increasing daily step totals from baseline by 3000 and 6000 steps a day. (Graphic adapted Mayo Clinic, *Mayo Clinic Health Lett,* 12(1), 1, 2008.)

ASSESSING BODY COMPOSITION WITH DUAL ENERGY X-RAY ABSORPTIOMETRY

Because of its high precision and reliability, low scanning time, and simplicity for the person being tested, the FDA-approved DXA technology is considered the "gold standard" for measuring total and regional bone density, fat, and lean mass. With the exception of the MRI, other "measures" of body composition, including hydrodensitometry, are not measures, but rather estimates. DXA actually x-rays tissue and bone; other techniques estimate these components. Its three-compartment measurement of total and regional fat, lean, and bone suggests that it is the preferred litmus test for assessing the safety and efficacy of weight loss interventions.

PRECISION AND RELIABILITY

In October 1995, the FDA approved the DXA test for the measurement of body composition (lean-to-fat ratios) and generated a plethora of studies over the next decade that led one reviewer to conclude that DXA is among the most critically analyzed body composition instruments available today [54]. DXA has been found to correlate with actual skeletal mass, total body calcium, and body fat as determined by neutron activation analysis [55]. DXA's typical precision error for total body bone mineral content is less than 1% [56]. It has been shown to be a precise method for assessing body composition [57–60], strongly correlating with underwater weighing [61], deuterium dilution [62], and total body potassium. DXA has been found to be an accurate and practical measurement of body composition in young children [63,64], the elderly [65], and obese subjects [66,67]. It has been shown to accurately detect small changes in body composition [65]. DXA's superiority over other assessments of body composition is due to the fact that it also provides actual measurements, not estimates, of total body and regional adipose tissue and BMD. Hydrodensitometry, dilutional methods, neutron activation analysis, bioelectrical impedance, infrared radiation, and skinfold calipers, in contrast, are based on assumptions that elemental composition remains constant and that the relative percentages of bone in FFM and of water in lean tissue are invariable—assumptions that have yet to be validated. One study measured the body composition of piglets weighing between 14 and 22 kg [64]. DXA's high reliability allows monitoring of the short-term effects of dietary and exercise interventions on regional and total body composition.

ASSESSMENT OF VISCERAL FAT

Although, as reviewed previously, total body fat is associated with a wide variety of disorders, abdominal or visceral fat (VF) may be an independent risk factor for many of these disorders. DXA provides an alternative to CT scans since DXA can accurately assess total and abdominal fat mass and has the advantages of being a low-cost and relatively quick procedure involving much less exposure to ionizing radiation. Compared with anthropological methods, DEXA has the advantage of being able to measure both total body and regional fat mass [58,68–70]. Although general obesity is an important risk factor for many diseases, human studies have demonstrated that VF accrual is most strongly related to many health conditions, including CVD [71] and insulin resistance [72], as well as increased death from all causes [73]. Another study reported a significant association between VF and inflammation concluding, "Our results suggest a relationship between central adiposity and inflammation process, irrespective of age and other potential confounders. This association was more prominent than the relationship between total obesity and inflammation. It could be hypothesized that a disproportionate accumulation of visceral fat mass could be partially associated with increased coronary risk, through inflammation process" [74]. Adiposity-related increases in arterial stiffness have also been reported as one of the potential pathways through which VF could lead to cardiovascular disease [75,76]. Epidemiologic studies have implicated abdominal obesity as a major risk factor for insulin resistance, type 2 diabetes, cardiovascular disease, stroke, metabolic syndrome, and death [77]. These researchers also report that "Increases in trunk mass and decreases in peripheral fat mass are associated with accelerated arterial stiffening. These findings emphasize the importance of assessing regional changes in body composition, because it may enable identification of individuals with an unrecognized increased cardiovascular disease risk."

SAFETY CONSIDERATIONS

A position paper released jointly by committees from the American College of Radiology (ACR) and the Radiological Society of North America [78] concluded that "There is always a slight chance of cancer from excessive exposure to radiation. However, the benefit of an accurate diagnosis far outweighs the risk. The effective radiation dose from this procedure is about 0.01 mSv, which is about the same as the average person receives from background radiation in one day. Women should always inform their physician or x-ray technologist if there is any possibility that they are pregnant. No complications are expected with the DXA procedure."

BENEFITS OF DXA TESTING

Informed consent forms list both risks and benefits that subjects are likely to experience during the study. They can affect subjects' willingness to participate and can influence the Institutional Review Boards' decisions as well. For some subjects, the benefit can be significant in view of the relatively high price of a DXA test that is often not covered by most third-party payers. Total body DXA measurements can, in some cases, make a profound contribution to subjects by providing a more realistic and achievable goal weight. Many overweight women have spent years attempting to achieve unrealistic goal weights due to the cultural pressure for thinness. For example, at the conclusion of a study, we provided a young woman with DXA results revealing a realistic goal weight of ~150 lb based on her high level of lean mass. She reported that throughout her teen age years she weighed between 170 and 180 lb and had been on several diets to achieve a recommended goal weight of 125 lb, consistent with her BMI. But on each diet, when she reached ~150 lb, she hit a plateau and almost no matter what she did, she could not lose any more. Her parents and coaches lost confidence in her, believing she had given up the diet and was being dishonest about her eating behavior and PA levels. The problem, as the DXA test revealed, was that 125 lb was an unrealistic goal weight based on her unusually high level of lean. A more realistic goal weight would have been 150—the point at which she "got stuck" and at which she was seen as being dishonest. Thus, she had spent her teenage years striving to reach an unrealistic "socially driven" goal weight instead of learning how to adjust to being a large woman in a society almost obsessed with thinness.

PARADIGM SHIFT IN THE CONCEPTUALIZATION OF OBESITY INTERVENTIONS

Traditional approaches to obesity interventions have typically encouraged dieters to modify food selection and portion sizes and to make lifestyle changes to achieve weight loss [79]. Yet, even highly motivated and nutritionally informed dieters often struggle to refrain from highly palatable, energy-dense foods available in the modern environment, and ultimately, only a small percentage of individuals achieve sustained weight loss through dietary modification [80–82]. Failed attempts at weight control are frustrating to dieters and health-care providers alike, both of whom frequently attribute obesity to the result of poor food choices and/or lack of discipline or willpower [83–85]. For example, a sample of British dietitians ranked "lack of willpower" as more important to the development of obesity than genetic factors [86] even though there is sufficient evidence that genetics contribute 55%–75% to adult body mass [87,88]. This not only stigmatizes the obese but has important effects on public policy and health-care insurance [89,90].

More recently, contrary to the willpower and lifestyle modification emphasis, there is increasing evidence to support metabolic and neurobiologically based explanations of behavior. With regard to metabolic changes, an increasing number of studies have identified physiological factors involved in overweight and obesity [91–102]. These studies suggest that the pleasure of eating has been traced to the brain's reward circuit similar to that found for engaging in compulsive sex, gambling, and substance abuse. Typical of this paradigm shift is the view expressed by a leading obesity researcher as cited earlier who has concluded that fat cells should be viewed as a type of endocrine cell and adipose tissue as an endocrine organ [40].

IMPACT OF INCLUSION/EXCLUSION CRITERIA

One challenge facing all studies is that the more extensive the inclusion/exclusion criteria, the less likely the results can be generalized to the population that is most likely to purchase the product or participate in the intervention being tested. Since the study is evaluating a product or intervention that often has never been studied before, there is no reliable evidence upon which to exclude or include subjects. Furthermore, when multiple ingredients are contained in the intervention being evaluated, it is even less likely that there is any evidence of interactive effects since the total effect can be greater, or less than, the sum of the parts. Absent this information, judgments are often made by excluding subjects who have health conditions that are thought to make participation unwise. However, this suggests that the study will be safe for subjects with pathologies that were not listed as exclusion criteria, which could result in enrolling high-risk subjects. Even if a physical is provided as an inclusion criterion, the physician conducting the physical rarely has sufficient medical information to make a judgment regarding inclusion. We have found a more effective method is to require subjects to review the study with their personal physician to ensure the subject has no preexisting conditions that would exclude participation.

PAYING FOR TRACKING/REPORTING INSTEAD OF PAYING INCENTIVES

Although payment of incentive fees is more likely to encourage compliance, it is not without its problems. Consideration must be given to whether or not the incentive payment is so high that it will encourage enrollment of high-risk subjects that would not otherwise enroll. It may also encourage subjects to remain in studies even though they are experiencing and not reporting adverse effects. It also may encourage dishonest reporting of violations of the study protocol. We have found that a more effective method of paying subjects is to pay for tracking or reporting fees under the conditions that the tracking fee will be paid irrespective of the subject's compliance with the research protocol. Subjects need to be told and reminded that the fee is for candid reporting and will allow for dose-related analyses, so even non- or partially compliant subjects will be contributing to the study. This candid reporting concept needs to be made clear throughout the study to ensure that subjects know that the emphasis is not on taking the product or following the protocol. Subjects should be reminded that the tracking fee will be paid even if they take less than or even none of the product being tested and even if they withdraw from the study as long as the subject reports that they have dropped, are no longer taking the product, and meet the requirements for completing the ending tests.

In one of our own studies, subjects were required to complete the ending tests to receive their tracking bonus irrespective of how well or poorly they adhered to the study protocol. Obviously, this increases the number of people who are willing to take these tests and allowed for a dose-related analysis between compliant and partially compliant subjects. However, when using this procedure, it is important that the required tests have minimal or no risk for subjects. When we used this procedure, we required that subjects complete a quality of life questionnaire, DXA test, and a 43-panel blood test. While the questionnaire is virtually risk-free, we have found the benefits from taking the DXA and blood test are much greater than the minimal risk posed by completing these tests. We have tested these assertions in post-study anonymous critiques, and, while some subjects reported that the tests were annoying and time consuming, the vast majority reported that they were aware of this requirement as it was stated in the informed consent and they agreed to participate with full knowledge of the requirement. Furthermore, the vast majority reported they thought that receiving the feedback from the test results was highly beneficial. None of the subjects reported that they were offended by the requirement or saw it as infringement on the rights as a subject.

COMPLIANCE/ADHERENCE: MAKING LEMONADE FROM LEMONS

There is considerable inconsistency in the use of the terms persistence, compliance, and adherence when describing the extent to which subjects prescribed follow protocols [103]. As used here, persistence is defined as following the intervention from the beginning to the end or for the recommended length of time. Compliance refers to following the timing, dose, and frequency of the intervention [104], and adherence is defined as encompassing both persistence and compliance. Adherence to medications is typically poor [105–108]. Although reasons for this lack of adherence vary, a number of studies have reported adherence is typically higher when the intervention produces short-term, for example, 90 days, [109] observable and measurable effects, such as in weight loss studies [110]. But weight loss studies face challenges that are often absent in many studies. For example, if the outcome measures are changes in lipids or other blood chemistries, subjects rarely know their measurements at baseline and virtually never take these tests on their own during the study period. However, subjects in weight loss studies typically weigh themselves at baseline and throughout the study period. If the intervention is designed to deplete fat while maintaining, or increasing, FFM, gains in lean can offset losses in fat, suggesting the intervention is failing when, in reality, it is succeeding. As will be discussed later, this becomes even more troublesome in placebo studies where a lack of sufficient changes in scale weight can lead subjects to incorrectly conclude that they have received the placebo. In our own research, post-study critiques revealed that among subjects who thought they had the placebo, over half of them were mistaken. Even more troublesome was that most of these subjects reported that they were convinced that they had the placebo.

USE OF A TRUSTEE

Recent concerns have been reported about undue influence sponsors may have on conclusions drawn from independent research. For example, an article in *Science Magazine* pointed out that

> An almost steady flow of articles have focused on the dangers or lack of efficacy of widely used drugs, along with allegations of hidden information, misinterpreted data, regulatory missteps, and corporate malfeasance. Many of these accounts involve analyses of research on human volunteers that had never been publicly disseminated. The uproar caused by an analysis of previously unpublished studies of the diabetes drug, Avandia, indicating that it may be harmful is one recent example. As a result, many question whether sufficient information about the safety and efficacy of medical interventions is available to the public [111].

Two years later, the U.S. Senate Finance Committee released a 334-page investigation of the RECORD trial of rosiglitazone and drug maker GlaxoSmithKline [112]. The Committee released documents and internal company e-mails that provided an extraordinary window into the conduct of an industry-sponsored clinical trial. The implications of these e-mails and other documents released by the Senate raised serious concerns as to the profound consequences by industry manipulating physician-scientists. The RECORD trial illustrates the consequences that an absence of independent access to all of the data in the trial may allow physician-scientists to be manipulated by the sponsor, resulting in a manuscript that does not provide the most accurate assessment of the risks and benefits of the therapy [113]. The use of an independent trustee/statistician from a local university who receives and stores all source data until the study is complete could help assuage these concerns [114]. Since the trustee is independent of the organization conducting the research, there is less chance of either conscious or unconscious bias. In our studies, we have used an independent university statistician as the principal investigator [115] and employed an attorney as a trustee who performed the same functions [116]. Both procedures seemed to allay the concerns about the integrity in industry-sponsored research.

CHALLENGES TO USING BLOOD CHEMISTRIES AS SAFETY MEASURES

Conducting baseline and ending multitest blood chemistry panels can provide an additional measure of safety that can prove valuable when evaluating untested weight loss products and plans. For some chemistries, increases or decreases will suggest positive or negative outcomes, for example, total cholesterol, LDL cholesterol, triglycerides, glucose, A1C, and HDL. For these chemistries, calculation of significant levels will provide meaningful safety data. But for many chemistries, changes are not as clear cut, and increases or decreases can both suggest either positive or negative outcomes, for example, white and red blood cell counts, albumin, and bilirubin. In these cases, it may be more appropriate to report the number of changes that were above or below the normal range at baseline and became either normal or abnormal during the study.

PLACEBO CHALLENGES

Placebo protocols have long been touted as the "gold standard" protocol. However, when used in weight loss studies, placebo protocols pose unique challenges. For example, when conducting a study on baseline-ending changes of lipid levels, there are no obvious or overt indications of how the lipids are changing during the study. Subjects rarely, if ever, have their lipids measured during the study, so subjects have virtually no idea how effective the intervention is. This is not the case with weight loss interventions where scale weights are readily available to subjects and they typically weigh themselves throughout the study and hypothesize about whether they have the active product or the placebo. Since scale weight can change for a variety of reasons unrelated to the product or plan, it is not uncommon for study participants to draw incorrect conclusions as to whether or not they are receiving a placebo that affects their motivation and compliance. In fact, when we had subjects complete anonymous questionnaires at the conclusion of a placebo study, over 80% said early in the study they hypothesized about having the placebo, and 30% said they were certain that their hypothesis was correct based on observed changes in their scale weight. Over 50% were wrong. It seems axiomatic that subjects who believe they are receiving a placebo will be less motivated and compliant than those who believe they are receiving the active product. This potential bias can be particularly troublesome when the plan is effective in improving lean-to-fat ratios. Gains in lean mass can mask losses of body fat, leaving scale weight virtually unchanged and creating the illusion that the plan is ineffective.

As with all studies, a potential bias exists from those who volunteer and those who do not, and the longer the trial, the more likely the bias. But the potential for bias seems to be greater in weight loss studies due to the motivational state of potential subjects. People often postpone dieting until something motivates them to start, for example, a reunion, a wedding, or a new boyfriend or girlfriend. Once they decide to do something about their weight and are highly motivated to start dieting or to participate in a research study, few of these highly motivated subjects are willing to run the risk of receiving a placebo. They will often choose not to participate, thus losing subjects who are likely to be the most compliant of all participants, thereby creating enrollment biases. In any case, it would seem prudent to query subjects at the conclusion of the study as to their beliefs about whether or not they received the placebo and how certain they are about their beliefs.

Compliance itself has a biasing effect since it does not affect placebo results as much as it does treatment results. Failure to take the product as prescribed has little effect on the placebo group since the placebo is inactive and failing to take something that would have no effect anyway is unlikely to distort the data. But failure to comply in the treatment group will attenuate the effect since the noncompliers will be taking less product.

Another difficulty when using placebos protocols is when the study involves drink mixes, chewables, nutrition bars, meal replacement shakes, etc. In these cases, it is almost impossible to match placebo products to the taste, texture, smell, and appearance of the active products.

In view of these challenges, alternative protocols need to be considered. One variety of these protocols is to complete baseline testing on the entire study participant population and then randomly assign participants to the treatment group or active control group. In the latter group, participants are asked to pursue any weight loss program of their own choosing and, at the end of the study period, return and complete the same end-of-study tests completed by the treatment group.

CER provides another alternative to placebo protocols and may have some added benefits as well as added challenges as we have discussed in a recent editorial [117]. CER is typically defined as the generation and synthesis of evidence comparing the benefits and risks of different interventions for preventing, diagnosing, treating, and monitoring health conditions under real-world patient conditions that typically confront physicians. CER shares some of the same characteristics of practical clinical trials that use real-world conditions to compare treatment choices practitioners face in patients drawn from their practice to allow them to decide between treatment options. CER is a marked departure from the efficacy and safety research typically used by the FDA to approve medications and devices where approval is often granted based on relatively small placebo studies conducted over relatively short periods under conditions unrepresentative of those encountered in daily practice. Typically, the only efficacy standard is that the new intervention outperforms placebo or randomized control groups. Thus, new interventions can be approved irrespective of whether they represent actual improvements in cost, safety, and efficacy over existing interventions. This informational vacuum can lead to approval of a number of "me too" interventions that ultimately rely more on the sponsor's ability to market the product to gain consumer acceptance that may be no better, less safe, or more costly than usual care but can be easily marketed. However, publication of the results of CER studies will also require a paradigm shift in the scientific community where the use of placebo or control groups in studies submitted for publication significantly increases the authors' chances of having their manuscript published.

CONCLUDING REMARKS

Obesity and overweight are obviously the result of complex interactions of multiple biological, biochemical, neurological, social, and unknown variables. However, at the risk of oversimplifying these complex processes, it seems to us that successful weight control is a function of two opposing and counteracting process—body fat and lean. The struggle for weight control seems to be heavily influenced by the countering effects of excess fat and metabolically active FFM, particularly muscle mass. We think there is abundant evidence that increases in fat mass have an adverse and self-perpetuating effect of accelerating the risk factors associated with most major degenerative diseases. We have also concluded that, for many people struggling with weight, this process is further aggravated by an addictive-like response to certain types of foods, particularly those containing simple carbohydrates such as sugar and refined flours. Increased fat also tends to make people more lethargic, making PA more difficult. Excess fat also has a negative effect on physical appearance exacerbated in the American culture that places a high social value on thinness. Thus, for some people, as fat increases, social activity decreases. Thus, excess fat becomes self-perpetuating—the fatter one is, the fatter one is likely to get. Conversely, FFM seems to have many opposite and opposing effects. It increases metabolism, reduces the risks for osteopenia and osteoporosis by preserving bone density, decreases sarcopenia (the age-related decline in muscle tissue) and improves physical appearance and energy levels.

It is the net result of these two opposing forces that determines effective weight control. The challenge for medicine and the weight loss industry is to develop products, technologies, and treatment plans that will improve body composition by reducing excess body fat without concomitant losses of FFM, and ideally, by facilitating gains in FFM. In our view, the pathway to safe and efficacious weight control is, simply put, improving body composition. Therefore, the BCI index should be one of the primary outcome measures for any intervention to improve body weight.

REFERENCES

1. U.S. Department of Health and Human Services. 2010. *The Surgeon General's Vision for a Healthy and Fit Nation*. Office of the Surgeon General, Rockville, MD.
2. Bennett WI. 1991. Obesity is not an eating disorder. *HMHL* 8:4–6.
3. Johns Hopkins Bloomberg School of Public Health. 2007. Obesity rates continue to climb in the United States. http://www.jhsph.edu/publichealthnews/pres_releases/2007/wang_adultobesity.html (accessed June 10, 2011).
4. Ogden CL, Carroll MD, Curtin LR et al. 2006. Prevalence of overweight and obesity in the United States, 1999–2004. *JAMA* 295:1549–1555.
5. Wang Y and Beydoun MA. 2007. The obesity epidemic in the United States—Gender, age, socioeconomic, racial/ethnic, and geographic characteristics: A systemic review and meta-regression analysis. *Epidemiol Rev* 29:6–28.
6. Centers for Disease Control. 2010. U.S. obesity trends by state 1985–2009. http://www.cdc.gov/obesity/data/trends.html (accessed November 2010).
7. Flegal KM, Carroll MD, Kuczmarski RJ et al. 1998. Overweight and obesity in the United States: Prevalence and trends, 1960–1994. *Int J Obes Relat Metab Disord* 22:39–47.
8. Flegal KM, Carroll MD, Ogden C et al. 2002. Prevalence and trends in obesity among US adults 1999–2000. *JAMA* 288:1728–1732.
9. Ryan DH and Kushner R. 2010. The state of obesity and obesity research. *JAMA* 304:1835–1836.
10. U.S. Department of Health and Human Services. 2003. The obesity crisis in America. Surgeon General's Website. http://www.surgeongeneral.gov/news/testimony/obesity07162003.html (accessed June 12, 2011).
11. Robert Wood Johnson Foundation. 2011. Adult obesity increases in 28 states. http://www.rwjf.org/newsroom/product.jsp?id=65468 (accessed August 8, 2011).
12. Wang YC, McPherson K, Marsh T et al. 2011. Health and economic burden of the projected obesity trends in the USA and the UK. *Lancet* 378:815–825.
13. Wang Y, Beydoun MA, Liang L et al. 2008. Will all Americans become overweight or obese? Estimating the progression and cost of the US obesity epidemic. *Obesity* 16:2323–2330.
14. Kopelman P, Jebb SA, and Butland B. 2007. Executive summary: Foresight 'Tackling Obesities: Future Choices' project. *Obes Rev* 8(Suppl 1):vi–ix.
15. Cawley, J and Meyerhoefer C. 2010. The medical care costs of obesity: An instrumental variables approach. NBER Working paper No. 16467 JEL No. D62,G22,H23,I1.
16. Finkelstein EA, Fiebelkorn IC, and Wang G. 2003. National medical spending attributable to overweight and obesity: How much, and who's paying? *Health Aff* Suppl Web Exclusives:W3-219–W3-226.
17. Finkelstein EA, Fiebelkorn IC, and Wang G. 2004. State-level estimates of annual medical expenditures attributable to obesity. *Obes Res* 12:18–24.
18. Finkelstein EA, Trogdon JG, Cohen JW et al. 2009. Annual medical spending attributable to obesity: Payer-and service-specific estimates. *Health Aff* 28:w822–w831.
19. Gorsky RD, Pamuk E, Williamson DF et al. 1996. The 25-year health care costs of women who remain overweight after 40 years of age. *Am J Prev Med* 12:388–394.
20. Jia H and Lubetkin EI. 2010. Obesity-related quality-adjusted life years lost in the U.S. from 1993 to 2008. *Am J Prev Med* 39:220–227.
21. Kortt MA, Langley PC, and Cox ER. 1998. A review of cost-of-illness studies on obesity. *Clin Ther* 20:772–779.
22. Machlin, S and Woodwell D. 2009. *Healthcare Expenses for Chronic Conditions among Non-Elderly Adults. Variations by Insurance Coverage, 2005–06 (Average Annual Estimates)*. MEPS Statistical Brief #243. Agency for Healthcare Research and Quality, Rockville, MD.
23. Roux L and Donaldson C. 2004. Economics and obesity: Costing the problem or evaluating solutions? *Obes Res* 12:173–179. Review.

24. Shiell A, Gerard K, and Donaldson C. 1987. Cost of illness studies: An aid to decision-making? *Health Policy* 8:317–323.
25. Hodgson TA. 1989. Cost of illness studies: No aid to decision making? Comments on the second opinion by Shiell et al. (Health Policy 8(1987) 317–323). *Health Policy* 11:57–60.
26. Thorpe KE, Florence CS, Howard DH et al. 2004. The impact of obesity on rising medical spending. *Health Aff* Suppl Web Exclusives:W4-480–W4-486.
27. Trasande L, Liu Y, Fryer G et al. 2009. Effects of childhood obesity on hospital care and costs, 1999–2005. *Health Aff* 28:w751–w760.
28. Trasande L. 2010. How much should we invest in preventing childhood obesity? *Health Aff* 29:372–378.
29. Dixon JB. 2010. The effect of obesity on health outcomes. *Mol Cell Endocrinol* 316:104–108.
30. Adami HO and Trichopoulos D. 2003. Obesity and mortality from cancer. *N Engl J Med* 348:1623–1624.
31. Seidell JC, Verschuren WM, van Leer EM et al. 1996. Underweight, overweight, and mortality: A prospective study of 48,287 men and women. *Arch Intern Med* 156:958–963.
32. Davey-Smith G, Sterne JA, Fraser A et al. 2009. The association between BMI and mortality using offspring BMI as an indicator of own BMI: Large intergenerational mortality study. *BMJ* 339:b5043.
33. Flegal KM, Graubard BI, Williamson DF et al. 2005. Excess deaths associated with underweight, overweight, and obesity. *JAMA* 293:1861–1867.
34. Allison DB, Fontaine KR, Manson JE et al. 1999. Annual deaths attributable to obesity in the United States. *JAMA* 282:1530–1538.
35. Mehta NK and Chang VW. 2009. Mortality attributable to obesity among middle-aged adults in the United States. *Demography* 46:851–872.
36. Oster G, Thompson D, Edelsberg J et al. 1999. Lifetime health and economic benefits of weight loss among obese persons. *Am J Public Health* 89:1536–1542.
37. Pi-Sunyer FX. 2002. Medical complications of obesity in adults. In: Fairburn CG and Brownell KD, *Eating Disorders and Obesity: A Comprehensive Handbook*, 2nd Edn. Guilford Press, New York.
38. U.S. Department of Health and Human Services. 2001. *The Surgeon General's Call to Action to Prevent and Decrease Overweight and Obesity*. U.S. Printing Office, Washington, DC.
39. National Institutes of Health. 1998. *Clinical Guidelines on the Identification, Evaluation and Treatment of Overweight and Obesity in Adults*. Publication 98-4083, Washington, DC.
40. Bray GA. 2004. Medical consequences of obesity. *J Clin Endocrinol Metab* 89:2583–2589.
41. Kline B and Tobias JL. 2008. The wages of BMI: Bayesian analysis of a skewed treatment-response model with nonparametric endogeneity. *J Appl Econometrics* 23:767–793.
42. Komlos J and Brabec M. 2010. The trend of mean BMI values of US adults, birth cohorts 1882–1986 indicates that the obesity epidemic began earlier than hitherto thought. *Am J Hum Biol* 22:631–638.
43. Burkhauser RV and Cawley J. 2008. Beyond BMI: The value of more accurate measures of fatness and obesity in social science research. *J Health Econ* 27:519–529.
44. Burkhauser RV, Cawley J, and Schmeiser MD. 2009. The timing of the rise in U.S. obesity varies with measure of fatness. *Econ Hum Biol* 7:307–318.
45. Gallagher D, Visser M, Sepulveda D et al. 1996. How useful is body mass index for comparisons of body fatness across age, sex, and ethnic groups? *Am J Epidemiol* 143:228–239.
46. Kragelund C and Omland T. 2005. A farewell to body-mass index? *Lancet* 366:1589–1591.
47. Kaats GR. 2008. *Restructuring Body Composition: How the Kind, Not the Amount, of Weight Loss Defines a Pathway to Optimal Health*. Taylor Publishing Company, Dallas, TX.
48. Preuss HG and Gottlieb B. 2007. *The Natural Fat Loss Pharmacy*. Broadway Books, New York. pp. 246–260.
49. U.S. Department of Health and Human Services. 2008. Physical activity and health. A report of the Surgeon General. Centers for Disease Control and Prevention, National Center for Chronic Disease Prevention, Atlanta, GA.
50. Pate RR, O'Neill JR, and Lobelo F. 2008. The evolving definition of "sedentary". *Exerc Sport Sci Rev* 36:173–178. http://www.acsm-essr.org (accessed September 2011).
51. U.S. Department of Health and Human Services. 2004. Bone health and osteoporosis. A report of the Surgeon General. Office of the Surgeon General, Washington, DC. http://surgeongeneral.gov/library/bonehealth/content.html (accessed June 2011).
52. Bowles DK and Laughlin MH. 2011. Mechanism of beneficial effects of physical activity on atherosclerosis and coronary heart disease. *J Appl Physiol* 111:308–310.
53. Mayo Clinic. 2008. Moderate exercise: A little goes a long way. *Mayo Clinic Health Letter* 12:1–2.
54. Pietrobelli A, Formica C, Wang Z et al. 1996. Dual-energy x-ray absorptiometry body composition model: Review of physical concepts. *Am J Physiol* 271:E941–E951.

55. Pierson RN Jr., Wang J, Thornton JC et al. 1995. Bone mineral and body fat measurements by two absorptiometry systems: Comparisons with neutron activation analysis. *Calcif Tissue Int* 56:93–98.

56. Friedl KE, DeLuca JP, Marchitelli LJ et al. 1991. Reliability of body-fat estimations from a four-compartment model by using density, body water and bone mineral measurements. *Am J Clin Nutr* 55:764–770.

57. Haarbo J, Gotfredsen A, Hassager C et al. 1991. Validation of body composition by dual energy x-ray absorptiometry (DEXA). *Clin Physiol* 11:331–341.

58. Svendsen OL, Hassager C, Skodt V et al. 1995. Impact of soft tissue on in vivo accuracy of bone mineral measurements in the spine, hip, and forearm: A human cadaver study. *J Bone Miner Res* 10:868–873.

59. Jebb SA and Elia M. 1993. Techniques for the measurement of body composition: A practical guide. *Int J Obes Relat Metab Disord* 17:611–621. Review.

60. Kohrt W. 1995. Body composition by DEXA: Tried and true? *Med Sci Sports Exer* 27:1349–1353.

61. Wang J, Heymsfield SB, Aulet M et al. 1989. Body fat from body density: Underwater weighing vs. dual-photon absorptiometry. *Am J Physiol* 256:E829–E834.

62. Jensen M, Kanaley J, Roust L et al. 1993. Assessment of body composition with use of dual-energy absorptriometry: Evaluation and comparison with other methods. *Mayo Clin Proc* 68:867–873.

63. Goran MI, Driscoll P, Johnson R et al. 1996. Cross-calibration of body-composition techniques against dual-energy x-ray absorptiometry in young children. *Am J Clin Nutr* 63:299–305.

64. Picaud JC, Rigo J, Nyamugabo K et al. 1996. Evaluation of dual-energy x-ray absorptiometry for body composition in piglets and term human neonates. *Am J Clin Nutr* 63:157–163.

65. Going SB, Massett MP, Hall MC et al. 1993. Detection of small changes in body composition by dual-energy x-ray absorptiometry. *Am J Clin Nutr* 57:845–850.

66. Tataranni PA and Ravussin E. 1995. Use of dual-energy x-ray absorptiometry in obese individuals. *Am J Clin Nutr* 62:730–734.

67. Van Loan MD, Keim NL, Berg K et al. 1995. Evaluation of body composition by dual energy x-ray absorptiometry with two different software packages. *Med Sci Sports Exerc* 27:587–591.

68. Glickman SG, Marn CS, Supiano MA et al. 2004. Validity and reliability of dual-energy x-ray absorptiometry for the assessment of abdominal adiposity. *J Appl Physiol* 97:509–514.

69. Park YW, Heymsfield SB, and Gallagher D. 2002. Are dual-energy x-ray absorptiometry regional estimates associated with visceral adipose tissue mass? *Int J Obes Relat Metab Disord* 26:978–983.

70. Snijder MB, Visser M, Dekker JM et al. 2002. The prediction of visceral fat by dual-energy x-ray absorptiometry in the elderly: A comparison with computed tomography and anthropometry. *Int J Obes Relat Metab Disord* 26:984–993.

71. Wiklund P, Toss F, Weinehall L et al. 2008. Abdominal and gynoid fat mass are associated with cardiovascular risk factors in men and women. *J Clin Endocrinol Metab* 93:4360–4366.

72. Snijder MB, Henry RM, Visser M et al. 2004. Regional body composition as a determinant of arterial stiffness in the elderly: The Hoorn study. *J Hypertens* 22:2339–2347.

73. Pischon T, Boeing H, Hoffmann K et al. 2008. General and abdominal adiposity and risk of death in Europe. *N Engl J Med* 359:2105–2120.

74. Panagiotakos DB, Pitsavos C, Yannakoulia M et al. 2005. The implication of obesity and central fat on markers of chronic inflammation: The ATTICA study. *Atherosclerosis* 183:308–315.

75. Safar ME, Czernichow S, and Blacher J. 2006. Obesity, arterial stiffness, and cardiovascular risk. *J Am Soc Nephrol* 17:S109–S111. Review.

76. Seals DR and Gates PE. 2005. Stiffening our resolve against adult weight gain. *Hypertension* 45:175–177.

77. Schouten F, Twisk JW, de Boer MR et al. 2011. Increases in central fat mass and decreases in peripheral fat mass are associated with accelerated arterial stiffening in healthy adults: The Amsterdam growth and health longitudinal study. *Am J Clin Nutr* 94(1):40–48.

78. Radiologyinfo. 2011. What is a bone density scan (DXA)? http://www.radiologyinfo.org & http://www.radiologyinfo.org (accessed June 2011).

79. Appelhans BM. 2009. Neurobehavioral inhibition of reward-driven feeding: Implications for dieting and obesity. *Obesity* 17:640–647.

80. Weiss EC, Galuska DA, and Kettel Khan L. 2007. Weight regain in U.S. adults who experienced substantial weight loss, 1999–2002. *Am J Prev Med* 33:34–40.

81. Dansinger ML, Tatsioni A, Wong JB et al. 2007. Meta-analysis: The effect of dietary counseling for weight loss. *Ann Intern Med* 147:41–50.

82. Franz MJ, VanWormer JJ, Crain AL et al. 2007. Weight-loss outcomes: A systematic review and meta-analysis of weight-loss clinical trials with a minimum 1-year follow-up. *J Am Diet Assoc* 107:1755–1767.

83. Mann T, Tomiyama AJ, Westling E et al. 2007. Medicare's search for effective obesity treatments: Diets are not the answer. *Am Psychol* 62:220–233.

84. Ogden J and Flanagan Z. 2008. Beliefs about the causes and solutions to obesity: A comparison of GPs and lay people. *Patient Educ Couns* 71:72–78.

85. McArthur LH and Ross JK. 1997. Attitudes of registered dieticians toward personal overweight and overweight clients. *J Am Diet Assoc* 97:63–66.

86. Harvey EL, Summerbell CD, Kirk SF et al. 2002. Dietitians' views of overweight and obese people and reported management practices. *J Hum Nutr Diet* 15:331–347.

87. Schousboe K, Visscher PM, Erbas B et al. 2004. Twin study of genetic and environmental influences on adult body size, shape, and composition. *Int J Obes Relat Metab Discord* 28:39–48.

88. Stunkard AJ, Foch TT, and Hrubec Z. 1986. A twin study of human obesity. *JAMA* 256:51–54.

89. Wikler D. 1987. Who should be blamed for being sick? *Health Educ Q* 14:11–25.

90. Dworkin G. 1981. Voluntary health risks and public policy. *Hasting Cent Rep* 11:26–31.

91. Wagner DM. 2002. *The Illusion of Conscious Will*. MIT Press, Cambridge, MA.

92. Roskies A. 2006. Neuroscientific challenges to free will and responsibility. *Trends Cogn Sci* 10:419–423.

93. Rangel A, Camerer C, and Montague PR. 2008. A framework for studying the neurobiology of value-based decision making. *Nat Rev Neurosci* 9:545–556.

94. Kuhn S, Haggard P, and Brass M. 2009. Intentional inhibition: How the "veto-area" exerts control. *Hum Brain Mapp* 30:2834–2843.

95. Haggard P. 2008. Human volition: Towards a neuroscience of will. *Nat Rev Neurosci* 9:934–946.

96. Zheng H, Lenard NR, Shin AC et al. 2009. Appetite control and energy balance regulation in the modern world: Reward-driven brain overrides repletion signals. *Int J Obes* 33:S8–S13.

97. Berridge KC, Ho CY, Richard JM et al. 2010. The tempted brain eats: Pleasure and desire circuits in obesity and eating disorders. *Brain Res* 350:43–64.

98. Fulton S. 2010. Appetite and reward. *Front Neuroendocrinol* 31:85–103.

99. Appelhans BM, Whited MC, Schneider KL et al. 2011. Time to abandon the notion of personal choice in dietary counseling for obesity? *J Am Diet Assoc* 111:1130–1136.

100. Epstein LH, Salvy SJ, Carr KA et al. Food reinforcement, delay discounting and obesity. *Physiol Behav* 100:438–445.

101. Davis C, Patte K, Curtis C et al. 2010. Immediate pleasure and future consequences: A neuropsychological study of binge eating and obesity. *Appetite* 54:208–213.

102. Dallman MF. 2010. Stress-induced obesity and the emotional nervous system. *Trends Endocrinol Metab* 21:159–165.

103. Osterberg L and Blaschke T. 2005. Adherence to medication. *N Engl J Med* 353:487–497.

104. Sabaté E. 2003. *Adherence to Long-Term Therapies: Evidence for Action*. WHO, Geneva, Switzerland.

105. Steiner JF and Earnest MA. 2000. The language of medication-taking. *Ann Intern Med* 132:926–930.

106. Lee JK, Grace KA, and Taylor AJ. 2006. Effect of a pharmacy care program on medication adherence and persistence, blood pressure, and low-density lipoprotein cholesterol: A randomized controlled trial. *JAMA* 296:2563–2571.

107. Winkler A, Teuscher AU, Mueller B et al. 2002. Monotoring adherence to prescribed medication in type 2 diabetic patients treated with sulfonylureas. *Swiss Med Wkly* 132:379–385.

108. Brown MT and Bussell JK. 2010. Medication adherence: WHO cares. *Mayo Clinic Proc* 86:304–314.

109. Kothawala P, Badamgarav E, Ryu S, Miller RM, and Halbert RJ. 2007. A systematic review and meta-analysis of real-world adherence to drug therapy for osteoporosis. *Mayo Clin Proc* 82(12):1493–1501.

110. Lespessailles E. 2007. A forgotten challenge when treating osteoporosis: Getting patients to take their meds. *Joint Bone Spine* 74:7–8.

111. U.S. Senate. 2010. Staff report on GlaxoSmithKline and the diabetes drug Avandia. http://finance.senate.gov/press/Gpress/2010/prg022010a.pdf (accessed August 2, 2011).

112. Nissen SE. 2010. Setting the RECORD straight. *JAMA* 303:1194–1195.

113. Moyer VA and First LR. 2011. To integrity and beyond. *Pediatrics* 127:776–778.

114. DeAngelis CD and Fontanarosa PB. 2010. Ensuring integrity in industry-sponsored research: Primum non nocere, revisited. *JAMA* 303:1196–1198.

115. Michalek JE, Preuss HG, Croft HA, Keith PL et al. 2011. Changes in total body bone mineral density following a common bone health plan with two versions of a unique bone health supplement: A comparative effectiveness research study. *Nutrition J* 10:32.

116. Kaats GR, Preuss HG, Croft HA, Keith SC et al. 2011. A comparative effectiveness study of bone density changes in women over 40 following three bone health plans containing variations of the same novel plant-sourced calcium. *Intl J Med Sci* 8:180–191.

117. Kaats GR, Preuss HG, and Leckie RB. 2009. Comparative effectiveness research (CER): Opportunities and challenges for the nutritional industry. *J Am Coll Nutr* 28:234–237.

Part VII

Child Obesity and Prevention

57 Obesity and Disordered Eating in Youth

Sarah S. Jaser, PhD

CONTENTS

INTRODUCTION

Youth today are experiencing food-related disorders at higher rates than any time in history. Understanding the health consequences, psychosocial correlates, and recommended treatments is increasingly important for practitioners working with youth.

PREVALENCE OF OBESITY

Obesity in youth has become a national problem; rates have tripled over the past few decades. Obesity in youth, defined as body mass index (BMI) $\geq$ 95th percentile adjusted for age and sex, has been tracked over time in a large, nationally representative study, the National Health and Nutrition Examination Survey. Findings from this study indicate that the rates of obesity have risen from 5% in 1970 to almost 17% for youth ages 2–19 in 2008.[1] Rates are lower among younger children (10.4% of children age 2–5 are obese), increase among middle childhood (19.6% of children 6–11 are obese), and level off in adolescents (18.1% of adolescents aged 12–19 are obese). Among minority youth, rates are even higher; Hispanic boys and non-Hispanic black girls are significantly more likely to be obese than non-Hispanic white youth, with rates of obesity as high as 29.2% for black girls aged 12–19.[1] In terms of gender, Hispanic boys are more likely to be obese than girls, but there are no significant gender differences between non-Hispanic white or non-Hispanic black youth.[1] These high rates of obesity have serious consequences for both the physical and psychosocial well-being of youth.

LIFESTYLE FACTORS

Availability of Healthy Food Options

Given the rapid increase in rates of obesity in youth over the past few decades, changes in lifestyle factors are important to consider. The lack of available healthy food options coupled with increased access and exposure to fast-food restaurants may be partially responsible for the increase in obesity. For example, the shortage of supermarkets in urban neighborhoods, or "food deserts," has been linked with obesity in low-income, urban neighborhoods.[2] More recently, efforts have been made to increase the availability of healthy foods in urban neighborhoods, such as farmers' markets in low-income neighborhoods in New York City and fresh produce in Walgreens stores in the Chicago area. There is little that health-care providers can do about this issue; it is likely that policy changes are needed on regional or national levels to increase access to healthy foods for those at highest risk for obesity.

On the other hand, fast-food restaurants are often clustered near schools, providing easy access for youth.[3] Furthermore, a recent report indicates that children's exposure to fast-food ads has increased and that 84% of parents reported taking their child to a fast-food restaurant at least once a week.[4] Analysis of fast-food choices indicated that only 17% of the items on fast-food menus qualified as healthy choices, and the unhealthy choices are the default (e.g., French fries vs. apple slices).[4] Frequent consumption of fast food may be a risk factor for obesity in youth, especially adolescents.[5] Again, policy-level changes may be needed to combat the pervasive advertising and availability of fast food for youth.

Physical Activity

Another factor implicated in the rising rates of obesity is the decrease in physical activity in youth. The Youth Risk Behavior Survey, which includes a large, nationally representative sample, showed that physical activity decreased each year in adolescents from 1993 to 2003.[6] In explaining this decrease, researchers point to the fact that physical education in schools has been reduced, and fewer students participate in after-school sports. Further, obese youth report decreased self-efficacy for physical activity.[7] There are also striking gender differences in levels of physical activity. Numerous studies have found that girls engage in less physical activity than males, within ethnic groups and across ages.[8] Specifically, activity levels in girls decline significantly between ages 9 and 19.[9] Taken together, these results suggest that increasing physical activity may be an important target for interventions aimed at preventing or treating obesity in youth and that such programs may need to be gender specific.

At the same time that physical activity has decreased, sedentary time has increased in youth. Another study that analyzed data from the Youth Risk Behavior Survey found that 30% of boys and 25% of girls watch more than 4 h of television a day.[10] When all forms of electronic media are included (e.g., music, computer, and video games), a recent study reported that youth age 8–18 spend an average of 7.5 h a day consuming media.[11] This study also found striking differences related to race/ethnicity engaging with media, with Hispanic and black youth averaging 13 h of media exposures a day, including 6 h a day of television time.[11] The extremely high number of hours of sedentary time may be related to a lack of parental restriction on access to media; a high percentage of youth (71%) report having a television in their room, and they report that parents are more likely to have rules about what they can watch, rather than how much time they can spend watching.[11] Such high levels of sedentary behavior have negative effects; among white and Hispanic girls, watching television for more than 2 h a day was associated with being overweight.[10] Therefore, reducing screen time by increasing parental awareness of the negative health effects may be an effective way to reduce the risk for obesity in youth.

Sugar-Sweetened Beverages

While consumption of 100% fruit juice is not associated with obesity, there is strong evidence that consumption of sugar-sweetened beverages (i.e., soda or fruit drinks) is linked with obesity in children.[5,12] One study found that each serving (e.g., can of soda) was associated with increased risk for obesity in youth.[13]

Further, studies show that these drinks are the main source of energy in the diets of children and adolescents.[14] Sugar-sweetened beverages may be an important target for interventions; a school-based intervention was successful in reducing the consumption of sugar-sweetened beverages in obese children over 12 months.[12] Decreasing intake of sugar-sweetened beverages may be a relatively simple lifestyle change to make with positive effects. Several states have eliminated sales of sugar-sweetened beverages in schools, and policymakers are promoting taxing such beverages to discourage their sales.[15]

Family Meals

Researchers have found that frequent family meals are associated with better nutrition and reduced risk of disordered eating behaviors. Much of what we know about the impact of family meals on adolescents' weight and eating habits comes from Project EAT, a longitudinal, population-based study with a large, ethnically and socioeconomically diverse sample. This study found that middle school students were more likely to have family meals than high school students, girls reported fewer family meals than boys, and higher socioeconomic status (SES) was associated with more frequent family meals.[16] Regular family meals (at least three times/week) were associated with better nutrition in adolescents (i.e., greater intake of vegetables, calcium-rich foods, and fiber and lower intake of soft drinks), and regular family meals in high school predicted better nutrition in young adulthood.[16] While these findings support the benefit of family meals, it is still unclear what it is about family meals that confers the beneficial effects, whether the entire family must be present for the positive effects to be realized, and whether the meal is important (i.e., dinner vs. breakfast).

Some problems must be acknowledged with promoting family meals as a way to prevent obesity. First, the direction of the positive effects of family meals is not yet clear—it is possible that families who are already engaging in healthy behaviors are more likely to eat together. For example, one study found that eating dinner together as a family was related to lower prevalence of overweight at the beginning of the study, but it was not predictive of youth becoming overweight over time.[17] Second, researchers note several barriers to families eating together, including parents' work schedules, adolescents' activities, and the desire of adolescents to be with friends rather than family. In Project EAT, 14% of adolescents reported never having family meals, and 19% reported having family meals only one to two times/week.[16] Despite these issues, the existing evidence supports that promotion of family meals may increase healthy eating and prevent obesity among youth.

HEALTH CONSEQUENCES OF OBESITY

Obesity in childhood and adolescence has been shown to be a strong predictor of obesity in early adulthood, increasing health risks.[18] One of the largest longitudinal studies to examine the long-term effects of childhood obesity, the Bogalusa Heath study, followed youth in Louisiana for several years. This study found that, of children with a BMI $\geq$ 95th percentile, 65% were obese and had excess adiposity as adults, and 39% had at least two cardiovascular risk factors.[19] Another study found that, for boys, childhood obesity predicted hypertension in young adulthood.[18] While these results suggest that childhood obesity is a direct risk factor for later cardiovascular disease, a recent review suggests this relationship is attenuated by adult BMI.[20] Thus, efforts to treat obesity in youth have the potential to reduce health risks in adulthood.

Obesity is also associated with serous metabolic abnormalities, including insulin resistance (IR), hyperinsulinemia, glucose intolerance, and dyslipidemia.[21] While the relationship between obesity, IR, and type 2 diabetes mellitus (T2DM) has been established in adults, it is becoming more evident in youth.[22] A study of overweight minority youth ages 5–10, for example, demonstrated a significant relationship between overweight and IR, particularly for African-American girls.[23] Research supports that obesity in youth increases risks for T2DM, resulting in significant morbidity and mortality.[7] These findings support that obesity in youth has serious immediate and long-term health consequences; thus, efforts to prevent and treat obesity and help youth maintain healthy weight may reduce their health risks both in adolescence and later in life.

PSYCHOSOCIAL CORRELATES

In addition to health problems, obesity in youth is also associated with increased risk for psycho-social problems, particularly depression.[24] Until recently, it was thought that depression was a consequence of obesity, as a result of peer rejection.[25,26] A large study using a nationally representative sample, however, found that adolescents who had higher depressive symptoms at baseline were twice as likely to be obese 1 year later.[27] Depressive symptoms were a significant predictor of later obesity in adolescents, even after controlling for self-esteem, physical activity, parental obesity, and parental education.[27] Another longitudinal study of adolescent girls also supports that depressive symptoms predict the onset of obesity; in this study, each additional depressive symptom was associated with a fourfold increase in the likelihood of becoming obese.[28] Depression in obese youth is also likely to have a negative impact on their motivation for healthy behaviors. For example, one study found that, among overweight and obese youth, depressive symptoms were related to lower levels of perceived support for physical activity and self-efficacy.[29] Since depressive symptoms may impact the ability to engage in healthy behavior changes, assessing and treating depression in obese youth may result in better quality of life and improve adherence to weight loss management programs.

In addition to depression, obese youth report significant psychosocial distress and poor quality of life. One study found that, among obese youth seeking treatment for weight loss management, 56% reported clinically significant levels of psychological distress.[30] Rates of distress among mothers of obese youth were also high, at 41%, and were strongly associated with psychological distress among youth.[30] Based on both parent- and self-report, quality of life in obese youth is significantly poorer than nonobese youth, regardless of race/ethnicity.[30] Poorer quality of life in obese youth is related to lower SES, lower perceived social support from peers, higher degree of overweight, and greater depressive symptoms.[30] Findings from a study of overweight and obese youth suggest that quality of life is also affected by parent distress and peer victimization.[24] These findings suggest the importance of assessing not only depressive symptoms and distress in obese youth but also in their parents. Cognitive-behavioral interventions aimed at reducing depressive symptoms[31] may have the potential to improve both quality of life and adherence to treatment recommendations for weight management.

TREATING/PREVENTING OBESITY IN YOUTH

Given the recent national attention to the problem of obesity, clinicians and public health officials are eager to find ways to prevent and treat obesity in youth. Two recent reviews have summarized these recommendations, with a focus on practical steps for health-care providers, as well as suggestions for community-level interventions.[32,33] First, health-care providers—particularly pediatricians and pediatric nurse practitioners—are encouraged to counsel *all* children of healthy weight to do the following: limit consumption of sugar-sweetened beverages, include fruits and vegetables in diet, limit screen time to 2 h/day or less and remove televisions and computers from children's rooms, eat breakfast, limit fast-food restaurants, limit portion sizes, engage in 60 min of exercise/day, and make family meals a priority[32] (see Table 57.1). For youth who are at or above BMI of 85, the recommendations are essentially the same, but experts recommend that health-care providers spend more time and intensity on recommendations and monitor progress every 3–6 months. For these children, the goal is weight maintenance, resulting in decreased BMI as children grow.[33] If this goal is not met, additional support and structure is needed, which requires additional training in behavioral counseling.[33] Pediatricians and family physicians are seen as the first line of defense, therefore, with the inclusion of dieticians and physical activity counselors as needed. In terms of community-level changes, experts suggest advocating for increased physical activity in schools, supporting efforts to use parks as safe areas for physical activity, including walking and bicycle paths.

TABLE 57.1

Evidence-Based Recommendations for Preventing Obesity in Youth

1. Limit consumption of sugar-sweetened beverages
2. Include fruits and vegetables in diet
3. Limit screen time to 2 h/day or less
4. Remove televisions and computers from children's rooms
5. Eat breakfast
6. Limit eating out (especially fast-food restaurants)
7. Limit portion sizes
8. Engage in 60 min of physical activity/day
9. Make family meals a priority

Source: Adapted from Spear, B.A. et al., *Pediatrics*, 120, S254, 2007.

While primary health-care providers are seen as the front line in the fight against obesity in youth, behavioral researchers have also taken on the challenge of developing effective programs to prevent and treat obesity. With so many recent trials, it is important to assess what has been successful and what needs improvement. A recent meta-analysis found that weight gain prevention studies have focused on four major types of interventions: (1) prevention programs that target obesity along with other cardiovascular risk factors (e.g., smoking), (2) prevention programs focused only on obesity or weight gain, (3) interventions focused only on increasing physical activity, and (4) eating disorder prevention programs that promote the use of healthy weight management. This study identified 64 programs, but only 21% had positive effects on weight.[34] Trials involving children and adolescents had larger effects on weight than trials with preadolescents. This difference may be due to the fact that adolescents have the cognitive skills needed to understand the material, and they are more likely than younger children to have control over their food and activity choices.[35] Programs for younger children may be more effective than those for preadolescents because they are more likely to include a parental component.[34] Larger effects were also found for female-only trials than for mixed-sex or male-only trials. This may be because females have greater society pressure to be thin than males, so they may be more invested in the program than males.[34] Effects were also larger for trials lasting 16 weeks or less, and interventions that targeted only weight change were more successful than those that targeted other behavioral changes. It is possible that more complex programs are too difficult for youth to incorporate; it seems that shorter and simpler programs are more effective.[34]

Several researchers have introduced school-based programs as a way to prevent obesity; 84% of the programs included in the meta-analysis were conducted in schools.[34] A review of the effects of school-based programs found that they were often successful in increasing self-reported knowledge, self-efficacy, and intentions but that they had only modest effects on weight.[36] These results may be due to the fact that most of these programs targeted individual changes, based on social cognitive theory,[37] rather than attempting to change the environment. Further, few school-based studies include parents.[36] It is important to note, however, that the meta-analysis of preventive interventions found parental involvement was not significantly related to effect sizes.[34] These findings suggest that school-based programs alone may not be effective in affecting weight in youth and that inclusion of the broader community may be necessary.

One of the few community-based interventions aimed at changing the environment to prevent obesity in children is the Shape Up Somerville study.[38] This study included parents, policy makers, restaurants, and the media to increase options for physical activity and the availability of healthy food in a culturally diverse, urban community. Children from the community that received the intervention (Somerville, MA) had significantly reduced BMI scores over 1 year, as compared to children from two control communities.[38] This type of community-level intervention may be what is required to significantly impact weight.

DISORDERED EATING

While the increase in obesity in youth has received much national attention, there is also increased interest in disordered eating behaviors in youth. The incidence of anorexia nervosa has increased over the past century until the 1990s, but it is still rare, with rates of about .3%, and it is most common among white girls.[39] Anorexia is notoriously difficult to treat and has a high mortality rate.[39] In contrast, rates of bulimia have decreased over the past few decades among both males and females.[40] Rather than focusing on these disorders, however, researchers have begun to study disordered eating behaviors more generally to capture the range of unhealthy eating behaviors. Disordered eating behaviors, including binging, purging, and unhealthy dieting, occur at much higher rates than the diagnosable disorders; a recent population-based study found that 11.6% of adolescents reported engaging in these behaviors.[41]

Research indicates that disordered eating behaviors put youth at risk for developing obesity. Binge eating, for example, may be a risk factor for obesity.[42] Similarly, adolescent girls who report frequently dieting are also at increased risk for developing obesity.[42] A study of adolescent girls found that self-reported dietary restraint (i.e., dieting behaviors) were three times more likely to become obese, and that girls who used weight-control behaviors (e.g., vomiting or laxative abuse) were five times more likely to become obese.[28] While these results may seem counterintuitive, this effect may be due to increased metabolic efficiency that results from such behaviors[43] or because such behaviors may be related to increases in binge eating.[44] These findings suggest that interventions targeting disordered eating behaviors in youth may also help to prevent obesity.

SHARED PREDICTORS OF DISORDERED EATING AND OBESITY IN YOUTH

The evidence suggesting that disordered eating may predict obesity has prompted researchers to examine shared risk and protective factors for disordered eating and obesity in adolescents. Findings are quite different for boys and girls (see Table 57.2). One study found that among girls, weight concern, weight-related teasing, and dieting predicted binge eating, purging (including vomiting and use of laxatives), and overweight.[45] For boys, however, weight concern and weight-control behaviors were associated with binge eating, purging, and overweight. A recent longitudinal analysis of the Growing Up Today study had similar findings. Specifically, concern with weight and dieting in girls predicted binging, purging, and overweight. Parental weight-related teasing predicted binge eating and overweight.[46] However, physical activity, fast-food intake, maternal dieting, eating breakfast, and television were not significant predictors. For boys, concern with weight predicted binge eating and overweight. None of the other predictors were significant for boys, but physical activity was positively associated with purging and negatively associated with overweight in cross-sectional analyses. These findings suggest that concern with weight was the strongest risk factor for boys and girls, and an integrated approach may address disordered eating and obesity within the same intervention.[46]

In contrast, regular family meals may serve as a protective factor against disordered eating behaviors, especially for girls. In the Growing Up Today study, frequent family meals predicted lower levels of binging, purging, and overweight in girls.[46] Another study found that regular family meals were associated with decreased use of weight-control behaviors in girls (e.g., self-induced vomiting and use of diet pills and laxatives), even after 5 years.[16] To help explain the protective effects of family meals, a recent study examined family factors among adolescents who ate frequent

TABLE 57.2
Shared Predictors of Disordered Eating Behavior and Obesity for Boys and Girls

Predictor	Girls	Boys
Concern with weight	Greater purging, binge eating, overweight	Greater binge eating, overweight
Weight-related teasing by parents	Greater binge eating, overweight	Not related
Dieting	Greater purging, binge eating, overweight	Not related
Family meals	Less purging, binge eating, overweight	Not related
Fast food	Not related	Not related
TV watching	Not related	Greater binge eating, overweight (cross-sectional only)
Eating breakfast	Not related	Not related
Physical activity	Not related	Greater purging, less overweight (cross-sectional only)

Source: Haines, J. et al., *Arch. Pediat. Adol. Med.,* 164, 336, 2010.

family meals.[47] These adolescents reported higher levels of family cohesion (i.e., feeling of closeness among family members) and higher levels of adaptive coping (e.g., problem solving), which mediated the relationship between frequency of family meals and adolescent disordered eating behaviors.[47] This provides an explanation for the positive effect of family meals on adolescents' healthy eating behaviors. Thus, promoting family meals may help to prevent not only obesity but also other disordered eating behaviors in youth. These shared risk and protective factors for disordered eating behaviors and obesity may provide the basis for an integrated approach to address the spectrum of weight problems in youth.

DIRECTIONS FOR FUTURE RESEARCH

Recent studies have provided valuable information about the modifiable behaviors related to obesity that are potential targets for interventions and provide the basis for recommendations. Some of these are obvious (e.g., increasing physical activity), while others are not so obvious (e.g., the protective factor of family meals). Other findings disprove previously held beliefs about contributors to obesity in youth (e.g., consumption of high-fat foods is not associated with obesity in youth).[5] Reviews of the programs aimed at reducing or preventing obesity in youth have several important messages. First, most of the programs that have been tested did *not* have a significant effect on weight. Future studies need to build on the programs that were effective, and replicate findings. Second, innovative ways are needed to reach the populations that had the smallest effects, including preadolescents and males.[34] Finally, there is a need for longer follow-up periods, since research with adults indicates that most people regain lost weight.[48] There is still a need for innovative programs that address the individual, family, and community levels in order to have a meaningful effect on obesity in youth.

ACKNOWLEDGMENTS

Dr. Jaser is supported by a career development award from the National Institute of Diabetes and Digestive and Kidney Diseases (K23 DK 088454-02).

REFERENCES

1. Ogden CL, Carroll MD, Curtin LR, Lamb MM, Flegal KM. Prevalence of high body mass index in US children and adolescents, 2007–2008. *JAMA—Journal of the American Medical Association*. 2010;303:242–249.
2. Jetter KM, Cassady DL. The availability and cost of healthier food alternatives. *American Journal of Preventive Medicine*. 2006;30:38–44.
3. Austin SB, Melly SJ, Sanchez BN, Patel A, Buka S, Gortmaker SL. Clustering of fast-food restaurants around schools: A novel application of spatial statistics to the study of food environments. *American Journal of Public Health*. 2005;95:1575–1581.
4. Harris JL, Schwartz MB, Brownell KD, Vishnudas S, Ustjanauskas A, Javadizadeh J, Weinberg M, Munsell C, Speers S. *Fast Food FACTS: Evaluating Fast Food Nutrition and Marketing to Youth: Rudd Center for Food Policy and Obesity*; November 2010.
5. American Dietetic Association. Pediatric overweight evidence analysis project. http://www.adaevidencelibrary.com/topic.cfm?cat=4102. Accessed December 6, 2010.
6. Brownson RC, Boehmer TK, Luke DA. Declining rates of physical activity in the United States: What are the contributors? *Annual Review of Public Health*. 2005;26:421–443.
7. Trost SG, Kerr LM, Ward DS, Pate RR. Physical activity and determinants of physical activity in obese and non-obese children. *International Journal of Obesity*. 2001;25:822–829.
8. Gordon-Larsen P, Adair L, Popkin BM. Ethnic differences in physical activity and inactivity patterns and overweight status. *Obesity Research*. 2002;10:141–149.
9. Kimm SY, Glynn N, Kriska A et al. Decline in physical activity in black girls and white girls during adolescence. *New England Journal of Medicine*. 2002;347:709–715.
10. Lowry R, Wechsler H, Galuska DA, Fulton JE, Kann L. Television viewing and its associations with overweight, sedentary lifestyle, and insufficient consumption of fruits and vegetables among US high school students: Differences by race, ethnicity, and gender. *Journal of School Health*. 2002;72:413–421.
11. Kaiser Family Foundation. Generation M2: Media in the lives of 8- to 18-year-olds. http://www.kff.org/entmedia/upload/8010.pdf. Accessed December 6, 2010.
12. Malik VS, Schulze MB, Hu FB. Intake of sugar-sweetened beverages and weight gain: A systematic review. *American Journal of Clinical Nutrition*. 2006;84:274–288.
13. Ludwig DS, Peterson KE, Gortmaker SL. Relation between consumption of sugar-sweetened drinks and childhood obesity: A prospective, observational analysis. *The Lancet*. 2001;357:505–508.
14. Reedy J, Krebs-Smith SM. Dietary sources of energy, solid fats, and added sugars among children and adolescents in the United States. *Journal of the American Dietetic Association*. 2010;110:1477–1484.
15. Brownell KD, Frieden TR. Ounces of prevention—The public policy case for taxes on sugared beverages. *New England Journal of Medicine*. 2009;360:1805–1808.
16. Neumark-Sztainer D, Larson NI, Fulkerson JA, Eisenberg ME. Family meals and adolescents: What have we learned from project EAT (Eating among teens)? *Public Health Nutrition*. 2010;13:1113–1121.
17. Taveras EM, Rifas-Shiman SL, Berkey CS et al. Family dinner and adolescent overweight. *Obesity Research*. 2005;13:900–906.
18. Field AE, Cook NR, Gillman MW. Weight status in childhood as a predictor of becoming overweight or hypertensive in early adulthood. *Obesity Research*. 2005;13:163–169.
19. Freedman DS, Mei Z, Srinivasan SR, Berenson GS, Dietz WH. Cardiovascular risk factors and excess adiposity among overweight children and adolescents: The bogalusa heart study. *Journal of Pediatrics*. 2007;150(1):12–17.e2.
20. Lloyd LJ, Langley-Evans SC, McMullen S. Childhood obesity and adult cardiovascular disease risk: A systematic review. *International Journal of Obesity*. 34:18–28.
21. Weiss R, Caprio S. The metabolic consequences of childhood obesity. *Best Practice and Research: Clinical Endocrinology and Metabolism*. 2005;19:405–419.
22. Bloomgarden ZT. Type 2 diabetes in the young: The evolving epidemic. *Diabetes Care*. 2004;27:998–1010.
23. Young-Hyman D, Schlundt DG, Herman L, DeLuca F, Counts D. Evaluation of the insulin resistance syndrome in 5 to 10 year old overweight/obese African American children. *Diabetes Care*. 2001;24:1357–1364.
24. Janicke DM, Marciel KK, Ingerski LM et al. Impact of psychosocial factors on quality of life in overweight youth. *Obesity*. 2007;15:1799–1807.
25. Erickson SJ, Robinson TN, Haydel KF, Killen JD. Are overweight children unhappy? Body mass index, depressive symptoms, and overweight concerns in elementary school children. *Archives of Pediatric Adolescent Medicine*. 2000;154:931–935.

26. Wallace WJ, Sheslow D, Hassink S. Obesity in children: A risk for depression. *Annals of the New York Academy of Science*. 1993;699:301–303.

27. Goodman E, Whitaker RC. A prospective study of the role of depression in the development and persistence of adolescent obesity. *Pediatrics*. 2002;110(3):497–504.

28. Stice E, Presnell K, Shaw H, Rohde P. Psychological and behavioral risk factors for obesity onset in adolescent girls: A prospective study. *Journal of Consulting and Clinical Psychology*. 2005;73:195–202.

29. Jaser SS, Holl MG, Jefferson V, Grey M. Correlates of depressive symptoms in Urban youth at risk for type 2 diabetes mellitus. *Journal of School Health*. 2009;79(6):286–292.

30. Zeller MH, Saelens BE, Roehrig H, Kirk S, Daniels SR. Psychological adjustment of obese youth presenting for weight management treatment. *Obesity Research*. 2004;12:1576–1586.

31. Clarke GN, Hornbrook M, Lynch F et al. A randomized trial of a group cognitive intervention for preventing depression in adolescent offspring of depressed parents. *Archives of General Psychiatry*. 2001;58(12):1127–1134.

32. Davis MM, Gance-Cleveland B, Hassink S, Johnson R, Paradis G, Resnicow K. Recommendations for prevention of childhood obesity. *Pediatrics*. 2007;120:S229–S253.

33. Spear BA, Barlow SE, Ervin C et al. Recommendations for treatment of child and adolescent overweight and obesity. *Pediatrics*. 2007;120:S254–S288.

34. Stice E, Shaw H, Marti CN. A meta-analytic review of the obesity prevention programs for children and adolescents: The skinny on interventions that work. *Psychological Bulletin*. 2006;132(5):667–691.

35. Baranowski T, Cullen KW, Nicklas T, Thompson D, Baranowski J. School-based obesity prevention: A blueprint for taming the epidemic. *American Journal of Health Behavior*. 2002;26:486–493.

36. Gittelson J, Kumar MB. Preventing childhood obesity and diabetes: Is it time to move out of the school? *Pediatric Diabetes*. 2007;8:55–69.

37. Bandura A. *Self-Efficacy: The Exercise of Control*. New York: W. H. Freeman; 1986.

38. Economos CD, Hyatt RR, Goldberg JP et al. A community intervention reduces BMI z-score in children: Shape up Somerville first year results. *Obesity*. 2007;15:1325–1336.

39. Hoek HW. Incidence, prevalence and mortality of anorexia nervosa and other eating disorders. *Current Opinion in Psychiatry*. 2006;19:389–394.

40. Keel PK, Heatherton TF, Dorer DJ, Joiner TE, Zalta AK. Point prevalence of bulimia nervosa in 1982, 1992, and 2002. *Psychological Medicine*. 2006;36:119–127.

41. Haley CC, Hedberg K, Leman RF. Disordered eating and unhealthy weight loss practices: Which adolescents are at highest risk? *Journal of Adolescent Health*. 2010;47:102–105.

42. Stice E, Cameron RP, Killen JD, Hayward C, Taylor CB. Naturalistic weight-reduction efforts prospectively predict growth in relative weight and onset of obesity among female adolescents. *Journal of Consulting and Clinical Psychology*. 1999;67:967–974.

43. Klesges RC, Isbell TR, Klesges LM. Relationship Between Dietary Restraint, Energy Intake, Physical Activity, and Body Weight: A Prospective Analysis. *Journal of Abnormal Psychology*. 1992;101:668–674.

44. Stice E, Presnell K, Spangler D. Risk factors for binge eating onset in adolescent girls: A 2-year prospective investigation. *Health Psychology*. 2002;21:131–138.

45. Neumark-Sztainer D, Wall MM, Haines J, Story MT, Sherwood NE, van den Berg PA. Shared risk and protective factors for overweight and disordered eating in adolescents. *American Journal of Preventive Medicine*. 2007;33:359–369.

46. Haines J, Kleinman KP, Rifas-Shiman SL, Field AE, Austin SB. Examination of shared risk and protective factors for overweight and disordered eating among adolescents. *Archives of Pediatric Adolescent Medicine*. 2010;164:336–343.

47. Franko DL, Thompson D, Affenito SG, Barton BA, Striegel-Moore RH. What mediates the relationship between family meals and adolescent health issues? *Health Psychology*. 2008;27:S109–S117.

48. Jeffery RW, Epstein LH, Wilson GT et al. Long-term maintenance of weight loss: Current status. *Health Psychology*. 2000;19:5–16.

58 Childhood Obesity
Exercise Physiologists' Viewpoints

Sang-Hoon Suh, PhD and Yu-Sik Kim, MS

CONTENTS

INTRODUCTION

LIMITED PHYSICAL ACTIVITY FOR THE SAKE OF CONVENIENCE CAUSES THE SPREAD OF OBESITY

Most industrialized countries during last decades have enjoyed a standard of living within well-nourished and sanitary environment. Our health-care system has provided us with drugs and technologies that cure illness and prolong lives and has made the world population largely free from the scourge of diseases suffered by hundreds of thousands in the past. The health problems dominating in the past, however, have been replaced by other diseases brought on by new environment within which we live. These include cardiovascular disease (CVD), cancer, stroke, nonalcoholic fatty liver disease, T2DM, respiratory diseases, orthopedic complications, and more; these may cause premature death and disability among all populations [1]. What is it meant by "new environment," and how does this contribute to this phenomenon of the shift in health problems? Today's transportation system and high personal vehicle penetration have provided us with convenient ways to move from places to places, labor-saving technologies have succeeded in reducing our physical demand remarkably, large food industries have supplied all kinds of grocery to the consumers conveniently with reasonable price helping prepare them for big meals at the end of the day, and development of entertainment system and contents has brought us to the couch in our living room and helped relax one's fatigued body from a hard day. Moreover, rapid development in computer and World-Wide-Web-based information technology has enabled anyone to do multiple tasks with minimal energy expenditure, even those who require his or her actual physical demand substantially such as shopping. Thanks to those who devoted themselves in building this new environment, it certainly has improved the quality of living to the extent where we cannot look forward to further convenience or improvement. However, while the developers were obsessed with building the *Laputa*, they did not take into account the importance of physical activity. For the sake of convenience, the developers tried to minimize energy expenditure by building the environment which limits physical activity.

We are now definitely well nourished than ever by providing high-energy-dense foods in the environment which favors lopsided energy balance with increased intake and decreased expenditure. We have traded convenience for our daily life with obesity; an explosive increase in obese population within last three decades, such that the prevalence of obese adult population (defined by BMI of $\geq 30 \text{kg/m}^2$) of the United States increased from 15% in 1980 to 32.2% in 2003 [2], the prevalence of obesity of Korea, a country which is traditionally considered to have a low obesity prevalence, increased from 26.2% in 1998 to 31.8% in 2005 according to International Obesity Task Force (IOTF)'s Asia-Pacific criteria of obesity, defined as a BMI $\geq 25 \text{kg/m}^2$ [3]. World Health Organization (WHO) estimated that 400 million worldwide were obese in 2005 and expects that this number will increase to 700 million by 2015 [4]. WHO in 2002 has changed its first declaration on obesity in 1998 from epidemic to pandemic that constituted one of the leading future threats to public health, and the conference chairs of the 10th International Congress on Obesity in 2006 announced that, for the first time in history, the global population of overweight outnumbered the famine [5]. This inexorable rise in the prevalence of obesity to such an extent together with changes in physical activity patterns is of great concern for its long-term implications on health as accruing evidence has linked obesity to morbidity and mortality from a wide variety of chronic diseases; in other words, obesity is rightly referred to as the major contributor to most predominant causes of recent adult-onset chronic diseases [1]. By not considering the fact that we may remain healthy as long as we maintain ourselves active during the pursuit of the development, humankind has sacrificed thousands of lives and wasted billions of dollars for medical treatment.

Obesogenic Environment Reduces Physical Activity and Increases Childhood Obesity

The late twentieth century's environment consists of many social and cultural characteristics that most developed countries accepted as normal parts of living which collectively contributed to the dramatic spread of the obesity pandemic; these include dining-out for calorie-dense meals, T.V. viewing for extended hours, and using automating systems that minimize physical demands. Children who were brought up in this environment are exposed to the potential to be obese for lifetime. The prevalence of overweight children has more than tripled during the last three decades; worldwide estimates identify 18,000,000 overweight children as of 2002 [6]; 1 in 3 U.S. children and adolescents (30.6%) aged 6 through 19 years is reported to be obese (defined by BMI of ≥ 30) based on the National Health and Nutrition Examination Survey (NHANES) [7]. Although childhood obesity seems to be less prevalent than adult obesity currently, its increasing rate among children is gathering pace superior to that of adults. The greater concern than this alarming increasing prevalence rate of childhood obesity is, however, the appearance of various metabolic complications that were traditionally known as adult-onset diseases among children and adolescents; type 2 diabetes is most salient among them [8]. Moreover, childhood obesity persists into adult life, where approximately 70% of obese adolescents grow up to become obese adults [9]. This gives concern for further increasing adult obesity prevalence in the future and higher risk for suffering from associated health problems for a lifetime. Beside its adverse consequences on physiological health, obesity is also known to be associated with significant psychological problems among children [10]. Most societies take a dim view of obese individuals and associate them with laziness, and obese students are often alienated from others or the victims of bullying at school. As a consequence, obese children often demonstrate lower levels of global self-esteem which may result in increased level of sadness, loneliness, nervousness, anxiety, disturbed body image, and likelihood of tobacco and alcohol consumption [11,12].

Obesity is a chronic energy imbalance condition resulting in the storing of excess energy as adipose tissue—not an acute, urgent, and hot topic disease like AIDS or H_1N_1 influenza—and is, therefore, likely to receive less attention. However, as described briefly earlier, worldwide spread of obesity, especially among children, gives cause for concern for its various and serious adverse effects on physiological and psychological health. Moreover, some insist that the problems of being obese are no longer solely those of increased risk for chronic diseases, but of the disease itself [13]. Thus, obesity constitutes a global health crisis, and it is generally assumed that modifying the current social, cultural, or environmental paradigms which provide risk factors for obesity is essential for reducing its prevalence. Recently, children definitely eat high-calorie junk foods and snacks, drink sweetened beverages more often, and are more physically inactive as compared to previous generations. The cause of pandemic of obesity among children is believed to be multifaceted by genetic and environmental factors, and it is widely acknowledged that being obese is, to some extent, "heritable" [14]. It is, however, definitely driven by aspects of this modern environment, or what is often termed an "obesogenic" environment, that encourage sedentary lifestyle and concomitant poor food choice. Now we know that the number of adipocytes for lean and obese individuals is set during childhood and adolescence and is subject to little variation during adulthood; therefore, substantial weight loss is difficult, and costly contemporary treatments of obesity during adulthood are only modestly effective [15]. Thus, this indicates that, to address this global health crisis, emphasis on successful prevention and early treatment before adulthood is necessary (Figure 58.1). Systemic reviews of interventions for the prevention

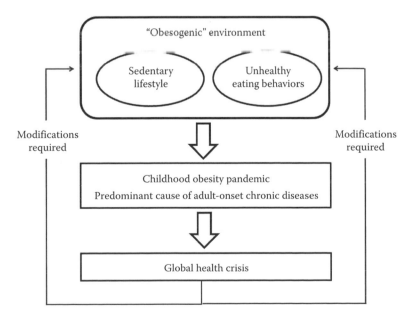

FIGURE 58.1   To address global health crisis of childhood obesity pandemic, emphasis on successful primary prevention focusing on changing "obesogenic" environment through lifestyle managements is necessary.

of childhood obesity showed that the most promising strategy for lowering obesity prevalence is to focus on increasing physical activity levels. In addition, there is a general consensus among experts in exercise science and health professionals that physical activity need not be of vigorous intensity for it to improve health or maintain healthy body weight [16]. In other words, considering the fact that obesity is a disease itself and, at the same time, is a preventable risk factor for various chronic diseases, health benefits from physical activity are achievable for most children and adolescents just by maintaining active lifestyle which favors energy expenditure.

In this chapter, we describe the problems associated with current physical activity levels during childhood and adolescence such as T2DM and CVDs and how physical activities can influence risk factors for those diseases including adiposity, insulin resistance (IR), dyslipidemia, hypertension, and inflammatory cytokines. We will also describe how it is important to be active parents to prevent childhood obesity and its related adverse outcomes and, more importantly, why physical activity during childhood and adolescence is primarily focused, rather than reducing caloric intake, to reduce obesity prevalence and improve overall health.

HOW PHYSICALLY ACTIVE ARE TODAY'S CHILDREN?

CURRENT PHYSICAL ACTIVITY LEVEL AMONG CHILDREN IS INSUFFICIENT

During the 1980s–1990s, when concern toward the initiation of era of obesity was raised, several comprehensive studies examined the impact of physical activity on body weight and obesity [17–20]. They reported lower weight, BMI, or adiposity among people with higher levels of self-rated physical activity and showed an inverse relationship between physical activity and weight gain. Previous studies mentioned earlier concluded that physical activity generally affects body composition and body weight favorably by promoting fat loss while preserving or increasing lean mass, and the rate of weight loss appears to be proportional to amount of physical activity; thus, any increase in physical activity levels adds some benefit to weight loss and its consequences on overall health. Physical activity is the most modifiable components of total energy expenditure [21]. Then how physically active are children these days? The majority studies examining physical activity levels among young people are subject to bias because they utilized self-reporting measurements such as questionnaires which provide only crude estimates. While over 90% and 70% of school age children and adolescents appeared to meet recommended daily accumulation of moderate physical activity suggested by Healthy People 2010 of United States [22] and the United Kingdom Expert Consensus Group guideline [23], respectively, other recent studies showed that only 42% of children (6–11 years of age) and 8% of adolescents (12–19 years of age) meet the U.S. Surgeon General's daily physical activity recommendation [24], and only one-third of adolescents meet the guidelines set by the United Kingdom Health Education Authority [25]. Although the accurate estimates of physical activity level among children are currently unavailable, it is assumed, from the current increase in the prevalence of childhood obesity, that current physical activity level is not sufficient to equalize energy balance to maintain healthy body weight and decrease the likelihood of associated medical conditions.

PHYSICAL ACTIVITY LEVELS DURING CHILDHOOD AND ADOLESCENCE
SOUNDLY AFFECT OVERALL HEALTH DURING ADULTHOOD

Being physically active during youth has critical consequences for later life as youth physical activity works toward overall health during adulthood by increasing the likelihood for adult physical activity levels [26,27]. This may be due to psychological "learning and liking" effect [28]. Therefore, making physical activity a natural and pleasant part of children's life through positive experiences from exercise is very important. Appropriate physical activities can take any form that increases heart rate and energy expenditure. Children can increase physical activity in many ways, just by playing, participating in organized physical activity programs provided by schools or community, or adopting active transport to school or neighbors. In order to do so, it requires a consolidated support of adults from all sectors, particularly parents, to influence the attitudes and behaviors of children toward increasing physical activity levels. It has been shown that shared environmental factors have a great influence on children's physical activity, and habitual physical activity established during the early years may provide the greatest impact on preventions of adulthood obesity and chronic diseases. According to Franks et al. [29], the familial resemblance in physical activity in children is explained predominantly by shared environmental factors and not by genetic variability; it is evidenced from the study with 100 twin pairs examining if free-living physical activity in children is attributable to genetic factors. However, as seen in concurrent trend in obesity prevalence and physical inactivity rate among adults, such that more than 60% of American adults are not regularly active and 25% are not active at all [24], adults have not succeeded in being role models to children. Despite the common knowledge that physical activity is an excellent tool for managing body weight and promoting health, its systemic effects are not clearly understood by most of others beside exercise physiologists and health professionals.

Therefore, clear understanding of the current and future health consequences of childhood obesity and of the effects of physical activity may help adults recognize that physical activity is conducive to a healthy lifestyle and prevention of obesity and its associated diseases. This may eventually prevent the spread of the epidemic of obesity by helping adults be role models to the children and develop the awareness of importance of being active during early years. Is physical activity really an effective treatment for obesity which predisposes children to other chronic diseases so that we may call it a panacea? The following sections will introduce a burgeoning interest in health issues related to childhood obesity, mainly focusing on T2DM and CVDs and how organized and unorganized physical activities, respectively, prevent and cause the aforementioned diseases and their complications.

PHYSICAL ACTIVITY CAN PREVENT DEVELOPING T2DM AMONG OBESE CHILDREN AND ADOLESCENTS

PHYSICAL INACTIVITY CAUSES OBESITY WHICH, IN TURN, CAUSES T2DM AMONG OBESE CHILDREN

The etiologic process in T2DM begins with obesity and IR, which, in turn, leads to inflammation and destruction of the insulin-secreting pancreatic β cells. An unprecedented rise in the prevalence of T2DM is emerging over the past 15 years among children and adolescents, and this has paralleled an inexorable increase in the prevalence of childhood obesity [30–32]. Sinha et al. [33] reported 25% and 4% incidence of impaired glucose tolerance (IGT) and T2DM, respectively, among obese youngsters, and Centers for Disease Control (CDC) estimated that one-third of the newborns born in 2000 will develop T2DM if the current obesity rate persists [34]. In the United States, T2DM, which is a gradual phenomenon that usually develops from IGT over 5–10 years [35], is reported to account for approximately 45% of new cases of diabetes in childhood [36]. This suggests an accelerated transition process from IGT to T2DM among children when compared to adults. This rapid deterioration from IGT to T2DM among obese children makes the window of opportunity to implement interventions limited unless early diagnosis is made. Although the etiology of this unwelcomed phenomenon is multifaceted, in today's youth, the major contributing factor is obesity [37]. Indeed, it has been noted that although researchers in genetic fields have succeeded in finding genes underlying chronic disease states such as T2DM, only 1%–2% of the incidence of T2DM can be attributed to genetic defect [38]. This points to the "obesogenic" environment rather than genetic error as the primary underlying cause of the current diabetic epidemics.

Physical Activity Reduces Obesity, Reverses IR, and Attenuates T2DM

Children tend to gain height and weight consistent with the growth pattern matching their age and gender, resulting in stable BMI scores. Children showing an exceeding rate of weight gain over growth in height, therefore having higher BMI score than others, are regarded as overweight or obese. Fortunately, T2DM among children and adolescents is reversible and potentially preventable if it is recognized and treated before permanent pancreatic β cell damage has occurred. The most effective and easiest treatment may be the lifestyle modification that encourages healthy body weight management. Weiss et al. [39] reported in the study with 102 obese young people that significant weight gain during 24 months follow-up is associated with the transition from normal glucose tolerance (NGT) to IGT and T2DM. However, what was worth noting in the study was the observation that the transition back from IGT to NGT was associated not with substantial weight loss but with minimal weight gain, suggesting that IGT in obese children can be reversed with proper weight management through physical activity.

In order to maintain a stable and ideal body weight during a period of active growth, energy consumed needs to equal energy expenditure. Physical activity is known as the most modifiable component of energy expenditure and, therefore, is an ideal tool for maintaining healthy body weight. Cross-sectional and retrospective studies in different ethnic groups have subsequently provided evidence that physical inactivity is strongly associated with IR and IGT. Retrospective studies showed that individuals with T2DM appeared to be currently less active and tended to have spent less time for physical activity over lifetime than those without T2DM [40–42]. In addition, cross-sectional studies showed that inactive individuals in the absence of T2DM had higher blood glucose [41,43,44] and serum insulin concentration [45,46] after an oral glucose tolerance test (OGTT) than active individuals. Results from aforementioned studies demonstrate that T2DM, or at least the risks for T2DM, can be prevented through healthy weight management by increasing physical activity. Savoye et al. [47] investigated how lifestyle intervention which encouraged changes in body weight and composition affected IR among 209 obese children of mixed ethnic groups at 6 and 12 months. Lifestyle intervention mainly comprised of two sessions per week of exercise physiologist–facilitated physical activity and one session per week of nutrition education class. This study reported the significant weight loss, improved body composition, and insulin sensitivity in intervention group. In another study with 26 obese Korean adolescents by Kim et al. [48], it was reported that 6 weeks of increased physical activity improved body composition and insulin sensitivity. Unpublished data from our laboratory also demonstrated that lifestyle intervention which encouraged vigorous physical activities for 12 weeks significantly lowered fasting glucose levels and improved body composition. Not only among children, studies with adult subjects also showed that changes in lifestyle favoring healthy weight management by increasing physical activity can delay or prevent the progression from IGT to T2DM [49,50].

These suggest that physical activity, which is the most modifiable component of total energy expenditure, mediated in maintaining a stable body weight and, thus, reducing the risk factors for T2DM. Moreover, physical activity directly influences physiological parameters related to IGT, mainly via promoting skeletomuscular health. IGT results mainly from IR, in which cellular mechanism to transport glucose in response to insulin action from blood into skeletal muscle cells is impaired when excess fat is accumulated in the body [37]. Physical activity controls fat mass by increasing its oxidation at the skeletal muscles, therefore reducing the potential risk factor for IR, and interacts with the insulin signaling pathway of glucose transporter 4 (GLUT4) translocation; these allow glucose homeostasis and a more potent insulin response independent of its effect on fat oxidation [51].

Weight Loss Is Not Essential in Managing T2DM

IR can be improved with moderate intensity of exercise regardless of substantial changes in body weight or body composition. An early review of the literature by Kelley and Goodpaster [52] suggested that exercise might improve glucose homeostasis and insulin action independent of body weight changes. Recently, Bell et al. [53] showed that the intervention comprised of 8 weeks of group circuit exercise program involving a total of 24 sessions significantly improved IR in obese children and adolescents at risk of the development of T2DM. Although change in fasting glucose level was not significant, IR that precedes the development of IGT and T2DM was significantly improved independent of significant changes in body composition. Another recent study that examined the effect of 12 weeks of aerobic exercise on insulin sensitivity among 19 overweight and obese girls also showed improved insulin sensitivity without changes in body weight and percent body fat [54]. The results of these studies suggest that increased physical activity may ameliorate the disease precursor, IR, of T2DM associated with obesity in young people. Although there was no significant change in body weight and composition, in both studies, the improvement in IR was associated with cardiorespiratory fitness improvement [55].

PHYSICAL ACTIVITY AIDS ENDOCRINAL FUNCTIONS TO IMPROVE T2DM

Contrary to the past knowledge that adipose tissue is only an inert energy-storage depot, it is now known as an important endocrine organ that secretes important adipokines, among which adiponectin is a physiologically active cytokine that enhances insulin-stimulated cascade for glucose uptake [56]. It appears to be associated with insulin sensitivity and inversely related to adiposity and insulin-resistant states such as T2DM independent of gender, age, and pubertal status [56–58]. Effect of exercise on weight loss and subsequent increase in adiponectin level was reported in many recent studies. Christiansen et al. [59] reported that weight loss achieved by exercise alone or in combination with hypocaloric diet significantly increased mRNA expression of adiponectin and adiponectin receptor in adipose tissue, and pronounced weight loss when combined with hypocaloric diet increased circulating adiponectin in 79 obese adult individuals. O'Leary et al. [60] also reported similar results from the study examining the effect of weight loss by endurance exercise alone and in combination with hypocaloric diet in 21 elderly subjects with IR. Effects of weight loss on circulating level of adiponectin and subsequent insulin sensitivity were confirmed with young people in recent studies [48,61,62], suggesting the adiponectin response to weight loss in all population.

Another aspect of positive influences of exercise on insulin sensitivity was suggested by O'Leary et al. [60] When adiponectin is secreted from adipose tissue into blood, it combines through its collagen domain to form three major oligomers—trimer (low molecular weight, LMW), hexamer (middle molecular weight, MMW), and 12~18 mer (high molecular weight, HMW) adiponectin [63], among which HMW adiponectin is known to be indicative of the most physiologically active adiponectin, is believed to play more important roles in glucose homeostasis, and is a better predictor for IR than other two [63,64]. While O'Leary et al. [60] reported improved insulin sensitivity, alterations in the ratio of high HMW/total adiponectin, which correlated with the percent change in insulin sensitivity even in individuals with metabolic abnormalities, Polak et al. [65] investigated the effect of weight loss induced only by calorie restriction in the absence of exercise intervention and failed to report favorable alteration in circulating adiponectin or multimer ratio. These data suggest the importance of physical activity rather than calorie restriction in the improvement of insulin sensitivity.

It is previously discussed in this chapter that insulin sensitivity can be improved with exercise in the absence of substantial change in body weight and body composition. However, other studies have demonstrated that visceral fat, independent of BMI, is associated with IR in children and adolescents; in other words, fat distribution is also another important contributing factor for IR and T2DM [66–68]. These studies consistently demonstrated that obese young people generally show higher level of visceral lipid deposition, lower level of circulating adiponectin, and less insulin sensitiveness. Adiponectin independent of adiposity contributes to the variability in insulin sensitivity, but its circulating level is definitely affected by adiposity. Kelly et al. [69] reported that exercise itself in the absence of weight loss appears to be insufficient to induce significant increase in adiponectin level. In this study, obese children who underwent 8-week-aerobic exercise program showed no differences for change in body weight and composition compared to sedentary children; adiponectin level was not different between groups. On the other hand, Esposito et al. [70] showed that mean of 14 kg reduction in body weight and decreased abdominal adiposity—a surrogate measure for visceral adiposity following 2 years of lifestyle intervention among healthy obese women—resulted in significant increase in adiponectin and reduction in IR compared to baseline and control group. Taken these evidences together, circulating adiponectin level seems to be more closely associated with adiposity than exercise itself. In addition, visceral adiposity in young people is associated with oxidative stress and endothelial dysfunction which appears to contribute T2DM [71]. According to the studies on physical activity and fat distribution in youth, physical activity can work on fat distribution by decreasing the proportion of visceral fat in abdominal region [72–74], in dose–response manner [72]. Therefore, accumulating calorie expenditure through regular exercise and/or lifestyle intervention encouraging negative energy balance to reduce visceral adiposity is necessary for reducing IR by adiponectin.

PARENTS' PHYSICAL ACTIVITY LEVELS' INFLUENCE ON OBESITY IN SUCCESSIVE GENERATION

PHYSICAL INACTIVITY DURING PREGNANCY CAUSES OBESITY AND T2DM AMONG CHILDREN AND ADOLESCENTS

Social network may be exploited to spread positive health behaviors, although the opposite is true; in this context, obesity appears to spread through social ties [75]. Parents' activeness or sedentarism can be more easily transmitted to their children as they are the closest social ties to each other; active children tend to be the children of active parents. Beyond this behavioral influence, parents, especially mothers-to-be, should be aware that their participation in regular physical activity during lifetime can physiologically influence their childhood obesity and early onset of offspring T2DM. A meta-analysis of 20 previous studies conducted to examine the prevalence of gestational diabetes mellitus (GDM), glucose intolerance with onset or first recognition during pregnancy, and risk of subsequent diabetes demonstrated that its prevalence among all ethnic groups has increased since the early 1990s; it currently occurs in 2.2%–8.8% of pregnancies, and 10%–31% of parous women with T2DM would have experienced a GDM pregnancy, depending on the ethnic groups and the criteria used for diagnosis [76]. This increase parallels the increase in obesity epidemic; thus, obesity, among multiple contributing factors, is considered to have most sound effect on it as in T2DM [77]. How does metabolic condition during pregnancy affect fetus and later life of newborns? Several previous large studies showed that existing diabetes before pregnancy and GDM were all associated with higher mean birth weight and with odds of macrosomia (birth weight > 4000 g) [77–80]. The relationship between maternal glucose and macrosomia is less clear among women who do not have GDM; even up to fourfold increase in incidence of macrosomia was reported among women with GDM [81].

Although exact causative mechanism is not yet determined, fuel-mediated teratogenesis, or fetal overnutrition, has been suggested as the most potential mechanism for the association currently [82]. Adverse effects of GDM are not limited only to greater difficulties during pregnancy, laboring pain, and over-breastfeeding during nurturing. A greater proportion of birth weight of newborns consists of fat mass, much of which is distributed to the abdomen region. The results of 10,591 mother–offspring pairs from the Avon Longitudinal Study of Parents and Children by Lawlor et al. [79] showed not only greater birth weight but also greater offspring mean BMI and waist circumference, and increased odds of general or central obesity at age 9–11. Other large studies on Pima Indians also reported a marked increase in risk of obesity at all ages from birth to 20 years among newborns to mothers who had experienced GDM during pregnancy when compared with those to mothers who developed postpregnancy diabetes later or mothers without history of any diabetic phenotypes during lifetime [83–85].

Although maternal metabolic conditions do have effects on fetus, paternal effects seem negligible. In a nuclear family study that investigated the effect of presence of diabetes of each parent, obesity appeared to be greater among newborns after mother had been diagnosed with GDM than among their siblings born before their mother's diagnosis. On the other hand, father's diagnosis with T2DM before and after the birth of the siblings did not appear to influence obesity among them [86]. Moreover, in the cohort study of 84 children with macrosomia and 95 normal children at ages 6, 7, 9, and 11, children with macrosomia of GDM or obese mothers appeared to be at 3.6-fold greater risk of developing metabolic syndrome (MS), a cluster of abdominal obesity, hypertension, dyslipidemia, and glucose intolerance, during childhood by 11 years [87]. The findings of these studies all together suggest that the exposure to maternal diabetes in utero (GDM) is another factor that predisposes newborns to obesity and risks of diabetic phenotype in later life in addition to genetic and shared familial factors. As history repeats itself, newborns who have been exposed to GDM are more likely to develop GDM during pregnancy, and the cycle continues. GDM is considered as a significant initiating factor in obesity and T2DM epidemic; therefore, prevention of GDM may have sound effects on prevention of the epidemic in successive generations [87].

PHYSICAL ACTIVITY DURING PREGNANCY PREVENTS CHILDHOOD OBESITY AND EARLY ONSET OF T2DM

Knowing the adverse outcomes of GDM on both pregnant women and newborns, it is the disease that must be prevented and treated. Once GDM is diagnosed, primary treatment by which potential harmful consequences do not accompany would be through nutritional management that is designed to achieve normal blood glucose concentration while maintain sufficient energy and nutrients for the needs of pregnancy. Recently, exercise has been advocated as an alternative therapeutic intervention in the management of the GDM as it controls not only blood glucose levels but also help overcoming a peripheral insulin resistance [88]. Now it is encouraged, by the American College of Obstetricians and Gynecologists (ACOG) Committee on Practice, that women with GDM maintain healthy lifestyle by continuing an exercise program approved for pregnancy not only to prevent chronic health conditions in women but also to benefit fetus by normalizing birth weight and decreasing the incidence of obesity and T2DM [88,89]. Positive association between physical activity, obesity, and T2DM has been repeatedly discussed in the previous sections; is physical activity an adjunctive treatment for GDM, and could it further prevent the risks and curb the incidence of obesity and T2DM in successive generations?

Several epidemiological studies on the physical activity during the pregnancy and GDM generally reported positive association between them. From the review of literature of interest, Dempsey et al. [90] stated that previous studies consistently reported that women who are active during pregnancy have approximately 50% reduction in the risk for developing GDM compared with inactive women. Here are some interesting studies of interest. An early study by Dye et al. [91] with 12,776 pregnant women in central New York during 1995–1996 showed that exercise did not appear to lower the GDM incidence among women with BMI of 33 or less. However, among those with BMI of higher than 33, approximately twofold decrease in GDM incidence was observed among relatively active women who participated at least 30 min of weekly exercise during pregnancy when compared to their sedentary counterparts. This study was noteworthy as it reflected an important underlying relation between adiposity and GDM and potential influence of physical activity on the relation. A more recent case-control study by Dempsey et al. [92] examining the relationship between recreational physical activities performed during the first 20 weeks of pregnancy and the risk of GDM with 155 GDM cases and 386 non-GDM pregnant controls reported a 48% reduction in risk of GDM among active women who participated in any recreational activity. Another interesting large study with 4813 women who reported physically inactive before pregnancy and no previous diabetes was conducted by Liu et al. [93] to examine whether physical activity during pregnancy reduced the risk of GDM among them. In this study, 11.8% of the subjects engaged in physical activity during the follow-up; these active subjects appeared to have 57% lower odds of developing GDM compared to those who were still sedentary during the follow-up. This study suggests that physical activity during pregnancy has positive effect in lowering incidence of GDM even in previously inactive women.

Then how much physical activity is required and how hard should pregnant women exert themselves during pregnancy? Unfortunately, it seems that there is no universally established guideline for exercise recommendations for women at risk for GDM or for prevention of GDM among nondiabetic pregnant women; even ACOG suggests vague recommendations that active lifestyle is encouraged. In addition, exercise prescriptions that optimize consequences of GDM women and the offspring are currently lacking. Weissgerber et al. [94] reviewed the current literatures to examine the relation between amount of physical activity and its consequences on GDM, and to compare the effectiveness of exercise intervention programs that were less than 55% of VO_{2max}. The studies reviewed did not consistently report the positive effects of exercise on the management of GDM, but the results suggest that women who were more active during the pregnancy had lower prevalence of GDM; lower exercise intensity would be more effective rather than moderate intensity, as exercising at moderate intensity is difficult for sedentary pregnant women, thus resulting in low compliance and continuity in the program.

Taken all together, the converging evidence suggests increasing physical activity levels during pregnancy. It may benefit pregnant women and the offspring by reducing the incidence of GDM and of obesity and diabetes during childhood among the offspring, therefore supporting the ACOG's recommendations that promote exercise during pregnancy. However, no prospective study that systemically examined the relation of physical activity during pregnancy, body weight and composition of pregnant woman, incidence of GDM, macrosomia, obesity, and MS among the offspring to GDM mothers during childhood, adolescence, and adulthood is currently available. Such investigation is necessary to examine the roles of physical activity during pregnancy on the offspring; even constant exertions of devoting researchers for a considerable amount of time are required. We, however, can assume from currently published literature that being active during pregnancy does help prevent, or at least attenuate, the spread of child obesity epidemic.

PHYSICAL ACTIVITY REDUCES OBESITY-RELATED CARDIOVASCULAR DISEASE DEVELOPMENT

OBESITY IS ASSOCIATED WITH CARDIOVASCULAR DISEASES

Obesity is a term applied to excess body weight with abnormal high degree of adiposity, and this disease predisposes individuals in all population with many other medical complications. The previous section discussed its contribution to the development of IR which is the major determinant for T2DM. What other complications are induced by obesity other than T2DM? Epidemiological studies have demonstrated that obesity is associated with an increased incidence of CVDs, particularly coronary heart disease and stroke [95,96]. A 26 year follow-up study by Hubert et al. [96] showed that the degree of obesity was an important long-term predictor of CVD incidence; particularly obesity among young people was associated with accelerated coronary atherosclerosis process, suggesting that leanness and avoidance of excess weight gain before adulthood are advisable goal in the prevention of CVD. This large cohort study demonstrated that the importance of weight management during childhood and adolescence is particularly important for the prevention of the diseases. There is a general consensus that the increased risk of CVD among obese individuals is primarily due to the coexistence of obesity-associated risk factors for CVD such as elevated blood pressure, dyslipidemia, high circulating inflammatory markers, adipokines, and so on [95–99], rather than the degree of obesity *per se*. It is, however, important to recognize that the common denominator for these risk factors is obesity itself, and these risk factors do not usually occur in isolation but are usually found concurrently.

The vast proportion of CVD develops from atherosclerosis, the condition in which an artery wall thickens as the result of the accumulation of lipids onto the arterial walls. Although CVD manifests clinically in middle and late adulthood, it is known that atherosclerosis, the predisposing factor for CVD, has a long asymptomatic phase of development, which begins early in life, often during childhood. In most children, atherosclerotic process is not common and can be minimized or prevented if early proper intervention is given. However, in some children, the process is accelerated in the exposure to the risk factors [100]. The possible pathophysiological mechanisms existing between obesity and CVD have not yet been completely understood; it is, however, now clear that inflammatory process precedes the development of atherosclerosis [101]. Thus, proinflammatory cytokines that initiate the inflammatory process may play critical roles in the initiation and progression of atherosclerosis by producing atherosclerotic plaques and, eventually, the development of CVD.

The secretion of the proinflammatory cytokines takes place in different tissues and cells, including the adipose tissue [102]. It is briefly discussed in the previous section that accumulated evidence has transformed the classic view on adipocytes as an energy-storage organ to an important endocrine organ that secretes a large variety of hormones, or adipokines, which may be relevant for the development of CVD. These include leptin, adiponectin, and the major proinflammatory cytokines—tumor necrosis factor-α (TNF-α) and interleukin-6 (IL-6) [103–105]. TNF-α and IL-6 are known to induce the secretion of C-reactive protein (CRP) from the liver; it has been found to play an active role in atherogenesis, thus contributing to CVD development, as evidenced by previous studies [106,107]. CRP has been shown to be the most consistently associated with the risk of CVD; therefore, its measurement is widely accepted as the best predictor of CVD among the proinflammatory cytokines up to date [108–110]. Leptin, another adipokine which is known to have effects on the regulation of the energy metabolism, is also found to play a role in the pathophysiology of CVD development; De Rosa et al. [97] demonstrated that leptin induces CRP mRNA transcription and synthesis of CRP. It is of particular interest that obese individuals frequently have elevated plasma levels of TNF-α, IL-6, leptin, and CRP—these variables are referred to as obesity biomarkers, as described by Pischon [101]. This suggests that the adipose tissue thereby actively participates in the development of CVD; in other words, it also suggests that reducing adipose tissue may prevent the development of CVD. In addition, fat distribution is another factor to consider, as visceral adipose tissue is metabolically more active and secretes more adipokines that are relevant for CVD compared with subcutaneous adipose tissue [103]. Though the aforementioned data linking these risk factors to cardiovascular events come mostly from the studies with adults, these risk factors have also been found to cause acceleration of atherosclerosis in children to the similar extent in adults.

Therefore, considering the fact that atherosclerosis has a long asymptomatic phase of development which begins during childhood [100] and the common denominator for risk factors for development of CVD is obesity, prevention of childhood obesity might be the primary intervention for preventing cardiovascular events during lifetime. It is discussed in previous section that the primary underlying cause for childhood obesity is the *surplus energy* due to physical inactivity rather than genetic determinants or disease status. The following sections will discuss if physical activity can improve the risk factors for CVD among children and adolescents.

PHYSICAL ACTIVITY REDUCES ADIPOSITY AND ITS RELATED FACTORS FOR CVD DEVELOPMENT

Previously, the fact that increased physical activity and reduction of body weight improve IR, therefore reducing the incidence of T2DM and improving T2DM among young people who were already diagnosed with T2DM, was described. As mentioned earlier, CVD and T2DM together are often clustered as MS as they usually share same risk factors. In this context, it may be assumed that CVD can also be improved by increasing physical activity and reducing body weight. Weight loss through lifestyle interventions through exercise training with caloric restriction does improve risk profiles such as inflammatory cytokines, dyslipidemia, and hypertension, all of which are related to CVD and lower mortality [111]. However, considering that some epidemiological studies showed that purposeful weight loss among those who are obese and with CVD may not be always beneficial and may even be detrimental, one should be aware that there are potential adverse effects of weight loss if it is not accompanied with exercise that preserves lean body mass [112–114].

Then, what would be the most appropriate recommendation for those who worry about CVD in the future of their children? Recalling from the previous section, atherosclerosis, the major determinant of developing CVD, begins to develop during childhood asymptomatically, and obesity is the common denominator for risk factors related to atherosclerosis and eventually CVD. Potential adverse effects of weight loss in obese people after diagnosis with CVD are suggested by large-scale studies. Taken all together, the answer to the question is simpler than anyone may think. Let us get children and adolescents out of couch and to be active, thereby lowering the degree of obesity before the progression of CVD accelerates. Exercise definitely decreases adiposity and improves adiposity-related risk factors contributing to the development of CVD.

Physical Activity Improves Dyslipidemia among Obese Children

Dyslipidemia is the term applied to the presence of increased or abnormal levels of lipids and/or lipoproteins such as decreased concentration of high-density lipoprotein cholesterol (HDL-C) and increased concentration of triglycerides (TG) and low-density lipoprotein cholesterol (LDL-C) in blood. Obese individuals regardless of age tend to have dyslipidemia [1], and accumulated evidence has shown that these conditions in children and adolescents are features of increased risk of CVD during adulthood [115,116].

Correlation between physical activity and dyslipidemia often appears to be very low and nonsignificant among children and adolescents, or inconsistent from study to study [115,117,118], mainly due to the inconsistency in the measurement of daily physical activity level. However, a study that used a multivariate approach on the data obtained from 610 children and adolescents and unified measuring method for physical activity levels by Katzmarzyk et al. [119] reported that physical activity is characterized by a negative association with LDL-C and TG, and a positive association with HDL-C, indicating that daily physical activity is associated with a favorable CVD risk profile. Then how does exercise-based intervention program reduce body weight and improve dyslipidemia, thus favoring CVD risk profile among obese young people? Reinehr et al. [120] studied changes in weight status and CVD risk factors in 240 obese children whose ages lie between 6 and 12 participating in 2 year intervention program targeted for reducing obesity primarily through exercise and health educations. The results of the study indicated that obese children had significantly higher BMI, LDL-C, and TG while having significantly lower HDL-C when compared to the counterparts; and the intervention resulted in the significant reduction in BMI which was accompanied by improved HDL-C, LDL-C and TG profile, and other risk factors for MS. Similar results have been reported from other smaller studies which showed that a reduction in BMI, the simple indicator of obesity, through the interventions which include exercise program leads to an improvement of CVD risk profile [121–123]. More important finding of these studies is that the improvement in CVD risk factors was sustained during 1 year follow-up period if reduced BMI during the intervention period was maintained. Furthermore, Reinehr and Andler [124,125] reported that greater weight loss over the period of time promotes greater improvement of atherogenic profile; these suggest that substantial improvement in dyslipidemia requires systemic and ongoing effort.

Physical Activity Improves Obesity-Related Hypertension among Children

Hypertension is a premature complication of obesity, and it is the term applied to a chronic medical condition in which the blood pressure is elevated, and can be classified as either primary or secondary. In primary hypertension, which is common and accounts for about 90%–95% of hypertension, no medical cause can be found to explain the raised blood pressure, while secondary hypertension indicates that the raised blood pressure is due to other conditions such as kidney failure [126].

The association between obesity and hypertension has been well established in most racial, ethnic, and socioeconomic groups, although the values vary, depending on age, gender, race, and so on. Primary hypertension in children was previously considered rare, but in recent years, it has become increasingly common in association with obesity. Obese children are at approximately a threefold higher risk for hypertension than nonobese children [127], and having hypertensive condition during childhood has been linked to increased carotid intima-media thickness (cIMT) and arterial stiffness which are indicative of accelerated atherosclerosis [100]. Furthermore, obese children tend to have lower flow-mediated dilation (FMD). When blood flow increases through a vessel, the vessel dilates in order to control blood pressure. Endothelium, the thin layer of cells that line the inner surface of blood vessels, participates in the regulation of blood flow in response to changes in tissue and organ perfusion. The fact that obese children have lower FMD suggests that they are in less favorable condition for normal blood pressure and atherosclerosis [128]. Obesity-induced hypertension has some unique characteristics with complicated pathophysiological mechanisms such as disturbances in autonomic function, abnormalities in cardiac and vascular structure and function, high blood volume, and inappropriate peripheral resistance [127,129,130]. Weight loss through caloric restriction and exercise is generally recommended in the prevention and improvement of hypertension. It is out of scope of this section to discuss how each of those mechanisms be altered through interventions for weight reduction; rather this section will introduce some studies examining the role of physical activities in reducing blood pressure and improving early markers of atherosclerosis in children.

Farpour-Lambert et al. [131] compared the early markers of atherosclerosis between obese and lean children and investigated the effects of 24 week exercise on the markers among obese children as well. In this study, it was reported that obese children had higher blood pressure, arterial stiffness, body weight, BMI, abdominal fat, IR indices, and CRP levels, and lower FMD, physical activity levels, and HDL-C levels than lean subjects, suggesting that obesity among children is the predisposing cause for atherosclerosis processes. This result shows that physical inactivity is the major risk factor for obesity and CVD. Moreover, it is interesting to see that exercise significantly reduces blood pressure, and this reduction was accompanied by the significant reduction in body weight, body fat, abdominal fat, and other atherosclerosis markers such as cIMT and arterial stiffness. As mentioned, having hypertensive condition during childhood is associated with accelerated atherosclerosis and eventually CVD; in this context, decreased blood pressure by increasing physical activity may reduce the presteps for developing CVD [131]. These results are in agreement with those of Meyer et al [132] who found significantly lower FMD and increased cIMT in obese children compared to lean children, and significant improvements in blood pressure with 6 month exercise. In this study, exercise-induced improvements in blood pressure were accompanied by favorable changes in cIMT, FMD, BMI, adiposity, waist/hip ratio, the levels of fasting insulin, TG, cholesterol profile, and CRP. Common reporting reviews on association between obesity and hypertension reveal that weight or BMI rather than age, gender, and height better predicts high blood pressure [133].

Obesity is a highly prevalent condition that causes or exacerbates other health problems, including hypertension. Achieving healthy body weight through regular exercise and/or physically active lifestyle is therefore an excellent and maybe the most efficient approach to prevent and improve hypertensive condition and CVD-related risk factors among children and all population. Thus, it is highly recommended especially for children to move out of couch and sweat themselves.

PHYSICAL ACTIVITY REDUCES OBESITY-INDUCED INFLAMMATORY CONDITION

As mentioned earlier, several prospective epidemiological studies have demonstrated that CRP is a predictor of the CVDs development [106–110] and has been consistently shown to be most associated with the risk of CVDs [108–110]. It is also briefly mentioned that CRP synthesis is mediated by the adipokines including leptin, IL-6, and TNF-α; therefore, adipocytes play a critical role in cardiovascular events [101,103–107]. What does having high or low level of CRP in the blood mean?

Among several functions of CRP, the most important is its ability to bind to cell membrane components, thus forming complexes that activate the classical complement pathway as well as removal of these structures from circulation only after membrane rupture. This property suggests an important role of CRP in the organism's defense system as it removes cell debris derived from necrotic cells or cells damaged during the inflammatory process, thus allowing tissue repair [134]. The increase in CRP concentration depends on the amount of protein that is required to effectively participate in the defense system; thus, its level is closely correlated with the extent of tissue damage [135]. It has also been demonstrated that CRP contributes to the formation of atherosclerotic plaques as it enhances clotting effect by increasing adhesion molecules that bind to plasma lipoproteins [136]. This is the reason why CRP has been intensively studied in the association with CVD. Considering the fact that obesity is a start of low grade of inflammation condition [95,96], it can be assumed that obese individuals are exposed to the inflammatory cytokines that are associated with CVD. Previous studies reported the association among obesity inflammatory cytokines and CVD among children and adolescents. For example, Semiz et al. [137] investigated an association between CRP, BMI, and cardiovascular risk factors in 28 obese children and adolescents and found the positive correlation between CRP and BMI, weight, blood pressure, and leptin concentration, supporting the relationship between CRP, obesity, and CVDs. This study also supports the previous finding that atherosclerotic process begins during childhood especially among obese children. In another study by Yoshinaga et al. [138] which was aimed to identify the adipokines that are predictive of the accumulation of CVD risk factors in 321 elementary school children, it was reported that leptin was the most sensitive marker for predicting the accumulation of CVD risk factors. Although CRP did not appear to be the most sensitive marker in this study, considering the fact that leptin which induces CRP mRNA transcription and synthesis of CRP, and its expression level in the blood is negatively related to adiposity, is the sensitive marker of CVD risks, it is assumed that adipocytes definitely play critical roles in the development of CVD by mediating inflammatory process [139].

Many studies investigated the association between obesity and inflammations generally conclude that obesity is a state of low-grade systemic inflammation. Forsythe et al. [140] reviewed the literature investigated the effects of weight loss on inflammatory profiles and concluded that the greatest improvements in obesity-related inflammatory cytokines are observed when at least 10% of weight loss was achieved among obese population; therefore, weight loss itself is capable of reversing the unfavorable inflammatory profile in the obese state.

In this context, as the primary prevention for CVD through mediating inflammatory cytokines, exercise seems to be a recommended intervention due to its regulatory effects on body weight. Exact mechanism for its anti-inflammatory is still unclear; inconsistent results on the down-regulatory effects of exercise have been reported. It is further complicated by the reports that some of inflammatory cytokines decrease [141–143] while the others increase [144–145] in response to regular exercise in children as the immune system is subject to developmental changes during childhood. However, many studies support that regular exercise can reduce basal or resting levels of inflammatory cytokines and can be useful as an anti-inflammatory intervention not only for the obese population but also for healthy individuals [146–148]. At least, considering the fact that obese individuals have higher basal levels of inflammatory cytokines, it is clear that prevention of childhood obesity by having children participate in regular exercise may help them to be free from a state of low-grade systemic inflammation which predisposes children to CVD. However, it is important to emphasize that exercise has to be performed in a safe manner where inflammatory cytokines are not further increased. Exercise *per se* exerts various effects on immune systems where both inflammatory and anti-inflammatory cytokines increase during and after a single bout of exercise, and this is more prominent when high-intensity exercise, especially anaerobic exercise, is performed [149–152]. On the other hand, low-intensity regular exercise not only reduces the basal or resting inflammatory cytokines but also blunts the inflammatory responses to acute exercise [152,153]. Therefore, sufficient low-intensity exercise would be required to lower the circulating inflammatory cytokine. However, these results are mostly from the studies with the subjects of adults, and the results from those with the children and adolescents often fail to come into the consistent conclusion. Unfortunately, until the very recent, no studies have investigated the effects of regular exercise on the chronic inflammatory cytokines among children in chronic inflammatory disease states [148]. It is also important to note that immunological responses to exercise among children are different than those of adults. This is of significance regarding the creation of exercise programs which are challenging, effective, and safe; therefore, further investigation on the effects of regular exercise as an anti-inflammatory intervention among children is required.

PHYSICAL ACTIVITY DOES MORE THAN LOWERING BODY WEIGHT AND IMPROVING CHRONIC DISEASES

BEING PHYSICALLY ACTIVE IS THE BEST MEDICINE TO REDUCE OBESITY AND ITS COMPLICATIONS

Two most common diseases that are of concern and derived from childhood obesity are T2DM and CVD, and the characteristics of each disease and the effects of weight loss through physical activity (or exercise) on the conditions were detailed separately in previous sections. Although major risk factors for each disease were discussed separately, what is interesting is that these diseases are not mutually exclusive from each other and each factor contributes to each disease. The MS is now a universal term which represents a cluster of obesity, IR, glucose intolerance, hypertension, and dyslipidemia; and each component of the MS is a common basis for the development of T2DM and CVD among all population [154,155]. In addition, inflammatory cytokines, especially CRP, also appear to be associated not only with CVD but also with T2DM [156–158]. Considering that profiles of these biomarkers are unfavorable among obese individuals, managing these components by reducing obesity during childhood and adolescence may prevent the development of both T2DM and CVD. As mentioned, obesity has been described as a multifactorial trait determined by genetic and environmental factors; at least as many as 250 obesity-associated genes have been identified [159], and the obesogenic environment causes predisposition to obesity. Up to date, gene manipulation technology has not been extended to the disease care for humans for various reasons, including ethical issues and risks of side effects. Medical treatments that are currently used to cure obesity and its related diseases are not completely free from the risks of side effects either. If genetic factors that determine obesity among children are not something that we can solve at this time, why aren't we doing something for changing the environmental factors to stop the obesity epidemic among children? It is not necessary to completely change the characteristics of obesogenic environment; instead, we just can simply be active with our children from day to day. We discussed that the characteristics of adulthood-onset diseases now appear among obese children, and these appearances become attenuated by weight reduction through physical activity. Some studies demonstrated that children who participate in more physical activities tend to remain more physically active during adulthood; others demonstrate that level of physical activity during childhood does not provide the protections for the chronic diseases if active lifestyle is not sustained in adulthood [134]. Having physically active habit during childhood and maintaining this habit is, therefore, critically important for reducing obesity and its metabolic complications for a lifetime.

PHYSICAL ACTIVITY IMPROVES ANOTHER CVD-ASSOCIATED FACTOR, PHYSICAL FITNESS

If weight loss is the key for reducing childhood obesity and its metabolic complications, what was the point of emphasizing the importance of physical activity or exercise throughout the chapter for weight loss rather than just low-calorie diet? In order to answer this question, it is necessary to consider another important point related to childhood obesity: there is significant association between fatness and fitness. In addition to biomarkers discussed in previous sections, poor physical fitness, especially cardiovascular fitness, has been demonstrated as a stronger risk factor for CVD and the development of IR in adults [160–164]. The associations between biomarkers for MS and poor physical fitness also have been reported among obese children [165,166]. The importance of physical fitness in the prevention of MS is supported by other studies. Lee et al. [167] showed that within a fatness category, better cardiovascular fitness attenuates the risk factors contributing to CVD; and Church et al. [168] reported that the greatest risk score for MS was found in the low-fitness obese group and the lowest score was found in the high-fitness normal weight group. In the latter study, it was also shown that within levels of fatness, risk score for MS was lower for the higher fitness groups. Brufani et al. [169] showed that poor cardiovascular fitness, IR, and components of MS were independently related to obesity among children; and Allen et al. [170] showed that in middle school students, levels of fitness were more closely related to measures of IR than percent body fat. Additionally, as reported by Nassis et al. [171], although exercise did not always decrease body weight and percent body fat, exercise was associated with beneficial changes in components of MS and physical fitness. From these aforementioned findings, we can assume that poor physical fitness may be an independent risk factor contributing to the development of T2DM and CVD; therefore, efforts to reduce the diseases should include exercise intervention sustained enough to improve physical fitness. Generally, obese children and adolescents are unfit except those who were born with a set of "good" genes [154]; lower fitness levels of obese young people further prevent their participation in physical activity; therefore, it is critically important to get children to be active to improve another risk factor for the development of T2DM and CVD.

It has been suggested that prevention of obesity in childhood and adolescence should emphasize increased physical activity rather than diet because of concerns relating to the adverse effects of inappropriate eating patterns, and dietary treatment of obesity is often reported to be relatively ineffective in all populations [172]. Some may raise doubts about the effect of physical activity on weight management since the energy expended during active periods will drive up hunger mechanism to compensate for the energy loss. However, studies show that interventions of a period of exercise generate little or no immediate effect on levels of hunger or daily energy intake [173]. Of course, healthy eating behavior is of particular importance in the management of childhood obesity, but as discussed earlier, more successful outcome is expected when the intervention combines focus on both weight loss and increasing physical fitness. It is a false belief that dietary treatment alone can facilitate weight loss and deterioration of risk factors for T2DM and CVD. Although it is not discussed in previous sections, most studies cited in this chapter which used the intervention comprised of various types of physical activity reported the concurrent decrease in the obesity and risk factors for its related metabolic complications, and the physical fitness, particularly the cardiovascular fitness. Beyond its beneficial effects on obesity-related medical complications and physical fitness, exercise is also shown to be helpful for relieving anxiety and stress, which brings a sense of well-being, therefore helping to maintain and promote overall health [174]. This way we know that physical activity is the component that cannot be disregarded in the prevention of obesity in all population (Figure 58.2).

How Much Should Children Be Physically Active?

In the beginning of this chapter, consistent conclusion from the review articles was discussed that physical activity promotes fat loss while preserving or increasing lean mass, and the rate of weight loss is proportional to the amount of physical activity; thus, every increase in activity adds some benefit to overall health. Sedentary lifestyle is an important risk factor for developing T2DM and CVD, but regular physical exercises are very important in the prevention and control of them by favorably influencing the primary risk factor, obesity, and other related risk factors including dyslipidemia, hypertension, and inflammatory cytokines. Now, how much physical activity is recommended for our children, and from when should they be active? The American Heart Association (AHA) establishes that the adoption of an active lifestyle should be encouraged from 2 year old and maintained throughout adolescence until adulthood to reduce risk factors for CVD [175], and as a general advice, healthy children should be encouraged to practice physical activities during leisure time or as organized physical sport activities at least 30 min per day, three to four times per week, to

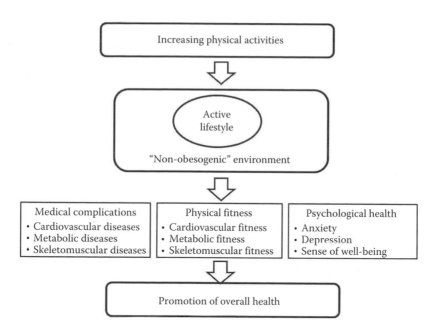

FIGURE 58.2 Having active lifestyle by increasing physical activity levels, obese individuals can improve medical complications, physical fitness, and psychological health as well. Physical activity thereby promotes overall health.

become physically fit [176]. Although suggestions are to prevent CVD development, when considering that the risk factors for CVD are the components of MS which are the underlying basis for both T2DM and CVD, it may be interpreted that adoption of active lifestyle from 2 year old is recommended to prevent early development of chronic diseases.

Different organizations have their own physical activity guidelines that focus on healthy body management and promotion of overall health. For example, minimum exercise guidelines by American College of Sports Medicine (ACSM) recommend 20–30 min of aerobic activity 3–5 days per week, and one set (8–12 repetitions) of 8–10 resistance exercises in moderate to vigorous intensity to train the major muscle groups 2 days per week to maintain healthy body weight and general health [177]. Physical activity guidelines of the Canadian Physical Activity, Fitness and Lifestyle Approach Protocol (CPAFLA) recommend participating in moderate physical activity and to increase it from 30 to 90 min progressively, and children and adolescents should participate in vigorous physical activity at least for one-third of their total physical activity time to maintain healthy body weight and promote overall health [178]. Although it appears that low-intensity aerobic exercise generates beneficial metabolic effects that would be similar to those produced by high-intensity exercise, high intensity is more likely to improve physical fitness, another associated cardiovascular risk factor for overall health, to the greater extent [179]. Therefore, once obese individuals succeed in managing weight and improving fitness level through long-term exercise interventions, it is recommended to gradually increase exercise intensity in order to achieve higher fitness level and promote overall health. No matter which exercise guideline or exercise intensity one chooses, what is more important is how one adopts an active lifestyle for lifetime and performs healthy behaviors to prevent obesity and to maintain and promote overall health.

SUMMARY

The spread of obesity pandemic, especially among children, gives causes for concern for its long-term implications on health as accruing evidence has linked obesity to morbidity and mortality from a wide variety of chronic diseases; in other words, obesity is rightly referred to as the major contributor to most predominant causes of recent adult-onset chronic diseases. These diseases include T2DM and CVDs. Moreover, childhood obesity persists into adult life; this gives concern for further increasing adult obesity prevalence in the future and higher risk for suffering from associated health problems for a lifetime. Beside its adverse consequences on physical and physiological health, obesity is also known to be associated with significant psychological and sociological problems among children. Insufficient physical activity levels during childhood and adolescence have been considered as one of the major causes of obesity pandemic. Therefore, the most promising strategy for lowering obesity prevalence is to focus on increasing physical activity levels. In this chapter, we have described how physical activities during childhood and adolescence can improve risk factors for T2DM and CVD, or the components of MS, including adiposity, IR, dyslipidemia, hypertension, and, in addition, inflammatory cytokines. We emphasized both physiological and behavioral roles of parents in the prevention of childhood obesity, and the solution for the prevention of childhood obesity lies in increasing physical activity levels rather than reducing calorie intake as physical activity not only reduces obesity prevalence but also promotes overall health. There are many exercise guidelines available to reduce obesity; more important thing than considering which guideline to choose is, however, to adopt an active lifestyle for lifetime and perform healthy behaviors as any positive lifestyle changes add some benefits to overall health.

REFERENCES

1. Regan, F. and Betts, P. (2006). A brief review of the health consequences of childhood obesity. In *Childhood Obesity*: *Contemporary Issues* (Cameron, N., Norgan, N.G., and Ellison, G.T.H., Eds), Chapter 3, pp. 25–38. Taylor & Francis Group, Boca Raton, FL.
2. Ogden, C.L., Carroll, M.D., Curtin, L.R., McDowell, M.A., Tabak, C.J., and Flegal, K.M. (2006). Prevalence of overweight and obesity in the United States, 1999–2004. *JAMA* **295(13)**, 1549 1555.
3. Lee, G.E., Park, H.S., Yun, K.E., Jun, S.H., Kim, H.K., Cho, S.I., and Kim, J.H. (2008). Association between BMI and metabolic syndrome and adenomatous colonic polyps in Korean men. *Obesity (Silver Spring)* **16(6)**, 1434–1439.
4. World Health Organization (WHO). (2006). Obesity and overweight. From http://www.who.int/mediacentre/factsheets/fs311/en/ (Retrieved on March 1, 2010).
5. N/A. (2006). Abstracts of the 10th international congress on obesity (ICO). September 3–8, 2006. Sydney, Australia. *Obes Rev* **7(Suppl 2)**, 1–352.
6. Ebbeling, C.B., Pawlak, D.B., and Ludwig, D.S. (2002). Childhood obesity: Public-health crisis, common sense cure. *Lancet* **360(9331)**, 473–482.
7. Hedley, A.A., Ogden, C.L., Johnson, C.L., Carroll, M.D., Curtin, L.R., and Flegal, K.M. (2004). Prevalence of overweight and obesity among US children, adolescents, and adults, 1999–2002. *JAMA* **291(23)**, 2847–2850.
8. Katz, L.L. and Abraham, M. (2006). Dominant western health care: Type 2 diabetes mellitus. *J Transcult Nurs* **17(3)**, 230–233.
9. Clarke, W.R. and Lauer, R.M. (1993). Does childhood obesity track into adulthood? *Crit Rev Food Sci Nutr* **33(4–5)**, 423–430.
10. Reilly, J.J., Methven, E., McDowell, Z.C., Hacking, B., Alexander, D., Stewart, L., and Kelnar, C.J. (2003). Health consequences of obesity. *Arch Dis Child* **88(9)**, 748–752.
11. Strauss, R.S. (2000). Childhood obesity and self-esteem. *Pediatrics* **105(1)**, e15.
12. Kimm, S.Y., Sweeney, C.G., Janosky, J.E., and MacMillan, J.P. (1991). Self-concept measures and childhood obesity: A descriptive analysis. *J Dev Behav Pediatr* **12(1)**, 19–24.
13. Kenchaiah, S., Evans, J.C., Levy, D., Wilson, P.W., Benjamin, E.J., Larson, M.G., Kannel, W.B., and Vasan, R.S. (2002). Obesity and the risk of heart failure. *N Engl J Med* **347(5)**, 305–313.
14. Crocker, M.K. and Yanovski, J.A. (2009). Pediatric obesity: Etiology and treatment. *Endocrinol Metab Clin North Am* **38(3)**, 525–548.
15. Dyer, R.G. (1994). Traditional treatment of obesity: Does it work? *Baillieres Clin Endocrinol Metab* **8(3)**, 661–688.
16. Centers for Disease Control and Prevention (CDC). (N/A). Physical activity and health: A report of the surgeon general executive summary. From http://www.fitness.gov/execsum/execsum.htm (Retrieved on March 1, 2010).

17. Stefanick, M.L. (1993). Exercise and weight control. *Exerc Sport Sci Rev* **21**, 363–396.

18. Epstein, L.H. and Wing, R.R. (1980). Aerobic exercise and weight. *Addict Behav* **5**, 371–388.

19. Ballor, D.L. and Keesey, R.E. (1991). A meta-analysis of the factors affecting exercise-induced changes in body mass, fat mass and fat-free mass in males and females. *Int J Obes* **15**, 717–726.

20. Wilmore, J.H. (1983). Body composition in sport and exercise: Directions for future research. *Med Sci Sports Exerc* **15**, 21–31.

21. Lagerros, Y.T. and Lagiou, P. (2007). Assessment of physical activity and energy expenditure in epidemiological research of chronic diseases. *Eur J Epidemiol* **22**, 353–362.

22. Pate, R.R., Freedson, P.S., Sallis, J.F., Taylor, W.C., Sirard, J., Trost, S.G., and Dowda, M. (2002). Compliance with physical activity guidelines: Prevalence in a population of children and youth. *Ann Epidemiol* **12**, 303–308.

23. Cooper, A.R., Page, A.S., Foster, L.J., and Qahwaji, D. (2003). Commuting to school: Are children who walk more physically active? *Am J Prev Med* **25**, 273–276.

24. Centers for Disease Control and Prevention. (N/A). Chapter Conclusions. From http://www.cdc.gov/NCCDPHP/SGR/chapcon.htm (Retrieved on March 1, 2010).

25. Logstrup, S. (2001). Children and young people—The importance of physical activity. Brussels: EHHI.

26. Tammelin, T., Näyhä, S., Hills, A.P., and Järvelin, M.R. (2003). Adolescent participation in sports and adult physical activity. *Am J Prev Med* **24**, 22–28.

27. Telama, R., Yang, X., Viikari, J., Välimäki, I., Wanne, O., and Raitakari, O. (2005). Physical activity from childhood to adulthood: A 21-year tracking study. *Am J Prev Med* **28**, 267–273.

28. Fogelholm, M. (2008). How physical activity can work? *Int J Pediatr Obes* **3(Suppl1)**, 10–14.

29. Franks, P.W., Ravussin, E., Hanson, R.L., Harper, I.T., Allison, D.B., Knowler, W.C., Tataranni, P.A., and Salbe, A.D. (2005). Habitual physical activity in children: The role of genes and the environment. *Am J Clin Nutr* **82**, 901–908.

30. Writing Group for the SEARCH for Diabetes in Youth Study Group, Dabelea, D., Bell, R.A., D'Agostino, R.B. Jr., Imperatore, G., Johansen, J.M., Linder, B., Liu, L.L., Loots, B., Marcovina, S., Mayer-Davis, E.J., Pettitt, D.J., and Waitzfelder, B. (2007). Incidence of diabetes in youth in the United States. *JAMA* **297**, 2716–2724.

31. Rosenbloom, A.L., Joe, J.R., Young, R.S., and Winter, W.E. (1999). Emerging epidemic of type 2 diabetes in youth. *Diabetes Care* **22**, 345–354.

32. Dabelea, D., Pettitt, D.J., Jones, K.L., and Arslanian, S.A. (1999). Type 2 diabetes mellitus in minority children and adolescents: An emerging problem. *Endocrinol Metab Clin North Am* **28**, 709–729.

33. Sinha, R., Fisch, G., Teague, B., Tamborlane, W.V., Banyas, B., Allen, K., Savoye, M., Rieger, V., Taksali, S., Barbetta, G., Sherwin, R.S., and Caprio, S. (2002). Prevalence of impaired glucose tolerance among children and adolescents with marked obesity. *N Engl J Med* **346(11)**, 802–810.

34. Narayan, K.M., Boyle, J.P., Thompson, T.J., Sorensen, S.W., and Williamson, D.F. (2003). Lifetime risk for diabetes mellitus in the United States. *JAMA* **290(14)**, 1884–1890.

35. Edelstein, S.L., Knowler, W.C., Bain, R.P., Andres, R., Barrett-Connor, E.L., Dowse, G.K., Haffner, S.M., Pettitt, D.J., Sorkin, J.D., Muller, D.C., Collins, V.R., and Hamman, R.F. (1997). Predictors of progression from impaired glucose tolerance to NIDDM: An analysis of six prospective studies. *Diabetes* **46**, 701–710.

36. Aye, T. and Levitsky, L. (2003). Type 2 diabetes: An epidemic disease in childhood. *Curr Opin Pediatr* **15(4)**, 411–415.

37. Kahn, B.B. and Flier, J.S. (2000). Obesity and insulin resistance. *J Clin Invest* **106**, 473–481.

38. Booth, F.W., Chakravarthy, M.V., Gordon, S.E., and Spangenburg, E.E. (2002). Waging war on physical inactivity: Using modern molecular ammunition against an ancient enemy. *J Appl Physiol* **93**, 3–30.

39. Weiss, R., Taksali, S.E., Tamborlane, W.V., Burgert, T.S., Savoye, M., and Caprio, S. (2005). Predictors of changes in glucose tolerance in obese youth. *Diabetes Care* **28**, 902–909.

40. Dowse, G.K., Gareeboo, H., Zimmet, P.Z., Alberti, K.G., Tuomilehto, J., Fareed, D., Brissonnette, L.G., and Finch, C.F. (1990). High prevalence of NIDDM and impaired glucose tolerance in Indian, Creole, and Chinese Mauritians. *Diabetes* **39**, 390–396.

41. Kriska, A.M., LaPorte, R.E., Pettitt, D.J., Charles, M.A., Nelson, R.G., Kuller, L.H., Bennett, P.H., and Knowler, W.C. (1993). The association of physical activity with obesity, fat distribution and glucose intolerance in Pima Indians. *Diabetologia* **36**, 863–869.

42. Taylor, R., Ram, P., Zimmet, P., Raper, L.R., and Ringrose, H. (1984). Physical activity and prevalence of diabetes in Melanesian and Indian men in Fiji. *Diabetologia* **27**, 578–582.

43. Cederholm, J. and Wibell, L. (1985). Glucose tolerance and physical activity in a health survey of middle-aged subjects. *Acta Med Scand* **217**, 373–378.

44. Pereira, M.A., Kriska, A.M., Joswiak, M.L., Dowse, G.K., Collins, V.R., Zimmet, P.Z., Gareeboo, H., Chitson, P., Hemraj, F., and Purran, A. (1995). Physical inactivity and glucose intolerance in the multiethnic island of Mauritius. *Med Sci Sports Exerc* **27**, 1626–1634.

45. Regensteiner, J.G., Shetterly, S.M., Mayer, E.J., Eckel, R.H., Haskell, W.L., Baxter, J., and Hamman, R.F. (1995). Relationship between habitual physical activity and insulin area among individuals with impaired glucose tolerance. The San Luis Valley Diabetes Study. *Diabetes Care* **18**, 490–497.

46. Wang, J.T., Ho, L.T., Tang, K.T., Wang, L.M., Chen, Y.D., and Reaven, G.M. (1989). Effect of habitual physical activity on age-related glucose intolerance. *J Am Geriatr Soc* **37**, 203–209.

47. Savoye, M., Shaw, M., Dziura, J., Tamborlane, W.V., Rose, P., Guandalini, C., Goldberg-Gell, R., Burgert, T.S., Cali, A.M., Weiss, R., and Caprio, S. (2007). Effects of a weight management program on body composition and metabolic parameters in overweight children: A randomized controlled trial. *JAMA* **297(24)**, 2697–2704.

48. Kim, E.S., Im, J.A., Kim, K.C., Park, J.H., Suh, S.H., Kang, E.S., Kim, S.H., Jekal, Y., Lee, C.W., Yoon, Y.J., Lee, H.C., and Jeon, J.Y. (2007). Improved insulin sensitivity and adiponectin level after exercise training in obese Korean youth. *Obesity (Silver Spring)* **15**, 3023–3030.

49. Tuomilehto, J., Lindström, J., Eriksson, J.G., Valle, T.T., Hämäläinen, H., Ilanne-Parikka, P., Keinänen-Kiukaanniemi, S., Laakso, M., Louheranta, A., Rastas, M., Salminen, V., Uusitupa, M., and Finnish Diabetes Prevention Study Group. (2001). Prevention of type 2 diabetes mellitus by changes in lifestyle among subjects with impaired glucose tolerance. *N Engl J Med* **344(18)**, 1343–1350.

50. Knowler, W.C., Barrett-Connor, E., Fowler, S.E., Hamman, R.F., Lachin, J.M., Walker, E.A., Nathan, D.M., and Diabetes Prevention Program Research Group. (2002). Reduction in the incidence of type 2 diabetes with lifestyle intervention or metformin. *N Engl J Med* **346(6)**, 393–403.

51. Maffeis, C. and Castellani, M. (2007). Physical activity: An effective way to control weight in children? *Nutr Metab Cardiovasc Dis* **17(5)**, 394–408.

52. Kelley, D.E. and Goodpaster, B.H. (1999). Effects of physical activity on insulin action and glucose tolerance in obesity. *Med Sci Sports Exerc* **3**, S619–S623.

53. Bell, L.M., Watts, K., Siafarikas, A., Thompson, A., Ratnam, N., Bulsara, M., Finn, J., O'Driscoll, G., Green, D.J., Jones, T.W., and Davis, E.A. (2007). Exercise alone reduces insulin resistance in obese children independently of changes in body composition. *J Clin Endocrinol Metab* **92(11)**, 4230–4235.

54. Nassis, G.P., Papantakou, K., Skenderi, K., Triandafillopoulou, M., Kavouras, S.A., Yannakoulia, M., Chrousos, G.P., and Sidossis, L.S. (2005). Aerobic exercise training improves insulin sensitivity without changes in body weight, body fat, adiponectin, and inflammatory markers in overweight and obese girls. *Metabolism* **54(11)**, 1472–1479.

55. Després, J.P., Lamarche, B., Mauriège, P., Cantin, B., Dagenais, G.R., Moorjani, S., and Lupien, P.J. (1996). Hyperinsulinemia as an independent risk factor for ischemic heart disease. *N Engl J Med* **334(15)**, 952–957.

56. Díez, J.J. and Iglesias, P. (2003). The role of the novel adipocyte-derived hormone adiponectin in human disease. *Eur J Endocrinol* **148**, 293–300.

57. Weiss, R., Dziura, J., Burgert, T.S., Tamborlane, W.V., Taksali, S.E., Yeckel, C.W., Allen, K., Lopes, M., Savoye, M., Morrison, J., Sherwin, R.S., and Caprio, S. (2004). Obesity and the metabolic syndrome in children and adolescents. *N Engl J Med* **350**, 2362–2374.

58. Winer, J.C., Zern, T.L., Taksali, S.E., Dziura, J., Cali, A.M., Wollschlager, M., Seyal, A.A., Weiss, R., Burgert, T.S., and Caprio, S. (2004). Adiponectin in childhood and adolescent obesity and its association with inflammatory markers and components of the metabolic syndrome. *J Clin Endocrinol Metab* **91**, 4415–4423.

59. Christiansen, T., Paulsen, S.K., Bruun, J.M., Ploug, T., Pedersen, S.B., and Richelsen, B. (2010). Diet-induced weight loss and exercise alone and in combination enhance the expression of adiponectin receptors in adipose tissue and skeletal muscle, but only diet-induced weight loss enhanced circulating adiponectin. *J Clin Endocrinol Metab* **95(2)**, 911–919.

60. O'Leary, V.B., Jorett, A.E., Marchetti, C.M., Gonzalez, F., Phillips, S.A., Ciaraldi, T.P., and Kirwan, J.P. (2007). Enhanced adiponectin multimer ratio and skeletal muscle adiponectin receptor expression following exercise training and diet in older insulin-resistant adults. *Am J Physiol Endocrinol Metab* **293(1)**, E421–E427.

61. Shalitin, S., Ashkenazi-Hoffnung, L., Yackobovitch-Gavan, M., Nagelberg, N., Karni, Y., Hershkovitz, E., Loewenthal, N., Shtaif, B., Gat-Yablonski, G., and Phillip, M. (2009). Effects of a twelve-week randomized intervention of exercise and/or diet on weight loss and weight maintenance, and other metabolic parameters in obese preadolescent children. *Horm Res* **72(5)**, 287–301.

62. Carrel, A.L., McVean, J.J., Clark, R.R., Peterson, S.E., Eickhoff, J.C., and Allen, D.B. (2009). School-based exercise improves fitness, body composition, insulin sensitivity, and markers of inflammation in non-obese children. *J Pediatr Endocrinol Metab* **22(5)**, 409–415.

63. Hara, K., Horikoshi, M., Yamauchi, T., Yago, H., Miyazaki, O., Ebinuma, H., Imai, Y., Nagai R., and Kadowaki, T. (2006). Measurement of the high–molecular weight form of adiponectin in plasma is useful for the prediction of insulin resistance and metabolic syndrome. *Diabetes Care* **29(6)**, 1357–1362.

64. Seino, Y., Hirose, H., Saito, I., and Itoh, H. (2009). High-molecular-weight adiponectin is a predictor of progression to metabolic syndrome: A population-based 6-year follow-up study in Japanese men. *Metabolism* **58**, 355–360.

65. Polak, J., Kovacova, Z., Holst, C., Verdich, C., Astrup, A., Blaak, E., Patel, K., Oppert, J.M., Langin, D., Martinez, J.A., Sørensen, T.I., and Stich, V. (2008). Total adiponectin and adiponectin multimeric complexes in relation to weight loss-induced improvements in insulin sensitivity in obese women: The NUGENOB study. *Eur J Endocrinol* **158(4)**, 533–541.

66. Bacha, F., Saad, R., Gungor, N., and Arslanian, S.A. (2006). Are obesity-related metabolic risk factors modulated by the degree of insulin resistance in adolescents. *Diabetes Care* **29(7)**, 1599–1604.

67. Weiss, R., Taksali, S.E., Dufour, S., Yeckel, C.W., Papademetris, X., Cline, G., Tamborlane, W.V., Dziura, J., Shulman, G.I., and Caprio, S. (2005). The "obese insulin-sensitive" adolescent: Importance of adiponectin and lipid partitioning. *J Clin Endocrinol Metab* **90(6)**, 3731–3737.

68. Stumvoll, M., Goldstein, B.J., and van Haeften, T.W. (2005). Type 2 diabetes: Principles of pathogenesis and therapy. *Lancet* **365(9467)**, 1333–1346.

69. Kelly, A.S., Steinberger, J., Olson, T.P., and Dengel, D.R. (2007). In the absence of weight loss, exercise training does not improve adipokines or oxidative stress in overweight children. *Metabolism* **56(7)**, 1005–1009.

70. Esposito, K., Pontillo, A., Di Palo, C., Giugliano, G., Masella, M., Marfella, R., and Giugliano, D. (2003). Effect of weight loss and lifestyle changes on vascular inflammatory markers in obese women: A randomized trial. *JAMA* **289(14)**, 1799–1804.

71. Lee, S., Gungor, N., Bacha, F., and Arslanian, S. (2007). Insulin resistance: Link to the components of the metabolic syndrome and biomarkers of endothelial dysfunction in youth. *Diabetes Care* **30(8)**, 2091–2097.

72. Klein-Platat, C., Oujaa, M., Wagner, A., Haan, M.C., Arveiler, D., Schlienger, J.L., and Simon, C. (2005). Physical activity is inversely related to waist circumference in 12-y-old French adolescents. *Int J Obes (Lond)* **29(1)**, 9–14.

73. Saelens, B.E., Seeley, R.J., van Schaick, K., Donnelly, L.F., and O'Brien, K.J. (2007). Visceral abdominal fat is correlated with whole-body fat and physical activity among 8-y-old children at risk of obesity. *Am J Clin Nutr* **85(1)**, 46–53.

74. Gutin, B., Barbeau, P., Owens, S., Lemmon, C.R., Bauman, M., Allison, J., Kang, H.S., and Litaker, M.S. (2002). Effects of exercise intensity on cardiovascular fitness, total body composition, and visceral adiposity of obese adolescents. *Am J Clin Nutr* **75(5)**, 818–826.

75. Christakis, N.A. and Fowler, J.H. (2007). The spread of obesity in a large social network over 32 years. *N Engl J Med* **357(4)**, 370–379.

76. Cheung, N.W. and Byth, K. (2003). The population health significance of gestational diabetes. *Diabetes Care* **26**, 2005–2009.

77. Jovanovic, L. and Pettitt, D.J. (2001). Gestational diabetes mellitus. *JAMA* **286**, 2516–2518.

78. Catalano, P.M., Thomas, A., Huston-Presley, L., and Amini, S.B. (2003). Increased fetal adiposity: A very sensitive marker of abnormal in utero development. *Am J Obstet Gynecol* **189**, 1698–1704.

79. Lawlor, D.A., Fraser, A., Lindsay, R.S., Ness, A., Dabelea, D., Catalano, P., Davey Smith, G., Sattar, N., and Nelson, S.M. (2010). Association of existing diabetes, gestational diabetes and glycosuria in pregnancy with macrosomia and offspring body mass index, waist and fat mass in later childhood: Findings from a prospective pregnancy cohort. *Diabetologia* **53(1)**, 89–97.

80. Hillier, T.A., Pedula, K.L., Vesco, K.K., Schmidt, M.M., Mullen, J.A., LeBlanc, E.S., and Pettitt, D.J. (2008). Excess gestational weight gain: Modifying fetal macrosomia risk associated with maternal glucose. *Obstet Gynecol* **112(5)**, 1007–1014.

81. Langer, O., Yogev, Y., Most, O., and Xenakis, E.M. (2005). Gestational diabetes: The consequences of not treating. *Am J Obstet Gynecol* **192(4)**, 989–997.

82. Freinkel, N. (1980). Banting Lecture of pregnancy and progeny. *Diabetes* **29**, 1023–1035.

83. Pettitt, D.J., Baird, H.R., Aleck, K.A., Bennett, P.H., and Knowler, W.C. (1983). Excessive obesity in offspring of Pima Indian women with diabetes during pregnancy. *N Engl J Med* **308**, 242–245.

84. Pettitt, D.J., Knowler, W.C., Bennett, P.H., Aleck, K.A., and Baird, H.R. (1987). Obesity in offspring of diabetic Pima Indian women despite normal birth weight. *Diabetes Care* **10**, 76–80.

85. Pettitt, D.J., Nelson, R.G., Saad, M.F., Bennett, P.H., and Knowler, W.C. (1993). Diabetes and obesity in the offspring of Pima Indian women with diabetes during pregnancy. *Diabetes Care* **16**, 310–314.

86. Dabelea, D., Hanson, R.L., Lindsay, R.S., Pettitt, D.J., Imperatore, G., Gabir, M.M., Roumain, J., Bennett, P.H., and Knowler, W.C. (2000). Intrauterine exposure to diabetes conveys risks for type 2 diabetes and obesity: A study of discordant sibships. *Diabetes* **49**, 2208–2211.

87. Boney, C.M., Verma, A., Tucker, R., and Vohr, B.R. (2005). Metabolic syndrome in childhood: Association with birth weight, maternal obesity, and gestational diabetes mellitus. *Pediatrics* **115(3)**, e290–e296.

88. American College of Obstetricians and Gynecologists Committee on Practice Bulletins—Obstetrics. (2001). ACOG practice bulletin. Clinical management guidelines for obstetrician-gynecologists. Number 30, September 2001 (replaces Technical Bulletin Number 200, December 1994). Gestational diabetes. *Obstet Gynecol* **98(3)**, 525–538.

89. Chatfield, J. (2001). ACOG issues guidelines on fetal macrosomia. American College of Gynecology. *Am Fam Physician* **64(1)**, 69–70.

90. Dempsey, J.C., Butler, C.L., and Williams, M.A. (2005). No need for a pregnant pause: Physical activity may reduce the occurrence of gestational diabetes mellitus and preeclampsia. *Exerc Sport Sci Rev* **33(3)**, 141–149.

91. Dye, T.D., Knox, K.L., Artal, R., Aubry, R.H., and Wojtowycz, M.A. (1997). Physical activity, obesity, and diabetes in pregnancy. *Am J Epidemiol* **146(11)**, 961–965.

92. Dempsey, J.C., Butler, C.L., Sorensen, T.K., Lee, I.M., Thompson, M.L., Miller, R.S., Frederick, I.O., and Williams, M.A. (2004). A case-control study of maternal recreational physical activity and risk of gestational diabetes mellitus. *Diabetes Res Clin Pract* **66(2)**, 203–215.

93. Liu, J., Laditka, J.N., Mayer-Davis, E.J., and Pate, R.R. (2008). Does physical activity during pregnancy reduce the risk of gestational diabetes among previously inactive women? *Birth* **35(3)**, 188–195.

94. Weissgerber, T.L., Wolfe, L.A., Davies, G.A., and Mottola, M.F. (2006). Exercise in the prevention and treatment of maternal-fetal disease: A review of the literature. *Appl Physiol Nutr Metab* **31(6)**, 661–674.

95. Sowers, J.R. (2003). Obesity as a cardiovascular risk factor. *Am J Med* **115**, 37–41.

96. Hubert, H.B., Feinleib, M., McNamara, P.M., and Castelli, W.P. (1983). Obesity as an independent risk factor for cardiovascular disease: A 26-year follow-up of participants in the Framingham Heart Study. *Circulation* **67**, 968–977.

97. De Rosa, S., Cirillo, P., Pacileo, M., Di Palma, V., Paglia, A., and Chiariello, M. (2009). Leptin stimulated C-reactive protein production by human coronary artery endothelial cells. *J Vasc Res* **46(6)**, 609–617.

98. Ross, R. (1999). Atherosclerosis-an inflammatory disease. *N Engl J Med* **340(2)**, 115–126.

99. Hansson, G.K. (2005). Inflammation, atherosclerosis, and coronary artery disease. *N Engl J Med* **352(16)**, 1685–1695.

100. Hong, Y.I. (2010). Atherosclerotic cardiovascular disease beginning in childhood. *Korean Circ J* **40**, 1–9.

101. Pischon, T. (2009). Use of obesity biomarkers in cardiovascular epidemiology. *Dis Markers* **26**, 247–263.

102. Soderberg, S., Ahren, B., Jansson, J.H., Johnson, O., Hallmans, G., Asplund, K., and Olsson, T. (1999). Leptin is associated with increased risk of myocardial infarction. *J Intern Med* **246**, 409–418.

103. Berg, A.H. and Scherer, P.E. (2005). Adipose tissue, inflammation, and cardiovascular disease. *Circ Res* **9**, 939–949.

104. Hotamisligil, G.S. (1999). The role of TNF alpha and TNF receptors in obesity and insulin resistance. *J Intern Med* **245(6)**, 621–625.

105. Kern, P.A., Ranganathan, S., Li, C., Wood, L., and Ranganathan, G. (2001). Adipose tissue tumor necrosis factor and interleukin-6 expression in human obesity and insulin resistance. *Am J Physiol Endocrinol Metab* **280(5)**, E745–E751.

106. Venugopal, S.K., Devaraj, S., Yuhanna, I., Shaul, P., and Jialal, I. (2002). Demonstration that C-reactive protein decreases eNOS expression and bioactivity in human aortic endothelial cells. *Circulation* **106**, 1439–1441.

107. Yasojima, K., Schwab, C., McGeer, E.G., and McGeer, P.L. (2001). Generation of C-reactive protein and complement components in atherosclerotic plaques. *Am J Pathol* **158**, 1039–1051.

108. Pai, J.K., Pischon, T., Ma, J., Manson, J.E., Hankinson, S.E., Joshipura, K., Curhan, G.C., Rifai, N., Cannuscio, C.C., Stampfer, M.J., and Rimm, E.B. (2004). Inflammatory markers and the risk of coronary heart disease in men and women. *N Engl J Med* **351(25)**, 2599–2610.

109. Ridker, P.M., Hennekens, C.H., Buring, J.E., and Rifai, N. (2000). C-reactive protein and other markers of inflammation in the prediction of cardiovascular disease in women. *N Engl J Med* **342(12)**, 836–843.

110. Ridker, P.M., Paynter, N.P., Rifai, N., Gaziano, J.M., and Cook, N.R. (2007). C-reactive protein and parental history improve global cardiovascular risk prediction: The Reynolds Risk Score for men. *Circulation* **118(22)**, 2243–2251.

111. Lavie, C.J., Milani, R.V., and Ventura, H.O. (2009). Obesity and cardiovascular disease: Risk factor, paradox, and impact of weight loss. *J Am Coll Cardiol* **53(21)**, 1925–1932.

112. Horwich, T.B., Fonarow, G.C., Hamilton, M.A., MacLellan, W.R., Woo, M.A., and Tillisch, J.H. (2001). The relationship between obesity and mortality in patients with heart failure. *J Am Coll Cardiol* **38(3)**, 789–795.

113. Allison, D.B., Zannolli, R., Faith, M.S., Heo, M., Pietrobelli, A., VanItallie, T.B., Pi-Sunyer, F.X., and Heymsfield, S.B. (1999). Weight loss increases and fat loss decreases all-cause mortality rate: Results from two independent cohort studies. *Int J Obes Relat Metab Disord* **23(6)**, 603–611.

114. Sierra-Johnson, J., Romero-Corral, A., Somers, V.K., Lopez-Jimenez, F., Thomas, R.J., Squires, R.W., and Allison, T.G. (2008). Prognostic importance of weight loss in patients with coronary heart disease regardless of initial body mass index. *Eur J Cardiovasc Prev Rehabil* **15(3)**, 336–340.

115. Kelley, G.A. and Kelley, K.S. (2008). Effects of aerobic exercise on non-HDL-C in children and adolescents: A meta-analysis of randomized controlled trials. *Prog Cardiovasc Nurs* **23(3)**, 128–132.

116. Thompson, G.R. (2004). Management of dyslipidemia. *Heart* **90**, 949–955.

117. Amstrong, N. and Simons-Morton, B. (1994). Physical activity and blood lipid in adolescents. *Pediatr Exerc Sci* **6**, 381–405.

118. Thomas, N.E., Baker, J.S., and Davies, B. (2003). Established and recently identified coronary heart disease risk factors in young people: The influence of physical activity and physical fitness. *Sports Med* **33(9)**, 633–650.

119. Katzmarzyk, P.T., Malina, R.M., and Bouchar, C. (1999). Physical activity, physical fitness, and coronary heart disease risk factors in youth: The Québec Family Study. *Prev Med* **29**, 555–562.

120. Reinehr, T., de Sousa, G., Toschke, A.M., and Andler, W. (2006). Long-term follow-up of cardiovascular disease risk factors in children after an obesity intervention. *Am J Clin Nutr* **84(3)**, 490–496.

121. Sung, R.Y., Yu, C.W., Chang, S.K., Mo, S.W., Woo, K.S., and Lam, C.W. (2002). Effects of dietary intervention and strength training on blood lipid level in obese children. *Arch Dis Child* **86(6)**, 407–410.

122. Knip, M. and Nuutinien, O. (1993). Long-term effects of weight reduction on serum lipids and plasma insulin in obese children. *Am J Clin Nutr* **57**, 490–493.

123. Wabitsch, M., Hauner, H., Heinze, E., Muche, R., Böckmann, A., Parthon, W., Mayer, H., and Teller, W. (1994). Body-fat distribution and changes in atherogenic risk-factor profile in obese adolescent girls during weight loss. *Am J Clin Nutr* **60**, 54–60.

124. Reinehr, T., Kiess, W., Kapellen, T., and Andler, W. (2004). Insulin sensitivity among obese children and adolescents, according to degree of weight loss. *Pediatrics* **114**, 1569–1573.

125. Reinehr, T. and Andler, W. (2004). Changes in the atherogenic risk-factor profile according to degree of weight loss. *Arch Dis Child* **89**, 419–422.

126. Carretero, O.A. and Oparil, S. (2000). Essential hypertension. Part I: Definition and etiology. *Circulation* **101(3)**, 329–335.

127. Sorof, J. and Daniels, S. (2002). Obesity hypertension in children: A problem of epidemic proportions. *Hypertension* **40**, 441–447.

128. Kelm, M. (2002). Flow-mediated dilatation in human circulation: Diagnostic and therapeutic aspects. *Am J Physiol Heart Circ Physiol* **282**, H1–H5.

129. Rocchini, A.P. (2002). Obesity and hypertension. *Am J Hypertens* **15**, 50S–52S.

130. Redon, J. (2001). Hypertension in obesity. *Nutr Metab Cardiovasc Dis* **11(5)**, 344–353.

131. Farpour-Lambert, N.J., Aggoun, Y., Marchand, L.M., Martin, X.E., Herrmann, F.R., and Beghetti, M. (2009). Physical activity reduces systemic blood pressure and improves early markers of atherosclerosis in pre-pubertal obese children. *J Am Coll Cardiol* **54(25)**, 2396–2406.

132. Meyer, A.A., Kundt, G., Lenschow, U., Schuff-Werner, P., and Kienast, W. (2006). Improvement of early vascular changes and cardiovascular risk factors in obese children after a six-month exercise program. *J Am Coll Cardiol* **48(9)**, 1865–1870.

133. Schiel, R., Beltschikow, W., Kramer, G., and Stein, G. (2006). Overweight, obesity and elevated blood pressure in children and adolescents. *Eur J Med Res* **11(3)**, 97–101.

134. Santos, M.G., Pegoraro, M., Sandrini, F., and Macuco, E.C. (2008). Risk factors for the development of atherosclerosis in childhood and adolescence. *Arq Bras Cardiol* **90(4)**, 276–283.

135. Mosca, L. (2002). C-reactive protein: To screen or not to screen? *N Engl J Med* **347**, 1615–1617.

136. Ridker, P.M. (2003). Clinical application of C-reactive protein for cardiovascular disease detection and prevention. *Circulation* **107**, 363–369.

137. Semiz, S., Rota, S., Ozdemir, O., Ozdemir, A., and Kaptanoğlu, B. (2008). Are C-reactive protein and homocysteine cardiovascular risk factors in obese children and adolescents? *Pediatr Int* **50(4)**, 419–423.

138. Yoshinaga, M., Sameshima, K., Tanaka, Y., Wada, A., Hashiguchi, J., Tahara, H., and Kono, Y. (2008). Adipokines and the prediction of the accumulation of cardiovascular risk factors or the presence of metabolic syndrome in elementary school children. *Circ J* **72(11)**, 1874–1878.

139. Afghani, A. and Goran, M.I. (2009). The interrelationships between abdominal adiposity, leptin and bone mineral content in overweight Latino children. *Horm Res* **72(2)**, 82–87.

140. Forsythe, L.K., Wallace, J.M., and Livingstone, M.B. (2008). Obesity and inflammation: The effects of weight loss. *Nutr Res Rev* **21(2)**, 117–33.

141. Boas, S.R., Joswiak, M.L., Nixon, P.A., Kurland, G., O'Connor, M.J., Bufalino, K., Orenstein, D.M., and Whiteside, T.L. (1996). Effects of anaerobic exercise on the immune system in eight to seventeen-year-old trained and untrained boys. *J Pediatr* **129**, 846–855.

142. Nemet, D., Oh, Y., Kim, H.S., Hill, M., and Cooper, D.M. (2002). Effect of intense exercise on inflammatory cytokines and growth mediators in adolescent boys. *Pediatrics* **110**, 681–689.

143. Scheett, T.P., Mills, P.J., Ziegler, M.G., Stoppani, J., and Cooper, D.M. (1999). Effect of exercise on cytokines and growth mediators in prepubertal children. *Pediatr Res* **46**, 429–434.

144. Scheett, T.P., Nemet, D., Stoppani, J., Maresh, C.M., Newcomb, R., and Cooper, D.M. (2002). The effect of endurance-type exercise training on growth mediators and inflammatory cytokines in pre-pubertal and early pubertal males. *Pediatr Res* **52**, 491–497.

145. Stewart, L.K., Flynn, M.G., Campbell, W.W., Craig, B.A., Robinson, J.P., Timmerman, K.L., McFarlin, B.K., Coen, P.M., and Talbert, E. (2007). The influence of exercise training on inflammatory cytokines and C-reactive protein. *Med Sci Sports Exerc* **39**, 1714–1719.

146. Petersen, A.M. and Pedersen, B.K. (2005). The anti-inflammatory effect of exercise. *J Appl Physiol* **98**, 1154–1162.

147. Timmons, B.W. (2005). Paediatric exercise immunology: Health and clinical applications. *Exerc Immunol Rev* **11**, 108–144.

148. Ploeger, H.E., Takken, T., de Greef, M.H., and Timmons, B.W. (2009). The effects of acute and chronic exercise on inflammatory markers in children and adults with a chronic inflammatory disease: A systematic review. *Exerc Immunol Rev* **15**, 6–41.

149. Moldoveanu, A.I., Shephard, R.J., and Shek, P.N. (2000). Exercise elevates plasma levels but not gene expression of IL-1beta, IL-6, and TNF-alpha in blood mononuclear cells. *J Appl Physiol* **89(4)**, 1499–1504.

150. Suzuki, K., Nakaji, S., Yamada, M., Totsuka, M., Sato, K., and Sugawara, K. (2002). Systemic inflammatory response to exhaustive exercise. Cytokine kinetics. *Exerc Immunol Rev* **8**, 6–48.

151. Woods, J., Lu, Q., Ceddia, M.A., and Lowder, T. (2000). Special feature for the Olympics: Effects of exercise on the immune system: Exercise-induced modulation of macrophage function. *Immunol Cell Biol* **78**, 545–553.

152. Gleeson, M. (2007). Immune function in sport and exercise. *J Appl Physiol* **103**, 693–699.

153. Gleeson, M. (2006). Immune system adaptation in elite athletes. *Curr Opin Clin Nutr Metab Care* **9**, 659–665.

154. Eisenmann, J.C. (2009). Aerobic fitness, fatness and the metabolic syndrome in children and adolescents. *Acta Paediatr* **96(12)**, 1723–1729.

155. Flynn, M.A., McNeil, D.A., Maloff, B., Mutasingwa, D., Wu, M., Ford, C., and Tough, S.C. (2006). Reducing obesity and related chronic disease risk in children and youth: A synthesis of evidence with "best practice" recommendations. *Obes Rev* **Suppl 1**, 7–66.

156. Pearson, T.A., Mensah, G.A., Alexander, R.W. Anderson, J.L., Cannon, R.O. 3rd, Criqui, M., Fadl, Y.Y., Fortmann, S.P., Hong, Y., Myers, G.L., Rifai, N., Smith, S.C. Jr. Taubert, K., Tracy, R.P., Vinicor, F., and Centers for Disease Control and Prevention; American Heart Association. (2003). Markers of inflammation and cardiovascular disease: Application to clinical and public health practice: A statement for healthcare professionals from the Centers for Disease Control and Prevention and the American Heart Association. *Circulation* **107(3)**, 499–511.

157. Pradhan, A.D., Manson, J.E., Rifai, N., Buring, J.E., and Ridker, P.M. (2001). C-Reactive protein, interleukin 6, and risk of developing type 2 diabetes mellitus. *JAMA* **286**, 327–334.

158. Festa, A., D'Agostino, R. Jr., Tracy, R.P., and Haffner, S.M. (2002). Elevated levels of acute-phase proteins and plasminogen activator inhibitor-1 predict the development of type 2 diabetes: The insulin resistance atherosclerosis study. *Diabetes* **51**, 1131–1137.

159. Rankinen, T., Perusse, L., Weisagel, S.J., Snyder, E.E., Chagnon, Y.C., and Bouchard, C. (2002). The human obesity gene map: The 2001 update. *Obes Res* **10**, 196–243.

160. Lee, C.D., Blair, S.N., and Jackson, A.S. (1999). Cardiorespiratory fitness, body composition, and all-cause and cardio-vascular disease mortality in men. *Am J Clin Nutr* **69**, 373–380.

161. Jebb, S.A. and Moore, M.S. (1999). Contribution of a sedentary lifestyle and inactivity to the etiology of overweight and obesity: Current evidence and research issues. *Med Sci Sports Exerc* **31**, S534–S541.

162. Blair, S.N., Cheng, Y., and Holder, J.S. (2001). Is physical activity or physical fitness more important than defining health benefits? *Med Sci Sports Exerc* **33**, S379–S399.

163. Church, T.S., Cheng, Y.J., Earnest, C.P., Barlow, C.E., Gibbons, L.W., Priest, E.L., and Blair, S.N. (2004). Exercise capacity and body composition as predictors of mortality among men with diabetes. *Diabetes Care* **27(1)**, 83–88.

164. Yoon, B.K., Kim, C.H., Lim, H.J., Kim, Y.S., Im, J.A., Paik, I.Y., Jeon, J.Y., Cho, H.S., Jeong, H.S., Jin, Y.S., and Suh, S.H. (2009). Association of physical performance and health-related factors among elderly Korean subjects. *ISMJ* **10(4)**, 205–215.

165. Kelly, A.S., Wetzsteon, R.J., Kaiser, D.R., Steinberger, J., Bank, A.J., and Dengel, D.R. (2004). Inflammation, insulin, and endo-thelial function in overweight children: The role of exercise. *J Pediatr* **145**, 731–736.

166. McVean, J.J., Carrel, A.L., Eickhoff, J.C., and Allen, D.B. (2009). Fitness level and body composition are associated with inflammation in non-obese children. *J Pediatr Endocrinol Metab* **22(2)**, 153–159.

167. Lee, S.L., Kuk, J.L., Katzmarzyk, P.T., Blair, S.N., Church, T.S., and Ross, R. (2005). Cardiorespiratory fitness attenuates metabolic risk independent of abdominal subcutaneous and visceral fat in men. *Diabetes Care* **28**, 895–901.

168. Church, T.S., Finley, C.E., Earnest, C.P., Kampert, J.B., Gibbons, L.W., and Blair, S.N. (2002). Relative associations of fitness and fatness to fibrinogen, white blood cell count, uric acid and metabolic syndrome. *Int J Obes Relat Metab Disord* **26**, 805–813.

169. Brufani, C., Grossi, A., Fintini, D., Fiori, R., Ubertini, G., Colabianchi, D., Ciampalini, P., Tozzi, A., Barbetti, F., and Cappa, M. (2008). Cardiovascular fitness, insulin resistance and metabolic syndrome in severely obese prepubertal Italian children. *Horm Res* **70(6)**, 349–356.

170. Allen, D.B., Clark, R.R., Peterson, S.E., Nemeth, B.A., Eickhoff, J., and Carrel, A.L. (2007). Fitness is a stronger predictor of fasting insulin than fatness in overweight male middle-school children. *J Pediatr* **150**, 383–387.

171. Nassis, G.P., Papantakou, K., Skenderi, K., Kavouras, S.A., Chrousos, G.P., and Sidossis, L.S. (2005). Aerobic exercise training improves insulin sensitivity without changes in body weight, body fat, adiponectin, and inflammatory markers in obese girls. *Metabolism* **54**, 1472–1479.

172. Watts, K., Jones, T.W., Davis, E.A., and Green, D. (2005). Exercise training in obese children and adolescents: Current concepts. *Sports Med* **35(5)**, 375–392.

173. Blundell, J.E., King, N.A., and Bryant, E. (2006). Interactions among physical activity, food choice, and appetite control: Health messages in physical activity and diet. In *Childhood Obesity: Contemporary Issues* (Cameron, N., Norgan, N.G., and Ellison, G.T.H., Eds), Chapter 10, pp. 135–147. Taylor & Francis Group, Boca Raton, FL.

174. Siddiqui, N.I., Nessa, A., and Hossain, M.A. (2010). Regular physical exercise: Way to healthy life. *Mymensingh Med* **19(1)**, 154–158.

175. Kavey, R.E.W., Daniels, S.R., Lauer, R.M., Atkins, D.L., Hayman, L.L., and Taubert, K. (2003). American heart association guidelines for primary prevention of atherosclerotic cardiovascular disease beginning in childhood. *Circulation* **107**, 1562–1566.

176. Williams, C.L., Hayman, L.L., Daniels, S.R., Robinson, T.N., Steinberger, J., Paridon, S., and Bazzarre, T. (2002). Cardiovascular health in childhood: A statement for health professionals from the committee on atherosclerosis, hypertension, and obesity in the young (AHOY) of the council on cardiovascular disease in the young, American Heart Association. *Circulation* **106**, 143–160.

177. American College of Sports Medicine (ACSM). (2007). Guidelines for healthy adults under age 65. From http://www.acsm.org/AM/Template.cfm?Section=Home_Page&TEMPLATE=CM/HTMLDisplay.cfm&CONTENTID=7764 (Retrieved on March 4, 2010).

178. Canadian Society for Exercise Physiology. (2002). Canada's physical activity guideline. The Canadian physical activity, fitness & lifestyle approach protocol (CPAFLA).

179. Poirier, P. and Després, J.P. (2001). Exercise in weight management of obesity. *Cardiol Clin* **19(3)**, 459–470.

59 Impact of Childhood Obesity on Musculoskeletal Growth, Development, and Disease

Lisa M. Esposito, MS, RD, CSSD, LN,
Paul W. Esposito, MD, and Archana Chatterjee, MD, PhD

CONTENTS

INTRODUCTION

There is extensive evidence of an increasing incidence of overweight as defined by body mass index (BMI) 85th–95th percentile matched for age and sex, and obesity as defined by a BMI over the 95th percentile matched for age and sex around the world. The many associated metabolic conditions such as diabetes and risk of heart disease are well recognized. Less clearly defined is the long-term impact of childhood obesity on musculoskeletal growth, development, and musculoskeletal disorders. Childhood musculoskeletal disorders such as slipped capital femoral epiphysis (SCFE), Blount's disease, and back pain are occurring at increasing rates, as well as at younger ages, over the past two decades.

Childhood deformities such as hip dysplasia have clearly been shown to lead to early arthritis and ongoing disability in adulthood. However, there is little, if any, ongoing research on the direct impact of these childhood obesity–related disorders on adult musculoskeletal problems. This chapter is an outgrowth of the authors' participation in the development of the efforts of the Strategic Planning Committee of the United States Bone and Joint Decade (USBJD), which is addressing the musculoskeletal impact of childhood obesity on children. The USBJD member organizations are concerned that the impact on the musculoskeletal system of childhood obesity needs to be recognized and included in education, advocacy, and research programs because of the significant long-term detrimental effects of these disorders [1–3]. It is also acknowledged that recognition of associated problems is important in combating childhood obesity and that the musculoskeletal impact of childhood obesity clearly interferes with the ability to perform healthy, physical activities [4].

PREVALENCE OF OBESITY

Obesity is a worldwide problem. Wang in 2006 demonstrated that with the exception of Russia and Poland in the 1990s, the prevalence of overweight and obesity has increased in almost all the countries studied [5]. This finding is most profound in economically developed countries and in urbanized populations. Kosti also showed significant prevalence of obesity not only in the United States but also in the European Union and throughout the world [6]. No area of the world is immune to this problem, with Chinese children showing the same metabolic abnormalities related to obesity as children in other parts of the world [7]. It has been reported that in some parts of Africa, obesity has become the major nutritional problem, rather than malnutrition [5,8].

Within the United States, there are large disparities in obesity prevalence between ethnic groups [9–11]. Increasing rates of childhood obesity have been noted in Native Americans and Alaska natives between 2003 and 2008. Prevalence was highest among Native Americans or Alaska natives (21.2%) and Hispanics (18.5%), while the rates were the lowest among whites (12.6%), Asian-Pacific Islanders (12.3%), and African American children (11.8%) [12]. The overall scope of musculoskeletal problems associated with the combined factors of obesity and ethnicity is not widely published. Anecdotally, the increase in childhood obesity in the black and Hispanic communities is well recognized by the medical community [13–15].

In the National Survey of Children's Health 2003, 36.4% of 5–17 year olds were ranked as "at risk for overweight" or "overweight" [16]. The terms "at risk for overweight" and "overweight" have been updated to "overweight" and "obese," respectively. This survey noted geographic variations in the prevalence of overweight and obesity. It was noted that among both girls and boys, the higher prevalence of obesity was in the southeast portion of the country. The lowest prevalence (22.4%–30%) of obesity was observed in the Rocky Mountain states (Utah, Colorado, and Wyoming), with the upper Midwest, Great Plains, and the Northwest in the second lowest category (30%–35%) [16].

SHORT-TERM IMPACT ON BONE HEALTH

PEAK BONE MASS

Ninety percent of bone mass is accrued during the first two decades of life, with peak bone mass attained during pubertal skeletal growth [17,18]. Adequate physical activity and proper nutrition are vital to maximizing bone formation and mineralization especially during this period of life [19]. The mechanical loading involved in physical activity stimulates increased bone mass [20–22]. Continuous suboptimal intake of calcium and vitamin D during the teenage years may create an irreversible deficit that cannot be reversed after reaching skeletal maturity. Inadequate dietary intake, coupled with reduced physical activity in childhood and adolescence, prevents maximal accumulation of peak bone mass. There is concern that prenatal hypovitaminosis may have a deleterious impact on childhood musculoskeletal development, but this has not been clearly shown [23].

PHYSICAL ACTIVITY

Physical activity during adolescence may have a stronger role on bone mass density (BMD) later in life than diet [20–22]. The lifestyles of adults, children, and adolescents have become increasingly sedentary in the United States [24], so that children and adolescents may not be maximizing bone accrual. In a study by Wosje et al. of preschoolers, the researchers observed that the greater the amount of time spent watching TV, the smaller gains in bone area and bone mass accounting for race, sex, and height [25]. The same study found that the higher the body fat mass at baseline, the smaller the increases in bone area and bone mass over the 3.5 years they were followed [25]. Exercise is a crucial component of bone accrual in children and adolescents; it is important to develop exercise programs for kids that do not cause pain and frustration. Programs designed to promote success and achievement and prevent children and adolescents from becoming discouraged about exercise must be a key component to their future health.

Physical activity influences not only bone accrual but also the development of lean muscle mass. In a study by Crabtree et al., the amount of lean muscle mass in children correlated more strongly with bone mineral content than relative fat mass [26].

Diet

Calcium

The largest concentration of the mineral calcium (99%) is found within the skeleton. If blood calcium levels decrease, parathyroid hormone (PTH) stimulates the resorption of calcium from bone to be released into the circulation. Continuous resorption without adequate dietary calcium to support bone re-formation and mineralization significantly reduces bone density. The current Dietary Reference Intake (DRI) for calcium is 500, 800, and 1300 mg for children 1–3 y/o, 4–8 y/o, and for 9–18 y/o, respectively [27]. Current average calcium intakes among children and adolescents consistently fall below the DRI. In particular, 3–10 year olds who avoid cow milk had average calcium intakes of 443 ± 230 mg in a study conducted by Black et al. [28]. This is very low considering the rate of growth and bone density accrual that occurs in childhood and adolescence.

Calcium absorption and utilization is regulated by the endocrine function of vitamin D. This function will be discussed further in the following section. Body weight is a strong predictor of bone mineral content in children [29,30]; however, dietary patterns and physical activity also play a significant role.

Dietary patterns aside from calcium intake play a role in calcium retention. Excessive intake of dietary protein, which is also key to normal growth and development, increases the amount of calcium excreted in the urine. An additional 6 mg of calcium is required to offset the losses due to the intake of 1 g of protein [31–33]. Excessive sodium intake, common in the American diet, may also increase the excretion of calcium in the urine. The evidence of this phenomenon is equivocal, and further research is needed. In several studies, for every 2300 mg of sodium excreted in the urine, 40–60 mg of calcium was also excreted (100 mmol:1 mmol) [34,35], whereas, in other studies, the losses are not significant [36].

Vitamin D

Vitamin D plays various roles in the human body; the endocrine function regulates calcium, while the noncalciotropic effects include cell differentiation and replication in many organs. Vitamin D also plays paracrine and endocrine roles in the immune system, endocrine pancreas, liver, skeletal muscle, and adipocytes [37]. The current recommended daily allowance (RDI) for vitamin D intake for all children and adolescents is 200 IU per day (5.0 mcg per day) [27,38]. Given the incidence of serum vitamin D insufficiency, the current RDI may not be adequate to meet the needs of the body, and further study to determine optimal intake in children needs to be considered.

There is no current consensus on the definition of vitamin D deficiency/insufficiency. Studies currently use a 25(OH)D measurement of <20 ng/mL (50 nmol/L) to define deficiency and <29 ng/mL (74.9 nmol/L) to define insufficiency [39–42]. Clinicians frequently promote a 25(OH)D level of >30 ng/ml [42,43]. In studies examining serum 25(OH)D levels, the occurrence of vitamin D insufficiency and deficiency ranged from 59% to 74%. Many factors influence vitamin D levels including dietary intake, ethnicity, exposure to the sun, season, and body fat mass. During the colder months, individuals living above the latitude 42°N cannot synthesize vitamin D (cholecalciferol) using UV light from sun exposure [44–46]. Ethnicity and skin pigmentation influence synthesis of vitamin D [47]. Increased sun exposure may be necessary for individuals with darker skin pigmentation in order to synthesize adequate amounts of vitamin D.

Hispanics and African Americans have a greater prevalence of vitamin D insufficiency and deficiency as well as lower dietary intake of vitamin D than Caucasians regardless of season [41,48–50]. That being said, 25(OH)D levels may play the strongest role in the BMD of Caucasians and be less of a factor for Hispanics and African Americans [51]. Kremer et al. reported that when comparing adolescent female Hispanics to Caucasians, the body fat mass of Hispanics played a stronger role in BMD than circulating 25(OH)D [39].

As a fat soluble vitamin, the human body sequesters vitamin D in body fat. Obese children and adults have lower circulating 25(OH)D [40,52–54], and several studies have reported a negative association of 25(OH)D with increased adiposity and higher BMI [39,41,55] with enhanced sequestration in body fat [56].

Vitamin D deficiency leads to secondary hyperparathyroidism. Hyperparathyroidism increases calcium resorption from the bone, furthering the deleterious effects to bone health during adolescence and into adulthood [49].

Phosphorus

Eighty percent of the mineral phosphorus is found in the skeleton and along with calcium forms hydroxyapatite, the principal building block of the skeleton. A balance of dietary calcium and phosphorus is important for maintenance and mineralization of healthy bone tissue. Wyshak et al. in two studies examined the effects of carbohydrate beverages, high in phosphoric acid and calcium intake on fracture risk in preadolescent and adolescent males and females. A strong association was seen between fracture risk and soda consumption in females, while adequate dietary calcium provided a protective effect. No significant association was found in males [57,58]. In growing children and adolescents, it is important that healthy sources of calcium and phosphorus not be offset for high-sugar carbonated beverages, both for bone health as well as body weight [59].

Magnesium

Sixty percent of the mineral magnesium is found in the skeleton and plays a role in BMD. Due to efficient homeostatic effects in the human body, a low dietary intake of magnesium does not cause a magnesium deficiency. Half of the magnesium found in the blood serum is bound to the protein albumin; therefore, children with malabsorption syndromes or protein-energy malnutrition may be at risk for hypomagnesemia [27,60].

FRACTURE

Distal radial and forearm fractures in children have been increasing in incidence over the past decades. It is unknown whether this is related to decreasing physical activity, decreased bone acquisition due to poor calcium and vitamin D intake, or other factors [61]. There is some suggestion that modifiable factors such as diet and exercise might decrease these rates [62]. Children with obesity also may be at higher risk of complications with fracture. However, the studies are small and limited, and the association of higher complications such as deep vein thrombosis (DVT) and decubiti following trauma in these children needs to be studied further [63,64]. It is unknown whether the higher incidence of fractures in children with obesity is a result of alterations of proprioception and balance, lower extremity malalignment, or a result of body habitus.

Overweight and obese children have been shown to have low bone mass and area for their weight than their peers [65]. Children with obesity also have a greater weight for height for age, advanced maturation, and a greater lean mass for height. Obesity is also associated with greater vertebral area bone mineral density for height, greater bone mineral density volume, and a greater vertebral bone mineral concentration (BMC) for bone area [59]. Obese children undergoing successful weight loss demonstrated that with ongoing growth, the unadjusted BMC increased among the obese adolescents, despite weight loss. They showed that after adjustment for height, the whole-body BMC did not change significantly [66]. There is further study being undertaken on bone loss of obese adolescents during weight loss. The relationship between childhood obesity and the accumulation of peak bone mass and risk of fractures, as well as the impact of weight loss on these variables, needs additional research.

PAIN

Musculoskeletal pain and postoperative complications are higher in obese adults, but strong linkage of back pain to obesity in adults has not been proven [67]. Increased pain associated with obesity has been shown to occur in children. The most common sites of discomfort in obese children were back pain in 39%, foot pain in 26%, and knee pain in 24%. The children with musculoskeletal pain in this study were older and taller, on average. Using BMI as the independent variable, Stovitz et al. noted that children with hip, knee, or ankle pain had a significantly higher BMI than those children without pain in those joints [68]. Forty-five percent of obese children reported back or lower extremity pain. This same group of researchers had previously shown a negative impact of obesity on quality of life in children and adolescents [69]. Children with ankle injuries, matched for age and sex, who had BMI of >85th percentile had 44% greater chance of persistent pain at 6 months postinjury, compared to 24% of children with a BMI of <85th percentile [70]. This increase in musculoskeletal pain in obese children and adolescents may perpetuate the cycle of ongoing obesity by decreasing their ability to participate in physical exercise [13,71]. Childhood obesity may result in extremity malalignment and joint changes, leading to continued, worsening, and persistent pain and increased potential for osteoarthritis in adults. Lifestyle factors such as exercise, learned during childhood, may also impact the risk of an obese child growing into an obese adult. Obesity in adults has been correlated with work-restricting pain of the knees and ankles [72].

CHILDHOOD MUSCULOSKELETAL OBESITY RELATED DISORDERS (FIGURES 59.1 THROUGH 59.4)

SLIPPED CAPITAL FEMORAL EPIPHYSIS

The etiology of SCFE is multifactorial, but obesity is associated with this disorder regardless of geography. Manoff et al. reviewed the relationships between BMI and the incidence of SCFE [73]. They showed that 81.1% of the individuals with SCFE had a BMI above the 95th percentile for age and sex, while the control group without SCFE averaged only 41.3%. They stated that lifestyle modifications may potentially decrease the incidence of not only SCFE but that of other illnesses related to obesity as well [6,73]. Exactly how obesity increases the risk of SCFE is unclear, but there is a higher incidence of decreased femoral anteversion in obese children, which may mechanically predispose them to this problem [74].

Lehman et al. compared data from the Kids' Inpatient Database and U.S. Census Bureau data for the years 1997 and 2000 to further define the epidemiology of SCFE [75]. The overall incidence of SCFE during those years was 10.8 cases/100,000 children. The relative incidence was 3.94 times higher in African American children and 2.53 times higher in Hispanic children than in Caucasian children. They also noted geographic differences in incidence, as well as a lower age of onset than had been previously reported, stating that this may suggest a downward trend in age of presentation [75]. Loder et al. noted in 2006 that bone age at presentation was essentially unchanged regardless of chronological age. He stated that this may be a reflection of children maturing physically at a younger chronologic age at presentation and that overweight may cause earlier maturation [76].

Benson et al. reported that the incidence of SCFE in New Mexico had doubled from between the 1960s and the time of their report in 2008. They correlated this to the tripling of the rates of childhood obesity between 1971 and the completion of their study [77]. The incidence of SCFE in Scotland also increased from 3.78/100,000 children in 1981 to 9.66/100,000 in 2000 [78]. This reflected a 2.5 times increase in incidence over two decades. These authors reported what had been reported in other studies, that SCFE was seen at progressively younger ages during the course of the study, with the average age at presentation decreasing from 13.4 to 12.6 years for boys and from 12.2 to 11.6 years of age for girls. More children with SCFE presented at less than 8 years of age in the decade prior to 2000 compared to the previous decade. They concluded that this change was related to the increase in childhood obesity over the preceding 20 years [78]. Bowen et al., in 2009, compared the associations among SCFE, Blount's disease, and type II juvenile diabetes [79]. They found the highest BMI in the children with Blount's disease, averaging 40.81, with the diabetes group at 35.76, and with the SCFE group at 29.08. There was no overlap of disease at initial presentation among any of the three disorders [79].

There have been no recent reports, however, of an increase in the incidence of endocrine problems associated with SCFE despite reports of an association in the past [80]. Loder et al. noted that of those children with hypothyroidism, no slips occurred after they had started hormone replacement therapy [81]. However, the slips in patients with growth hormone deficiency usually have the endocrinopathy diagnosed before the slip is diagnosed. All of the hypothyroid patients developed their first slip before or during hormonal supplementation, while 92% of the growth hormone deficient children developed a slip during or after supplementation [81]. They recommended prophylactic treatment of the opposite radiographically normal hip in children with hormonal abnormalities because of the eventual 61% incidence of bilaterality in this group [81].

Blount's Disease

Although there is no significant information on what the long-term effects of altered gait secondary to obesity will have as these children become adults, there is concern that lower extremity malalignment related to obesity may lead to degenerative arthritis and debilitating pain [82,83]. It is of great concern that obese children and adolescents are already presenting with significant pain and malalignments at a very young age.

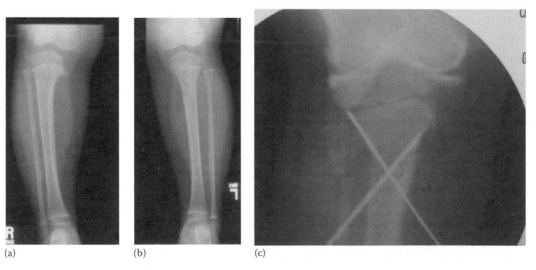

(a)   (b)   (c)

FIGURE 59.1   (a and b) Preoperative right knee x-ray of a 3 year 6-month-old female with progressive Blount's disease despite weight bearing bracing with normal left leg x-ray for comparison. Infantile Blount's disease is associated with childhood obesity. (c) Intraoperative arthrogram following corrective osteotomy to transfer the compressive stresses from the medial tibia, demonstrating the significant deformity of the tibial plateau caused at least partially by excessive compression of the medial physis in a toddler with excessive weight on top of persistent neonatal genu varum.

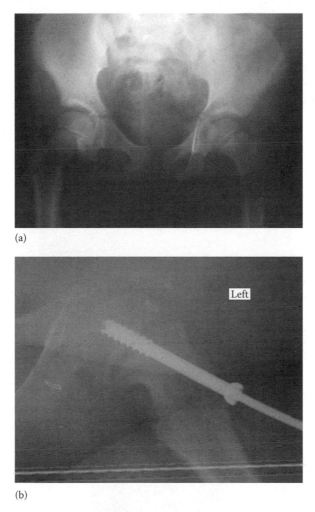

(a)

(b)

FIGURE 59.2 (a) Significant SCFE of the left hip with negative work-up for thyroid disease and other metabolic disorders in the same child as in Figure 59.1 at age 6. (b) She subsequently required percutaneous screw stabilization of both hips. SCFE historically has been rare without significant underlying disease such as hypothyroidism or genital irradiation in children under the age of 10, but is now occurring more frequently in otherwise normal children who are significantly overweight and/or obese.

Varus loading of the knee, which may be related to large thighs, places excessive compressive stress on the medial side of the knee. This may predispose to the development of Blount's disease [83,84] as well as degenerative changes of the knee [85]. There are data that show that the underlying static varus malalignment is not necessarily a prerequisite for the development of adolescent tibia vara and that the dynamic gait deviation is secondary to the obesity, which was referred to as the "fat thigh gait" and is significant in the development of Blount's [85,86]. Symptomatic progressive genu valgum can also be associated with obesity.

LONG-TERM IMPACT

Obesity in children has a strong genetic link. An overweight or obese child with a familial history of excessive weight gain has a high risk of obesity in adulthood [87–89]; the risk that the child will remain overweight or obese increases with age [90–92]. In twin studies examining monozygotic and dizygotic male twins, genetics played a significant role in obesity as the subjects aged, even in twins

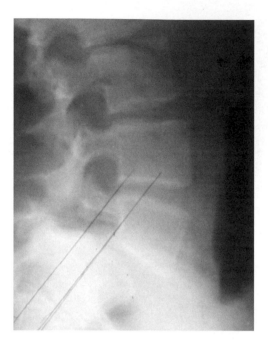

FIGURE 59.3   Same child as in Figures 59.1 and 59.4 at age 10 when she presented with low back pain and was diagnosed with spondylolysis and listhesis. This has remained stable and her back pain has resolved with a weight reduction and fitness program. This combination of disorders in one child is extremely rare.

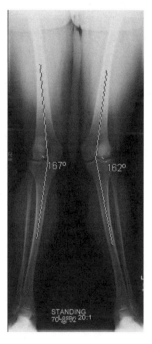

FIGURE 59.4   Otherwise healthy 120 kg 17-year-old female with progressive knock knee (genu valgum) related to her weight. If recognized early, this can be treated with hemi-epiphyseodesis. In this skeletally mature individual, who is already demonstrating degenerative changes and cyst formation in her lateral compartments, osteotomy is necessary to normalize the weight bearing axis. It is unknown, however, if this process is totally reversible. This is also being seen more commonly, and is related to the size of the patient's thighs as well as the patient's weight on the growing physis. This is being encountered more frequently in adolescents, along with an increase in the incidence of adolescent Blount's disease.

reared in separate homes [93,94]. In adoption studies, where children were raised by nonbiological parents, the genetics played a role in their subsequent body weight [95].

Dietary habits and preferences are developed at an early age, and the home environment significantly impacts the risk for developing childhood overweight or obesity [96–99]. Modeling of healthy eating and exercise behaviors by parents, as well as providing an environment conducive to those behaviors, is important for the development of health habits children will carry into adulthood.

FUTURE DIRECTIONS

The relationship of childhood obesity to metabolic diseases such as diabetes and heart disease cannot be emphasized enough. This does not, however, lessen the importance of the associated musculoskeletal problems. Clinicians are recognizing that obese children and adolescents are presenting with significant long-term musculoskeletal abnormalities, especially pain and developmental issues of the lower extremities, and a higher rate of fractures. There are also significant musculoskeletal problems associated with the opposite end of the spectrum; these are the eating disorders. It is important that these children be included in efforts related to maintaining a healthy lifestyle, as the impact of eating disorders may be equally as devastating as obesity.

There is also relatively little documentation of the chronic joint problems and chronic pain syndromes with which these children present. The long-term implication of significant obesity and/or overweight on joint function and overall musculoskeletal health as these individuals enter adulthood is unclear. However, the association of bone and joint diseases and malalignment with obesity is clearly described in adults. It is unfathomable that obese children with significant malalignment and significant increased joint reactive forces will not develop degenerative changes at a relatively early age.

The ideal daily intake of vitamin D and mineral supplementation is also not clear in children and requires further areas of emphasis and research. It is becoming increasingly recognized that many children are vitamin D deficient, both from a dietary as well as a sun-exposure standpoint [48–51]. This obviously has implications long-term not only for musculoskeletal health but also for many other potential medical conditions.

There are many resources at this time to help clinicians as well as families deal with childhood obesity [46]. There are also many resources easily available to encourage healthy lifestyles, public fitness, and musculoskeletal activity [1,2]. There needs to be increasing awareness of the significant short- and long-term impact of childhood obesity and lifestyle issues on musculoskeletal health, as well as availability and coordination of existing resources to children, parents, schools, and social and sports organizations to intervene to reverse this trend.

REFERENCES

1. United States Bone and Joint Decade. 2011. Available from: http://www.usbjd.org/. Accessed February 14, 2011.
2. American Academy of Pediatrics. 2010. Available from: http://www.aap.org/healthtopics/overweight.cfm. Accessed February 14, 2011.
3. The Pediatric Orthopaedic Society of North America. 2011. Available from: www.posna.org. Accessed February 14, 2011.
4. Shultz, S.P., J. Anner, and A.P. Hills. 2009. Paediatric obesity, physical activity and the musculoskeletal system. *Obes Rev* 10(5):576–582.
5. Wang, Y. and T. Lobstein. 2006. Worldwide trends in childhood overweight and obesity. *Int J Pediatr Obes* 1(1):11–25.
6. Kosti, R.I. and D.B. Panagiotakos. 2006. The epidemic of obesity in children and adolescents in the world. *Cent Eur J Public Health* 14(4):151–159.
7. Li, Y.P. et al. 2005. Disease risks of childhood obesity in China. *Biomed Environ Sci* 18(6):401–410.

8. Miller, J., A. Rosenbloom, and J. Silverstein. 2004. Childhood obesity. *J Clin Endocrinol Metab* 89(9):4211–4218.

9. Ogden, C.L. et al. 2006. Prevalence of overweight and obesity in the United States, 1999–2004. *JAMA* 295(13):1549–1555.

10. Wang, Y. and Q. Zhang. 2006. Are American children and adolescents of low socioeconomic status at increased risk of obesity? Changes in the association between overweight and family income between 1971 and 2002. *Am J Clin Nutr* 84(4):707–716.

11. Wang, Y. and M.A. Beydoun. 2007. The obesity epidemic in the United States—Gender, age, socioeconomic, racial/ethnic, and geographic characteristics: A systematic review and meta-regression analysis. *Epidemiol Rev* 29:6–28.

12. Centers for Disease Control and Prevention. 2011. Obesity prevalence among low-income, preschool-aged children 1998–2008. Overweight and Obesity. Available from: http://www.cdc.gov/obesity/childhood/lowincome.html. Accessed February 27, 2011.

13. Taylor, E.D. et al. 2006. Orthopedic complications of overweight in children and adolescents. *Pediatrics* 117(6):2167–2174.

14. Wills, M. 2004. Orthopedic complications of childhood obesity. *Pediatr Phys Ther* 16(4):230–235.

15. Live Well Omaha Kids. 2010. Available from: http://www.livewellomahakids.org/index2.html. Accessed February 27, 2011.

16. Tudor-Locke, C. et al. 2007. A geographical comparison of prevalence of overweight school-aged children: The National Survey of Children's Health 2003. *Pediatrics* 120(4):e1043–e1050.

17. Fournier, P.E. et al. 1997. Asynchrony between the rates of standing height gain and bone mass accumulation during puberty. *Osteoporos Int* 7(6):525–532.

18. Theintz, G. et al. 1992. Longitudinal monitoring of bone mass accumulation in healthy adolescents: Evidence for a marked reduction after 16 years of age at the levels of lumbar spine and femoral neck in female subjects. *J Clin Endocrinol Metab* 75(4):1060–1065.

19. Specker, B.L., L. Mulligan, and M. Ho. 1999. Longitudinal study of calcium intake, physical activity, and bone mineral content in infants 6–18 months of age. *J Bone Miner Res* 14(4):569–576.

20. Lloyd, T. et al. 2002. Modifiable determinants of bone status in young women. *Bone* 30(2):416–421.

21. Lloyd, T. et al. 2000. Adult female hip bone density reflects teenage sports-exercise patterns but not teenage calcium intake. *Pediatrics* 106(1 Pt 1):40–44.

22. Nieves, J.W., J.A. Grisso, and J.L. Kelsey. 1992. A case-control study of hip fracture: Evaluation of selected dietary variables and teenage physical activity. *Osteoporos Int* 2(3):122–127.

23. Pasco, J.A. et al. 2008. Maternal vitamin D in pregnancy may influence not only offspring bone mass but other aspects of musculoskeletal health and adiposity. *Med Hypotheses* 71(2):266–269.

24. McCracken, M., R. Jiles, and H.M. Blanck. 2007. Health behaviors of the young adult U.S. population: Behavioral risk factor surveillance system, 2003. *Prev Chronic Dis* 4(2):A25.

25. Wosje, K.S. et al. 2009. Adiposity and TV viewing are related to less bone accrual in young children. *J Pediatr* 154(1):79–85.e2.

26. Crabtree, N.J. et al. 2004. The relationship between lean body mass and bone mineral content in paediatric health and disease. *Bone* 35(4):965–972.

27. Dietary Reference Intakes for Calcium, Phosphorus, Magnesium, Vitamin D, and Fluoride. 1997. *Food and Nutrition Board. Institute of Medicine, Editor*. National Academy Press: Washington, DC.

28. Black, R.E. et al. 2002. Children who avoid drinking cow milk have low dietary calcium intakes and poor bone health. *Am J Clin Nutr* 76(3):675–680.

29. Du, X.Q. et al. 2002. Milk consumption and bone mineral content in Chinese adolescent girls. *Bone* 30(3):521–528.

30. Moro, M. et al. 1996. Body mass is the primary determinant of midfemoral bone acquisition during adolescent growth. *Bone* 19(5):519–526.

31. Breslau, N.A. et al. 1988. Relationship of animal protein-rich diet to kidney stone formation and calcium metabolism. *J Clin Endocrinol Metab* 66(1):140–146.

32. Heaney, R.P. and R.R. Recker. 1982. Effects of nitrogen, phosphorus, and caffeine on calcium balance in women. *J Lab Clin Med* 99(1):46–55.

33. Weaver, C.M., W.R. Proulx, and R. Heaney. 1999. Choices for achieving adequate dietary calcium with a vegetarian diet. *Am J Clin Nutr* 70(3 Suppl):543S–548S.

34. Matkovic, V. et al. 1995. Urinary calcium, sodium, and bone mass of young females. *Am J Clin Nutr* 62(2):417–425.

35. Nordin, B.E. et al. 1993. The nature and significance of the relationship between urinary sodium and urinary calcium in women. *J Nutr* 123(9):1615–1622.

36. Jones, G., M.D. Riley, and S. Whiting. 2001. Association between urinary potassium, urinary sodium, current diet, and bone density in prepubertal children. *Am J Clin Nutr* 73(4):839–844.
37. Reis, A.F., O.M. Hauache, and G. Velho. 2005. Vitamin D endocrine system and the genetic susceptibility to diabetes, obesity and vascular disease. A review of evidence. *Diabetes Metab* 31(4 Pt 1):318–325.
38. Gartner, L.M. and F.R. Greer. 2003. Prevention of rickets and vitamin D deficiency: New guidelines for vitamin D intake. *Pediatrics* 111(4 Pt 1):908–910.
39. Kremer, R. et al. 2009. Vitamin D status and its relationship to body fat, final height, and peak bone mass in young women. *J Clin Endocrinol Metab* 94(1):67–73.
40. Lenders, C.M. et al. 2009. Relation of body fat indexes to vitamin D status and deficiency among obese adolescents. *Am J Clin Nutr* 90(3):459–467.
41. Alemzadeh, R. et al. 2008. Hypovitaminosis D in obese children and adolescents: Relationship with adiposity, insulin sensitivity, ethnicity, and season. *Metabolism* 57(2):183–191.
42. Holick, M.F. 2009. Vitamin D status: Measurement, interpretation, and clinical application. *Ann Epidemiol* 19(2):73–78.
43. Holick, M.F. 2007. Vitamin D deficiency. *N Engl J Med* 357(3):266–281.
44. Norman, A.W. 1998. Sunlight, season, skin pigmentation, vitamin D, and 25-hydroxyvitamin D: Integral components of the vitamin D endocrine system. *Am J Clin Nutr* 67(6):1108–1110.
45. Holick, M.F. 2003. Vitamin D: A millenium perspective. *J Cell Biochem* 88(2):296–307.
46. Looker, A.C. et al. 2002. Serum 25-hydroxyvitamin D status of adolescents and adults in two seasonal subpopulations from NHANES III. *Bone* 30(5):771–777.
47. Weng, F.L. et al. 2007. Risk factors for low serum 25-hydroxyvitamin D concentrations in otherwise healthy children and adolescents. *Am J Clin Nutr* 86(1):150–158.
48. Gordon, C.M. et al. 2004. Prevalence of vitamin D deficiency among healthy adolescents. *Arch Pediatr Adolesc Med* 158(6):531–537.
49. Outila, T.A., M.U. Karkkainen, and C.J. Lamberg-Allardt. 2001. Vitamin D status affects serum parathyroid hormone concentrations during winter in female adolescents: Associations with forearm bone mineral density. *Am J Clin Nutr* 74(2):206–210.
50. Rajakumar, K. et al. 2005. Vitamin D insufficiency in preadolescent African-American children. *Clin Pediatr* 44(8):683–692.
51. Hannan, M.T. et al. 2008. Serum 25-hydroxyvitamin D and bone mineral density in a racially and ethnically diverse group of men. *J Clin Endocrinol Metab* 93(1):40–46.
52. Parikh, S.J. et al. 2004. The relationship between obesity and serum 1,25-dihydroxy vitamin D concentrations in healthy adults. *J Clin Endocrinol Metab* 89(3):1196–1199.
53. Peterlik, M. and H.S. Cross. 2005. Vitamin D and calcium deficits predispose for multiple chronic diseases. *Eur J Clin Invest* 35(5):290–304.
54. Rockell, J.E. et al. 2005. Season and ethnicity are determinants of serum 25-hydroxyvitamin D concentrations in New Zealand children aged 5–14 y. *J Nutr* 135(11):2602–2608.
55. Liel, Y. et al. 1988. Low circulating vitamin D in obesity. *Calcif Tissue Int* 43(4):199–201.
56. Wortsman, J. et al. 2000. Decreased bioavailability of vitamin D in obesity. *Am J Clin Nutr* 72(3):690–693.
57. Wyshak, G. 2000. Teenaged girls, carbonated beverage consumption, and bone fractures. *Arch Pediatr Adolesc Med* 154(6):610–613.
58. Wyshak, G. and R.E. Frisch. 1994. Carbonated beverages, dietary calcium, the dietary calcium/phosphorus ratio, and bone fractures in girls and boys. *J Adolesc Health* 15(3):210–215.
59. Mahmood, M. et al. 2008. Health effects of soda drinking in adolescent girls in the United Arab Emirates. *J Crit Care* 23(3):434–440.
60. Rude, R.K. 1998. Magnesium deficiency: A cause of heterogeneous disease in humans. *J Bone Miner Res* 13(4):749–758.
61. Khosla, S. et al. 2003. Incidence of childhood distal forearm fractures over 30 years: A population-based study. *JAMA* 290(11):1479–1485.
62. Rana, A.R. et al. 2009. Childhood obesity: A risk factor for injuries observed at a level-1 trauma center. *J Pediatr Surg* 44(8):1601–1605.
63. Leet, A.I., C.P. Pichard, and M.C. Ain. 2005. Surgical treatment of femoral fractures in obese children: Does excessive body weight increase the rate of complications? *J Bone Joint Surg Am* 87(12):2609–2613.
64. Lubicky, J.P. 2006. Surgical treatment of femoral fractures in obese children. *J Bone Joint Surg Am* 88(8):1890–1891; author reply 1891–1892.
65. Goulding, A. et al. 2000. Overweight and obese children have low bone mass and area for their weight. *Int J Obes Relat Metab Disord* 24(5):627–632.

66. Stettler, N. et al. 2008. Observational study of bone accretion during successful weight loss in obese adolescents. *Obesity* 16(1):96–101.

67. Leboeuf-Yde, C. 2000. Body weight and low back pain. A systematic literature review of 56 journal articles reporting on 65 epidemiologic studies. *Spine* 25(2):226–237.

68. Stovitz, S.D. et al. 2008. Musculoskeletal pain in obese children and adolescents. *Acta Paediatr* 97(4):489–493.

69. Schwimmer, J.B., T.M. Burwinkle, and J.W. Varni. 2003. Health-related quality of life of severely obese children and adolescents. *JAMA* 289(14):1813–1819.

70. Timm, N.L., J. Grupp-Phelan, and M.L. Ho. 2005. Chronic ankle morbidity in obese children following an acute ankle injury. *Arch Pediatr Adolesc Med* 159(1):33–36.

71. Chan, G. and C.T. Chen. 2009. Musculoskeletal effects of obesity. *Curr Opin Pediatr* 21(1):65–70.

72. Peltonen, M., A.K. Lindroos, and J.S. Torgerson. 2003. Musculoskeletal pain in the obese: A comparison with a general population and long-term changes after conventional and surgical obesity treatment. *Pain* 104(3):549–557.

73. Manoff, E.M., M.B. Banffy, and J.J. Winell. 2005. Relationship between Body Mass Index and slipped capital femoral epiphysis. *J Pediatr Orthop* 25(6):744–746.

74. Galbraith, R.T. et al. 1987. Obesity and decreased femoral anteversion in adolescence. *J Orthop Res* 5(4):523–528.

75. Lehmann, C.L. et al. 2006. The epidemiology of slipped capital femoral epiphysis: An update. *J Pediatr Orthop* 26(3):286–290.

76. Loder, R.T., T. Starnes, and G. Dikos. 2006. The narrow window of bone age in children with slipped capital femoral epiphysis: A reassessment one decade later. *J Pediatr Orthop* 26(3):300–306.

77. Benson, E.C. et al. 2008. A new look at the incidence of slipped capital femoral epiphysis in new Mexico. *J Pediatr Orthop* 28(5):529–533.

78. Murray, A.W. and N.I. Wilson. 2008. Changing incidence of slipped capital femoral epiphysis: A relationship with obesity? *J Bone Joint Surg Br* 90(1):92–94.

79. Bowen, J.R. et al. 2009. Associations among slipped capital femoral epiphysis, tibia vara, and type 2 juvenile diabetes. *J Pediatr Orthop* 29(4):341–344.

80. Rappaport, E.B. and D. Fife. 1985. Slipped capital femoral epiphysis in growth hormone-deficient patients. *Am J Dis Child* 139(4):396–399.

81. Loder, R.T., B. Wittenberg, and G. DeSilva. 1995. Slipped capital femoral epiphysis associated with endocrine disorders. *J Pediatr Orthop* 15(3):349–356.

82. Daniels, S.R. 2006. The consequences of childhood overweight and obesity. *Future Child* 16(1):47–67.

83. Dietz, W.H., Jr., W.L. Gross, and J.A. Kirkpatrick, Jr. 1982. Blount disease (tibia vara): Another skeletal disorder associated with childhood obesity. *J Pediatr* 101(5):735–737.

84. Sabharwal, S. 2009. Blount disease. *J Bone Joint Surg Am* 91(7):1758–1776.

85. Davids, J.R., M. Huskamp, and A.M. Bagley. 1996. A dynamic biomechanical analysis of the etiology of adolescent tibia vara. *J Pediatr Orthop* 16(4):461–468.

86. Hills, A.P. 1994. Locomotor characteristics of obese children. In *Exercise and Obesity*. Eds. A.P. Hills and M.L. Wahlqvist, pp. 141–150. Smith-Gordon: London, U.K.

87. Davison, K.K. and L.L. Birch. 2001. Child and parent characteristics as predictors of change in girls' body mass index. *Int J Obes Relat Metab Disord* 25(12):1834–1842.

88. Treuth, M.S., N.F. Butte, and J.D. Sorkin. 2003. Predictors of body fat gain in nonobese girls with a familial predisposition to obesity. *Am J Clin Nutr* 78(6):1212–1218.

89. Whitaker, R.C. et al. 1997. Predicting obesity in young adulthood from childhood and parental obesity. *N Engl J Med* 337(13):869–873.

90. Freedman, D.S. et al. 2005. The relation of childhood BMI to adult adiposity: The Bogalusa Heart Study. *Pediatrics* 115(1):22–27.

91. Guo, S.S. et al. 2002. Predicting overweight and obesity in adulthood from body mass index values in childhood and adolescence. *Am J Clin Nutr* 76(3):653–658.

92. Whitlock, E.P. et al. 2005. Screening and interventions for childhood overweight: A summary of evidence for the US Preventive Services Task Force. *Pediatrics* 116(1):e125–e144.

93. Stunkard, A.J., T.T. Foch, and Z. Hrubec. 1986. A twin study of human obesity. *JAMA* 256(1):51–54.

94. Stunkard, A.J. et al. 1990. The body-mass index of twins who have been reared apart. *N Engl J Med* 322(21):1483–1487.

95. Stunkard, A.J. et al. 1986. An adoption study of human obesity. *N Engl J Med* 314(4):193–198.

96. Golan, M. and S. Crow. 2004. Parents are key players in the prevention and treatment of weight-related problems. *Nutr Rev* 62(1):39–50.
97. Golan, M. and S. Crow. 2004. Targeting parents exclusively in the treatment of childhood obesity: Long-term results. *Obes Res* 12(2):357–361.
98. Daniels, S.R. et al. 2005. Overweight in children and adolescents: Pathophysiology, consequences, prevention, and treatment. *Circulation* 111(15):1999–2012.
99. Lindsay, A.C. et al. 2006. The role of parents in preventing childhood obesity. *Future Child* 16(1):169–186.

60 New Directions in Childhood Obesity

Fernando Zapata, MD, Ruben E. Quiros-Tejeira, MD, Cristina Fernandez, MD, Karla Lester, MD, Archana Chatterjee, MD, PhD, and Sandra G. Hassink, MD

CONTENTS

INTRODUCTION

The obesity epidemic has become a major global focus of the medical and public health communities. Millions of dollars are lost each year due to the consequences of obesity [1]. The alarming prevalence of obesity in the pediatric age group and the fact that an obese child has a 70% chance of becoming an obese adult has led to the need for and development of preventive strategies in childhood. Complications of obesity include cardiovascular disease (CVD) which is the leading cause of death and morbidity in the United States [2]. The indirect costs of obesity (absenteeism, disability, premature mortality, and workers' compensation) are related to long-term disease and have increased to two billion dollars [3]. The life expectancy of the current generation is lower than that of their parents and related to the effects of obesity [4,5]. The purpose of this chapter is to introduce, recognize, and summarize the epidemiology, definition, management, and complications of childhood obesity and evaluate different strategies to combat this problem.

DEFINITIONS

Body mass index (BMI) is recommended as the international standard measurement of adiposity in children 2 years of age and older. BMI is weight in kilograms divided by height in meters squared. BMI in children must be correlated with their BMI for age (Centers for Disease Control and Prevention [CDC]-derived normative percentiles) to determine their weight status category. *Overweight* is when the BMI percentile is between the 85th to less than 95th percentile for age. *Obesity* is when the BMI percentile is equal to or greater than the 95th percentile for age. *Morbid obesity* is when the BMI percentile is greater than the 99th percentile for age. An increased BMI is related to morbidity and mortality in adults. Elevated BMI and waist circumference in adults have been correlated with CVD risk factors in Mexican, African American, and white, non-Hispanic populations. Adults experience increased health risks if their BMI is over $30 \, kg/m^2$, which is about the 95th percentile of BMI at 19½ years of age [6]. Children's standard BMI charts for age also show a correlation of BMI and morbidity [6]. However, the BMI may be imprecise in children who are 4 years of age or younger. Clinicians may want to consider correlating the BMI-for-age curve with the weight and height percentile charts in young children.

A definition of *metabolic syndrome* (MS) (a consequence of obesity) continues to be extensively debated in the pediatric literature. No single definition has been reached by the National Institute for Children's Health and Development. Several definitions have been reported recently in the literature, but they have not been validated.

EPIDEMIOLOGY/PRIOR TRIALS

In 2007–2008, the prevalence of obesity was 32.2% among adult men and 35.5% among adult women, as reported by the National Health and Nutrition Examination Survey (NHANES) [7]. The increases in the prevalence of obesity previously observed from 1976 to 1980 and 1988 to 1994 were statistically significant in both genders and all age groups [8].

The prevalence of childhood obesity has doubled since the 1980s. A review by NHANES in 2003–2006 demonstrates that 11.3% of children and adolescents aged 2–19 years were at or above the 97th percentile of the 2000 BMI-for-age growth charts, 16.3% were at or above the 95th percentile, and 31.9% were above the 85th percentile [1]. The prevalence of high BMI for age among children and adolescents showed no significant changes between 2003–2004 and 2005–2006 and no significant trends between 1999 and 2006 [5].

Obesity also has disproportionately affected certain ethnic groups. Recent data show that 22% of Latino and 20% of African American adolescents (12–19 years old) are overweight and obese, while the prevalence in Caucasians is at about 14% [1]. In children, 6–11 years old, 22% of Mexican American, 20% of African American, and 14% of non-Hispanic white children were overweight [1]. A survey of Native American children shows that 39% of children between 5 and 18 years old are overweight or obese [1].

ETIOLOGY

Obesity is the result of genetic, environmental, physiological, social, and cultural factors that result in an energy imbalance and promote excessive fat deposition. Multiple studies indicate that the interaction between environmental and behavioral factors is primarily responsible. The dramatic increase of childhood obesity in the last few decades is associated with maternal diabetes, being born small for gestational age, parental obesity, maternal weight gain during pregnancy, and lack of breastfeeding.

Genetics and Energy Imbalance

Mouse genetics has made enormous contributions to theoretical models explaining how to balance energy intake and expenditure. The *ob* gene and its gene product leptin were identified in the early 1990s by Friedman et al. [9]. Leptin deficiency causes severe obesity in mice and humans. Leptin was proposed to regulate energy homeostasis, to suppress appetite, and to increase energy expenditure. Recent studies suggest that leptin is physiologically more important as an indicator of energy deficiency, rather than energy excess, and may moderate adaptations driving food intake and direct neuroendocrine functions that regulate energy balance. Leptin is secreted mainly by white adipose tissue, and levels have a positive correlation with the amount of body fat. Leptin binds to specific leptin receptors (LRs) to activate several signal transduction pathways including a Janus kinase signal that is important for the activation of the phosphatidylinositol 3-kinase (PI3'-K) pathway, which in turn regulates food intake and glucose homeostasis [10].

Ghrelin, a 28-amino-acid peptide, has been identified from the stomach as the first endogenous ligand for the growth hormone secretagogue receptor [11]. Ghrelin levels increase before meals and decrease after meals. It is considered the counterpart of the hormone leptin [12].

Variations in fat mass and obesity are also associated with a gene called FTO in the phenotypic obese Caucasian population [13].

Twin studies have shown significant genetic influence on body fat apart from BMI. In one classic study, concordance rates for different degrees of overweight were twice as high for monozygotic twins as for dizygotic twins [14]. Genetic factors alone can also play a role in specific rare cases of obesity, such as Prader–Willi syndrome (partial deletion of chromosome 15q 11–13), Alstrom syndrome, Cohen syndrome, Albright's hereditary osteodystrophy, Carpenter syndrome, MOMO syndrome (comprising macrosomia [excessive birth weight], obesity, macrocephaly [excessive head size], and ocular abnormalities), maternal uniparental disomy of chromosome 14, fragile X syndrome, and Borjeson–Forssman–Lehmann syndrome [15].

Environment

Genetics alone, however, cannot explain the increased rate of childhood obesity. Environmental factors such as poor nutrition, use of sweetened beverages, energy-dense foods, large portions, increased screen time, decreased physical activity, change in eating patterns, ordering out of food, and lower-income families with food insecurity have impacted the rapid rise of childhood obesity in the last few decades [11]. Increased consumption of calories and decreased physical activity are the keys to increased weight. The availability, per capita, of numbers of ready-to-eat food places and food dollars spent away from home play important roles in obesity [16]. Overweight children are more likely to skip breakfast and consume a few large meals, per day, than their leaner counterparts that are more likely to consume smaller, more frequent meals [11]. The Cardiovascular Health in Children Study (CHIC-1) was able to improve physiological outcomes by decreasing body fat and cholesterol concentration through increased moderate-to-vigorous physical activity in schools [17].

Family

Differences in feeding practices between lower- and upper-income mothers have been documented, but there is no proof that either approach is related to the risk of the child being overweight. Some studies demonstrate that upper-income mothers restricted more unhealthy foods and lower-income mothers permitted more snacking, if the children ate their main meal [18,19]. Low-income mothers are three times more likely to be obese than upper-income mothers [18]. Breastfeeding behavior also has a clear correlation in reducing infant mortality and protecting against obesity. Breastfeeding mothers have lower maternal weight [18]. Parent–child interactions and the home environment can affect the behavior of children related to calorie intake and physical activity. Parents are role models for their children who are likely to develop habits similar to their parents. Family meals provide a venue for parents to show model behavior [18,19].

Cultural Influences

African American, Mexican, and Cuban heritage families recognize overweight as a positive symbol [20]. Research shows that the association of minority groups with low income and obesity is bidirectional (including habits, media, genetic factors, earlier puberty, and the preference of larger bodies).

CLINICAL AND LABORATORY EVALUATION

Obesity is a chronic disease that does not represent a failure on the part of the patient or family and should not result in guilt. Lifestyle intervention is the hallmark of therapy, involving the physician, family, and patient to enhance behavior change.

History and Physical Examination

It is very important to evaluate the patient when they start gaining weight and elicit symptoms associated with obesity, such as anxiety, school avoidance, social isolation, headache, shortness of breath, exercise intolerance, snoring, apnea, daytime sleepiness, abdominal pain, leg pain, irregular menses, amenorrhea, polyuria, polydipsia, enuresis, or tobacco use. It is necessary to review the patient's nutritional practices such as consumption of meals outside the home, intake of sweetened beverages, portion sizes, breakfast habits, consumption of food with high energy density, intake of fruits and vegetables, and the quality and frequency of meals and snacks. Physical activity and inactivity also need to be documented, including school activities. Anthropometric measures including BMI percentile, as well as a history of obesity, overweight, or normal weight, physical examination to include blood pressure, acanthosis nigricans, hirsutism, striae, goiter, wheezing, abdominal tenderness, hepatomegaly, Tanner stage, gait, and range of motion of extremities, should be evaluated.

Algorithm for Assessment

In June 2007, the Expert Committee of the Childhood Obesity Action Network published guidelines for the assessment and prevention of childhood obesity [16].

Recommendations include the following:

- Assess ALL children, aged 2–18, for obesity at well care visits
- Use % BMI for age to screen for obesity
- Assess behaviors (diet and activity) and attitudes (readiness for change and concerns)
- Give consistent evidence-based messages for all children regardless of weight
- Advocate for improved access to fresh fruits and vegetables and safe physical activity in the community and school
- Identify and promote community services that encourage healthy eating and physical activity (Figures 60.1 and 60.2)

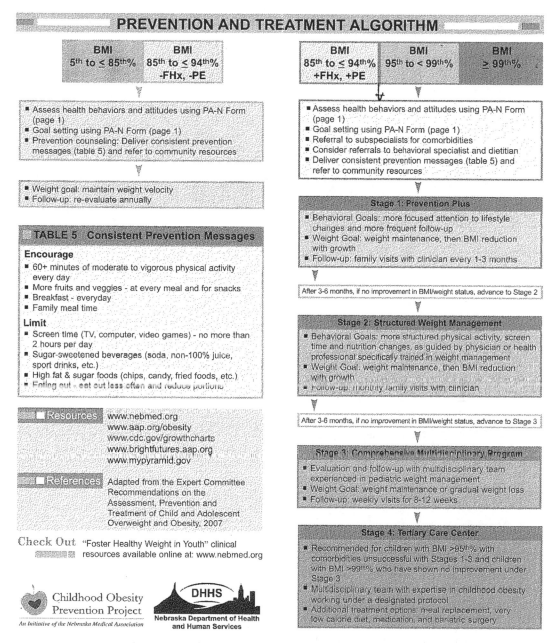

FIGURE 60.1 It presents an algorithm that illustrates the steps necessary to prevent and treat obesity, overweight, and unhealthy habits. (Modified from the Expert Committee Guidelines.) In the state of Nebraska, United States, the Department of Health and Human Services has approved a prescription for its use at each health-care visit.

How Much Physical Activity Each Day?

Youth Physical Activity and Nutrition Assessment   DHHS / NEBRASKA

Youth's Name: _____ Age: _____ Date: ___ / ___ / ___

Physical Activity	Current Activity	Activity Goal
1. Daily Physical Activity Moderate-Vigorous Intensity Ex: Active play, jumping, biking brisk walking, running, sports	1. _____ min/day _____ days/wk	1. _____ min/day _____ days/wk
Do not complete questions 2 & 3 for children aged 2-5 years old. Go to question 4.		
2. High-Intensity Activity Activities that cause fast breathing and sweating	2. _____ days/wk	2. _____ days/wk
3. Strengthening Activity Bone & muscle strengthening Ex: Jumping, climbing, lifting	3. _____ days/wk	3. _____ days/wk
4. Screen Time (outside of the school day) Ex: TV, video games, computer	4. _____ hours/day	4. _____ hours/day

Nutrition	Current Nutrition	Nutrition Goal
1. Breakfast Eating within 2 hours of waking	1. _____ days/wk	1. _____ days/wk
2. Fruits & Veggies • fresh, canned, dried, frozen 1 cup = 1 large potato or orange 1/2 cup = 4 strawberries, 6 baby carrots, beans (whole or refried)	2. Fruits: _____ cups per Circle: **DAY or WEEK** Veggies: _____ cups per Circle: **DAY or WEEK**	2. Fruits: _____ cups/day Veggies: _____ cups/day
3. Milk or Milk Products 1 cup = 8 oz milk, yogurt or 2 slices of cheese (1 1/2 oz)	3. _____ cups/day	3. _____ cups/day* *fat free or low fat
4. Whole Grains Whole grain cereal, oatmeal, whole wheat bread, brown rice	4. _____ times/day	4. _____ times/day
5. High Fat and Sugary Foods "Junk Foods" - chips, candy, fried foods, ice cream	5. _____ times/day	5. _____ times/day
6. Sugar-Sweetened Drinks Regular soda, lemonade, fruit punch, non-100% juice	6. _____ times/day	6. _____ times/day
7. Eating Out Meals eaten out of home or school	7. _____ days/wk	7. _____ days/wk

Comments

Note to Clinician: Have youth set only 1-2 behavioral goals at a time. Goals should be specific and measurable.

Goal Tracker

Check a box each day you meet your nutrition and activity goal(s).

I MET MY GOAL!

Week #1: ☐☐☐☐ ☐☐☐
Week #2: ☐☐☐☐ ☐☐☐
Week #3: ☐☐☐☐ ☐☐☐
Week #4: ☐☐☐☐ ☐☐☐
Week #5: ☐☐☐☐ ☐☐☐
Week #6: ☐☐☐☐ ☐☐☐
Week #7: ☐☐☐☐ ☐☐☐
Week #8: ☐☐☐☐ ☐☐☐

Way To Go!

If you've met your goal, keep it up and set a new activity or nutrition goal. Use another sheet to continue tracking your goals.

On a scale of 1–5 with 1 being not ready and 5 being very ready—How ready or interested are you in changing any of the behaviors above?

Not ready — 1   2   3   4   5 —Very ready

Referral:

Follow-up:

Complete after form is discussed:
I, _____ (youth or parent signature), agree to the goal(s) set above and understand how important nutrition and activity are to staying healthy.
Clinician's signature: _____

FIGURE 60.2 The Youth Physical Activity and Nutrition Assessment (PA-N) is a useful tool to educate and guide parents and patients to make a positive change in nonhealthy behaviors using motivational interviewing techniques. The parents and patient fill out the first column together, and with the use of motivational tools, the clinician assesses the readiness for change. Together a change of one or two behaviors is made. The recommendation is to change no more than 20% of each behavior. Small changes and big rewards are key to starting to make a difference. (From Barlow, S.E. and Expert Committee, *Pediatrics,* 120(Suppl 4), S164, 2007.)

Physical Activity Basics

How Much Physical Activity Each Day?

Type of Activity	Definition	Examples
Moderate aerobic activity	Activities that increase the heart rate, warm the body and cause a light sweat	Brisk walking, active play, bike riding, rollerblading, hiking
Vigorous aerobic activity	More challenging activity that increases the heart rate and causes fast breathing and more sweating	Running, active games (tag), sports such as soccer, swimming, tennis, martial arts
Muscle strengthening	Activities that create a force or overload on muscles	Climbing, push-ups, sit-ups, weight lifting
Bone strengthening	Activities that create a force or impact on bones that promotes bone growth and strength	Jumping, skipping, hopscotch, running, gymnastics

For more physical activity information visit: www.cdc.gov/physical activity.

FIGURE 60.2 (continued)

Comments

2–5 Years	6–18 Years
60+ min of activity every day Get 60 min day with: Structured play (planned activity) Unstructured play (free play) Focus on movement and coordination skills.	60+ min of activity every day Add up to 60 min day with: Moderate aerobic activity: Daily Vigorous aerobic activity: 3 times/week Muscle/bone strengthening activities: 3 times/week
Less than 2 h of screen time a day. (TV, video games, computer)	Less than 2 h of screen time a day. (TV, video games, computer)

*Note: Long periods of continuous, vigorous activity are not recommended for youth ages 6–12 unless chosen by the youth and not forced by an adult.

How Much Food Each Day?**

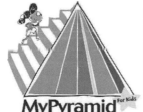

2-3 years	4-8 years	9-13 years	14-18 years
1 cup fruit	1 - 1.5 cups fruit	1.5 cups fruit	1.5 - 2 cups fruit
1 cup veggies	1.5 cups veggies	2 - 2.5 cups veggies	2.5 - 3 cups veggies
3 oz of grains	4-5 oz grains	5-6 oz grains	6-7 oz grains
2 cups milk	2 cups milk	3 cups milk	3 cups milk
2 oz meat/beans	3-4 oz meat/beans	5 oz meat/beans	5-6 oz meat/beans

**Food intake based on estimated calorie needs for boys and girls that get light physical activity.

MyPyramid For Kids
Eat Right. Exercise. Have Fun.

Healthy Eating Basics

Fruits Focus on fruits	Veggies Vary your veggies	Grains Make half your grains whole	Milk Get your calcium-rich foods	Meats and Beans Go lean with protein
Fruits are nature's treats - sweet and delicious. Eat them at meals, and at snack time, too. Choose fresh, frozen, canned, or dried. Go easy on juice and make sure it's 100%.	Color your plate with all kinds of great-tasting veggies. What's green and orange and tastes good? Veggies! Go dark green with broccoli and spinach or try orange veggies like carrots and sweet potatoes.	Just because bread is brown doesn't mean it's a whole grain. Look for the word "whole" to top the label ingredient list. Did you know, 1 ounce of whole-grain = a slice of whole-wheat bread, 1/2 cup of oatmeal, brown rice, or 1 cup whole-grain cereal.	Move to the milk group to get your calcium. Calcium builds strong bones. Look at the carton or container to make sure your milk, yogurt or cheese is low-fat or fat-free!	Eat lean or lowfat meat, chicken, turkey and fish. Bake, broil or grill meat instead of frying. A deck of cards = 3 ounces of meat. Nuts, seeds, peas, and beans are all great sources of protein, too!

Change your oil. We all need oil. Get yours from fish, nuts, and liquid oils such as canola, corn, soybean, and olive oil.

Don't sugarcoat it. Choose foods and beverages that do not have sugar and caloric sweeteners as one of the first ingredients. Added sugars contribute calories with few, if any, nutrients.

For more nutrition information visit: www. MyPyramid.gov

The Expert Committee further recommends that the following laboratory tests be considered in the evaluation of a child identified as overweight or obese:

If the BMI for age and sex is between the 85th and 94th percentiles with no risk factors, a fasting lipid profile should be performed.

For a BMI between the 85th and 94th percentiles with risk factors, a fasting glucose, aspartate aminotransferase (AST), and alanine aminotransferase (ALT) need to be performed biannually.

For a BMI greater than the 95th percentile, even in the absence of risk factors, all of the tests listed earlier plus blood urea nitrogen (BUN), creatinine, and other testing as clinically indicated should be performed [16,21].

CONSEQUENCES OF OBESITY AND OVERWEIGHT IN CHILDHOOD

Childhood obesity and overweight are associated with various health-related consequences.

EARLY EMERGENCY COMPLICATIONS

Severe obesity-related complications are now being seen more frequently in emergency rooms.

Hyperglycemic hyperosmolar syndrome is one of the complications of type 2 diabetes. Patients present with vomiting, abdominal pain, dizziness, polyuria, polydipsia, weight loss, and diarrhea. The criteria to make the diagnosis are glucose >600 mg/dL, serum CO_2 > 15 mmol/L, small ketonuria, serum osmolarity >320 mOsm/kg, and stupor or coma [22].

Diabetic ketoacidosis (DKA) can be manifested in patients with type 2 diabetes. Their basal insulin level is low, and there is an increased susceptibility to relative insulin deficiency. Symptoms and signs are ketonemia, acidosis, polyuria, polydipsia, dehydration, and coma.

Pulmonary embolism has been reported in obese adolescents. Patients present with dyspnea, chest pain, hypoxia, and hemoptysis. Risk factors include obesity, obesity hypoventilation syndrome, and coagulation disorder (V Leiden) [23].

LONG-TERM COMPLICATIONS

Cardiomyopathy of obesity is due to the high metabolic activity of excessive fat, increasing total blood volume and cardiac output. This produces left ventricular dysfunction [24].

Pseudotumor cerebri requires immediate attention due to an increase of intracranial pressure with papilledema and normal cerebrospinal fluid in the absence of ventricular enlargement. Patients present with headache, vomiting, blurred vision, or diplopia. It can lead to blindness, loss of peripheral visual fields, and reduction in visual acuity. This occurs in 30%–80% of obese children. The treatment includes acetazolamide and lumboperitoneal shunt. If the patient loses weight, the symptoms do resolve [25].

Slipped capital femoral epiphysis (SCFE) needs to be suspected in any limping, obese adolescent because 50%–70% of the patients with SCFE are obese. Associated symptoms can be groin, thigh, or knee pain. Diagnosis at physical examination is clear with limited motion of the hip in abduction and internal rotation. X-ray finalizes the diagnosis, and surgical intervention is needed [26].

Blount's disease is bowing of the tibia and femur unilaterally or bilaterally. In this group, two-third of the patients are obese. Weight loss and sometimes orthopedic correction are needed.

Obstructive sleep apnea (OSA) is defined as a prolonged partial or complete upper airway obstruction. Children with OSA demonstrate significant decrease in learning and memory, attention deficit, pulmonary hypertension, and right heart failure. Symptoms are nighttime awakening, restless sleep, and difficulty waking in the morning, daytime somnolence, napping, decreased concentration, and poor school performance. Definitive treatment includes weight loss; tonsillectomy/adenoidectomy; and, in severe cases, continuous positive airway pressure (CPAP), uvulopharyngopalatoplasty, craniofacial surgery, and tracheotomy [27].

Asthma has a strong association with obesity. Obesity contributes to the severity of asthma. Patients present with respiratory distress and history of gastroesophageal reflux, altered activity patterns, and dropping out of sports. Leptin is associated with obesity and asthma [28].

Nonalcoholic fatty liver disease (NAFLD) has a wide spectrum presentation. It ranges from simple steatosis to steatohepatitis to cirrhosis and finally end-stage liver disease. Diagnosis is suspected with evidence of elevation of liver enzymes and confirmed by liver biopsy. Predictive risk factors are male gender, Hispanic ethnicity, and elevated BMI. Treatment includes weight reduction and, at some centers, the use of medications such as vitamin E or metformin [29]. NAFLD refers to the presence of hepatic steatosis in the absence of significant ethanol consumption, underlying liver disease, or inborn error of metabolism. NAFLD is likely part of a continuum of disease beginning with asymptomatic changes of steatosis on liver biopsy, to active liver inflammation termed nonalcoholic steatohepatitis (NASH), which can eventually result in frank hepatic necrosis with cirrhosis. NAFLD most commonly occurs in obese individuals. Although NAFLD can be present in the absence of obesity, up to 90% of children with NAFLD are overweight or obese. Children with NAFLD also typically have evidence for insulin resistance (IR), even when controlling for BMI. There is also a high prevalence of other features of the MS in children with NAFLD including elevated triglycerides, an atherogenic lipid profile, and elevated blood pressure. NAFLD causes few if any symptoms, even in the presence of markedly abnormal liver pathology. However, it has been argued that liver biopsy is not appropriate for general screening. Alternative proposed diagnostic criteria include elevated transaminase levels (ALT > AST) coupled with characteristic findings on ultrasound in the absence of other causes of liver disease. The prevalence of this disorder has been increasing alongside that of the obesity epidemic. Rates from the NHANES data are consistent with autopsy studies where histologically proven NAFLD has been found in 9.6% of 2–19 year old children [30]. Others have reported prevalence rates among obese youth of 14%–24%. Autopsy data have demonstrated rates among obese youth of 38% [30].

Cholelithiasis presents with abdominal pain and abnormal ultrasound. Obesity is correlated with gallbladder stones in 8%–33% of patients [31].

IR and acanthosis nigricans are associated with future type 2 diabetes.

MS in pediatrics has the characteristics of an abnormal lipid profile [31], impaired glucose tolerance, BMI >95% for age and sex, and elevated blood pressure [29]. Obesity, specifically visceral adiposity, is directly linked to IR in both adults and children. The resistance to insulin action at the cellular level requires increasing insulin secretion to maintain normal rates of glucose uptake. Not surprisingly, obese children are more insulin resistant than children with normal BMI. MS refers to a clustering of clinical findings and metabolic disturbances including abdominal obesity, hypertension, dyslipidemia, and IR. Obesity and IR predispose to the other metabolic abnormalities observed in MS.

Type 2 diabetes is diagnosed with elevated fasting insulin and hyperglycemia. One-third of the new type 2 diabetics present between the ages of 10 and 19 years. African Americans, Hispanics, and Native Americans have a higher chance of developing type 2 diabetes.

Polycystic ovarian syndrome (PCOS) presents with the classic hyperandrogenism, amenorrhea, hirsutism, acne, polycystic ovaries, and eventually infertility [32]. Girls with premature adrenarche are at increased risk for PCOS and need to be followed longitudinally. PCOS is one of the most common endocrine disorders encountered in females, occurring in 3%–10% of women. PCOS is characterized clinically by anovulatory menstrual cycles and hirsutism or biochemical hyperandrogenism.

TABLE 60.1

Lipid Treatment Thresholds and Dietary Strategies for Dyslipidemia in Obese Children

Lipid Thresholds

- Total cholesterol >200 mg/dL
- LDL cholesterol >130 mg/dL
- Triglycerides >150 mg/dL
- HDL <35 HDL

Dietary Strategies

- Reduce total fat intake to <25% of total calories
- Reduce saturated fat intake to <7% of total calories
- Eliminate trans fats (<1% of total calories)
- Increase soluble fiber: dose of 5–20 g per day
- Initiate omega-3 fatty acids (1–2 g per day)
- Use products containing plant stanols or sterols

Typical laboratory abnormalities in PCOS include elevations in free testosterone and dehydroepi-androsterone sulfate (DHEAS) and decreases in sex hormone binding globulin. There also is growing evidence that PCOS is strongly associated with features of the MS and markers for subclinical CVD. The diagnosis of PCOS is exclusive to reproductively mature females, but childhood associations and risk factors have emerged. Prepubertal characteristics, including being small for gestational age and having a history of precocious pubarche, are proposed risk factors for later PCOS and MS. The etiology of PCOS is not completely understood, but it is likely multifactorial with both genetic and environmental influences playing key roles along with severe IR.

Hypertension is associated with an elevated BMI in 60% of the adolescent population. Hypertrophic left ventricle, CVD, and stroke are associated with uncontrolled hypertension [31,33]. Hypertension is a known risk factor for CVD, and management of hypertension is an essential component of preventative care in adults. Children who develop hypertension are more likely to have hypertension as an adult. The presence of hypertension in childhood is one of the risk factors associated with early atherosclerotic change. Obesity is a well-established risk factor for hypertension in children, and increases in measures of adiposity during childhood increase the risk of hypertension as a young adult. In general, secondary forms of hypertension are more common in the pediatric population. However, the increased rates of pediatric obesity have been a proposed factor in the increasing rates of primary hypertension in children [31].

Hyperlipidemia is associated with obesity due to an increase of fat distribution and hyperinsulinemia [31]. A clear association between an atherogenic lipid profile (elevated LDL cholesterol and triglycerides with low HDL cholesterol) and obesity in children has been well established. An atherogenic lipid profile is a known risk factor for development of fatty streaks in the aorta. Lipid profiles track from childhood into adulthood. Obesity is listed as a risk factor to screen for lipid abnormalities in the most recent policy statement adopted by the American Academy of Pediatrics [6]. Up to 46% of a referral population of overweight 7–12 year old children had evidence of abnormalities in the lipid profile when compared to population-based norms [6]. The dyslipidemia seen in pediatric obesity has both genetic and environmental origins. However, a key risk factor for development for lipid abnormalities is concomitant IR. For the same BMI, adolescents with evidence for IR are more likely to have an abnormal lipid profile. See Table 60.1 for lipid treatment thresholds and dietary strategies.

Psychological morbidity in obesity is associated with depression, anxiety, low self-esteem, bullying, binge eating disorder, and depression [34].

INTERVENTIONS

Multiple studies have been published highlighting promising research in childhood obesity prevention and treatment strategies; however, only a few interventions have been designed to investigate the underlying metabolic abnormalities. Conventional approaches, targeting weight management in children, have resulted in positive outcomes over 12 months. Some studies show success in reducing the BMI, BMI SD score, or percentage overweight that resulted from weight loss or weight gain prevention interventions [35]. Comprehensive treatment that consists of counseling for diet, physical activity, and instruction in, and support for, the use of behavioral management techniques to sustain the changes is effective [31]. These low-intensity interventions were more effective in the primary care setting than other low-intensity interventions such as a structured group model (family, parent-only, child-only instructions), use of the Internet, or social support.

TRIALS

Systematic monitoring of BMI is essential and needs to be continuous. BMI screening is recommended by the Expert Committee on the Prevention and Treatment of Childhood Obesity at all well care visits [16]. The need for research into effective intervention and prevention should continue to be a priority. There are limited quality data to recommend one treatment program over another. However, combined, multidisciplinary, behavioral, and lifestyle interventions compared to standard care or self-help can produce a significant and clinically meaningful reduction in overweight children and adolescents. In obese adolescents, the use of orlistat or sibutramine with lifestyle interventions should be carefully considered as adverse effects of these medications may be significant [36]. Combined diet and physical activity through school-based interventions may help prevent children from becoming overweight in the long term [37,38]. Physical activity interventions particularly for girls in primary schools may help prevent overweight in the short term [38]. A meta-analysis showed that school-based interventions were effective in the short term in reducing the prevalence of childhood obesity [38]. However, longer programs were more effective than shorter programs [38].

It should be noted that the Endocrine Expert Committee recommends referral to genetics for testing for the MC4R gene in children with excessive weight gain in early infancy when weight has risen above the 97th percentile by 3 years of age [11]. However, this test is only positive in 2%–4% of children and does not alter treatment. Other reasons for referral include those who have obesity associated with neurodevelopmental abnormalities and short stature [11].

PREVENTION

There are multiple recommendations from the AAP and Expert Committee on the prevention of obesity and overweight in children [11,16]. The Nebraska Department of Health and Human Services developed a toolkit for health-care providers as part of the "Foster Healthy Weight in Youth" program [39] using the Youth PA-N Form, which is an objective assessment tool that facilitates the conversation between health-care providers and patients around weight, nutrition, and activity habits. The Youth PA-N Form also is infused with consistent prevention messages and is a tool that integrates the Expert Committee recommendations in the clinic setting.

Youth PA-N Form highlights include the following:

1. Target population.
   To be used in ALL children 2–18 years, regardless of BMI status.
2. Eleven health behaviors are assessed.
   The front of the form assesses current information regarding the top 11 health behaviors associated with recommended activity and eating patterns that promote healthy weight and optimal growth and development.

3. Organized in more vs. less healthy behaviors.
   It is organized so the healthy behaviors are listed first and the less healthy behaviors are in the lower part of the section.
4. Quick reference.
   Age-specific physical activity and nutrition tables are on the back of the form. Circling the age specific column can help guide parents to understand their child's specific needs.
5. Assesses attitudes and motivation.
   The bottom of the form has a numerical scale that assesses the patient and/or parent's readiness to change any one of the behaviors assessed on the Youth PA-N Form.
6. Goal setting and tracker sections.
   A separate column is provided for setting 1–2 goals with the patient, and a goal tracker section helps patients monitor their health behaviors.
7. Contractual signature box.
   The contractual signature box is to be signed by the provider and patient to affirm commitment to goals set.

The purpose for providers is to

- Use as a prevention and treatment tool: structure discussion around healthy lifestyle behaviors
- Use language that is reflective of national guidelines (consistent messaging)
- Set individualized, measureable goals
- Encourage follow-up and serve as a critical referral point
- Educate and raise awareness among families on the importance of nutrition and activity for lifelong health

The purpose for parents/patients is to

- Assess current activity and nutrition behaviors
- Understand the recommended amounts of activity needed for health
- Understand age-specific eating patterns needed to meet nutritional adequacy and promote healthy growth patterns
- Give parents and youth a chance to share concerns

The following components are included in the Youth PA-N Form:

PHYSICAL ACTIVITY BEHAVIORS

Daily physical activity includes moderate and/or vigorous intensity activities such as active play, biking, brisk walking, running, etc. The Youth PA-N Form collects total minutes per day and days per week. The goal for daily physical activity is 60 min per day, 7 days per week.

High-intensity activity is a vigorous activity that is challenging, and causes increased heart rate, fast breathing, and sweating. Any activity can be done at a high intensity. High-intensity activities are a part of the recommended 60 min per day, but the goal is to get high-intensity activity at least 3 days per week. Because national guidelines do not provide specific recommendations for 2–5 year olds on high-intensity and strengthening activities, those behaviors should only be collected on patients age 6 or older.

Strengthening activity is an activity such as jumping, skipping, climbing, gymnastics, running, and weightlifting. The recommendation for strengthening activity is 3 days per week and can also be a part of the total daily physical activity time of 60 min per day.

Screen time should be assessed for all patients and includes time spent watching TV, playing video games, and computer times. Screen time is assessed in hours/day, and the recommendation is that children 2 or older spend no more than 2 h per day at a screen.

NUTRITION BEHAVIORS

Breakfast is defined as eating within 2 h of waking, and the recommendation is to eat breakfast every day.

Fruit and vegetable intake is assessed in amount of cups per day or week and not servings. All forms should be counted: fresh, frozen, dried, or canned. It is recommended that children get 1–2 cups of fruit per day and 1–3 cups of vegetables, with overall intake based on the child's age.

Milk or milk products—the recommendation is 2–3 cups per day of fat-free or low-fat milk, yogurt, and/or cheese.

Whole grains are assessed in frequency by times per day. Whole grains include whole wheat, oatmeal, brown rice, etc. Whole grains are recommended at 2–3 times per day.

High fat and sugar foods include foods high in added fats and sugars, such as chips, candy, fried foods, ice cream, etc. These foods are also assessed in frequency by times per day. The recommendation is to limit the consumption of foods high in fat and sugar to 0 to 1 time per day.

Sugar-sweetened drinks are those beverages with added sugar and include regular soda, lemonade, fruit punch, sports drinks, and non-100% juice. These drinks are assessed in frequency by times per day. The recommendation is to limit the consumption of sugar-sweetened beverages to 0–1 time/day.

Eating out includes those meals consumed out of the home or school and is assessed by days per week. The recommendation is to limit eating out to 0–2 days/week.

ASSESS ATTITUDES AND MOTIVATION

- The readiness scale at the bottom of the Youth PA-N Form is used to assess the patient's readiness for change.
- If the patient/parent is not ready (3 or below), feedback is given: *"Sounds like you aren't quite ready to make any changes now. We will follow up at your child's next visit."* Or *"Although you aren't ready to make changes today, you might want to think about your child's weight gain and the importance of lowering his diabetes risk."*
- If the patient/parent is ready to change (4 or above), they may advance to goal setting.

For a number of reasons, it can be difficult to counsel children and families on such a touchy subject as obesity. Listed as follows are the "ABCs" of counseling and motivating overweight children and families:

Ask open-ended questions:

- How do you feel about us talking about your physical activity, TV watching, and eating today?
- How concerned are you about your child's weight? Why?
- What are some of the things you might like to change?

Body language:

- Put patient at ease.
- Use eye contact without barriers.
- Convey respect.
- Counsel in a private setting.

Care and empathy:

- Do not criticize.
- Acknowledge patient's feelings.
- Answer questions without sign of judgment.
- Use language that is nonjudgmental.
  "Healthier" food vs. "bad" food
  "Healthier" weight vs. "ideal" weight

Simple acronyms, such as "OARS," can help as well:

- Ask open-ended questions.
- Give affirmations.
- Be reflective of patient's/parent comments.
- Give summarizations that include patient/parent comments.

It is important to know whether to set goals with the parent, the patient, or both. For children less than 12 years of age, parents or guardians control the foods coming into the home and access to physical activity, television, and other screen time. Thus, goals should be set for this age group with parents/guardians. For children 12–14 years of age, parents/guardians need to be included, but the teen should be interviewed individually and asked about his/her goals separately as well. High school–aged teens can be counseled in confidence. The teen's permission should be sought as to whether or not they want to involve the parent.

The following stages of intervention are recommended:

Stage 1

If the patient has a normal BMI between the 5th percentile and ≤85th percentile or a BMI of the 85th to ≤94th percentile with a normal family history and a normal physical examination:

- Assess health behaviors and attitudes using the Youth (PA-N) Form.
- Use the goal setting portion of the Youth PA-N Form.
- Deliver consistent prevention messages and refer to a community resource.

The plan is to maintain weight velocity and follow up with the patient annually. Consistent prevention messages are those that have been identified by the Expert Committee [16] and the CDC [40] to prevent obesity and are unlikely to cause harm. Delivering one or two consistent prevention messages at each visit can positively reinforce goals and behaviors. Consistent prevention messages include the following:

- Encourage 60+ minutes of moderate-to-vigorous physical activity every day.
- Encourage more fruits and vegetables—at every meal and for snacks.
- Encourage breakfast—everyday.
- Encourage family meal time.
- Limit screen time (TV, computer, video games) to no more than 2 h per day.
- Limit sugar-sweetened beverages (soda, non-100% juice, sports drinks, etc.).
- Limit high fat and sugar foods (chips, candy, fried foods, etc.).
- Limit eating out and reduce portions.

Stage 2

If the patient has a BMI between the 85th percentile and ≤94th percentile, the plan includes setting behavioral goals for a more focused attention to lifestyle changes and more frequent follow-ups, setting a weight goal for weight maintenance and then BMI reduction with growth, as well as follow-up with family visits with the clinician every 1–3 months. If there is no improvement in BMI/weight status after 3–6 months, advance to stage 3.

Stage 3

In a patient with a BMI between the 95th percentile and 99th percentile, the plan includes evaluation and follow-up with a multidisciplinary team experienced in pediatric weight management, setting a weight goal for weight maintenance and gradual weight loss with weekly follow-up visits for 8–12 weeks.

Stage 4

This stage is recommended for children with a BMI > 95th percentile with comorbidities, unsuccessful stages 1–3 interventions, and children with a BMI > 99th percentile who have shown no improvement under stage 3. Follow-up with a multidisciplinary team with expertise in childhood obesity working under a designated protocol is recommended. Additional treatment options include meal replacement, very low calorie diet, medication, and bariatric surgery.

In conclusion, obesity and overweight are an increasing problem in childhood. In this chapter, we have reviewed the definition of these terms, as well as the epidemiology, etiology, clinical and laboratory evaluation, management, and complications of childhood obesity.

REFERENCES

1. Ogden, C. and M. Carroll. 2010. Prevalence of obesity among children and adolescents: United States, trends 1963–1965 through 2007–2008. Available at: http://www.cdc.gov/nchs/data/hestat/obesity_child_07_08/obesity_child_07_08.pdf (accessed February 27, 2011).
2. Singh, A. S. et al. 2008. Tracking of childhood overweight into adulthood: A systematic review of the literature. *Obes Rev* 9:474–488.
3. Finkelstein, E. A., Rohm, C. S., and K. M. Kosa. 2005. Economic causes and consequences of obesity. *Annu Rev Public Health* 26:239–257.
4. Trogdon, J. G. et al. 2008. Indirect cost of obesity: A review of the current literature. *Obes Rev* 9:489–500.
5. Ogden, C. L., Carrol, M. D., and K. Flegal. 2008. High body mass index for age among US children and adolescents, 2003–2006. *JAMA* 299(20):2401–2405.
6. Wake, M. 2009. Issues in obesity monitoring, screening and subsequent treatment. *Curr Opin Pediatr* 21(6):811–816.
7. Flegal, K. M. et al. 2010. Prevalence and trends in obesity among US adults, 1999–2008. *JAMA* 303(3):235–241.
8. Land, I. A. et al. 2011. Variation in childhood and adolescent obesity prevalence defined by international and country-specific criteria in England and the United States. *Eur J Clin Nutr* 65(2):143–150.
9. Friedman, J. M. 2009. Leptin at 14 y of age: An ongoing story. *Am J Clin Nutr* 89(3):973S–979S.
10. Myers, M. G. 2004. Leptin receptor signaling and the regulation of mammalian physiology. *Recent Prog Horm Res* 59:287–304.
11. August, G. et al. 2008. Prevention and treatment of pediatric obesity: An endocrine society clinical practice guideline based on expert opinion. *J Clin Endocrinol Metab* 93(12):4576–4599.
12. Klok, M. D., Jakobsdottir, S., and M. L. Drent. 2007. The role of leptin and ghrelin in the regulation of food intake and body weight in humans: A review. *Obes Rev* 8(1):21–34.
13. Frayling, T. M. et al. 2007. A common variant in the FTO gene is associated with body mass index and predisposes to childhood and adult obesity. *Science* 316(5826):889–894.
14. Stunkard, A. J., Foch, T. T., and Z. Hrubec. 1986. A twin study of human obesity. *JAMA* 256(1):51–54.
15. Gunay-Aygun, M., Cassidy, S. D., and R. D. Nicholls. 1997. Prader-Willi and other syndromes associated with obesity and mental retardation. *Behav Genet* 27:307–324.
16. Barlow, S. E. and Expert Committee. 2007. Expert committee recommendations regarding the prevention, assessment, and treatment of child and adolescent overweight and obesity: Summary report. *Pediatrics* 120(Suppl 4):S164–S192.
17. Harrell, J. S. et al. 1999. A public health vs. a risk-based intervention to improve cardiovascular health in elementary school children: The Cardiovascular Health in Children Study. *Am J Public Health* 89(10):1529–1535.

18. Feinson, J., Atkinson, A., and S. Hassink. 2010. How a primary care quality improvement initiative is implementing the expert recommendations on childhood obesity. *Del Med J* 82(2):57–65.

19. Kumanyika, S. and S. Grier. 2006. Targeting interventions for ethnic minority and low-income populations. *Future Child* 16(1):187–207.

20. Denney, J. T. et al. 2004. Race/ethnic and sex differentials in body mass among US adults. *Ethn Dis* 14(3):389–398.

21. Daniels, S. R., Greer. F., and the Committee on Nutrition. 2008. Lipid screening and cardiovascular health in childhood. *Pediatrics* 122(1):198–208.

22. Morales, A. and A. Rosenbloom. 2004. Death caused by hyperglycemic hyperosmolar state at the onset of type 2 diabetes. *J Pediatr* 144(2):270–273.

23. Sugeiman, H. et al. 2003. Pulmonary embolism. *J Gastrointest Surg* 7(1):102–107.

24. Alpert, M. A. 2001. Obesity cardiomyopathy: Pathophysiology and evolution of the clinical syndrome. *Am J Med Sci* 321(4):225–236.

25. Baker, R. S. et al. 1985. Visual loss in pseudotumor cerebri of childhood. A follow-up study. *Arch Ophthalmol* 103(11):1681–1686.

26. Wilcox, P. G., Weiner, D. S., and B. Leighley. 1988. Maturation factors in slipped capital femoral epiphysis. *J Pediatr Orthop* 8:196–200.

27. Schechter, M. S., The Section on Pediatric Pulmonology, and Subcommittee on Obstructive Sleep Apnea Syndrome. 2002. Technical report: Diagnosis and management of childhood obstructive sleep apnea syndrome. *Pediatrics* 109(4):e69–e79.

28. Guler, N. et al. 2004. Leptin: Does it have any role in childhood asthma? *J Allergy Clin Immunol* 114(2):254–259.

29. Harrison, S. A. and A. M. Diehl. 2002. Fat and the liver- a molecular overview. *Sem Gastrointest Dis* 13(1):3–16.

30. Schwimmer, J.B., Deutsch, R., Kahen, T., Lavine, J.E., Stanley, C., and C. Behling. 2006. Prevalence of fatty liver in children and adolescents. *Pediatrics* 118(4):1388–1393.

31. Hassink, S. 2008. Obesity in adolescents: Part 1. Adolescent health update. *AAP News* 21(1):1–8.

32. Glueck, C. J. et al. 2011. Sex hormone-binding globulin, oligomenorrhea, polycystic ovary syndrome, and childhood insulin at age 14 years predict metabolic syndrome and class III obesity at age 24 years. *J Pediatr* 159(2):308–313.

33. Sorof, J. and S. Daniels. 2002. Obesity hypertension in children: A problem of epidemic proportions. *Hypertension* 40:441–447.

34. Sjoberg, R. et al. 2005. Obesity, shame and depression in school-aged children: A population based study. *Pediatrics* 116(3):e389–e392.

35. Kamath, C. C. et al. 2008. Clinical review: Behavioral interventions to prevent childhood obesity: A systematic review and meta-analysis of randomized trials. *J Clin Endocrinol Metab* 93(12):4606–4615.

36. Luttikhuis, H. O. et al. 2009. Interventions for treating obesity in children. *Cochrane Database of Syst Rev* 3:1–57.

37. Brown, T. and C. Summerbell. 2009. Systematic review of school-based interventions that focus on changing dietary intake and physical activity levels to prevent childhood obesity: An update to the obesity guidance produced by the National Institute for Health and Clinical Excellence. *Obes Rev* 10(1):110–141.

38. Gonzales-Suarez, C. et al. 2009. School-based interventions on childhood obesity: A meta-analysis. *Am J Prev Med* 37(5):418–427.

39. Lester, K., Fernandez, C., and H. Dingman. 2010. Foster healthy weight in youth, Nebraska's clinical childhood obesity model. Available at http://www.hhs.state.ne.us/hew/hpe/NAFH/fosterhealthyweighti-nyouth.htm (accessed March 6, 2011).

40. US Preventive Services Task Force. and M. Barton. 2010. Screening for obesity in children and adolescents: US Preventive Services Task Force recommendation statement. *Pediatrics* 125(2):361–367.

61 Thinking Outside the Box
The TEEEN Program, a Primary Care Approach to Address the Public Health Concern of Pediatric Obesity

Shirley Gonzalez, MD, FAAP
and Betsy Ramsey, MS, RD, CDE, LDN

CONTENTS

INTRODUCTION

EXPERIENCES OF A PEDIATRICIAN: 2003

Pediatric obesity is a major public health concern that is seen everyday in primary care pediatrics. In 2003, it became apparent to a pediatrician that too many adolescents from multiethnic backgrounds were already heading down the path predicted to result in progressive obesity and the associated health, socioeconomic, and emotional problems related to obesity. It seemed that their lives needed to change course now before their problems escalated. The social situation varied for each of the adolescents seen, but many lacked direction and did not have positive role models in their lives. Health disparities and deficiencies in the area of health literacy were noticed. The families of these children often reported facing economic barriers, concerns of safety in their neighborhoods, and time constraints. Various caregivers may have realized that their children should exercise more but could not arrange for safe opportunities for them to be physically active. Parents also indicated that they did not feel safe walking around their neighborhood with their children after getting home from work at night. Financial limitations led to frequent inexpensive meals and limited daily consumption of fresh fruits and vegetables. Parents often reported having limited time to participate with their children in activities promoting increased physical activity. In terms of health literacy, some families did not know the significance of the problem of pediatric obesity and its comorbidities, did not see a need to learn to change, or felt helpless if they did see a need. Some of the reasons for the insufficient consumption of healthy foods were insufficient health literacy or financial difficulties. This pediatrician wanted to do something to help improve this situation by concentrating her efforts in launching these young men and women onto a path of good health, truth, and professional development, so they could be all that they were made to be by showing them their value and by empowering them to value themselves. The pediatrician knew that this would take more than just a few minutes in the office and would involve more than just writing a prescription. Thinking outside the box, her vision was to offer a program in a nonclinical setting where they could learn how to do what they were told to do in the doctor's office. They were taught, in a hands-on way, how to exercise safely and effectively, the benefit of trying new foods, and what to notice on food labels as a start. Health equity was a concern. Could they overcome the barriers they faced and achieve their full health potential? Could the quality of their lives be as great as those of children who did not face the same barriers?

PROBLEM OF PEDIATRIC OBESITY

Among children and adolescents 2–19 years, during the time period of 2007–2008, 31.7% were at or above the 85% of BMI for age.[1] During this time frame, Hispanic boys had significantly higher odds of having high BMI compared with non-Hispanic white boys. Non-Hispanic black girls were significantly more likely than non-Hispanic white girls to have high BMI.[1] Looking at the trends between 1999–2000 and 2007–2008 among 6–19 year old children and adolescents, there was a statistically significant increasing trend for boys at or above the 97th percentile for the total population and for non-Hispanic white boys.[1] Factors leading to obesity include an increase in sedentary lifestyles, a reduction in physical activity, a decrease in consumption of foods with high nutritional value, and an accompanying increase in consumption of unhealthy foods. According to the Youth Risk Behavior Surveillance (YRBS) United States, among high school students nationwide, during 2007, 35.4% had watched television 3 h or more/day on an average school day.[2] Excessive time spent watching television has been shown to be associated with an increase in BMI.[3,4] Nationwide, results from the YRBS showed that during the 7 days before the survey, 78.6% of high school students had not eaten fruits and vegetables five or more times per day, 33.8% had consumed soda or pop at least one time per day, 14.1% had consumed three or more glasses/day of milk, and 65.3% had not met recommended levels of physical activity.[2] NHANES data showed an increase in per capita daily caloric contribution from sugar-sweetened beverages and 100% juice from 242 kcal/day in 1988–1994 to 270 kcal/day in 1999–2004 among children and adolescents (aged 2–19 years) in the United States.[5]

NHANES data from 1999 to 2004 demonstrated that soda contributed around 67% of all sugar-sweetened beverage calories among adolescents, and fruit drinks contributed more than half of the sugar-sweetened beverage calories consumed by preschool-aged children.[5]

Notable comorbidities that may be seen with obesity include type 2 diabetes mellitus, nonalcoholic fatty liver disease, dyslipidemia, hypertension, arthritis, obstructive sleep apnea, and vitamin D deficiency.[6,7] The incidence of type 2 diabetes in childhood in the United States has increased over the past two decades.[8] Coronary heart disease may become a disease of young adulthood.[9] Life expectancy of people with diabetes may be close to 13 years less than that of people without diabetes.[10] Obesity has also been associated with an increased incidence of and mortality from a number of cancers.[11] The quality of life of an obese adolescent may be comparable to that observed in a patient with cancer.[12,13] Studies have shown that the effects of obesity may track into adulthood.[14,15] Adults with elevated body weight in adolescence have an increased risk of morbidity and mortality independent of adult weight.[16] Men with excessive weight during adolescence have an increased risk of mortality.[16] Men and women with excessive weight during adolescence have an increased risk of morbidity from coronary heart disease and atherosclerosis.[16] Excessive weight in adolescent girls leads to compromised functional capacity in adulthood.[16] These increased risks were independent of adult BMI.[16] Adolescent weight control is a high priority. One of the objectives of Healthy People 2020 DPHHS is to reduce the proportion of children and adolescents who are overweight/obese.[17]

A study done to estimate the expected years of life lost (YLL) due to overweight and obesity showed that obesity appears to lessen life expectancy especially among younger adults.[18]

It is estimated that the prevalence of obesity in children may nearly double by 2030 and that the total health-care costs associated with obesity/overweight may double every decade to 860.7–956.9 billion U.S. dollars by 2030.[19] This would represent 16%–18% of total U.S. health-care costs.[19]

There is an urgent need for everyone to be doing something. This problem is unlikely to yield to just one single policy intervention, so it is important to pursue multiple opportunities to achieve incremental gains. There is a need to achieve health equity as indicated by the Centers for Disease Control (CDC) (2007).[20] Health disparities exist at many levels, especially in the areas of access to safe places to play and be physically active, to good education, to affordable healthy food items, and to positive role models.

HISTORY OF THE TEEEN PROGRAM (TEENS, EMPOWERMENT, EXERCISE, EDUCATION, NUTRITION)

The TEEEN program started in 2003 in response to what was seen in a pediatric office. The participants in the program voted for the title of the program, the logo, its colors, and the t-shirt design. This symbolizes the philosophy of what was envisioned back in 2003: a program that motivated the participants and their families to take the steps needed toward a healthy lifestyle through empowerment. The pediatrician wanted a supportive environment to raise awareness of healthier choices and wanted to think outside the box, in terms of what a pediatrician is supposed to do. One of the goals was to show the participants and their families how much fun it would be to be physically active or try a new fruit. The message is obvious but how it was to be conveyed is different. The goal was to reverse the trend before they started developing comorbidities such as type 2 diabetes mellitus. Patience was required since necessary change would take time. It was understood that since it took a few years for them to reach their current status, it likely would take a few years before the intervention would yield results.

The program started in a small room using an aerobics video followed by a series of talks on healthy eating and exercise. Gradually, a curriculum was developed and educational games were designed. Medical students were enlisted, and outside speakers were invited to contribute to the program. Colleagues in the field of pediatric endocrinology, pediatrics, and family medicine provided encouragement and support for this endeavor. This led to a systematic arrangement of various components and simultaneous evaluation/research to determine its effectiveness. Other areas of investigation include quality of life and food label knowledge acquisition.

WHY THIS PROGRAM IS DIFFERENT: MULTIFACETED

The TEEEN program is unique in its design because it incorporates many individually effective components into one program of intervention. Empowerment, caretaker involvement, multiethnic appeal, education, exercise, a nonclinical approach, and primary care leadership are some of the unique aspects of the program.

Empowerment is promoted in all phases. The program is led by a pediatrician, a dietitian, and medical students. Participants are empowered in many ways. They are encouraged to lead some of the exercises, to ask questions, and to present findings from food labels to teach the group what they have learned. As they actively participate month after month, they are empowered to do the exercises on their own at home. As future leaders, they learn leadership skills and are empowered to practice these skills in other settings. The medical students experience firsthand exposure to the problem of pediatric obesity and are empowered to do something about it. The medical students themselves may be different practitioners because of this experience and will have a different frame of reference for the future. Children and parents/caregivers are taught to think for themselves about how to make changes in their lives and are empowered with the tools they need to modify their diet and lifestyles. Individuals are challenged to keep food records and to evaluate their own diets via 24 h food recalls in the group setting.

Caretaker involvement is actively pursued. Parents are invited to participate in exercise, didactic events, and presentations. As they join in the educational lectures, exercise, activities, and games with their children, they are empowered to be helpful resources to their families. The dietitian meets with the parents separately, while the children are doing an activity. This provides them with an opportunity to learn how to offer healthy foods for their families and to understand the nutritional needs of their children. Questions are encouraged, and the group of parents is supportive of one another. Having separate activities for caretakers is important since family-centered interventions that incorporate a separate curriculum for caretakers have shown promising results.[21]

From the beginning, participants have come from many ethnic backgrounds. A key component of the program has been minority receptivity and acceptance. The program offers a culturally sensitive place for them to ask questions like the following: "What is it about this food that is healthy?" "How can I change my behavior?" When their questions are answered, they gain the knowledge necessary to make better decisions.

Nutrition education occurs at various levels. The participants are offered new fruits and vegetables to try and bottled water to drink after exercise sessions. Activities are designed to practice finding a healthy choice on a restaurant menu or finding a snack that is sufficiently palatable but lower in calories. Other didactic sessions give opportunities to evaluate common food portions, eating habits, and choice of beverages. They thus learn to try different foods, may learn to like the new foods, and may continue to have healthier foods as a regular part of their diet. Food label education is provided during every session. Participants and their families learn to understand facts on food labels during lectures and through presentations by participants and their caretakers.

The education curriculum only mentions weight and obesity twice. Information is given with a positive focus emphasizing fun, empowerment, exercise, education, and hands-on learning. It is a program that is health centered not weight centered. Through all the educational activities, which include games and projects, participants are encouraged to have fun. This may contribute to the number of participants who keep coming in subsequent years.

Exercise is a crucial element of the program. Research shows that exercise is an important component, and engagement in physical activity is a critical intervention in obesity prevention and weight management programs.[22] Participation promotes self-efficacy and positive cues toward sense of achievement regarding their physical selves. Participants learn to measure their heart rate before and after exercise to learn about the effect of exercise on their bodies. All leaders participate in the exercise component. The exercises are fun for all ages and are not difficult to complete. Thus, everyone can think of himself or herself as an active person.

For many, this maybe the first time they have done any formal exercise. They achieve self-confidence through the experience and learn that exercising regularly can be feasible and affordable. Thus, self-efficacy in the area of physical activity is promoted. Each participant's self-image now includes being an active person. Participants envision themselves being physically active throughout their lives. The exercises require minimal equipment, and participants are taught how to make their own equipment from things they have at home, such as milk containers filled with sand, or cans. Each child is given a Thera-Band, a pair of sneakers, and a pedometer, as incentives to continue the exercises at home. They may also be given other equipment as rewards for completing a project.

Other factors contribute to making this a unique program. The setting is different. It is not in a clinic. Thus, it is primary care outside the office: It is thinking outside the box. It is a meeting of primary health care and public health. Also, the program follows a continuous care model. Participants attend the program for 1 year. After this year, they are invited to come back as leaders and thus continue to be exposed to all the elements of the program, but now as leaders. This provides the leaders with ongoing education in an indirect way. All of the leaders become positive role models for the participants at multiple levels.

Indeed, through coordinated goals among various professionals, the TEEEN program teaches self-regulation, models behaviors related to nutrition and exercise, facilitates problem-solving techniques at all levels, and promotes parental knowledge acquisition.

TEEEN PROGRAM SESSIONS

This is a skeletal outline of what an observer might see during a regular TEEEN session. The group attends monthly, pediatrician-led, 4 h sessions for 1 year. Each session is conducted in a hospital auditorium and consists of the following:

1. Tracking of sedentary behaviors and food choices (1 h):

    *   Completion of a 24 h food and beverage recall used to monitor progress and to aid discussions during sessions
    *   Documentation of physical activity using a validated questionnaire for adolescents (PDPAR or previous day physical activity recall) to calculate metabolic equivalents (Mets)[23,24]
    *   Documentation of sedentary behaviors: television, computer, video games
    *   Documentation of type of liquid choices (water, juice, soda) and quantity (oz/day) of each one using standard models

2. Exercise (1 h):

    *   Strength and endurance training routine designed with the help of an exercise physiologist using aids such as Thera-Bands, medicine balls, and free weights
    *   Exercise testing conducted every 3 months to assess endurance, agility, balance, curl ups/min, power

3. Education (1 h):
Interactive and educational presentations on topics such as human physiology and pathophysiology of obesity, food label literacy, nutrition science, healthy eating strategies, physical activity, strategies for a healthier lifestyle, and social changes precipitating/sustaining the obesity epidemic are presented during this hour.

The education curriculum consists of three sets of interactive lectures. These sets are repeated twice during the course of 1 year:

1. Medical lectures: This set includes the topics of pediatric obesity, comorbidities associated with pediatric obesity, lipid metabolism, and muscle groups used during exercise.
2. Nutritional information lectures: This set presents information on portion control, food selection, eating habits, preparation of foods, planning a balanced diet, eating out, and how to achieve and maintain a healthy weight.
3. Nutritional environment lectures: This set presents information on how to increase physical activity, read food labels, understand liquid calories, interpret fast-food menus, and understand popular diets.

4. Projects/games (1 h):

The use of glucometers to aid understanding of postprandial glucose metabolism, TEEEN quiz game, a pedometer project, and the use of resources in hospital library.

Motivational interviewing is conducted to assess subjects' behaviors and readiness to change.[25]

Incentives: Thera-Bands, pedometers, a pair of sneakers, certificates (for participation, leading exercises, presenting food labels), and prizes (for completing take-home assignments) are offered to stimulate participation and compliance with visits.

WHAT HAS BEEN SEEN: THE IMPACT OF THE PROGRAM

The impact this program would have on these patients would not have been imagined by those involved in its inception. The participants themselves confirmed the effect of the program on their lives. One would hope that time spent teaching and encouraging children about nutrition, exercise, and healthy lifestyles would promote healthy futures for these children. The team has also witnessed the exciting changes in other areas of these lives as well.

Some have become involved in sports, resulting in afternoons spent developing athletic skills instead of playing video games at home after school. Another participant has shared her experiences of providing nutritional guidance to the others on her sport teams and asks for nutrition information at restaurants when the team stops for meals to decide on the healthiest choice.

Several of the participants are leading others in their immediate family in their quest for healthier diets and lifestyles. One of the mothers learned valuable information from her child who attended the TEEEN program that helped her during treatments for cancer. Many children are inviting their friends and grandparents to the sessions.

While initially hesitant to stand up in front of the group, quite a few of the participants have become comfortable as speakers. Some are now actively involved in school and willing to speak to the class, having practiced public speaking at the TEEEN sessions. This enhanced self-confidence has resulted in the teens' growth as leaders in their schools.

One girl, who found weight loss especially trying, has persevered and is an avid leader looking for chances to speak to the group and to others to encourage them to persevere in the struggle with weight control. This participant relates her story of transforming her sedentary self to an active person which started by walking to school. This process led to a desire to train for a marathon.

There are adolescents who are the first in their families to go to college. With the help of her pediatrician and encouragement from the medical students, a participant is now enrolled in a local college and thriving. This participant mentioned that the positive feedback received in the TEEEN program was the first time positive feedback had been given to her after speaking in public. A few participants are enrolled in premed programs as a direct result of the positive role models they witnessed in the TEEEN program sessions.

The student-leaders have developed some new topics for sessions from their own experiences and ask to speak about them to the rest of the group. One wanted to speak about the negative consequences of watching too much television. Another wanted to bring her violin and play for the group as an example of what one can do instead of watching television.

Many other participants have developed social skills over the years of their attendance, such as obedience, self-respect, and respect for others. Some participants had trouble living with limits initially but over time have shown an ability to thrive within the boundaries necessary to be part of a community of others.

DIETITIAN'S PERSPECTIVE

The dietitian has seen an increase in the prevalence of pediatric obesity during the past 25 years. A significant reason for this has to do with sedentary lifestyles. There may not be opportunities for active play that are affordable and accessible for children outside of school. Computers, televisions, video games, and other sedentary activities have taken the place that active play used to have in the lives of healthy children and adolescents. When individuals of any age are less active, they require fewer calories. However, many of these less active children are not eating fewer calories and may in fact be eating more. The result is weight gain, which is continued for as long as the calories consumed are in excess of the calories required. If children and adolescents remain primarily sedentary as they age, they may not learn how to exercise safely and effectively. They may also tend to conserve energy throughout their lives, by avoiding physically active opportunities.

Additionally, parents of today's children were often fed fast food meals, convenience food meals, and had soda instead of milk to drink when they were children. Parents often lament not knowing how to cook meals for themselves and their families. Parents and children want to know what foods are good for them and are confused by the plethora of mixed messages about healthy diets. The hidden calories, simple sugars, and fats in many fast foods, convenience foods, and beverages contribute to a typical diet of surplus calories for many families of today. Without fiber, balanced meals, and guidelines for appropriate portions to meet, but not exceed, a person's nutritional needs, it is difficult for parents and children not to overeat. When parents do not like to eat fruits, vegetables, and whole grains, nor drink low fat milk, the children may not be taught or encouraged to consume these healthy dietary components either. They may lack the guidance necessary to choose a healthy diet. The TEEEN Program, conducted at St. Elizabeth's Medical Center in Boston, Massachusetts, has been effectively providing this essential guidance to parents and adolescents for the past few years. Through the active involvement of the leading pediatrician, a rotation of skilled and personable medical students, a concerned registered dietitian, and graduates of the program, children are learning to eat better and exercise more with resultant statistically significant improvements in BMI.

Children learn they have choices about what they eat and how they spend their time. They are taught that the portions they eat are important and that even healthy foods can be unhealthy if consumed in excess. They learn that their diets should include fruits, vegetables, milk, and whole grains. Many of them were not familiar with these healthy foods, having primarily soft drinks, fast foods, and other high-calorie low-nutrient foods often. They begin to learn that they need to eat breakfast every day and practice finding meal options that are nutritious as well as enjoyable. School lunch presents challenges to children, and discussions in the TEEEN program are designed to help them make good choices. After-school snacking, especially if no adult is supervising, can lead to excessive calorie consumption also. Children learn that it may sometimes be their responsibility to make good food choices when parents are not making the decisions for them.

Parents also are interested in learning about food and nutrition, as well as providing affordable, healthy options for their children. Discussions between the dietitian and the parents yield questions and concerns about the eating habits in the household. Support from other parents in these discussions and information provided by the dietitian are regarded as helpful by those attending. Parents often express frustration with issues such as limited time with their children because of work schedules, limited financial resources to offer their children healthier foods, and conflict in the home when limits of foods or changes in foods offered are made. Parents are urged to have a collaborative role with their children in selection and preparation of new foods. Concepts such as limit setting are discussed in general and in the food consumption scenario specifically. Parents note that they also need to make changes in their own diets and levels of physical activity. In families where there is positive parental involvement, both parents and children describe improvements in diet and increased physical activity.

In the course of parental discussions with the dietitian, it was noted that many parents had not been raised with healthy diets. Some stated they had eating habit issues that led to obesity and weight issues themselves. Frequent themes included erratic meals; the ambivalence about including vegetables and fruits in their diets; the use of soft drinks, either diet or regular, on a daily basis; and the absence of daily milk consumption. Some of the parents had been diagnosed with hyperlipidemia and type 2 diabetes at younger ages than their own parents. Many voiced misconceptions about healthy eating because of previous weight-loss dieting. Parents who intend to offer healthy diets to their families may not understand the basics of adequate nutrition for children or for themselves. Some take the opportunity of an individual consultation with the registered dietitian for individualized dietary guidelines and answers to their questions.

This program has grown in scope and practice and continues to meet monthly on Saturday afternoons. Most of the professionals donate their time for the sessions. Instead of the continuation of unhealthy eating practices, children and families could begin to see the possibilities of healthier diets. Instead of children continuing to be inactive throughout their lives into adulthood, they could become knowledgeable and confident in physically active endeavors. With healthier diets and active lifestyles, the trend of earlier diagnosis of medical problems related to obesity would likely be reversed.

REPRODUCIBLE

Programs following the protocol of the TEEEN program could be offered anywhere there are children, parents, and caring professionals who are willing to give back to their community. A manual with the information pertaining to the program provides the skeleton of lectures and activities conducted in the TEEEN program. This skeleton allows for the opportunity for exploration and self-expression.

The TEEEN program has shown acceptability and short-term promising results of a multicomponent intervention for adolescent weight control beginning in primary care using a hands-on and fun approach. Any pediatrician with the help of medical students and a dietitian can start this continuous care model of obesity intervention. It is within the scope of primary care pediatric physicians.

FUTURE

The program staff plans to expand the program. Even if pediatric obesity disappears, there will always be a need to promote good health and to empower adolescents. The TEEEN program is designed in a way that it could achieve both of these aims.

Immediate action and continuous research are not mutually exclusive. Nonrandomized and randomized controlled studies to evaluate the effects of attending the TEEEN program on BMI have been conducted, and these have demonstrated promising results. More subjects in the intervention group (group that attended the TEEEN program) had a reduction in BMI compared to the control group (group that did not attend the TEEEN program), and this was statistically significant.

We are currently doing a quality of life study to objectively measure the subjective findings we have seen related to improvements in participants' lives. It is important to evaluate the quality of life since weight management programs have been shown to improve aspects of quality of life in children.[26] We are also conducting a food label knowledge acquisition study.

Another area that needs more research involves studying how to best approach each particular ethnic group in terms of effectiveness research. There is also a need to identify behavioral, environmental, and biological factors contributing to the sustaining of the problem of pediatric obesity as well as effective interventions.[1]

CONCLUSION

The approach used for these patients is holistic: one which offers awe and respect of the patients' possibilities. Scientific rigor, medical knowledge, and honesty, especially regarding healthier lifestyles, are used. The hope is to challenge patients and their families to enable them to take their place in society and to use accurate and timely medical care in combination with inspiring role models, so patients can see the truth about life.

During the past years, the pediatrician who directs the TEEEN program has seen the rewards of this program. This pediatrician has seen adolescents develop autonomy and competencies; learn about health in the context of family, friends, and community; and get involved in organized sports. Many participants desire to pursue a career in medicine and pediatrics. Adolescents will always need positive role models, empowerment, and direction. The TEEEN program aims to provide a microcosm that promotes these.

The original goal was that patients would take their place in society with maximum health and confidence as leaders and become an inspiration to others. Simply put, that they can become all that they were made to be.

REFERENCES

1. Ogden, C.L., Carroll, M.D., Curtin, L.R., Lamb, M.M., and Flegal, K.M. (2009). Prevalence of high body mass index in US children and adolescents, 2007–2008. *JAMA* 303(3), 242–249.
2. Eaton, D.K., Kann, L., Kinchen, S., Shanklin, S., Ross, J., Hawkins, J., Harris, W.A., Lowry, R., McManus, T., Chyen, D., Lim, C., Brener, N.D., and Wechsler, H. (June 6, 2008). Youth risk behavior surveillance—United States, 2007. *MMWR Surveillance Summaries* 57(SS-4), 1–131.
3. Robinson, T.N. (1999). Reducing children's television viewing to prevent obesity: A randomized controlled trial. *JAMA* 282(16), 1561–1567.
4. Gortmaker, S.L., Must, A., Sobol, A.M., Peterson, K., Colditz, G.A., and Dietz, W.H. (1996). Television viewing as a cause of increasing obesity among children in the United States, 1986–1990. *Arch Pediatr Adolesc Med* 150, 356–362.
5. Wang, Y.C., Bleich, S.N., and Gortmaker, S.L. (2008). Increasing caloric contribution from sugar-sweetened beverages and 100% fruit juices among US children and adolescents, 1988–2004. *Pediatrics* 121(6), e1604–e1614.
6. Daniels, S.R., Arnett, D.K., Eckel, R.H., Gidding, S.S., Hayman, L.L., Kumanyika, S., Robinson, T.N., Scott, B.J., St. Jeor, S., and Williams, C.L. (2005). Overweight in children and adolescents: Pathophysiology, consequences, prevention, and treatment. *Circulation* 111, 1999–2012.
7. Alemzadeh, R., Kichler, J., Babar, G., and Calhoun, M. (2008). Hypovitaminosis D in obese children and adolescents: Relationship with adiposity, insulin sensitivity, ethnicity, and season. *Metabolism* 57(2), 183–191.
8. Fagot-Campagna, A., Pettitt, D.J., Engelgau, M.M., Burrows, N.R., Rios, N., Geiss, L.S., Valdez, R., Beckles, G.L.A., Saaddine, J., Gregg, E.W., Williamson, D.F., and Narayan, K.M.V. (2000). Type 2 diabetes among North American children and adolescents: An epidemiologic review and a public health perspective. *J Pediatr* 136(5), 664–672.
9. Ludwig, D.S. and Ebbeling, C.B. (2001). Type 2 diabetes mellitus in children. *JAMA* 286(12), 1427–1430.
10. Manuel, D.G. and Schultz, S.E. (2004). Health-related quality of life and health-adjusted life expectancy of people with diabetes in Ontario, Canada, 1996–1997. *Diabetes Care* 27(2), 407–414.
11. Giovannucci, E. and Michaud, D. (2007). The role of obesity and related metabolic disturbances in cancers of the colon, prostate, and pancreas. *Gastroenterology* 132(6), 2208–2225.
12. Swallen, K.C., Reither, E.N., Haas, S.A., and Meier, A.M. (2005). Overweight, obesity, and health related quality of life among adolescents: The national longitudinal study of adolescent health. *Pediatrics* 115(2), 340–347.
13. Schwimmer, J.B., Burwinkle, T.M., and Varni, J.W. (2003). Health related quality of life of severely obese children and adolescents. *JAMA* 289(14), 1813–1819.
14. Freedman, D.S., Khan, L.K., Dietz, W.H., Srinivasan, S.R., and Berenson, G.S. (2001). Relationship of childhood obesity to coronary heart disease risk factors in adulthood: The Bogalusa Heart Study. *Pediatrics* 108(3), 712–718.
15. Lauer, R.M., Lee, J., and Clarke, W.R. (1998). Factors affecting the relationship between childhood and adult cholesterol levels: The Muscatine Study. *Pediatrics* 82(3), 309–318.
16. Must, A., Jacques, P.F., Dallal, G.E., Bajema, C.J., and Dietz, W.H. (1992). Long-term morbidity and mortality of overweight adolescents: A follow-up of the Harvard Growth Study of 1922 to 1935. *NEJM* 327(19), 1350–1355.

17. www.healthypeople.gov/hp2020/objectives (last accessed 1/11/10).

18. Fontaine, K.R., Redden, D.T., Wang, C., Westfall, A.O., and Allison, D.B. (2003). Years of life lost due to obesity. *JAMA* 289(2), 187–193.

19. Wang, Y., Beydoun, M.A., Liang, L., Caballero, B., and Kumanyika, S.K. (2008). Will all Americans become overweight or obese? Estimating the progression and cost of the US obesity epidemic. *Obesity* 16(10), 2323–2330.

20. www.cdc.gov/chronicdisease/healthequity (last accessed 1/11/10).

21. Kalavainen, M.P., Korppi, M.O., and Nuutinen, O.M. (2007). Clinical efficacy of group-based treatment for childhood obesity compared with routinely given individual counseling. *Int J Obes* 31, 1500–1508.

22. Flynn, M.A., McNeil, D.A., Maloff, B., Mutasingwa, D., Wu, M., Ford, C., and Tough, S.C. (2006). Reducing obesity and related chronic disease risk in children and youth: A synthesis of evidence with 'Best Practice' recommendations. *Obes Rev* 7(Suppl.1), 7–66.

23. Ainsworth, B.E., Haskell, W.L., Leon, A.S., Jacobs, D.R. Jr., Montoye, H.J., Sallis, J.F., and Paffenbarger, R.S. Jr. (1993). Compendium of physical activities: Classification of energy costs of human physical activities. *Med Sci Sports Exerc* 25(1), 71–80.

24. Weston, A.T., Petosa, R., and Pate, R.R. (1997). Validation of an instrument for measurement of physical activity in youth. *Med Sci Sports Exerc* 29(1), 138–143.

25. Prochaska, J.O., DiClemente, C.C., and Norcross, J.C. (1992). In search of how people change: Applications to addictive behaviors. *Am Psychol* 47(9), 1102–1114.

26. Fullerton, G., Tyler, C., Johnston, C.A., Vincent, J.P., Harris, G.E., and Foreyt, J.P. (2007). Quality of life in Mexican-American children following a weight management program. *Obesity* 15(11), 2553–2556.

Part VIII

Bariatric Surgery in Weight
Management

62 Bariatric Surgery and Reversal of Metabolic Disorders

Melania Manco, MD, PhD, FACN

CONTENTS

INTRODUCTION

Bariatric surgery is increasingly regarded as a treatment of morbidly obese patients who fail on medical and/or behavioral weight reduction therapies and/or, particularly, have serious comorbidities. In 1991, the National Institutes of Health Consensus Conference made a recommendation for surgery in patients having a body mass index (BMI) >40 kg/m² and exhibiting a strong desire for substantial weight loss to improve quality of life, or a BMI >35 kg/m² plus serious comorbidities [1]. More recently, the delegates from the Diabetes Surgery Summit recognized the legitimacy of surgical approaches to treat type 2 diabetes mellitus (T2DM) among comorbidities even in patients with a BMI ≥30 kg/m², but carefully selected [2]. Indeed, bariatric surgery is emerging as a valuable therapeutic approach for T2DM and much effort has been devoted to understand the mechanisms of diabetes resolution. Nevertheless, bariatric surgery can be curative of most of the other comorbidities, which accompany obesity such as hypertension, dyslipidemia, nonalcoholic fatty liver disease (NAFLD), polycystic ovary syndrome (PCOS), sleep apnea, obesity-hypoventilation syndrome, cardiac dysfunction, reflux esophagitis, arthritis, infertility, stress incontinence, and venous stasis ulcers.

So far, several surgical procedures have been developed. Traditional approaches include gastric banding, vertical banded gastroplasty (VBG), Roux-en-Y gastric bypass (RYGB), and biliopancreatic diversion (BPD) (Figure 62.1, Panels from A to D) [3]. BPD was, for a long time, regarded as the only purely malabsorptive procedure, while other techniques were considered as prevalently restrictive.

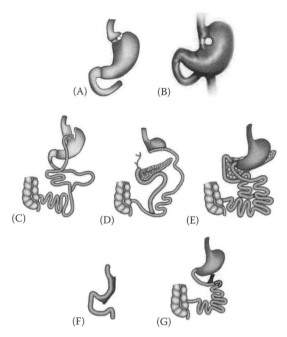

FIGURE 62.1 Schematic representation of common bariatric procedure: gastric banding (Panel A), VBG (Panel B), RYGB (Panel C), BPD (Panel D), DJB (Panel E), SG (Panel F), and ileal interposition (IIT) (Panel G).

Nowadays, such distinction into malabsorptive or restrictive procedure seems being outdated in front of newer experimental procedures developed during the last decade. Such procedures were designed with the particular aim of ameliorating glucose metabolism independently of weight loss. Indeed researchers have speculated that the rearrangement in the anatomy of the gastrointestinal tract can influence glucose homeostasis by largely unknown mechanisms, which are behind the weight loss [4–8]. In keeping with this hypothesis, RYGB has been experimentally performed in selected patients with BMI $\leq$35 kg/m^2 to explore its effects on the control of plasma glucose and lipids (elegantly reviewed in [2]). Newer techniques consist of duodenal-jejunal-bypass (DJB), sleeve gastrectomy (SG), and ileal interposition (IIT) (Figure 62.1 Panels from E to G) [2].

Evidence for the successful reversal of T2DM in severely obese individuals following bariatric surgery is robust, but what is impressive is how early after surgery and independently of weight loss, amelioration of glucose homeostasis occurs [6,9–23].

SURGICAL TECHNIQUES AND WEIGHT LOSS

Surgery induces weight loss by two expected mechanisms, the intestinal malabsorption and the gastric restriction. Probably and more importantly, surgery may also alter the gut-brain neuroendocrine axis, which modulates food intake, and the neurohormonal pathways, which regulate glucose homeostasis [2,24].

Laparoscopical adjustable gastric banding (LAGB, Figure 62.1, Panel A) involves placement of a prosthetic band around the upper stomach to partition it into a small, proximal pouch and a large, distal remnant connected through a narrow constriction [25,26]. Weight loss after gastric banding is usually less than that expected from RYGB [22].

Gastroplasty (Figure 62.1, Panel B) implicates placing a horizontal staple line. A small, proximal pouch is separated from the large distal remnant, and the two parts are connected through a narrow stoma [27]. To avoid the dilation of the stoma and/or proximal pouch, or dehiscence of the horizontal gastroplasty, Mason modified this procedure [28] into the VGB, in which the partitioning line extends upward from the angle of His. A polypropylene band supports the stoma. Although VBG effectively limits the amount of food that can be consumed at one sitting and causes ~30%–50% reduction of excess body weight within the first 1–2 years, long-term results are disappointing, showing a nearly 80% failure rate after 10 years [22,29]. Patients often accommodate to gastric restriction by frequently eating small meals and calorie-dense foods [30].

RYGB (Figure 62.1, Panel C) is the most effective restrictive procedure to induce and maintain weight loss [27–30]. The stomach is divided into a small, proximal pouch and a separate, large, distal remnant. The upper pouch is joined to the proximal jejunum through a narrow gastrojejunal anastomosis. The storage capacity of the stomach is reduced to approximately 5% of its normal volume, and ingested food bypasses approximately 95% of the stomach, the entire duodenum, and a small portion (15–20 cm) of the proximal jejunum. Patients lose ~35%–40% of total body weight, and most of this effect is maintained for at least 15 years [12,21,22].

BPD (Figure 62.1, Panel D) is the malabsorptive procedure carried out prevalently. It allows patients to eat as much as they want, acting through predominant lipid malabsorption. Malabsorption occurs because pancreatic and biliary secretions are diverted to the distal approximately 50 cm of the ileum. Some authors do not perform BPD since they judge that this procedure causes an increased rate of life-threatening complications [22].

Rubino and Marescaux [31] described in mouse models the DJB, whose safety and efficacy have been successively tested in humans by Cohen [32] (Figure 62.1, Panel E). The procedure consists of a stomach-sparing bypass of a short portion of the proximal intestine, comparable to that performed in the RYGB. Variants of this experimental procedure include techniques that preserve the pylorus (duodenal-JEJUNAL anastomosis) or do not (gastrojejunal anastomosis) [2]. DJB may be combined with a sleeve resection of the stomach to reduce the likelihood of marginal ulcerations and increase potential for weight loss [2].

Sleeve gastrectomy (Figure 62.1, Panel F) can precede the duodenal-ileostomy and ileo-ileostomy, which are performed successively as a second stage a few months later [2]. This technique may be valuable in terms of weight loss as it eliminates the ghrelin-rich gastric fundus, probably contributing to reduce appetite [2].

The ileal transposition or interposition (Figure 62.1, Panel G) was first described in rodents as well [33]. The ileal transposition involves the surgical insertion of a small segment of ileum, with its neurovascular supply intact, into the proximal intestine, increasing its exposure to ingested nutrients. The exaggerated release of glucagon-like peptide 1 (GLP1) and peptide YY in response to nutrient load observed in animal studies of IIT may lead to the significant reduction in food intake and, consequently, body weight [34].

The endoluminal duodenal-jejunal sleeve is a flexible plastic sleeve that excludes the proximal intestine from the alimentary flow, analogous to the surgical bypass in the routinely RYGB or DJB, but the device can be implanted endoscopically without disrupting bowel continuity [2].

MALNUTRITION

Bypassing of stomach and duodenum impairs absorption of micronutrients such as iron, calcium, thiamine, vitamin B_{12}, and various vitamins. Those intestinal bypass procedures that avoid duodenum and part of jejunum can cause deficiencies in iron, calcium, and vitamin D unless proper postoperative nutritional supplementation is taken. BPD or long-limb RYGB (with an alimentary limb >150 cm) is more frequently associated with protein malnutrition [22]. In patients who undergo RYGB, the incidence of iron deficiency is described as high as 6%–33%, while calcium and vitamin D deficiency range from 10% to 51% [35,36] and can cause decreased bone mass and secondary hyperparathyroidism. Vitamin B12 and folate deficiency is as high as 33% and 63%, respectively [37]. Deficiencies in fat-soluble vitamins are more common after BPD [38,39]. Up to 68% of patients undergoing BPD develop vitamin K deficiency, despite clinical manifestations being infrequent [2].

In our experience, mostly in patients following BPD, they are admitted to the care unit monthly during the first 6 months of follow-up, every 3 months, and then, after the first year, every 6 months. A dietary recall diary is required to check the daily energy intake. Patients are prescribed oral supplementation of sulfate iron (525–1050 mg/die), calcium carbonate 1 g/die, multivitamins, and ergocalciferol (400,000–160,000 UI i.m. monthly). Despite ergocalciferol supplementation, prevalence of hypovitaminosis D ranges from 89% to 91% in women 10 years after BPD [40]. Intravenous iron supplementation may be required mostly in fertile women.

Following BPD, patients are prescribed to eat largely and frequently as compared with those who underwent RYGB, who must restrain consumption of calorie-dense foods, including fats, refined carbohydrates, ice cream, and sweetened beverages. Proteins should be consumed daily at least twice a day in patients following either BPD or RYGB. Protein deficiency, when it occurs, represents a serious complication and should be treated with diet modifications and, in more severe cases, total parenteral nutrition [41]. Such figures rise from older studies, but with the growing recognition of bariatric surgery as valuable therapeutic approach for obesity and comorbidities, much attention is paid to prevention of nutrient deficiency in these patients.

Periodic monitoring for deficiencies is required, and micronutrients should be supplemented daily.

POSTOPERATIVE MORBIDITY AND MORTALITY

We strongly believe that operative risk and postoperative and late complications must be measured against the medical benefits of massive weight loss and amelioration of comorbidities. Operative risk is reported to be approximately 1%, but it may be further lowered by experienced surgeons. Postoperative complications, which are recalled in Table 62.1, occur in approximately 10%. Cholecystectomy is strongly recommended to avoid gallstone formation with rapid weight loss [21,22,30]. In our experience, operative and late complications may be prevented by close surveillance and follow-up of patients.

It is remarkable to note that overall annual mortality is lower in obese patients who undergo bariatric surgery than in morbidly obese people who refuse to undergo surgery for personal reasons [18,42]. In a large case-control study involving 7925 patients undergoing RYGB versus 7925 matched nonoperated individuals, at a mean follow-up of 8.4 years, surgery reduced all-cause mortality by 56%, cancer mortality by 60%, and, remarkably, diabetes-related mortality by 92% [43].

TABLE 62.1
Main Surgical Complications of RYGB and BPD

	RYGB	BPD
Deep venous thrombosis	Yes	Yes
Anastomotic leaks	Yes	Yes
Internal hernias	Yes	Yes
Gastrointestinal bleeding	Yes	Yes
Intestinal obstruction	Yes	Yes
Wound complications	Yes	Yes
Staple-line disruption	Yes	Yes
Ulcers	Yes	Yes
Torsion or volvulus of the roux limb	Yes	
Stomal stenosis	Yes	
Biliopancreatic limb obstruction and pancreatitis		Yes
Closed loop obstruction	Yes	

Moreover, contrary to some popular misconception, bariatric surgery confers low operative mortality. In a meta-analysis of 361 studies on 85,048 patients, total mortality was 0.28% in the first postoperative month and 0.35% between the second month and 2 years [44].

On the other hand, we must point out that, hitherto, no consensus has been stated on management, therapy, and follow-up required after surgery. Thus, the success of each surgical procedure in terms of weigh loss and low incidence of any complication depends on the ability of surgeons, physicians, and nurses in selecting patients for bariatric surgery and taking care of them after that.

WEIGHT LOSS AND ENERGY EXPENDITURE

Nonsurgical methods are notoriously ineffective at achieving major, long-term weight reduction. On the contrary, surgery is the most effective method to obtain major, long-term weight loss [22,30]. In individuals genetically prone to develop obesity, any attempt to reduce body fat stores by conventional weight-losing programs triggers compensatory changes in appetite and energy expenditure that resist weight change [45]. Physiological regulation of the body weight developed as mechanism to defend against malnutrition in times of famine, and therefore, the adaptive responses to weight loss seem to be stronger than are those to weight gain. The so-called adipostat regulates body weight in a manner analogous to that by which a thermostat controls ambient temperature. No more than 5%–10% of body weight is lost through dieting and exercise. Recidivism after dietary weight reduction is very common [46–49]. Bariatric surgery is able to reduce body weight by ~35%–40%. Most of this effect is maintained for at least 10 years or longer [12,21,22]. Surgery imposes a fixed cut on energy intake, which represents a declining proportion of energy requirements as subjects lose largely fat mass but also, to a lesser extent, fat-free mass. The decline in body weight after surgery is a nonlinear function of time [50]. The resting energy expenditure (REE) is a function of the fat-free mass, which represents the mass of metabolically active tissues [51]. The total amount of energy expenditure results basically from REE; energy expenditure related to physical activity; nonexercise activity thermogenesis (NEAT), which is the energy required to fidget, to maintain posture, and to do other activities of daily living [52]; and diet-induced thermogenesis (DIT), which is the energy consumed for absorbing, digesting, processing, and storing nutrients. In dieting obese individuals, REE decreases inappropriately to body size [53,54], DIT is blunted, thermogenesis is defective [55–60], and fat oxidation is decreased [61,62]. Such impairment in metabolism can contribute to weight regain after diet. On the contrary, after surgery, energy intake is constantly reduced or unchanged, while energy expenditure and metabolic efficiency are both increased. In post-BPD patients, the amount of metabolizable energy per kg of fat-free mass, which is defined as total energy intake minus fecal and urinary losses, is not different before and after surgery [63], but the energy required for absorption and digestion processes is greater [64]. Surgery is likely to positively influence also NEAT since body agility is improved after massive weight loss. The average daily oxidation of lipids is improved from ~69% before to 97% of metabolized fats after BPD [64], meaning that the metabolic efficiency in oxidation of absorbed lipid is significantly increased by surgery-induced weight loss.

NORMALIZATION OF METABOLIC INFLEXIBILITY

The higher efficiency in substrate oxidation suggests that the metabolic inflexibility may partially reverse after BPD. Metabolic inflexibility, which characterizes obesity, is defined as the pathological incapacity to utilize lipid and carbohydrate fuels as needed and switch between them [65,66]. Inflexibility includes (i) impairment of the cephalic phase of the insulin secretion, (ii) failure of muscle tissue to correctly oxidize lipids at fasting and carbohydrate in the insulin-stimulated prandial state, and (iii) impaired transition of fatty acid efflux from storage in response to a meal. Major weight loss following bariatric surgery is able to restore the early phase of insulin secretion by T2DM patients [19]. Insulin secretion in response to a meal is normalized and postobese subjects are able to oxidize lipids or carbohydrates as they need [67]. Oxidation of lipid substrates is more efficient in the fasting status, while glucose oxidation is increased in the insulin-stimulated condition during a euglycemic hyperinsulinemic clamp [68].

As far as circulating free fatty acids (FFAs) are concerned, after-surgery levels of FFAs are significantly lowered. In post-BPD, this effect is largely due to the massive lipid malabsorption. In RYGB subjects, changes in eating behavior occur for unknown reasons, and these patients voluntary reduce the intake of calorie-dense foods, including fats [11].

First, we hypothesized that the massive reduction in dietary fats induces the dramatic reduction in circulating and intramyocyte fat depots [68], which is associated with the reversal of insulin resistance 6 months after surgery [68]. Abolishment of lipotoxicity and normalization of lipid-fuel sensing inside the cells translate into the amelioration of insulin action, with enhanced glucose oxidation, and appropriate shift from lipid to glucose metabolism [69,70]. Insulin sensitivity improves in proportion to weight loss with use of predominantly restrictive procedures but is completely reversed by predominantly malabsorptive approaches long before normalization of body weight [50,71]. Full normalization of insulin action occurs in parallel with achievement of ideal body weight [9,12], but it is astonishing that normalization results also in patients who do not achieve a normal BMI [67,68]. The amount of weight loss may not be the only determinant of the metabolic improvement, and the surgical strategy used to achieve weight reduction may have an independent effect. Despite the degree and time course of weight reduction (average weight loss of 53 kg) being almost identical after BPD and RYGB [50], patients who underwent BPD achieve levels of insulin sensitivity that are double than those of patients following RYGB. Normalization of insulin action may be not complete after RYGB despite substantial weight reduction [72]. After RYGB, the improvement in insulin sensitivity is of the exact magnitude predicted by the general relation between glucose disposal and BMI, which is described in healthy normal-weight individuals [50]. In contrast, in post-BPD patients, levels of insulin sensitivity were almost normal at 6 months, when their BMI averages 39 kg/m². A further loss of approximately 15 kg over the following 18 months increased insulin sensitivity up to levels higher than those observed in lean controls [71].

INSULIN ACTION AND SECRETION

In people with normal glucose tolerance, a decrease in insulin action is accompanied by the upregulation of insulin secretion and vice versa [71]. A compensatory increase of insulin secretion maintains normoglycemia despite decreased insulin sensitivity. After being algebraically transformed, insulin secretion and sensitivity are commonly represented as a hyperbola describing the acute insulin response (AIR) as a function of insulin sensitivity [72]. The hyperbola reflects the natural relationship between beta cell function and insulin sensitivity, taking into the account the beta cell compensation for the insulin resistance. The so-called disposition index represents the mathematical product of the insulin action for the beta cell function, and it simplifies the concept of the hyperbola [73]. The disposition index is a way of measuring the ability of the beta cells to compensate for insulin resistance. This compensation is thought to be perfect when the disposition index remains constant in the face of decreasing insulin action. Thus, it seems to be intuitive that beta cell function is modified in normotolerant individuals for every significant change in peripheral insulin sensitivity to ensure normal glycemia. Surprisingly, this is true for obese patients following BPD, but not in T2DM patients after hypocaloric diet, or in those who undergo RYGB or gastroplasty [50].

The normalization in beta cell function and insulin action, which occurs in T2DM patients within 1 week following BPD, does not occur in obese subjects who undergo abdominal surgery for gallstones, despite both groups of patients consuming no food in the immediate period after surgery [23]. This observation excludes that the early improvement of diabetes may be related to the diminished meal-induced challenge of beta cells and does not depend upon the amount of weight loss. This observation reinforces the concept of an unknown incretin effect related to the gastrointestinal surgery. Abolished lipotoxicity due to the preferential malabsorption of lipids may contribute to control glucose homeostasis.

Contrary to what is observed in patients after BPD, in those patients following RYGB, a paradoxical rise in insulin secretion is observed after surgery. Such phenomenon is commonly regarded as the result of removing the toxic effect of chronic hyperglycemia on beta cell function [74–76]. Alternatively, as postulated for BPD, it may be the effect of a different hormonal milieu (glucose-dependent increase in insulin secretion also termed as "incretin effect") caused by the anatomical rearrangement of the intestinal tract [2]. Of note, long-term hyperactivity of the beta cells in patients following RYGB may lead to nesiodioblastosis in prone individuals, decades after the surgery [77].

"INCRETIN" EFFECT

The effects of gastrointestinal surgery on glucose metabolism represent a clinically impressive and scientifically interesting phenomenon, which can result in identifying new targets for diabetes medications. The gastrointestinal tract produces dozens of biologically active peptides [78] and rearrangement of the gut anatomy may activate pathways acting on glucose homeostasis which differ and, thus, may cause gradient of efficacy among procedures varying from mild remission to overt disappearance of diabetes (see Table 62.2).

Gastrointestinal bypass procedures connect two otherwise separated segments of the gastrointestinal tract, thereby allowing nutrients to reach the distal portion of the small intestine more rapidly than usual and preventing the contact of nutrients with much of the stomach, the entire duodenum, and part of the jejunum, depending on the type of surgery. Among the different hypotheses postulated to explain the surgery-induced amelioration of glucose homeostasis (schematically resumed in Table 62.3), the "lower intestinal hypothesis," also known as hindgut hypothesis (reviewed in 25), postulated that the rapid delivery of nutrients to the lower intestine increases stimulation of L cells. In turn, such stimulation results in increased secretion of gastrointestinal factors that decrease insulin secretion and/or promote insulin resistance (i.e., the gastric inhibitory *peptide* [GIP] and/or GLP1). Although the proximal and the distal hypotheses are often conceptualized in terms of the release of hormones, they are also

TABLE 62.2

Graded Antidiabetes Effect of the Most Frequently Performed Bariatric Procedure

	LAGB	RYGB	BPD
Resolution of T2DM	48	84	98
Resolution of hypertension	43	68	83
Improvement of hyperlipidemia	59	97	99
Percent excess weight loss	47	62	70

Percent Remission from Ref. [85].

TABLE 62.3

Supposed Weight-Independent Antidiabetes Mechanisms of Gastrointestinal Surgery

1. Increased postprandial secretion of L-cell peptides such as GLP1 or unknown hormones from enhanced distal intestinal nutrient delivery (known as "incretin effects")

2. Exclusion of the proximal small intestine from nutrient flow possibly downregulating unidentified anti-incretin factors

3. Impaired ghrelin secretion

4. Changes in intestinal nutrient sensing mechanisms regulating insulin sensitivity

5. Bile acid perturbations

compatible with the theory that altered nutrient flow triggers neural signaling rather than hormone release. Both mechanisms cannot be elusive and both contribute to resolution of diabetes.

In RYGB, enhanced GLP1 release is due to earlier delivery of food to lower segments of the gut. This effect is likely to occur also after BPD. GLP1 and GIP seem to be attractive candidates to explain amelioration of glucose metabolism after bariatric surgery.

GIP is synthesized and released in the duodenum and proximal jejunum especially in response to glucose and fat ingestion. It acts as an insulinotropic agent with a stimulatory effect on insulin release and synthesis [79]. Defects in its signaling pathways are considered among the most critical alterations underlying T2DM. The incretin effect of GIP is characteristically attenuated in T2DM [80], and the expression of GIP receptor (GIPR) is also decreased [81].

After RYGB, levels of GIP have been found to be decreased [82], and GLP1, released by the L cells of the distal ileum and colon, increased [4,83] or unchanged [84]. Rubino [82] et al. found an exaggerated GLP1 response following a 420 kcal meal in gastric bypass subjects. The authors speculated that in susceptible individuals, such as diabetic patients, chronic exaggerated stimulation of the proximal gut with fat and carbohydrates may induce overproduction of an unknown factor that causes impairment of GIPR expression or GIP/GIPR interaction, leading to an insufficient or inappropriate insulin secretion. The duodenal-jejunal exclusion might resolve this aberration by reestablishing normal GIPR sensitivity and reducing GIP secretion. Unlike GIP, GLP1 has been shown to significantly improve or even restore normal glucose-induced insulin secretion in diabetic patients [86]. Moreover, although changes in GLP1 levels did not reach statistical significance in the Rubino's study, the author did not exclude a role of GLP1 in restoring glucose homeostasis [82].

REVERSAL OF T2DM

Randomized controlled [6,39,43,87], observational [12], and meta-analyses studies [6,88] support strongly the efficacy of bariatric surgery in the reversal of T2DM.

One randomized trial [39] and a long-term, well-designed comparative study (Swedish Obese Subjects, Study SOS) showed that surgery is superior to conventional management of T2DM in severely obese subjects, yielding better glycemic control and improving survival [43,89]. The Greenville study [12] demonstrated that 82% of 165 patients with T2DM stably remitted from diabetes after an average 14 years follow-up. In a systematic review and meta-analysis of the data reported in the literature on bariatric surgery from 22,094 patients, Buchwald et al. [6] found a gradation of effects from 99% in patients after BPD or duodenal switch to 84% for RYGB, 72% for gastroplasty, and 48% for gastric banding, with an overall 77% remission of T2DM after bariatric surgery. An antidiabetes efficacy gradient probably exists among bariatric operations (BPD > RYGB > LAGB) [6]. In a randomized controlled trial that compared SG and gastric bypass, greater rates of T2DM remission were found among patients treated with gastric bypass than among those treated with SG, despite equivalent weight loss in both groups [90]. Scopinaro et al. retrospectively analyzed data of 201 patients with T2DM following BPD. Fasting glycemia normalized in 97% of cases at 10 years after surgery [91].

RESOLUTION OF HYPERTENSION

Even a modest weight loss can lower blood pressure significantly. It is commonly assumed that a decrease of 1% in body weight reduces systolic blood pressure by 1 mmHg and diastolic blood pressure by 2 mmHg [91–94]. The meta-analysis by Buchwald et al. [6] shows that hypertension significantly improves in morbidly obese subjects after bariatric surgery with a graded improvement depending on the type of surgery (Table 62.2). The percentage of patients in the total population whose hypertension fully resolved was ~62%, and the percentage rose to 78% when resolution and development were both considered [6].

RESOLUTION OF DYSLIPIDEMIA

Hypercholesterolemia and hypertriglyceridemia improved significantly after bariatric surgery in 70% of patients. The major improvement is achieved in patients after BPD, duodenal switch, or RYGB [6]. Total cholesterol may be decreased by a mean value of 33 mg, very-low-density lipoproteins by ~29 mg, and triglycerides by ~80 mg. Surprisingly, high-density lipoproteins (HDL) are improved after RYGB (by ~4.63 mg) or gastroplasty (by ~5 mg). In particular, after BPD, HDL levels increase significantly, leading to the overall reduction of cardiovascular risk [94]. In the late 1990s, a couple of studies proposed bariatric surgery as a therapeutic option for severe dyslipidemia [9,10]. Two sisters affected by a familiar deficit of lipoprotein lipase and T2DM underwent BPD. The rationale for surgery, despite BMI being within the normal range, was reducing the absorption of lipids [9].

PCOS AND ENDOCRINE-RELATED DISEASES

The etiology of the PCOS is still largely unknown. The primary defect consists of increased androgen synthesis and secretion by ovarian thecal cells [95,96], which is worsened by hyperinsulinemia and insulin resistance [96]. Obesity is commonly associated with PCOS and hyperandrogenism [97]. Compared with nonhyperandrogenic women with morbid obesity, PCOS and hyperandrogenic patients with regular menstrual cycles present with similarly increased total and free testosterone levels, but insulin resistance is present only in the PCOS group [98,99]. We and others [100,101] showed that surgery-induced massive weight loss is able to ameliorate or resolve signs and symptoms of hyperandrogenism. Moreover, the sustained and marked weight loss achieved either after RYGB or BPD leads to the almost complete resolution of PCOS [6]. Patients recover regular ovulatory menstrual cycles after weight loss in parallel with a marked improvement in the indexes of insulin resistance [6].

RESOLUTION OF NONALCOHOLIC STEATOHEPATITIS

NAFLD is a common condition that may progress to end-stage liver disease. NAFLD ranges from fat depot in the liver, known as simple steatosis, to nonalcoholic steatohepatitis (NASH) or fat with inflammation and/or fibrosis to advanced fibrosis and cirrhosis, when fat may no longer be present. NAFLD is closely associated with obesity and insulin resistance. NALFD is estimated to occur in 30%–100% of obese adults. The majority of obese patients have ultrasonographic evidence of fatty liver, but 30% have histologically proved NASH. Up to 25% of obese patients with NASH may progress to cirrhosis [101]. The exact mechanisms leading to NAFLD and/or fibrosis are incompletely understood. Hyperinsulinemia and insulin resistance are clearly important, acting to increased influx of FFAs into the liver and driving the hepatic production of triglycerides via upregulated *de novo* lipogenesis. Lipid export from the liver may be impaired because of defective incorporation of triglyceride into apolipoprotein B (apoB) or reduced apoB synthesis or excretion [102,103]. Hepatic triglyceride accumulation aggravates subsequent hepatic insulin resistance in a vicious manner by interfering with tyrosine phosphorylation of insulin receptor substrates 1 and 2 [104,105]. Hepatic lipid accumulation does not universally result in hepatocellular injury, indicating that additional secondary insults are important [106]. Day et al. [106] initially proposed a "two-hit" model to explain the progression of NAFLD. The "first hit" constitutes the deposition of triglycerides into the hepatocyte cytoplasm. The disease does not progress unless additional cellular events occur (the "second hit"), thus promoting inflammation, cell death, and fibrosis. To date, surgical solutions for morbid obesity have proven to be effective in the treatment of NAFLD, despite some of these studies being confounded by unexplained progression of disease occurring after surgery in few patients [107–109]. Mattar et al. [109] demonstrated significant and widespread improvement up to the resolution of NAFLD and NASH after laparoscopic weight loss procedures, which included gastric bypass, SG, and laparoscopic banding in 70 obese patients. More than one-third of the patients had postoperative liver biopsies that showed resolution of steatosis and inflammation, and 20% of the patients had at least some reversal of fibrosis. No patient experienced a progression of abnormal liver morphology or a deterioration of hepatic function, as indicated by persistently normal liver enzymes. The beneficial effects of weight loss are believed to be mediated primarily via improved insulin sensitivity. After surgery, circulating levels of glucose, insulin, and leptin are decreased, contributing to the decrease in fatty liver infiltration and inflammation [110]. Amelioration of liver histology as well as of other metabolic abnormalities may also be due to changes in the gut microbiota, induced by the anatomical rearrangement of the gastrointestinal tract [111], or to reduced inflammation [112] and reduced activity of innate immune system [113]. Nevertheless, it cannot be ruled out that rapid weight loss may aggravate liver function and histology as a result of increased FFA level derived from extensive fat mobilization or that additional factor, such as toxins from bacterial overgrowth or nutritional challenge, may represent a "second hit" in susceptible livers. Luyckx et al. [108] confirmed this observation in patients after RYGB. Initially, steatosis improved and inflammation transiently worsened. Then liver inflammation improved over time in accordance with resolution of other metabolic abnormalities [108]. Dixon et al. [107] demonstrated major improvement in liver disease in patients who achieved significant weight loss with gastric banding. After BPD, a remarkable reversal of fibrosis and macroscopic liver appearance was found in 60% of cirrhotic patients. In nearly 40%, fibrosis increased and *de novo* cirrhosis developed few cases [110].

CONCLUSION

Gastrointestinal surgery is effective in the resolution of metabolic comorbidities associated with severe obesity. Diabetes, hypertension, dyslipidemia, NAFLD, and PCOS ameliorate significantly or resolve completely. Nevertheless, it must point out that (i) mechanisms by which bariatric surgery acts to ameliorate metabolic comorbidities are still unclear; (ii) severe morbidity is resolved by inducing a different pathological status, which requires a close follow-up and continuous medication; and (iii) no consensus has been achieved on the treatment and the follow-up of these patients, despite the widespread diffusion of surgery as therapeutic option for severe obesity and metabolic comorbidities. Indeed, no standard criteria exist to judge the best surgical option for each patient and to evaluate the success of surgery for morbid obesity in terms of weight loss.

Therefore, long-term complications of bariatric surgery must be carefully weighted against beneficial effects. Surgery must represent the last therapeutic option following the failure of any other feasible treatment.

REFERENCES

1. NIH Consensus Development Panel. 1991. Gastrointestinal surgery for severe obesity. *Ann Intern Med* 115:956–961.
2. Rubino F, Kaplan LM, Schauer PR, Cummings DE, Diabetes Surgery Summit Delegates. 2010. The Diabetes Surgery Summit consensus conference: Recommendations for the evaluation and use of gastrointestinal surgery to treat type 2 diabetes mellitus. *Ann Surg* 251:399–405.
3. The American Society for Bariatric Surgery. http://www.bariatric-surgery.info/types-of-weight-loss-surgery.htm (accessed on February 2, 2012).
4. Rubino F, Gagner M, Gentileschi P, Kini S, Fukuyama S, Feng J, Diamond E. 2004. The early effect of the Roux-en-Y gastric bypass on hormones involved in body weight regulation and glucose metabolism. *Ann Surg* 240:236–242.
5. Thaler JP, Cummings DE. 2009. Minireview: Hormonal and metabolic mechanisms of diabetes remission after gastrointestinal surgery. *Endocrinology* 150:2518–2525.
6. Buchwald H, Avidor Y, Braunwald E, Jensen MD, Pories W, Fahrbach K, Schoelles K. 2004. Bariatric surgery: A systematic review and meta-analysis. *JAMA* 292:1724–1737.
7. de Paula AL, Macedo AL, Prudente AS, Queiroz L, Schraibman V, Pinus J. 2006. Laparoscopic sleeve gastrectomy with ileal interposition ("neuroendocrine brake")—Pilot study of a new operation. *Surg Obes Relat Dis* 2:464–467.

8. Ramos A, Galvao Neto M, Galvao M, Evangelista LF, Campos JM, Ferraz A. 2010. Laparoscopic greater curvature plication: Initial results of an alternative restrictive bariatric procedure. *Obes Surg* 20:913–918.

9. Mingrone G, Henriksen FL, Greco AV, Krogh LN, Capristo E, Gastaldelli A, Castagneto M, Ferrannini E, Gasbarrini G, Beck-Nielsen H. 1999. Triglyceride-induced diabetes associated with familial lipoprotein lipase deficiency. *Diabetes* 48:1258–1263.

10. Mingrone G, DeGaetano A, Greco AV, Capristo E, Benedetti G, Castagneto M, Gasbarrini G. 1997. Reversibility of insulin resistance in obese diabetic patients: Role of plasma lipids. *Diabetologia* 40:599–605.

11. Cummings DE, Overduin J, Foster-Shubert KE. 2004. Gastric Bypass for obesity: Mechanisms of weight loss and diabetes resolution. *J Clin Endocrinol Metab* 89:2608–2615.

12. Pories WJ, Swanson MS, MacDonald KG, Long SB, Morris PG, Brown BM, Barakat HA, deRamon RA, Israel G, Dolezal JM. 1995. Who would have thought it? An operation proves to be the most effective therapy for adult-onset diabetes mellitus. *Ann Surg* 222:339–352.

13. Schauer PR, Burguera B, Ikramuddin S, Cottam D, Gourash W, Hamad G, Eid GM, Mattar S, Ramanathan R, Barinas-Mitchel E, Rao RH, Kuller L, Kelley D. 2003. Effect of laparoscopic Roux-en Y gastric bypass on type 2 diabetes mellitus. *Ann Surg* 238:467–484; discussion 84–85.

14. Sugerman HJ, Wolfe LG, Sica DA, Clore JN. 2003. Diabetes and hypertension in severe obesity and effects of gastric bypass-induced weight loss. *Ann Surg* 237:751–756; discussion 757–758.

15. Wittgrove AC, Clark GW. 2000. Laparoscopic gastric bypass, Roux-en-Y-500 patients: Technique and results, with 3–60 month follow-up. *Obes Surg* 10:233–239.

16. Schauer PR, Ikramuddin S, Gourash W, Ramanathan R, Luketich J. 2000. Outcomes after laparoscopic Roux-en-Y gastric bypass for morbid obesity. *Ann Surg* 232:515–529.

17. Long SD, O'Brien K, MacDonald Jr KG, Leggett-Frazier N, Swanson MS, Pories WJ, Caro JF. 1994. Weight loss in severely obese subjects prevents the progression of impaired glucose tolerance to type II diabetes. A longitudinal interventional study. *Diabetes Care* 17:372–375.

18. Pories WJ. 2004. Diabetes: The evolution of a new paradigm. *Ann Surg* 239:12–13.

19. Polyzogopoulou EV, Kalfarentzos F, Vagenakis AG, Alexandrides TK. 2003. Restoration of euglycemia and normal acute insulin response to glucose in obese subjects with type 2 diabetes following bariatric surgery. *Diabetes* 52:1098–1103.

20. Sjostrom L, Lindroos AK, Peltonen M, Torgerson J, Bouchard C, Carlsson B, Dahlgren S, Larsson B, Narbro K, Sjostrom CD, Sullivan M, Wedel H. 2004. Lifestyle, diabetes, and cardiovascular risk factors 10 years after bariatric surgery. *N Engl J Med* 351:2683–2693.

21. Kopelman PG. 2000. Obesity as a medical problem. *Nature* 404:635–643.

22. Brolin RE. 2002. Bariatric surgery and long-term control of morbid obesity. *JAMA* 288:2793–2796.

23. Guidone C, Manco M, Valera-Mora E, Iaconelli A, Gniuli D, Mari A, Nanni G, Castagneto M, Calvani M, Mingrone G. 2006. Mechanisms of recovery from type 2 diabetes after malabsorptive bariatric surgery. *Diabetes* 55:2025–2031.

24. Rubino F, R'bibo SL, del Genio F, Mazumdar M, McGraw TE. 2010. Metabolic surgery: The role of the gastrointestinal tract in diabetes mellitus. *Nat Rev Endocrinol* 6:102–109.

25. Bo O, Modalsli O. 1983. Gastric banding, a surgical method of treating morbid obesity: Preliminary report. *Int J Obes* 7:493–499.

26. Kuzmak L. 1992. Stoma adjustable silicone gastric banding. *Prob Gen Surg* 9:298–317.

27. Pace WG, Martin EW, Tetrick T, Fabri PJ, Carey LC. 1979. Gastric partitioning for morbid obesity. *Ann Surg* 190:392–400.

28. Howard L, Malone M, Michalek A, Carter J, Alger S, Van Woert J. 1995. Gastric bypass and vertical banded gastroplasty—A prospective randomized comparison and 5-year follow-up. *Obes Surg* 5:55–60.

29. Sugerman HJ, Starkey J, Birkenhauer R. 1987. A randomized prospective trial of gastric bypass versus vertical banded gastroplasty for morbid obesity and their effects on sweets versus non-sweets eaters. *Ann Surg* 205:613–624.

30. Naslund I. 1986. A prospective randomized comparison of gastric bypass and gastroplasty. *Acta Chir Scand* 152:681–689.

31. Rubino F, Marescaux J. 2004. Effect of duodenal-jejunal exclusion in a non-obese animal model of type 2 diabetes: A new perspective for an old disease. *Ann Surg* 239:1–11.

32. Cohen RV, Schiavon CA, Pinheiro JS, Correa JL, Rubino F. 2007. Duodenal-jejunal bypass for the treatment of type 2 diabetes in patients with body mass index of 22–34 kg/m^2: A report of 2 cases. *Surg Obes Relat Dis* 3:195–197.

33. Koopmans HS, Sclafani A, Fichtner C, Aravich PF. 1982. The effects of ileal transposition on food intake and body weight loss in VMH-obese rats. *Am J Clin Nutr* 35:284–293.

34. Strader AD, Vahl TP, Jandacek RJ, Wods SC, D'Alessio DA, Seeley RJ. 2005. Weight loss through ileal transposition is accompanied by increased ileal hormone secretion and synthesis in rats. *Am J Physiol Endocrinol Metab* 288:E447–E453.

35. Brolin RE, Gorman RC, Milgrim LM, Kenler HA. 1991. Multivitamin prophylaxis in prevention of post-gastric bypass vitamin and mineral deficiencies. *Int J Obes* 15:661–667.

36. Halverson JD. 1986. Micronutrient deficiencies after gastric bypass for morbid obesity. *Am Surg* 52:594–598.

37. le Roux CW, Welbourn R, Werling M, Osborne A, Kokkinos A, Laurenius A, Lönroth H, Fändriks L, Ghatei MA, Bloom SR, Olbers T. 2007. Gut hormones as mediators of appetite and weight loss after Roux-en-Y gastric bypass. *Ann Surg* 246:780–785.

38. Marceau P, Hould FS, Simard S, Lebel S, Bourque RA, Potvin M, Biron S. 1998. Biliopancreatic diversion with duodenal switch. *World J Surg* 22:947–954.

39. Dixon JB, O'Brien PE, Playfair J, Chapman L, Schachter LM, Skinner S, Proietto J, Bailey M, Anderson M. 2008. Adjustable gastric banding and conventional therapy for type 2 diabetes: A randomized controlled trial. *JAMA* 23;299:316–323.

40. Manco M, Calvani M, Nanni G, Greco AV, Iaconelli A, Gasbarrini G, Castagneto M, Mingrone G. 2005. Low 25-hydroxyvitamin D does not affect Insulin Sensitivity in obese women after bariatric surgery. *Obes Res* 13:1692–1700.

41. Bloomberg RD, Fleishman A, Nalle JE, Herron DM, Kini S. 2005. Nutritional deficiencies following bariatric surgery: What have we learned? *Obes Surg* 15:145–154.

42. MacDonald Jr KG, Long SD, Swanson MS, Brown BM, Morris P, Dohm GL, Pories WJ. 1997. The gastric bypass operation reduces the progression and mortality of non-insulin-dependent diabetes mellitus. *J Gastrointest Surg* 1:213–220.

43. Adams TD, Gress RE, Smith SC, Halverson RC, Simper SC, Rosamond WD, Lamonte MJ, Stroup AM, Hunt SC. 2007. Long-term mortality after gastric bypass surgery. *N Engl J Med* 357:753–761.

44. Buchwald H, Estok R, Fahrbach K, Banel D, Sledge I. 2007. Trends in mortality in bariatric surgery: A systematic review and meta-analysis. *Surgery* 142:621–632.

45. Cummings DE, Schwartz MW. 2003. Genetics and pathophysiology of human obesity. *Annu Rev Med* 54:453–471.

46. Yanovski SZ, Yanovski JA. 2002. Obesity. *N Engl J Med* 346:591–602.

47. Bray GA, Tartaglia LA. 2000. Medicinal strategies in the treatment of obesity. *Nature* 404:672–677.

48. McTigue KM, Harris R, Hemphill B, Lux L, Sutton S, Bunton AJ, Lohr KN. 2003. Screening and interventions for obesity in adults: Summary of the evidence for the US Prevention Services Task Force. *Ann Intern Med* 139:933–949.

49. Safer DJ. 1991. Diet, behavior modification, and exercise: A review of obesity treatments from a long-term perspective. *Southern Med J* 84:1470–1474.

50. Muscelli E, Mingrone G, Camastra S, Manco M, Pereira JA, Pareja JC, Ferrannini E. 2005. Differential effect of weight loss on insulin resistance in surgically treated obese patients. *Am J Med* 118:51–57.

51. Pereira JA, Lazarin MACT, Pareja JC. 2003. Insulin resistance and hyperinsulinemia in non-diabetic morbidly obese patients (effect of weight loss induced by bariatric surgery). *Obes Res* 11:1495–1501.

52. Astrup A, Anderson T, Christensen NJ, Bülow J, Madsen J, Breum L, Quaade F. 1990. Impaired glucose-induced thermogenesis and arterial norepinephrine response persist after weight reduction in obese humans. *Am J Clin Nutr* 51:331–337.

53. Leibel RL, Rosenbaum M, Hirsch J. 1995. Changes in energy expenditure resulting from altered body weight. *N Engl J Med* 332:621–628.

54. Bessard T, Schutz Y, Jéquier E. 1983. Energy expenditure and postprandial thermogenesis in obese women before and after weight loss. *Am J Clin Nutr* 38:680–693.

55. Katzeff HL, Danforth E. 1989. Decreased thermic effect of a mixed meal during overnutrition in human obesity. *Am J Clin Nutr* 50:15–21.

56. Swaminathan R, King RFGJ, Holmfield J, Siwek RA, Baker M, Wales JK. 1985. Thermic effect of feeding carbohydrate, fat, protein and mixed meal in lean and obese subjects. *Am J Clin Nutr* 42:177–181.

57. Felig P, Cunningham J, Levitt M, Hendler R, Nadel E. 1983. Energy expenditure in obesity, in fasting and postprandial state. *Am J Physiol* 244:E45–E51.

58. Nair KS, Halliday D, Garrow JS. 1983. Thermic response to isoenergetic protein, carbohydrate or fat meals in lean and obese subjects. *Clin Sci* 65:307–312.

59. Welle SL, Campbell RG. 1983. Normal thermic effect of glucose in obese women. *Am J Clin Nutr* 37:87–92.

60. Astrup A, Buemann B, Christensen NJ, Toubro S. 1994. Failure to increase lipid oxidation in response to increasing dietary fat content in formerly obese women. *Am J Physiol* 266:E592–E599.

61. Larson DE, Ferraro RT, Robertson DS, Ravussin E. 1995. Energy metabolism in weight stable post-obese individuals. *Am J Clin Nutr* 62:735–739.

62. Sims EAH, Danforth E Jr, Horton ES, Bray GA, Glennon JA, Salans LB. 1973. Endocrine and metabolic effects of experimental obesity in man. *Recent Prog Horm Res* 29:457–496.

63. Mingrone G, Manco M, Granato L, Calvani M, Scarfone A, Valera Mora E, Greco AV, Vidal H, Castagneto M, Ferrannini E. 2005. Leptin pulsatility in formerly obese women. *FASEB J* 19:1380–1385.

64. Tataranni A, Larson DE, Snitker S, Ravussin E. 1995. Thermic effect of food in humans: Methods and results from use of a respiratory chamber. *Am J Clin Nutr* 61:1013–1019.

65. Kelley DE, He J, Menshikova EV, Ritov VB. 2002. Dysfunction of mitochondria in human skeletal muscle in type 2 diabetes. *Diabetes* 51:2944–2950.

66. Kelley DE. 2005. Skeletal muscle fat oxidation: Timing and flexibility are everything. *J Clin Invest* 115:1699–1702.

67. Letiexhe MR, Desaive C, Lefebvre PJ, Scheen AJ. 2004. Cross-talk between insulin secretion and insulin action after postgastroplasty recovery of ideal body weight in severely obese patients. *Int J Obes Relat Metab Disord* 28:821–823.

68. Greco AV, Mingrone G, Giancaterini A, Manco M, Morroni M, Cinti S, Granzotto M, Vettor R, Camastra S, Ferranini E. 2002. Insulin resistance in morbid obesity: Reversal with intramyocellular fat depletion. *Diabetes* 51:1–8.

69. Unger RH. 1995. Lipotoxicity in the pathogenesis of obesity-dependent NIDDM. Genetic and clinical implications. *Diabetes* 44:863–870.

70. Manco M, Calvani M, Mingrone G. 2004. Effects of dietary fatty acids on insulin sensitivity and secretion. *Obes Diabetes Metab* 6:402–413.

71. Ferrannini E, Camastra S, Gastaldelli A, Maria Sironi A, Natali A, Muscelli E, Mingrone G, Mari A. 2004. Beta-cell function in obesity: Effects of weight loss. *Diabetes* 53:S26–S33.

72. Burstein R, Epstein Y, Charuzi I, Suessholz A, Karnieli E, Shapiro Y. 1995. Glucose utilization in morbidly obese subjects before and after weight loss by gastric bypass operation. *Int J Obes Relat Metab Disord* 19:558–561.

73. Bergman RN. 1989. Toward physiological understanding of glucose tolerance. Minimal-model approach. Lilly lecture. *Diabetes* 38:1512–1527.

74. Valensi P, Moura I, Le Magoarou M, Paries J, Perret G, Attali JR. 1997. Short-term effects of continuous subcutaneous insulin infusion treatment on insulin secretion in non-insulin-dependent overweight patients with poor glycaemic control despite maximal oral anti-diabetic treatment. *Diabete Metab* 23:515–517.

75. Jimenez J, Zuniga-Guajardo S, Zinman B, Angel A. 1987. Effects of weight loss in massive obesity on insulin and C-peptide dynamics: Sequential changes in insulin production, clearance, and sensitivity. *J Clin Endocrinol Metab* 64:661–668.

76. Guldstrand M, Ahrén B, Adamson U. 2003. Improved ß-cell function after standardized weight loss in severely obese subjects. *Am J Physiol Endocrinol Metab* 284:E557–E565.

77. Carpenter T, Trautmann ME, Baron AD. 2005. Hyperinsulinemic hypoglycemia with nesidioblastosis after gastric-bypass surgery. *N Engl J Med* 353:2192–2194.

78. Rehfeld JF. 2004. A centenary of gastrointestinal endocrinology. *Horm Metab Res* 36:735–741.

79. Pederson RA. 1993. Gastric inhibitory polypeptide. In: Walsh JH, Dockray GJ, eds., *Gut Peptides: Biochemistry and Physiology*. New York: Raven Press, pp. 217–259.

80. Miyawaki K, Yamada Y, Yano H, Niwa H, Ban N, Ihara Y, Kubota A, Fujimoto S, Kajikawa M, Kuroe A, Tsuda K, Hashimoto H, Yamashita T, Jomori T, Tashiro F, Miyazaki J, Seino Y. 1999. Glucose intolerance caused by a defect in the entero-insular axis: A study in gastric inhibitory polypeptide receptor knockout mice. *Proc Natl Acad Sci USA* 96:14843–1484.

81. Sirinek KR, O'Dorisio TM, Hill D, McFee AS. 1986. Hyperinsulinism, glucose-dependent insulinotropic polypeptide, and the enteroinsular axis in morbidly obese patients before and after gastric bypass. *Surgery* 100:781–787.

82. MacDonald PE, El-koly M, Riedel MJ. 2002. The multiple actions of GLP-1 on the process of glucose-stimulated insulin secretion. *Diabetes* 51:S434–S442.

83. Mason EE. 1999. Ilial transposition and enteroglucagon/GLP-1 in obesity (and diabetic?) surgery. *Obes Surg* 9:223–228.

84. Naslund E, Gryback P, Hellstrom PM. 1997. Gastrointestinal hormones and gastric emptying 20 years after jejunoileal bypass for massive obesity. *Int J Obes Relat Metab Disord* 21:387–392.

85. Rubino F, Schauer PR, Kaplan LM, Cummings DE. 2010. Metabolic surgery to treat type 2 diabetes: Clinical outcomes and mechanisms of action. *Annu Rev Med* 61:393–411.

86. Hickey MS, Pories WJ, MacDonald KG. 1998. A new paradigm for type 2 diabetes mellitus: Could it be a disease of the foregut? *Ann Surg* 227:637–643; discussion 643–644.

87. Nauck MA, Heimesaat MM, Orskov C, Holst JJ, Ebert R, Creutzfeldt W. 1993. Preserved incretin activity of glucagon-like peptide 1 [7–36 amide] but not of synthetic human gastric inhibitory polypeptide in patients with type-2 diabetes mellitus. *J Clin Invest* 91:301–307.

88. Buchwald H, Estok R, Fahrbach K, Banel D, Jensen MD, Pories WJ, Bantle JP, Sledge I. 2009. Weight and type 2 diabetes after bariatric surgery: Systematic review and meta-analysis. *Am J Med Mar* 122:248–256.e5.

89. Sjöström L, Narbro K, Sjöström CD, Karason K, Larsson B, Wedel H, Lystig T, Sullivan M, Bouchard C, Ca rlsson B, Bengtsson C, Dahlgren S, Gummesson A, Jacobson P, Karlsson J, Lindroos AK, Lönroth H, Näslund I, Olbers T, Stenlöf K, Torgerson J, Agren G, Carlsson LM, Swedish Obese Subjects Study. 2007. Effects of bariatric surgery on mortality in Swedish obese subjects. *N Engl J Med* 357:741–752.

90. Vidal J, Ibarzabal A, Romero F, Delgado S, Momblán D, Flores L, Lacy A. 2008. Type 2 diabetes mellitus and the metabolic syndrome following sleeve gastrectomy in severely obese subjects. *Obes Surg* 18:1077–1082.

91. Scopinaro N, Marinari GM, Camerini GB, Papadia FS, Adami GF. 2005. Specific effects of biliopancreatic diversion on the major components of metabolic syndrome: A long-term follow-up study. *Diabetes Care* 28:2406–2411.

92. Dornfeld LP, Maxwell MH, Waks AU, Schroth P, Tuck ML. 1985. Obesity and hypertension: Long-term effects of weight reduction on blood pressure. *Int J Obes* 9:381–389.

93. Hypertension Prevention Treatment Group. 1990. The hypertension prevention trial: Three year effects of dietary changes on blood pressure. *Arch Intern Med* 150:153–162.

94. Reisin E, Frohilic ED. 1982. Effect of weight reduction on arterial pressure. *J Chronic dis* 35:887–891.

95. Nelson VL, Legro RS, Strauss III JF, McAllister JM. 1999. Augmented androgen production is a stable steroidogenic phenotype of propagated theca cells from polycystic ovaries. *Mol Endocrinol* 13:946–957.

96. Nelson VL, Qin KN, Rosenfield RL, Wood JR, Penning TM, Legro RS, Strauss JF, McAllister JN. 2001. The biochemical basis for increased testosterone production in theca cells propagated from patients with polycystic ovary syndrome. *J Clin Endocrinol Metab* 86:5925–5933.

97. Dunaif A. 1997. Insulin resistance and the polycystic ovary syndrome: Mechanism and implications for pathogenesis. *Endocr Rev* 18:774–800.

98. Gambineri A, Pelusi C, Vicennati V, Pagotto U, Pasquali R. 2002. Obesity and the polycystic ovary syndrome. *Int J Obes Relat Metab Disord* 26:883–896.

99. Asunción M, Calvo RM, San Millán JL, Sancho J, Avila S, Escobar-Morreale HF. 2000. A prospective study of the prevalence of the polycystic ovary syndrome in unselected Caucasian women from Spain. *J Clin Endocrinol Metab* 85:2434–2438.

100. Manco M, Castagneto M, Nanni G, Guidone C, Tondolo V, Greco AV, Gasbarrini G, Mingrone G. 2005. Biliopancreatic diversion as a novel approach to the HAIR-AN syndrome. *Obesity Surgery* 15:286–289.

101. Escobar-Morreale HF, Botella-Carretero JI, Álvarez-Blasco F, Sancho J, San Millán JL. 2006. The polycystic ovary syndrome associated with morbid obesity may resolve after weight loss induced by bariatric surgery. *J Clin Endocrinol Metab* 90:6364–6369.

102. Blackburn GL, Mun EC. 2004. Effects of weight loss surgeries on liver disease. *Semin Liver Dis* 24:371–379.

103. Charlton M, Sreekumar R, Rasmussen D, Lindor K, Nair KS. 2002. Apolipoprotein synthesis in non-alcoholic steatohepatitis. *Hepatology* 35:898–904.

104. Samuel VT, Liu ZX, Qu X, Elder BD, Bilz S, Befroy D. 2004. Mechanism of hepatic insulin resistance in non-alcoholic fatty liver disease. *J Biol Chem* 279:32345–32353.

105. Schattenberg JM, Wang Y, Singh R, Rigoli RM, Czaja MJ. 2005. Hepatocyte CYP2E1 overexpression and steatohepatitis lead to impaired hepatic insulin signaling. *J Biol Chem* 280:9887–9894.

106. Day CP, James OF. 1998. Steatohepatitis: A tale of two 'hits'? *Gastroenterology* 114:842–845.

107. Dixon JB, Bhathal PS, Hughes NR. 2004. Nonalcoholic fatty liver disease: Improvement in liver histological analysis with weight loss. *Hepatology* 39:1647–1654.

108. Luyckx FH, Desaive C, Thiry A. 1998. Liver abnormalities in severely obese subjects: Effect of drastic weight loss after gastroplasty. *Int J Obes Relat Metab Disord* 22:222–226.

109. Mattar SG, Velcu LM, Rabinovitz M, Demetris AJ, Krasinskas AM, Barinas-Mitchell E, Eid GM, Ramanathan R, Taylor DS, Schauer PR. 2005. Surgically-induced weight loss significantly improves nonalcoholic fatty liver disease and the metabolic syndrome. *Ann Surg* 242:610–620.

110. Kral JG, Thung SN, Biron S, Hould FS, Lebel S, Marceau S, Simard S, Marceau P. 2004. Effects of surgical treatment of the metabolic syndrome on liver fibrosis and cirrhosis. *Surgery* 135:48–58.
111. Manco M, Fernandez-Real JM, Vecchio FM, Vellone V, Moreno JM, Tondolo V, Bottazzo G, Nanni G, Mingrone G. 2010.The decrease of serum levels of human neutrophil alpha-defensins parallels with the surgery- induced amelioration of NASH in obesity. *Obes Surg* 20:1682–1689.
112. Manco M, Putignani L, Bottazzo GF. 2010. Gut microbiota, lipopolysaccharides, and innate immunity in the pathogenesis of obesity and cardiovascular risk. *Endocr Rev* 31:817–844.
113. Manco M, Fernandez-Real JM, Equitani F, Vendrell J, Valera Mora ME, Nanni G, Tondolo V, Calvani M, Ricart W, Castagneto M, Mingrone G. 2007. Effect of massive weight loss on inflammatory adipocytokines and the innate immune system in morbidly obese women. *J Clin Endocrinol Metab* 92:483–490.

63 Bariatric Surgery in Pediatric Weight Management

Anand Dusad, MD, Cristina Fernandez, MD,
Geetanjali Rathore, MD, Sumeet K. Mittal, MD,
and Archana Chatterjee, MD, PhD

CONTENTS

INTRODUCTION

Obesity was recognized as a global epidemic by WHO in 1997.[1] Obesity among children and adolescents is particularly alarming due to its clearly recognized serious, immediate, and long-term health and financial consequences. Childhood and adolescent obesity is an established, independent risk factor for adult morbidity and premature mortality.[2,3] Adolescence is a period of significant growth and maturation both physically and emotionally and thus has its unique issues. The rapid physiological changes occurring during this period make obesity in adolescents difficult to treat. A carefully designed approach to weight management in adolescents is essential. This chapter focuses on the consequences of adolescent obesity, indications for bariatric surgery, the various procedures commonly used, and the pre- and postoperative management. It also describes the role of these approaches in the resolution of the metabolic consequences of obesity.

DEFINITION

Obesity is a term that refers to the condition of having excess body fat. Body mass index (BMI, kg/m^2) is widely used as a measure of adiposity because it can be easily used as a screening tool in clinical settings.[4,5] Adults with a BMI >25 kg/m^2 are considered overweight, whereas those with BMI $\geq$30 kg/m^2 are considered obese. In children and adolescents, physiologic increases in adiposity, height, and weight during growth are expected. Therefore, a single BMI value cannot be used to make accurate predictions about adiposity.[6] Instead, growth charts and BMI percentiles are used to determine overweight and obesity for age and sex in children and adolescents.

In this context, pediatric obesity is defined as BMI >95th percentile for age and sex. Overweight has been defined as a BMI >85th percentile.[7,8] However, for very severe categories of obesity in adolescents who might be candidates for bariatric surgery, these percentile definitions become unreliable. This is because currently the National Health and Nutrition Examination Survey (NHANES) has no reliable data on children and adolescents with BMI >40 kg/m^2. Currently, most authors use BMI >40 kg/m^2 as a threshold for defining morbid obesity in children and adolescents, extrapolating the WHO definition of morbid obesity in adults.

EPIDEMIOLOGY AND RISK FACTORS

Children and adolescents are the fastest growing segment of the population affected by obesity. The proportion of obese children in the age group 6–19 years tripled between 1980 and 2002.[9,10] In the United States, studies estimate 17% of children and adolescents to be obese.[11] Hispanic and

African American communities are noted to have especially high rates of obesity.[11–14] Obesity is a complex multifactorial phenotype influenced by the interaction of genetic, psychological, cultural, and environmental factors. The variables that have been shown to be risk factors include parental obesity,[15] diabetic mother, bottle feeding, socioeconomic status, and hours spent watching television.[16] Insight into these risk factors helps identify those individuals who might be least likely to manage obesity with conventional measures and those who may benefit most from early surgical therapy.

CONSEQUENCES AND COMORBIDITIES

With the marked increase in pediatric obesity, there is also an increase in obesity-related chronic diseases at a younger age and an increased risk for long-term adult morbidity and mortality. Pediatric obesity is a multisystemic disease with a large number of health consequences (Table 63.1).

As the overall prevalence of obesity increases, there is an accompanied increase in comorbid diseases attributable to obesity. In addition to medical issues, childhood obesity also has adverse social and economic consequences.

METABOLIC SYNDROME

The constellation of upper-body obesity, hypertriglyceridemia, hypertension, and glucose intolerance is called metabolic syndrome, syndrome X, or insulin resistance metabolic syndrome of

---

TABLE 63.1
Comorbidities of Adolescent Obesity

Endocrine	Gastrointestinal
Type 2 diabetes mellitus	Gallstones
Insulin resistance	Steatohepatitis
Metabolic syndrome	Gastroesophageal reflux disease
Precocious puberty	Musculoskeletal
Polycystic ovary syndrome	Slipped capital femoral epiphysis
Hypogonadism (boys)	Blount's disease (tibia vara)
Cardiovascular	Forearm fractures
Dyslipidemia	Flat feet (pes planus)
Hypertension	Osteoarthritis
Coagulopathy	Scoliosis
Endothelial dysfunction	Spondylolisthesis
Venous stasis disease	Dermatologic
Chronic inflammation	Acanthosis nigricans
Pulmonary	Intertriginous candidiasis
OSA	Psychosocial
Pickwickian syndrome	Depression
Asthma and exercise intolerance	Eating disorders
Renal	Low self-esteem
Glomerulosclerosis	Discrimination, prejudice, social marginalization
Neurological	Poor quality of life, impairment of daily activities
Pseudotumor cerebri	

---

obesity. According to the National Cholesterol Education Program Adult Treatment Panel III, the guidelines for defining metabolic syndrome require three out of the five given criteria:

* Central adiposity: waist circumference ≥102 cm in men and ≥88 cm in women
* High blood pressure, ≥130/85 mmHg
* HDL cholesterol, <40 mg/dL in men and <50 mg/dL in women
* Hypertriglyceridemia, >150 mg/dL
* High fasting glucose, ≥110 mg/dL

The International Diabetes Federation (IDF) criteria are the same except the waist circumference cutoff points (≥94 cm in men and ≥80 cm in women). The defining criteria for metabolic syndrome in children and adolescents are still controversial, and there are no universally accepted criteria at present. Recently, the IDF has published a set of guidelines to define metabolic syndrome in children from age 10 to 16, which state that all must have central adiposity (waist circumference ≥ the 90th percentile for age and gender), along with at least two out of the following four criteria:

* High blood pressure, ≥130/85 mmHg
* HDL cholesterol, <40 mg/dL
* Hypertriglyceridemia, >150 mg/dL
* High fasting glucose, ≥110 mg/dL or known type 2 diabetes

The IDF recommends avoiding these criteria to define metabolic syndrome for children less than 10 years of age. For adolescents above age 16, the adult IDF criteria can be used. According to the data from the 1999 to 2000 NHANES, the prevalence of metabolic syndrome among U.S. adolescents has been estimated to be 6.4%, with prevalence as high as 32.1% in obese teens.[10]

Type 2 Diabetes Mellitus

There has been a dramatic increase in the prevalence of type 2 diabetes in children. Pinhas-Hamiel et al. showed a 10-fold increase in the incidence of type 2 diabetes in adolescents diagnosed from 1982 to 1994.[17] In 2007, more than 2 million adolescents and more than 16% of overweight teens in the United States had prediabetes.[18] The prevalence was even higher in females and Hispanics.[19] Prediabetes is defined as the intermediate steps of impaired glucose tolerance and impaired fasting glycemia prior to the development of frank diabetes. Serum glucose and glycosylated hemoglobin levels in these patients are within normal limits. Classification using fasting plasma and the oral glucose tolerance test is given in Table 63.2.[20] In children and adolescents, obesity and family history are strongly associated with type 2 diabetes, and more than 95% cases of type 2 diabetes are associated with obesity. Thus, obesity acts as an "accelerator" to the development of type 2 diabetes in children and adolescents.

Obese individuals require higher levels of insulin than nonobese individuals to maintain euglycemia in both fasting and postprandial states.[21] Normally on a cellular level, insulin binds to its receptor on the surface of target cells, triggering tyrosine autophosphorylation and consequent

TABLE 63.2

Classification of Prediabetes and Diabetes

	Normal	Impaired	Diabetes
Fasting plasma glucose	<100 mg/dL	100–125 mg/dL	>125 mg/dL
Oral glucose tolerance test (2 h postload)	<140 mg/dL	140–199 mg/dL	>200 mg/dL

intracellular signaling. This leads to cellular responses such as translocation of glucose transporters to the cell surface to allow glucose uptake for use in glycogen storage. Insulin resistance can be due to genetic defects or metabolic consequences of obesity, such as improper insulin signaling and actions, which include impaired generation of the second messenger, reduced glucose transport in skeletal muscle, and abnormality in enzymatic steps involved in glucose use. Increased levels of free fatty acids found in obese individuals also contribute to defects in glucose use and storage, especially in patients with central obesity. The homeostasis model assessment of insulin resistance (HOMA-IR) is another useful indicator of impaired carbohydrate metabolism.[22] It is calculated by dividing the product of fasting insulin levels (in μU/mL) and glucose levels (in mg/dL) by 402, which gives an index of insulin resistance. The cutoff values for insulin resistance in adults have been defined as 2.5, but there are no cutoff values of HOMA-IR for adolescents.[22]

Hypertension

Classification of elevated blood pressure in the pediatric population is based on percentiles[23]:

1. Prehypertension: ≥90th and ≤95th percentile or ≥120/80 in adolescents
2. Hypertension: ≥95th percentile
   a. Stage 1 hypertension: 95th to 99th percentile +5 mmHg
   b. Stage 2 hypertension: ≥99th percentile +5 mmHg

The majority of hypertension in the pediatric population is primary, often associated with risk factors such as family history, hyperlipidemia, diabetes, and obstructive sleep apnea (OSA). However, screening for renal disease should be done in a child whose BP is persistently ≥95th percentile for secondary causes of hypertension.

Dyslipidemia and Atherosclerosis

Autopsy studies in children and adolescents have shown correlation of atherosclerotic lesions with various risk factors such as hyperlipidemia, hypertension, total cholesterol, LDL cholesterol, triglycerides, and increased BMI.[24,25] According to a prospective study in severely obese children, abdominal fat and insulin levels are correlated with increased vascular stiffness and endothelial dysfunction.[26] Weight loss does reverse the endothelial dysfunction [27]

Nonalcoholic Fatty Liver Disease/Steatohepatitis

Ludwig in 1980 termed a liver disease with histopathologic changes such as hepatic steatosis, inflammation, and fibrosis as nonalcoholic steatohepatitis (NASH), which was associated with obesity, hyperlipidemia, and type 2 diabetes.[28] The population prevalence of fatty liver disease was shown to be 9.6% in children and 38% in obese children by Schwimmer.[29] The various factors that increase the risk of NAFLD in children and adolescents are visceral obesity, insulin resistance, metabolic syndrome, and ethnicity.[29] Hepatic ultrasound is used as the noninvasive screening test for NAFLD, whereas liver biopsy remains the gold standard for diagnosing NAFLD.

Polycystic Ovarian Disease

In 1990, the National Institutes of Health (NIH) set the diagnostic criteria for PCOD which necessitates the presence of both chronic anovulation and hyperandrogenicity. Using the NIH criteria, the baseline prevalence of PCOD is between 6.5% and 8%, with up to 66% of PCOD patients being either overweight or obese.[30] PCOD is commonly associated with hirsutism, acne, obesity, metabolic syndrome, infertility, and menstrual dysfunction.[31]

OBSTRUCTIVE SLEEP APNEA

OSA involves increased airflow resistance in upper airways, decreased airflow, snoring, and multiple episodes of apnea (brief cessation of breathing during sleep). Various symptoms of OSA include snoring, increased daytime sleepiness, poor school performance, enuresis, and hyperactivity. The prevalence of OSA in obese children and adolescents is between 30% and 50%.[32,33]

PSEUDOTUMOR CEREBRI

Also known as benign intracranial hypertension, the condition should be suspected in obese adolescent females presenting with persistent headache, visual disturbance, and papilledema. Ophthalmologic examination is mandatory as the compression on the optic nerve can lead to visual impairment.

PSYCHOSOCIAL

It is quite clear that obesity does cause psychological complications in obese children and adolescents, but there are insufficient data on the long-term psychosocial sequelae of childhood obesity. Psychosocial complications are believed to be the earliest set of complications associated with obesity in children and adolescents. According to a study by Erermis et al., various mental disorders such as anxiety, depression, hyperactivity, and binge eating were found to be significantly higher in obese adolescents than their normal weight counterparts.[34]

MANAGEMENT

NONOPERATIVE

The various medical and psychosocial consequences and comorbidities associated with obesity, which significantly increase morbidity and mortality in adulthood, make it imperative to counter the long-term implications by early evaluation and treatment of obesity in this age group via multidisciplinary interventions led by pediatric care providers. According to the recent guidelines for the treatment of childhood obesity by the American Medical Association, a staged approach that takes into account the child's age, BMI percentile, family history, and related comorbidities should be used.

Stage 1 care is provided by the primary care physician with focus on early intervention in dietary habits and physical activity such as limiting sugar-sweetened beverage intake, increased intake of fruit and vegetables, encouraging >1 h physical activity, and reducing TV time <2 h daily.

Stage 2 interventions should be implemented if very little or no improvement is seen after 3–6 months of stage 1 interventions. This stage is also provided in the primary care setting with the help of other health-care professionals such as dieticians for more structured weight management. The goal is to maintain weight or lose up to 1 lb per week. Behavioral counseling with focus on diet and activity behaviors is an integral part.

Stage 3 includes a more intensive and multidisciplinary approach to weight management. It can take place in primary care settings with provision for appropriate specialized referrals. The behavioral approach in this stage includes setting individualized goals with positive reinforcement via rewards on achievement of the set goals.

Stage 4 is also a multidisciplinary approach carried out in referral tertiary care settings and includes a team of pediatricians experienced in weight management, dieticians trained in behavioral pediatric weight management, pediatric psychologist, physiotherapist, and often a pediatric bariatric surgeon. The team should also have access to pediatric subspecialists such as endocrinologists, pulmonologists, cardiologists, gastroenterologists, etc., who can evaluate and treat comorbid conditions associated with obesity. This is the most intensive approach using strategies such as very-low-calorie diets and drug therapy, with an option of bariatric surgery. Due to the aggressive nature of this stage, standard protocols recommended by expert committees should be followed for patient selection, evaluation, and treatment.

Currently, only two drugs, orlistat and sibutramine, have been approved by the U.S. Food and Drug Administration (FDA) for long-term use in pediatric obesity. Effective behavioral changes are essential for the success of all the four stages mentioned earlier. Behavioral family-based treatment approaches have been shown to be the most effective for the nonsurgical management of childhood obesity.[35-37]

SURGICAL

Although successful weight loss is possible through behavioral modification and dietary changes, it requires great effort and commitment and is associated with high attrition rates, poor weight loss, and weight regain. Bariatric surgery is becoming more popular as a treatment modality for pediatric obesity due to evidence suggesting long-lasting success (>1 year).[38] Sugerman et al.[39] have reported that weight loss surgery in adolescents is associated with significant weight loss and correction of comorbidities associated with obesity. It is reported to be safe in adolescents and has been shown to improve self-image and social interactions. Thus, for morbidly obese adolescents who have failed the nonsurgical approach for maintaining weight loss or for those who have serious comorbidities, bariatric surgery provides a practical alternative.

Guidelines for Bariatric Surgery in Adolescents

Recommendations specific for bariatric surgery in adolescents have been proposed by a panel of experts in pediatric obesity, suggesting guidelines for patient selection, timing of surgery, and program requirements.

Patient Selection Criteria

The unique metabolic, developmental, and psychological needs of adolescents have to be kept in mind while selecting candidates for weight loss surgery. The inclusion and exclusion criteria to be considered while selecting adolescent candidates for bariatric surgery recommended by Inge and colleagues are given in the following text.[40]

Criteria for Adolescent Bariatric Surgery

- Failure of ≥6 months of organized weight loss attempts
- Attainment of physiological maturity
- BMI ≥40 kg/m² with serious obesity-related comorbidities
- BMI ≥50 kg/m² with less serious obesity-related comorbidities
- Commitment to comprehensive medical and psychological evaluations before and after surgery
- Commitment to medical and nutritional recommendations postoperatively
- Ability to provide informed consent for surgical treatment
- Cognitive maturity and decision-making capacity
- Supportive family environment

Contraindications to Adolescent Bariatric Surgery
- Medically correctable cause of obesity
- Substance abuse problem within preceding year
- Medical, psychiatric, or cognitive condition that would impair the patient's ability to adhere to dietary or medication regimen

- Current lactation
- Current pregnancy or planned pregnancy within 2 years after surgery
- Inability to comprehend or refusal to participate in lifelong medical surveillance

In 1991, the NIH published guidelines that suggest that it is reasonable to consider weight loss surgery for adults with BMI of $\geq$35 kg/m^2 with comorbidities or BMI $\geq$40 kg/m^2 with or without comorbidities.[41] Performing bariatric surgery in adolescents with severe obesity or severe comorbidities may result in higher rates of complications and lower success rates. The American Society for Bariatric Surgery (ASBS) emphasizes the importance of offering surgical therapy earlier to prevent comorbidities rather than waiting for them to develop in this patient population.[42] It does not support a strict BMI cutoff of 40 kg/m^2 for morbidly obese adolescents to qualify for bariatric surgery and suggests applying the same criteria as in adults.

Timing of Surgery

Adolescence is a period of both physical and emotional growth and maturation. Bariatric procedures during this period may have a marked impact on the growth and development of adolescents. Thus, physical and psychological maturation of the candidate influences the timing of the surgery.

Physical Maturation

By Tanner, stage 4 physiologic maturation is usually complete. Skeletal maturation which determines the adult stature is normally attained by the age of 13–14 years in girls and 15–16 years in boys.[43] Obese children generally attain puberty earlier than nonobese children of the same age and are more likely to be taller with advanced bone age. For adolescents who have attained >95% of their adult stature, bariatric procedures are unlikely to have a marked impact on the completion of their linear growth.[44] For those who have not yet reached their predicted adult stature, the risk of growth delay due to the nutritional implications of bariatric surgery should be weighed against potentially more significant risk of progression of comorbid conditions if surgery is delayed. Bone age can be used by radiography of the hand and wrist if there is uncertainty about the status of skeletal maturation.

Psychological Maturation

Before the decision for surgical treatment is made, each adolescent and family needs to be extensively evaluated by a team with experience and specialized knowledge in pediatric obesity. The knowledge, motivation, and compliance of the adolescent and at least one parent or legal guardian should be assessed.

Goals of this evaluation include the following:

- To determine whether the adolescent is able to comprehend the consequences of the surgery, provide informed consent, and comply with medical care and lifestyle changes required pre- and postsurgery
- To identify past and present psychiatric, emotional, behavioral or eating disorders, substance or sexual abuse, cigarette smoking, etc., which may be contraindications to bariatric surgery or interfere with treatment
- To define potential support for, or barriers to, regimen compliance
- To evaluate family readiness for surgical treatment and required lifestyle changes and family stability and identify stressors or conflicts within the family
- To assess whether the expectations about the outcome are reasonable

A comprehensive psychological assessment by a multidisciplinary team helps identify a good candidate for bariatric surgery. In summary, the attributes of a good candidate for adolescent bariatric surgery are as follows.

Suggested Attributes of a Good Adolescent Bariatric Candidate

- Patient is motivated and has good insight.
- Patient has realistic expectations.
- Family support and commitment are present.
- Patient is compliant with health-care commitments.
- Family and patient understand that long-term lifestyle changes are needed.
- Patient agrees to long-term follow-up.
- Decisional capacity is present.
- Weight loss attempts are well documented and at least temporarily successful.
- No major psychiatric disorder is evident that may complicate postoperative regimen adherence.
- No major conduct/behavioral problems are noted.
- No substance abuse has occurred in the preceding year.
- No plans for pregnancy in the upcoming 2 years.

Medical Evaluation

Preoperative investigations should be performed to rule out endogenous causes of obesity that may be reversible by medical treatment and also identify health complications related to obesity. The preoperative panel includes

1. Blood tests
   a. Serum electrolytes, albumin, calcium, uric acid, liver function tests
   b. Serum transferrin, homocysteine, iron, folate, vitamin A, B1, B6, B12, D, E, K levels
   c. Lipid profile, fasting blood sugar, fasting insulin, HbA1c, thyroid function tests
   d. Complete blood count, PT, PTT, INR
2. Urine analysis
3. Pregnancy test in females
4. Echocardiogram and electrocardiogram
5. Abdominal ultrasound
6. Polysomnography for patients with symptoms of OSA
7. Pulmonary function tests
8. Anthropometrics: height, weight, waist and hip circumference, and DEXA scan (or bioelectric impedance in patients >300 lb)

All the previously mentioned blood tests are repeated 3, 6, 9, and 12 months postoperatively, then yearly. The DEXA scan allows for the measurement of relative amounts of fat and lean body mass loss and changes in bone mineral density.

Bariatric Programs for Adolescents

Patients being considered for bariatric surgery should be referred to a specialized bariatric center equipped for making difficult patient selection decisions and providing long-term follow-up and management of the unique challenges posed by severely obese adolescents.

Guidelines established by the ASBS and the American College of Surgeons require the team to include specialists in obesity evaluation and management, nutrition, physical therapy, psychology, and a bariatric surgical team.[42] Additional expertise in general pediatrics, adolescent medicine, endocrinology, pulmonology, gastroenterology, orthopedics, and cardiology should be readily available, depending on the individual needs of the patient. Pediatric surgeons are eligible for credentialing in bariatric surgery. The multidisciplinary team provides a specific treatment plan, individually tailored for the patient.

Surgical Options

There is no procedure of choice as yet for bariatric surgery in adolescents due to lack of data. Some of the limitations of the available studies in adolescents include small sample size; lack of consistency across programs, surgeons, and procedures; and a short average length of follow-up. However, a large number of studies have been done on the adult population, which have significant statistical and clinically relevant data. Selected components of outcomes from these studies can be safely extrapolated to the adolescent population.

In this new era of surgical approaches in bariatric surgery, an open surgical approach is less preferred or almost obsolete in comparison to the laparoscopic approach by surgeons all over the world. The major advantage of the laparoscopic approach, according to the ASBS and the Society of American Gastrointestinal and Endoscopic Surgeons (SAGES), especially in morbidly obese individuals with lack of adequate vascularization, is that it significantly reduces wound complications such as infections, hernias, and dehiscence.[45] The majority of the available bariatric surgical procedures can be broadly classified into either purely restrictive or restrictive/malabsorptive.

Roux-en-Y Gastric Bypass

Roux-en-Y gastric bypass (RYGB) is the gold standard bariatric surgical procedure in the United States.[39] It involves creation of

- A gastric pouch
- A jejunojejunostomy (Roux limb)
- End to side gastrojejunostomy

The biliopancreatic limb constitutes the excluded part of the stomach, duodenum, and proximal jejunum. This drains bile, digestive enzymes, and gastric secretions. The midjejunum anastomosed to the gastric pouch carries the ingested food. The digestive enzymes are mixed with the food at the level of the jejunojejunostomy and absorption takes place in the common channel. The Roux limb is a short bypass; therefore, this procedure is mainly restrictive with a small component of malabsorption. The advantages of this procedure are excellent long-term weight loss, decreased oral intake with early satiety, and aversion to sweets. Disadvantages include greater risk of perioperative mortality among adults (0.5%) compared to those with adjustable gastric banding (0.05%). It also has more complications such as intestinal leakage, thromboembolism, dumping syndrome, cholelithiasis, gastric distention, gastrojejunal stoma stenosis, small bowel obstruction, protein-calorie malnutrition, and micronutrient deficiency (iron, calcium, and vitamin B12).

Laparoscopic Adjustable Gastric Banding

This is a purely restrictive procedure in which an adjustable balloon band is placed encircling the most proximal part of the stomach, creating a smaller pouch above the band and the larger section below with a constricting stoma. The major advantages of laparoscopic adjustable gastric banding (LAGB) are ease and safety of placement, lower morbidity and mortality compared to RYGB, reversibility, and the possibility of adjusting the band stoma size. The weight loss is gradual and has been satisfactory in adults. Because it is less likely to affect micronutrient absorption, it is a safer alternative with fewer nutritional risks in adolescents. Disadvantages include foreign body infection, band erosion, pouch dilation, pouch slippage/prolapse, device malfunction or malposition, and the need for multiple adjustments. Adolescent patients may need to undergo replacement due to the limited lifespan of the prosthesis.

The LAGB procedure is currently not approved by the FDA for use in patients younger than 18 years of age, but studies from Australia and Europe and in adults have shown promising outcomes.

Vertical banded gastroplasty is another restrictive procedure used in the past but has been displaced by RYGB and LAGB.[46]

Laparoscopic Vertical Sleeve Gastrectomy

This is also a purely restrictive procedure in which a major portion of the greater curvature of the stomach is excised, leaving a tubularized stomach. A small gastric reservoir is created, leading to early satiety with small amounts of food. Serum levels of ghrelin, a hunger regulating hormone mainly produced in the fundus of the stomach, are much lower after this procedure. This may also explain the mechanism by which laparoscopic vertical sleeve gastrectomy (LVSG) helps resolve comorbidities such as insulin resistance and diabetes. Advantages include significant initial weight loss with lower operative risk, avoiding device-related long-term adverse effects of LAGB, and fewer nutritional risks. However, revision surgery without transection cannot be performed as in LAGB.

Biliopancreatic Diversion with Duodenal Switch

The biliopancreatic diversion with duodenal switch (BPD-DS) procedure consists of creating a lesser curvature tube with resection of the greater curvature of stomach. The duodenum distal to the pylorus is divided and anastomosed to the distal ileum. The distal duodenal stump is closed to form the biliopancreatic limb which is anastomosed to the distal ileum. This procedure is primarily malabsorptive with a restrictive component. The procedure results in excellent weight loss in adults but has higher risks of operative complications and postoperative nutritional risks such as diarrhea, anemia, vitamin and mineral deficiencies, bone demineralization, etc.

Newer Techniques

- Gastric pacing using implantable gastric stimulation (IGS)
- Intragastric balloon (IGB): (a) Garren-Edwards gastric bubble (GEGB)
  (b) Bioenteric intragastric balloon (BIB)
- Endoluminal and transgastric bariatric surgery also referred to as natural orifice translumenal endoscopic surgery (NOTES)

POSTOPERATIVE

COMPLICATIONS

Postoperatively, patients require close monitoring for fever, tachycardia, tachypnea, increased oxygen requirement, worsening abdominal pain, and acute alteration in mental status. These may suggest early complications such as

- Respiratory obstruction, atelectasis, pneumonia
- Pulmonary embolism
- Bowel obstruction
- Fistula
- Dehiscence and evisceration
- Gastrointestinal leakage
- Acute gastric pouch dilation with impending rupture
- Peritonitis
- Sepsis and multiple organ failure

While the late complications specific to individual bariatric procedures have been mentioned earlier, procedure-independent late complications are as follows:

- Ventral/incisional hernia, more common in open surgical procedures
- Internal hernia, more common in laparoscopic procedures
- Intestinal obstructions (adhesions), more common in open procedures

MANAGEMENT

On postoperative day 1, an upper GI water-soluble contrast study is done to look for satisfactory passage of contrast. Subsequently, the patient is begun on clear liquids with advancing high-protein liquid diet. The diet is slowly advanced introducing a new food every 2–3 days, increasing the complexity of foods gradually according to the patient's recovery. The goal is a well-balanced, small-volume, high-protein diet (1 g protein/kg of the ideal weight). In order to minimize adverse reactions to introduction of food, such as "dumping syndrome," foods rich in fat and sugars are avoided. Dumping syndrome, characterized by bloating, cramping, sweating, tachycardia, vomiting, and diarrhea, occurs due to rapid passage of food from the new gastric pouch to the intestine.

Postoperative follow-up requires close monitoring to verify adherence to diet and supplementation to avoid nutritional complications. Often, follow-up visits are scheduled weekly for the first month, monthly for 6 months, quarterly until the first 12 months, and yearly thereafter. Serum chemistries, complete blood count, and vitamin B complex levels are obtained at 6 and 12 months postoperatively and then yearly.

Strict adherence to procedure-specific diet and supplementation is required to avoid nutritional complications. RYGB requires very low calorie intake, thus necessitating adequate protein intake (0.5–1 g/kg per day) to minimize lean body mass loss during the weight loss phase. Iron, calcium, folate, and vitamin B12 supplementation is required after gastric bypass due to impaired absorption.

There is rapid skeletal mineral accretion in adolescence which may be negatively impacted post–bariatric surgery due to impaired absorption of both vitamin D and calcium. Thus, it is essential to closely monitor bone mineral density in these patients by performing DEXA scans annually.

Postoperatively, adolescents are at increased risk of gallstones and peptic ulcers following gastric bypass and are therefore prescribed ursodiol and proton pump inhibitors. NSAIDs are avoided due to risk of ulceration and bleeding. All females and their caregivers are informed about increased fertility and likelihood of risk-taking behavior after weight loss. The physicians caring for adolescent girls undergoing bariatric surgery must provide daily folate and vitamin B complex supplements as a majority of these adolescents may want to be mothers in the future. Pregnancy is contraindicated for 2 years postsurgery.

COMPLIANCE

Long-term success with bariatric surgery depends on strict compliance with health care and dietary recommendations, which is usually very poor in adolescents. This is a period of rebellion and risk-taking behavior, often leading to noncompliance due to low self-esteem, poor cognitive abilities, and insufficient support. Studies have suggested that continued behavioral therapy improves adolescent adherence to strict regimens.[46]

The adolescent's compliance may be enhanced by

- Repetitive reinforcement
- Goal setting and incentives for achievement of these goals
- Visual aids for recommended diet
- Encouraging self-monitoring and participation in self-management
- Focus on immediate benefits
- Enlisting peer and family support

FOLLOW-UP

The NIH Consensus Development Conference on Gastrointestinal Surgery for Severe Obesity in 1991 recommended: "Postoperative care, nutritional counseling, and surveillance should continue for an indefinitely long period. The surveillance should include the monitoring of indices of inadequate nutrition and of amelioration of any preoperative disorders such as diabetes, hypertension, and dyslipidemia. The monitoring should include not only indices of macronutrients but also of mineral and vitamin nutrition."[41] The ASBS has developed two sets of guidelines for postoperative follow-up care:

1. For postoperative follow-up care, the recommendations are visits during the immediate postoperative period, then within 3 months of the operation, at 6 months, then yearly for 3 years, at 5 years, then at 5 year intervals for life, with additional visits as indicated by the patient's condition.[47]
2. For length of follow-up necessary based on a classification of results, it defined results as preliminary (<2 years of follow-up), intermediate (2–5 years), long-term (5–10 years), very long-term (>10 years).[48]

OUTCOMES

WEIGHT LOSS

Various studies have been done to demonstrate weight loss after bariatric surgery including two systematic reviews, and meta-analyses have been performed. The first study focused on the comorbid conditions associated with obesity including type 2 diabetes, hyperlipidemia, hypertension, and OSA[49]; but the second one focused only on type 2 diabetes.[50] It was observed in these studies that weight loss was proportional to the severity of the procedure, progressively increasing from laparoscopic gastric banding to the duodenal switch. These studies, however, show only the short-term follow-up results, as no long-term follow-up studies for weight loss are available. Sugerman et al. reviewed the results of RYGBP in adolescents over the last 20 years and showed results similar to those obtained from adult studies.[39]

NUTRITION

Weight loss in bariatric surgery is achieved by restricting either the intake or absorption of nutrients, thus creating a potential for nutritional deficiency. There may be a deficiency of macronutrients (proteins, essential fatty acids), micronutrients (iron, calcium, zinc, magnesium), and vitamins (B12, B6, B1, A, E, D, and K) as well as increased levels of homocysteine. The extent of nutrient deficiency greatly depends on the surgical procedure performed. The most severe iron and vitamin B12 deficiency is seen with RYGB while calcium, fatty acid, and fat-soluble vitamin (A, D, E, and K) deficiency is seen with BPD with duodenal switch. The best preventive measure is appropriate vitamin and mineral supplementation in addition to a diet rich in micronutrients. Lifetime periodic laboratory monitoring is essential post–bariatric surgery.

RESOLUTION OF COMORBIDITIES

Many of the comorbid diseases associated with obesity are cured or reversed up to a significant extent after bariatric surgery. The comorbid conditions where reversal or improvement has been proven are type 2 diabetes, hyperlipidemia, hypertension, OSA, asthma, gastroesophageal reflux disease, nonalcoholic fatty liver disease and cirrhosis, polycystic ovarian syndrome, pseudotumor cerebri, depression, and orthopedic complications.[51] The resolution of these diseases depends on factors such as duration and severity of disease, postsurgical weight loss, and the net effect of obesity on the disease. Different surgical procedures have different impacts on obesity-associated comorbid conditions because their effects depend on factors such as postoperative weight loss, hormonal changes, and surgery-induced malabsorption.

Type 2 Diabetes Mellitus and Insulin Resistance

Type 2 diabetes mellitus is especially resistant to conservative nonsurgical weight loss management.[52] Significant weight loss results in marked decrease in insulin resistance and hence lower insulin requirements to maintain normal blood sugar levels. There are several possible mechanisms for reduction in blood sugar levels after bariatric surgery. Reduced caloric intake by limiting the amount of food intake, early satiety, and delayed gastric emptying following gastric bypass surgery lead to lower blood sugar levels. Changes in the composition of diet post–bariatric surgery also play a role in inducing euglycemia, e.g., patients avoid sweets due to fear of the dumping syndrome and eat fiber-rich foods. Gastric bypass surgery changes the gut hormone milieu. The reduction in calories passing through the gut after a bypass reduces gut hormone secretion influencing the mechanism of type 2 diabetes mellitus. It was observed that within days of gastric bypass, manifestations of type 2 diabetes can totally clear even before any significant weight loss occurs.[53–55] The hypothesis mentioned earlier was further substantiated by Rubino ct al. who demonstrated euglycemia in diabetic rats by performing bypass of the duodenum and upper jejunum in the absence of weight loss.[56]

A meta-analysis of comorbidities in 2007 demonstrated complete resolution of type 2 diabetes in 78% and improvement in 87% of patients undergoing bariatric surgery.[50] These findings were confirmed by reduction in HbA1c and fasting blood sugar levels. In most cases, after discharge from the hospital, no pharmacological treatment is required to maintain blood sugars <180 mg/dL. Usually by 1 month postoperatively, blood sugar levels are normalized (sometimes even low).

Polycystic Ovarian Disease

If PCOD is not due to a genetic abnormality, weight loss cures this syndrome. Insulin levels drop, which leads to decrease in fat mass and normalization of the menstrual cycle. Hirsutism may persist for a longer duration because once the hair follicles are stimulated, they are slow to regress.

Hyperlipidemia

Secondary forms of hypercholesterolemia and hyperlipidemia are cured by weight loss and dietary changes secondary to bariatric surgery. For those with primary hyperlipidemias exacerbated by obesity, better control may be achieved by bariatric surgery. In a report by the Program on Surgical Control of the Hyperlipidemias (POSCH) in 1990, levels of total and low-density lipoprotein cholesterol were shown to be 23% and 38% lower, respectively, after distal ileal malabsorptive surgery.[57] In 2004, a meta-analysis showed improvement in 70% of patients with hyperlipidemia.[49] Greater reduction in cholesterol levels is seen after BPD-DS due to interruption of enterohepatic circulation, leading to increased *de novo* synthesis of bile acids from cholesterol.

Hypertension

Hypertension related to obesity is multifactorial with complex interrelated mechanisms including insulin resistance, hyperinsulinemia, central adiposity, and renin-angiotensin-aldosterone system and sympathetic nervous system stimulation. Weight loss has shown improvement in hypertension with greater loss showing increased benefit. In general, 1% decrease in body weight decreases systolic BP by 1 mmHg and diastolic BP by 2 mmHg. A meta-analysis showed 62% resolution of hypertension and 79% improvement postoperatively.[49] Besides depending upon the amount of weight loss and type of procedure performed, the effect on hypertension also depends upon duration and exposure to other risk factors such as diabetes. Presence of comorbidities such as diabetes increases the likelihood of irreversibility due to permanent end organ damage.[58,59]

OSA

The treatment for OSA in morbid obesity is weight loss. Improvement occurs in over 80% of patients.[49] In addition to improvement in clinical findings, there is also increase in arterial oxygen content and decrease in arterial carbon dioxide.[60–62] The reduction in intra-abdominal pressure after bariatric surgery improves diaphragmatic excursion which facilitates the favorable blood gas changes mentioned earlier.

QUALITY OF LIFE

Losing a significant amount of excess weight and resolution of debilitating comorbidities, with subsequent improvement in self-esteem, energy levels, and physical activities, are all positive outcomes of bariatric surgery. This helps adolescents to become more socially active and results in a definite improvement in the quality of life. There are several instruments that have been developed over time to evaluate a patient's quality of life. However, there is no standardized tool that is universally accepted. Any tool used should be reliable, valid, and sensitive and should be able to detect changes over time. Irrespective of the methods of analysis, over time all bariatric surgery patients have shown significant improvement in subjective quality of life. Postoperative changes in BMI are linear and inversely proportional to subjective improvement in quality of life.

FUTURE RESEARCH

In spite of having comprehensive literature on adult bariatric surgery, sufficient data and long-term studies in pediatric bariatric surgery are lacking. All efforts should be made to develop a comprehensive centralized data collection system in order to determine how outcomes in adolescents may differ from adults. After bariatric surgery is performed on adolescent patients, they should be assessed for the quality of care and outcomes. Data sources and specific interventions need to be evaluated critically in order to compare short- and long-term outcomes. This is necessary for the advancement of the field, improvement in patient management, and prediction of outcomes.

REFERENCES

1. Caballero B. The global epidemics of obesity: An overview. *Epidemiol Rev* 2007;29:1–5.
2. Reilly JJ, Methven E, McDowell ZC et al. Health consequences of obesity. *Arch Dis Child* 2003;88(9):748–752.
3. Freedman DS, Khan LK, Dietz WH et al. Relationship of childhood obesity to coronary heart disease risk factors in adulthood: The Bogalusa Heart Study. *Pediatrics* 2001,108(3).712–718.
4. Dietz WH and Robinson TN. Use of the body mass index (BMI) as a measure of overweight in children and adolescents. *J Pediatr* 1998;132:191–193.
5. Pietrobelli A, Faith MS, Allison DB et al. Body mass index as a measure of adiposity among children and adolescents: A validation study. *J Pediatr* 1998;132:204–210.
6. Himes JH and Dietz WH. Guidelines for overweight in adolescent preventive services; recommendations from an expert committee. The Expert Committee on Clinical Guidelines for Overweight in Adolescent Preventive Services. *Am J Clin Nutr* 1994;59:309–316.
7. Yanovski JA. Pediatric obesity. *Rev Endocr Metab Disord* 2001;2(4):371–383.
8. Strauss RS and Pollack HA. Epidemic increase in childhood overweight. 1986–1998. *JAMA* 2001;286:2845–2848.
9. Hedley AA, Ogden CL, Johnson CL et al. Prevalence of overweight and obesity among US children, adolescents, and adults, 1999–2002. *JAMA* 2004;291(23):2847–2850.
10. Ogden CL, Flegal KM, Carroll MD, and Johnson CL. Prevalence and trends in overweight among US children and adolescents, 1999–2000. *JAMA* 2002;288(14):1728–1732.
11. Ogden CL, Carroll MD, Curtin LR et al. Prevalence of overweight and obesity in the United States, 1999–2004. *JAMA* 2006;295(13):1549–1555.
12. Dwyer JT, Stone EJ, Yang M et al. Prevalence of marked overweight and obesity in a multiethnic pediatric population: Findings from the Child and Adolescent Trial for Cardiovascular Health (CATCH) study. *J Am Diet Assoc* 2000;100(10):1149–1156.
13. Kimm SYS, Barton BA, Obarzanek E et al. Obesity development during adolescence in a biracial cohort: The NHLBI Growth and Health study. *Pediatrics* 2002;110(5):e54.

14. Freedman DS, Khan LK, Serdula MK et al. Racial and ethnic differences in secular trends for childhood BMI, weight, and height. *Obesity* 2006;14(2):301–308.
15. Whitaker RC, Wright JA, Pepe MS et al. Predicting obesity in young adulthood from childhood and parental obesity. *N Engl J Med* 1997;337(13):869–873.
16. Burke V, Beilin LJ, Simmer K et al. Predictors of body mass index and associations with cardiovascular risk factors in Australian children: A prospective cohort study. *Int J Obes* 2005;29(1):15–23.
17. Pinhas-Hamiel O, Dolan LM, Daniels SR et al. Increased incidence of non-insulin-dependent diabetes mellitus among adolescents. *J Pediatr* 1996;128:608–615.
18. ADA Factsheet. Total Prevalence of Diabetes and Pre-diabetes. American Diabetes Association, 2007. Was available at: diabetes.org/diabetes-statistics/prevalence.jsp (accessed August 16, 2007).
19. Narayan KM, Boyle JP, Thompson TJ et al. Lifetime risk of diabetes mellitus in the United States. *JAMA* 2003;290(14):1884–1890.
20. Craig ME, Hattersley A, and Donaghue K. ISPAD Clinical Practice Consensus Guidelines 2006–2007. Definition, epidemiology and classification. *Pediatr Diabetes* 2006;7(6):343–351.
21. Pi-Sunyer FX. The obesity epidemic: Pathophysiology and consequences of obesity. *Obes Res* 2002;10:97S–104S.
22. Mattews DR, Hosker JP, Rudenski AS et al. Homeostasis model assessment: Insulin resistance and beta-cell function from fasting plasma glucose and insulin concentrations in man. *Diabetologia* 1985;28(7):412–419.
23. National High Blood Pressure Education Program Working Group on High Blood Pressure in Children and Adolescents. The fourth report on the diagnosis, evaluation, and treatment of high blood pressure in children and adolescents. *Pediatrics* 2004;114(2 suppl):555–576.
24. Relationship of atherosclerosis in young men to serum lipoprotein cholesterol concentration and smoking. A preliminary report from the Pathobiological Determinants of Atherosclerosis in Youth (PDAY) Research Group. *JAMA* 1990;264(23):3018–3024.
25. Berenson GS, Srinivasan SR, Bao W et al. Association between multiple cardiovascular risk factors and atherosclerosis in children and young adults. The Bogalusa Heart Study. *N Engl J Med* 1998;338(23):1650–1656.
26. Tounian P, Aggoun Y, Dubern B et al. Presence of increased stiffness in the common carotid artery and endothelial dysfunction in severely obese children: A prospective study. *Lancet* 2001;358:1400–1404.
27. Skilton MR and Celermajer DS. Endothelial dysfunction and arterial abnormalities in childhood obesity. *Int J Obes* 2006;30:1–8.
28. Ludwig J, Viggiano TR, McGill DB et al. Nonalcoholic steatohepatitis: Mayo Clinic experiences with a hitherto unnamed disease. *Mayo Clin Proc* 1980;55(7):434–438.
29. Schwimmer JB. Definitive diagnosis and assessment of risk for non-alcoholic fatty liver disease in children and adolescents. *Semin Liver Dis* 2007;27:312–318.
30. Azziz R, Woods KS, Reyna R et al. The prevalence and features of the polycystic ovary syndrome in an unselected population. *J Clin Endocrinol Metab* 2004;89(6):2745–2749.
31. Norman RJ, Dewailly D, Legro RS et al. Polycystic ovary syndrome. *Lancet* 2007;370(9588):685–697.
32. Dubern B, Tounian P, Medjadhi N, Maingot L, Girardet JP, and Boule M. Pulmonary function and sleep-related breathing disorders in severely obese children. *Clin Nutr* 2006;2:803–809.
33. Verhulst SL, Schrauwen N, Haentjens D et al. Sleep-disordered breathing in overweight and obese children and adolescents: Prevalence, characteristics and the role of fat distribution. *Arch Dis Child* 2007;92:205–208.
34. Erermis S, Cetin N, Tamar M, Bukusoglu N, Akdeniz F, and Goksen D. Is obesity a risk factor for psychopathology among adolescents? *Pediatr Int* 2004;46(3):296–301.
35. Jelalian E and Saelens BE. Empirically supported treatments in pediatric psychology: Pediatric obesity. *J Pediatr Psychol* 1999;24(3):223–248.
36. Epstein LH, Myers MD, Raynor HA, and Saelens BE. Treatment of pediatric obesity. *Pediatrics* 1998;101(3 Pt 2):554–570.
37. Kirk S, Zeller M, Claytor R et al. The relationship of health outcomes to improvement in BMI in children and adolescents. *Obes Res* 2005;13(5):876–882.
38. Yanovski JA. Intensive therapies for pediatric obesity. *Pediatr Clin North Am* 2001;48(4):1041–1053.
39. Sugerman HJ, Sugerman EL, DeMaria EJ et al. Bariatric surgery for severely obese adolescents. *J Gastrointest Surg* 2003;7:102–107.
40. Inge TH, Krebs NF, Garcia VF et al. Bariatric surgery for severely overweight adolescents: Concerns and recommendations. *Pediatrics* 2004;114(1):217–223.

41. National Institutes of Health Consensus Development Panel: National Institutes of Health Consensus Development Conference Statement, Gastrointestinal surgery for severe obesity. *Ann Intern Med* 1991;115:956–961.

42. Buchwald H. Consensus Conference Panel. Consensus conference statement bariatric surgery for morbid obesity: Health implications for patients, health professionals, and third-party payers. *Surg Obes Relat Dis* 2005;1(3):371–381.

43. Marshall WA and Tanner JM. Variations in the pattern of pubertal changes in boys. *Arch Dis Child* 1970;45:13–23.

44. Tanner JM. *Assessment of Skeletal Maturity and Prediction of Adult Height (TW2 Method)*. San Diego, CA, Academic Press, 1983.

45. Guidelines for Laparoscopic and Open Surgical Treatment of Morbid Obesity. (Document adopted by the American Society for Bariatric Surgery and the Society of American Gastrointestinal Endoscopic Surgeons, June 2000.) *Obes Surg* 2000;10:378–379.

46. Nadler EP and Kane TD. Bariatric surgery. In: Langer JC and Albanese CT (eds.), *Pediatric Minimal Access Surgery*. Boca Raton, FL, Taylor & Francis, 2005, pp. 319–330.

47. Mason EE, Amaral JF, Cowan GSM et al. Guidelines for selection of patients for surgical treatment of obesity. *Obes Surg* 1993;3:429.

48. American Society for Bariatric Surgery: Standards Committee Statement on length and percentage of follow up. *Obes Surg* 2000;10:1.

49. Buchwald H, Avidor Y, Braunwald E et al. Bariatric Surgery: A systematic review and meta-analysis. *JAMA* 2004;1724–1737.

50. Buchwald H, Estok R, Fahrbach K et al. Weight and type 2 diabetes after bariatric surgery: Systemic review and meta-analysis. *Am J Med* 2009;122:248–256.

51. Buchwald H. Overview of bariatric surgery. *J Am Coll Surg* 2002;194:367–375.

52. Greenway SE, Greenway FL, and Klein S. Effects of obesity surgery on non-insulin-dependent diabetes mellitus. *Arch Surg* 2002;137(10):1109–1117.

53. Pories WJ, Swanson MS, MacDonald KG et al. Who would have thought it? An operation proves to be the most effective therapy for adult-onset diabetes mellitus. *Ann Surg* 1995;222:339–352.

54. Pories WJ and Albrecht RJ. Etiology of type II diabetes mellitus: Role of the foregut. *World J Surg* 2001;25:527–531.

55. Hickey MS, Pories WJ, MacDonald KG et al. A new paradigm for type 2 diabetes mellitus: Could it be a disease of the foregut? *Ann Surg* 1998;227:637–643.

56. Rubino F, Forgione A, Cummings DE et al. The mechanism of diabetes control after gastrointestinal bypass surgery reveals a role of the proximal small intestine in the pathophysiology of type 2 diabetes. *Ann Surg* 2006;244:741–749.

57. Buchwald H, Varco RL, Matts JP et al. Effect of partial ileal bypass surgery on mortality and morbidity from coronary heart disease in patients with hypercholesterolemia. Report of the Program on the Surgical Control of the Hyperlipidemias (POSCH). *New Engl J Med* 1990;323:946–955.

58. Lapidus L, Bengtsson C, Larsson B et al. Distribution of adipose tissue and risk of cardiovascular death: A 12-year follow up of participants in the population study of women in Gothenburg, Sweden. *BMJ* 1984;289:1257–1261.

59. Kral JG. Morbidity of severe obesity. *Surg Clin North Am* 2001;81:1039–1061.

60. Nachmany I, Szold A, Klausner J, and Abu-Abeid S. Resolution of bariatric comorbidities: Sleep apnea. In: Buchwald H, Pories W, and Cowan GM Jr. (eds.), *Surgical Management of Obesity*. Philadelphia, PA, Elsevier, 2007, pp. 377–382.

61. Rajala R, Partinen M, Sane T et al. Obstructive sleep apnea syndrome in morbidly obese patients. *J Intern Med* 1991;230:125–129.

62. Rasheid S, Banasiak M, Gallagher SF et al. Gastric bypass is an effective treatment for obstructive sleep apnea in patients with clinically significant obesity. *Obes Surg* 2003;13:58–61.

Index

O